Stedman's

OB-GYN & PEDIATRIC WORDS

INCLUDES NEONATOLOGY

FOURTH EDITION

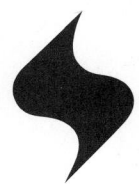

Stedman's

OB-GYN & PEDIATRIC WORDS

INCLUDES NEONATOLOGY

FOURTH EDITION

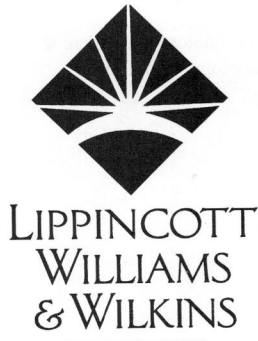

LIPPINCOTT
WILLIAMS
& WILKINS

Publisher: Julie K. Stegman
Senior Product Manager: Eric Branger
Associate Managing Editor: Steve Lichtenstein
Production Coordinator: Jason Delaney
Typesetter: Peirce Graphic Services, LLC.
Printer & Binder: Malloy Litho, Inc.

Copyright © 2005 Lippincott Williams & Wilkins
351 West Camden Street
Baltimore, Maryland 21201-2436

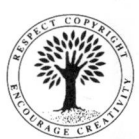

Printed in the United States of America

Fourth Edition, 2005

Library of Congress Cataloging-in-Publication Data

Stedman's OB-GYN & pediatric words, includes neonatology.— 4th ed.
    p. ; cm. — (Stedman's word books)
    Combination of: Stedman's OB-GYN & genetics words and Stedman's
pediatric words includes neonatology.
    Includes bibliographical references.
    ISBN 0-7817-5449-6
    1. Gynecology—Terminology. 2. Obstetrics—Terminology. 3. Pediatrics—
Terminology. 4. Neonatology—Terminology. I. Title: OB-GYN & pediatric words,
includes neonatology. II. Title: Stedman's OB-GYN and pediatric words, includes
neonatology. III. Stedman, Thomas Lathrop, 1853–1938. IV. Lippincott Williams &
Wilkins. V. Stedman's OB-GYN & genetics words. VI. Stedman's pediatric words
includes neonatology. VII. Series.
    [DNLM: 1. Obstetrics—Terminology—English. 2. Gynecology—Terminology—
English. 3. Pediatrics—Terminology—English.
WQ 15 S812 2005]
RG47.S74 2005
618'.014—dc22

2004011735

04 05 06
1 2 3 4 5 6 7 8 9 10

Contents

Acknowledgments

An important part of our editorial process is the involvement of medical transcriptionists—as advisors, reviewers, and editors.

We extend special thanks to Ellen Atwood, R. Jo-Ann Clarke, and Jeanne Bock, CSR, MT, for editing the manuscript, helping to resolve many difficult content questions, and contributing material for the appendix sections. We also extend special thanks to Helen Littrell, CMT, for performing the final prepublication review.

We are grateful, as well, to our MT Editorial Advisory Board members, including Marty Cantu, CMT; Patricia Gibson; Nancy Hill, MT; Heather Little, CMT; Wendy Ryan, ART; and Sandra Wideburg, CMT. These medical transcriptionists and medical language specialists served as important editors and advisors.

Other important contributors to this edition include Robin Koza, Nicole Peck, CMT, and Mary Chiara Zaratkiewicz.

Lisa Fahnestock played an integral role in the process by reviewing the files for format, updating the content, and providing a final quality check. Special thanks also to Barb Ferretti for her timely advice and problem-solving skills.

As with all our *Stedman's* word references, this resource incorporates the suggestions and expertise of our many contacts in the medical transcriptionist community. Thanks to all of our advisory board participants, reviewers, and editors; AAMT meeting attendees; and others who have written us with requests and comments—keep talking, and we'll keep listening.

Editor's Preface

A century ago the population of the United States was about 83 million. Now it is 293 million or so. Shifting population via immigration accounts for a small percentage, but in the same period the world population has swollen from a mere 1.6 billion to well over 6 billion people.

What is astonishing about these numbers is that, in the intervening 100 years, we have had history's worst pandemic (flu of 1918) with mortality in the United States alone rivaling or exceeding that of the Black Death of the Middle Ages. This was closely followed by two World Wars with astronomical carnage from battle, collateral damage, The Holocaust, and aftermath. A quarter century ago a new killer arrived; AIDS, with its ongoing massive mortality. An unusual fact unifies these causes of population decrease: All have had the highest mortality among the young, robust, reproductive age groups.

Less than half a century ago, reliable ways to prevent conception became readily available. But, since the introduction of The Pill in the 1960s, the populations of the United States and of the world have nearly doubled, even though the rate of increase has been cut by more than half. Some estimate that there are more people alive in the world right now than cumulatively in recorded history!

Why does the population continue to increase? Mathematicians undoubtedly can produce elegant equations to explicate this explosion. The urge to multiply and increase has been examined with theories from the lofty to the pragmatic to the highly emotional, but they all boil down to: Babies are our promise for the future, and they are so very appealing.

In the 21st century, even though babies are still (mostly) conceived and gestated in the old-fashioned way, medical technological management of all phases of pregnancy and birth are the norm in the English-speaking world. Accompanying all these advances and all these new people in the world are scads of words, many newly coined, describing genes, procedures, and even diseases that either did not exist or were unknown a century—or a decade—ago. Just as medical practitioners require specialized knowledge, so too do medical language specialists require this knowledge.

Fetuses, neonates, infants, children, and teens all have unique medical and health care concerns. These are largely intertwined with their mothers' health and medical care. At puberty, young girls may need both a pediatrician and a gynecologist. Statistics about teen pregnancy indicate that many require the attention of an obstetrician as well. Although children and women also have health concerns and conditions that involve all systems of the body, some areas are specific to gender and age.

Men have become more integrally involved in the gestation, birth, and care of young children. Assisted reproduction and genetic counseling both require male-specific information and terminology. Reproductive technology has made some amazing advances, but to my knowledge, scientists have not devoted time to finding ways for men to actually be pregnant or give birth, despite a couple of comic movies exploring the possibility. Only women can conceive, carry a pregnancy, and give birth. Women's physiology, function, and health are inseparably involved in either preparation for conception and pregnancy, or in dealing with the lack of it. Fortunately, we have come a long way from the time when menstruation was described as "the weeping of a disappointed womb."

A book incorporating all of the medical aspects of men's genetic and reproductive health, women's reproductive and gender-specific health, along with infants' and children's growth, development and health through myriad phases would encompass all of general medicine as well as most of the specialties. Trying to do this would produce a "word boom" similar to the population statistics above. This is neither feasible in the *Stedman's Word Book* format, nor would it be helpful.

All of these various stages and phases have many things in common: Anatomy is essentially the same after birth as it will be through adulthood. Adverse conditions affecting human beings are also fairly consistent. Winnowing out these general terms that are available in other books in the *Stedman's* series, we were still faced with what degree of specialization would be appropriate. Does a myocardial infarction belong to gynecology or cardiology? Sperm production is important in assisted reproduction, but does prostatitis affect conception or pregnancy? Infants regurgitate regularly, but if their vomiting becomes severe, they need to see a gastroenterologist or a pediatric subspecialist. Obstetricians are surgeons, but they do not perform general surgery. Breast cancer is of highest concern to women, yet its course of treatment is supervised by oncologists. Congenital conditions, once diagnosed, are usually attended to by the pertinent specialist.

Thus, we have kept the content of this book narrowed to the specialized language necessary for female-specific health (gynecology) not addressed by general or reproductive medicine; fertility, conception, pregnancy, and birth (obstetrics); and areas affecting growth, development, and health of offspring from conception to age 18 (pediatrics). These are vast fields by themselves. Such focus will assist you in finding that specialized word or piece of equipment quickly, a key ingredient for medical transcription accuracy and production.

We hope that our selections, which include fetology, fetal surgery, neonatology, pediatrics, adolescent medicine, genetics, assisted reproduction, obstetrics, gynecology, and associated surgeries, tests, and drugs, along with a smattering of psychology, will prove useful.

Jo-Ann Clarke did the lion's share of the background work on this combined OB-GYN and Pediatrics book. I am grateful for her contributions. Thanks also to Jeanne Bock for her review and recommendations for the appendices. There are many freelancers and employees involved in bringing a book to the shelf; they all have my appreciation. We are all honored by medical transcriptionists, who continue to choose *Stedman's* books.

Ellen Atwood
May 9, 2004

Publisher's Preface

Stedman's OB-GYN & Pediatric Words, Includes Neonatology, Fourth Edition, offers an authoritative assurance of quality and exactness to the wordsmiths of the healthcare professions—medical transcriptionists, medical editors and copyeditors, health information management personnel, court reporters, and the many other users and producers of medical documentation.

In *Stedman's OB-GYN & Pediatric Words, Includes Neonatology, Fourth Edition,* users will find thousands of words related to gynecology, pediatrics, maternal-fetal medicine, endocrinology, infertility, ART, neonatology, and medical genetics. Users will also find terms for diagnostic and therapeutic procedures, new techniques, and lab tests, as well as equipment names and abbreviations with their expansions. The appendix sections provide anatomical illustrations with useful captions and labels; sample reports; common terms by procedure; and drugs listed by indication. For quick reference, we have also included tables of Apgar scores, common poisonings, biophysical profile scores, and normal lab values.

This compilation of more than 100,000 entries, fully cross-indexed for quick access developed from *Stedman's Medical Dictionary, 27th Edition,* and supplemented by terminology found in current medical literature (please see list of References on page xix).

We at Lippincott Williams & Wilkins strive to provide you with the most up-to-date and accurate word references available. Your use of this Word Book will prompt new editions, which we will publish as often as updates and revisions justify. We welcome your suggestions for improvements, changes, corrections, and additions—whatever will make this *Stedman's* product more useful to you. Please complete the postpaid card at the back of this book or complete the Got a Good Word submission on www.stedmans.com.

Explanatory Notes

Medical transcription is an art as well as a science. Both approaches are needed to correctly interpret the dictation of a physician, whose language is a product of education, training, and experience. This variety in medical language means that there are several acceptable ways to express certain terms, including jargon. *Stedman's OB-GYN & Pediatric Words, Includes Neonatology, Fourth Edition,* provides variant spellings and phrasings for many terms. These elements, in addition to complete cross-indexing, make *Stedman's OB-GYN & Pediatric Words, Includes Neonatology, Fourth Edition,* a valuable resource for determining the validity of terms as they are encountered.

Alphabetical Organization
Alphabetization of main entries is letter by letter as spelled, ignoring punctuation, spaces, prefixed numbers, or other special characters. For example:

umbilical
>   u. coiling index (UCI)
>   10-mm u. port
>   u. vein catheter (UVC)

Terms beginning with Greek letters show the Greek letter spelled out and listed alphabetically. For example:

beta, β
>   b. carotene
>   estrogen receptor b.
>   b. thalassemia

In subentry alphabetization, the abbreviated singular form or the spelled-out plural form of the noun main entry word is ignored.

Format and Style
All main entries are in **boldface** to expedite locating a sought-after term, to enhance distinction between main entries and subentries, and to relieve the textual density of the pages. Most main entries included are singular; exceptions to this rule are noted below. Plural subentries are noted by the convention of adding 's. This does not imply possessive, nor does it indicate preferred spelling:

activity
    a.'s of daily living

Plural, Preferred, Variants

English terms or Anglicized Latin terms are shown in American English spelling. Exceptions include publications, studies, or other titles, which may carry the British spelling, or spelling of the language of origin.

United States Pharmacopeia
British Pharmacopoeia
bacille Calmette-Guérin

Irregular plurals and variant spellings are shown on the same line as the singular or preferred form of the word. For example:

os, pl. **ora**
anulus, annulus

Terms typically used in the plural are listed with the plural first:

criteria, sing. **criterion**
adnexa, sing. **adnexum**

Hyphenation

As a rule of style, multiple eponyms (e.g., Counsellor-Davis artificial vagina operation) are hyphenated. Also, hyphens have been added between a manufacturer and one or more eponyms (e.g., Vital-Metzenbaum dissecting scissors). Please note that in many cases, hyphenation is a question of style, not of accuracy, and thus is a matter of choice.

Eponyms and Possessives

The possessive form of eponyms (**Down's syndrome**) has been dropped (**Down syndrome**) in this reference for the sake of consistency and conformance with the guidelines of the American Association for Medical Transcription (AAMT) and other groups.

Possessive forms of common nouns are still used:

witch's milk
footballer's migraine

Please note, however, that in many cases, retaining the possessive, like hyphenating, is a question of style, not of accuracy, and thus is a matter of choice. To form the possessive of a word, simply add the apostrophe or apostrophe "s" to the end of the word. The style convention of adding 's to plural subentries, explained above, does not imply possessive.

Trademarks and Manufacturers Names

Every effort is made to verify accurate representation of manufacturer's preferred spelling and style for equipment and proprietary names. We no longer use all capital letter forms of equipment or drug names, and do not use symbols such as ® or ™. Irregular capitalization is used as required. You may find a term in this book with spelling identical to, but capitalization differing from, another main entry or book in this series. This occurs if the two entries are different terms, designed for these specialties, or are from a different manufacturer.

Genus and Species

Genus and species names of bacteria, fungi, and plants are italicized, with genus capitalized.

Staphylococcus aureus
Streptococcus viridans

Common bacteria and fungus names used as modifiers, or in a general way, are lower case, regular font:

beta hemolytic staphylococcus
strep throat

Cross-indexing

The word list is in an index-like main entry-subentry format that contains two combined alphabetical listings:

(1) A *noun* main entry-subentry organization, which is typical of the A-Z section of medical dictionaries like *Stedman's*:

septum
  membranous s.
  nasal s.
  uterine s.

transfusion
  autologous t.
  intrauterine maternofetal t.
  twin-to-twin t.

(2) An *adjective* main entry-subentry organization, which lists words and phrases as you hear them. The main entries are the adjectives or modifiers in a multiword term. The subentries are the nouns around which the terms are constructed and to which the adjectives or modifiers pertain:

neonatal
    n. encephalopathy (NE)
    n. hemochromatosis (NH)
    n. intensive care unit (NICU)

severe
    s. chronic neutropenia (SCN)
    s. combined immunodeficiency disorder (SCID)
    s. ovarian hyperstimulation syndrome (SOHS)

This format provides the user with more than one way to locate and identify a multiword term. For example:

sequencing
    gene s.

gene
    g. sequencing

diabetic
    d. fetopathy

fetopathy
    diabetic f.

It also allows the user to see together all terms that contain a particular descriptor, as well as all types, kinds, or variations of a noun entity. For example:

serum
    fetal s.
    s. inhibitory titer (SIT)
    maternal s.

failure
    fertility f.
    growth f.
    f. to thrive (FTT)

Wherever possible, abbreviations are separately defined and cross-referenced. For example:

GIFT
    gamete intrafallopian transfer

gamete
    g. intrafallopian transfer (GIFT)

transfer
    gamete intrafallopian t. (GIFT)

References

In addition to the manufacturers' literature we gather at various medical meetings, scientific reports from hospitals, and the lists created by our MT Editorial Advisory Board members from their daily transcription work, we used the following sources for new terms in *Stedman's OB-GYN & Pediatric Words, Includes Neonatology, Fourth Edition*:

Books

Bankowski BJ, ed. The Johns Hopkins Manual of Gynecology and Obstetrics. 2nd Edition. Philadelphia: Lippincott Williams & Wilkins, 2002.

Bernstein D, Shelov SP, eds. Pediatrics for Medical Students. 2nd Edition. Philadelphia: Lippincott Williams & Wilkins, 2003.

Boynton RW, ed. Manual of Ambulatory Pediatrics. 5th Edition. London: Lippincott Williams & Wilkins, 2003.

Dorland's Obstetrics Gynecology Word Book for Medical Transcriptionists. Philadelphia: WB Saunders Co, 2002.

Havens CS, Sullivan ND, eds. Manual of Outpatient Gynecology. 4th Edition. Philadelphia: Lippincott Williams & Wilkins, 2002.

Hill WC, ed. Ambulatory Obstetrics. Philadelphia: Lippincott Williams & Wilkins, 2002.

Lance LL. 2003 Quick Look Drug Book. Baltimore: Lippincott Williams & Wilkins, 2003.

MacDonald MG, Ramasethu J, eds. Atlas of Procedures in Neonatology. Philadelphia: Lippincott Williams & Wilkins, 2002.

Migita DS, Christakis DA, eds. The Saint-Frances Guide to Pediatrics. Baltimore: Lippincott Williams & Wilkins, 2003.

Morgan G, Hamilton C, eds. Practice Guidelines for Obstetrics & Gynecology. 2nd Edition. Philadelphia: Lippincott Williams & Wilkins, 2003.

Peter G, ed. 1997 Red Book: Report of the Committee on Infectious Diseases. 24th Edition. Elk Grove Village, IL: American Academy of Pediatrics, 1997.

Pitman SC, ed. OB-GYN and Genitourinary Words and Phrases. Modesto, CA: Health Professions Institute, 2002

Pyle V. Current Medical Terminology, 9th Edition. Modesto, CA: Health Professions Institute, 2003.

Reece EA, Hobbins JC, eds. Medicine of the Fetus and Mother, 2nd Edition. Philadelphia: Lippincott-Raven Publishers, 1999.

Rhodes S, ed. Dorland's Pediatrics Word Book for Medical Transcriptionists. Philadelphia: WB Saunders Co, 2004.

Rock JA, Jones HW III, eds. Te Linde's Operative Gynecology. 9th Edition. Philadelphia: Lippincott Williams & Wilkins, 2003.

Sabella C, Cunningham RJ, Moodie DS, eds. The Cleveland Clinic Intensive Review of Pediatrics. Philadelphia: Lippincott Williams & Wilkins, 2002.

Schwartz MW, ed. Clinical Handbook of Pediatrics. 3rd Edition. Philadelphia: Lippincott Williams & Wilkins, 2003.

Scott JR, Gibbs RS, Karlan BY, Haney AF, eds. Danforth's Obstetrics and Gynecology. 9th Edition. Philadelphia: Lippincott Williams & Wilkins, 2003.

Stedman's Medical Dictionary, 27th Edition. Baltimore: Lippincott Williams & Wilkins, 2000.

Images

Agur, AMR, Lee, MJ. Grant's Atlas of Anatomy, 10th edition. Baltimore: Lippincott Williams & Wilkins, 1999.

Fuller J, Schaller-Ayers J. Health Assessment: A Nursing Approach. 3rd Edition. Baltimore: Lippincott Williams & Wilkins, 2000.

Hardy NO. Westport, CT. Stedman's Medical Dictionary, 27th edition. Baltimore: Lippincott Williams & Wilkins, 2000.

LifeART Nursing 1, CD-ROM. Baltimore: Lippincott Williams & Wilkins.

LifeART Nursing 2, CD-ROM. Baltimore: Lippincott Williams & Wilkins.

LifeART Nursing 3, CD-ROM. Baltimore: Lippincott Williams & Wilkins.

LifeART Pediatrics 1, CD-ROM. Baltimore: Lippincott Williams & Wilkins.

LifeART Super Anatomy Collection 9, CD-ROM. Baltimore: Lippincott Williams & Wilkins.

MediClip Clinical Cardiopilmonary Images, CD-ROM. Baltimore: Lippincott Williams & Wilkins.

MediClip Clinical OB/GYN Images, CD-ROM. Baltimore: Lippincott Williams & Wilkins.

MediClip Color Anatomy 2 Images, CD-ROM. Baltimore: Lippincott Williams & Wilkins.

Nettina SM. The Lippincott Manual of Nursing Practice. 6th Edition. Baltimore: Lippincott Williams & Wilkins, 1996.

Pillitteri A. Maternal & Child Health Nursing: Care of the Childbearing & Childrearing Family. Baltimore: Lippincott Williams & Wilkins, 2002.

Roche Lexikon Medizin, 3rd edition. Munich, Germany: Urban & Schwarzenberg, 1993.

Sauerland, EK. Grant's Dissector,12th edition. Baltimore: Lippincott Williams & Wilkins, 1999.

Schenk S. Jackson, MS. Stedman's Medical Dictionary, 27th edition. Baltimore: Lippincott Williams & Wilkins, 2000.

Smeltzer SC, Bare BG. Textbook of Medical-Surgical Nursing, 9th Ed. Philadelphia: Lippincott Williams & Wilkins, 2000.

Journals

Contemporary OB/GYN. Montvale, NJ: Medical Economics, 2002–2004.

Contemporary Pediatrics. Montvale, NJ: Medical Economics, 2002–2004.

Journal of Pediatric Gastroenterology and Nutrition. Baltimore: Lippincott Williams & Wilkins, 2002–2004.

OBGYN News. Morristown, NJ: International Medical News Group, 2002–2004.

OBGYN Clinical Alert. Atlanta: American Health Consultants, 2002–2004.

Obstetrical and Gynecological Survey. Baltimore: Lippincott Williams & Wilkins, 2002–2004.

Pediatric Emergency Care. Baltimore: Lippincott Williams & Wilkins, 2002–2004.

Stedman's WordWatcher. Baltimore: Lippincott Williams & Wilkins, 1995–2004.

The Female Patient. Chatham, NJ: Quadratn HealthCom, 2002–2004.

The Journal of Pediatrics. St. Louis: Mosby, 2002–2004.

The Pediatric Infectious Disease Journal. Baltimore: Lippincott Williams & Wilkins, 2002–2004.

Websites

http://asrm.abstracts.org/1997TOC.HTM

http://generalpediatrics.com/

http://genomics.phrma.org

http://home.coqui.net/myrna/

http://news.bmn.com/hmsbeagle

http://pediatrics.about.com/health/pediatrics/

http://pedsccm.wustl.edu/

http://ww2.med.jhu.edu/peds/neonatology/

http://www.acog.com

http://www.ama-assn.org/insight/h_focus/wom_hlth/wom_hlth.htm

http://www.ama-assn.org/special/womh/womh.htm

http://www.amwa-doc.org

http://www.cdc.gov/genetics/update/current.htm

http://www.cdc.gov/nip/recs/child-schedule.PDF

http://www.centerwatch.com/studies/LISTING.HTM

http://www.fpnotebook.com/NIC.htm

http://www.geneticalliance.org

http://www.hpisum.com

http://www.hum-molgen.de

http://www.icondata.com/health/pedbase/

http://www.mayohealth.org/mayo/0003/htm/hrt.htm

http://www.mcg.edu/PedsOnL/ForHealthProf/HealthProfMenu.html

http://www.medscape.com

http://www.mtdesk.com

http://www.mtmonthly.com

http://www.neonatology.org/

http://www.nhgri.nih.gov

http://www.nichd.nih.gov/

http://www.nlm.nih.gov/mesh/jablonski/syndrome_title.html

http://www.obgyn.net/medical.asp

http://www.pedinfo.org/welcome.html

http://www.sph.uth.tmc.edu/retnet/what-dis.htm

http://www.thebody.com/apla/july99/immunize.html

http://www.utoronto.ca/kids/

http://www.virtualdrugstore.com

http://www.womens-health.org

α (*var. of* alpha)
A
  abortus
  alveolar
    A antigen
    A and D Ointment
A2
  thromboxane A2
A$_4$
  androstenedione
A$_2$
  hemoglobin A. (HbA$_2$)
  phospholipase A.
a
  arterial
A-200 Shampoo
AA
  acetabular anteversion
  acute appendicitis
  atlantoaxial
    AA genotype
A-a
  alveolar-arterial
    A-a gradient
a-A
  arterial to alveolar
AAA
  achalasia-addisonianism-alacrimia
    AAA syndrome
AABR, A-ABR
  automated auditory brainstem response
    AABR hearing screening
AAC
  augmentative and alternative
    communication
AACAP
  American Academy of Child and
    Adolescent Psychiatry
AAD
  antibiotic-associated diarrhea
AADH
  alopecia, anosmia, deafness,
    hypogonadism
    AADH syndrome
Aagenaes syndrome
AAI
  axial acetabular index
AAM
  aggressive angiomyxoma
AAMD
  American Association on Mental
    Deficiency
    AAMD Adaptive Behavior Scale
    for Children and Adults

AAMR
  American Association on Mental
    Retardation
AAP
  American Academy of Pediatrics
AAPCC
  American Association of Poison Control
    Centers
Aarskog-Scott syndrome (ASS)
Aarskog syndrome
Aase-Smith syndrome
Aase syndrome
AASH
  adrenal androgen-stimulating hormone
AAST
  American Association for the Surgery of
    Trauma
    AAST Organ Injury Scaling of
      vulva, vagina, bladder, urethral,
      rectal injury (grade I–V)
AAT
  animal-assisted therapy
AB
  abdominal
  abortion
  abortus
A&B
  apnea and bradycardia
    A&B spell
ABA
  applied behavior analysis
abacavir
ABAER
  automated brainstem auditory evoked
    response
abandonment
abarelix depot-F, -M
Abate
Abbe-McIndoe
  A.-M. procedure
  A.-M. vaginal reconstruction
Abbe-McIndoe-Williams procedure
Abbe vaginal construction
Abbe-Wharton-McIndoe procedure
Abbokinase
Abbot LCx Uriprobe assay
**Abbott LifeCare PCA Plus II infusion
system**
ABC
  absolute band count
  airway, breathing, circulation
  argon beam coagulator
  aspiration biopsy cytology

ABCDE
> airway, breathing, circulation and control
> bleeding, disability, exposure
>> ABCDE assessment

Abderhalden-Fanconi syndrome

abdomen
> acute a.
> bloated a.
> distended a.
> milk lines of a.
> pendulous a.
> scaphoid a.
> tympanitic a.

abdominal (AB)
> a. actinomycosis
> a. adhesion
> a. approach
> a. auscultation
> a. ballottement
> a. binder
> a. breathing
> a. bruit
> a. cavity
> a. circumference (AC)
> a. coarctation
> a. compartment syndrome (ACS)
> a. crisis
> a. delivery
> a. distention
> a. dystocia
> a. enlargement
> a. epilepsy
> a. examination
> a. fetal echocardiography
> a. fetal electrocardiography
> a. free-fluid sign
> a. girth
> a. hernia
> a. heterotaxy
> a. hysterectomy
> a. hysteropexy
> a. hysterotomy
> a. incision
> a. irradiation
> a. leak point pressure (ALPP)
> a. mass
> a. metroplasty
> a. migraine
> a. muscle deficiency
> a. muscle deficiency anomalad
> a. muscle deficiency syndrome
> a. muscular deficiency
> a. musculature aplasia syndrome
> a. myomectomy
> a. neurofibroma
> a. ostium
> a. pain
> a. paravaginal repair
> a. percussion

> a. peritoneum
> a. pregnancy
> a. radiograph
> a. rectopexy
> a. rescue
> a. sacral colpoperineopexy
> a. sacral colpopexy
> a. sacrocolpopexy
> a. sacropexy
> a. sacrospinous ligament
>> colposuspension
> a. salpingo-oophorectomy
> a. salpingotomy
> a. sheath
> a. stria
> a. strip radiotherapy
> a. tenderness
> a. trauma
> a. tuberculosis
> a. ultrasound
> a. wall

abdominis
> a. muscle
> rectus a.

abdominocyesis
abdominocystic
abdominogenital
abdominohysterectomy
abdominohysterotomy
abdominopelvic
> a. CT scan
> a. irradiation
> a. pain
> a. procedure
> a. scan

abdominoperineal resection
abdominoscrotal hydrocele
abdominovaginal hysterectomy
abducens
> a. facial paralysis
> a. nerve
> a. palsy

abducent palsy
abducted thumbs syndrome
abduction
> a. cast
> defective eye a.
> forefoot a.
> resisted a.
> a. splint

abductor lurch
Abelcet
abembryonic
Aberdeen knot
Aberfeld syndrome
aberrancy
> puberal a.

aberrant
> a. coronary artery

a. course
a. course of testicular descent
a. regeneration
a. right subclavian artery (ARSA)
a. subclavian artery
a. supraventricular tachycardia
a. systemic feeding artery
a. vitamin D metabolism

aberration
chromosomal a.
chromosome a.
fetal growth a.
G-banded cytogenetic a.
heterosomal a.
newtonian a.
penta-X chromosomal a.
sex chromosome a.
steroidogenic a.
tetra-X chromosomal a.
triple-X chromosomal a.

abetalipoproteinemia (ABL)

ABG
arterial blood gas

ABI
ABI model 373, 377 sequencing gel system
ABI model 377 sequencing gel system
ABI PRISM Dye Terminator Cycle Sequencing Ready Reaction Kit

ability
cognitive a.
Illinois Test of Psycholinguistic A.'s (IPTA)
McCarthy Scales of Children's A.'s
Revised Tests of Cognitive A.

Abiotrophia
A. defectiva
A. elegans

abiotrophy
Leber a.

abirritant

Abitrate

ABL
abetalipoproteinemia

ablactation

ablation
balloon endometrial a.
endometrial a.
endometrial resection and a. (ERA)
hysteroscopic endometrial a.
laser a.

laser uterosacral nerve a. (LUNA)
microwave endometrial a. (MEA)
mucosal intact laser tonsillar a. (MILTA)
Nd:YAG laser a.
ovarian a.
partial rollerball endometrial a.
percutaneous transluminal coronary rotational a. (PTCRA)
radiofrequency catheter a.
rectoscopic endometrial a.
rollerball endometrial a. (REA)
rollerbar-loop-rollerbar a.
stellate ganglion a.
thermal balloon a.
transurethral a.
uterosacral nerve a.
valve a.

ablatio placentae

ablative
a. surgery
a. therapy with bone marrow rescue

ablator
endometrial a.

ablepharon-macrostomia syndrome (AMS)

ABM
adult bone marrow

aBMD
areal bone mineral density

abnormal
a. aortic valve attachment
a. cortical visual input
a. cortisol secretion
a. deceleration
a. dysfluency
a. embryo
a. face
a. facies
a. feedback signal
a. fetal development
a. gastric emptying
a. gene expression
a. gestational sac
a. glucosylceramide storage
a. head size
A. Involuntary Movement Scale (AIMS)
a. karyotype
a. labor
a. laxity of upper airway

NOTES

3

abnormal *(continued)*
    a. lie
    a. menstruation
    a. mitochondrion
    a. opacity
    a. palate
    a. palpebral fissure
    a. penile curvature
    a. phonation
    a. placentation
    a. puberty
    a. respiratory pattern
    a. response
    a. transit
    a. uterine bleeding (AUB)
    a. vaginal bleeding
    a. vasculature flow pattern
abnormality
    acral dysostosis with facial and
      genital a.'s
    cardiac a.
    central serotonin a.
    cervical a.
    chromosomal structural a.
    coagulation a.
    congenital enamel a.
    conotruncal a.
    cord a.
    cortical gyral a.
    deflexion a.
    dermatoglyphic a.
    electrographic background a.
    electroretinal a.
    epithelial cell a.
    extracardiac a.
    Fairbank skeletal a.
    fetal chromosome a.
    fetal postural a.
    fetal thoracic a.
    fibrinogen a.
    fishmouth a.
    genetic a.
    genitourinary a.
    gestational a.
    gyral a.
    hemodynamic a.
    histologic a.
    hormonal a.
    hypogonadism, alopecia, diabetes
      mellitus, mental retardation,
      deafness and ECG a.'s
    immune-mediated a.
    intrapartum fetal heart rate a.
    macrosomia, obesity, macrocephaly,
      ocular a. (MOMO)
    mammographic a.
    metabolic a.
    midbrain a.
    müllerian a.

    multiple endocrine a.'s (MEA)
    neurobehavioral a.
    neurologic a.
    nonpalpable a.
    oral-facial-digital syndrome with
      retinal a.'s
    ovarian a.
    palpable bony a.
    parental chromosomal a.
    parental chromosome a.
    perisylvian a.
    placental a.
    placentation a.
    platelet a.
    possible migrational a.
    posterior fossa malformation,
      hemangiomas, arterial anomalies,
      coarctation of aorta and cardiac
      defects, eye a.'s (PHACE)
    regional wall motion a.
    reproductive tract a.
    Ribbing skeletal a.
    sex chromosomal a.
    sex chromosome a.
    single-gene a.
    situs a.
    skeletal a.
    skeletal abnormalities, cutis laxa,
      craniostenosis, psychomotor
      retardation, facial a.'s (SCARF)
    soft tissue a.
    spinal cord injury without
      radiographic a. (SCIWORA)
    sporadic chromosome a.
    ST-segment a.
    ST-T wave a.
    tuberous breast a.
    T-wave a.
    umbilical artery waveform
      notching a.
    urinary tract a.
    uterine a.
    vaginal epithelial a.
    X-chromosome a.
**abnormally wide splitting of second
heart sound**
ABO
    ABO antigen
    ABO blood group system
    ABO erythroblastosis
    ABO hemolytic disease
    ABO hemolytic disease of the
      newborn
    ABO incompatibility
aboral flow
abort
aborted ectopic pregnancy
aborter
    habitual a.

abortient
abortifacient
abortigenic
abortion (AB)
    Aburel a.
    accidental a.
    ampullar a.
    aneuploid a.
    complete a.
    a. complication
    criminal a.
    Csapo a.
    elective a.
    euploid a.
    habitual a.
    idiopathic a.
    imminent a.
    incipient a.
    incomplete a.
    induced a.
    inevitable a.
    infected a.
    justifiable a.
    menstrual extraction a.
    missed a.
    recurrent euploidic a.
    recurrent spontaneous a. (RSA)
    repeated a.
    saline a.
    selective a.
    septic a.
    spontaneous a. (SAB)
    surgically-induced a.
    therapeutic a. (TA, TAB)
    threatened a.
    tubal a.
abortionist
abortive poliomyelitis
abortus (A, AB)
Aboulker stent
ABP
    ambulatory blood pressure
    arterial blood pressure
ABPA
    allergic bronchopulmonary aspergillosis
ABPM
    ambulatory blood pressure monitoring
ABPN
    American Board of Psychiatry and
     Neurology
ABQ
    attitude behavior questionnaire

ABR
    auditory brainstem response
abrachia
abrachiocephalia
Abramson classification
abrasion
    corneal a.
    pleural a.
abrogated neonatal alveolization
abruption
    placental a.
    sinus a.
abruptio placentae (AP)
ABS
    arterial blood sample
abscess
    amebic hepatic a.
    amebic liver a.
    appendiceal a.
    auricular a.
    Bartholin gland a.
    Bezold a.
    biliary a.
    breast a.
    Brodie a.
    a. cavity
    cold a.
    cranial epidural a.
    crypt a.
    dental a.
    Douglas a.
    Dubois a.
    embolic a.
    epidural a.
    extradural a.
    a. formation
    intermuscular a.
    intersphincteric a.
    intraabdominal a.
    intramedullary spinal a.
    ischiorectal a.
    lung a.
    metastatic tuberculous a.
    milk a.
    myocardial a.
    neonatal scalp a.
    orbital subperiosteal a.
    otogenic brain a.
    ovarian a.
    parametritic a.
    parapharyngeal a.
    parauterine a.

NOTES

abscess *(continued)*
paravertebral a.
parenchymal a.
pelvic a.
perianal a.
periappendiceal a.
perinephric a.
perirectal a.
perirenal a.
peritonsillar a.
premammary a.
psoas a.
pyogenic a.
retroesophageal a.
retropharyngeal a.
retrotonsillar a.
spinal epidural a.
stitch a.
subareolar a.
subdural a.
subperiosteal a.
subphrenic a.
supralevator a.
tuberculous a.
tuboovarian a. (TOA)
visceral a.

abscessus
Mycobacterium a.

absence
a. of abdominal muscle syndrome
a. attack
atypical a.
a. of branch pulmonary artery
congenital a.
a. defect
a. epilepsy
myoclonic a.
protein-induced vitamin K a.
(PIVKA)
a. of rectal muscles
a. seizure
a. status
a. status epilepticus
testicular a.
uterine a.
vaginal a.

absent
ankle reflexes a.
a. antihelical fold
a. cerebellum
a. menses
a. patella
a. prostate
a. pulmonary valve syndrome
a. radius
a. splenium
a. tears
a. testes

Absolok endoscopic clip applicator

absolute
a. band count (ABC)
a. cardiac dullness
a. CD4 count
a. length gain
a. lymphocyte count
a. neutrophil count
a. nucleated red blood cell
(ANRBC)
a. shunt
a. sterility
a. temperature
a. weight gain

absorbable
a. gelatin sponge
a. staple
a. suture

absorbance
time-of-flight and a. (TOFA)

absorbed
rabies vaccine, a. (RVA)

absorbent gelling material (AGM)

Absorbine Jr. Antifungal

absorptiometer
Hologic 1000 QDR dual-energy a.
Lunar DPX dual-energy a.

absorptiometry
dual-energy photon a.
dual-energy x-ray a. (DEXA,
DXA)
dual-photon a.
radiographic a.
single-energy photon a.
single-photon a.
x-ray a.

absorption
calcium a.
coefficient of fat a.
defective tryptophan a.
fat a.
a. fever
fluorescent treponemal antibody a.
(FTA-ABS)

absorptive hypercalciuria

ABSR
auditory brainstem response

abstinence
a. score
a. syndrome

abstract thinking

ABT
alternating breath test

Abt-Letterer-Siwe syndrome

Aburel abortion

abuse
alcohol a.
CAGE test for alcohol a.
child a. (CA)
child physical a. (CPA)

child sexual a. (CSA)
domestic a.
a. dwarfism syndrome
emotional a.
mandated reporter (of child a.)
maternal drug a.
maternal substance a.
physical a.
physical sexual a. (PSA)
psychological a.
sexual a.
a., sexuality, safety assessment
spousal a.
substance a.
verbal a.

abuser
child of substance a. (COSA)

ABVD
Adriamycin (doxorubicin), bleomycin, vinblastine, dacarbazine

AC
abdominal circumference
acromioclavicular
AC joint

A1c
hemoglobin A1c

ACA
anticentromere antibody

acalculous cholecystitis
acalvaria
Acanthamoeba
A. *castellani*
A. *culbertsoni*
A. keratitis
A. polyphagia
A. *rhysodes*

acanthocyte
acanthocytosis
acantholysis bullosa
acanthosis
a. nigricans
paraductal a.

ACAPI
anterior cerebral artery pulsatility index

acarbose
acardia
acardiac fetus
acardiacus
fetus a.

acardius
acephalus a.

fetus a.
a. myelacephalus

Acarosan
ACAT
automated computerized axial tomography

acatalasemia
acatalasia
accelerate
accelerated
a. atherosclerosis
a. hypertension
a. junctional ectopic tachycardia
a. painless labor (APL)
a. rejection
a. skeletal maturation, Marshall-Smith type
a. starvation

acceleration
FHR a.
a. injury
a. phase

acceleration-deceleration force
accelerator
betatron electron a.
linear a.

accentuation
perifollicular a.

acceptance stage
access
fetoplacental a.
transcervical tubal a.
uterine a.

accessory
a. auricle
BabyFace 3-D surface rendering a.
a. breast
a. chromosome
a. lobe of placenta
a. müllerian funnel
a. muscle
a. muscle retraction
a. navicular
a. nerve
a. nipple
a. ovarian tissue
a. ovary
a. placenta
a. protein
a. sex gland
a. soleus
a. spleen

NOTES

accessory *(continued)*
    a. tragus
    a. yolk
accident
    cerebrovascular a. (CVA)
    cord a.
    neonatal vascular a.
    obstetric a.
    umbilical cord a.
accidental
    a. abortion
    a. caustic ingestion
    a. dural puncture
    a. fetal injury
    a. hemorrhage
    a. penetration
    a. poisoning
    a. pregnancy
Accolate
accommodation
    gastric a.
accommodative esotropia
accompanying mood state
accouchement forcé
accoucheur
accreditation
accreta
    placenta a.
accretio cordis
accretion
    bone a.
    mass a.
    neural tissue a.
Accu-Chek
    A.-C. Easy glucose monitor
    A.-C. II Freedom blood glucose monitor
    A.-C. II glucometer
    A.-C. test
AccuLevel
accumbens
    nucleus a.
accumulation
    dermatan sulfate a.
    glycogen a.
    heparan sulfate a.
    ketoacid a.
    lipid a.
Accupep HPF enteral formula
accuracy
    assay a.
    diagnostic a.
Accurbron
    A. Aerolate III
Accurette
    A. endometrial suction curette
    A. microcurettage
Accuscope II
AccuSite injectable gel

AccuSpan tissue expander
AccuStat
    A. hCG pregnancy test
    A. Strep A assay
accustimulation
    electrical a.
Accutane
    A. dysmorphic syndrome
    A. effect
ACD
    alopecia, contracture, dwarfism
    area of cardiac dullness
    ACD level
    ACD mental retardation syndrome
ACE
    angiotensin-converting enzyme
    antegrade continence enema
    ACE genotype
    ACE inhibitor
    ACE procedure
acebutolol
Acel-Imune
    A.-I. HibTITER
    A.-I. vaccine
acellular
    a. pertussis
    a. pertussis vaccine
acentric chromosome
acephalia *(var. of* acephalus)
acephalobrachia
acephalocardia
acephalochiria
acephalogaster
acephalogastria
acephalopodia
acephalorrhachia
acephalostomia
acephalostomus
acephalothoracia
acephalothorus
acephalous
acephalus, acephalia
    a. acardius
Acephen
aceruloplasminemia
Aceta
acetabula (*pl. of* acetabulum)
acetabular
    a. anteversion (AA)
    a. dysplasia
    a. index (AI)
    a. labrum
    a. roof
acetabuloplasty
    Pemberton a.
acetabulum, gen. acetabuli, pl. acetabula
    protrusio acetabuli
    shallow a.

acetamide
    modafinil a.
acetaminophen
    hydrocodone and a.
    oxycodone and a.
    propoxyphene and a.
    a. toxicity
    a. Uniserts
Acetasol HC otic
acetate
    aluminum a.
    calcium a.
    cellulose a. (CA)
    Cortone A.
    cyproterone a.
    depomedroxyprogesterone a.
     (DMPA)
    depot medroxyprogesterone a.
     (DMPA)
    desmopressin a.
    estradiol cypionate and
     medroxyprogesterone a.
    estradiol/norethindrone a.
    flecainide a.
    Florinef A.
    ganirelix a.
    glatiramer a.
    gonadorelin a.
    goserelin a.
    histrelin a.
    leuprolide a.
    leuprorelin a.
    m-cresyl a.
    medroxyprogesterone a. (MPA)
    megestrol a.
    methylprednisolone a.
    nafarelin a.
    norethindrone a.
    octreotide a.
    quingestanol a.
    sermorelin a.
    sodium a.
acetazolamide
acetic acid
acetoacetate
acetohexamide
acetone
acetonide
    fluocinolone a.
    triamcinolone a.
acetonuria
acetophenazine

acetophenetidin
acetophenide
    dihydroxyprogesterone a.
acetowhite
    a. epithelium
    a. lesion
    a. reaction
acetoxyprogesterone derivative
    17-α-acetoxyprogesterone derivative
acetylcholine chloride
acetylcholinesterase (ACHE, AchE)
    a. histochemical stain
acetyl-CoA
    a.-CoA carboxylase
    a.-CoA dehydrogenase
acetylcysteine drug
acetyldigitoxin
acetylsalicylic acid (ASA)
ACF
    asymmetric crying facies
    ACF syndrome
ACGME
    American College of Graduate Medical
     Education
achalasia
    familial a.
    infantile a.
achalasia-addisonianism-alacrimia (AAA)
achalasia-microcephaly syndrome
Achard syndrome
Achard-Thiers syndrome
ACHE, AchE
    acetylcholinesterase
ache
    stomach a.
acheilia
acheiria, achiria
acheiropody, achiropody
Achenbach
    A. Child Behavior Checklist
    A. questionnaire
achievable
    as low as reasonably a. (ALARA)
achievement
    Kaufman Test of Educational A.
     (K-TEA)
    Woodcock-Johnson Tests of A.
Achilles
    A. tendon
    A. tendon insertion
    A. tendon lengthening
    A. tendon xanthoma

NOTES

Achillis
    tendo A.
achiria (*var. of* acheiria)
achiropody (*var. of* acheiropody)
achlorhydria
acholic stool
achondrogenesis syndrome
achondroplasia
    homozygous a.
    a. syndrome
achondroplastic dwarfism
achromasia
achromia
achromians
    incontinentia pigmenti a.
achromic nevus
Achromobacter
    A. *lwoffi*
    A. *xylosoxidans*
Achromycin
    A. Ophthalmic
    A. Topical
    A. V
acid
    acetic a.
    acetylsalicylic a. (ASA)
    all-*trans*-retinoic a.
    alpha-aminoadipic a.
    alpha-ketoadipic a.
    alpha-linolenic a. (ALA)
    amino a.
    D-amino a.
    L-amino a.
    aminocaproic a.
    5-aminosalicylic a.
    amoxicillin-clavulanic a.
    antideoxyribonucleic a. (anti-DNA)
    arachidic a.
    arachidonic a.
    arginine-glycine-aspartic a. (arg-gly-asp)
    argininosuccinic a.
    arylalkanoic a.
    arylcarboxylic a.
    arylpropionic a.
    ascorbic a.
    aspartic a.
    a. aspiration syndrome
    bichloracetic a.
    bicinchonic a. (BCA)
    bile a.
    boric a.
    branched-chain amino a.
    branched-chain fatty a. (BCFA)
    branched deoxyribonucleic a. (bDNA)
    carbonic a.
    a. ceramidase deficiency
    9-cis-retinoic a.

    citrate and citric a.
    clavulanic a.
    complementary deoxyribonucleic a. (cDNA)
    conjugated linoleic a. (CLA)
    C-palmitic a.
    deoxyadenylic a. (dAMP)
    deoxycytidylic a. (dCMP)
    deoxyguanylic a. (dGMP)
    deoxyribonucleic a. (DNA)
    deoxythymidylic a. (dTMP)
    dibasic amino a.
    dichloroacetic a.
    diethylenetriaminepentaacetic a. (DTPA)
    diisopropyl iminodiacetic a. (DISIDA)
    dimercaptosuccinic a.
    docosahexaenoic a. (DHA)
    docosapentaenoic a.
    eicosapentaenoic a.
    elevated bile a.
    a. elution test
    epsilon-aminocaproic a. (EACA)
    erucic a.
    essential amino a.
    essential fatty a. (EFA)
    ethacrynic a.
    ethylenediaminetetraacetic a. (EDTA)
    excitotoxic amino a. (EAA)
    fatty a.
    flufenamic a.
    folic a.
    folinic a.
    formic a.
    formiminoglutamic a. (FIGLU)
    free fatty a.
    fusaric a.
    gamma-aminobutyric a. (GABA)
    glutamic a.
    gossypol acetic a. (GAA)
    homovanillic a. (HVA)
    hydriodic a.
    hydroxybenzoic a. (HABA)
    hydroxyeicosatetraenoic a.
    5-hydroxyindoleacetic a. (5-HIAA)
    21-hydroxyindoleacetic a. (21-HIAA)
    hypochlorous a.
    iduronic a.
    imino a.
    iocetamic a.
    iopanoic a.
    isobutyric a.
    isovaleric a.
    kinetoplast deoxyribonucleic a. (kDNA)
    lactic a.

linoleic a.
linolenic a.
a. lipase deficiency disease
lipid-associated sialic a.
lipoic a.
long-chain fatty a.
long-chain polyunsaturated fatty a.
  (LCPUFA)
lysergic a.
a. maltase
a. maltase deficiency (AMD)
mandelic a.
a. mantle
medium-chain fatty a. (MCFA)
mefenamic a.
messenger ribonucleic a. (mRNA)
methylmalonic a.
methylsuccinic a.
mitochondrial deoxyribonucleic a.
  (mtDNA)
mycophenolic a.
N-acetylaspartic a.
N-acetylneuraminic a. (NANA)
nalidixic a.
neuraminic a.
N-[2-hydroxyethyl]piperazine N'-[2-
  ethanesulfonic a.] (HEPES)
nicotinic a.
noncarbonic a.
nonessential amino a.
nonvolatile a.
nucleic a.
omega fatty a.
omega-3 fatty a.
orotic a.
palmitic a.
pantothenic a.
paraaminomethylbenzoic a.
  (PAMBA)
paraaminosalicylic a. (PAS)
a. peptic disease
phenylacetic a.
phenylpyruvic a.
a. phosphatase
phytanic a.
plasma linoleic a.
plasma very-long-chain fatty a.
polyglycolic a.
polyunsaturated fatty a. (PUFA)
pteroylglutamic a.
pyruvic a.
quinolinic a.

a. reflux
retinoic a.
ribonucleic a. (RNA)
salicylic a.
salicylsalicylic a.
serum amino a.
serum uric a.
short-chain fatty a. (SCFA)
short-chain polyunsaturated fatty a.
  (SCPUFA)
sialic a.
Slow Fe with folic a.
sodium citrate with citric a.
sulfur and salicylic a.
thioctic a.
ticarcillin/clavulanic a.
tolfenamic a.
tranexamic a.
trans fatty a. (tFA)
transfer ribonucleic a. (tRNA)
trichloroacetic a. (TCA)
2,4,5-trichlorophenoxyacetic a.
umbilical venous plasma amino a.
undecylenic a.
unsaturated linolenic a.
uric a.
urinary orotic a.
urine organic a.
urine vanillylmandelic a.
urocanic a.
ursodeoxycholic a.
valproic a.
vanillylmandelic a. (VMA)
very long chain fatty a. (VLCFA)
volatile a.
xanthurenic a.

acid-base
  a.-b. balance
  a.-b. disorder
  a.-b. equilibrium
  a.-b. measurement
  a.-b. problem
  a.-b. status
  a.-b. value
acidemia
  branched-chain amino a.
  fetal a.
  glutaric a. (type I, II)
  hyperpipecolic a.
  isovaleric a.
  lactic a.
  metabolic a.

NOTES

acidemia *(continued)*
    methylmalonic a.
    mevalonic a.
    mixed umbilical arterial a.
    organic a.
    orotic a.
    pipecolic a.
    propionic a.
    pyroglutamic a.
    trihydroxycoprostanic a.
acid-fast
    a.-f. bacillus
    a.-f. sputum smear
    a.-f. stain
acidic fibroblast growth factor (FGFa)
acidification
    disordered renal a.
    renal a.
    vaginal a.
acidified serum lysis test
acidity
    fecal a.
acid-loaded infant
acidophilus
    Lactobacillus a.
acidosis
    chronic respiratory a.
    congenital lactic a.
    cord blood a.
    diabetic a.
    fetal a.
    hyperchloremic metabolic a.
    hyperchloremic renal a.
    hyperchromic a.
    hypokalemic a.
    lactic a.
    metabolic a.
    nonanion gap metabolic a.
    organic a.
    perinatal a.
    primary lactic a.
    renal tubular a. (RTA)
    respiratory a.
    transient respiratory a.
acid-Schiff
    periodic a.-S. (PAS)
    a.-S. staining
aciduria
    alpha-aminoadipic a.
    alpha-ketoadipic a.
    argininosuccinic a.
    beta-aminoisobutyric a.
    ethylmalonic-adipic a.
    glutaric a. (type I, II)
    hereditary orotic a.
    HMG a.
    3-hydroxy-3-methylglutaric a.
    isovaleric a.
    3-methylglutaconic a.

    methylmalonic a. (MMA)
    mevalonic a.
    organic a.
    orotic a.
    paradoxical a.
    urocanic a.
    xanthurenic a.
Aci-Jel vaginal jelly
acinar artery
Acinetobacter
    A. baumannii
    A. lwoffi
acinic cell carcinoma
ACIP
    Advisory Committee on Immunization Practices
Aciphex
acitretin
ACL
    anterior cruciate ligament
aCL
    anticardiolipin antibody
aclasis
    diaphysial a.
Aclovate Topical
ACLS
    advanced cardiac life support
acne
    acute febrile ulcerative a.
    a. conglobata
    cosmetic a.
    a. cyst
    drug-induced a.
    a. fulminans
    a. (grade I–IV)
    gram-negative a.
    halogen a.
    neonatal a.
    a. neonatorum
    occupational a.
    a. rosacea
    steroid a.
    toddler-age nodulocystic a.
    truncal a.
    a. vulgaris
acnes
    Propionibacterium a.
acorn cannula
Acosta classification
acoustic
    a. admittance
    a. blink reflex
    a. enhancement
    a. impedance
    a. meningioma
    a. nerve
    a. neuroma
    a. reflectometry
    a. reflex test

a. respiratory motion sensor (ARMS)
a. schwannoma
a. shadow
a. stimulation study
a. stimulation test (AST)
a. trauma
acoustical interference
ACPS
  acrocephalopolysyndactyly
acquired
a. abducens palsy
a. agammaglobulinemia
a. angioedema (type I, II)
a. antithrombin III deficiency
a. ascending undescended testis
a. C1 INH deficiency
a. conjunctivitis
a. cutis laxa
a. epileptic aphasia
a. growth hormone deficiency
a. heart disease
a. hemolytic anemia
a. hemophilia
a. hydrocephalus
a. hypogammaglobulinemia
a. hypothalamic lesion
a. hypothyroidism
a. immune deficiency syndrome (AIDS)
a. immunodeficiency
a. immunodeficiency syndrome (AIDS)
a. immunodeficiency syndrome-related virus (ARV)
a. inflammatory Brown syndrome
a. melanocytic nevus (AMN)
nosocomially a. (NA)
a. nystagmus
a. PAP
a. platelet disorder
a. pneumonia
a. protein C, S deficiency
a. 6th nerve palsy
a. torticollis
a. urticaria
acquisita
  epidermolysis bullosa a.
acquisition
  intrauterine a.
  multiple gated a. (MUGA)

acral
a. cyanosis
a. demineralization
a. dysostosis with facial and genital abnormalities
a. keratotic papule
a. skin lesion
acral-renal-mandibular syndrome
acrania
acridine orange stain
acrid odor
acrivastine
acroblast
acrobrachycephaly
acrocallosal syndrome (ACS)
acrocentric chromosome
acrocephalopolysyndactyly (ACPS)
acrocephalosyndactyly (type I–V) (ACS)
acrocephaly
acrochordon
acrocraniofacial dysostosis
acrocyanosis
  peripheral a.
acrodermatitis
a. chronica atrophicans
a. enteropathica
papular a.
papular a. of childhood (PAC)
papulovesicular a.
acrodynia
acrodysgenital syndrome
acrodysostosis syndrome
acrodysplasia
acrodysplasia-dysostosis syndrome
acrofacial
a. dysostosis
a. dysostosis with postaxial defects syndrome
acrofrontofacionasal (AFFN)
acrokeratosis paraneoplastica
acromastitis
acromegaloid-cutis verticis gyrata-leukoma syndrome
acromegaloid facial appearance (AFA)
acromegaly
acromelic
a. frontonasal dysplasia
a. shortening
acromesomelia
acromesomelic
a. dwarfism
a. dysplasia

NOTES

acromial dimple
acromicric dysplasia
acromioclavicular (AC)
    a. ligament
acromion
    a. presentation
    a. process
acroosteolysis
    cranioskeletal dysplasia with a.
    hereditary osteodysplasia with a.
    a. syndrome
    a. with osteoporosis and changes
      in skull and mandible
acropectorovertebral dysplasia
acropustulosis
    a. of infancy
    infantile a.
acrorenal syndrome
acrorenomandibular syndrome
acrorenoocular syndrome
acrosin
acrosomal cap
acrosome
    a. reaction
    a. reaction with ionophore
      challenge (ARIC)
acrosome-intact sperm
acrosphenosyndactyly
acrosyndactyly
acrotism
acrylic splint
ACS
    abdominal compartment syndrome
    acrocallosal syndrome
    acrocephalosyndactyly (type I–V)
    acute chest syndrome
    American Cancer Society
    anterior cricoid split
      ACS procedure
ACT
    activated clotting time
act
    Americans with Disabilities A.
      (ADA)
    Child Abuse Prevention and
      Treatment A. (CAPTA)
    Education for All Handicapped
      Children A.
    Family Medical Leave A. (FMLA)
    Individuals with Disabilities
      Education A. (IDEA)
    self-harming a.
Actamin
act-FU-Cy
    actinomycin D, 5-fluorouracil,
    cyclophosphamide
ACTH
    adrenocorticotropic hormone
    ACTH deficiency

    ACTH gel
    ACTH insufficiency
    ACTH stimulation
    ACTH stimulation test
    ACTH unresponsiveness
Acthar gel
ActHIB vaccine
Acticin Cream
Acticort Topical
Actidose-Aqua
Actidose with Sorbitol
Actifed Allergy Tablet
Actigall
actigraphy
    limb a.
Actimmune
actin
    muscle a.
actinic prurigo
actin-myosin interaction
Actinobacillus actinomycetemcomitans
Actinomadura madurae
Actinomyces
    A. georgiae
    A. gerencseriae
    A. graevenitzii
    A. israelii
    A. meyeri
    A. naeslundii
    A. neuii
    A. odontolyticus
    A. pyogenes
    A. viscosus
actinomycetemcomitans
    Actinobacillus a.
actinomycin
    a. D
    a. D, 5-fluorouracil,
      cyclophosphamide (act-FU-Cy)
actinomycosis
    abdominal a.
    cervicofacial a.
    genital a.
    pelvic a.
action
    discoordinated uterine a.
    excessive insulin a.
    fetal heart a.
    gene a.
    law of mass a.
    luteolytic a.
    mediating a.
    muscarinic a.
    self-priming a.
    uterine a.
Actiprofen
activate
activated
    a. charcoal

a. clotting factor X
a. clotting time (ACT)
a. estrogen receptor
a. partial thromboplastin time
   (APTT)
a. partial thromboplastin time
   coagulation test
a. protein C (APC)
a. protein C resistance (APCR)
a. T cell

activation
egg a.
embryonic genome a.
endothelial cell a.
genome a.
polyclonal B cell a.

activator
gli family zinc-finger
   transcriptional a.'s
lymphocyte a.
plasminogen a. (PA)
Platelin Plus A.
recombinant tissue type
   plasminogen a. (rt-PA)
tissue plasminogen a. (t-PA)
urokinase plasminogen a. (u-PA)

active
a. bowel sounds
Free & A.
a. ignoring
a. immunization
Immunization Monitoring
   Program, A. (IMPACT)
a. and intense crying state
a. learner
a. phase
a. phase arrest
a. phase of labor
a. range of motion (AROM)
a. sleep
a. specific immunotherapy (ASI)
a. third-stage management

Activella, Activelle
activin A
activity
antigen a.
antigravity a.
aspartoacylase hydrolytic a.
breech-born with delayed fetal a.
cause-and-effect a.
ceramidase a.
colony-stimulating a. (CSA)

conjugation a.
daily a.
a.'s of daily living (ADL)
elevated enzyme a.
endometrial cycling a.
enzyme a.
epileptiform a.
fetal cardiac a.
fetal heart a.
fetal somatic a.
functional brain a.
high-voltage slow a. (HVSA)
H and Lewis blood group a.
low-voltage electrocortical a. (LV
   ECoG, LVECoG)
lupus anticoagulant a.
lymphotoxin antitumor a.
Manning score of fetal a.
mitogenic a.
opioid a.
ovarian a.
oxidative-reductase a.
peripheral androgen a.
phospholipase a.
PK a.
plasma renin a.
play a.
progestational a.
proline aminopeptidase a.
pulseless electrical a.
ristocetin cofactor a.
sexual a.
tonic-clonic seizure a.
tonicoclonic seizure a.
uterine a.
vagal a.
withdrawal-like a.

actometer
Actonel
Actron
actuarial survival
acuity
baseline visual a.
hearing a.
VEP a.
visual a.

Acular Ophthalmic
acuminata
acuminate
a. papule
a. plaque

NOTES

acuminatum
  condyloma a.
  giant anorectal condyloma a.
acupuncture for dysmenorrhea
Acuson
  A. color Doppler
  A. computed sonography
  A. 128 Doppler ultrasound
  A. Model 128XP machine
  A. 128XP-10 scanner
  A. 128XP ultrasound
  A. 128XP-10 ultrasound
acuta
  pityriasis lichenoides et
    varioliformis a. (PLEVA)
  pustulosis vacciniformis a.
acute
  a. abdomen
  a. abdominal series
  a. acalculous cholecystitis
  a. acquired neutrophilia
  a. adrenal crisis
  a. anaphylaxis
  a. angle closure glaucoma
  a. anterior uveitis
  a. appendicitis (AA)
  a. ascending radiculomyelitis
  a. aseptic meningitis syndrome
  a. atherosis
  a. atrophic candidiasis
  a. bacterial endocarditis
  a. barotitis
  a. bronchiolitis
  a. cerebellar ataxia
  a. cerebellar ataxia of unknown
    cause
  a. cerebellitis
  a. chagasic encephalitis
  a. chest syndrome (ACS)
  a. childhood ataxia
  a. childhood ITP
  a. circulatory collapse
  a. coalescent mastoiditis
  a. confusional migraine
  a. cystitis
  a. dacryocystitis
  a. disseminated encephalomyelitis
    (ADEM)
  a. disseminated histiocytosis
  a. disseminated histiocytosis X
  a. epidemic conjunctivitis
  a. epiglottitis
  a. eruptive lichen planus
  a. exudative tonsillitis
  a. fatty liver
  a. fatty liver of pregnancy (AFLP)
  a. febrile neurophilic dermatosis
  a. febrile ulcerative acne
  a. fibrinous pericarditis

  a. flaccid paralysis
  a. follicular tonsillitis
  a. fulminant colitis
  a. fulminant disease
  a. glomerulonephritis
  a. graft versus host disease
    (AGVHD, aGVHD)
  a. headache
  a. hemarthrosis
  a. hematogenous osteomyelitis
  a. hemorrhagic conjunctivitis
  a. hemorrhagic edema of infancy
    (AHEI)
  a. hemorrhagic pancreatitis
  a. hydrocephalus
  a. illness
  A. Illness Observation Scale
    (AIOS)
  a. infantile hemiplegia
  a. infectious colitis
  a. infectious polyneuritis
  a. inflammatory demyelinating
    polyneuropathy (AIDP)
  a. influenza A encephalitis
  a. injury
  a. insulin response
  a. intermittent porphyria (AIP)
  a. interpersonal loss
  a. interstitial myocarditis
  a. interstitial nephritis
  a. interstitial pneumonia
  a. intrapartum transfusion
  a. iridocyclitis
  a. iron poisoning
  a. labyrinthitis
  a. laryngotracheal bronchitis
  a. life-threatening event (ALTE)
  a. lower respiratory infection
    (ALRI)
  a. lower respiratory tract infection
    (ALRTI)
  a. lymphatic leukemia
  a. lymphoblastic leukemia (ALL)
  a. lymphocytic leukemia (ALL)
  a. lymphonodular pharyngitis
  a. mastoid osteitis
  a. megakaryoblastic leukemia
  a. meningoencephalitis syndrome
  a. motor-axonal neuropathy
    (AMAN)
  a. motor-sensory axonal neuropathy
    (AMSAN)
  a. mountain sickness (AMS)
  a. MS
  a. myeloblastic leukemia
  a. myelogenous leukemia
  a. myeloid leukemia (AML)
  a. myeloradiculitis
  a. myocardial infarction (AMI)

a. necrotizing ulcerative gingivitis (ANUG)
a. neonatal herpes
a. neuritis
a. neuronopathic Gaucher disease
a. nonlymphoblastic leukemia (ANLL)
a. nonlymphocytic leukemia
a. otitis media (AOM)
a. pancarditis
a. parotitis
a. pericoronitis
a. perinatal conjunctivitis
a. perinatal transfusion
A. Physiology and Chronic Health Evaluation (APACHE)
a. pneumonitis
a. postinfectious glomerulonephritis (APGN)
a. postinfectious nephritis
a. poststreptococcal glomerulonephritis (APSGN)
a. pseudomembranous candidiasis
a. purulent conjunctivitis
a. pyelonephritis
a. radiation syndrome
a. recurrent ataxia
a. rejection
a. renal failure (ARF)
a. renal parenchymal inflammation
a. respiratory disease (ARD)
a. respiratory distress syndrome (ARDS)
a. respiratory infection (ARI)
a. retroviral syndrome
a. rheumatic carditis
a. rheumatic fever (ARF)
a. schistosomiasis
a. scombroid intoxication
a. secondary localized peritonitis
a. sera
a. sinusitis
a. spasmodic laryngitis
a. spastic paraparesis
a. splenic sequestration
a. splenic sequestration crisis
a. streptococcal gangrene
a. stress disorder (ASD)
a. subdural hematoma
a. subglottic stenosis
a. suppurative cervical lymphadenopathy

a. suppurative otitis media
a. suppurative thyroiditis
a. surgical mastoiditis
a. syphilitic leptomeningitis
a. tocolysis
a. torticollis
a. total asphyxia
a. tracheitis
a. transfusion reaction
a. transverse myelitis
a. traumatic compartment syndrome
a. tubular necrosis (ATN)
a. urethral syndrome
a. urticaria
a. uterine inversion
acute-on-chronic
a.-o.-c. SCFE
a.-o.-c. tissue hypoxemia
acute-phase
a.-p. attrition
a.-p. reactant
a.-p. serum study
AcuTrainer device
Acutrim
A. II
A. Late Day
A. Precision Release
acyanotic
a. cardiac anomaly
a. congenital cardiac defect
a. congenital heart disease
a. lesion
a. tetralogy of Fallot
acyclic pelvic pain
acyclovir
acyesis
acylcarnitine
a. analysis
a. profile
acystia
A-D
Imodium A-D
ad
ad lib feeding
ad libitum diet
ADA
adenosine deaminase
American Diabetes Association
Americans with Disabilities Act
ADA diet
adactylia, adactyly
Adagen

NOTES

Adair-Dighton syndrome
Adair-Veress needle
Adalat CC
Adam
    A. complex
    A. position
adamantinoma
Adamkiewicz
    artery of A.
Adams
    A. advancement
    A. advancement of round ligaments
    A. forward-bending test
    A. test for scoliosis
Adams-Oliver syndrome
Adams-Stokes syndrome
adapalene
Adapin
adaptability
    poor a.
adaptation
    bowel a.
    immediate extrauterine a.
    maternal ocular a.
    uterine artery hemodynamic a.
adapter
    Briggs T a.
    side-port a.
adaptive
    a. behavior
    a. chair
    a. delay
    a. development
    a. domain
    a. immunity
    a. landscape
    a. peak
    a. radiation
    a. surface
    a. switch
    a. value
ADB
    anti-DNase B
    ADB antibody
    ADB titer
ADC
    AIDS dementia complex
    ADC Medicut shears
ADCC
    antibody-dependent cell-mediated
     cytotoxicity
Adcon-L anti-adhesion barrier
ADD
    attention deficit disorder
add-back
    a.-b. regimen
    a.-b. therapy
    a.-b. treatment
Adderall

addiction
    alcohol a.
    cocaine a.
    drug a.
    opioid a.
Addison
    A. disease
    A. disease-cerebral sclerosis
     syndrome
    A. disease-spastic paraplegia
     syndrome
addisonian
    a. crisis
    a. pernicious anemia
    a. syndrome
Addison-Schilder syndrome
additive genetic variance
additivity
adducted
    a. great toe
    a. thumb-clubfoot syndrome
    a. thumbs-mental retardation
     syndrome
    a. thumbs syndrome
adduction
    a. deformity
    eye retraction with a.
    forefoot a.
adductor
    a. angle
    a. interosseous compartment
    a. spasm
adductus
    a. clubfoot
    congenital metatarsus a.
    forefoot a.
    metatarsus a. (MA)
    simple metatarsus a.
adefovir dipivoxil
adelomorphous
ADEM
    acute disseminated encephalomyelitis
    recurrent ADEM
adenine
    a. arabinoside
    a. nucleotide
    a. phosphoribosyltransferase
adenitis
    bacterial cervical a.
    cervical a.
    inguinal a.
    mesenteric a.
    periodic fever, aphthous stomatitis,
     pharyngitis, cervical a. (PFAPA)
    salivary a.
    sclerosing a.
    tuberculous a.
    vestibular a.

adenoacanthoma
    endometrial a.
    lymph node endometriotic a.
adenocarcinoma
    cervical clear cell a.
    ciliated cell endometrial a.
    clear cell a.
    endometrial clear cell a.
    endometrial secretory a.
    a. of infantile testis
    mesonephric a.
    metastatic a.
    microinvasive a.
    minimal deviation a.
    ovarian clear cell a.
    papillary a.
    secretory a.
    serous a.
    a. in situ
    vaginal clear cell a.
    vulvar adenocystic a.
    vulvar adenoid cystic a.
Adenocard
adenocystic carcinoma
adenofibroma
adenofibromyoma
adenofibrosis
adenohypophysis
adenohypophysitis
    lymphocytic a.
adenoidal hypertrophy
adenoid cystic carcinoma
adenoidectomy
    tonsillectomy and a. (T&A)
adenoiditis
adenoleiomyofibroma
adenoma
    apocrine a.
    benign hepatic a.
    beta cell a.
    chromophobic a.
    ductal a.
    eosinophilic a.
    growth hormone-secreting a.
    islet cell a.
    lactating a.
    a. malignum
    a. of nipple
    ovarian tubular a.
    parathyroid a.
    pituitary a.
    prolactin-producing a.

    prolactin-secreting a.
    a. sebaceum
    suspected pituitary a.
    testosterone-secreting adrenal a.
    thyrotropin-secreting pituitary a.
    virilizing a.
adenomatoid
    a. malformation
    a. oviduct tumor
adenomatosis
    beta cell a.
    erosive a. of nipple
    familial multiple endocrine a.
    fibrosing a.
    islet cell a.
    multiple endocrine a. (MEA)
adenomatous
    a. colonic polyposis
    a. endometrial hyperplasia
    a. hyperplasia (AH)
    a. polyp
adenomegaly
adenomere
adenomyoma
adenomyomatosis
adenomyosis
    stromal a.
    a. uteri
adenopathy
    axillary a.
    cervical a.
    inguinal a.
    phenytoin-associated a.
    postinflammatory a.
    preauricular a.
    reactive a.
adenosalpingitis
adenosarcoma
    müllerian a.
adenosine
    a. deaminase (ADA)
    a. deaminase deficiency
    a. monophosphate (AMP)
    a. phosphate
    a. triphosphatase (ATPase)
    a. triphosphate (ATP)
adenosis
    blunt duct a.
    congenital vaginal a.
    fibrosing a.
    mammary sclerosing a.
    microglandular a.

NOTES

adenosis *(continued)*
    sclerosing a.
    a. vaginae
    vaginal a.
adenosquamous
    a. carcinoma
    a. sarcoma
adenosylcobalamin
adenosyltransferase
    cobalamin a.
adenotomy
adenotonsillar hypertrophy
adenotonsillectomy
adenotonsillitis
adenoviral
    a. pneumonia
    a. tonsillitis
adenovirus
    a. 7
    enteric a.
    epidemic keratoconjunctivitis a.
    a. infection
    a. type 3
adenylate cyclase
adenyl cyclase
adenylosuccinate
    a. deficiency
    a. lyase deficiency (ASLD)
adequate caliber of anus
adermia
adermogenesis
ADH
    antidiuretic hormone
    atypical ductal hyperplasia
adhalin gene
ADHD
    attention deficit hyperactivity disorder
    Girls, Ritalin LA, and ADHD
      (GRACE)
adherens
    fascia a.
    zonula a.
adherent
    a. placenta
    a. pseudomembrane
    a. vaginal discharge
adhesiolysis
adhesion
    abdominal a.
    amniotic a.
    banjo-string a.
    cell-extracellular matrix a.
    dense a.
    endometrial a.
    fiddle-string a.
    filmy a.
    fimbrial a.
    intracervical a.
    intrauterine a.

    labial a.
    lysis of a.
    a. molecule
    omental a.
    paraovarian a.
    peritubal a.
    piano-wire a.
    platelet a.
    A. Scoring Group (ASG)
    serosal a.
    sperm-egg a.
    tongue-lip a.
    vaginal cuff a.
adhesiotherapy
adhesive
    a. band
    Biobrane a.
    a. disease
    a. endometriosis
    a. otitis
    Testoderm with A.
    a. vaginitis
    a. vulvitis
ADI
    atlantodens interval
    Autism Diagnostic Interview
adiabatic effect
adiadochokinesia
Adie
    A. chronic pupillary syndrome
    A. pupil
Adipex-P
adipocyte
adiponecrosis subcutanea neonatorum
adipose tissue
adiposity
adiposogenital syndrome
adipsia
ADI-R
    Autism Diagnostic Interview-Revised
aditus ad antrum
adjunctive treatment
adjusted gestational age
adjustment
    a. disorder
    psychosocial a.
adjuvant
    a. chemoradiation therapy
    a. chemotherapy
    Freund a.
    a. radiotherapy
ADL
    activities of daily living
    Amsterdam Depression List
ADMCKD
    autosomal dominant medullary cystic
      kidney disease
administration
    exogenous estrogen a.

A

Food and Drug A. (FDA)
Health Care Financing A. (HCFA)
oral a.
oxytocin a.
parenteral a.
pulsatile GnRH a.
rectal a.
RSV immunoglobulin for
intravenous a. (RSV-IGIV, RSV-IVIG)
sequential a.
silver nitrate a.
surfactant a.
transdermal a.
transnasal a.
vaginal a.

admission
antenatal a.

admittance
acoustic a.
peak a.
static a.

adnata
alopecia a.

adnatum
filiform a.

adnexa, sing. **adnexum**
ocular a.
a. oculi
transposed a.
a. uteri

adnexal
a. adhesion classification system
a. cyst
a. infection
a. involvement
a. mass
a. metastasis
a. torsion
a. tumor

adnexectomy
adnexitis
adnexopexy
adnexum (*sing. of* adnexa)
ADOD
arthrodentoosteodysplasia
adolescence
early a.
late a.
middle a.
adolescent
a. breast

a. bunion
Computerized Diagnostic Interview
for Children and A.'s (cDICA)
Functional Impairment Scale for
Children and A.'s (FISCA)
a. gynecology
a. idiopathic scoliosis (AIS)
Interview Schedule for Children
and A.'s (ISCA)
a. medicine
a. obesity
A. and Pediatric Pain Tool
(APPT)
Pictorial Instrument for Children
and A.'s (PICA)
a. pregnancy
a. scoliosis
a. seborrhea
Service Assessment for Children
and A.'s (SACA)
a. sterility
a. stretch syncope
a. tibia vara
a. vulvovaginitis

adolescentis
Bifidobacterium a.
adolescent-onset patient
adoption
adoptive immunotherapy
ADOS
Autism Diagnostic Observation Schedule
autosomal dominant Opitz syndrome
ADPKD
autosomal dominant polycystic kidney
disease
ADR
adverse drug reaction
ataxia-deafness-retardation
ADR syndrome
ADR syndrome with ketoaciduria
adrenal
a. androgen
a. androgen secretion
a. androgen-stimulating hormone
(AASH)
a. axis dysfunction
a. calcification
a. cell rest tumor
a. cortex
a. cortical carcinoma
a. crisis
a. excess

NOTES

21

adrenal *(continued)*
    a. gland
    a. gland morphology
    a. hematoma
    a. hemorrhage
    a. hyperandrogenism
    a. hyperandrogenism marker
    a. hyperplasia
    a. hypofunction
    a. hypoplasia
    a. hypoplasia congenita
    a. insufficiency
    a. leukodystrophy
    Marchand a.'s
    a. maturation
    a. medulla
    a. morphologic consideration
    a. neoplasm
    a. reticularis
    a. steroid
    a. steroidogenesis
    a. suppression
    a. virilism
    a. virilizing syndrome
adrenalectomy
Adrenalin Chloride
adrenaline injection
adrenalitis
    autoimmune a.
    necrotizing a.
adrenarche
    idiopathic premature a.
    precocious a.
    premature a.
adrenergic
    a. blocker
    a. drug
    a. receptor
    a. stimulator
adrenocortical
    a. atrophy-cerebral sclerosis syndrome
    a. function
    a. hormone
    a. hyperplasia
    a. insufficiency
    a. steroid
    a. steroidogenesis
    a. stress
adrenocorticotropic, adrenocorticotrophic
    a. hormone (ACTH)
    a. hormone deficiency
    a. hormone insufficiency
adrenocorticotropin
    chorionic a.
adrenogenital syndrome (AGS)
adrenoleukodystrophy (ALD)

    neonatal a.
    X-linked a.
adrenoleukomyeloneuropathy (ALMN)
adrenomedullary
adrenomegaly
adrenomyeloneuropathy (AMN)
adrenomyodystrophy
Adriamycin
    cisplatin, Cytoxan, A. (CISCA)
    cisplatin, etoposide, Cytoxan, A. (CECA)
    A. (doxorubicin), bleomycin, vinblastine, dacarbazine (ABVD)
    A., fluorouracil, methotrexate (AFM)
    A., Oncovin, prednisone, etoposide (AOPE)
    A. PFS
    A. RDF
adRP
    autosomal dominant retinitis pigmentosa
Adrucil Injection
ADS
    anonymous donor sperm
Adson
    A. forceps
    A. ganglion scissors
    A. pickups
adult
    AAMD Adaptive Behavior Scale for Children and A.'s
    a. bone marrow (ABM)
    a. generalized gangliosidosis
    a. granulosa cell tumor (AGCT)
    a. NCL
    a. polycystic disease
    a. progeria
    a. pseudohypertrophic muscular dystrophy
    a. Refsum disease
    a. respiratory distress syndrome (ARDS)
    a. T-cell leukemia/lymphoma (ATLL)
adult-directed instruction
adulthood
adult-onset
    a.-o. congenital adrenal hyperplasia
    a.-o. diabetes mellitus (AODM)
    a.-o. hypogammaglobulinemia
    a.-o. polycystic kidney disease
    a.-o. polyglandular syndrome
    a.-o. spinocerebellar ataxia
adultorum
    scleredema a.
Advair Diskus
advance
    a. directive
    A. formula

advanced
- a. carcinoma
- a. cardiac life support (ACLS)
- A. Collection breast pump
- a. epithelial ovarian cancer
- Imodium A.
- a. life support (ALS)
- a. maternal age
- a. oxidation protein product
- a. pediatric life support (APLS)
- a. trauma life support (ATLS)

advanced-stage disease

advancement
- Adams a.
- mandibular a.
- maxillary a.
- vaginal a.

advantage
- A. 24 bio-adhesive contraceptive gel
- A. ultrasound

adventitia

adventitious
- a. breath sounds
- a. choreiform movement
- a. deafness

Advera formula

adverse
- a. drug reaction (ADR)
- a. food reaction
- a. maternal effect
- a. outcome

Advil Cold & Sinus Caplets

Advisory Committee on Immunization Practices (ACIP)

advocacy
- protection and a. (P&A)

advocate

adynamia episodica hereditaria

adynamic ileus

adysplasia
- hereditary renal a.
- hereditary urogenital a.

AEA
- antiendomysium antibody

AEC
- ankyloblepharon, ectodermal dysplasia, clefting
- AEC syndrome

AED
- antiepileptic drug

Aedes triseriatus

aEEG
- amplitude-integrated electroencephalogram

AEGIS sonography management system

AENNS
- Albert Einstein Neonatal Developmental Scale

AEP
- auditory evoked potential

aequales

Aequitron 9200 apnea monitor

AER
- aldosterone excretion rate
- auditory evoked response

aeration
- lung a.
- unequal a.

aeroallergen

aerobe

aerobic
- digital auditory a.'s (DAA)
- a. metabolism
- water a.'s

AeroBid-M Oral Aerosol Inhaler

AeroBid Oral Aerosol Inhaler

AeroChamber spacer device

aerocolpos

aerodigestive tract

Aerolate
- Accurbron A. III
- A. III
- A. JR
- A. SR S

Aeromonas hydrophila

aerophagia

aerophore

Aeroseb-Dex Topical Aerosol

Aeroseb-HC Topical

aerosol
- Aeroseb-Dex Topical A.
- Breezee Mist A.
- Bronkometer A.
- cromolyn sodium inhalation a.
- Dexacort Phosphate Turbinaire Intranasal A.
- Nasalide Nasal A.
- a. therapy
- Tilade Inhalation A.
- Virazole A.

aerosolization

aerosolized
- a. amphotericin B

NOTES

aerosolized *(continued)*
  a. medication
  a. racemic epinephrine
  a. ribavirin
aerotitis
aeruginosa
  Pseudomonas a.
aestivale
  hydroa a.
AF
  amniotic fluid
  SSD AF
AFA
  acromegaloid facial appearance
  AFA syndrome
AFAFP
  amniotic fluid alpha fetoprotein
AFDC
  Aid to Families with Dependent Children
AFE
  amniotic fluid embolism
afebrile
  a. bacteremia
  a. convulsion
  a. pneumonia syndrome
  a. seizure
afetal
affect
  a. attunement
  Eating Disorders Inventory Score
    for Interoceptive Awareness A.
  flat a.
affective
  a. disorder
  a. storm
affectivity
  negative a.
afferent vessel
Affinity bed
Affirm
  A. VPIII test
  A. VP microbial identification
    system
AFFN
  acrofrontofacionasal
  AFFN dysostosis syndrome 1
affricate
Affymetrix GeneChip system
AFI
  amniotic fluid index
afibrinogenemia
  congenital a.
Afipia felis
Afko-Lube
aflatoxin poisoning
AFLP
  acute fatty liver of pregnancy
AFM
  Adriamycin, fluorouracil, methotrexate

AFO
  ankle-foot orthosis
AFP
  alpha-fetoprotein
  AFP X-tra
AFP-EIA
  alpha-fetoprotein enzyme immunoassay
AFRAX
  autism-fragile X syndrome
africae
  Rickettsia a.
African
  A. American variant galactosemia
  A. Burkitt lymphoma
  A. tick bite fever
  A. trypanosomiasis
africanum
  Mycobacterium a.
Afrin
Afrinol
AFS
  American Fertility Society
  AFS adhesion scoring system
  AFS Revised Classification of
    Endometriosis
Aftate
afterbirth pain
afterload
  a. applicator
  a. colpostat
  LV a.
  a. reduction therapy
  ventricular a.
afterpain
AFUD
  American Foundation of Urologic
  Diseases
  AFUD classification
AFV
  amniotic fluid volume
afzelii
  Borrelia a.
A/G
  albumin-globulin ratio
AGA
  antigliadin antibody
  appropriate for gestational age
  aspartylglucosamine
  average for gestational age
  AGA deficiency
  postterm AGA
  term AGA
agalactia
agalactiae
  Streptococcus a.
agalactorrhea
agalactosis
agalactous

agammaglobulinemia
    acquired a.
    Bruton a.
    X-linked a. (XLA)
aganglionic
    a. bowel
    a. colon
    a. megacolon
    a. rectum
    a. sphincter
aganglionosis
    colonic a.
    congenital intestinal a.
    intestinal a.
    long-segment a.
    total colonic a.
    zonal a.
agar
    BiGGY a.
    blood a.
    charcoal a.
    chocolate a.
    a. gel precipitation technique
    Hektoen a.
    a. immunoprecipitin technique
    MacConkey II a.
    nalidixic acid a.
    Novy-McNeal-Nicolle biphasic
      blood a.
    a. plate
    Ryan a.
    Thayer-Martin a.
    xylose lysine deaminase a.
AGCT
    adult granulosa cell tumor
AGCUS, AGUS
    atypical glandular cells of uncertain
      significance
    atypical glandular cells of undetermined
      significance
age
    adjusted gestational a.
    advanced maternal a.
    appropriate for gestational a.
      (AGA)
    average for gestational a. (AGA)
    birth weight for gestational a.
      (BWGA)
    bone a.
    childbearing a.
    chronological a.
    coital a.

    conception a.
    corrected gestational a.
    delayed bone a.
    developmental a. (DA)
    Dubowitz/Ballard Exam for
      Gestational A.
    estimated gestational a. (EGA)
    estimation of gestational a.
    fertilization a.
    fetal a.
    functional a.
    gestational a. (GA)
    Greulich and Pyle bone a.
    growth-adjusted sonographic a.
      (GASA)
    hand-wrist bone a.
    a. index
    large for gestational a. (LGA)
    maternal a.
    mean a.
    menstrual a.
    mental a.
    ovulatory a.
    paternal a.
    postconceptional a. (PCA)
    postnatal a.
    postovulatory a.
    premenarchal a.
    reproductive a.
    small for gestational a. (SGA)
    A.'s and Stages Questionnaire
      (ASQ)
age-adjusted obesity
agency
    child protective a.
    lead a.
    local education a. (LEA)
    protective service a.
Agenerase
agenesia corticalis
agenesis
    anorectal a.
    bilateral facial a.
    callosal a.
    caudal a.
    cerebellar vermis a.
    a. of cerebellar vermis
    cervical a.
    a. of corpus callosum
    a. of corpus callosum-mental
      retardation-osseous lesions
      syndrome

NOTES

agenesis *(continued)*
    corpus callosum partial a.
    a. of corpus callosum with
      stenogyria
    cortical a.
    diaphragmatic a.
    gonadal a.
    hereditary renal a.
    lumbosacral a.
    a. of lung
    müllerian a.
    nuclear a.
    ovarian a.
    pancreatic a.
    partial a.
    penile a.
    pulmonary a.
    renal a.
    sacral a.
    septum pellucidum a.
    thymic a.
    thyroid and pituitary a.
    unilateral renal a.
    uterine a.
    vaginal a.
agenitalism
agent
    alkylating a.
    alpha-adrenergic a.
    AngioMark MRI contrast a.
    anthelminthic a.
    antianxiety a.
    anticancer a.
    antidysrhythmic a.
    antifibrinolytic a.
    antifolic a.
    antimicrobial a.
    antineoplastic a.
    antiplatelet a.
    antiprostaglandin a.
    antistaphylococcal a.
    anxiolytic a.
    beta-adrenergic a.
    beta-2-adrenergic a.
    betamimetic a.
    butenafine antifungal a.
    cervical-priming a.
    chemotactic a.
    chemotherapeutic a.
    Combidex MRI contrast a.
    cycle-nonspecific a.
    cycle-specific a.
    cytotoxic a.
    delta a.
    emetic a.
    fertility a.
    fibrinolytic a.
    Hawaii a.
    hyperosmotic a.

    infertility a.
    myelosuppressive a.
    neuromuscular blocking a.
    nonalkylating a.
    nondepolarizing paralyzing a.
    Norwalk a.
    A. Orange
    pressor a.
    progestational a.
    prokinetic a.
    satumomab pendetite imaging a.
    sclerosing a.
    Snow Mountain a.
    teratogenic a.
    tocolytic a.
    TWAR a.
    uterine contractile a.
age-related
    a.-r. pharmacodynamic response
    a.-r. risk
age-to-dose pattern
agglomeration schedule
agglutination
    a. assay
    febrile antigen a. (FAA)
    head-to-head sperm a. (H-H)
    head-to-tail sperm a. (H-T)
    a. inhibition
    a. inhibition test
    labial a.
    latex a. (LA)
    latex particle a.
    pediatric labial a.
    rickettsial a.
agglutinin
    cold a.
    Lens culinaris a.
aggregated mucopolysaccharide
**Aggregate Neurobehavioral Student
  Health & Education Review System**
aggregation
    defective primary platelet a.
    platelet a.
aggression
    inattention-overactivity with a.
    (IOWA)
aggressive
    a. angiomyxoma (AAM)
    a. behavior
    a. conduct disorder
aging
    a. gamete
    premature a.
agitated depression
agitation
aglossia-adactylia syndrome
aglossia congenita
aglossostomia

AGM
    absorbent gelling material
agminated lentigo
agnathia
agnogenic myeloid metaplasia (AMM)
agnosia
    auditory a.
    finger a.
    verbal-auditory a. (VAA)
agonadal
agonadism, mental retardation, short stature, retarded bone age syndrome
agonal respirations
agonist
    beta-2 a.
    beta-adrenergic a.
    beta receptor a.
    calcium a.
    cholinergic a.
    dopamine receptor a.
    dopaminergic a.
    estrogen a.
    GnRH a. (GNRHa)
    gonadotropin-releasing hormone a. (GnRHa)
    inhaled beta-2 a.
    motilin receptor a.
agoraphobia
agouti protein
AGR
    aniridia, ambiguous genitalia, mental retardation
    AGR syndrome
    AGR triad
agranulocytosis
    congenital a.
    infantile a.
    Kostmann infantile a.
AGS
    adrenogenital syndrome
AGT
    aminoglutethimide
AGU
    aspartylglucosaminuria
AGUS (*var. of* AGCUS)
AGVHD, aGVHD
    acute graft versus host disease
agyria
agyria-pachygyria
    a.-p. band
    a.-p. cortical dysplasia
    a.-p. syndrome

AH
    adenomatous hyperplasia
    assisted hatching
    AH antibody
    AH titer
AHA
    American Heart Association
    AHA Step One Diet
AHD
    arteriohepatic dysplasia
AHDS
    Allan-Herndon-Dudley syndrome
AHEI
    acute hemorrhagic edema of infancy
AHF
    antihemophilic factor
Ahlfeld sign (I, II)
AHO
    Albright hereditary osteodystrophy
A-hydroCort Injection
AI
    acetabular index
    anal index
    artificial insemination
    AI 5200 S Open Color Doppler imaging system
Aicardi-Goutières syndrome
Aicardi syndrome
AID
    artificial insemination by donor
    artificial insemination donor
aid
    communication a.
    Compoz Nighttime Sleep A.
    crawling a.
    electronic communication a.
    A. to Families with Dependent Children (AFDC)
    Foille Medicated First A.
    hearing a.
    low-vision a.
    mobility a.
    Sensability breast self-examination a.
    Swim-Ear water drying a.
    vibrotactile hearing a.
AIDP
    acute inflammatory demyelinating polyneuropathy
AIDS
    acquired immune deficiency syndrome
    acquired immunodeficiency syndrome

NOTES

AIDS *(continued)*
    AIDS Clinical Trials Group
    AIDS Clinical Trials Group
      protocol
    AIDS dementia complex (ADC)
    AIDS encephalopathy
    AIDS gastropathy
    transfusion-related AIDS (TRAIDS)
AIDS-related
    AIDS-r. complex (ARC)
    AIDS-r. lymphoma
AIE
    autoimmune enteropathy
AIH
    artificial insemination by husband
AIHA
    autoimmune hemolytic anemia
AIM
    area of interest magnification
AIMS
    Abnormal Involuntary Movement Scale
    Alberta Infant Motor Scale
AIN
    anal intraepithelial neoplasia
    autoimmune neutropenia
AIOS
    Acute Illness Observation Scale
AIP
    acute intermittent porphyria
air
    a. arthrogram
    a. bronchogram
    a. embolism
    a. embolus
    a. enema
    a. evacuation
    extrapulmonary extravasation of a.
    free peritoneal a.
    high-efficiency particulate a.
      (HEPA)
    humidified a.
    a. hunger
    a. leak
    a. leak syndrome
    a. leak test
    a. pollution
    a. reduction
    reflux of a.
    room a.
    A. Shields incubator
    subdiaphragmatic a.
    a. swallowing
    a. trapping
airbag injury
airborne allergen
air-contrast barium enema
AIRE
    autoimmune regulator

    AIRE gene
    AIRE promoter
Airet
air-filled heart
airflow
    laminar a.
    turbulent a.
air-fluid level
Airlift balloon retractor
AirPacks backpack
airplane glue
Airshields
    A. Isolette
    A. jaundice meter
airspace
Airtec ergonomic backpack
airway
    abnormal laxity of upper a.
    a. branching
    a., breathing, circulation (ABC)
    a., breathing, circulation and
      control bleeding, disability,
      exposure (ABCDE)
    a. and cervical spine precautions
    a. compromise
    a. conductance
    a. control
    double-lumen a.
    a. epithelium
    extrinsic compression of a.
    a. fluoroscopy
    laryngeal mask a. (LMA)
    a. malformation
    a. management
    a. obstruction
    a. obstruction syndrome
    a. occlusion
    a. opening pressure (P_{ao})
    a. protection
    reactive a.
    a. reactivity testing
    a. resistance
    reversible obstructive a.
    a. smooth muscle
    a. suction
    a. transmural pressure
AIS
    adolescent idiopathic scoliosis
AIT
    auditory integration thinking
    auditory integration training
AITP
    autoimmune thrombocytopenic purpura
AIUM
    American Institute of Ultrasound in
      Medicine
akari
    Rickettsia a.
Akarpine Ophthalmic

akathisia
AK-Con Ophthalmic
AK-Dex Ophthalmic
AK-Dilate Ophthalmic Solution
Akesson
akinesia algera
akinetic
    a. mutism
    a. seizure
Akineton
akiyami
AK-Mycin
AK-NaCl
AK-Nefrin Ophthalmic Solution
Akne-Mycin
AK-Pentolate
AK-Poly-Bac Ophthalmic
AK-Pred Ophthalmic
AK-Sulf
AKTob Ophthalmic
AK-Tracin Ophthalmic
AK-Trol Ophthalmic
ALA
    alpha lactalbumin
    alpha-linolenic acid
ala, pl. alae
    nasal a.
    a. nasi
Ala-Cort Topical
alacrima
    a., achalasia, adrenal insufficiency
    a. congenita
Aladdin Infant Flow System
alae (pl. of ala)
Alagille syndrome
Alagille-Watson syndrome (AWS)
Alajouanine syndrome
Alamast ophthalmic solution
alanine
    a. aminotransferase (ALT)
    a. transaminase (ALT)
alaninuria
ALARA
    as low as reasonably achievable
    ALARA principle
alar flaring
alarm
    Nite Train'r A.
    Sioux a.
Ala-Scalp Topical
Alateen

alba
    cutis marmorata a.
    linea a.
    pityriasis a.
    pneumonia a.
Albalon Liquifilm Ophthalmic
albendazole
Albers-Schönberg
    A.-S. disease
    A.-S. syndrome
Alberta Infant Motor Scale (AIMS)
Albert Einstein Neonatal Developmental
    Scale (AENNS)
Albert-Smith pessary
albescens
    retinopathy punctata a.
albicans
    Candida a.
Albini nodule
albinism
    cutaneous a.
    Forsius-Eriksson type ocular a.
    generalized a.
    localized a.
    Nettleship-Falls ocular a.
    ocular a. (OA)
    oculocutaneous a. (OCA)
    partial oculocutaneous a.
    tyrosinase-negative
      oculocutaneous a.
    tyrosinase-positive oculocutaneous a.
albinism-deafness syndrome
albinismus circumscriptus
albipunctatus
    fundus a.
albopapuloid
    a. epidermolysis bullosa variant
    a. Pasini form of dominant
      dystrophic epidermolysis bullosa
Albright
    A. disease
    A. hereditary osteodystrophy (AHO)
    A. syndrome
albuginea
    tunica a.
albumin
    a. gradient
    plasma a.
    serum a.
Albuminar
albumin-bound toxin
albumin-globulin ratio (A/G)

NOTES

29

albuminocytologic dissociation
albuminuria
Albutein
albuterol
    sustained-release a.
Alcaine
Alcaligenes xylosoxidans
ALCAPA
    anomalous left coronary artery from
      pulmonary artery
      ALCAPA syndrome
alcaptonuria
Alcare formula
alclometasone
Alcock canal
alcohol
    a. abuse
    a. addiction
    benzyl a.
    blood a.
    cetyl a.
    ethyl a. (EtOH)
    fetal effects of a.
    a. ingestion
    isopropyl a.
    nicotinyl a.
    a. and other drugs (AOD)
    a. related (AR)
    a., tobacco, and other drugs
      (ATOD)
    A. Use Disorders Identification
      Test (AUDIT)
alcoholic
    child of a. (COA)
    children of a. (COA)
    a. embryopathy
    a. tincture
    a. tincture of opium
alcoholica
    embryopathy a.
alcoholism
    maternal a.
alcohol-related neurodevelopmental
  disorder (ARND)
ALD
    adrenoleukodystrophy
Aldactazide
Aldactone
Aldara cream
Alder anomaly
Alder-Reilly anomaly
aldolase
Aldomet
Aldoril
aldosterone
    a. deficiency
    a. excretion rate (AER)
    a. replacement therapy

aldosteronism
    juvenile a.
aldosteronism-normal blood pressure
  syndrome
Aldred syndrome
Aldrich
    hypoganglionic segment of A.
    A. syndrome
Aldridge
    A. rectus fascia sling
    A. sling procedure
Aldridge-Studdefort urethral suspension
ALEC
    artificial lung-expanding compound
Ale-Calo syndrome
alendronate sodium
alert inactivity
alertness
    quiet a.
    a., response to voice, response to
      pain, unresponsive (AVPU)
    state of a.
Alesse
aleukia
    congenital a.
Aleve
Alexander
    A. anomaly
    A. aplasia
    A. disease
    A. operation
    A. syndrome
    A. unit
Alexander-Adams
    A.-A. hysteropexy
    A.-A. uterine suspension
alexandrite laser
alexithymia
alfa (*See* alpha)
    choriogonadotropin a.
    dornase a.
    epoetin a.
    poractant a.
alfalfa
Alfenta
alfentanil
Alferon N
AL 110 formula
ALFW
    anterolateral free wall
algae
    blue-green a.
algal oil
algera
    akinesia a.
algesiometer
    vulvar a.

alginate
    calcium a.
    a. wound dressing
AlgiSite dressing
alglucerase
algodystrophy
algomenorrhea
Algo newborn hearing screener
ALGO 1-plus
Algosteril dressing
Alice in Wonderland syndrome
alignment
    body a.
    ocular a.
    torsional a.
alimentary
alimentation
    intravenous a.
    parenteral a.
Alimentum
    A. feeding
    A. formula
A-line
    arterial line
aliphatic hydrocarbon
aliquot
Alitraq formula
Alkaban-AQ
Alka-Butazolidin
alkalemia
alkalemic
alkali
    a. burn
    a. infusion
    a. therapy
    a. toxicity
alkaline
    a. diuresis
    a. phosphatase (ALP)
    a. reflux
alkalinization
alkaloid
    levorotatory a.
    plant a.
    Veratrum a.
    Vinca a.
alkalosis
    cerebral lactic a.
    diet-induced hypochloremic metabolic a.
    hypochloremic metabolic a.
    hypokalemic a.
    metabolic a.
    respiratory a.
Alka-Mints
alkaptonuria
Alka-Seltzer Plus Children's Cold Medicine
Alkeran
alkylating
    a. agent
    a. chemotherapy
ALL
    acute lymphoblastic leukemia
    acute lymphocytic leukemia
Allan-Herndon-Dudley syndrome (AHDS)
Allan-Herndon syndrome
allantoic
    a. artery
    a. cyst
    a. duct
    a. sac
    a. stalk
allantoidoangiopagous twins
allantoidoangiopagus
allantois
Allegra
Allegra-D
allele
    fixed a.
    a. frequency
    multiple a.'s
    mutant a.
    papG a.
    premutation a.
    recessive a.
    silent a.
    a. specific associated primer
    a. specific oligo
    wild-type a.
    Z a.
allele-specific
    a.-s. oligonucleotide hybridization
    a.-s. PCR
allelic
    a. exclusion
    a. gene
    a. heterogeneity
allelism
Allemann syndrome
Allen
    A. and Capute neonatal neurodevelopmental examination
    A. chart

NOTES

Allen *(continued)*
    A. fetal stethoscope
    A. Kindergarten Picture Cards
    A. laparoscopic stirrups
    A. picture test
Allen-Doisy test
Allen-Masters syndrome
Allerest
    A. Children's Tablets
    A. Headache Strength
    A. Maximum Strength
allergen
    airborne a.
    contact a.
    A. Ear Drops
    food a.
    a. immunotherapy
allergenic
allergen-induced asthma
allergic
    a. anlage
    a. bowel disease
    a. bronchopulmonary aspergillosis (ABPA)
    a. colitis
    a. conjunctivitis
    a. contact dermatitis
    a. coryza
    a. crease
    a. diaper rash
    a. encephalitis
    a. encephalomyelitis
    a. enterocolitis
    a. eosinophilic gastroenteritis
    a. esophagitis
    a. gape
    a. gastroenteropathy
    a. inflammatory response
    a. polyp
    a. rhinitis
    a. rhinitis perennial
    a. rhinoconjunctivitis
    a. salute
    a. shiner
    a. sinusitis
    a. vulvitis
allergy
    barley a.
    cow's milk a. (CMA)
    cow's milk protein a.
    fire ant a.
    gluten a.
    honeybee a.
    milk a.
    milk-protein a.
    milk/soy-protein a.
    non-IgE-mediated food a.
    pollen a.
    soy-protein a.
    sperm a.
    stinging insect a.
    a. treatment
    vespid a.
    wasp a.
    yellow jacket a.
AllerMax Oral
Allerphed
Allevyn dressing
all-fours
    a.-f. maneuver
    a.-f. maneuver for shoulder dystocia
Allgrove syndrome
alligator
    a. forceps
    a. skin
Allis
    A. clamp
    A. forceps
Allis-Abramson
    A.-A. breast biopsy
    A.-A. breast biopsy forceps
alloantibody
alloantigen
allodiploid
alloenzyme
allogenic, allogeneic
    a. antigen
    a. BMT
    a. bone marrow transplantation
    a. disease
    a. fetal graft
    a. stem cell transplantation
allogenicity
allograft
    composite a.
    cryopreserved valved a.
    dura mater a.
    fascia lata a.
    a. membrane
    a. rejection
    a. survival
alloimmune
    a. disease
    a. factor
    a. mechanism
    a. neonatal neutropenia (ANN)
    a. neonatal thrombocytopenic purpura
    a. thrombocytopenia
alloimmunity
alloimmunization
    antepartum a.
    Kell a.
alloimmunize
Alloiococcus otitis
alloisoleucine
alloploidy

allopolyploidy
allopurinol
all-or-none phenomenon
allosome
    paired a.
allosyndesis
allotetraploidy
allothreonine
allotropism
allotype
allowance
    recommended daily a. (RDA)
    recommended dietary a. (RDA)
allozygote
Allport retractor
all-progestin contraceptive
all-terrain vehicle (ATV)
all-*trans*-retinoic acid
allylamine
ALMN
    adrenoleukomyeloneuropathy
Almora
alobar holoprosencephaly
Alocril
Aloka
    A. 650 CL ultrasound
    A. OB/GYN ultrasound
    A. 650 scanner
    A. SD ultrasound system
    A. SSD-720 real-time scanner
Alomide
alopecia
    a. adnata
    androgenic a.
    a., anosmia, deafness, hypogonadism (AADH)
    a., anosmia, deafness, hypogonadism syndrome
    a. areata
    cicatricial a.
    a. congenitalis
    a., contracture, dwarfism (ACD)
    a., contracture, dwarfism, mental retardation syndrome
    a., epilepsy, oligophrenia syndrome
    generalized a.
    a. hereditaria
    marginal a.
    a., mental retardation, epilepsy, microcephaly syndrome
    pyoderma a.
    secondary a.
    a. totalis congenita
    toxic a.
    traction a.
    traumatic a.
    a. universalis
    a. universalis totalis
    a. universalis with mental retardation
alopecia-mental
    a.-m. retardation (AMR)
Alora
    A. Transdermal
    A. Transdermal patch
ALP
    alkaline phosphatase
    bone ALP
Alpern-Boll Developmental Profile
Alpers
    A. disease
    A. syndrome
alpha, α
    a. antitrypsin level
    Curosurf poractant a.
    a. dimeric protein
    a. error
    estrogen receptor a. (Er alpha)
    follitropin a.
    a. helix
    a. interferon
    interferon a.
    A. Keri soap
    a. lactalbumin (ALA)
    macrophage inflammatory protein-1 a. (MIP-1 alpha)
    a. particle
    a. Proteobacteria
    a. thalassemia
    transforming growth factor a. (TGF alpha)
alpha-1
    a.-1-antitrypsin
    a.-1 antitrypsin deficiency
    a.-1 antitrypsin disease
    a.-1 PI
    a.-1 protease inhibitor
    a.-1 proteinase inhibitor (A1PI, a1PI)
    a.-1 thymosin product
alpha-2
    a.-2 antiplasmin
    a.-2 antiplasmin coagulation inhibitor

NOTES

alpha-2 *(continued)*
    a.-2 antitrypsin inhibitor
    a.-2 macroglobulin
    a.-2 macroglobulin coagulation
      inhibitor
alpha-2a
    interferon a.-2a
alpha-adrenergic
    a.-a. agent
    a.-a. blocker
    a.-a. receptor
    a.-a. stimulator
alpha-aminoadipic
    a.-a. acid
    a.-a. aciduria
3 alpha-androstanediol glucuronide
alpha-antilysin deficiency
alpha-2AP coagulation inhibitor
alpha-2AT coagulation inhibitor
alpha-2b
    interferon a.-2b
alphabet
    manual a.
alpha-chain disorder
alpha-chemokine receptor
Alphaderm
5alpha-dihydroprogesterone
20alpha-dihydroprogestin dehydrogenase
17-alpha-ethinyl testosterone
alpha-fetoprotein (AFP)
    a.-f. elevation
    a.-f. enzyme immunoassay (AFP-
      EIA)
alpha-glucosidase
    a.-g. deficiency
    a.-g. inhibitor
alpha-granule
    giant platelet a.-g.
17alpha-hydroxypregnenolone
17alpha-hydroxyprogesterone caproate
alpha-ketoadipic
    a.-k. acid
    a.-k. aciduria
alpha-L-fucosidase (FUCA)
alpha-L-iduronidase (IDA, IDUA)
alpha-linolenic acid (ALA)
alpha-lipoprotein deficiency
alpha-mannosidosis (type I, II)
alpha-2M coagulation inhibitor
alpha-melanocyte-stimulating hormone
    (alpha-MSH)
alpha-melanotrophin
alpha-methylcrotonyl-coenzyme A
    carboxylase
alpha-methyl-para-tyrosine (AMPT)
Alphamine
alpha-MSH
    alpha-melanocyte-stimulating hormone

alpha-N-acetylgalactosaminidase
    deficiency
Alphanate
AlphaNine SD
alphaprodine
alpha-recombinant interferon
alpha-reductase
    a.-r. deficiency
    15 a.-r. deficiency
5-alpha reductase
Alpha-Tamoxifen
alpha-thalassemia
    a.-t./mental retardation (ATR)
    a.-t./mental retardation syndrome,
      deletion type (ATR1, ATR-16)
    a.-t./mental retardation syndrome,
      nondeletion type (ATR2, ATR,
      nondeletion)
alpha-tocopherol concentration
Alphatrex Topical
alphavirus
Alport
    A. syndrome
    A. syndrome-like nephritis
ALPP
    abdominal leak point pressure
alprazolam
alprostadil
ALPS
    autoimmune lymphoproliferative
      syndrome
ALRI
    acute lower respiratory infection
ALRTI
    acute lower respiratory tract infection
ALS
    advanced life support
    amyotrophic lateral sclerosis
Alsoy 1, 2 formula
Alström
    A. sign
    A. syndrome
Alström-Hallgren syndrome
ALT
    alanine aminotransferase
    alanine transaminase
ALTE
    acute life-threatening event
    apparent life-threatening event
Altemeier
    A. perineal rectosigmoidectomy
    A. procedure
alteration
    uterine activity a.
altered
    a. gastric motility
    a. sensorium
    a. state of consciousness (ASC)

alternans
  electrical a.
  pulsus a.
  strabismus convergens a.
Alternaria
alternate-cover test
alternating
  a. breath test (ABT)
  a. hemiplegia
  a. hemiplegia of childhood
alternative
  a. birthing position
  a. communication device
  a. hypothesis
  a. system
  a. therapy
Alteromonas putrefaciens
altretamine
altruism
Aludrine
aluminum
  a. acetate
  a. acetate solution
  a. chloride
  a. hydroxide
  a. intoxication
  a. toxicity
Alupent
Alurate
aluteal
alveolar (A)
  arterial to a. (a-A)
  a. capillary dysplasia
  a. consolidation
  a. cyst
  a. echinococcosis
  a. fibrinous exudate
  a. hydatidosis
  a. hypoxia
  a. lavage
  a. lymphangioma
  a. myofibroblast differentiation
  a. notch
  a. osteitis
  a. partial pressure (PA)
  a. proteinosis
  a. recruitment
  a. ridge
  a. RMS
  a. saccule formation
  a. sarcoid
  a. soft part sarcoma

  a. stage
  a. stage of lung development
  a. ventilation
alveolar-arterial (A-a)
  a.-a. oxygen diffusing capacity
  a.-a. oxygen gradient
  a.-a. pressure gradient
alveoli (*pl. of* alveolus)
alveolitis
  cryptogenic fibrosing a.
  extrinsic alveolar a.
alveolization
  abrogated neonatal a.
alveolus, pl. **alveoli**
  functional a.
  pulmonary a.
alymphocytosis
alymphoplasia
  thymic a.
Alzate catheter
Alzheimer
  A. disease
  A. II cell
amalonaticus
  Citrobacter a.
AMAN
  acute motor-axonal neuropathy
Amanita
  A. mushroom
  A. phalloides
amantadine
amastia
amaurosis
  a. congenita
  a. fugax
  Leber congenital a. (LCA)
  Leber congenital retinal a.
  recessive Leber congenital a.
amaurotic familial idiocy
amazia
Amazon thorax
AmBd
  amphotericin B deoxycholate
ambenonium
Ambien
ambient
  a. light
  a. oxygen concentration
  a. sound
  a. temperature
ambiguity
  frank a.

NOTES

ambiguity *(continued)*
 genital a.
 sexual a.
ambiguous
 a. external genitalia
 a. reference
ambiguus
 situs a.
AmBisome
amblyogenic stimulus
Amblyomma americanum
amblyopia
 ametropic a.
 anisometropic a.
 deprivation a.
 disuse a.
 image-degradation a.
 isoametropic a.
 occlusion a.
 strabismic a.
 transient a.
amblyopic eye
amboceptor
ambosexual area
Ambras syndrome
Ambu
 A. bag
 A. infant resuscitator
 A. respirator
ambulate
ambulation
ambulatory
 a. antibiotic treatment
 a. anticoagulation
 a. anticoagulation therapy
 a. blood pressure (ABP)
 a. blood pressure monitoring
  (ABPM)
 a. monitoring
 a. obstetric care
 a. obstetrics
 a. polysomnography
 a. testing
 a. urodynamic monitoring (AUM)
 a. uterine contraction test
AMC
 arthrogryposis multiplex congenita
 ataxia-microcephaly-cataract
 AMC syndrome
Amcill
amcinonide
AMD
 acid maltase deficiency
AME
 apparent mineralocorticoid excess
 congenital AME
amebiasis
 cerebral a.
 hepatic a.

amebic
 a. colitis
 a. dysentery
 a. hepatic abscess
 a. liver abscess
 a. meningoencephalitis
 a. vaginitis
amelia
 upper limb a.
ameliorate
amelioration
ameloblastoma
amelogenesis imperfecta
ameloonychohypohidrotic syndrome
amendment
 Education of the Handicapped A.'s
  of 1986
amenia
amenorrhea
 athletic a.
 ballet dancer's secondary a.
 dietary a.
 emotional a.
 eugonadal a.
 eugonadotropic a.
 exercise-induced a.
 hypergonadotropic a.
 hyperprolactinemic a.
 hypogonadotropic a.
 hypophysial a.
 hypothalamic a.
 hypothalamic-pituitary a.
 jogger's a.
 lactation a.
 ovarian a.
 pathologic a.
 physiologic a.
 postmenopausal a.
 postpartum a.
 postpill a.
 primary a.
 secondary a.
 traumatic a.
amenorrhea-galactorrhea syndrome
amenorrheic, amenorrheal
 a. patient
 a. woman
amentia
 nevoid a.
Amerge
Americaine
American
 A. Academy of Child and
  Adolescent Psychiatry (AACAP)
 A. Academy of Pediatrics (AAP)
 A. Association on Mental
  Deficiency (AAMD)
 A. Association on Mental
  Retardation (AAMR)

A. Association of Poison Control Centers (AAPCC)
A. Association for the Surgery of Trauma (AAST)
A. Board of Psychiatry and Neurology (ABPN)
A. Burkitt lymphoma
A. Cancer Society (ACS)
A. Cancer Society procedure
A. College of Graduate Medical Education (ACGME)
A. College of Nurse Midwives
A. College of Obstetrics & Gynecology network
A. Diabetes Association (ADA)
A. Diabetes Association diet
A. Fertility Society (AFS)
A. Foundation of Urologic Diseases (AFUD)
A. Foundation of Urologic Diseases classification
A. Heart Association (AHA)
A. Heart Association Step One Diet
A. Institute of Ultrasound in Medicine (AIUM)
A. Sign Language (ASL)
A. Sleep Disorders Association (ASDA)
A. trypanosomiasis
A. Urogynecologic Society
A.'s with Disabilities Act (ADA)
americanum
  Amblyomma a.
americanus
  Ancylostoma a.
  Necator a.
A-methaPred Injection
amethocaine gel
amethopterin
Ametop gel
ametria
ametropic amblyopia
AMF
  autocrine motility factor
AMH
  antimüllerian hormone
AMI
  acute myocardial infarction
  non-Q-wave AMI
Amicar
amicrobic pyuria

Amiel-Tison test
amifostine
amikacin sulfate
Amikin
amiloride
amine
  a. odor
  sympathomimetic a.
  a. test
amino
  a. acid
  a. acid analyzer
  a. acid chromatography
  a. acid metabolism
  a. acid screening
  a. acid transport defect
aminoacetic analog
aminoacidemia
aminoacidopathy
aminoaciduria
  dibasic a.
  generalized a.
  renal a.
aminocaproic acid
Amino-Cerv pH 5.5 cervical Cream
aminoglutethimide (AGT)
aminoglycoside
  antimicrobial a.
  a. nephrotoxicity
aminogram
  plasma a.
aminoguanidine
Amino-Opti-E
aminopenicillin
aminopeptidase
  leucine a.
aminophospholipid
Aminophyllin
aminophylline
aminopterin
  aminopterin syndrome sine a. (ASSAS)
  a. embryopathy syndrome
aminopterin-like embryopathy syndrome
aminopyrine
5-aminosalicylic acid
Aminosyn-PF supplement
amino-terminal peptide
aminotransferase
  alanine a. (ALT)
  aspartate a. (AST)
  branched-chain a.

NOTES

aminotransferase *(continued)*
> serum a.
> tyrosine a. (TAT)

amiodarone

Amipaque

AMIS
> antibody-mediated immune suppression

Amish brittle hair syndrome

amisulpride

Amitid

Amitone

Amitril

amitriptyline

AML
> acute myeloid leukemia

AMLA
> antimyolemmal antibody

AMM
> agnogenic myeloid metaplasia

Ammon
> A. fissure
> A. horn sclerosis

ammonemia, ammoniemia

ammonia
> a. metabolism
> plasma a.
> serum a.

ammoniac
> sal a.

ammoniemia *(var. of* ammonemia)

ammonium
> a. bromide
> a. chloride
> a. lactate

AMN
> acquired melanocytic nevus
> adrenomyeloneuropathy

amnesia
> hysterical a.
> posttraumatic a.
> retrograde a.

amnesic
> a. response
> a. shellfish poisoning

amniocentesis
> early a. (EA)
> genetic a.
> second-trimester a.

amniochorion

amniocyte

amniogenesis

amniogenic cell

amniogram

amniography in hydatidiform mole

Amniohook

amnioinfusion
> a. therapy
> transabdominal a.

amnioma

amnion
> inner a.
> a. nodosum
> a. ring
> a. rupture

amnion-chorion separation

amnionic *(var. of* amniotic)

amnionicity

amnionitis
> silent a.

amniopatch

amnioreduction

amniorrhea

amniorrhexis

amnioscope

amnioscopy

AmnioStat-FLM
> A.-FLM maturity screening
> A.-FLM test

amniotic, amnionic
> a. adhesion
> a. band anomalad
> a. band disruption sequence
> a. banding
> a. banding syndrome
> a. band limb amputation
> a. band syndrome
> a. caruncle
> a. cavity
> a. constriction band
> a. debris
> a. fluid (AF)
> a. fluid alpha fetoprotein (AFAFP)
> a. fluid aspiration
> a. fluid assessment
> a. fluid bilirubin
> a. fluid cell culture
> a. fluid embolism (AFE)
> a. fluid embolism syndrome
> a. fluid embolus
> a. fluid embolus syndrome
> a. fluid fluorescence polarization
> a. fluid index (AFI)
> a. fluid infection
> a. fluid level
> a. fluid pocket
> a. fluid quantitation
> a. fluid supernatant
> a. fluid volume (AFV)
> a. fluid volume disorder
> a. fluid white blood cell count
> a. infection syndrome
> a. infection syndrome of Blane
> a. membrane
> a. sheet

amniotic-chorionic surface

amniotome
> Baylor a.

amniotomy plus oxytocin method

amobarbital
A-mode
    A-m. echocardiography
    A-m. ultrasound
amorphous
    a. breast calcification
    a. fetus
    a. inspissation
amorphus
    fetus a.
amotio placentae
amotivational syndrome
amoxapine
amoxicillin
amoxicillin-clavulanate
amoxicillin-clavulanic acid
Amoxil
AMP
    adenosine monophosphate
    assisted medical procreation
AmpErase electrocautery
amphetamine
    a. aspartate
    a. sulfate
amphidiploidy
amphigonous inheritance
amphimixis
Amphojel
Amphotec
amphotericin
    aerosolized a. B
    a. B
    a. B cholesteryl sulfate complex
    a. B deoxycholate (AmBd)
    a. B lipid complex
ampicillin
    a. rash
    a. resistant
    a. sodium/sulbactam sodium
    a. and sulbactam
    a. trihydrate
ampicillin-resistant *Escherichia coli*
ampicillin/sulbactam
Ampicin
Amplatz catheter
Amplatzer
    A. device
    A. septal occluder
Amplicor
    A. Chlamydia assay
    A. HIV-1 test kit
    A. PCR diagnostics

    A. PCR kit
    A. typing kit
amplification
    DNA a.
    gene a.
    nucleic acid a. (NAA)
    nucleic acid sequence-based a.
     (NASBA)
    transcription-mediated a. (TMA)
    Y-specific DNA a.
amplified fragment length polymorphism
AmpliTaq DNA polymerase FS
amplitude
    oscillation a.
amplitude-integrated
    a.-i. EEG
    a.-i. electroencephalogram (aEEG)
AMPT
    alpha-methyl-para-tyrosine
ampulla, pl. **ampullae**
    a. of oviduct
    a. of Vater
ampullar
    a. abortion
    a. pregnancy
amputation
    amniotic band limb a.
    birth a.
    cervical a.
    congenital a.
    intrauterine a.
    Jaboulay a.
    spontaneous a.
    Syme a.
    traumatic a.
AMR
    alopecia-mental retardation
    AMR syndrome
Amreich vaginal extirpation
amrinone lactate
AMS
    ablepharon-macrostomia syndrome
    acute mountain sickness
    AMS 800 artificial urethral
     sphincter
amsacrine
AMSAN
    acute motor-sensory axonal neuropathy
Amsel criteria
amstelodamensis
    typus degenerativus a.

NOTES

Amsterdam
    A. Depression List (ADL)
    A. dwarfism
    A. infant ventilator
    A. type
amyelencephalia
amyelencephalic, amyelencephalous
amyelia
amyeloid leukemia
amyelous
amygdala, pl. **amygdalae**
amygdalin
amygdalohippocampectomy
Amyl
    A. Nitrate Vaporole
    A. Nitrite Aspirols
amylase
    human pancreatic a. (HPA)
    salivary a.
    serum a.
amylobarbitone
amyloidosis
    paraneoplastic a.
    secondary a.
amyloidosis
amylopectinosis
    branching enzyme deficiency a.
amylophagia
amyopathic
    a. JDM
    a. juvenile dermatomyositis
amyoplasia
    bimelic a.
    a. congenita
    oculomelic a.
    segmental a.
amyotonia congenita
amyotrophic
    a. lateral sclerosis (ALS)
    a. lateral sclerosis-Parkinson-
        dementia complex
amyotrophy
Amytal
AN
    anorexia nervosa
ANA
    antinuclear antibody
    ANA seropositive
anabolic androgenic steroid
Anabolin
anabolism
anacatadidymus, anakatadidymus
Anacin
anaclitic
    a. depression
    a. depression of infancy
anadidymus
anadysplasia
    metaphysial a.

anaerobe
anaerobic
    a. bacteria
    a. cellulitis
    a. streptococcus
    a. vaginosis
anaerobius
    Peptococcus a.
Anafranil
anagen effluvium
anagenesis
anakatadidymus (*var. of* anacatadidymus)
Ana-Kit
anal
    a. atresia
    a. canal
    a. condyloma
    a. dimple
    a. EMG PerryMeter sensor
    a. fissure
    a. incontinence
    a. index (AI)
    a. intercourse
    a. intraepithelial neoplasia (AIN)
    a. manometry
    a. margin
    a. Pap smear
    a. penetration
    a. pruritus
    a. sphincter
    a. sphincter cinedefecography
    a. sphincter disruption
    a. sphincter dysplasia
    a. sphincter electromyography
    a. sphincter laceration
    a. sphincter oscillation
    a. sphincter paralysis
    a. sphincter tone
    a. squamous intraepithelial lesion
        (ASIL)
    a. stenosis
    a. thrombosis
    a. verge
    a. wink
    a. wink reflex
analbuminemic patient
**anal-ear-renal-radial malfunction
    syndrome**
analeptic
analgesia
    caudal a.
    conduction a.
    congenital a.
    continuous epidural a.
    epidural a.
    labor a.
    narcotic a.
    obstetric a.
    patient-controlled a. (PCA)

peridural a.
perineal a.
procedural sedation and a. (PSA)
regional a.
segmental epidural a.
spinal a.
subarachnoid a.
analgesic
narcotic a.
analgesic-rebound headache
analog, analogue
aminoacetic a.
gonadotropin-releasing hormone a.
 (GnRHa)
LH-RH a.
luteinizing hormone-releasing
 hormone a.
nucleoside a.
oxytocin a.
prostaglandin E a.
tetracycline a.
vasopressin a.
analysis, pl. analyses
acylcarnitine a.
applied behavior a. (ABA)
aqueous a.
automated multiple a.
base sequence a.
bioelectrical impedance a. (BIA)
bioimpedance a.
blood chromosome a.
blood gas a.
bulked segregant a.
capillary electrophoresis/frontal a.
 (CE/FA)
cell block a.
chorionic villus haplotype a.
chromosomal a.
chromosome a.
clinicopathological a.
computer-assisted semen a. (CASA)
cytogenetic a.
cytologic a.
deoxyribonucleic acid a.
DNA a.
endonuclease a.
fat a.
FISH a.
flow cytometric a.
flow cytometry a.
fluorescence depolarization a.
fragile X a.

genetic bit a.
genetic linkage a.
hair cotinine a.
heart rate power spectral a.
 (HRSA)
heteroduplex a.
induced sputum a. (ISA)
karyotype a.
latent class a. (LCA)
linkage a.
molecular genetic a.
oligonucleotide probe a.
photometric a.
pleural fluid a.
postoperative symptom a.
power spectral a. (PSA)
prenatal cytogenetic a.
restriction endonuclease a.
RFLP a.
risk-benefit a.
saturation a.
semen a.
seminal fluid a. (SFA)
sequential multiple a. (SMA)
spectophotometrical a.
spectral power a.
synovial fluid a.
toxicologic a.
transgenerational a.
Trauma Score and Injury Severity
 Score A. (TRISS)
white blood cell lysosomal
 enzyme a.
analyte
serum a.
analyzer
amino acid a.
AVL 9110 pH a.
Bayer DCA2000 a.
BiliCheck bilirubin a.
BRACAnalyzer gene a.
Clinitek 50 urine chemistry a.
Cobas fast centrifugal a.
computer-assisted semen a. (CASA)
cooximeter a.
CO-stat end tidal breath a.
Coulter Channelyser cell a.
Elecsys 1010 a.
HemoCue blood glucose a.
HemoCue blood hemoglobin a.
LeadCare handheld blood lead a.
Multichannel discrete a. (MDA)

NOTES

analyzer *(continued)*
    NE-8000 a.
    Osteomeasure computer-assisted
      image a.
    Serono SR1 FSH a.
    Sonoclot coagulation a.
    SRI automated immunoassay a.
    STA a.
anamnestic immune response
Anandron
ANA-negative lupus
anaphase
    a. I, II
    a. lag
anaphylactic
    a. purpura
    a. reaction
    a. shock
anaphylactoid
    a. purpura
    a. reaction
    a. shock
    a. syndrome of pregnancy
anaphylatoxin
anaphylaxis
    acute a.
    biphasic a.
    cold a.
    drug-related a.
    gastrointestinal a.
    recurrent a.
anaplasia
anaplastic
    a. carcinoma
    a. large cell lymphoma
    a. oligodendroglioma
    a. pathology
    a. pilocytic astrocytoma
Anaprox-DS
anarthria
anasarca
    fetal a.
    fetoplacental a.
anaspadias
Anaspaz
anastomosis, pl. **anastomoses**
    arteriovenous a.
    circular end-to-end a. (CEEA)
    Clado a.
    colorectal a.
    cornual a.
    Damus-Kaye-Stansel a.
    descending aorta a.
    end-to-side a.
    esophageal a.
    extended end-to-end a.
    extracardiac conduit
      cavopulmonary a.
    gastrointestinal a. (GIA)

    Glenn a.
    ileal pouch-anal a. (IPAA)
    ileoanal a. (IAA)
    ileoileal a.
    intrarenal a.
    isthmointerstitial a.
    jejunojejunal a.
    LAT cavopulmonary a.
    microsurgical tubocornual a.
    onlay patch a.
    placental vascular a.
    primary a.
    Roux-en-Y a.
    side-to-end a.
    staple a.
    total cavopulmonary a.
    tubocornual a.
    ureterotubal a.
    ureteroureteral a.
    Waterston aortopulmonary a.
anastrozole
anatomic
    a. asplenia
    a. conjugate
    a. profile (AP)
    a. shunt
    a. support defect
anatomy
    fetal intracranial a.
    immune system a.
    intracranial a.
Anavar
Anbesol Maximum Strength
AN-BP
    anorexia nervosa with binging and
      purging
ANCA
    antineutrophil cytoplasmic antibody
      ANCA titer
Ancef
ancestor
    leading a.
anchor
    bone a.
    Mainstay urologic soft tissue a.
    Mitex GII/mini a.
    press-in bone a.
anchoring
    a. fibril
    a. villus
Ancobon
Ancotil
Ancylostoma
    A. americanus
    A. braziliense
    A. caninum
    A. ceylanicum
    A. duodenale
ancylostomiasis

Andermann syndrome
Andernach ossicle
Andersen
    A. deficiency
    A. disease
    A. syndrome
Anderson
    A. disease
    A. marker
    A. syndrome
Anderson-Fabry disease
andersoni
    Dermacentor a.
Andogsky syndrome
Andrews infant laryngoscope
Andro
androblastoma
Androcur Depot
Andro-Cyp
Androderm Transdermal System
Andro/Fem
androgen
    adrenal a.
    a. antagonist
    attenuated a.
    a. binding
    a. dynamics
    a. excess
    excess a.
    a. excess disorder
    a. insensitivity
    a. insensitivity syndrome
    a. interaction
    a. metabolism
    a. receptor
    a. resistance
    a. resistance syndrome
    a. secretion
    a. synthesis defect
androgen-dependent carcinoma
androgenesis
androgenic
    a. alopecia
    a. steroid
androgenicity
androgenized woman
androgenous
androgen-producing tumor
androgynism
androgynous
androgyny

android
    a. obesity
    a. pattern
    a. pelvis
Android-F
andrology
Androlone
    A. 50
    A.-D
Andronate
Andropository-200
androstane
androstenediol
androstenedione (A_4)
androsterone glucuronide
Androvite
anechoic
    a. space
    a. tissue
anectasis
Anectine Chloride
anejaculation
anembryonic
    a. gestation
    a. pregnancy
anemia
    acquired hemolytic a.
    addisonian pernicious a.
    angiopathic hemolytic a.
    anti-Kell a.
    aplastic a.
    aregenerative a.
    autoimmune acquired hemolytic a.
    autoimmune hemolytic a. (AIHA)
    Benjamin a.
    Blackfan-Diamond a.
    blood-loss a.
    B_6-responsive a.
    cardiac hemolytic a.
    chronic nonspherocytic hemolytic a.
    congenital aplastic a.
    congenital dyserythropoietic a.
      (CDA)
    congenital Heinz body a.
    congenital hypoplastic a.
    congenital nonregenerative a.
    congenital nonspherocytic
      hemolytic a.
    congenital pernicious a.
    congenital sideroblastic a.
    Cooley a.

NOTES

43

anemia *(continued)*
  Coombs-negative autoimmune hemolytic a.
  Coombs-positive isoimmune hemolytic a.
  copper deficiency a.
  crescent cell a.
  a. of CRF
  Czerny a.
  Diamond-Blackfan a. (DBA)
  Diamond-Blackfan congenital hypoplastic a.
  Diamond-Blackfan juvenile pernicious a.
  dilutional a.
  drug-induced hemolytic a.
  elliptocytic a.
  erythroblastic a.
  familial erythroblastic a.
  Fanconi a. (FA)
  Fanconi aplastic a.
  fetal a.
  globe cell a.
  Heinz body hemolytic a.
  hemolytic a.
  hereditary hemolytic a.
  hereditary nonspherocytic a.
  Herrick a.
  homozygous sickle cell a.
  a. hypochromica sideroachrestica hereditaria
  hypochromic microcytic a.
  hypoplastic a.
  hypoproliferative a.
  iatrogenic a.
  idiopathic acquired sideroblastic a. (IASA)
  iron deficiency a. (IDA)
  isoimmune a.
  Jaksch a.
  juvenile pernicious a.
  Larzel a.
  macrocytic megaloblastic a.
  macrocytic a. of pregnancy
  Mediterranean a.
  megaloblastic a.
  microangiopathic hemolytic a.
  microcytic a.
  mild a.
  mitochondrial myopathy and sideroblastic a. (MLASA)
  mixed iron and folate deficiency a.
  myopathy, lactic acidosis, sideroblastic a.
  neonatal isoimmune hemolytic a.
  a. neonatorum
  nonspherocytic a.
  normochromic a.
  normocytic a.
  ovalocytary a.
  pernicious a. (PA)
  PGK hereditary nonspherocytic a.
  physiologic a.
  posthepatic aplastic a.
  pregnancy-associated hypoplastic a.
  a. of prematurity
  a. pseudoleukemica infantum
  pyridoxine-refractory sideroblastic a.
  pyridoxine-responsive a.
  refractory dyserythropoietic a.
  Runeberg a.
  schistocytic hemolytic a.
  severe megaloblastic a.
  sickle cell a.
  sideroblastic a.
  a. syndrome
  thiamin-response sideroblastic a.
  von Jaksch a.
  X-linked pyridoxine-responsive sideroblastic a.

anemic effect

anemicus
  nevus a.

anencephalic, anencephalous

anencephaly, anencephalia

anergy

Anestacon Topical Solution

anesthesia
  a. bag
  caudal a.
  conduction a.
  CSE a.
  epidural a.
  extradural a.
  general endotracheal a.
  hypotensive a.
  inhalation a.
  local a.
  lumbar epidural a.
  mask inhalation a.
  maternal a.
  neuraxial a.
  obstetric a.
  office laparoscopy under local a. (OLULA)
  paracervical a.
  peridural a.
  perineal a.
  pudendal a.
  regional block a.
  saddle block a.
  spinal a.

anesthesia-related maternal mortality

anesthesiologist
  pediatric a.

anesthetic
  eutectic mixture of local a.'s (EMLA)

gas a.
a. gas exposure
local a.
a. skin lesion
volatile a.
walking epidural a.

anesthetist
certified registered nurse a.

anestrous
anetoderma of prematurity
aneugamy
aneuploid abortion
aneuploidy
atypical a.
fetal a.
a. infant
mosaic a.
Pallister mosaic a.
recurrent a.
segmental a.
X chromosome a.
XXXXY a.

aneurysm
aortic a.
arterial a.
berry a.
cerebral artery a.
circle of Willis a.
cirsoid a.
CNS a.
congenital cerebral a.
coronary a.
coronary artery a. (CAA)
dissecting aortic a.
fusiform a.
giant coronary artery a.
intracerebral a.
intracranial arterial a.
intrauterine cirsoid a.
left ventricular apical a.
mycotic a.
ruptured cerebral a.
ruptured sinus of Valsalva a.
saccular a.
splenic artery a.
vein of Galen a.
a. of vein of Galen
ventricular a.

aneurysmal bone cyst
AneuVysion Assay prenatal genetic test
Anexsia

ANF
atrial natriuretic factor
Angelman syndrome
angel-shaped phalangoepiphyseal dysplasia (ASPED)
angel's kiss
anger
A. Expression Scale
a. stage
angiectatic skin rash
angiitic luminal compromise
angiitis
granulomatous a.
hypersensitivity a.
leukoclastic a.
leukocytoclastic a.
lupus a.
angina
bowel a.
Ludwig a.
nocturnal a.
Vincent a.
angiocardiogram
Elema a.
Angiocath catheter
angiocatheter
angiodysplasia
angioedema
acquired a. (type I, II)
episodic a.
hereditary a. (type I)
recurrent a.
angiofibroma
juvenile nasopharyngeal a.
angiofollicular lymph node hyperplasia
angiogenesis
placental adaptive a.
angiogenic growth factor
angiogram
superior mesenteric a.
angiographic embolization
angiography
catheter a.
cerebral a.
digital subtraction a.
fluorescein fundus a.
magnetic resonance a. (MRA)
pulmonary a.
radioisotope a.
selective a.
angiokeratoma
a. circumscriptum

NOTES

45

angiokeratoma *(continued)*
 a. corporis diffusum
 Mibelli a.
 a. of Mibelli
 vulvar a.
angiolysis
angioma
 a. capillare et venosum calcificans
 capillary a.
 cavernous venous a.
 cerebral a.
 cutaneocerebral a.
 cutaneous a.
 dural spinal a.
 facial a.
 intradural spinal a.
 leptomeningeal a.
 port-wine stained a.
 retinal a.
 spider a.
 spinal a.
 subependymal cryptic a.
 venous a.
AngioMark MRI contrast agent
angiomatoid tumor
angiomatosis
 bacillary a. (BA)
 cerebrocutaneous a.
 cutaneomeningospinal a.
 encephalocraniofacial a.
 encephalofacial a.
 a. encephalofacialis
 encephalotrigeminal a.
 leptomeningeal a.
 meningeal capillary a.
 meningooculofacial a.
 a. meningoulofacialis
 neurooculocutaneous a.
 Sturge-Weber a.
angiomatosis-oculo-orbito-thalamo-
 encephalic syndrome
angiomatous involuting nevus
angiomyofibroblastoma
angiomyolipoma rupture
angiomyoma of oviduct
angiomyxoma
 aggressive a. (AAM)
angioneurotic edema
angioosteohypertrophy syndrome
angiopathic hemolytic anemia
angiopathy
 vulvar congenital dysplastic a.
angioplasty
 percutaneous transluminal a. (PTA)
 pulmonary artery a.
angiosarcoma
 uterine a.
angiosonography
angiostrongyliasis

Angiostrongylus cantonensis
angiotensin-converting
 a.-c. enzyme (ACE)
 a.-c. enzyme inhibitor
angiotensin (I, II, III)
angiotensinogen
angle
 adductor a.
 anterior chamber a.
 calcaneotibial a.
 center edge a.
 A. classification
 A. classification of occlusion
 corneoscleral a.
 costovertebral a. (CVA)
 decreased talocalcaneal a.
 femoral-tibial a.
 foot-progression a. (FPA)
 hip-knee-ankle a.
 a. of His
 knee a.
 metaphysial-diaphysial a.
 neck-shaft a. (NSA)
 popliteal a.
 Q a.
 talar to first metatarsal a.
 talocalcaneal a. (TCA)
 thigh-foot a. (TFA)
 thigh-leg a. (TLA)
 transmalleolar axis a. (TMA)
 urethral a.
 urethrovesical a.
angular
 a. cheilitis
 a. cheilosis
 a. deformity
 a. movement
 a. stomatitis
angulation
 congenital anterolateral tibial a.
 congenital posteromedial tibial a.
 flow a.
 metaphysis a.
 volar a.
anhedonia
anhidrosis
 ipsilateral a.
 neuropathic a.
anhidrotic
 a. ectodermal dysplasia
 a. sweating
anhydramnion
anhydremia
anhydrohydroxyprogesterone
Anhydron
anhydrotic ectodermal dysplasia
anhydrous
 betaine a.
 a. magnesium sulfate

ANI
    autoimmune neutropenia of infancy
ani (*pl. of* anus)
anicteric
    a. hepatitis
    a. leptospirosis
anideus
    embryonic a.
anileridine
aniline dye
animal
    a. antisera
    a. bite
    a. dander
    a. scabies
animal-assisted therapy (AAT)
anion
    competing a.
    a. gap
aniridia
    a., ambiguous genitalia, mental
        retardation (AGR)
    a., cerebellar ataxia-oligophrenia
        syndrome
    nonfamilial a.
    sporadic a.
    a., Wilms tumor association
        (AWTA)
    a., Wilms tumor association
        syndrome
    a., Wilms tumor, gonadoblastoma
        syndrome
anisindione
anismus
anisocoria
    ipsilateral a.
    simple central a.
anisocytosis
anisodactyly
anisomastia
anisomelia
anisometropia
anisometropic amblyopia
anisotropic
anisotropine
ankle
    a. clonus
    dancer's a.
    a. equinus
    jogger's a.
    a. reflexes absent
    a. stability
    a. stirrup splint
ankle-foot orthosis (AFO)
ankyloblepharon
    a., ectodermal dysplasia, clefting
        (AEC)
    a., ectodermal dysplasia, clefting
        syndrome
ankylocheilia
ankylocolpos
ankylodactyly
ankyloglossia superior syndrome
ankyloproctia
ankylosing
    a. spondylitis
    a. spondyloarthropathy
ankylosis
    artificial a.
    interbody a.
ankyrin
anlage, pl. **anlagen**
    allergic a.
    anlagen of the auditory ossicle
    fibrous a.
    ventral pancreatic a.
ANLL
    acute nonlymphoblastic leukemia
ANN
    alloimmune neonatal neutropenia
Ann Arbor Staging System
anneal
annexectomy
annexin
annexitis
annexopexy
annual
    a. goal
    a. review
annular (*var. of* anular)
annulare
    granuloma a.
    perforating granuloma a.
    subcutaneous granuloma a.
annulati (*var. of* anulati)
annuloaortic ectasia
annuloplasty
    De Vega tricuspid a.
annulus (*var. of* anulus)
ano
    fissure in a.
anococcygeal raphe
anocutaneous reflex

NOTES

anodontia
anogenital wart
anomalad
  abdominal muscle deficiency a.
  amniotic band a.
  facioauriculovertebral a.
  holoprosencephaly a.
  Poland a.
  Robin a.
  Sturge-Weber a.
anomalous
  a. coronary artery
  a. left coronary artery from
    pulmonary artery (ALCAPA)
  a. left coronary artery from
    pulmonary artery syndrome
  a. left pulmonary artery
  a. pulmonary vein
  a. pulmonary venous connection
  a. pulmonary venous drainage
  a. right pulmonary vein
    dextroposition
  a. uterus
anomaly
  acyanotic cardiac a.
  Alder a.
  Alder-Reilly a.
  Alexander a.
  aortic arch a.
  Arnold-Chiari a.
  arthrogryposis-like hand a.
  Axenfeld a.
  Axenfeld-Rieger a.
  birth a.
  body stalk a.
  branchial cleft a.
  cardiac a.
  cervical a.
  Chédiak-Higashi a.
  Chiari a.
  chromosomal a.
  cloacal plate a.
  congenital a.
  conotruncal facial a.
  craniofacial a.
  DiGeorge a.
  Duane a.
  duplication a.
  ear a.
  Ebstein a.
  extracardiac a.
  facial a.
  fetal skeletal a.
  fetal vascular a.
  genetic a.
  Greig cephalopolysyndactyly a.
  gyral a.
  immunodeficiency, centromeric
    instability, facial a.'s (ICF)
  imperforate anus, hand, and
    foot a.'s
  intracranial dural vascular a.
  intraspinous vascular a.
  iridogoniodysgenesis with
    somatic a.'s
  May-Hegglin a.
  Michel a.
  microcephaly-cervical spine
    fusion a.'s
  microphthalmia or anophthalmos
    with associated a.'s (MAA)
  Möbius a.
  Mondini a.
  morning glory disc a.
  müllerian duct a.
  multiple congenital a.'s
  Nager a.
  orthopaedic a.
  pancreaticobiliary a.
  partial DiGeorge a.
  Pelger-Huet a.
  Peters a.
  Poland a.
  Rieger a.
  Scheibe a.
  sex chromosomal a.
  Shone a.
  skeletal a.
  sling a.
  spondylar changes-nasal a.-striated-
    metaphyses (sponastrime)
  Sprengel a.
  structural a.
  Taussig-Bing a.
  thymic hypoplasia a.
  Uhl a.
  umbilical a.
  umbilical cord a.
  Undritz a.
  urinary tract a.
  urogenital congenital a.
  uterine a.
  vaginal a.
  valvuloplasty and angioplasty of
    congenital a.'s (VACA)
  vascular a.
  vertebral a.'s, anal atresia, cardiac
    defects, tracheoesophageal fistula,
    renal, and limb a.'s (VACTERL)
  X-linked mental-retardation-bilateral
    clasp thumb a.
  X-linked mental retardation/multiple
    congenital a. (XLMR/MCA)
anomeric
anonychia
anonychia-ectrodactyly
anonychia-onychodystrophy
anonymous donor sperm (ADS)

anophthalmia, anophthalmos
    a., hand-foot defects, mental
      retardation syndrome
anophthalmia-limb anomalies syndrome
anophthalmia-syndactyly syndrome
anophthalmia-Waardenburg syndrome
anophthalmos (*var. of* anophthalmia)
anoplasty
anorchia
anorchism
anorectal
    a. agenesis
    a. incontinence
    a. perfusion manometry
    a. plug
    a. stenosis
    a. syndrome
anorectic, anoretic
    a. reaction
anorectoplasty
    anterior sagittal a.
    laparoscopically assisted a.
    Pena midsagittal a.
    posterior sagittal a.
anorectum
anoretic (*var. of* anorectic)
Anorex
anorexia
    a. athletica
    infantile a.
    a. nervosa (AN)
    a. nervosa with binging and
      purging (AN-BP)
anorgasmia, anorgasmy
anorgasmic
anosmia
    congenital a.
    hypogonadotropic hypogonadism, a.
anosteogenesis
anotia
anovarianism
anovular menstruation
anovulation
    chronic a.
    hyperandrogenic a. (HA)
    hyperandrogenic chronic a.
    persistent a.
anovulatory
    a. bleeding
    a. infertility
    a. patient

anoxia
    cerebral a.
    fetal a.
    a. neonatorum
    tissue a.
anoxic-ischemic
    a.-i. encephalopathy
    a.-i. injury
anoxic seizure
ANP
    atrial natriuretic peptide
ANRBC
    absolute nucleated red blood cell
ANS
    antenatal corticosteroid treatment
    autonomic nervous system
Ansaid Oral
Ansaldo AU560 ultrasound
ANSD
    autonomic nervous system dysfunction
anserinus
    pes a.
Anspor
Answer Plus
Antabuse
antacid
antagonism
antagonist
    androgen a.
    bradykinin a.
    calcium channel a.
    coactivated a.'s
    estrogen a.
    folate a.
    folic acid a.
    FSH a.
    gonadotropin-releasing hormone a.
    GRH a.
    leukotriene receptor a. (LTRA)
    narcotic a.
    opioid receptor a.
    progesterone a.
    proton pump a.
    serotonin receptor a.
antagonistic muscle
antagonist-induced gonadotropin
  deprivation
antalgic
    a. gait
    a. limp

NOTES

antecedent
> cerebral palsy a.
> plasma thromboplastin a. (PTA)

antecedent-behavior-consequence
relationship

antecubital
> a. space
> a. vein

anteflexed
> anteverted and a. (AV/AF)

anteflexion

antegrade
> a. continence enema (ACE)
> a. continence enema procedure

antenatal
> a. admission
> a. anti-D immunoglobulin
> a. assessment
> a. complication
> a. corticosteroid
> a. corticosteroid therapy
> a. corticosteroid treatment (ANS)
> a. diagnosis
> a. disease process
> a. fetofetal transfusion
> a. management
> a. morbidity
> a. patient
> a. phenobarbital treatment
> a. screening
> a. steroid
> a. testing
> a. testing unit
> a. thyrotropin releasing hormone
> a. ultrasound

antepartum
> a. alloimmunization
> a. asphyxia
> a. bed rest
> a. bleeding
> a. care
> a. complication
> a. dosage
> a. fetal assessment
> a. fetal BPP
> a. fetal CST
> a. fetal NST
> a. fetal surveillance
> a. fetal testing
> a. hemorrhage
> a. home care
> a. hospital bed rest
> a. hospitalization
> a. management
> a. monitor
> a. period
> a. pyelonephritis
> a. Rh isoimmunization
> a. steroid therapy

> a. stress
> a. support group
> a. surveillance program
> a. unit

anteposition

anterior
> a. abdominal wall
> a. apical vault defect
> a. asynclitism
> a. cerebral artery pulsatility index (ACAPI)
> a. chamber
> a. chamber angle
> a. chamber cleavage syndrome
> a. chamber dysgenesis syndrome
> a. colporrhaphy
> a. commissure
> a. cord syndrome
> a. cricoid split (ACS)
> a. cricoid split procedure
> a. cruciate ligament (ACL)
> a. drawer test
> dysgenesis mesostromalis a.
> a. enterocele
> a. ethmoidal sinusitis
> a. exenteration
> a. fontanelle
> a. head cap
> a. horn cell degeneration
> a. horn cell disease
> a. hypospadias
> a. labial arteries of vulva
> a. labial nerves
> a. lenticonus
> a. lie
> a. lip of the cervix
> a. microphthalmia
> a. nasal packing
> a. nasal septum
> a. neural tube closure
> a. neural tube defect
> occiput a. (OA)
> a. pelvic exenteration
> a. pituitary disorder
> a. pituitary-like hormone
> a. and posterior (A&P)
> a. and posterior repair
> a. rectoperineal fistula
> a. rectus sheath
> a. resection rectopexy
> a. retrosternal hernia of Morgagni
> a. sagittal anorectoplasty
> a. spinal fusion
> a. spinal instrumentation
> a. superior iliac spine
> a. synechia
> a. talofibular ligament (ATFL)
> a. thoracic wall
> a. tibial bowing

a. tibialis transfer
a. translation
a. translation of knee
a. urethritis
a. vagina
a. vaginotomy
anteriorly displaced anus
anterolateral
a. fontanelle
a. free wall (ALFW)
a. tibial bowing
anteroposterior (AP)
a. colporrhaphy
a. diameter of the pelvic inlet
a. laxity
a. view
antetorsion
femoral a.
anteversion
acetabular a. (AA)
bilateral increased femoral a.
femoral a. (FA)
increased femoral a.
anteverted
a. and anteflexed (AV/AF)
a. naris
a. nostril
a. pinna
anthelix
anthelminthic, anthelmintic
a. agent
a. drug
anthracycline
anthrax
cutaneous a.
pulmonary a.
anthropi
Ochrobactrum a.
anthropoid pelvis
anthropometric
a. measure
a. measurement
anthropometry
anthropomorphic measurement
anti-A, anti-B isohemagglutinin
anti-ACh antibody
antiadrenal antibody
antiandrogen receptor blocker
antiangiogenic therapy
antiannexin V antibody

antianxiety
a. agent
a. drug
antiarrhythmic
antiasthmatic
antibacterial
a. drug
a. therapy
antibasement membrane antibody
antibiotic
antitumor a.
beta-lactam a.
beta-lactamase-resistant
antistaphylococcal a.
broad-spectrum a.
a. drug
a. infusion therapy
preventive a.
prophylactic a.
a. prophylaxis
a. resistance
a. treatment
antibiotic-associated
a.-a. colitis
a.-a. diarrhea (AAD)
AntibiOtic Otic
antibiotic-resistant gram-negative organism (ARGNO)
antibody
ADB a.
AH a.
anti-ACh a.
antiadrenal a.
antiannexin V a.
antibasement membrane a.
anticardiolipin a. (aCL)
anticardiolipin a.-positive
anticentromere a. (ACA)
anticholera toxin a.
anti-CMV a.
anticytomegalovirus a.
anti-D a.
anti-DNase B a.
antidrug IgE a.
anti-EBNA a.
antiendomysium a. (AEA)
anti-Epstein-Barr nuclear antigen a.
antiferritin a.
anti-GBM a.
antigliadin a. (AGA)
antihistone a.
anti-*Histoplasma* a.

NOTES

antibody *(continued)*
  anti-HIV a.
  antihyaluronidase a.
  antiidiotype a.
  antiinsulin a.
  anti-Kell a.
  anti-La a.
  anti-Lewis a.
  anti-M a.
  antimitochondrial a.
  antimyolemmal a. (AMLA)
  antineutrophil a.
  antineutrophil cytoplasmic a.
   (ANCA)
  antinuclear a. (ANA)
  antiovarian a.
  antipaternal antileukocytotoxic a.
  antiphospholipid a. (aPL)
  antiplatelet IgG a.
  antireticulin a.
  antiribosomal P a.
  anti-Ro a.
  anti-*Saccharomyces cerevisiae* a.
  anti-smooth-muscle a.
  antisperm a.
  anti-SS-A a.
  anti-SS-B a.
  antithyroid a.
  anti-TNF a.
  antitoxocaral a.
  ASO a.
  blood group a.
  celiac a.
  circulating platelet a.
  cold a.
  complement-fixing serum a.
  conjugated antichlamydial
   monoclonal a.
  Coombs a.
  cytophilic a.
  a. deficiency
  direct fluorescent a. (DFA)
  endomysium a. (EMA)
  fluorescent treponemal a. (FTA)
  Frei a.
  genus-specific monoclonal a.
  glutamic acid decarboxylase a.
  hantavirus immunoglobulin M a.
  hemagglutination inhibition a. (HIA)
  a. to hepatitis A virus (anti-HAV)
  hepatitis B core a. (HBcAb)
  a. to hepatitis B core antigen
   (anti-HBcAg)
  hepatitis B early a. (HBeAb)
  hepatitis B surface a. (HBsAb)
  a. to hepatitis B surface antigen
   (anti-HBsAg, anti-HBs)
  heterophil a.
  HI a.

HPV type 16 capsid a.
humoral a.
IgA antiendomysium a.
IgA antireticulin a.
IgD a.
IgE a.
IgG a.
IgM a.
immunofluorescent a. (IFA)
immunoglobulin a.
indirect fluorescent a. (IFA)
indirect hemagglutination a. (IHA)
a. induction therapy
intrathecal anti-HIV a.
islet cell a. (ICA)
Jo-1 a.
Kell a.'s
Ki67 a.
Kveim a.
link a.
lupus anticoagulant a.
maternal antiplatelet a.
maternal antithyroid a.
maternal-fetal transmission of a.
maternal IgG a.
maternal sperm a.
monoclonal a. (MAb)
monoclonal antiendotoxin a.
monoclonal anti-IgE a.
mycoplasmal a.
natural a.
neurofilament a.
OncoScint CR103 monoclonal a.
ovarian a.
parietal cell a.
perinuclear antineutrophil
  cytoplasmic a. (pANCA)
phospholipid a.
platelet-associated a.
polyclonal antiendotoxin anticore a.
polyclonal-monoclonal a.
a. production assay
a. reaction site
a. replacement therapy
a. response
Rh a.
rhesus a.
Rh-negative a.
Rh-positive a.
RSV monoclonal a.
S-100 a.
a. screening
serum a.
serum antienterocyte a.
species-specific a.
sperm surface a.
streptococcal a.
tissue-specific a.
titer of anti-ragweed IgE a.

transglutaminase a.
a. transplacental transfer
Treponema pallidum a.
vibriocidal a.
virus-neutralizing a. (VNA)
VZV-specific IgM a.
warm a.
xenogeneic a.
antibody-dependent cell-mediated cytotoxicity (ADCC)
antibody-mediated
a.-m. hemolysis
a.-m. immune suppression (AMIS)
antibody-secreting cell (ASC)
anticancer agent
anticardiolipin
a. antibody (aCL)
a. antibody-positive
anticentromere antibody (ACA)
anticholera toxin antibody
anticholinergic
a. drug
a. plant
a. poisoning
anticholinesterase medication
anticipated
a. behavioral milestone
a. developmental milestone
anticipation
evidence of a.
anticipatory
a. anxiety
a. grief
anti-CMV antibody
anticoagulant
circulating a.
lupus a. (LAC)
anticoagulation
ambulatory a.
outpatient a.
peripartal heparin a.
therapeutic a.
a. therapy
anticodon
anticonvulsant
a. drug
a. hypersensitivity syndrome
a. intoxication
a. treatment
anticus
saccus a.
anticysticercal therapy

anticytomegalovirus antibody
anti-D
a.-D antibody
a.-D autoantibody
a.-D globulin treatment
a.-D immune globulin
a.-D immunoglobulin
a.-D therapy
antide
antideoxyribonucleic acid (anti-DNA)
antidepressant
a. drug
heterocyclic a.
a. poisoning
a. therapy
tricyclic a. (TCA)
antidiarrheal
antidiuresis
antidiuretic hormone (ADH)
anti-DNA
antideoxyribonucleic acid
anti-DNA antitopoisomerase 1
anti-DNase
a.-DNase B (ADB)
a.-DNase B antibody
a.-DNase B titer
antidromic conduction
antidrug IgE antibody
antidysrhythmic agent
anti-EBNA antibody
antiembolism stocking
antiemetic
a. medication
a. therapy
antiendometriotic effect
antiendomysial
IgA a.
antiendomysium antibody (AEA)
antiepileptic drug (AED)
anti-Epstein-Barr nuclear antigen antibody
antiestrogen effect
antiestrogenic effect
antiferritin antibody
antifibrinolytic agent
antifolic agent
antifungal
Absorbine Jr. A.
a. azole
a. drug
a. drug therapy
antigalactagogue

NOTES

antigalactic
Anti-Gas
    Maalox A.-G.
anti-GBM antibody
antigen
    A a.
    ABO a.
    a. activity
    allogenic a.
    antibody to hepatitis B core a.
      (anti-HBcAg)
    antibody to hepatitis B surface a.
      (anti-HBsAg, anti-HBs)
    antigen-specific a.
    antiproliferating cell nuclear a.
      (anti-PCNA)
    anular erythema a.
    Australia a.
    a. binding site
    CA 125 a.
    carcinoembryonic a. (CEA)
    carcinoembryonic a. 125 (CEA 125)
    carcinoma a.
    cell surface a.
    chorioembryonic a.
    cryptococcal a.
    a. detection test
    a. determinant
    direct fluorescent a. (DFA)
    Duffy a.
    E a.
    epithelial membrane a. (EMA)
    Epstein-Barr nuclear a. (EBNA)
    fetal histocompatibility a.
    fluorescent antibody against
      membrane a. (FAMA)
    Forssman a.
    glomerular basement membrane a.
    hepatitis B a. (HBAg)
    hepatitis B surface a. (HBsAg)
    heterophil a.
    histocompatibility locus a.
    histone a.
    HIV-1 p24 a.
    HLA-B27 a.
    human leukocyte a. (HLA)
    H-Y a.
    incompatible blood group a.
    Kell a.
    La/SSB a.
    Lewis a.
    lipoglycan a.
    M a.
    major histocompatibility a.
    melanoma specific a.
    MHC a.
    nuclear a.
    O a.

    oncofetal a.
    ovarian carcinoma a.
    pancreatic oncofetal a. (POA)
    platelet a.
    Pm-Scl a.
    polysaccharide group-specific a.
    RBC P a.
    red blood cell a.
    respiratory syncytial virus a.
    Rh a.
    rhesus a.
    ribonucleoprotein a.
    Ro/SSA a.
    RSV a.
    sclerodermatomyositis a.
    a. screen
    sialylated Lewis A a.
    sialyl Tn a.
    Sm a.
    surface a.
    surface a. (subtype ayw1–ayw4)
    Thomsen-Friedenreich a.
    thymic lymphocyte a. (TL)
    T-independent a.
    a. tolerance
    Toxoplasma a.
    transplantation a.
    Treponema pallidum a.
    tumor a.
    tumor-associated a. (TAA)
    tumor-specific transplantation a.
      (TSTA)
    viral capsid a. (VCA)
    von Willebrand factor a.
    vWF a.
antigen-antibody complex
antigenemia
antigenic
    a. mimicry
    a. modulation
    a. paralysis
    a. stimulus
antigenicity
    tumor a.
antigen-presenting cell (APC)
antigen-sensitive cell
antigen-specific antigen
antigenuria
antigliadin
    a. antibody (AGA)
    IgA a.
antiglobulin test
antiglomerular basement membrane
  antibody disease
antigonadotropin
antigravity
    a. activity
    a. position

anti-HAV
    antibody to hepatitis A virus
      IgG anti-HAV
anti-HBcAg
    antibody to hepatitis B core antigen
anti-HBsAg, anti-HBs
    antibody to hepatitis B surface antigen
      a.-H. concentration
antihelical fold
antihelix
antihelminthic therapy
antihemophilic factor (AHF)
antihistamine
    a. drug
    histamine 1 a.
Antihist-D
antihistone antibody
anti-*Histoplasma* antibody
anti-HIV antibody
antihyaluronidase
    a. antibody
    a. titer
antihypertensive
    a. drug
    a. therapy
antiicteric
antiidiotype antibody
antiimmunoglobulin reagent
antiincontinence
antiinflammatory
    a. effect
    a. intervention
    a. therapy
    a. treatment
antiinhibitor coagulant complex
antiinsulin antibody
anti-Jo1
anti-Kell
    a.-K. anemia
    a.-K. antibody
    a.-K. sensitization
anti-La antibody
antileukemic therapy
anti-Lewis antibody
antilewisite
    British a. (BAL)
antilipolysis
antiluteogenic
antilymphocyte
    a. globulin
    a. sera

antimalarial
    a. drug
    a. poisoning
antimanic treatment
anti-M antibody
antimesenteric surface
antimetabolite
antimicrobial
    a. agent
    a. aminoglycoside
    beta-lactam a.
    a. prophylaxis
    a. susceptibility testing
    a. therapy
    a. treatment
antimicrosomal
antimitochondrial antibody
antimongolism
antimongoloid
    a. deformity
    a. eye slant
    a. obliquity
    a. palpebral fissure
antimüllerian hormone (AMH)
antimycobacterial
antimycoplasma titer
antimyolemmal antibody (AMLA)
antinauseant poisoning
antineoplastic
    a. agent
    a. drug
antineutrophil
    a. antibody
    a. cytoplasmic antibody (ANCA)
antinuclear antibody (ANA)
anti-O-specific polysaccharide
antiovarian antibody
antioxidant
    chain-breaking a.
    a. enzyme
    preventive a.
    a. therapy
antiparasitic drug therapy
antipaternal antileukocytotoxic antibody
anti-PCNA
    antiproliferating cell nuclear antigen
antiperistaltic intestinal interposition
antiphospholipid
    a. antibody (aPL)
    a. antibody syndrome
    a. syndrome (APS)
antiplasmin (AP)

NOTES

antiplasmin *(continued)*
    alpha-2 antiplasmin
    a. deficiency
antiplatelet
    a. agent
    a. IgG antibody
    a. therapy
antiprogesterone
antiprogestin
antiprogestogen
antiproliferating cell nuclear antigen (anti-PCNA)
antiprostaglandin agent
antipruritic medication
antipsychotic
    a. drug
    a. poisoning
antipyretic therapy
antipyrine and benzocaine
antirabies serum
antireceptor
antireticulin antibody
antiretroviral
    a. medication
    a. resistance
    a. therapy
anti-Rh gamma globulin
anti-Rho(D)
    a. globulin
    a. titer
antiribosomal P antibody
anti-Ro antibody
anti-RSV
anti-*Saccharomyces cerevisiae* antibody
anti-Scl-70 autoantibody
antisense
    a. nucleotide
    a. oligodeoxynucleotide
    a. oligonucleotide
    a. strand
antiseptic
    Avagard instant hand a.
antiserum, pl. **antisera**
    animal antisera
    SB-6 a.
    tetanus a.
antishock trousers
antisialagogue
antisiphon device
anti-smooth-muscle antibody
antisocial
    a. behavior
    a. personality disorder (ASPD)
Antispas Injection
antispasmodic poisoning
antispastic
    a. drug
    a. medication
antisperm antibody

anti-SS-A antibody
anti-SS-B antibody
anti-ssDNA
antistaphylococcal
    a. agent
    a. IgE
    a. penicillin
antistreptolysin O (ASO)
antithrombin (AT)
    a. III (AT3)
    a. III coagulation inhibitor
    a. III deficiency
    a. I, II, III
    protein S a.
antithymocyte globulin
antithyroglobulin
antithyroid
    a. antibody
    a. drug
    a. drug therapy
anti-TNF antibody
antitoxin
    botulinum a. (type A, B, E)
    diphtheria a.
    equine a.
    scarlatina a.
    tetanus a. (TAT)
antitoxocaral antibody
anti-*Toxoplasma*
    serum immunoglobulin G a.-*T.*
antitragus
antitreponemal test
antitrypsin
antituberculosis chemotherapy
antituberculous therapy
antitumor antibiotic
antitussive medication
antivenin (Crotalidae) polyvalent
antivenom
Antivert
antivesicuoreteral reflux surgery
antiviral therapy
Antizol
Antley-Bixler syndrome
Antopol disease
antra (*pl. of* antrum)
antral
    a. choanal polyp
    a. follicle
    a. gastritis
    a. lavage
    a. stenosis
    a. washout
Antrizine
antrum, pl. **antra**
    aditus ad a.
    nasal a.
anucleate fragment

ANUG
  acute necrotizing ulcerative gingivitis
anular, annular
  a. band
  a. erythema antigen
  a. lesion
  a. pancreas
  a. placenta
  a. stenosis
  a. testis
  a. tubule
anular-array transducer
anulati, annulati
  pili a.
  pseudopili a.
anulus, annulus
Anumed
anuria
anuric
anus, pl. **ani**
  adequate caliber of a.
  anteriorly displaced a.
  arcus tendineus levator ani
  ectopic a.
  high imperforate a.
  imperforate a.
  levator ani
  low imperforate a.
  Paget disease of a.
  patent a.
  pruritus ani
  a. of Rusconi
  spastic levator ani
  supralevator imperforate a.
  translevator imperforate a.
  vaginal ectopic a.
  vestibular a.
  vulvovaginal a.
anus-hand-ear syndrome
Anusol
  A. HC-1 Topical
  A. HC-2.5% Topical
Anusol-HC Suppository
anvil
anxiety
  anticipatory a.
  childhood a.
  a. depression
  a. disorder
  A. Disorder Interview for Children
  a. management
  a. rating for children (ARC)

  a. sensitivity index (ASI)
  separation a.
  stranger a.
anxiety-withdrawal scale
anxiogenic
anxiolytic
  a. agent
  a. drug
  a. medication
anxious look
Anzemet
AO
  arthroophthalmopathy
AOD
  alcohol and other drugs
AODM
  adult-onset diabetes mellitus
AOM
  acute otitis media
  arthroophthalmopathy
AOP
  apnea of prematurity
AOPA
  Ara-C, Oncovin, prednisone,
    asparaginase
AOPE
  Adriamycin, Oncovin, prednisone,
    etoposide
aorta, pl. **aortae**
  coarctation of a.
  descending a.
  a. dilation
  fetal a.
  hypoplastic a. (HA)
  overriding a.
  traumatic rupture of thoracic a.
    (TRA)
aortic
  a. aneurysm
  a. arch
  a. arch anomaly
  a. arch anomaly, peculiar facies,
    mental retardation syndrome
  a. arch coarctation (CoA)
  a. arch malformation
  a. arch rupture
  a. bifurcation
  a. blood flow velocity waveform
  a. blood pressure
  a. bruit
  a. bud
  a. coarctation

NOTES

57

aortic *(continued)*
  a. cusp prolapse
  a. dissection
  a. ejection click
  a. ejection murmur
  a. knob
  a. laceration
  a. node
  a. node metastasis
  a. oxygen content
  a. regurgitation
  a. root
  a. root diameter
  a. runoff
  a. sac
  a. stenosis, corneal clouding, growth and mental retardation syndrome
  a. valve
  a. valve atresia
  a. valve disease
  a. valve insufficiency
  a. valve stenosis
  a. valvotomy
aorticopulmonary
  a. septation
  a. window defect
aortic-to-pulmonary shunt
aortitis
aortogram
  thoracic a.
aortography
aortopexy
aortoplasty
  prosthetic patch a.
  subclavian flap a. (SFA)
aortopulmonary
  a. collateral coil embolization
  a. septum
  a. shunt
  a. transposition
  a. window
AP
  abruptio placentae
  anatomic profile
  anteroposterior
  antiplasmin
  appendiceal perforation
  AP diameter
A&P
  anterior and posterior
  A&P repair
Apacet
APACHE
  Acute Physiology and Chronic Health Evaluation
Apak syndrome
apareunia
apathy

APC
  activated protein C
  antigen-presenting cell
  atrial premature contraction
APCR
  activated protein C resistance
APE
  Ara-C, Platinol, etoposide
APECED
  autoimmune polyendocrinopathy, candidiasis, ectodermal dystrophy
ape hand
Apert
  A. disease
  A. syndrome
Apert-Crouzon
  A.-C. disease
  A.-C. syndrome
aperture
  supraglottic a.
apex, pl. **apices**
  a. of intussusception
  a. linguae
  prolapsing a.
  a. of vagina
  vaginal a.
Apgar
  A. rating
  A. scale
  A. score
  A. scoring system
  A. timer
APGN
  acute postinfectious glomerulonephritis
aphakia
  pediatric a.
aphasia
  acquired epileptic a.
  Broca a.
  expressive a.
  global a.
  infantile acquired a.
  migraine with a.
  receptive a.
  thymic a.
  Wernicke a.
apheresis
  LDL a.
aphonia
aphrodisiac
aphrophilus
  Haemophilus a.
aphtha, pl. **aphthae**
  Bednar aphthae
aphthosis
  perianal a.
aphthous
  a. stomatitis

a. ulcer
a. ulceration
A1PI, a1PI
alpha-1 proteinase inhibitor
APIB
Assessment of Preterm Infants' Behavior
apical
a. ectodermal ridge
a. four-chamber view
a. heave
a. impulse
a. pleural stripping
a. presystolic murmur
a. pulse
a. vertebra
apices (*pl. of* apex)
apista
Pandoraea a.
APL
accelerated painless labor
aPL
antiphospholipid antibody
aplasia
Alexander a.
a. axialis extracorticalis congenita
bone marrow a.
cerebellar vermis a.
complete cerebellar a.
complete radial a.
congenital cutis a.
congenital RBC a.
congenital skin a.
congenital vaginal a.
a. cutis
a. cutis congenita
extracortical axial a.
gonadal a.
heminasal a.
hereditary retinal a.
idiosyncratic marrow a.
Leydig cell a.
Michel a.
Mondini a.
nuclear a.
optic nerve a.
ovarian a.
parvovirus B19-induced red blood cell a.
parvovirus B19 red blood cell a.
pulmonary acinar a.
pure red blood cell a.

radial ray a.
retinal a.
Scheibe a.
selective a.
thymic a.
thymic-parathyroid a.
thyroid a.
vas deferens a.
aplastic
a. abdominal muscle syndrome
a. anemia
a. crisis
a. leukemia
a. pancytopenia
a. patella
Apley compression test
APLS
advanced pediatric life support
APLS model
apnea
a. alarm mattress
a. and bradycardia (A&B)
central sleep a.
expiratory a.
hyperreflexic a.
idiopathic a.
a. of infancy
infantile sleep a.
initial a.
late a.
mixed sleep a.
a. monitor
neonatal a.
a. neonatorum
obstructive a.
obstructive sleep a. (OSA)
pathologic a.
pathological a.
postanesthetic a.
postoperative a.
posttussive a.
a. of prematurity (AOP)
prolonged expiratory a.
secondary a.
sleep a.
unrecognized a.
vasovagal reflex a.
apnea-bradycardia
apnea-hypopnea combination
apnea/hypoventilation
obstructive sleep a./h. (OSA/H)

NOTES

apneic
>   a. event
>   a. seizure

apneustic center

APO, Apo
>   apolipoprotein

Apo-
>   Apo-Amoxi
>   Apo-Ampi
>   Apo-Cephalex
>   Apo-Cimetidine
>   Apo-Cloxi
>   Apo-Diazepam
>   Apo-Diclo
>   Apo-Diflunisal
>   Apo-Doxy
>   Apo-Doxy Tabs
>   Apo-Flurbiprofen
>   Apo-Naproxen
>   Apo-Pen VK
>   Apo-Piroxicam
>   Apo-Ranitidine
>   Apo-Sulfamethoxazole
>   Apo-Sulfatrim
>   Apo-Tamox
>   Apo-Terfenadine
>   Apo-Tetra
>   Apo-Zidovudine

apoB
>   apobetalipoprotein
>   apoB gene

apobetalipoprotein (apoB)

apocrine
>   a. adenoma
>   a. chromhidrosis
>   a. cyst
>   a. cystadenoma
>   a. duct
>   a. gland of Moll
>   a. hydrocystoma
>   a. metaplasia
>   a. miliaria
>   a. sweat gland

apodia

apoenzyme deficiency

apoferritin

apogamy

Apogee 800 ultrasound system

apolipoprotein (APO, Apo)
>   familial defective a. B-100
>   serum a.

aponeurosis
>   epicranial a.
>   gastrocnemius a.

apophysial, apophyseal
>   a. space

apophysis, pl. **apophyses**

apophysitis
>   calcaneal a.

iliac crest a.
olecranon a.
traction a.

apoplectic

apoplexy
>   parturient a.
>   uteroplacental a.

apoprotein

ApopTag Plus kit

apoptosis
>   neutrophil a.
>   postasphyxial a.
>   spinal a.
>   spontaneous a.

apoptotic cell death

apotransferrin infusion

apparatus, pl. **apparatus**
>   Barcroft/Haldane a.
>   figure-of-eight a.
>   Golgi a.
>   Heyns abdominal decompression a.
>   vestibular a.

apparent
>   a. exophthalmos
>   a. life-threatening event (ALTE)
>   a. mineralocorticoid excess (AME)
>   a. paresis

appearance
>   acromegaloid facial a. (AFA)
>   apple-peel a.
>   bag of worms a.
>   bat wing a.
>   bird's beak a.
>   bread-and-butter a.
>   bull's eye sonographic a.
>   cobblestone a.
>   copper-wire a.
>   corkscrew a.
>   cushingoid a.
>   drooping lily a.
>   Erlenmeyer flask a.
>   ground-glass a.
>   hair-on-end a.
>   hatchet face a.
>   honeycombed a.
>   Hurler-like facial a.
>   lamellated a.
>   meconium ileus a.
>   onion-skin a.
>   peau d'orange a.
>   powder-burn visual a.
>   puppetlike a.
>   salt and pepper a.
>   silver-wire a.
>   slapped cheek a.
>   snowstorm a.
>   soap-bubble a.
>   sporotrichoid a.
>   stacked-coin a.

strawberry a.
sunburst a.
toxic a.
water bottle a.
wing-beating a.
worried facial a.
Appelt-Gerkin-Lenz syndrome
appendage
testicular a.
a. torsion
appendectomy
inversion-ligation a.
appendiceal
a. abscess
a. fecalith
a. intussusception
a. inversion
a. lumen
a. perforation (AP)
a. structure
a. stump
appendices (*pl. of* appendix)
appendicitis
acute a. (AA)
gangrenous a.
pelvic a.
perforated a.
ruptured a.
suppurative a.
appendicolith
calcified a.
appendicostomy
appendicovesicostomy
Mitrofanoff a.
appendicular artery
appendix, pl. **appendices**
a. epididymis
ligation of a.
obstruction of a.
a. testis
a. testis torsion
torsion of a.
vascularized a.
vermiform a.
apperception
appetite
decreased a.
apple
A. Medical bipolar forceps
a. pattern

apple-peel
a.-p. appearance
a.-p. atresia
appliance
dental speech a.
lingual a.
orthodontic a.
orthopedic a.
application
bioelectromagnetic a.
nonionizing nonthermal a.
silicone band a.
spring clip a.
topical iodine a.
applicator
Absolok endoscopic clip a.
afterload a.
benzoin a.
Bloedorn a.
cotton-tipped a.
Falope ring a.
Filshie clip a.
Fletcher-Suit a.
radioactive a.
ring a.
applied behavior analysis (ABA)
applier
LDS clip a.
vascular clip a.
appointment
prenatal a.
appositional ossification
apposition of skull suture
apprehension
a. sign
a. test
approach
abdominal a.
family-centered a.
hysteroscopic a.
Kahn a.
staircase a.
transrectal a.
appropriate
a. blood pressure cuff size
a. for gestational age (AGA)
a. learning experience
APPT
Adolescent and Pediatric Pain Tool
apraxia
ataxia-oculomotor a.
buccolingual a.

NOTES

apraxia *(continued)*
    congenital ocular motor a. (COMA)
    congenital ocular motor a. (type Cogan) (COMA)
    gait a.
    oculomotor a.
    sensory a.
apraxia-ataxia-mental deficiency syndrome
apraxia-oculomotor contracture-muscle atrophy syndrome
apraxic
Apresoline
    A. Injection
    A. Oral
aprobarbital
aproctia
Aprodine
apron
    Hottentot a.
    perineal surgical a.
    pudendal a.
aprosencephaly-atelencephaly syndrome
aprosencephaly syndrome
aprosopia
aprotinin
APS
    antiphospholipid syndrome
APSGN
    acute poststreptococcal glomerulonephritis
APT-Downey test
aptitude
    Detroit Test of Learning A. 2
APTT
    activated partial thromboplastin time
       APTT coagulation test
aP vaccine
AQ
    Beconase AQ
    Nasacort AQ
    Vancenase AQ
Aqua
    A. Glycolic
    A. Tar
Aquacel dressing
Aquachloral Supprettes
Aquacort
Aquaflex ultrasound gel pad
Aquagel lubricating gel
AquaMEPHYTON Injection
Aquaphor gauze
AquaSens FMS 1000 Fluid Monitoring System
Aquasol
    A. A, E
    A. E Oral

Aquasonic 100 ultrasound transmission gel
Aquasorb dressing
Aquaspirillum itersonii
Aquatensen
aqueduct
    cochlear a.
    a. of Sylvius
aqueductal
    a. forking
    a. gliosis
    a. stenosis
aqueous
    a. analysis
    A. AVP
    a. beclomethasone
    a. crystalline penicillin
    a. crystalline penicillin G
    a. humor
    a. penicillin sodium
    a. phase
AR
    alcohol related
    autosomal recessive
arabinoside
    adenine a.
    cytosine a.
arabinosylcytosine (Ara-C, araC)
    cyclophosphamide, Oncovin, methotrexate, a. (COMA)
Ara-C, araC
    arabinosylcytosine
       Ara-C, Oncovin, prednisone, asparaginase (AOPA)
       Ara-C, Platinol, etoposide (APE)
arachidic
    a. acid
    a. bronchitis
arachidonic
    a. acid
    a. acid level
    a. acid metabolite
arachnid envenomation
arachnidism
    necrotic a.
arachnodactyly
    congenital contractural a. (CCA)
arachnoid
    a. cyst
    a. granulation
    a. villus
arachnoiditis
    chronic adhesive a.
    obliterative a.
    posterior fossa a.
    spinal a.
    tuberculous spinal a.
aragonite precipitation
Arakawa syndrome

Aralen
Aramine
Aran-Duchenne
    A.-D. disease
    A.-D. muscular dystrophy
araneus
    nevus a.
ARAS
    ascending reticular activating system
arbitrarily
    a. primed polymerase chain
      reaction
    a. primer
arborization
    dendritic a.
    pulmonary a.
    vaginal fluid a.
arbor vitae
arboviral encephalitis
arbovirus
ARC
    AIDS-related complex
    anxiety rating for children
    Association for Retarded Citizens
arc
    xenon a.
arcade
    mitral a.
Arcanobacterium haemolyticum
arch
    aortic a.
    branchial a.
    double aortic a. (DAA)
    hypoplastic zygomatic a.
    a. insole pad
    interrupted aortic a. (type A, B)
    medial longitudinal a.
    narrow pubic a.
    neural a.
    pubic a.
    right aortic a. (RAA)
    tendinous a.
    vertebral laminar a.
    zygomatic a.
archencephalon
archenteron
archenteronoma
archiblast
archigastrula
architectural disturbance
architecture
    cortical a.

    crypt-villus a.
    dysplastic cortical a.
    histologic a.
    lobular a.
    mixed cystic/solid a.
    pelvic a.
    sleep a.
arciform lesion
arcing spring diaphragm
Arcoxia
ARCS
    azoospermia, renal anomaly,
      cervicothoracic spine dysplasia
    ARCS syndrome
arcuate
    a. artery
    a. ligament of pubis
    a. line
    a. nucleus
    a. uterus
arcus
    a. corneae
    a. juvenilis
    a. tendineus
    a. tendineus fasciae pelvis
    a. tendineus levator ani
ARD
    acute respiratory disease
ARDS
    acute respiratory distress syndrome
    adult respiratory distress syndrome
area
    ambosexual a.
    body surface a. (BSA)
    Broca a.
    a. of cardiac dullness (ACD)
    delivery a.
    developmental a.
    echolucent a.
    flexural a.
    frontal pole a.
    hypoechogenic a.
    infraclavicular a.
    inguinal a.
    a. of interest magnification (AIM)
    intertriginous a.
    Kiesselbach a.
    Little a.
    paracervical a.
    pudendal a.
    skip a.
    social-emotional developmental a.

NOTES

area *(continued)*
    subpannicular a.
    subpulmonic a.
    total body surface a. (TBSA)
    Wernicke a.
areal bone mineral density (aBMD)
areata
    alopecia a.
Aredia
areflexia
areflexic paraparesis
aregenerative anemia
Arenavirus
areola, pl. **areolae**
    nevoid hyperkeratosis of the nipple
      and a.
    a. umbilicus
areolar enlargement
Arey rule
ARF
    acute renal failure
    acute rheumatic fever
      nonoliguric ARF
      oliguric ARF
      postrenal ARF
      prerenal ARF
ArF excimer laser
Arfonad Injection
Argentine hemorrhagic fever
Argesic-SA
arg-gly-asp
    arginine-glycine-aspartic acid
arginase deficiency
arginine
    a. glutamate
    a. hydrochloride
    plasma a.
    a. tolerance test (ATT)
    a. vasopressin (AVP)
    a. vasopressin regulation
    a. vasotocin
arginine-glycine-aspartic acid (arg-gly-asp)
arginine-insulin
    a.-i. stimulation test
    a.-i. tolerance test
argininemia
argininosuccinic
    a. acid
    a. acid synthetase deficiency
    a. aciduria
argininosuccinicacidemia
argininosuccinicaciduria
ARGNO
    antibiotic-resistant gram-negative
    organism
argon
    a. beam coagulation
    a. beam coagulator (ABC)
    a. diode
    a. laser
Argonz-Del Castillo syndrome
Argyle arterial catheter
Argyll Robertson pupil
argyrophilic granule
arhinencephaly, arrhinencephalia, arrhinencephaly
arhinia, arrhinia
    a., choanal atresia, microphthalmia
    syndrome
ARI
    acute respiratory infection
Arias-Stella
    A.-S. effect
    A.-S. phenomenon
    A.-S. reaction
ariboflavinosis
ARIC
    acrosome reaction with ionophore
    challenge
Aries-Pitanguy procedure
Arimidex
Aristocort
    A. A Topical
    A. Forte Injection
    A. Intralesional Injection
    A. Oral
Aristospan
    A. Intraarticular Injection
    A. Intralesional Injection
arithmetic method
Arkless-Graham syndrome
ARM
    artificial rupture of membranes
arm
    a. board
    a. of chromosome
    a. circumference
    a. dysfunction
    nuchal a.
    parallel study a.
    a. position
    a. presentation
    a. recoil
    sling a.
    a. span
armamentarium
ARMS
    acoustic respiratory motion sensor
Army-Navy retractor
ARND
    alcohol-related neurodevelopmental
    disorder
Arnold-Chiari
    A.-C. anomaly
    A.-C. deformity
    A.-C. malformation
    A.-C. syndrome

AROM
    active range of motion
    artificial rupture of membranes
Aromasin
aromatase inhibitor
aromatherapy
aromatization
arousal
    a. center
    confusional a.
    a. disorder
    a. level
    sexual a.
ARPKD
    autosomal recessive polycystic kidney
    disease
ARPTH
    autosomal recessive renal proximal
    tubulopathy and hypercalciuria
array
    density spectral a.
    superficial linear a. (SLA)
arrayed library
arrest
    active phase a.
    cardiac a.
    circulatory a.
    deep hypothermia and total
      circulatory a. (DHCA)
    deep hypothermic circulatory a.
    deep transverse a.
    a. disorder
    follicular development a.
    growth a.
    a. of labor
    physial a.
    preterm labor a.
    puberal a.
    respiratory a.
    sinus a.
    transverse a.
arrest/akinetic fit
arrested
    a. development
    a. hydrocephalus
arrhenoblastoma
arrhinencephalia (*var. of* arhinencephaly)
arrhinencephaly (*var. of* arhinencephaly)
arrhinia (*var. of* arhinia)
arrhythmia
    cardiac a.
    clinically significant a. (CSA)

    digitalis-induced a.
    fetal a.
    late a.
    malignant a.
    nonspecific a. (NSA)
    primary cardiac a.
    respiratory sinus a.
    sinus a.
    Xylocaine HCl I.V. Injection for
      Cardiac A.'s
arrhythmic twitching
arrhythmogenesis
arrhythmogenic
    a. right ventricular dysplasia
      (ARVD)
    a. syncope
arrival
    born on a. (BOA)
Arrow catheter
Arruga-Nicetic capsule forceps
ARSA
    aberrant right subclavian artery
arsenic
    a. nickel silicon
    a. poisoning
arsenical
    organic a.
ART
    assisted reproductive technology
    automated reagin test
    ART treatment
art
    arterial
    art line
Artane
Artemisinin
arterenol
arterial (a, art)
    a. to alveolar (a-A)
    a. to alveolar oxygen tension ratio
    a. aneurysm
    a. banding
    a. blood gas (ABG)
    a. blood pressure (ABP)
    a. blood sample (ABS)
    a. calcification
    a. cannulation
    a. catheter
    a. ectasia
    a. embolization
    a. fibrosing sclerosis
    a. lactate

NOTES

arterial *(continued)*
  a. ligation
  a. line (A-line, artline)
  a. linear density
  a. line flush solution
  a. obstruction
  a. occlusive disease
  a. partial pressure (Pa)
  a. pressure
  a. puncture
  a. retransposition
  a. rupture
  a. spasm
  a. stick
  a. supply
  a. switch operation
  a. switch procedure
  a. thrombosis
  a. transposition
  a. vascular bed
  a. vascular disease
  a. waveform
arterial-ascitic fluid pH gradient
arterialized blood
arteriogram
  pelvic a.
  pulmonary a.
arteriography
  selective pulmonary a.
arteriohepatic dysplasia (AHD)
arteriolar occlusion
arteriole
  pulmonary a.
arteriolitis
  necrotizing a.
arteriolopathy
  decidual a.
arteriomesenteric duodenal compression syndrome
arteriopathy
arterioplasty
arterioportal fistula
arteriosclerosis
  infantile a.
arteriosus
  ductus a. (DA)
  machinery murmur in patent ductus a.
  patent ductus a. (PDA)
  right ductus a. (RDA)
  truncus a.
  Van Praagh classification of truncus a.
arteriovenous (AV)
  a. anastomosis
  a. canal defect
  a. fistula
  a. fistula malformation (AVFM)
  a. malformation (AVM)

  a. oxygen difference
  a. shunt
arteritis
  familial granulomatous a.
  giant cell a.
  inflammatory a.
  necrotizing a.
  Takayasu a. (TA)
  a. umbilicalis
artery
  aberrant coronary a.
  aberrant right subclavian a. (ARSA)
  aberrant subclavian a.
  aberrant systemic feeding a.
  absence of branch pulmonary a.
  acinar a.
  a. of Adamkiewicz
  allantoic a.
  anomalous coronary a.
  anomalous left coronary artery from pulmonary a. (ALCAPA)
  anomalous left pulmonary a.
  appendicular a.
  arcuate a.
  azygos a. of vagina
  basal a.
  brachial a.
  caliber-persistent a.
  carotid a.
  celiac a.
  central retinal a.
  cervical a.
  circumflex a.
  coiled a.
  colic a.
  complete transposition of great a.'s
  deep circumflex iliac a.
  discordant umbilical a.'s
  D-transposition of great a.'s (D-TGA)
  endometrial spiral a.
  epigastric a.
  external iliac a.
  femoral circumflex a.
  fetal cranial a.
  a. forceps
  gastroepiploic a. (GEA)
  great a.'s
  hemorrhoidal a.
  hypogastric a.
  ileocolic a.
  iliac a.
  iliofemoral a.
  inferior epigastric a.
  inferior mesenteric a.
  innominate a.
  internal iliac a.
  left main coronary a.

A

L-transposition of great a.'s (L-TGA)
lumbar a.
major aortopulmonary collateral a. (MAPCA)
mesenteric a.
middle cerebral a. (MCA)
middle sacral a.
obliterated umbilical a.
obturator a.
omphalomesenteric a.
ovarian a.
Parrot a.
pelvic a.
posterior inferior cerebellar a. (PICA)
proximal pulmonary a.
pudendal a.
pulmonary a. (PA)
radial a.
right common carotid a. (RCCA)
right femoral a. (RFA)
a. of Sampson
sinoatrial node a.
spiral endometrial a.
subclavian a.
superficial circumflex iliac a.
superficial epigastric a.
superficial external pudendal a. (SEPA)
superior epigastric a.
superior mesenteric a.
thalamostriatal a.
transposition of great a.'s (TGA)
umbilical a. (UA)
uterine a.
vaginal a.
vertebral a.

arthralgia
psychogenic a.

arthritis, pl. **arthritides**
candidal a.
chronic juvenile a.
degenerative a.
gonococcal a.
gouty a.
hematogenous septic a.
idiopathic chronic a.
infectious a.
juvenile a. (JA)
juvenile chronic a.
juvenile idiopathic a. (JIA)
juvenile idiopathic polyarticular a.
juvenile psoriatic a.
juvenile rheumatoid a. (type I, II) (JRA)
Lyme a.
migratory peripheral a.
monarticular a.
mumps a.
neonatal septic a.
oligoarticular a.
pauciarticular juvenile chronic a.
pauciarticular-onset juvenile a.
peripheral a.
polyarticular juvenile chronic a.
postdysenteric a.
postenteritis a.
postinfectious a.
poststreptococcal reactive a.
Pseudomonas septic a.
psoriasis-associated a.
psoriatic a.
purulent a.
pyogenic a.
reactive a.
a. of rheumatic fever
rheumatoid a. (RA)
septic a.
spondylitis, enthesitis, a. (SEA)
suppurative a.
systemic juvenile chronic a.
systemic-onset juvenile rheumatoid a.
viral a.
Yersinia a.

arthritis-dermatitis syndrome
Arthrobacter globiformis
arthrocentesis
arthrochalasis
a. multiplex congenita
a. multiplex congenita Ehlers-Danlos syndrome
arthrodentoosteodysplasia (ADOD)
arthrodesis
Dennyson-Fulford extraarticular subtalar a.
triple a.
arthrogram
air a.
arthrography
arthrogryposis
distal a. (type I, II)

NOTES

arthrogryposis *(continued)*
  a., ectodermal dysplasia, cleft lip/palate developmental delay syndrome
  fetal a.
  a. multiplex
  a. multiplex congenita (AMC)
  skeletal a.
arthrogryposis-like hand anomaly
arthrogrypotic clubfoot
arthroophthalmopathia hereditaria
arthroophthalmopathy (AO, AOM)
  hereditary progressive a.
Arthropan
arthropathy
  hemophilic a.
  human parvovirus a.
  sensory a.
  seronegativity, enthesopathy, a. (SEA)
arthropod-borne virus
arthropod-induced blister
arthrosis
Arthus reaction
articular
articulate
articulation
  calcaneonavicular a.
  compensatory a.
  cricoarytenoid a.
  a. disorder
artifact
  cultural a.
  deodorant a.
  point-spread a.
  technical a.
artificial
  a. anal sphincter
  a. ankylosis
  a. chromosome
  a. erection
  a. fever
  a. insemination (AI)
  a. insemination by donor (AID)
  a. insemination donor (AID)
  a. insemination by husband (AIH)
  a. insemination with donor sperm
  a. intravaginal insemination
  a. lung-expanding compound (ALEC)
  a. pacemaker
  a. respiration
  a. rupture of membranes (ARM, AROM)
  a. spermatocele
  a. temperature
  a. urethral sphincter (AUS)
  a. urinary sphincter

  a. vagina
  a. vaginal epithelium
Arts syndrome
ARV
  acquired immunodeficiency syndrome-related virus
ARVD
  arrhythmogenic right ventricular dysplasia
Arvee model 2400 infant apnea monitor
aryepiglottic fold
arylalkanoic acid
arylcarboxylic acid
arylpropionic acid
arylsulfatase
arylsulfatase-activator deficiency
arytenoid
AS
  Asperger syndrome
    Duracillin AS
    Pentids-P AS
as
  as low as reasonably achievable (ALARA)
ASA
  acetylsalicylic acid
  5-ASA
  MSD Enteric Coated ASA
asaccharolyticus
  Peptococcus a.
Asacol Oral
ASB
  asymptomatic bacteriuria
    ASB syndrome
ASC
  altered state of consciousness
  antibody-secreting cell
  asthma symptom checklist
  atypical squamous cell
A-scan
ascariasis
  pulmonary a.
Ascaris
  A. lumbricoides
ascending
  a. cholangiopathy
  a. cholangitis
  a. colon
  a. intrauterine infection
  a. radiculomyelitis
  a. reticular activating system (ARAS)
  a. venography
ascensus
ascertainment
  total a.

Ascher syndrome
Aschheim-Zondek (AZ)
    A.-Z. test
aschistodactylia
Aschoff
    A. body
    A. nodule
ascites
    biliary a.
    chylous a.
    culture-negative neutrocytic a.
    eosinophilic a.
    exudative a.
    fetal a.
    lues a.
    massive a.
    refractory a.
    tense a.
    tumor a.
ascitic fluid
ascorbate
ascorbic
    a. acid
    a. acid deficiency
Ascriptin A/D
ASCUS
    atypical squamous cells of undetermined
    significance
        ASCUS smear
ASCUS/AGUS
    atypical squamous cells of undetermined
    significance/atypical glandular cells of
    undetermined significance
ASD
    acute stress disorder
    atrial septal defect
    autism spectrum disorder
    autistic spectrum disorder
        canal type ASD
        ostium primum ASD
        ostium secundum ASD
        ostium venosus ASD
ASDA
    American Sleep Disorders Association
aseptic
    a. fever
    a. meningitis
    a. meningitis syndrome
    a. meningoencephalitis
    a. necrosis
    a. necrosis of bone

    a. preparation
    a. temperature
Asepto syringe
asexual dwarfism
ASG
    Adhesion Scoring Group
    ASG system
Asherman syndrome
Ashkenazi
    A. Jew
    A. Jewish heritage
ash-leaf
    a.-l. macule
    a.-l. spot
Ashworth
    A. score
    A. score of spasticity
ASI
    active specific immunotherapy
    anxiety sensitivity index
ASIL
    anal squamous intraepithelial lesion
Askanazy cell
Askin tumor
Ask-Upmark kidney
ASL
    American Sign Language
Aslan
    A. endoscopic scissors
    A. 2 mm minilaparoscope
ASLD
    adenylosuccinate lyase deficiency
ASO
    antistreptolysin O
        ASO antibody
        ASO assay
        ASO titer
asoma
asparaginase
    Ara-C, Oncovin, prednisone, a.
    (AOPA)
asparagine
aspartate
    a. aminotransferase (AST)
    amphetamine a.
    a. transaminase (AST)
aspartic acid
aspartoacylase hydrolytic activity
aspartylglucosamine (AGA)
aspartylglucosaminidase
aspartylglucosaminuria (AGU)
A-Spas S/L

NOTES

ASPD
  antisocial personality disorder
ASPED
  angel-shaped phalangoepiphyseal
    dysplasia
Aspen
  A. laparoscopy electrode
  A. ultrasound platform
AspenVac smoke evacuation system
Asperger
  A. disorder
  A. syndrome (AS)
aspergilloma
aspergillosis
  allergic bronchopulmonary a.
    (ABPA)
  bronchopulmonary a.
  cerebral a.
  fatal cutaneous a.
  ocular a.
  pulmonary a.
Aspergillus
  A. *flavus*
  A. *fumigatus*
  A. *nidulans*
  A. *niger*
  A. *terreus*
Aspergum
aspermatogenesis
aspermia
asphyctic infant
asphyxia
  acute total a.
  antepartum a.
  asphyxia, bacterial meningitis,
    congenital perinatal infection
    (cytomegalovirus, rubella, herpes,
    toxoplasmosis, syphilis), defects of
    head or neck, elevated bilirubin
    exceeding indications for
    exchange, family history of
    childhood hearing impairment,
    gram birth weight ≤500 g
  autoerotic a.
  birth a.
  blue a.
  fetal a.
  intrapartum a.
  intrauterine a.
  a. livida
  neonatal a.
  a. neonatorum
  a. pallida
  perinatal a.
  prenatal a.
  prolonged partial a.
  sexual a.
asphyxial
  a. birth injury

  a. brain injury
  a. event
asphyxiating
  a. thoracic chondrodystrophy
  a. thoracic dysplasia
  a. thoracic dysplasia syndrome
  a. thoracic dystrophy (ATD)
  a. thoracodystrophy syndrome
asphyxiation
  intrapartum a.
aspiny interneuron
aspirate
  blood-flecked gastric a.
  bone marrow a. (BMA)
  bubo a.
  nasogastric a.
  nasopharyngeal a. (NPA)
  surveillance tracheal a.
  tracheal a.
  tracheobronchial a.
aspiration
  amniotic fluid a.
  a. biopsy
  a. biopsy cytology (ABC)
  bone marrow a.
  caustic a.
  chronic a.
  cyst a.
  electric vacuum a.
  epididymal sperm a.
  fine-needle a. (FNA)
  foreign body a.
  a. of gastric contents
  gastric fluid a.
  a. of mature oocyte
  maxillary sinus a.
  meconium a.
  menstrual a.
  metaphysial a.
  microsurgical epididymal sperm a.
    (MESA)
  needle a.
  percutaneous cyst a.
  percutaneous epididymal sperm a.
    (PESA)
  a. pneumonia
  a. pneumonitis
  a. prophylaxis
  pulmonary a.
  rete testis a. (RETA)
  sperm a.
  subperiosteal a.
  suprapubic bladder a.
  a. syndrome
  testicular sperm a. (TESA)
  transtracheal a.
  Vabra a.
  vacuum a.
aspiration-tulip device

aspirator
- Aspirette endocervical a.
- blunt a.
- Cavitron ultrasonic surgical a. (CUSA)
- Cook a.
- electric vacuum a.
- Endo-Assist sponge a.
- endocervical a.
- endometrial a.
- GynoSampler endometrial a.
- manual vacuum a.
- mucus a.
- Nezhat-Dorsey a.
- Sharplan USA ultrasonic surgical a.
- Vabra cervical a.
- vacuum a.

Aspirette endocervical aspirator

aspirin
- Bayer A.
- oxycodone and a.
- a. triad

Aspirols
- Amyl Nitrite A.

asplenia
- anatomic a.
- congenital a.
- functional a.
- surgical a.
- a. syndrome

asplenic

ASQ
- Ages and Stages Questionnaire

ASS
- Aarskog-Scott syndrome
- Asthma Severity Score

ASSAS
- aminopterin syndrome sine aminopterin

assault
- sexual a.

assaultive
- verbally a.

assay
- Abbott LCx Uriprobe a.
- a. accuracy
- AccuStat Strep A a.
- agglutination a.
- Amplicor Chlamydia a.
- antibody production a.
- ASO a.

automated
- immunochemiluminometric insulin a.
- BCA protein a.
- Bethesda a.
- biologic a.
- CA 125 a.
- CH_{50} a.
- Chiron branched DNA a.
- Clinitest a.
- clonogenic a.
- Coat-A-Count a.
- C1q a.
- cytomegalovirus total immunoglobulin a.
- Detect HIV-1 a.
- Digene HPV A.
- DNA hybridization a.
- dot immunobinding a. (DIA)
- electrophoretic mobility shift a. (EMSA)
- ELISpot a.
- enzyme a.
- enzyme immunosorbent a. (EIA)
- enzyme-linked immunofiltration a. (ELIFA)
- enzyme-linked immunosorbent a. (ELISA)
- estradiol a.
- factor Xa inhibition a.
- FAMA a.
- fetal fibronectin a.
- FSH MAIAclone immunoradiometric a.
- genotypic a.
- Gen-Probe amplified CT a.
- hamster egg penetration a.
- hemagglutinin enzyme-linked immunosorbent a. (H(c)ELISA)
- hemizona a. (HZA)
- HemoQuant a.
- Heptest Xa a.
- HIV-1 RNA PCR a.
- hormone a.
- Hybrid Capture DNA A.
- 5-hydroxyindoleacetic a.
- IIF a.
- immunoblot a.
- immunochemiluminometric insulin a.
- immunofluorescent a. (IFA)
- immunofunctional a.
- immunologic a.

NOTES

assay *(continued)*
    immunoradiometric a. (IRMA)
    immunosorbent agglutination a.
     (ISAGA)
    IMx Estradiol A.
    IVAP a.
    latex agglutination a.
    LCR a.
    ligase chain reaction a.
    limulus amebocyte lysate a.
    luciferase a.
    lysosomal hydrolase enzyme a.
    a. marker
    measles virus enzyme-linked
     immunosorbent a. (MV(c)ELISA)
    microhemagglutination a. (MHA)
    NucliSens a.
    PCR a.
    PIVKA-II a.
    prostacyclin a.
    Pyrilinks-D a.
    quantitative Bethesda a.
    quantitative serum drug a.
    radioantigen-binding a. (RABA)
    radioimmunoprecipitation a. (RIPA)
    radioreceptor a.
    Raji cell a.
    RAMP hCG a.
    receptor a.
    Recombigen a.
    recombinant immunosorbent a.
     (RIBA)
    respiratory burst a.
    Roche Amplicor Monitor a.
    salivary cortisol a.
    sandwich a.
    a. sensitivity
    serum a.
    serum hexosaminidase a.
    solid-phase enzyme-linked
     immunospot a.
    a. specificity
    sperm penetration a. (SPA)
    stem cell a.
    TDxFLM A.
    TDxFLx A.
    tetrazolium dye a.
    Thomsen-Friedenreich antigen a.
    thyroid-stimulating hormone a.
    TMA a.
    transcription-mediated
     amplification a.
    tumor-cloning a.
    TUNEL a.
    ultrasensitive a.
    Vidas varicella zoster a.
    ViraType HPV DNA typing a.
    virologic a.

assembly
    brush border a.
    infant nasal cannula a. (INCA)
assertive
assessment
    ABCDE a.
    abuse, sexuality, safety a.
    amniotic fluid a.
    antenatal a.
    antepartum fetal a.
    Ballard gestational a.
    behavioral a.
    child and adolescent burden a.
     (CABA)
    Child and Adolescent
     Psychiatric A. (CAPA)
    Child and Adolescent Services A.
     (CASA)
    clinical risk a. (CRA)
    developmental a.
    Dubowitz Neurological A.
    Erhardt developmental prehension a.
    fetal movement a.
    four-quadrant a.
    gestational age a.
    high-risk pregnancy a.
    HRQOL a.
    A. in Infancy Ordinal Scales of
     Psychological Development
    Lund and Browder chart for
     burn a.
    maternal a.
    morphologic a.
    neonatal a.
    neurodevelopmental a.
    neuromuscular maturity a.
    nutritional a.
    perinatal a.
    periodic patient a.
    phallometric a.
    preconception risk a.
    preschool-age psychiatric a. (PAPA)
    A. of Preterm Infants' Behavior
     (APIB)
    projective a.
    psychometric a.
    quadrant a.
    qualitative developmental a.
    risk a.
    Scanlon A.
    school, home, activities,
     depression/self-esteem, substance
     abuse, sexuality, safety a.
    sonographic a.
    TOVA ADD/ADHD a.
    ultrasonographic a.
    ultrasound a.
    young adult psychiatric a. (YAPA)
ASSI bipolar coagulating forceps

assignment
    gender a.
    sex a.
assimilation
    atlas a.
    a. pelvis
assistant
    Carter Tubal A.
assist control ventilation
assisted
    a. breech
    a. breech delivery
    a. cephalic delivery
    a. conception
    a. fertilization
    a. hatching (AH)
    a. medical procreation (AMP)
    a. reproduction
    a. reproductive technology (ART)
    a. spontaneous vaginal delivery
    a. ventilation (AV)
    a. zona hatching (AZH)
assistive technology (AT)
association
    American Diabetes A. (ADA)
    American Heart A. (AHA)
    American Sleep Disorders A. (ASDA)
    aniridia, Wilms tumor a. (AWTA)
    CHARGE a.
    a. constant
    New York Heart A. (NYHA)
    a. reaction
    A. for Retarded Citizens (ARC)
    VACTERL a.
    A. of Women's Health, Obstetrics, and Neonatal Nursing (AWHONN)
assortative mating
ASSQ
    autism spectrum screening questionnaire
assurance
    National Committee for Quality A. (NCQA)
AST
    acoustic stimulation test
    aspartate aminotransferase
    aspartate transaminase
astasia-abasia
astatic seizure
asteatotic eczema
Astech Peak Flow Meter

Astelin Nasal Spray
astemizole
asterixis
asteroid body
asteroides
    Nocardia a.
asthenia
asthenospermia
asthenozoospermia
asthma
    A. Action Plan
    allergen-induced a.
    atopic a.
    bronchial a.
    cardiac a.
    chronic a.
    a. exacerbation
    exercise-induced a. (EIA)
    infantile a.
    intrinsic a.
    labile a.
    maternal a.
    a. morbidity
    nocturnal a.
    perennial a.
    seasonal a.
    A. Severity Score (ASS)
    a. symptom checklist (ASC)
    thymic a.
    a. with vasculitis
asthmatic
    a. bronchitis
    a. response
asthmaticus
    status a.
astigmatism
Astler-Coller modification of Dukes classification
astomia
astragalus
Astramorph
    A. PF
    A. PF Injection
Astrand 30-beat stopwatch method
astrocyte
    fibrinoid degeneration of a.'s
    a. footplate
astrocytic gliosis
astrocytoma
    anaplastic pilocytic a.
    chiasmatic pilocytic a.
    diffuse a.

NOTES

astrocytoma *(continued)*
    fibrillary a.
    a. (grade I–IV)
    juvenile pilocytic a.
    low-grade diffuse a.
    low-grade fibrillary a.
    malignant pilocytic a.
    pilocytic fibrillary a.
Astroglide personal lubricant
astrogliosis
astrovirus
    human a. type 1 (HAstV-1)
    a. infection
Astrup blood gas value
asymbolia for pain
asymmetric
    a. crying facies (ACF)
    a. growth restriction
    a. hyperopia
    a. IUGR
    a. muscle imbalance
    a. nystagmus
    a. palatal paresis
    a. short stature syndrome
    a. small foramen magnum
    a. tonic neck reflex (ATNR)
asymmetrical conjoined twins
asymmetrically
asymmetros
    syncephalus a.
asymmetrus
    janiceps a.
asymmetry
    a. of face
    facial a.
    left/right a.
    nasolabial fold a.
    truncal a.
asymptomatic
    a. bacteriuria (ASB)
    a. dehiscence
    a. infection
    a. infertility
    a. mild endometriosis
    a. myoma
    a. urinary tract infection (AUTI)
    a. viral shedding
asynapsis
asynchronous
    a. birth
    a. multifetal delivery
    a. puberty
asynchronously
asynchrony
    marked a.
asynclitic
    a. position
    a. position of fetus

asynclitism
    anterior a.
    posterior a.
asynergia
    cerebellar a.
asystole
AT
    antithrombin
    assistive technology
    ataxia-telangiectasia
AT1, AT2 receptor
AT3
    antithrombin III
        AT3 coagulation inhibitor
        AT3 deficiency (types I, II)
        AT3 type II PE, RS
atactic *(var. of* ataxic)
atactica
    heredopathia a.
Atad Ripener device
Atarax
ataxia
    acute cerebellar a.
    acute childhood a.
    acute recurrent a.
    adult-onset spinocerebellar a.
    cerebellar a.
    chronic progressive a.
    congenital a.
    dominant recurrent a.
    episodic a. (1, 2)
    fixed-deficit a.
    Friedreich a.
    gait a.
    hereditary paroxysmal a.
    infantile-onset spinocerebellar a.
    Machado-Joseph a.
    myoclonic a.
    a., myoclonic encephalopathy,
      macular degeneration, recurrent
      infections syndrome
    spastic a.
    spinocerebellar a. (type 1–7) (SCA)
    a. telangiectasia
    transient cerebellar a.
    truncal a.
    a. with isolated vitamin E
      deficiency
    X-linked cerebellar a. (CLA)
ataxia-deafness-retardation (ADR)
    a.-d.-r. syndrome with ketoaciduria
ataxia-deafness syndrome
ataxia-microcephaly-cataract (AMC)
ataxia-oculomotor apraxia
ataxia-telangiectasia (AT)
    a.-t. syndrome
ataxic, atactic
    a. cerebral palsy
    a. gait

ATD
  asphyxiating thoracic dystrophy
atelectasis
  congenital a.
  linear a.
  massive a.
  obstructive a.
  plate-like a.
  primary a.
  resorption a.
  secondary a.
  subsegmental a.
atelectatic
atelectrauma
atelencephalia, atelencephaly
atelencephalic syndrome
atelia
ateliosis
ateliotic dwarfism
atelocardia
atelocephaly
atelocephaly
atelocheiria
ateloglossia
atelognathia
atelomyelia
atelopodia
atelosteogenesis
atelostomia
atenolol
ATFL
  anterior talofibular ligament
Atgam
athelia
atheosis
atherectomy
  directional coronary a. (DCA)
atherogenesis
atherogenic
atherosclerosis
  accelerated a.
atherosis
  acute a.
  decidual arteriolar a.
athetoid
  a. cerebral palsy
  a. movement
athetosis
  congenital a.
athetotic
  a. movement disorder
  a. posturing

athlete's foot
athletica
  anorexia a.
athletic amenorrhea
at-home activity restriction
athyreotic (*var. of* athyrotic)
athyroid
athyroidism, athyrea
athyrotic, athyreotic
  a. cretinism
  a. hypothyroidism
  a. neonate
Ativan
Atkin-Flaitz-Patil syndrome
Atkin-Flaitz syndrome
Atkins diet
ATL
  ATL HDI 3000 ultrasound system
  ATL Ultramark 4,8,9 ultrasound
Atlanta Scottish Rite Hospital orthosis
atlantoaxial (AA)
  a. dislocation
  a. instability
  a. rotary subluxation
atlantodens interval (ADI)
atlantodidymus
atlantooccipital dislocation
atlas
  a. assimilation
  Greulich and Pyle radiographic a.
ATLL
  adult T-cell leukemia/lymphoma
ATLS
  advanced trauma life support
ATN
  acute tubular necrosis
ATNR
  asymmetric tonic neck reflex
ATOD
  alcohol, tobacco, and other drugs
atomic
  a. absorption spectrometer
  a. absorption spectrophotometry
  a. absorption spectroscopy
  a. milk
Atomlab 200 dose calibrator
atonic
  a. astatic diplegia
  a. cerebral palsy
  a. seizure
atony
  bowel a.

NOTES

75

atony *(continued)*
    diaphragmatic a.
    gastric a.
    uterine a.
atopic
    a. asthma
    a. child
    a. dermatitis
    a. diaper rash
    a. eczema
    a. erythroderma
    a. triad
atopy
atosiban
atovaquone
ATP
    adenosine triphosphate
    deoxy ATP
ATPase
    adenosine triphosphatase
ATR
    alpha-thalassemia/mental retardation
ATR1
    alpha-thalassemia/mental retardation
    syndrome, deletion type
ATR2
    alpha-thalassemia/mental retardation
    syndrome, nondeletion type
ATR-16
    alpha-thalassemia/mental retardation
    syndrome, deletion type
atra
    Stachybotrys a.
atracurium besylate
atransferrinemia
    congenital a.
atraumatic forceps
atresia
    anal a.
    aortic valve a.
    apple-peel a.
    aural a.
    bilateral a.
    biliary a. (BA)
    bronchial a.
    cervical a.
    a. choanae
    choanal a.
    congenital aural a.
    congenital duodenal a.
    de la Cruz classification of
    congenital aural a.
    distal esophageal a.
    duodenal a.
    esophageal a. (EA)
    extrahepatic biliary a.
    a. folliculi
    a. of the foramina of Luschka and
    Magendie

    functional pulmonary a.
    gastrointestinal a.
    ileal a.
    intestinal a.
    intrahepatic biliary a.
    jejunal a.
    jejunal-ileal a.
    jejunoileal a.
    laryngeal a.
    a. of larynx
    mitral valve a.
    oocyte a.
    primary repair of esophageal a.
    pulmonary artery a.
    pure esophageal a.
    pyloric a.
    Schuknecht classification of
    congenital aural a. (type A–D)
    small bowel a.
    tracheal a.
    tracheoesophageal a.
    tricuspid a.
    urethral a.
    vaginal a.
atretic
    a. cervix
    a. extrahepatic bile duct resection
    a. follicle
    a. gallbladder
    a. ureter
    a. vagina
atretocormus
atretocystia
atretogastria
atria (*pl. of* atrium)
atrial
    a. bigeminy
    a. contraction
    a. fibrillation
    a. flutter
    a. hypertrophy
    a. inversion procedure
    a. natriuretic factor (ANF)
    a. natriuretic hormone
    a. natriuretic peptide (ANP)
    a. premature contraction (APC)
    a. premature depolarization
    a. septal defect (ASD)
    a. septectomy
    a. septoplasty procedure
    a. septostomy
    a. septostomy procedure
    a. septostomy via balloon
    a. septum excision
    a. shunt
    a. switch operation
    a. switch procedure
    a. tachyarrhythmia
    a. tachycardia

atriodigital dysplasia
atriotomy
atrioventricular (AV)
    a. block
    a. canal
    a. canal defect
    a. conduction delay
    a. discordance
    a. dissociation
    a. nodal reentrant tachycardia
    (AVNRT)
    a. node
    a. node function
    a. reciprocating tachycardia (AVRT)
    a. septal defect
    a. septum
    a. shunt
    a. valve
at-risk
    a.-r. infant
    a.-r. pregnancy
atrium, pl. **atria**
    common a.
    left a.
    ventricles to a.
ATR, nondeletion
    alpha-thalassemia/mental retardation
    syndrome, nondeletion type
atrophia bulborum hereditaria
atrophic
    a. change
    a. endometrium
    a. patch
    a. vaginal mucosa
    a. vaginitis
atrophicae
    striae a.
atrophicans
    acrodermatitis chronica a.
atrophicus
    lichen sclerosus et a. (LS)
atrophy
    Behr optic a.
    brain a.
    central a.
    cerebral a.
    congenital microvillus a.
    cortical a.
    corticosteroid-induced a.
    cutaneous a.
    Dejerine-Sottas a.
    dentatorubral a.

    dentatorubral-pallidoluysian a.
    (DRPLA)
    diabetes insipidus, diabetes mellitus,
    optic a. (DIDMO)
    disuse muscular a.
    endometrial a.
    epithelial a.
    familial muscular a.
    familial olivopontocerebellar a.
    Fazio-Londe a.
    focal a.
    frontotemporal cortical a.
    gastric a.
    generalized gray matter a.
    generalized white matter a.
    genitourinary a.
    gyral a.
    gyrate a.
    hereditary optic neuron a.
    hereditary spinal muscular a.
    infantile cerebellooptic a.
    infantile progressive spinal
    muscular a. (type I–III)
    infantile spinal muscular a.
    intestinal villous a.
    juvenile spinal muscular a.
    Kjer-type dominant optic a.
    Leber hereditary a.
    leg a.
    Leydig cell a.
    limb girdle muscular weakness
    and a.
    linear a.
    macular a.
    microvillus a. (MVA)
    muscle a.
    muscular a.
    neurogenic a.
    olivopontocerebellar a. (OPCA)
    optic nerve a.
    Parrot a.
    Parrot a. of newborn
    partial villus a.
    perifascicular a.
    peroneal muscle a.
    peroneal muscular a.
    postmenopausal a.
    primary macular a.
    progressive encephalopathy, edema,
    hypsarrhythmia, optic a. (PEHO)
    secondary macular a.
    skin a.

NOTES

atrophy *(continued)*
    spinal muscle a.
    spinal muscular a. (SMA)
    Sudeck a.
    syndrome of cerebral a.
    testicular a.
    total villous a.
    traction a.
    tubular a.
    urogenital a. (UGA)
    vaginal a.
    villous a.
    vulvar a.
    Werdnig-Hoffmann muscular a.

atropine
    a. cromolyn
    diphenoxylate and a.
    a. sulfate

Atropine-Care Ophthalmic
Atropisol Ophthalmic
Atrovent
    A. Aerosol Inhalation
    A. Inhalation Solution
    A. Nasal Spray

ATRX
    X-linked alpha-thalassemia/mental
    retardation
    ATRX syndrome

A/T/S Topical
ATT
    arginine tolerance test

attaching process
attachment
    abnormal aortic valve a.
    dismissing a.
    a. disorder
    disturbance of a.
    gubernacular a.
    maternal-infant a.
    nonautonomous a.
    a. parenting
    prosthetic a.
    secure a.
    testicular a.

attack
    absence a.
    cataplectic a.
    drop a.
    grand mal a.
    lightning a.
    migrainous a.
    narcoleptic a.
    panic a.
    paroxysmal hypercyanotic a.
    petit mal a.
    shuddering a.
    sleep a.
    Stokes-Adams a.
    transient ischemic a. (TIA)

attapulgite
attempted suicide
attending skill
attention
    a. deficit
    a. deficit disorder (ADD)
    A. Deficit Disorders Evaluation
    Scale
    a. deficit hyperactivity disorder
    (ADHD)
    joint a.
    a. span
    Test of Variables of A. (TOVA)

attentional difficulty
attention-distractibility problem
attenuated
    a. androgen
    live a.
    a. pyloric canal

attenuating tissue
attenuation
Attenuvax
attitude
    a. behavior questionnaire (ABQ)
    fetal a.
    postpartum a.

attorney
    durable power of a.

attrition
    acute-phase a.
    follicular a.
    a. rate scale
    sperm a.

attunement
    affect a.

Attwood staining method
ATV
    all-terrain vehicle

atypia
    bowenoid a.
    cervical a.
    cytologic a.
    glandular a.
    koilocytic a.
    koilocytotic a.
    nuclear a.
    vulvar a.

atypica
    Veillonella a.

atypical
    a. absence
    a. absence seizure
    a. adenomatous hyperplasia
    a. aneuploidy
    a. cell
    a. chondrodystrophy
    a. depression
    a. ductal hyperplasia (ADH)
    a. endosalpingiosis

a. epithelium
a. febrile seizure
a. glandular cells of uncertain
significance (AGCUS, AGUS)
a. glandular cells of undetermined
significance (AGCUS, AGUS)
a. hemolytic uremia syndrome
a. interest
a. karyotype
a. Kawasaki disease
a. lobular hyperplasia
a. measles
a. melanocytic nevus
a. mycobacteria
a. petit mal seizure
a. squamous cell (ASC)
a. squamous cells of undetermined
significance (ASCUS)
a. squamous cells of undetermined
significance/atypical glandular cells
of undetermined significance
(ASCUS/AGUS)
a. teratoid/rhabdoid tumor
a. teratoid tumor
a. teratoma
a. vasculature
a. vessel colposcopic pattern
¹⁹⁸Au
gold-198
AUB
abnormal uterine bleeding
**Auchincloss modified radical
mastectomy**
audible stridor
Audio Doppler D920
audiogram
audiological testing
audiologist
audiology
audiometer
Pilot a.
audiometric
a. evaluation
a. examination
a. testing
audiometry
behavioral a.
behavioral observation a. (BOA)
brainstem evoked response a.
(BSERA)
conditioned play a.
evoked response a. (ERA)

impedance a.
visual reinforcement a. (VRA)
visual response a. (VRA)
AudioScope
Welch Allyn A.
AUDIT
Alcohol Use Disorders Identification Test
auditory
a. agnosia
a. brainstem response (ABR,
ABSR)
a. canal
a. discrimination
a. dysfunction
a. evoked potential (AEP)
a. evoked response (AER)
a. impairment
integrated visual and a. (IVA)
a. integration thinking (AIT)
a. integration training (AIT)
a. learner
a. meatus
a. nerve
a. ossicles
a. response to bell
a. response cradle
a. training
audouinii
Microsporum a.
Auerbach plexus
Aufricht nasal retractor
augmentation
bladder a.
colocecal bladder a.
a. cystoplasty
intestinal bladder a.
labor a.
a. mammaplasty
oxytocin a.
Pitocin a.
submucosal urethral a.
transumbilical breast a. (TUBA)
a. ureterocystoplasty
Wise areola mastopexy breast a.
(WAMBA)
augmentative
a. and alternative communication
(AAC)
a. communication device
augmented breast
Augmentin ES
augnathus

NOTES

AUM
    ambulatory urodynamic monitoring
aura
    epileptic a.
    migraine with a.
    migraine without a.
    somatosensory a.
    viscerosensory a.
    visual a.
aural
    a. atresia
    a. atresia and microtia
    a. polyp
    a. temperature
Auralgan
auramine
auramine-rhodamine stain
auranofin
aureus
    borderline-resistant
        Staphylococcus a. (BRSA)
    community-acquired methicillin-
        resistant *Staphylococcus a.*
        (CAMRSA)
    methicillin-resistant
        Staphylococcus a. (MRSA)
    Staphylococcus a.
    Streptococcus a.
    vancomycin intermediate resistant
        Staphylococcus a. (VISA)
    vancomycin-resistant
        Staphylococcus a. (VRSA)
auricle
    accessory a.
auricular
    a. abscess
    a. hematoma
    a. seroma
auriculoosteodysplasia
aurocephalosyndactyly
Auro Ear Drops
Aurolate
Aurora MR breast imaging system
aurothioglucose
Auroto
AUS
    artificial urethral sphincter
auscultation
    abdominal a.
    chest percussion and a.
    obstetric a.
    periodic a.
Austin
    A. Flint murmur
    A. syndrome
Australia antigen
australis
    Rickettsia a.

authority
    Human Fertilization and
        Embryology A. (HFEA)
AUTI
    asymptomatic urinary tract infection
autism
    a., dementia, ataxia, loss of
        purposeful hand use syndrome
    A. Diagnostic Interview (ADI)
    A. Diagnostic Interview-Revised
        (ADI-R)
    A. Diagnostic Observation Schedule
        (ADOS)
    early infantile a.
    a.-fragile X syndrome (AFRAX)
    high-functioning a. (HFA)
    infantile a.
    a. spectrum disorder (ASD)
    a. spectrum screening questionnaire
        (ASSQ)
autism-fragile X syndrome (AFRAX)
autistic
    a. behavior
    a. disorder
    a. enterocolitis
    a. spectrum disorder (ASD)
    a. syndrome
autistic-like behavior
Auto
    A. Suture ABBI system
    A. Suture Multifire Endo GIA 30
        stapler
    A. Syringe
autoamputate
autoamputation of ovary
autoantibody
    anti-D a.
    anti-Scl-70 a.
    E a.
    Kell a.
    thyroid a.
    typhoid a.
    warm a.
autoantigen
    La (SS-B) a.
    Ro/SSA a.
autoaugmentation
    laparoscopic laser-assisted a.
autobiographical memory
auto-brewery syndrome
autochthonous tumor
autoclave
autocrine
    a. communication
    a. motility factor (AMF)
autocrine-acting growth factor
autocrine/paracrine-acting growth factor
AutoCyte System

AutoDELFIA
> A. PRL molecule kit
> A. unconjugated E3 kit

autodilation
> Frank nonsurgical perineal a.

autoeczematization

autoerotic asphyxia

autofluorescent

autogamy

autogenous vaccine

autograft
> free tracheal a.

AutoGuard catheter

autohemolysis

autoimmune
> a. acquired hemolytic anemia
> a. adrenalitis
> a. chronic acute hepatitis
> a. cytopenia
> a. disease
> a. disease of the vulva
> a. enteropathy (AIE)
> a. factor
> a. glomerulonephritis
> a. hemolytic anemia (AIHA)
> a. interstitial nephritis
> a. lymphoproliferative syndrome (ALPS)
> a. mechanism
> a. myasthenia gravis
> a. neutropenia (AIN)
> a. neutropenia of infancy (ANI)
> a. oophoritis
> a. polyendocrine syndrome
> a. polyendocrinopathy, candidiasis, ectodermal dystrophy (APECED)
> a. polyglandular syndrome
> a. regulator (AIRE)
> a. regulator gene
> a. thrombocytopenia
> a. thrombocytopenic purpura (AITP)
> a. thyroiditis

autoimmune-associated congenital heart block

autoimmunity

autoinfarction

Auto-Injector

autoinoculation

autologous
> a. blood donation
> a. blood transfusion
> a. BMT

> a. bone marrow reinfusion
> a. bone marrow transplantation
> a. cord blood
> a. ovarian transplant
> a. reconstruction
> a. stem cell transplantation

autolysis

automated
> a. auditory brainstem response (AABR, A-ABR)
> a. brainstem auditory evoked response (ABAER)
> a. computerized axial tomography (ACAT)
> a. hematocrit
> a. immunochemiluminometric insulin assay
> a. multiple analysis
> a. radiometric technique
> a. reagin test (ART)

automatic
> a. atrial tachycardia
> a. karyotype system database
> a. movement reaction
> a. reflex
> a. walking

automaticity

automatism
> motor a.

autonomic
> a. crisis
> a. dysregulation
> a. innervation
> a. nerve tumor
> a. nervous system (ANS)
> a. nervous system dysfunction (ANSD)
> a. neuropathy
> a. seizure
> a. walking reflex

autonomous
> a. ovarian follicular cyst
> a. replication sequence

autonomy

AutoPap
> A. 300
> A. automated screening device
> A. 300 QC system
> A. reader

auto-PEEP (*var. of* intrinsic PEEP)
> auto-positive end-expiratory pressure

Autoplex T

NOTES

autopolyploid
autopolyploidy
auto-positive end-expiratory pressure (auto-PEEP)
autoprothrombin (I, II, IIA, III)
autopsy
autoradiograph
autoradiography
autoreaction
Autoread centrifuge hematology system
autoregulation
autosite
autosomal
    a. chromosome disorder
    a. congenital tubular dysgenesis
    a. deletion
    a. dominant
    a. dominant genetic disorder
    a. dominant inheritance
    a. dominant macrocephaly syndrome
    a. dominant medullary cystic kidney disease (ADMCKD)
    a. dominant nonsyndromic hearing loss (DFNA3)
    a. dominant Opitz syndrome (ADOS)
    a. dominant polycystic disease
    a. dominant polycystic kidney disease (ADPKD)
    a. dominant retinitis pigmentosa (adRP)
    a. dominant trait
    a. gene
    a. heredity
    a. monosomy
    a. recessive (AR)
    a. recessive disorder
    a. recessive inheritance
    a. recessive muscular dystrophy
    a. recessive mutation
    a. recessive nonsyndromic hearing loss (DFNB1)
    a. recessive ocular Ehlers-Danlos syndrome
    a. recessive polycystic kidney disease (ARPKD)
    a. recessive renal proximal tubulopathy and hypercalciuria (ARPTH)
    a. recessive trait
    a. trisomy
autosome
    balanced rearrangement of a.
    group C a.
    a. translocation
autosplenectomized
autosplenectomy
autostapling device
autotransfusion

autozygote
Auvard speculum
auxiliary orthotopic liver transplantation
auxometry
auxotyping
AV
    arteriovenous
    assisted ventilation
    atrioventricular
        AV malformation
        AV nodal reentry tachycardia
        AV node dysfunction
        AV shunt
AV/AF
    anteverted and anteflexed
        AV/AF uterus
Avagard instant hand antiseptic
avascular
    a. necrosis (AVN)
    a. space of Graves
avascularity
    periungual a.
AVC
    AVC Cream
    AVC suppository
Aveeno Cleansing Bar
Aventyl Hydrochloride
average
    a. blood loss
    a. for gestational age (AGA)
    pure-tone a. (PTA)
    a. radiation dose
aversive
AVFM
    arteriovenous fistula malformation
Aviane-28 tablet
Avicidin
Avina female urethral plug
Avirax
Avita
Avitene hemostatic material
avium
    Mycobacterium a.
avium-intracellulare
    Mycobacterium a.-i. (MAI)
Aviva mammography system
AVL 9110 pH analyzer
AVM
    arteriovenous malformation
AVN
    avascular necrosis
AVNRT
    atrioventricular nodal reentrant tachycardia
avoidance
    a. behavior
    phobic a.
    school a.
avoidant disorder

Avonex
AVP
arginine vasopressin
Aqueous AVP
AVPU
alertness, response to voice, response to
pain, unresponsive
AVRT
atrioventricular reciprocating tachycardia
avulse
avulsion
dental a.
a. fracture
a. injury
avuncular relationship
awake and active state
awareness
inadequate body a.
phonemic a.
AWHONN
Association of Women's Health,
Obstetrics, and Neonatal Nursing
AWS
Alagille-Watson syndrome
AWTA
aniridia, Wilms tumor association
AWTA syndrome
Axenfeld
A. anomaly
A. syndrome
Axenfeld-Rieger
A.-R. anomaly
A.-R. syndrome
axes (*pl. of* axis)
axetil
cefuroxime a. (CAE)
axial
a. acetabular index (AAI)
a. hypertonia
a. load
a. mesodermal dysplasia complex
a. resolution
a. traction
Axid AR Acid Reducer
axilla, pl. **axillae**
axillary
a. adenopathy
a. freckling
a. hair
a. hair development
a. hematoma
a. irradiation

a. irradiation therapy
a. lymphadenopathy
a. lymph node
a. node dissection
a. node sampling
a. skin lesion
a. tail
a. tail of Spence
a. temperature
a. vein
a. vein insertion site
a. view
axis, pl. **axes**
celiac a.
conjugate a.
a. deviation
embryonic a.
gonadal a.
HPA a.
HPO a.
hypothalamic-hypophysial-ovarian-
endometrial a.
hypothalamic-pituitary a. (HPA)
hypothalamic-pituitary-gonadal a.
long a.
neural a.
pelvic a.
a. of pelvis
pituitary a.
P-wave a.
reproductive a.
short a.
thigh-foot a.
a. traction
transmalleolar a.
T-wave a.
axis-traction forceps
axonal
a. degeneration
a. injury
a. retraction ball
a. type
axonotmesis
axon reflex
axon-reflex function
Axotal
Ayercillin
Aygestin
Aylesbury spatula
Ayr
A. Nasal

NOTES

Ayr *(continued)*
    A. saline drops
    A. saline nasal mist
Ayre
    A. spatula
    A. spatula-Zelsmyr Cytobrush
    technique
AZ
    Aschheim-Zondek
Azactam
5-azacytidine
azar
    kala a.
azasteroid
azatadine
azathioprine
azelastine
AZF
    azoospermia factor
AZFa region of Yq
AZFb region of Yq
AZFc region of Yq
AZH
    assisted zona hatching
azidothymidine (AZT)
azithromycin dihydrate
azlocillin
Azmacort Oral Inhaler
azo dye
Azo-Gamazole
Azo Gantrisin

azole
    antifungal a.
    a. therapy
azoospermia
    deleted in a. (DAZ)
    a. factor (AZF)
    obstructive a.
    a., renal anomaly, cervicothoracic
    spine dysplasia (ARCS)
azoospermic man
Azorean disease
Azo-Standard
azotemia
    prerenal a.
azotemic osteodystrophy
AZT
    azidothymidine
Aztec
    A. ear
    A. idiocy
aztreonam
Azulfidine EN-tabs
azygos
    a. artery of vagina
    a. continuation of inferior vena
    cava
    a. fissure
    a. lobe of right lung
    a. vein
azygous

β (*var. of* beta)

B
> B cell
> B chromosome
> B complex vitamins
> B lymphocyte
> B symptoms

B19
> HPV B19
> parvovirus B19

B$_6$
> B$_6$ deficiency
> vitamin B$_6$

B$_{12}$
> vitamin B$_{12}$

BA
> bacillary angiomatosis
> biliary atresia

babbling

Babcock
> B. clamp
> B. forceps

BABE
> B. OB ultrasound reporting system
> B. ultrasound
> B. ultrasound report software

Babee Teething

Babesia
> *B. divergens*
> *B. microti*
> B. WA1 type

babesiosis

Babinski
> B. reflex
> B. response
> B. sign

Babinski-Fröhlich syndrome

Babkin reflex

Babson chart

baby
> B. Air mesh netting
> blue b.
> blueberry muffin b.
> boarder b.
> bottle-fed b.
> b. bottle syndrome
> breast-fed b.
> breech b.
> bronze b.
> B. CareLink system
> Clinical Risk Index for B.'s (CRIB)
> cocaine b.
> collodion b.

> crack b.
> B. Doe regulations
> B. Dopplex 4000
> B. Dopplex 3000 antepartum fetal monitor
> drug b.
> febrile b.
> giant b.
> gray b.
> jittery b.
> juice b.
> nipple-fed b.
> B. Sense monitor
> sling b.
> b. teeth
> test-tube b.
> b. Tischler biopsy punch
> well-hydrated b.
> well-oxygenated b.
> well-perfused b.

BABYbird
> B. II ventilator
> B. respirator

BabyFace 3-D surface rendering accessory

babygram

Babylog
> B. 8000 oscillator
> B. 8000 respirator

baby's day diary

Babytherm IC

BAC
> bacterial artificial chromosome
> blood alcohol concentration

bacampicillin

Bacarate

Bacid

Baciguent Topical

Baci-IM Injection

bacillary
> b. angiomatosis (BA)
> b. dysentery
> enteric gram-negative b. (EGNB)
> b. meningitis
> b. peliosis
> b. peliosis hepatis

bacille
> b. bilié de Calmette-Guérin (BCG)
> b. Calmette-Guérin vaccine

bacilli (*pl. of* bacillus)

bacilliformis
> *Bartonella b.*

Bacillus
> *B. cereus*

Bacillus (continued)
  B. megaterium
  B. subtilis
bacillus, pl. **bacilli**
  acid-fast b.
  b. Calmette-Guérin (BCG)
  b. Calmette-Guérin vaccine
  Döderlein b.
  Ducrey b.
  gram-negative bacilli
  gram-positive bacilli
bacitracin
  neomycin, polymyxin B, b.
  b. and polymyxin B
back
  b. board
  b. clamp
  flat b.
backache
backcross mating
background
  dirty b.
Backhaus clamp
back-knee deformity
backpack
  AirPacks b.
  Airtec ergonomic b.
backscatter
  dipyridamole stress integrated b.
back-selected T cell
back-up position
backward chaining
backwardness
  general reading b. (GRB)
backwash ileitis
baclofen
Bacon-Babcock operation
Bactec blood-culturing system
bacteremia
  afebrile b.
  catheter-associated b.
  clostridial b.
  coagulase-negative b.
  CoNS b.
  occult b.
  polymicrobial b.
  streptococcal b.
bacteremia-associated pneumococcal pneumonia (BAPP)
bacteremic shock
bacteria (*pl. of* bacterium)
bacterial
  b. artificial chromosome (BAC)
  b. artificial chromosome probe
  b. cervical adenitis
  b. conjunctivitis
  b. contamination
  b. count
  b. cystitis

  b. endocarditis
  b. enteritis
  b. exanthem
  b. growth
  b. homeostasis
  b. infection
  b. inhibition assay method of Guthrie
  b. keratitis
  b. labyrinthitis
  b. laryngotracheobronchitis
  b. meningitis
  b. meningoencephalitis
  b. overgrowth syndrome
  b. parotitis
  b. pericarditis
  b. peritonitis
  b. pharyngitis
  b. plaque
  b. pneumonia
  b. recovery
  b. rhinosinusitis
  b. sepsis
  b. sinusitis
  b. soilage
  b. toxin
  b. tracheitis
  b. translocation
  b. vaginitis
  b. vaginosis (BV)
bactericidal, bacteriocidal
  b. drug
bactericidal/permeability-increasing protein (BPI)
bacteriologic
bacteriology
bacteriophage
bacteriostatic drug
bacteriotoxic endometritis
bacterium, pl. **bacteria**
  anaerobic bacteria
  coccobacillary bacteria
  coliform bacteria
  gas-forming bacteria
  gram-negative bacteria
  gram-positive bacteria
  intracerebral seeding of bacteria
  occasional bacteria
  pathogenic bacteria
  pyogenic bacteria
  Salmonella bacteria
  Shigella bacteria
  Streptococcus bacteria
bacteriuria
  asymptomatic b. (ASB)
  rapid filter testing for b.
bacteroide
Bacteroides
  B. capillosus

B

B. corrodens
B. distasonis
B. fragilis
B. gingivalis
B. melaninogenicus
B. ovatus
B. thetaiotaomicron
bacteroidosis
Bactine Hydrocortisone
BactoShield
Bactrim DS
Bactroban cream
Bact-T-Screen
Badenoch urethroplasty
Baden procedure
BADS
  black locks with albinism and deafness
    syndrome
BAEP
  brainstem auditory evoked potential
BAER
  brainstem auditory evoked response
    BAER test
Baer cavity
bag
  Ambu b.
  anesthesia b.
  B. balm
  Barnes b.
  Cardiff resuscitation b.
  Champetier de Ribes b.
  Douglas b.
  Endopouch Pro specimen-
    retrieval b.
  Hope resuscitation b.
  intestinal b.
  manual ventilation b. (MVB)
  b. and mask
  b. and mask resuscitation
  b. and mask ventilation
  passenger air b. (PAB)
  Rusch b.
  sterile isolation b.
  b., valve, mask (BVM)
  Vi-Drape bowel b.
  Void-Ease urine collection b.
  Voorhees b.
  b. of waters (BOW)
  b. of worms appearance
  zinc-free plastic b.
bagged urinalysis
Baggish hysteroscope

Bagshawe protocol
Bailey Physical Development Index
Bailey-Williamson forceps
Baird forceps
Bair Hugger patient warming system
Bakchaus towel forceps
Bakelite cystoscopy sheath
Baker
  B. cyst
  B. punch
baker's leg
baking soda sitz bath
BAL
  blood alcohol level
  British antilewisite
  bronchoalveolar lavage
    BAL fluid
    BAL in Oil
Balamuthia
  B. mandrillaris
  B. meningoencephalitis
balance
  acid-base b.
  electrolyte b.
  fetal acid-base b.
  macronutrient b.
  negative b.
  b. reaction
  sodium b.
  transcapillary fluid b.
balanced
  b. chromosome rearrangement
  b. rearrangement of autosome
  b. translocation
balancing
  soft tissue b.
balanic, balanitic
  b. hypospadias
balanitis
  b. circinata
  circinate b.
  b. circumscripta plasmacellularis
  plasma cell b.
  b. of Zoon
balanoposthitis
Balantidium coli
balding
  temporal b.
baldness
  frontal b.
Baldy operation

NOTES

Baldy-Webster
  B.-W. procedure
  B.-W. uterine suspension
Balfour
  B. bladder blade
  B. retractor
ball
  axonal retraction b.
  Bichat fat b.
  birthing b.
  cauterizing b.
  b. electrode
  fungal b.
  fungus b.
  B. operation
  B. pelvimetry technique
  Prader b.'s
  renal fungus b.
  TheraGym exercise b.
  tissue link floating b.
Ballantine clamp
Ballantyne-Runge syndrome
Ballantyne-Smith syndrome
Ballard
  B. Assessment Score (BAS)
  B. chart
  B. examination
  B. gestational assessment
  B. score
  B. test
Ball-Burch procedure
Baller-Gerold syndrome (BGS)
ballet dancer's secondary amenorrhea
Ballinger-Wallace syndrome
ballismus
balloon
  b. atrial septostomy (BAS)
  atrial septostomy via b.
  b. catheter technique
  electrode b.
  b. endometrial ablation
  French Foley b.
  24 French Foley b.
  gastric b.
  b. heating therapy
  Origin b.
  pediatric b.
  b. pulmonary valvuloplasty
  Rashkind b.
  Rigiflex b.
  b. septostomy
  b. septostomy catheter
  Soft-Wand atraumatic tissue
    manipulator b.
  b. tamponade
  B. Therapy System
  b. thermoplasty
  transurethral self-detachable b.
  b. tuboplasty

  b. valvotomy
  b. valvulotomy
ballooning
balloon-tipped catheter
ballottable
ballottement
  abdominal b.
  uterine b.
ball-valve effect
balm
  Bag b.
  Butt B.
  lemon b.
Balmex cream
Balminil Decongestant
Baló disease
Baloser hysteroscope
balsa vaginal form
BALT
  bronchus-associated lymphoid tissue
Balthazar Scales of Adaptive Behavior
Baltic myoclonus
Bamberger fluid
bamboo
  b. hair
  b. spine
bambooing of digit
Bamforth syndrome
BAMO
  behavioral, anxiety, mood, and other
    types of disorders
  BAMO scale
banana
  Kanana B.
  b.'s, rice, applesauce, tea, toast
    (BRATT)
  b.'s, rice cereal, applesauce, toast
    (BRAT)
  b. sign
Bancap HC
band
  adhesive b.
  agyria-pachygyria b.
  amniotic constriction b.
  anular b.
  BB b.
  C b.
  b. cell
  chorioamnionic b.
  congenital intestinal b.
  congenital peritoneal b.
  cytological b.
  dense b.
  b. form neutrophil
  G b.
  b. heterotopia
  hymenal b.
  iliotibial b.
  b. keratopathy

Ladd b.
limbic b.'s
lucent b.
MM b.
myocardial b. (MB)
oligoclonal b.'s
pelvic b.
Q b.
R b.
Silastic b.
b. stage
Streeter b.
T b.
vitreous b.
Z b.

bandage
Kerlix gauze b.
Kling b.
b. scissors
Tubigrip b.
tumescent absorbent b.
Velpeau b.
Webril b.

bandaging
elastic b.

Band-Aid operation

bandemia

banding
amniotic b.
arterial b.
centromeric b.
chromosomal b.
chromosome b.
Giemsa b.
high-resolution b.
low-resolution b.
b. pattern
proximal pulmonary artery b.
pulmonary arterial b.
pulmonary artery b.
quinacrine b.
reverse b.
tubal b.

Bandl
pathologic retraction ring of B.
B. ring

banging
head b.

banjo curette

banjo-string adhesion

bank, banking
clone b.

cord blood b.
sperm b.
umbilical cord blood b.

Bankart lesion

banked breast milk

banking (*var. of* bank)

Banki syndrome

Bannayan-Riley-Ruvalcaba syndrome (BRRS)

Bannayan syndrome

Bannayan-Zonana syndrome (BZS)

Bannwarth syndrome

Banthine

Banti syndrome

BAP
bone alkaline phosphatase

BAPP
bacteremia-associated pneumococcal pneumonia

bar
Aveeno Cleansing B.
bilateral b.'s
Bill traction b.
calcaneonavicular b.
Denis Browne b.
Fostex B.
hyoid b.
Mercier b.
PanOxyl B.
pectus b.
stabilizing b.
syndet cleaning b.
talocalcaneal b.
unilateral b.

Baraitser-Burn syndrome

Baraitser-Winter syndrome

barbae
sycosis b.

Barbero-Marcial
B.-M. classification
B.-M. procedure

Barber-Say syndrome

Barbilixir

barbiturate
b. intoxication
b. poisoning

barbotage

Barcroft/Haldane apparatus

Bard
B. Biopty cut needle
B. Biopty gun

B

NOTES

Bard *(continued)*
  B. cervical cannula
  B. PDA Umbrella
Bardet-Biedl syndrome (BBS)
Bard-Parker blade
bare lymphocyte syndrome
bargaining stage
Baridium
barium
  b. contrast
  b. enema
  b. esophagogram
  b. esophagography
  b. esophagram
  b. study
  b. swallow
barium-impregnated plastic intrauterine device
Barkan infant lens
Barker low birth weight hypothesis
barking cough
barley
  b. allergy
  b. malt
Barlow
  B. disease
  B. hip dysplasia test
  B. maneuver
  B. mitral regurgitation repair technique
  B. and Ortolani test
  B. sign
  B. syndrome
Barnes
  B. Akathisia Scale (BAS)
  B. bag
  B. cerclage
  B. curve
  B. zone
baromacrometer
Barophen
baroreceptor
baroreflex response
barotitis
  acute b.
barotrauma
barovolutrauma
Barr body
barrel
  b. cervix
  b. chest
  b. chest deformity
barrel-shaped
  b.-s. cervix
  b.-s. chest
  b.-s. lesion
  b.-s. upper central incisor
barren
Barré sign

Barrett esophagus
barrier
  Adcon-L anti-adhesion b.
  blood-brain b. (BBB)
  blood-testis b.
  b. contraceptive
  ferric hyaluronate adhesion b.
  b. gown
  Interceed TC7 absorbable adhesion b.
  b. laparoscopy drape
  b. method
  b. method of contraception
  b. pack
  placental b.
  Sil-K OB b.
  TC7 adhesion b.
Barron pump
Barrow solution soak
Bart
  hemoglobin B.
  B. syndrome
Bartholin
  B. cystectomy
  B. duct
  B. gland
  B. gland abscess
  B. gland carcinoma
  B. gland cyst
  B., urethral, Skene (BUS)
bartholinitis
Bartholin-Patau syndrome
Bartholomew rule of fourths
Barth syndrome
Bartonella
  B. bacilliformis
  B. henselae
  B. henselae infection
  B. quintana
Barton forceps
Bartsocaas-Papas syndrome
Bartter syndrome (BS)
barymazia
BAS
  Ballard Assessment Score
  balloon atrial septostomy
  Barnes Akathisia Scale
basal
  b. arterial occlusion
  b. artery
  b. body temperature (BBT)
  b. body thermometer
  b. cell carcinoma
  b. cell epithelioma
  b. cell hyperplasia
  b. cell nevus syndrome (BCNS)
  b. cistern
  b. ganglia calcification
  b. ganglia disorder

b. ganglia necrosis
b. ganglion
b. ganglion disorder-mental retardation (BGMR)
b. lamina
b. membrane (BM)
b. metabolic rate (BMR)
b. perivillous fibrin
b. plate
b. skull fracture

basalis
decidua b.
zona b.

BASC
Behavioral Assessment Scale for Children
BASC monitor

base
broad nasal b.
b. deficit
b. excess
hydrocortisone b.
b. medication
methylprednisolone b.
nitrogenous b.
b. pair
b. sequence
b. sequence analysis
thickened b.

baseball
b. finger
b. stitch

baseline
b. fetal bradycardia
b. fetal heart rate
b. fetal tachycardia
FHR b.
b. tonus
b. value
b. variability of fetal heart rate
b. visual acuity
zero-voltage b.

basement
b. membrane
b. membrane zone (BMZ)

bases (*pl. of* basis)

bas-fond

basic
b. fibroblast growth factor (bFGF)
b. life support (BLS)
b. skill

basicaryoplastin

basichromatin
basicranial flexure
basicranium
basilar
b. artery migraine
b. consolidation
b. impression
b. invagination
b. meningitis
b. skull fracture
basilemma
basis, pl. **bases**
B. breast pump
b. pontis
B. soap
basket cell
basolateral membrane transport system
basophil
basophilia
basophilic
b. leukemia
b. stippling
Bassen-Kornzweig
B.-K. disease
B.-K. syndrome
Basset radical vulvectomy
bassinet
bastard
Bastiaanse-Chiricuta procedure
bat
b. ear
b. wing appearance
bath
baking soda sitz b.
belly b.
hexachlorophene b.
pHisoHex b.
B. respirator
b. seat
sitz b.
sponge b.
bathing trunk nevus
bathrocephaly
batrachian position
Battelle Developmental Inventory (BDI)
Batten-Bielschowsky
B.-B. type
B.-B. type of late infantile and juvenile amaurotic idiocy
Batten disease
Batten-Mayou disease
Batten-Turner congenital myopathy

NOTES

battered
- b. buttock syndrome
- b. child syndrome
- b. fetus syndrome
- b. wife syndrome
- b. woman

battering cycle

battery
- MacArthur Story Stem B. (MSSB)
- Vulpe Assessment B.
- Woodcock-Johnson Psychoeducational B.

battery-operated breast pump

battle
- b. neurosis
- B. sign

battledore placenta

Baudelocque
- B. diameter
- B. operation
- B. uterine circle

baumannii
- *Acinetobacter b.*

Baxa oral dispenser

Bayer
- B. Aspirin
- B. DCA2000 analyzer
- B. Timed-Release Arthritic Pain Formula

bayesian hypothesis

Bayley
- B. cognitive outcome
- B. Mental Developmental index
- B. Mental Scale
- B. Motor Score
- B. and Pinneau height-predicting method
- B. Psychomotor Developmental Index
- B. Scales of Infant Development (BSID)
- B. Scales of Infant Development-II (BSID-II)
- B. Scales of Infant Development-Motor, 2nd Edition

Bayley-Pinneau table

Baylisascaris procyonis

Baylor
- B. amniotic perforator
- B. amniotome

Bayne Pap Brush

bayonet
- b. forceps
- b. leg

bazedoxifine

Bazett formula

Bazex-Dupré-Christol syndrome

Bazex syndrome

Bazin
- erythema induration of B. (EIB)

BBB
- blood-brain barrier
- bundle branch block
- BBB syndrome

BB band

BBS
- Bardet-Biedl syndrome

BBT
- basal body temperature
- BBT chart

BCA
- bicinchonic acid
- BCA protein assay

BCAVD
- bilateral congenital absence of vas deferens

BCC
- benign cellular changes

BC Cold Powder Non-Drowsy Formula

BCD
- blepharocheilodontic
- BCD syndrome

BCDDP
- Breast Cancer Detection Demonstration Project

BCDL
- Brachmann-Cornelia de Lange

BCDLS
- Brachmann-Cornelia de Lange syndrome

BCE
- bone collagen equivalent unit

B-cell
- B-c. dysfunction
- B-c. lineage
- B-c. lymphoma

BCFA
- branched-chain fatty acid

BCG
- bacille bilié de Calmette-Guérin
- bacillus Calmette-Guérin
- BCG live
- Tice BCG
- BCG vaccine

BCI
- blunt cardiac injury

Bcl-2
- B. oncogene
- B. protein

BCNS
- basal cell nevus syndrome

BCNU
- bis-chloroethylnitrosourea

BCP
- birth control pill

BCPT
- breast cancer prevention trial

bcr
    breakpoint cluster region
BCT
    benign cystic teratoma
    breast conservation therapy
    breast-conserving therapy
BD
        BD Sensability breast self-
          examination
        BD syndrome
        BD test
BDD
    body dysmorphic disorder
B$_6$-dependent convulsion
BDI
    Battelle Developmental Inventory
    Beck Depression Inventory
        BDI score
bDNA
    branched deoxyribonucleic acid
BDNF
    brain-derived neurotrophic factor
BDProbeTec ET system
bead
        Chelex b.
        DEAE b.'s
        medical worry b.'s
beading
beak
        medial metaphyseal b.
beaked
        b. nose
        b. pelvis
beaking
BEAM
    brain electrical activity map
    brain electrical activity mapping
bean
        cassava b.
        castor b.
        fava b.
        b. gum
        jelly b.
bear
        B. Cub infant ventilator
        B. Hugger warming blanket
        InterMed B.
        B. NUM-1 tidal volume monitor
        B. respirator
        b. tracks
        b. walk
beard ringworm

Beare-Stevenson cutis gyrata syndrome
Beare syndrome
bearing down
bearing-down pain
beat
        dropped b.
        escape b.'s
        left ventricular paced b.
        b.'s per minute (bpm)
Beath pin
Beatson ovariotomy
beat-to-beat
        b.-t.-b. continuous blood pressure
          monitoring
        b.-t.-b. variability
        b.-t.-b. variability of fetal heart
          rate
Beau line
beaveri
        Brugia b.
Beben
Because vaginal foam
Beccaria sign
Beck
        B. Depression Inventory (BDI)
        B. disease
        B. triad
Becker
        B. breast prosthesis
        B. disease
        B. melanosis
        B. muscular dystrophy (BMD)
        B. nevus
        B. pseudohypertrophic muscular
          dystrophy
        B. tissue expander
        B. type progressive muscular
          dystrophy
Becker-Kiener muscular dystrophy
Beckwith syndrome
Beckwith-Wiedemann syndrome (BWS)
Béclard nucleus
Becloforte
beclomethasone
        aqueous b.
        b. dipropionate
        b. propionate
Beclovent Oral Inhaler
Beconase
        B. AQ
        B. AQ Nasal Inhaler

NOTES

BED
    binge eating disorder
bed
    Affinity b.
    arterial vascular b.
    bumper b.
    hypoplastic pulmonary vascular b.
    Ohio b.
    oversewing placental b.
    placental b.
    pulmonary vascular b.
    b. rest
    b. rest checklist
    B. Rest Helpline
    b. rest support program
    vascular b.
Bednar aphthae
bedwetting
beef insulin
Beemer-Langer syndrome
Beemer lethal malformation syndrome
Beesix
bee sting challenge
Begeer syndrome
Béguez César disease
behavior
    adaptive b.
    aggressive b.
    antisocial b.
    Assessment of Preterm Infants' B.
      (APIB)
    B. Assessment System for Children
      monitor
    autistic b.
    autistic-like b.
    avoidance b.
    Balthazar Scales of Adaptive B.
    catatonic b.
    cognitive b.
    b. contract
    b. contract system
    defiant b.
    disorganized b.
    dysregulated b.
    externalizing b.
    fire-setting b.
    functional b.
    heterosexual high risk b.
    hypersexual b.
    immature social b.
    b. modification
    neuropsychiatric b.
    obsessive-compulsive b. (OCB)
    b. pattern
    B. Problem Inventory (BPI)
    B. Rating Scale (BRS)
    risk b.
    risk-taking b.
    risky b.

    self-comforting b.
    self-injurious b. (SIB)
    self-mutilating b.
    social b.
    stereotypic b.
    withdrawn b.
behavioral
    b., anxiety, mood, and other types
      of disorders (BAMO)
    b. assessment
    B. Assessment Scale for Children
      (BASC)
    b. audiometry
    b. disturbance
    B. and Emotional Rating Scale
      (BERS)
    b. family systems therapy (BFST)
    b. genetics
    b. inhibition
    b. intervention
    b. management
    b. milestone
    b. observation audiometry (BOA)
    b. pediatrics
    b. rebound
    b. state
    b. stress
    b. therapy
Behçet
    B. disease
    B. syndrome
Behr
    B. disease
    B. optic atrophy
    B. syndrome
BEI
    bioelectrical impedance
beigelii
    Trichosporon b.
Beighton criteria
bejel
belching
Belgian type mental retardation
bell
    auditory response to b.
    Gomco b.
    B. palsy
    B. staging criteria
    b. stethoscope
belladonna
Bell-Buettner hysterectomy
bell-clapper deformity
Bellergal
belli
    Isospora b.
Bellucci alligator forceps
belly
    b. bath
    b. bath therapy

B

b. crawl
prune b.
Bel-Phen-Ergot S
belt
b. mark
Marsupial b.
belt-position booster seat
BEMP
bleomycin, Eldisine, mitomycin, Platinol
Benadryl
B. Decongestant Allergy Tablet
B. Injection
B. Oral
B. Topical
Bence Jones protein
bend
deep-knee b.
b. deformity
b. fracture
Bendectin
Bender Visual Motor Gestalt Test
Bendopa
bendroflumethiazide
beneficence
BeneFix
Benelli mastopexy
benign
b. breast disease
b. breast examination
b. cellular changes (BCC)
b. childhood epilepsy
b. congenital hypotonia
b. cystic ovarian teratoma
b. cystic teratoma (BCT)
b. epilepsy of childhood
b. external hydrocephalus
b. familial chronic pemphigus
b. familial hematuria (BFH)
b. familial macrocephaly (BFM)
b. familial megalencephaly
b. familial neonatal convulsion
  (BFNC)
b. familial neonatal seizure
b. familial recurrent cholestasis
b. focal epilepsy
b. fructosuria
b. hepatic adenoma
b. hyperphenylalaninemia
b. idiopathic neonatal convulsion
b. implant
b. infantile familial convulsion
  (BIFC)

b. infantile hypotonia
b. intracranial hypertension
b. jaundice
b. juvenile melanoma
b. lesion
b. lymphoid hyperplasia
b. mass
b. maturation delay
b. mesothelioma of genital tract
b. migratory glossitis
b. mucinous cystadenoma
b. myoclonic epilepsy
b. myoclonus of infancy
b. nasopharyngeal fibroma
b. neonatal epilepsy
b. neutropenia
b. nevus
b. nonprogressive familial chorea
b. nonprolapsed uterus
b. ovarian neoplasm
b. papillomatosis
b. papillomavirus infection
b. paroxysmal torticollis
b. paroxysmal torticollis of infancy
b. paroxysmal vertigo (BPV)
b. partial epilepsy
b. partial epilepsy with
  centrotemporal spike (BPEC)
b. pineal cyst
b. recurrent hematuria
b. rolandic epilepsy (BRE)
b. transient gynecomastia
b. transient optic disc edema
b. tumor
b. vascular neoplasm
b. venous hum
b. X-linked recessive muscular
  dystrophy
Benisone
Benjamin
B. anemia
B. syndrome
Bennett
B. PR-2 ventilator
B. respirator
B. small corpuscles
Benoxyl
Benson baby pylorus separator
bent finger
Benton Visual Retention Test

NOTES

Bentyl
- B. Hydrochloride Injection
- B. Hydrochloride Oral

Benylin
- B. Expectorant
- B. Pediatric

Benzac
- B. AC Gel
- B. AC, W Wash
- B. W Gel

BenzaClin topical gel
5-Benzagel
10-Benzagel
Benzamycin
benzathine
- b. benzylpenicillin
- b. penicillin
- penicillin G b.
- b. penicillin G (BPG)

Benzedrine
benzene
benzimidazole
benzoate
- benzyl b.
- sodium phenylacetate and sodium b.

benzocaine
- antipyrine and b.
- b. lozenge

Benzodent
benzodiazepine
benzoin applicator
benzothiophene-derived selective estrogen receptor modulator
benzoyl peroxide
benzthiazide
benztropine mesylate
benzyl
- b. alcohol
- b. benzoate

benzylpenicillin
benzylpenicilloyl-polylysine
BEP
- bleomycin, etoposide, cisplatin
- bleomycin, etoposide, Platinol
- BEP therapy

bepridil
beractant surfactant
Berardinelli-Seip-Lawrence syndrome
Berardinelli-Seip syndrome
Berardinelli syndrome
Berdon syndrome
Berens 3-character test
Berger
- B. paresthesia
- B. renal disease

bergeriae
- *Gemella b.*

Bergia syndrome

Bergmeister papilla
beriberi
- infantile b.
- Shoshin b.

Berkeley
- B. suction curette
- B. suction machine
- B. Vacurette

Berkeley-Bonney retractor
Berkow formula for burns
Berkson-Gage
- B.-G. calculation
- B.-G. test/assay

Berlin
- B. breakage syndrome
- B. edema
- B. score

Bernard-Soulier syndrome
Bernay uterine packer
Berne criteria
Bernoulli trial
Bernstein test
berry
- b. aneurysm
- B. syndrome

Berry-Kravis and Israel syndrome
Berry-Treacher Collins syndrome
BERS
- Behavioral and Emotional Rating Scale

Bertini syndrome
Berwick dye
Besnier prurigo of pregnancy
Best disease
bestiality
besylate
- atracurium b.

beta, β
- b. blocker
- b. carotene
- b. cell adenoma
- b. cell adenomatosis
- b. chain
- b. error
- estrogen receptor b. (Er beta)
- b. FGF-stimulated cell proliferation
- follitropin b.
- b. interferon
- b. lactamase
- b. phase
- b. ray
- b. receptor
- b. receptor agonist
- b. subunit
- b. thalassemia
- transforming growth factor b. (TGF beta)

beta-2
- b. agonist
- b. microglobulin

beta-adrenergic
    b.-a. agent
    b.-a. agonist
    b.-a. blockade
    b.-a. drug
    b.-a. receptor
beta-2-adrenergic agent
beta-aminoisobutyric aciduria
beta-chemokine receptor
Betacort
3beta-dehydrogenase deficiency
Betaderm
Betadine PrepStick Plus
beta-endorphin
17beta-estradiol dehydrogenase
beta-galactosidase
beta-galactosidase-1 (GLB-1)
    b.-g.-1 deficiency
beta-glucuronidase (GUSB)
    b.-g. deficiency
        mucopolysaccharidosis
beta-hCG, beta-HCG
    beta-human chorionic gonadotropin
    beta-hCG discriminatory zone
beta-hemolytic
    b.-h. streptococcal coinfection
    b.-h. *Streptococcus*
3betaHSD
    3beta-hydroxysteroid dehydrogenase
11-beta-HSD2 deficiency
beta-human chorionic gonadotropin
    (beta-hCG, beta-HCG)
3beta-hydroxysteroid dehydrogenase
    (3betaHSD)
11-beta-hydroxysteroid dehydrogenase
    type 2 deficiency
betaine
    b. anhydrous
    b. hydrochloride
beta-1, -2 integrin
beta-lactam
    b.-l. antibiotic
    b.-l. antimicrobial
beta-lactamase-resistant
    antistaphylococcal antibiotic
beta-lactamase-stable drug
beta-lipotrophin
Betaloc
betamethasone
    b. dipropionate
    b. valerate
betamimetic agent

17beta-ol-dehydrogenase
5beta-pregnane-3,20-dione
Betasept
Betaseron
beta-spectrin
betasympathomimetic
beta-synthase
    cystathionine b.-s. (CBS)
beta-thalassemia
    HbE b-t.
    sickle b-t.
Betatrex Topical
betatron electron accelerator
Betaxin
bethanechol chloride
Bethesda
    B. assay
    B. 2001 cervical cytology
        classification
    B. classification system
    B. II system
    B. System guidelines
    B. System Pap smear classification
    B. unit
Bethlem myopathy
Betke-Kleihauer test
Betke stain
Betnelan
Betnesol
Betnovate
Betz cell
Beuren syndrome
Bevan incision
Beverly-Douglas lip-tongue adhesion
    technique
BeWo cell
bexarotene
Bexophene
Bextra tablet
bezafibrate
Bezalip
bezoar
Bezold abscess
Bezold-Jarisch reflex
bFGF
    basic fibroblast growth factor
BFH
    benign familial hematuria
BFL
    Börjeson-Forssman-Lehmann
BFLS
    Börjeson-Forssman-Lehmann syndrome

B

NOTES

BFLUTS
  Bristol Female Lower Urinary Tract
    Symptoms
      BFLUTS questionnaire
BFM
  benign familial macrocephaly
BFNC
  benign familial neonatal convulsion
BFST
  behavioral family systems therapy
BF-STS
  biological false-positive serologic test for
    syphilis
BFU-E
  burst-forming units-erythroid
bG
  Chemstrip bG
BGMR
  basal ganglion disorder-mental
    retardation
      BGMR syndrome
BGS
  Baller-Gerold syndrome
BH$_4$
  tetrahydrobiopterin cofactor
      BH$_4$ loading test
BHS
  Bogalusa Heart Study
BIA
  bioelectrical impedance analysis
biallelic marker
Bianchine-Lewis syndrome
biatriatum
  cor triloculare b.
Biaxin
bibasilar
BICAP
  BICAP cautery
  BICAP probe
bicap
bicarbonate (HCO$_3$)
  b. concentration
  b. infusion
  plasma b. (PHCO$_3$)
  sodium b. (NaHCO$_3$)
  b. wasting
bicarbonate-carbonic acid system
bicarbonaturia
bicephalus
biceps
  b. femoris muscle
  b. reflex
Bichat fat ball
bichloracetic acid
bichorial pregnancy
Bicillin
  B. C-R

B. C-R 900/300
B. L-A
bicinchonic acid (BCA)
bicipital tuberosity
Bicitra
Bickers-Adams syndrome
BiCNU
BiCoag forceps
biconcave vertebra
bicornuate, bicornate, bicornous
  b. uterus
bicuculline-induced seizure
bicuspid
  b. aortic valve
  first b.
  second b.
bicycle ergometer
bicycling movement
bidet
bidirectional
  b. Glenn procedure
  b. Glenn shunt
  b. PDA
  b. shunting
bidiscoidal placenta
BIDS
  brittle hair, intellectual impairment,
    decreased fertility, short stature
      BIDS syndrome
Biederman sign
Bielschowsky-Jansky disease
Bielschowsky syndrome
Biemond syndrome 1, 2
bieneusi
  Enterocytozoon b.
Bierer ovum forceps
Bieri scale
bifascicular block
BIFC
  benign infantile familial convulsion
bifid
  b. cervix
  b. clitoris
  b. earlobe
  b. exencephalia
  b. nose
  b. pelvis
  b. scrotum
  b. spinal cord
  b. uterus
  b. uvula
  b. xiphoid
bifida
  spina b.
Bifidobacterium
  B. adolescentis
  B. bifidum
  B. breve
  B. catenulatum

B

B. infantis
B. longum
bifidum
    Bifidobacterium b.
    cranium b.
bifidus
    b. factor
    Lactobacillus b.
biforate uterus
bifurcate
bifurcation
    aortic b.
bigeminal pregnancy
bigeminy
    atrial b.
Biggers medium
BiGGY
    bismuth sulfite, glucose, glycine, yeast
    BiGGY agar
Biglieri syndrome
biguanide
    polyhexamethyl b. (PHMB)
biischial diameter
bikini cut incision
bikinin (HI-30)
bilabial
    b. closure
    b. speech sound
bilaminar blastoderm
BiLAP bipolar laparoscopic probe
bilateral
    b. acoustic neurofibromatosis
    b. acoustic neuromas
    b. atresia
    b. atresia of external auditory
      meatus
    b. bars
    b. breast pump
    b. cephalhematomas
    b. cerebral ventriculomegaly
    b. choreoathetosis
    b. choroid plexus cyst
    b. club feet
    b. congenital absence of vas
      deferens (BCAVD)
    b. congenital ptosis
    b. conjunctivitis
    b. corticobulbar disruption
    b. cryptorchidism
    b. ductus
    b. ectopic pregnancy
    b. facial agenesis

    b. flank masses
    b. gonadal failure
    b. hearing impairment
    b. increased femoral anteversion
    b. left-sidedness
    b. lung hypoplasia
    b. mediolateral episiotomies
    b. myocutaneous graft
    b. myringotomy tubes (BMT)
    b. optic nerve hypoplasia
    b. optic neuritis
    b. otitis media with effusion
      (BOME)
    b. ovarian neoplasm
    b. PC-IOL implantation
    b. periventricular nodular
      heterotopia
    b. pyramidal tract signs
    b. retinoblastomas
    b. salpingo-oophorectomy (BSO)
    b. schizencephalic cleft
    b. simultaneous tubal pregnancies
    b. slowing
    b. spasticity
    b. stocking hypesthesia
    b. subcostal incisions
    b. tubal ligation (BTL)
    b. ureteral diversion
    b. ureteral obstruction (BUO)
    b. uropathy
bile
    b. acid
    b. acid flux
    b. acid malabsorption
    b. acid sequestration
    b. acid synthesis
    b. chenodeoxycholic acid level
    b. duct
    b. duct catheter
    b. duct paucity
    b. duct resection
    b. duct stenosis
    b. ductule
    inspissated b.
    milk of calcium b.
    b. peritonitis
    b. pigment
    b. salt
    b. salt-stimulated lipase (BSSL)
    b. stasis
    supersaturation of b.
bile-plug syndrome

NOTES

bile-stained emesis
bilevel positive airway pressure (BiPAP, B-PAP)
bili
 b. light
 B. mask phototherapy eye cover
biliary
 b. abscess
 b. ascites
 b. atresia (BA)
 b. cirrhosis
 b. colic
 b. hypoplasia
 b. lithiasis
 b. microhamartoma
 b. microlithiasis
 b. neonatal hepatitis
 b. perforation
BiliBed phototherapy unit
BiliBlanket Plus phototherapy system
BiliBottoms
BiliCheck bilirubin analyzer
bililights
bilineal category
bilingual
biliopancreatic diversion
bilious
 b. emesis
 b. vomiting
 b. vomitus
bilirubin
 amniotic fluid b.
 b. blanket
 conjugated b.
 cord blood b.
 direct b.
 direct-reacting b.
 elevated conjugated b.
 b. encephalopathy
 hour-specific total serum b.
 indirect b.
 b. infarction
 b. lights
 serum b.
 total b.
 total serum b. (TSB)
 transcutaneous b. (TcB)
 unconjugated b.
bilirubin-albumin binding
bilirubin-induced neurologic dysfunction (BIND)
bilirubinometer
 BiliTest transcutaneous b.
bilirubinometry
BiliTest transcutaneous bilirubinometer
Bili-Timer
Bill
 B. maneuver
 B. traction bar
 B. traction handle forceps
Billings method
Billroth tumor forceps
biloba
 ginkgo b.
 placenta b.
bilobate placenta
bilobed placenta
biloculare
 cor b.
biloma
Bilopaque
Biloptin
Biltricide
bimanual
 b. massage
 b. pelvic examination
 b. version
bimelic amyoplasia
bimodal pattern
binary process
binasal prongs
BIND
 bilirubin-induced neurologic dysfunction
 BIND score
binder
 abdominal b.
 breast b.
 Dale abdominal b.
 obstetric b.
 Scultetus b.
 B. syndrome
binding
 androgen b.
 bilirubin-albumin b.
 breast b.
 C1q b.
 fragment antigen b.
 ligand b.
 protein b.
 b. protein
 b. protein-2 insulinlike growth factor
 b. protein-3 insulinlike growth factor
 b. site
 sperm-zona pellucida b.
binge drinking
binge-eating
 b.-e. disorder (BED)
 b.-e. syndrome
bingeing
binocular
 b. function
 b. vision
binomial
binovular twins
bioactive hormone

B

bioactivity
bioassay
BioBands bracelet
biobehavioral shift
bioblast
Biobrane adhesive
Biobrane/HF dressing
Biocef
Biocell RTV saline-filled breast implant
Biocept-5 pregnancy test
Biocept-G pregnancy test
biochemical
    b. defect
    b. genetics
    b. pregnancy
    b. study
biochemistry
Bioclate
biocompatibility
bioelectrical
    b. impedance (BEI)
    b. impedance analysis (BIA)
bioelectromagnetic application
biofeedback
    b. technique
    b. therapy
biofield therapeutics
biofilm
bioflavonoid
Biogel
    B. Reveal glove
    B. Reveal puncture indication system
bioimpedance analysis
bioinformatics
Biojector 2000
biologic
    b. assay
    b. response modifier (BRM)
    b. satiation curve
    b. treatment
biological
    b. false-positive serologic test for syphilis (BF-STS)
    b. risk
    b. sampling
biologically plastic femora
biology
biomedical factor
Biomerica
BioMerieux Vitek system
biometric profile

biometry
    fetal b.
biomicroscopy
    slit-lamp b.
Biomydrin
Biopatch dressing
biophysical
    b. profile (BPP)
    b. profile score
biopsy
    Allis-Abramson breast b.
    aspiration b.
    bone marrow b.
    cervical cone b.
    chorionic villus b. (CVB)
    ciliary b.
    coin b.
    cold cup b.
    cold knife b.
    cold knife cone b.
    cone b.
    core b.
    core needle b. (CNB)
    cul-de-sac b.
    b. dating
    embryo b.
    endometrial b.
    endomyocardial b.
    excisional b.
    fetal tissue b.
    fine-needle aspiration b. (FNAB)
    b. forceps
    frozen b.
    full-thickness bowel b.
    full-thickness intestinal b.
    hot b.
    image-guided breast b.
    jejunal b.
    Kevorkian punch b.
    Keyes punch b.
    kidney b.
    laparoscopic full-thickness intestinal b.
    liver b.
    lymph node b.
    mirror image breast b.
    mucosal b.
    muscle b.
    needle localization breast b.
    negative punch b.
    omental b.
    open b.

NOTES

biopsy *(continued)*
> open lung b. (OLB)
> out-of-phase endometrial b.
> percutaneous renal b.
> peritoneal b.
> Pipelle b.
> pleural b.
> b. probe
> punch skin b.
> quadriceps femoris muscle b.
> renal b.
> sentinel lymph node b.
> single cell b.
> skeletal muscle b.
> skin b.
> skinny-needle b.
> small bowel b.
> stereotactic breast b.
> sural nerve b.
> synovial b.
> timed endometrial b.
> transanal rectal b.
> transvaginal fine-needle b.
> trophectoderm b.
> vulvar b.

biopsychosocial syndrome
biopterin
Biopty cut needle
biosampler
Bioself fertility indicator
BioStar
> B. Flu OIA
> B. Flu optical immunoassay
> B. Strep A OIA test

biosynthesis
> inborn error of bile acid b.
> prostaglandin b.
> steroid b.

biosynthetic defect
biotechnology
biotin
> b. factor
> B. Forte
> B. Forte Extra Strength

biotinidase deficiency
biotinylated
Biotirmone
biotyping
BIP
> bleomycin, ifosfamide, Platinol

BiPAP, B-PAP
> bilevel positive airway pressure
> BiPAP machine

biparental inheritance
biparietal
> b. bulge
> b. diameter (BPD)
> b. diameter level

bipartita
> placenta b.

bipartite
> b. patella
> b. uterus

bipedal
> b. lymphangiography
> b. posture

biperiden
biphasic
> b. anaphylactic reaction
> b. anaphylaxis
> b. fever
> b. response
> b. stridor
> b. temperature pattern

biphenyl
> polychlorinated b.

biplane
> b. cineangiocardiography
> b. cineangiography
> b. intracavitary probe
> b. seriography

bipolar
> b. cautery
> B. Circumactive Probe
> b. cutting loop
> b. depression
> b. diathermy coagulation
> b. disorder (type 1, 2) (BPD)
> b. electrocautery
> b. electrode
> b. laparoscopic forceps
> b. taxis
> b. urological loop
> b. vaporization
> b. version

bipolarity
> prepuberal-onset b.

bipotential
bipotentiality
Bipp paste
bipronucleate
Birbeck
> B. granule
> B. granule-positive cell

birch tree pollen
Bird
> B. Mark 8 respirator
> B. OP cup
> B. vacuum extractor

bird-beak jaw
bird-headed
> b.-h. dwarfism
> b.-h. dwarf of Seckel
> b.-h. dwarf syndrome

birdlike
> b. face syndrome
> b. facies

bird's beak appearance
Birnberg bow
birth
- b. amputation
- b. anomaly
- b. asphyxia
- asynchronous b.
- breech b.
- b. canal
- b. canal laceration
- b. care center
- b. certificate
- b. control
- b. control pill (BCP)
- b. cushion
- date of b. (DOB)
- b. defect
- dry b.
- b. fracture
- gravida, para, multiple births, abortions, live b.'s (GPMAL)
- head b.
- higher-order b.
- home b.
- b. injury
- b. length
- live b.
- multiple b.'s
- b. paralysis
- premature b.
- preterm b.
- b. rate
- spontaneous preterm b. (SPTB)
- b. trauma
- b. trauma theory
- twin b.
- b. weight (BW)
- b. weight discordance
- b. weight for gestational age (BWGA)
- b. weight Z score
- wrongful b.
- year of b. (YOB)

birthing
- b. ball
- b. chair
- b. position
- b. room

birthmark
- vascular b.

BIS
- budesonide inhalation suspension

Bisac-Evac
bisacodyl
- b. suppository
- b. tablet
- b. Uniserts

bis-chloroethylnitrosourea (BCNU)
biscoumacetate
- ethyl b.

Bi-Set catheter
bisexual
- gay, lesbian, b. (GLB)
- b. relationship

bisexuality
bisferiens
- pulsus b.

Bishop
- B. pelvic scoring system
- B. Prelabor Scoring System
- B. score
- B. score of cervical ripening

Bishop-Harmon forceps
Bishop-Koop
- B.-K. ileostomy
- B.-K. procedure

bishydroxycoumarin
Bismatrol
bismuth
- b. subsalicylate
- b. sulfite, glucose, glycine, yeast (BiGGY)
- b. toxicity

bisphosphonate therapy
bis(piareloyloxymethyl) (bis-POM)
bis-POM
- bis(piareloyloxymethyl)

Biswas Silastic vaginal pessary
bitartrate
- dihydrocodeine b.

bite
- animal b.
- black widow spider b.
- cat b.
- b. cell
- chigger b.
- closed b.
- dog b.
- human b.
- insect b.
- open b.
- b. reflex
- spider b.

B

NOTES

bite *(continued)*
   stork b.
   tick b.
bitemporal
   b. aplasia cutis congenita
   b. diameter
   b. forceps marks syndrome
   b. hemianopia
bithionol
biting
   tongue b.
bitolterol
Bitot spot
bitterling pregnancy test
bivalent chromosome
bivalved cast
bivalve speculum
bivalving of the uterus
bivariate
biventricular hypertrophy
bivia
   Prevotella b.
Bixler
   B. hypertelorism
   B. syndrome
Björnstad syndrome
BK
   human papovavirus BK
BL
  Burkitt lymphoma
black
   b. dot
   b. dot ringworm
   B. Draught
   b. hairy tongue
   b. jaundice
   b. line
   b. locks with albinism and deafness syndrome (BADS)
   b. measles
   b. pigmentation
   b. spot
   b. widow spider
   b. widow spider bite
blackened speculum
Blackfan-Diamond
   B.-D. anemia
   B.-D. syndrome
blackhead
blackout
   weight-lifter b.
blackwater fever
bladder
   b. augmentation
   b. blade
   b. bubble
   b. capacity
   b. catheter
   b. catheterization

Christmas tree b.
b. control
defunctionalized b.
b. diverticulum
b. dysfunction
b. emptying
b. exstrophy
exstrophy of the b.
b. filling
b. flap
b. function
b. habit
b. hypotonia
hypotonic b.
iatrogenic b.
b. injury
b. instability
b. instrumentation
kidneys, ureters, b. (KUB)
b. laceration
low pressure b.
b. muscle stress test
b. neck
b. neck elevation test
b. neck mobility
b. neck obstruction
b. neck stenosis
b. neck surgery
b. neck suspension
neurogenic b.
neuropathic b.
nonneurogenic neurogenic b.
occult neurogenic b.
b. outlet syndrome
overactive b. (OAB)
b. pillar
b. pressure
psychologic nonneuropathic b.
radiolucent circular shadow in b.
b. reflection
b. retractor
b. retraining
b. retraining drill
b. sphincter paralysis
stammering b.
b. stretching
b. tap
b. tumor
uninhibited b.
unstable b.
urinary b.
in utero drainage of fetal b.
b. wall
walnut-shaped b.
BladderManager portable ultrasound scanner
BladderScan BVI2500
bladder-stretching exercise

blade
- #15 b.
- Balfour bladder b.
- Bard-Parker b.
- bladder b.
- E-Mac laryngoscope b.
- Endo-Assist retractable b.
- laryngoscope b.
- Miller b. (#0, #1)
- Orbit b.

Blair-Brown procedure

Blaivas classification of urinary incontinence

Blake closure of peritoneum

Blalock-Hanlon
- B.-H. atrial septostomy procedure
- B.-H. operation

Blalock-Taussig
- B.-T. operation
- B.-T. shunt
- B.-T. shunt procedure

blanch

blanching
- cutaneous b.
- episodic b.
- laser b.
- b. macule
- b. pallor
- b. wheal and flare lesion

bland cytology

Bland-Garland-White syndrome

Blane
- amniotic infection syndrome of B.

blanket
- Bear Hugger warming b.
- bilirubin b.
- cooling b.
- forced-air b.
- plastic b.
- space b.
- b. swinging

Blaschko line

blast
- b. crisis
- leukemic b.

blastema
- metanephric b.
- renal b.

blastemic

blastocele

blastocyst
- b. hatching

- b. implantation
- b. splitting
- b. transfer

Blastocystis hominis

blastocyte

blastoderm
- bilaminar b.
- embryonic b.
- trilaminar b.

blastodisk

blastogenesis

blastogenic period

blastolysis

blastoma
- nodular renal b.
- pleuropulmonary b. (PPB)
- primitive b.

blastomere
- b. cell
- b. separation

Blastomyces dermatitidis

blastomycosis
- Brazilian b.
- Lutz-Splendore-Almeida b.
- South American b.

blastomycosis-like pyoderma

blastotomy

blastula

blastysis
- trichorrhexis b.

Blaustein classification

bleb
- pulmonary b.
- subpleural b.
- venous b.

bleed
- brain b.
- extraembryonic b.
- fetomaternal b.
- herald b.
- intraparenchymal b.
- intraventricular b.
- joint b.
- physiologic neonatal withdrawal b.

bleed-back valve

bleeding
- abnormal uterine b. (AUB)
- abnormal vaginal b.
- anovulatory b.
- antepartum b.
- breakthrough b. (BTB)
- catastrophic b.

NOTES

bleeding *(continued)*
cyclic uterine b.
b. diathesis
dysfunctional uterine b. (DUB)
estrogen breakthrough b.
estrogen-progesterone withdrawal b.
estrogen withdrawal b.
GI b.
gum b.
implantation b.
intermenstrual b.
intracranial b.
intractable uterine b.
mucocutaneous b.
mucosal b.
pelvic b.
placental b.
postcoital b.
postdouching b.
postmenarchal b.
postmenopausal b. (PMB)
preadolescent vaginal b.
progesterone breakthrough b.
progesterone withdrawal b.
b. scan
self-limited b.
severe gastrointestinal b. (SGIB)
b. site
b. site ligation
space of Retzius b.
subependymal b.
third trimester b.
b. time
uterine withdrawal b.
vaginal b.
withdrawal b.
Bleier clip
blennorrhagia
blennorrhagic
blennorrhagicum
keratoderma b.
blennorrhea
blennorrheal
Blenoxane
bleomycin
cisplatin, vinblastine, and b.
b., Eldisine, mitomycin, Platinol (BEMP)
b., etoposide, cisplatin (BEP)
b., etoposide, Platinol (BEP)
b., ifosfamide, Platinol (BIP)
b. sulfate
Bleph-10
blepharitis
seborrheic b.
simple squamous b.
staphylococcal b.
ulcerative b.

blepharochalasis
blepharocheilodontic (BCD)
b. syndrome
blepharoconjunctivitis
blepharonasofacial malformation syndrome
blepharophimosis
b., ptosis, epicanthus inversus (BPEI)
b., ptosis, epicanthus inversus syndrome (BPEIS)
b., ptosis, epicanthus inversus, telecanthus complex
b., ptosis, syndactyly, short stature syndrome
b. sequence
blepharoptosis, blepharophimosis, epicanthus inversus, telecanthus syndrome
blepharospasm
blepharostenosis
BLES
bovine lavage extract surfactant
Blessig groove
blighted ovum
blind
legally b.
b. loop syndrome
b. trachea
b. vagina
b. vaginal pouch
blinded challenge
blind-ending vagina
blindness
congenital retinitis b. (CRB)
congenital stationary night b.
cortical b.
Episkopi b.
night b.
transient cortical b.
blinking
paroxysmal b.
rapid b.
blink reflex
BLIS
breast leakage inhibitor system
blister
arthropod-induced b.
b. cell
fever b.
intraepidermal b.
recurrent b.
rosettelike b.
subepidermal b.
sucking b.
suprabasal b.
tense b.
BlisterFilm dressing

B

blistering
    b. disease
    b. distal dactylitis
    b. sunburn
Blistik
Blizzard syndrome
BLL
    blood lead level
        capillary BLL
BLM
    borderline malignancy
bloat
    gas b.
bloated abdomen
bloc
    en b.
Bloch-Siemens syndrome
Bloch-Sulzberger
    B.-S. melanoblastoma
    B.-S. syndrome
block
    atrioventricular b.
    autoimmune-associated congenital heart b.
    bifascicular b.
    bundle branch b. (BBB)
    Cerrobend b.
    complete atrioventricular b.
    complete fetal heart b.
    congenital complete AV b.
    congenital complete heart b. (CCHB)
    congenital heart b.
    b. design test
    dorsal penile nerve b. (DPNB)
    enzymatic b.
    extradural b.
    field b.
    first-degree AV b.
    heart b.
    iatrogenic complete heart b.
    intramuscular b.
    lead b.
    left bundle branch b.
    Mobitz (I, II) b.
    nerve b.
    paracervical b.
    peripheral nerve b.
    pudendal b.
    radial nerve b.
    regional nerve b.
    right bundle branch b. (RBBB)
    saddle b.
    second-degree heart b.
    sinoatrial b.
    spinal subarachnoid b.
    subarachnoid b.
    supraorbital nerve b.
    third-degree AV b.
    ulnar nerve b.
    b. vertebra
    Wenckebach b.
blockade
    beta-adrenergic b.
    neuromuscular b.
    paracervical b.
    serotonergic reuptake b.
    serotonin receptor b.
    spinal b.
    sympathetic b.
blockage
    epiglottal b.
    neuromuscular b.
    proximal tubal b.
    shunt b.
blocked
    b. duct
    b. premature atrial complex
blocker
    adrenergic b.
    alpha-adrenergic b.
    antiandrogen receptor b.
    beta b.
    calcium channel b.
    cyproheptadine receptor b.
    ganglionic b.
    H_2 b.
    serotonin reuptake b.
blocking factor
Block-Sulzberger incontinentia pigmenti
Bloedorn applicator
blood
    b. agar
    b. alcohol
    b. alcohol concentration (BAC)
    b. alcohol level (BAL)
    b. ammonia level
    arterialized b.
    autologous cord b.
    b. cell indices
    b. chimerism
    b. chromosome analysis
    b. component
    b. component therapy

NOTES

blood (*continued*)
    cord b.
    b. count
    b. culture
    designated donor b.
    donor-specific b.
    b. dyscrasia
    b. ethanol
    b. extravasation
    fetal cord b.
    b. flow (Q̇)
    b. gas
    b. gas analysis
    b. gas determination
    b. glucose
    b. glycine
    b. group
    b. group antibody
    b. group D variant equivalent to
      Rh-negative (Du)
    b. group immunization
    b. group incompatibility
    b. grouping
    b. group isoimmunization
    intervillous b.
    b. lactate
    b. lead
    b. lead level (BLL)
    b. loss
    maternal peripheral b.
    b. mole
    occult b.
    oxygenated fetal b.
    b. patch
    peripheral b.
    b. PHE
    b. pigment stain
    b. pressure (BP)
    b. pressure cuff size
    b. pressure gradient
    b. pressure measurement
    b. pressure monitor
    b. pressure transducer
    b. product
    b. relationship
    b. relative
    b. sample
    b. sampling
    b. smear
    b. spot
    b. sugar
    b. sugar monitoring
    swallowed maternal b.
    b. transfusion
    b. type A, AB, B, O
    b. typing
    b. urea nitrogen (BUN)
    b. vessel
    b. vessel elasticity
    b. vessel formation
    b. vessel transillumination
    b. volume
    whole b.
blood-borne pathogen
blood-brain barrier (BBB)
blood-flecked gastric aspirate
Bloodgood
    B. disease
    B. syndrome
blood-loss anemia
bloodstream infection (BSI)
blood-testis barrier
blood-type test
bloody
    b. CSF
    b. diarrhea
    b. show
Bloom syndrome
blot, blotting
    Eastern b.
    enzyme-linked immunotransfer b.
      (EITB)
    Northern b.
    serum enzyme-linked
      immunoelectrotransfer b.
    Southern b.
    Western b.
Blount
    B. disease
    B. syndrome
blow-by
    b.-b. oxygen
    b.-b. through tubing
blowing decrescendo diastolic murmur
blowout
    b. fracture
    b. injury
    orbital b.
BLS
    basic life support
Bluboro powder
blue
    b. asphyxia
    b. baby
    b. baby syndrome
    b. cone monochromatism
    b. diaper syndrome
    b. dome cyst
    b. dome syndrome
    b. dot sign
    b. histiocyte syndrome
    maternity b.'s
    methylene b.
    b. navel
    b. papule
    postpartum b.'s
    b. ring pessary
    b. rubber bleb nevus

b. rubber bleb nevus syndrome
(BRBNS)
b. sclera
b. scleral hue
b. spell
b. spot
toluidine b.
blueberry
b. muffin baby
b. muffin nodule
b. muffin rash
b. muffin skin lesion
b. muffin spot
b. muffin syndrome
blue-cell sarcoma
blue-green algae
bluish-black macule
bluish discoloration of flank
Blumberg sign
Blumer shelf
blunt
b. aspirator
b. cardiac injury (BCI)
b. cardiac trauma
b. chest trauma
b. curettage
b. duct adenosis
b. probe
b. and sharp dissection
Bluntport disposable trocar
blurred vision
blurring of left psoas margin
blush
ciliary b.
erythematous b.
terminal b.
tumor b.
BM
basal membrane
BMA
bone marrow aspirate
BMC
bone mineral content
BMD
Becker muscular dystrophy
bone mineral density
BMI
body mass index
BMI Z-score
BMM
bone mineral mass
B-mode ultrasound

BMR
basal metabolic rate
BMT
bilateral myringotomy tubes
bone marrow transplant
bone marrow transplantation
allogenic BMT
autologous BMT
BMZ
basement membrane zone
BN
bulimia nervosa
BNBAS
Brazelton Neonatal Behavioral
Assessment Scale
BN-NP
bulimia nervosa nonpurging
BOA
behavioral observation audiometry
born on arrival
board
arm b.
back b.
communication b.
papoose b.
prone b.
recumbent infant b.
scooter b.
vestibular b.
boarder baby
Boari flap
Bobath
B. physical therapy
B. response
bobbing
head b.
ocular b.
bobble-head doll syndrome
Bochdalek
congenital diaphragmatic hernia
of B.
B. hernia
Bockhart impetigo
BOD
brachymorphism, onychodysplasia,
dysphalangism
BOD syndrome
Bodian-Schwachman syndrome
body
b. alignment
Aschoff b.
asteroid b.

NOTES

109

body *(continued)*
    Barr b.
    b. body
    Call-Exner b.
    b. coils of cord
    b. composition
    b. conscious
    Cowdry types A, B inclusion b.
    Creola b.
    cytoid b.
    dense b.
    Döhle b.
    Donovan b.
    b. dysmorphic disorder (BDD)
    esophageal foreign b.
    extracranial foreign b.
    b. fat
    b. fluid
    foreign b.
    Golgi b.
    b. habitus
    Heinz b.
    b. homeostasis
    Howell-Jolly b.
    hyaline b.
    b. image
    inclusion b.
    intracranial foreign b.
    intranuclear inclusion b.
    b. jacket
    ketone b.
    Lafora b.
    lamellar b. (LB)
    lamellar inclusion b.
    b. language
    lateral geniculate b.
    b. lead burden
    loose b.
    Lostorfer b.
    b. louse
    lyssa b.
    b. mass index (BMI)
    b. mass index nomogram
    b. morphometrics
    Negri b.
    Nissl b.'s
    osmiophilic b.
    owl's eye inclusion b.
    perineal b.
    b. phenotype
    pineal b.
    polar b.
    b. proportion measurement
    psammoma b.
    refractile b.
    retained foreign b.
    b. ringworm
    b. rocking
    Schaumann b.
    Schiller-Duvall b.
    b. shell
    b. size
    b. stalk
    b. stalk anomaly
    b. stalk malformation
    striate b.
    b. surface area (BSA)
    b. surface area calculation
    b. temperature
    vaginal foreign b.
    vertebral b.
    vitreous b.
    Weibel-Palade b.
    b. weight
    Winkler b.
    zebra b.

bodybuilding
body-image distortion
BOF
    branchiooculofacial
BOFS
    branchiooculofacial syndrome
Bogalusa Heart Study (BHS)
boggy
    b. synovial effusion
    b. uterus
Bogros space
Bohn
    B. epithelial pearls
    B. nodule
Bohr effect
Bohring syndrome
Boix-Ochoa
    B.-O. GER score (BOS)
    B.-O. procedure
Bolivian hemorrhagic fever
bolster
bolt
    subarachnoid b.
bolus
    b. dose
    fecal b.
    fluid b.
    b. fluid therapy
    isotonic b.
    b. tube feeding
Bombay erythrocyte phenotype
BOME
    bilateral otitis media with effusion
Bonamine
bond
    hydrogen b.
bonding
    maternal-infant b.
    mother-infant b.
bone
    b. accretion
    b. age

b. age determination
b. age standard of Greulich and Pyle
b. alkaline phosphatase (BAP)
b. ALP
b. anchor
aseptic necrosis of b.
b. attenuation coefficient
b. avascular necrosis
brittle b.'s
capitate b.
b. collagen equivalent unit (BCE)
cortical b.
craniobasal b.
cuneiform b.
b. demineralization
b. densitometry
b. density
b. density measurement
dwarfism and cortical thickening of tubular b.'s
b. dysplasia
ethmoid b.
fiber b.
flat frontal b.
b. formation
fragmentation of necrotic b.
b. graft
b. hemangioma
high frontal b.
hyoid b.
b. infection
innominate b.
ivory b.'s
lacrimal b.
lamellar b.
long b.
b. loss
marble b.'s
b. marrow
b. marrow aplasia
b. marrow aspirate (BMA)
b. marrow aspiration
b. marrow biopsy
b. marrow cytogenetics
b. marrow dysfunction
b. marrow failure
b. marrow hypoplasia
b. marrow infiltration
b. marrow puncture
b. marrow relapse
b. marrow stem cell

b. marrow suppression
b. marrow toxicity
b. marrow transplant (BMT)
b. marrow transplantation (BMT)
b. mass
b. matrix
maxillary b.
b. mineral
b. mineral content (BMC)
b. mineral density (BMD)
b. mineral mass (BMM)
b. mineral measurement
b. mineral metabolism
b. mineral uptake
nasal b.
navicular b.
omovertebral b.
b. pain
parietal b.
b. quantitative ultrasound velocity
b. remodeling
b. resorption
round iliac b.
b. scan
b. sclerosis
short metacarpal b.
small maxillary b.
sphenoid b.
b. stippling
b. strength measurement
b. tissue mineralization
tubular b.
b. tumor
turbinate b.
b. turnover
weightbearing b.
wormian b.'s
woven b.
zygomatic b.
bone-age determination method
bone-specific alkaline phosphatase
Bonine
Bonnaire method
Bonnano catheter
Bonneau syndrome
Bonnet-Dechaume-Blanc syndrome
Bonnevie-Ullrich syndrome
Bonney
  B. abdominal hysterectomy
  B. blue stress incontinence test
Bontril

NOTES

111

bony
>   b. dysplasia
>   b. enlargement
>   b. erosion
>   b. metastasis
>   b. projection
>   b. spur

book
>   communication b.

Bookwalter retractor
boomerang
>   b. dysplasia
>   b. syndrome

Boom syndrome
BOOP
>   bronchiolitis obliterans organizing
>   pneumonia

Boost
>   B. nutritional drink
>   B. nutritional supplement

booster
>   tetanus toxoid b.

boot-shaped heart
BOR
>   branchiootorenal
>   BOR dysplasia
>   BOR syndrome

borborygmus, pl. **borborygmi**
border
>   serpiginous b.
>   shaggy heart b.

borderline
>   b. amniotic fluid index
>   Child Version of the Retrospective
>   Diagnostic Interview for B.'s
>   b. diabetes
>   b. epithelial ovarian carcinoma
>   b. epithelial ovarian neoplasm
>   b. epithelial ovarian tumor
>   b. intelligence
>   b. lepromatous leprosy
>   b. malignancy (BLM)
>   b. malignant epithelial neoplasm
>   b. personality disorder
>   b. tuberculoid
>   b. tuberculoid leprosy

borderline-resistant *Staphylococcus*
>   *aureus* (BRSA)
Bordetella
>   *B. bronchiseptica*
>   *B. parapertussis*
>   *B. pertussis*

Bordet-Gengoi medium
boredom
Borg
>   B. Perceived Exertion Scale
>   B. Physical Activity Scale

boric
>   b. acid
>   b. acid capsule

Börjeson-Forssman-Lehmann (BFL)
>   B.-F.-L. syndrome (BFLS)

Börjeson syndrome
Borna disease virus
borne
Bornholm disease
born on arrival (BOA)
boron
Boropak
Borrelia
>   *B. afzelii*
>   *B. burgdorferi*
>   *B. burgdorferi* sensu lato
>   *B. burgdorferi* sensu stricto
>   *B. garinii*
>   *B. recurrentis*

borreliosis
Borsieri sign
BOS
>   Boix-Ochoa GER score

Bosma Henkin Christiansen syndrome
bosselated
bossing
>   frontal b.
>   occipital b.

Boston
>   B. exanthem
>   B. Naming Test
>   B. orthosis

Boston-type craniosynostosis
Botox
botryoid
>   b. pseudosarcoma
>   b. sarcoma

botryoides
>   sarcoma b.

Botryomycosis
bottle
>   disposable b.
>   b. fed
>   b. feed
>   Mead Johnson b.
>   Nursette prefilled disposable b.
>   prefilled disposable b.
>   b. propping
>   b. tooth decay
>   transgrow b.

bottle-fed baby
botulinum
>   b. antitoxin (type A, B, E)
>   *Clostridium b.*
>   b. immune globulin
>   b. toxin
>   b. toxin A (BTA)

botulinus
    b. intoxication
    b. neurotoxin
botulism
    Clostridium b.
    infantile b. (IB)
    b. toxin
    wound b.
Bouchut respiration
Boudreaux's
    B's Butt balm
    B's Butt paste
bougie
    b. dilator
    Holinger infant b.
bougienage
Bouin solution
boulardii
    Saccharomyces b.
bouncing
bound
    b. estradiol
    b. testosterone
bounding pulse
Bourneville
    B. disease
    B. syndrome
Bourneville-Brissaud disease
Bourneville-Pringle syndrome
Bourns
    B. infant respirator
    B. LS104-150 infant ventilator
boutonneuse fever
boutonnière
    b. finger
    b. incision
Bovie
    B. cauterization
    B. cautery
    B. unit
bovina
    facies b.
bovine
    b. dermal collagen
    b. face
    b. facies
    b. lavage extract surfactant (BLES)
    b. mucus penetration test
    pegademase b.
    b. pericardium patch
    b. spongiform encephalopathy
      (BSE)

    b. surfactant
    b. tuberculosis
bovis
    Mycobacterium b.
    Streptococcus b.
BOW
    bag of waters
bow
    Birnberg b.
    cupid's b.
    posteromedial b.
bowel
    b. adaptation
    aganglionic b.
    b. angina
    b. atony
    b. clean-out
    b. duplication
    echogenic fetal b.
    b. function
    b. habit
    hyperechoic b.
    impacted b.
    b. infarction
    b. injury
    invaginated b.
    b. irrigation
    b. lengthening procedure
    b. loop resection
    malrotation of b.
    neurogenic b.
    b. obstruction
    perforated b.
    b. preparation
    proximal b.
    b. segment resection
    short small-b. (SSB)
    b. sounds
    b. stasis
Bowen
    B. double-bladed scalpel
    B. Hutterite syndrome
Bowen-Conradi syndrome
bowenoid
    b. atypia
    b. papulosis
bowing
    anterior tibial b.
    anterolateral tibial b.
    congenital posteromedial b.
    b. deformity
    b. fracture

NOTES

bowing *(continued)*
    lateral tibial b.
    posteromedial tibial b.
    b. reflex
    tibial b.
    traumatic b.
bowleg
    physiologic b.
bowleggedness
bowl of pelvis
Bowman
    B. capsule
    B. layer
    B. space
bowstringing of tendon
box
    head b.
    Hogness b.
    negative-pressure b.
    paired b.
    Pribnow b.
boxer's fracture
boydii
    Pseudallescheria b.
Boyle uterine elevator
Bozeman
    B. operation
    B. position
    B. uterine dressing forceps
Bozeman-Fritsch catheter
BP
    blood pressure
B-PAP *(var. of* BiPAP)
BPD
    biparietal diameter
    bipolar disorder (type 1, 2)
    bronchopulmonary dysplasia
BPEC
    benign partial epilepsy with
      centrotemporal spike
BPEI
    blepharophimosis, ptosis, epicanthus
      inversus
BPEIS
    blepharophimosis, ptosis, epicanthus
      inversus syndrome
BPF
    bronchopulmonary fistula
BPG
    benzathine penicillin G
BPI
    bactericidal/permeability-increasing
      protein
    Behavior Problem Inventory
    brachial plexus injury
bpm
    beats per minute
    breaths per minute

BPP
    biophysical profile
      antepartum fetal BPP
      fetal BPP
      modified BPP
      BPP score
BPS
    bronchopulmonary sequestration
BPV
    benign paroxysmal vertigo
bra
    lead b.
braakii
    Citrobacter b.
BRACA, BRCA
    BRCA1 and BRCA2
      multisite BRACA
      BRACA mutation test
      single site BRACA
BRACAnalyzer gene analyzer
brace
    cast boot b.
    Charleston b.
    Cruiser hip abduction b.
    Friedman Splint b.
    b. management
    Milwaukee b.
    Rhino Triangle b.
    Risser b.
    b. treatment
bracelet
    BioBands b.
    MedicAlert b.
brachial
    b. artery
    b. birth palsy
    b. plexopathy
    b. plexus
    b. plexus injury (BPI)
    b. plexus palsy
    b. plexus stretching
brachiocephalic vessel
brachioradialis reflex
brachioskeletogenital (BSG)
Brachmann-Cornelia
    B.-C. de Lange (BCDL)
    B.-C. de Lange syndrome
      (BCDLS)
Bracht maneuver
brachycamptodactyly
brachycephalic configuration
brachycephalosyndactyly
brachycephaly, deafness, cataract, microstomia, mental retardation syndrome
brachydactyly
    b., dwarfism, hearing loss,
      microcephaly, mental retardation
      syndrome

b., mesomelia, mental retardation,
aortic dilation, mitral valve
prolapse, characteristic facies
syndrome
b., nystagmus, cerebellar ataxia
syndrome
Pitt-Williams b.
Sugarman b.
brachydactyly-distal symphalangism
syndrome
brachydactyly-ectrodactyly
brachygnathia
brachymelia
rhizomelic b.
brachymesomelia-renal syndrome
brachymesophalangy,
brachymesophalangism
brachymetacarpalia, brachymetacarpalism
b., cataract, mesiodens syndrome
brachymetacarpy
brachymetatarsus IV
brachymorphism, onychodysplasia,
dysphalangism (BOD)
brachyolmia
brachypelvic, brachypellic
brachysyndactyly
brachytelephalangy
brachytelomesophalangy
brachytherapy
interstitial b.
intracavitary b.
remote afterloading b. (RAB)
Bradley
B. childbirth education
B. method
B. method of prepared childbirth
bradyarrhythmia
bradycardia
apnea and b. (A&B)
baseline fetal b.
feeding b.
fetal b.
post cordocentesis b.
prolonged b.
sinus b.
vagotonic b.
bradycardiac
bradycardia-tachycardia syndrome
bradygenesis
bradykinin antagonist
bradylexia
bradymenorrhea

bradyspermatism
bradytocia
Bragg-Paul respirator
Bragg peak
Brailsford
B. disease
B. syndrome
brain
b. atrophy
b. bleed
butterfly b.
coning of b.
b. damage
b. death
b. disorder
b. dysfunction
b. edema
b. electrical activity map (BEAM)
b. electrical activity mapping
(BEAM)
fetal b.
b. function
b. herniation
b. imaging technique
b. injury
b. lesion
b. mapping
b. metabolism
b. peptide
b. sparing
b. swelling
b. tumor
b. vesicle
b. wart
water on b.
b. wave
brain-death syndrome
brain-derived neurotrophic factor
(BDNF)
brain-sparing effect
brainstem, brain stem
b. auditory evoked potential
(BAEP)
b. auditory evoked response
(BAER, BSAER)
b. auditory tract
b. compression
b. encephalitis
b. evoked response (BSER)
b. evoked response audiometry
(BSERA)
b. function

NOTES

brainstem *(continued)*
>   b. glioma
>   b. herniation
>   b. lesion

2-Br-alpha-ergocryptine mesylate
branched
>   b. deoxyribonucleic acid (bDNA)
>   b. DNA

branched-chain
>   b.-c. amino acid
>   b.-c. amino acidemia
>   b.-c. aminotransferase
>   b.-c. fatty acid (BCFA)
>   b.-c. ketoacid
>   b.-c. ketoaciduria
>   b.-c. ketonuria

brancher deficiency
branchial
>   b. arch
>   b. arch syndrome
>   b. cleft
>   b. cleft anomaly
>   b. cleft cyst
>   b. cleft fistula
>   b. cleft remnant
>   b. cleft sinus
>   b. clefts-lip pseudocleft syndrome
>   b. ducts
>   b. plexus
>   b. pouch

branching
>   airway b.
>   b. enzyme deficiency
>   b. enzyme deficiency
>   amylopectinosis
>   fetal capillary b.
>   b. morphogenesis
>   b. pattern
>   b. snowflake test

branchiomere
branchiooculofacial (BOF)
>   b. syndrome (BOFS)

branchiootic syndrome
branchiootorenal (BOR)
Brandt-Andrews maneuver
Brandt syndrome
Branhamella catarrhalis
brash
>   weaning b.

brasiliensis
>   *Nocardia b.*
>   *Paracoccidioides b.*

brassy cough
BRAT
>   bananas, rice cereal, applesauce, toast
>   BRAT diet

BRATT
>   bananas, rice, applesauce, tea, toast
>   BRATT diet

Bratton-Marshall test
Braun
>   B. episiotomy scissors
>   B. tympanic thermometer

Braune canal
Braun-Schroeder single-tooth tenaculum
Bravelle
brawny
>   b. dermatitis
>   b. edema
>   b. hyperpigmentation
>   b. scaling

Braxton
>   B. Hicks contraction
>   B. Hicks sign
>   B. Hicks version

**Brazelton Neonatal Behavioral
  Assessment Scale (BNBAS)**
Brazilian blastomycosis
braziliense
>   *Ancylostoma b.*

braziliensis
>   *Leishmania b.*

BRBNS
>   blue rubber bleb nevus syndrome

BRCA *(var. of* BRACA*)*
BRCA1
>   breast cancer gene 1
>   BRCA1 gene mutation

BRCA2
>   breast cancer gene 2
>   BRCA2 gene mutation

BRCA1 and BRCA2 (BRACA, BRCA)
>   breast cancer gene 1

BRE
>   benign rolandic epilepsy

bread-and-butter appearance
breakage
>   catheter b.
>   chromosome b.

BreakAway dressing
breakdown
>   endometrial b.
>   germinal vesicle b. (GVBD)
>   skin b.
>   wound b.

breakpoint cluster region (bcr)
breakthrough
>   b. bleeding (BTB)
>   b. varicella

breast
>   b. abscess
>   accessory b.
>   adolescent b.
>   augmented b.
>   b. binder
>   b. binding
>   b. biopsy tissue
>   b. bud

caked b.
b. cancer
B. Cancer Detection Demonstration
  Project (BCDDP)
b. cancer gene 1 (BRCA1,
  BRCA1 and BRCA2)
b. cancer gene 2 (BRCA2)
b. cancer prevention trial (BCPT)
B. Cancer System 2100
b. carcinoma
b. care
b. change
childhood b.
b. conservation
b. conservation therapy (BCT)
Contour Profile anatomically shaped
  silicone b.
Cooper irritable b.
b. cyst
b. development
b. disease
b. embryology
engorged b.
b. engorgement
b. enlargement
fibrocystic b.
b. flush
b. implant
irritable b.
keeled b.
lactating b.
b. leakage inhibitor system (BLIS)
b. macrocalcification
b. malignancy
b. milk
b. milk jaundice
nonlactating b.
Paget disease of b.
peau d'orange appearance of
  the b.
pendulous b.
pigeon b.
b. plate
proemial b.
b. prosthesis
b. pump
sclerosing adenosis of b.
b. secretion
b. self-examination (BSE)
shotty b.
b. stimulation contraction test
  (BSCT)

supernumerary b.
Trilucent b.
true accessory b.
**BreastAlert differential temperature
  sensor**
BreastCheck
breast-conserving therapy (BCT)
BreastExam
breast-fed, breastfed
    breast-fed baby
breast-feed
breast-feeding
    failed b.
    b. jaundice
breast/ovarian familial cancer syndrome
breast-preserving therapy
breaststroker's knee
breath
    fetid b.
    b. holding
    b. H$_2$ test
    b. hydrogen excretion test
    b. hydrogen study
    malodorous b.
    b.'s per minute (bpm)
    b. sounds
    strep b.
    b. testing
    B. Tracker
    uriniferous b.
**breath-by-breath method of gas
  collection**
Breathe
    B. Easy foam pad
    B. Free
    B. Right
breath-holding spell
breath-hold MR cholangiography
breathing
    abdominal b.
    fetal b.
    intermittent positive pressure b.
      (IPPB)
    mouth b.
    mouth-to-mask b.
    paradoxical b.
    b. pattern
    patterned b.
    periodic b.
    rescue b.
    seesaw b.
    sleep-disordered b.

NOTES

breathing *(continued)*
    spontaneous periodic b.
    stridulous b.
    synchronous b.
    tidal b.
    tubular b.
    upper airway sleep-disordered b.
    work of b.
breathing-related sleep disorder
Breathmobile mobile asthma testing lab
Brecht feeder
breech
    assisted b.
    b. baby
    b. birth
    b. deformation sequence
    b. extraction
    frank b.
    b. head
    b. location
    b. location out of pelvis
    midfoot b.
    nonfrank b.
    b. position
    b. presentation
    b. singleton
    spontaneous b.
    b. type
    b. vaginal delivery
breech-born with delayed fetal activity
breech-first twin
breed
breeding
    cross b.
    b. line
Breeze
    B. respirator
    B. ventilator
Breezee Mist Aerosol
bregma
bregmatodymia
bregmocardiac reflex
Breisky-Navratil retractor
Brennen biosynthetic surgical mesh
Brenner tumor
Brentano syndrome
brephic
brephoplastic
brephotrophic
brequinar
Breslow-Day test
Breslow microstaging system
B$_6$-responsive anemia
Brethine
Brett
    B. epileptogenic encephalopathy
    B. syndrome
bretylium tosylate

Breuer-Hering inflation reflex
Breus mole
breve
    Bifidobacterium b.
Brevibloc
Brevicon
Brevi-Kath epidural catheter
brevis
    Demodex b.
Brevital Sodium
Brewster retractor
Briard-Evans syndrome
Bricker
    B. procedure
    B. ureteroileostomy
bridge
    flat nasal b.
    low nasal b.
    membrane b.
    nasal b.
    physial b.
    B. Reading Program
bridging
    b. cross
    b. flap
    b. physis
    b. vein
brief
    b. reactive psychosis
    b., small, abundant motor-unit action potential (BSAP)
    b. tonic seizure
Brigance Diagnostic Inventory of Early Development
Briggs T adapter
bright
    b. thalamus syndrome
    b. white light therapy for postpartum depression
Brill disease
Brill-Zinsser disease
brim
    pelvic b.
    b. sign
brine flotation method
bring-your-own medical record
bris
Brissaud
    B. dwarfism
    B. infantilism
    B. syndrome
Bristol Female Lower Urinary Tract Symptoms (BFLUTS)
British antilewisite (BAL)
brittle
    b. bones
    b. diabetes
    b. hair

b. hair, intellectual impairment, decreased fertility, short stature (BIDS)
b. hair-mental deficit syndrome
b. nail
brittle-bone disease
BRM
   biologic response modifier
broad
   b. débridement
   b. flat nose
   b. forehead
   b. ligament
   b. ligament fold
   b. ligament hernia
   b. ligament pregnancy
   b. ligament tear syndrome
   b. nasal base
   b. nasal root
   b. physis
   b. thumb
   b. thumb-hallux syndrome
   b. thumb-mental retardation syndrome
   b. toe
broad-band scale
broad-based gait
broad-spectrum
   b.-s. antibiotic
   b.-s. antibiotic therapy
   b.-s. white light
Broca
   B. aphasia
   B. area
   B. pouch
Brockenbrough transseptal catheterization technique
Broders index
Brodie abscess
Brodie-Trendelenburg test
Brofed Elixir
Bromaline Elixir
Bromanate Elixir
Bromatapp
bromelin method
Bromfed
   B. Syrup
   B. Tablet
Bromfenex PD
bromhidrosis
   eccrine b.
   plantar eccrine b.

bromide
   ammonium b.
   calcium b.
   cyanogen b. (CNBr)
   diphenyl tetrazolium b.
   distigmine b.
   ipratropium b.
   mepenzolate b.
   methantheline b.
   pancuronium b.
   Peacock b.
   potassium b.
   pyridostigmine b.
   sodium b.
   strontium b.
   triple b.
   vecuronium b.
bromium
bromocriptine
   Apo-B.
   injectable b.
   b. mesylate
   b. prolactinoma
   b. rebound
   b. resistance
   b. therapy
bromocriptine-resistant prolactinoma
bromodeoxyuridine (BUdR)
bromodiphenhydramine
bromomenorrhea
bromopheniramine
   b. maleate
   b. and phenylpropanolamine
bromsulfophthalein (BSP)
Bronalide
bronchi (*pl. of* bronchus)
bronchial
   b. asthma
   b. atresia
   b. breath sounds
   b. bud
   b. challenge test
   b. hyperactivity
   b. mucous cast
   b. provocation
   b. provocation challenge
   b. provocation testing
   b. tree
   b. tube
   b. wall thickening
bronchiectasis
   congenital b.

B

NOTES

bronchiolar thickening
bronchiole
    ruptured b.
    terminal b.
bronchiolectasia
bronchiolitis
    acute b.
    b. obliterans
    b. obliterans organizing pneumonia
      (BOOP)
    obliterative fibroproliferative b.
    respiratory syncytial virus b.
      (RSVB)
    RSV b.
    viral necrotizing b.
bronchiseptica
    Bordetella b.
bronchitis
    acute laryngotracheal b.
    arachidic b.
    asthmatic b.
    chronic obstructive b.
    epidemic capillary b.
    follicular b.
    obliterative b.
    plastic b.
    wheezy b.
bronchoalveolar
    b. fluid
    b. lavage (BAL)
bronchobiliary fistula
bronchoconstriction
bronchodilation
bronchodilator
    b. drug
    inhaled b.
    oral b.
    short-acting beta-2 agonist b.
bronchoesophageal fistula
bronchogenic cyst
bronchogram
    air b.
bronchomalacia
bronchomotor tone
bronchophony
bronchopleural fistula
bronchopneumonia
bronchopulmonary
    b. aspergillosis
    b. dysplasia (BPD)
    b. fistula (BPF)
    b. lavage
    b. malformation
    b. sequestration (BPS)
bronchorrhea
bronchoscope
    Holinger infant b.
    Storz infant b.

bronchoscopy
    fiberoptic b.
    flexible fiberoptic b.
    open-tube b.
    pediatric b.
    virtual b.
bronchospasm
    exercise-induced b. (EIB)
bronchospastic cough
bronchovesicular breath sounds
bronchus, pl. **bronchi**
    elastic recoil of the b.
    main b.
bronchus-associated lymphoid tissue
   (BALT)
Bronkaid
Bronkometer Aerosol
Bronson chewable prenatal vitamins
Brontex
bronze
    b. baby
    b. baby syndrome
    b. diabetes
    b. Schilder disease
Brooks syndrome
Brooks-Wisniewski-Brown syndrome
Broselow
    B. chart
    B. tape
broth
    b. culture
    Lim b.
    Todd-Hewitt b.
Brouha test
Broviac catheter
brow
    olympian b.
    b. position
    b. presentation
brow-anterior position
brow-down
    b.-d. position
    b.-d. presentation
brown
    b. baby syndrome
    b. fat nonshivering thermogenesis
    B. and Harris interview
    B. nodule
    b. recluse spider
    b. skin lesion
    B. superior oblique tendon sheath
      syndrome
    B. uvula retractor
    B. vertical retraction syndrome
Brown-Adson tissue forceps
Browne
    testis within superficial inguinal
      pouch of Denis B.
Brown-Hopp tissue Gram stain

Brown-Séquard syndrome
Brown-Symmers disease
Brown-Vialetto-Van Laere syndrome
Brown-Wickham urethral pressure
   profilometry technique
brow-posterior position
brow-up position
Broxidine
broxuridine
Brozek body fat percentage formula
BRRS
   Bannayan-Riley-Ruvalcaba syndrome
BRS
   Behavior Rating Scale
BRSA
   borderline-resistant *Staphylococcus*
   aureus
brucei
   Trypanosoma b.
Brucella
   B. agar plate
   B. canis
   B. melitensis
   B. suis
brucellosis
Bruck-de Lange syndrome
Bruckner pupillary light reflex test
Brudzinski sign
Brugada syndrome
Brugia
   B. beaveri
   B. lepori
Bruhat
   B. laser fimbrioplasty
   B. technique
Bruininks-Oseretsky
   B.-O. test
   B.-O. Test of Motor Proficiency
bruisability
   easy b.
bruit
   abdominal b.
   aortic b.
   carotid b.
   cranial b.
   b. placentaire
   placental b.
Brun
   layer of B.
Brunner
   B. gland
   B. syndrome

Brusa-Toricelli syndrome
brush
   Bayne Pap B.
   b. border assembly
   cytology b.
   b. cytology
   endocervical sampling b.
   FoamCare double scrub b.
   Stormby b.
Brushfield spot
Brushfield-Wyatt syndrome
brushing
   colposcopically directed b.
Bruton
   B. agammaglobulinemia
   B. disease
Bruton/B-cell tyrosine kinase gene
bruxism
   sleep b.
Bryan-Leishman stain
Bryant traction
Bryce-Teacher ovum
BS
   Bartter syndrome
BSA
   body surface area
BSAER
   brainstem auditory evoked response
BSAP
   brief, small, abundant motor-unit action
   potential
B-scanner
   real-time B-s.
   static B-s.
BSCT
   breast stimulation contraction test
BSE
   bovine spongiform encephalopathy
   breast self-examination
BSER
   brainstem evoked response
BSERA
   brainstem evoked response audiometry
BSG
   brachioskeletogenital
   BSG syndrome
BSI
   bloodstream infection
BSID
   Bayley Scales of Infant Development
BSID-II
   Bayley Scales of Infant Development-II

NOTES

B

BSO
bilateral salpingo-oophorectomy
BSP
bromsulfophthalein
BSSL
bile salt-stimulated lipase
BTA
botulinum toxin A
BTA stat test
BTB
breakthrough bleeding
BTL
bilateral tubal ligation
bubble
bladder b.
b. boy disease
extraluminal gas b.
gastric b.
b. gum cytoplasm
b. isolation unit
b. isolette
b. stability test
stomach b.
bubbler humidifier
bubbly
b. crackle
b. lungs
b. lung syndrome
bubo, pl. **buboes**
b. aspirate
bullet b.
chancroidal b.
climatic b.
primary b.
tropical b.
venereal b.
virulent b.
bubonic
bucca, pl. **buccae**
buccal
b. cellulitis
b. fat pad
b. feeding technique
b. mucosa
b. mucosa graft
Nitrogard B.
buccolingual apraxia
buccomandibular dystonia
bucket-handle fracture
buckle fracture
buckshot calcification
buclizine
bucrylate
bud
aortic b.
breast b.
bronchial b.
distal tongue b.
end b.

epithelial b.
hair b.
limb b.
liver b.
metanephric b.
pulmonary b.
syncytial b.
tail b.
taste b.
tooth b.
ureteric b.
Budd-Chiari syndrome
Buddhalike habitus
Buddha stance
budding
buddy taping
budesonide
controlled ileal release b.
b. inhalation suspension (BIS)
b. therapy
b. Turbuhaler
Budin rule
BUdR
bromodeoxyuridine
Buenos Aires type mental retardation
buffalo hump
Buffaprin
buffer
buffered
b. aspirin
b. lidocaine
Bufferin
Buffinol
buffy
b. coat
b. coat component
b. coat examination
b. coat layer
Bugbee electrode
Buhl disease
Buist method
bulb
femoral b.
phototherapy b.
Rouget b.
sinovaginal b.
b. suction
b. suctioning
b. syringe
vaginal b.
vestibular b.
b. of vestibule of vagina
vestibulovaginal b.
bulbar
b. conjunctiva
b. conjunctival injection
b. hereditary motor neuropathy
(type I, II)
b. palsy

b. paralysis
b. polioencephalitis
b. poliomyelitis
bulbitis
bulbocavernosus
b. fat flap
b. muscle
b. reflex
bulbocavernous reflex
bulbospinal poliomyelitis
bulbospongiosus muscle
bulbourethral gland
bulbous nasal tip
bulboventricular foramen
bulbus
b. cordis
b. penis
b. pili
b. urethrae
b. vestibuli vaginae
bulgaricus
Lactobacillus b.
bulge
biparietal b.
parietal b.
precordial b.
bulging
b. flank
b. fontanelle
bulimia
b. nervosa (BN)
b. nervosa nonpurging (BN-NP)
bulimorexia
bulk
b. flow
Modane B.
muscle b.
b. selection
bulked segregant analysis
bulk-forming laxative
bulky carcinoma
bulla, pl. **bullae**
sausage-shaped b.
scaling b.
transparent b.
bulldog syndrome
bullet bubo
bullosa
acantholysis b.
albopapuloid Pasini form of
dominant dystrophic
epidermolysis b.

Cockayne-Touraine variant of
dominant dystrophic
epidermolysis b.
concha b.
dermolysis b.
dominant dystrophic
epidermolysis b.
dystrophic epidermolysis b.
epidermolysis b. (EB)
generalized atrophic benign
epidermolysis b. (GABEB)
hereditary macular epidermolysis b.
junctional epidermolysis b.
recessive dystrophic
epidermolysis b. (RDEB)
varicella b.
bullous
b. congenital ichthyosiform
erythroderma
b. dermatosis
b. drug eruption
b. erythema multiforme
b. impetigo
b. mastocytosis
b. myringitis
b. pemphigoid
b. reaction
b. varicella
bull's eye sonographic appearance
bumetanide
Bumex
Buminate
Bumm curette
bump
Bumpa Bed crib bumper pad
bumper bed
BUN
blood urea nitrogen
bundle
b. branch block (BBB)
b. of His
hypertrophic b.
papillomacular b.
b. of Probst
bungarotoxin
bunion
adolescent b.
dorsal b.
bunionette deformity
bunny hopping
Bunostomum phlebotomum
Bunyaviridae

NOTES

Bunyavirus
BUO
    bilateral ureteral obstruction
Buphenyl
buphthalmia, buphthalmos
bupivacaine
buprenorphine
bupropion hydrochloride
Burch
    B. colposuspension
    B. colpourethropexy
    B. modification
    B. procedure
    B. retropubic urethropexy
burden
    body lead b.
    b. of care interview for children
    genetic b.
    tumor b.
burgdorferi
    Borrelia b.
Burger triangle
buried
    b. penis
    b. vaginal island procedure
Burkholderia
    B. cepacia
    B. cepacia genomovar (III)
    B. gladioli
    B. mallei
    B. multivorans
    B. multivorans genomovar (II)
    B. norimbergensis
    B. pickettii
    B. pseudomallei
    B. vietnamiensis
Burkitt
    B. lymphoma (BL)
    B. sarcoma
    B. tumor cell
burn
    alkali b.
    Berkow formula for b.'s
    circumferential b.
    deep partial-thickness b.
    dry chemical b.
    electrical b.
    b. encephalopathy
    first-degree b.
    flame b.
    fourth-degree b.
    full-thickness b.
    immersion b.
    b. management
    partial-thickness b.
    second-degree b.
    splash b.
    thermal b.
    third-degree b.

burned
    TBSA b.
burner
Burnet acquired immunity
burnetii
    Coxiella b.
burning
    b. vulva syndrome
    vulvovaginal b.
burnlike dermatitis
Burn-McKeown syndrome
burnout
    mother b.
Burow solution
burp
    wet b.
burping
burrow
    pus b.
burr-shaped erythrocyte
bursa, pl. **bursae**
    b. of Fabricius
    gastrocnemius-semimembranosus b.
    greater trochanteric b.
    iliopectineal b.
bursa-dependent system
bursitis
    pes anserina b.
    prepatellar b.
    septic b.
    suppurative b.
burst
    suppression b.
burst-forming units-erythroid (BFU-E)
bursting fracture
burst-suppression pattern
Burton gum lead line
Burt Word Reading Test
BUS
    Bartholin, urethral, Skene
    BUS glands
Busacca iris nodule
Buschke
    scleredema of B.
Buschke-Ollendorf syndrome
buserelin
BuSpar
buspirone hydrochloride
bus transport
busulfan, busulphan
butabarbital
Butalan
butalbital
Butalgen
Butanefrine
butaperazine
Butazolidin
Butazone
butenafine antifungal agent

butoconazole
    b. 2% cream
    b. nitrate
butorphanol
    b. tartrate
    b. tartrate nasal spray
butoxide
    piperonyl b.
    pyrethrins and piperonyl b.
butriptyline hydrochloride
Butschli granule
Butt
    B. Balm
    B. paste
butterbur
butterfly
    b. brain
    b. distribution
    b. drain
    b. flap
    b. rash
    b. scalp vein needle
    b. vertebrae
button
    gastrostomy b.
    peritoneal b.
buttonhole incision
buttonholing
buttonpexy fixation
buttress
    facial b.
    mechanical b.
    b. response
butyrate
    hydrocortisone b.
    b. therapy

butyrophenone
Buxton clamp
BV
    bacterial vaginosis
BVI2500
    BladderScan B.
BVM
    bag, valve, mask
    BVM device
    BVM ventilation
BW
    birth weight
BWGA
    birth weight for gestational age
BWS
    Beckwith-Wiedemann syndrome
by
    by mouth feeding
    by way of rectum (p.r.)
Byers flap
Byler
    B. disease
    B. syndrome
bypass
    cardiopulmonary b.
    b. continence mechanism
    gastric b.
    jejunoileal b.
    low-flow cardiopulmonary b.
    b. surgery
    ventricular b.
bystander effect
BZS
    Bannayan-Zonana syndrome

NOTES

C

C band
C syndrome

C1

C1 to C2 dislocation
C1 esterase inhibitor
C1 esterase inhibitor deficiency

3C

craniocerebellocardiac
3C dysplasia
3C syndrome

C-500

Optimox C.

C_{21}

C_{21} progestin
C_{21} progestogen

C_4

leukotriene C_4 (LTC_4)

C1INH coagulation inhibitor
C1r deficiency
C2–C9 deficiency
CA

carcinoma
cardiac-apnea
cellulose acetate
child abuse
chorioamnionitis
community-acquired
CA 15-3
CA 125 antigen
CA 125 assay
CA 15-3 breast cancer marker
CA 125 endometrial cancer marker
CA monitor
CA 549 tumor marker

Ca

calcium

CAA

coronary artery aneurysm

CABA

child and adolescent burden assessment

cabbage leaves
cabergoline
CaBF

carotid blood flow

cable

twister c.

Cabot

C. cannula
C. trocar

CAC

cisplatin, Ara-C, caffeine

cachectic infantilism
cachectin

cachexia

cancer c.

cacogenesis
cacomelia
Ca:Cr

calcium-creatinine ratio

CAD

computer-aided diagnosis

cadaveric donor
CADD-Prizm pain control system
cadence
CAE

cefuroxime axetil

caeruleus

locus c.
noradrenergic locus c.

CAF

cell adhesion factor
coronary artery fistula
cyclophosphamide, doxorubicin, and 5-fluorouracil
Cytoxan, Adriamycin, fluorouracil

CAFAS

Child and Adolescent Functional Assessment Scale

Cafatine
Cafcit
café au lait (CAL)

café au lait spot

Cafergot
caffeine

cisplatin, Ara-C, c. (CAC)
c. citrate
citrated c.
c. terbutaline
c. therapy

caffeinism
Caffey

C. disease
C. pseudo-Hurler syndrome

Caffey-Kenny disease
Caffey-Silverman syndrome
Caffey-Smyth-Roske syndrome
CAFMHS

child, adolescent, and family mental health service

CAFTH

Cytoxan, Adriamycin, fluorouracil, tamoxifen, Halotestin

CAGE

cutting, annoyance, guilt, eye-opener
CAGE test
CAGE test for alcohol abuse

cage

manual splinting of thoracic c.

C

127

CAH
congenital adrenal hyperplasia
CAHMR
cataract, hypertrichosis, mental
retardation
CAHMR syndrome
CAIS
complete androgen insensitivity
syndrome
Caisson disease
Caitlin mark
CAIV
cold-adapted influenza vaccine
CAIV-T
trivalent live cold-adapted influenza
vaccine
Cajal-Retzius neuron
cake
omental c.
caked breast
CAL
café au lait
coronary artery lesion
cal
calorie
Calabro syndrome
Caladryl for Kids
calamine lotion
Calan SR
calcaneal
c. apophysitis
c. compartment
c. fracture
c. prominence
c. tendon
c. view
calcanei (*pl. of* calcaneus)
calcaneocuboid ligament
calcaneofibular ligament (CFL)
calcaneonavicular (CN)
c. articulation
c. bar
c. coalition
c. fusion
calcaneotibial angle
calcaneovalgus
c. deformity
c. flatfoot
c. foot
talipes c.
calcaneovarus
talipes c.
calcaneus, pl. **calcanei**
talipes c.
Cal Carb-HD
Calci-Chew
calcidiol
calcifediol
calciferol

calcificans
angioma capillare et venosum c.
chondrodystrophia fetalis c.
calcification
adrenal c.
amorphous breast c.
arterial c.
basal ganglia c.
buckshot c.
cardiovascular c.
cervical disc space c.
coarse c.
dystrophic c.
granulomatous c.
hepatic capsular c.
intervertebral disc c. (IDC)
intracranial c.
malignant c.
perivascular c.
popcorn-like c.
provisional c.
skin c.
subcutaneous c.
sutural c.
vascular c.
zone of preparatory c. (ZPC)
calcific vasopathy
calcified
c. appendicolith
c. bacterial plaque
c. exostosis
c. fecalith
c. fetus
c. mass
c. matrix
c. myoma
c. outline of cyst
c. phleboliths in pelvis
c. uterine fibroid
calcifying epithelioma
Calcijex
Calci-Mix
calcineurin inhibitor
calcinosis
c., Raynaud phenomenon,
esophageal dysmotility,
sclerodactyly, telangiectasia
(CREST)
c., Raynaud phenomenon,
sclerodactyly, telangiectasia
(CRST)
calciotropic
Calciparine
calcipotriene
calcitonin
c. receptor
c. salmon
calcitriol

calcitropic hormone
calcium (Ca)
> c. absorption
> c. acetate
> c. agonist
> c. alginate
> c. alginate swab
> c. bromide
> c. carbonate
> c. channel antagonist
> c. channel blocker
> c. chloride
> cisplatin, 5-fluorouracil,
>   leucovorin c. (CFL)
> c. citrate
> c. crystal
> c. cyclamate
> death by c.
> c. deficiency
> C. Disodium Versenate
> docusate c.
> c. glubionate
> c. gluconate
> c. heparin
> c. indicator rhod-2
> intracellular c.
> c. ion
> ionized c. (iCa)
> c. leukovorin
> c. pantothenate
> c. phosphate
> c. polycarbophil
> c. rich
> c. salt
> c. supplement
> c. supplementation
calcium-creatinine ratio (Ca:Cr)
calcivirus
calcofluor white stain
calculation
> Berkson-Gage c.
> body surface area c.
> free water c.
> population-attributable risk c. (PAR)
> water deficit c.
calculus, pl. **calculi**
> indinavir calculi
> lacteal c.
> mammary c.
> renal c.
> urate c.

> urinary c.
> uterine c.
CaldeCort
> C. Anti-Itch Topical Spray
> C. Topical
Calderol
Caldesene Topical
Caldwell-Moloy
> C.-M. classification
> C.-M. pelvis types
Caldwell view
CALF
> Cytoxan, Adriamycin, leucovorin,
>   calcium, fluorouracil
calf
> c. compression unit
> c. lung surfactant extract (CLSE)
calfactant
CALF-E
> Cytoxan, Adriamycin, leucovorin,
>   calcium, fluorouracil, ethinyl estradiol
Calgiswab
caliber
caliber-persistent artery
calibrated
calibration
calibrator
> Atomlab 200 dose c.
calicivirus
> human c. (HuCV)
> C. infection
caliectasis
California
> coast of C. café au lait spots
> C. encephalitis
> C. Verbal Learning Test-Children's
>   Version
californium-252 (^{252}Cf)
calipers
> Harpenden c.
> Tenzel c.
cal/kg/day, cal/kg day
> calorie per kilogram per day
Calkins sign
Call-Exner body
callosal
> c. agenesis
> c. inhibition
callosum
> agenesis of corpus c.
> congenital thrombocytopenia, Robin
>   sequence, agenesis of corpus c.,

NOTES

C

callosum *(continued)*
>   distinctive facies, developmental
>   delay syndrome
> corpus c.
> hereditary agenesis of corpus c.
> X-linked mental retardation-seizures-
>   acquired microcephaly-agenesis of
>   corpus c.

callus
> exuberant c.

Calmers
> Robitussin Cough C.
> Sucrets Cough C.

Calmette-Guérin
> bacille bilié de C.-G. (BCG)
> bacillus C.-G. (BCG)

calmodulin
Calmol 4
Calmoseptine ointment
Calm-X Oral
calomel
caloric
> c. challenge
> c. insufficiency
> c. intake
> c. method

calorie (cal)
> c. per kilogram per day
>   (cal/kg/day, cal/kg day)
> c. per ounce (cal/oz)

24-calorie formula
20-calorie formula
calorimeter
> Deltatrac II indirect c.

calorimetry
> indirect c.
> infrared thermographic c. (ITC)
> resting c.

cal/oz
> calorie per ounce

calpainopathy
calprotectin
> fecal c.
> median fecal c.

Caltrate 600
calusterone
calvarial
> c. hyperostosis
> c. osteomyelitis

calvarium
Calvé-Legg-Perthes syndrome
Calvé-Perthes disease
Calymmatobacterium granulomatis
calyx, pl. **calyces**
> obstructed c.
> renal c.

CAM
> cell adhesion molecule
> child-adult mist

chorioallantoic membrane
complementary and alternative medicine
cystic adenomatoid malformation
cystic adenomatous malformation
> CAM tent

CAMAK
> cataract, microcephaly, arthrogryposis,
>   kyphosis
> CAMAK syndrome

Camalax
Cameco
> C. syringe holder
> C. syringe pistol aspiration device

camera
> video c.

Cameron-Myers vaginoscope
Camey
> C. ileocystoplasty
> C. reservoir

CAMFAK
> cataract, microcephaly, failure to thrive,
>   kyphoscoliosis
> CAMFAK syndrome

Camino monitor
CAMP
> Childhood Asthma Management Program

cAMP
> cyclic adenosine monophosphate
> cAMP test

Campbell Soup kid facies
Camper
> C. fascia
> C. fascia of vulva

campesterol
camphor
camphorated oil
camplodactyly (*var. of* camptodactyly)
**CAMP-specific phosphodiesterase
 inhibitor**
camptobrachydactyly
**camptodactyly, camplodactyly,
 camptodactylia**
camptomelia
camptomelic
> c. dwarfism
> c. dysplasia
> c. syndrome

Camptosar
Campylobacter
> C. coli
> C. concisus
> C. cryaerophilia
> C. curvus
> C. enteritis
> C. fetus
> C. fetus intestinalis
> C. fetus jejuni
> C. gastroenteritis
> C. gracilis

C. *hyointestinalis*
C. infection
C. *jejuni*
C. *jejuni* subspecies *doylei*
C. *lari*
C. *mucosalis*
C. *pylori*
C. *sputorum*
C. *upsaliensis*

CAMRSA
community-acquired methicillin-resistant
Staphylococcus aureus

camsylate
trimethaphan c.

Camurati-Englemann syndrome

Canadian
C. Acute Respiratory Illness and
Flu Scale (CARIFS)
C. Crohn Relapse Prevention Trial

canal
Alcock c.
anal c.
atrioventricular c.
attenuated pyloric c.
auditory c.
birth c.
Braune c.
cervical c.
complete atrioventricular c.
ear c.
elastic c.
endocervical c.
external auditory c.
Hunter c.
inguinal c.
Kohn c.
Kovalevsky c.
medullary c.
neurenteric c.
Nuck c.
c. of Nuck
obstetric c.
omphalomesenteric c.
parturient c.
Petit c.'s
pudendal c.
rectal c.
Schlemm c.
semicircular c.
Steiner c.
c. type ASD

uterovaginal c.
vesicourethral c.

canalicular
c. period
c. stage
c. stage of lung development
c. testis

canaliculus, pl. **canaliculi**
pili trianguli et canaliculi

Canavan disease

Canavan-van Bogaert-Bertrand disease

Cancell

cancer
advanced epithelial ovarian c.
c. antigen 125
c. antigen 125 test
breast c.
c. cachexia
cervical stump c.
c. chemotherapy
clear cell vaginal c.
Collaborative Group on Hormonal
Factors in Breast C.
colorectal c.
C. Committee of College of
American Pathologists
endometrial c.
epithelial c.
epithelial ovarian c. (stage I–IV)
familial ovarian c.
c. family syndrome
gynecologic c.
hereditary nonpolyposis colorectal c.
hereditary ovarian c.
inflammatory breast c. (IBC)
intraductal c.
intraepithelial endometrial c.
invasive c. (IC)
invasive cervical c.
lung c.
microinvasive cervical c.
mucinous c.
c. nest
occult c.
ovarian c.
ovarian epithelial c. (OEC)
c. predisposition syndrome
rectal c.
SGO classification of c.
site-specific familial ovarian c.
stage I–IV epithelial ovarian c.
c. and steroid hormone (CASH)

C

NOTES

cancer *(continued)*
    testicular c.
    c. therapy
    thyroid c.
    tubular c.
    vaginal c.
cancericidal dose
Candela laser
candicidin
candida
    C. albicans
    c. colonization
    C. diaper dermatitis
    C. dubliniensis
    eczematous c.
    C. glabrata
    C. guilliermondi
    C. krusei
    C. meningitis
    C. parapsilosis
    C. paratropicalis
    C. pseudotropicalis
    recurrent c.
    C. skin test
    C. stellatoides
    C. tropicalis
candidal
    c. arthritis
    c. diaper dermatitis
    c. diaper rash
    c. glossitis
    c. onychomycosis
    c. paronychia
    c. vaginitis
    c. vulvovaginitis
candidate
    gene c.
    c. gene
candidemia
    transient c.
candidiasis
    acute atrophic c.
    acute pseudomembranous c.
    chronic mucocutaneous c.
    congenital c.
    cutaneous c.
    disseminated c.
    esophageal c.
    hepatosplenic c.
    intertriginous c.
    invasive c.
    mucocutaneous c.
    neonatal c.
    oral c.
    oropharyngeal c. (OPC)
    renal c.
    systemic c.
    vaginal c.
    vulvovaginal c. (VVC)

candidosis
    congenital cutaneous c.
    interdigital c.
    intertriginous c.
    mucocutaneous c.
    oral c.
    perianal c.
    vaginal c.
candiduria
Candistatin
candle
    cesium c.
    c. dripping
    urethral c.
    vaginal c.
candlestick sign
candy-cane stirrups
Canesten
    C. Topical
    C. Vaginal
canicola
    Leptospira c.
canimorsus
    Capnocytophaga c.
canine
    c. distemper
    c. scabies
    c. tooth
caninum
    Ancylostoma c.
canis
    Brucella c.
    Microsporum c.
    Pasteurella c.
    Toxocara c.
canker sore
Cannabis sativa
cannonball lesion
cannula
    acorn c.
    Bard cervical c.
    Cabot c.
    cervical c.
    Circon-ACMI c.
    Cohen uterine c.
    Core Dynamics disposable c.
    Dexide disposable c.
    endometrial c.
    Ethicon disposable c.
    Genitor mini-intrauterine
      insemination c.
    Gesco c.
    Hasson c.
    high-flow nasal c.
    Hunt-Reich c.
    indwelling c.
    intrauterine balloon-type c.
    intrauterine insemination c.
    IUI disposable c.

Jacobs c.
Jarit disposable c.
Kahn c.
Karman c.
KDF-2.3 intrauterine
  insemination c.
LaparoSAC single-use obturator
  and c.
Lübke uterine vacuum c.
Marlow disposable c.
nasal c.
Olympus disposable c.
Rubin c.
Scott c.
Semm uterine vacuum c.
Solos disposable c.
stable access c.
stepdown c.
Storz disposable c.
trumpet c.
Vabra c.
vacuum c.
Vancaillie uterine c.
Weck disposable c.
Wisap disposable c.
Wolf disposable c.
Ximed disposable c.

cannulate
cannulated screw
cannulation
arterial c.
jugular venous c.
peripheral arterial c.
posterior tibial artery c.
venoarterial c.
venovenous c.

canopy
surgical overhead c. (SOC)

cantharidin
cantharis, pl. **cantharides**
canthi (*pl. of* canthus)
canthomeatal line
canthorum
dystopia c.

canthus, pl. **canthi**
heterochromia of inner c.
inner c.
lateral displacement of inner c.
outer c.

Cantil
cantonensis
Angiostrongylus c.

Cantor tube
Cantrell
pentalogy of C.
C. syndrome

Cantú syndrome
Cantwell-Ransley repair
CAP
cyclophosphamide, Adriamycin, cisplatin

cap
acrosomal c.
anterior head c.
cervical c.
Compoz Gel C.'s
cradle c.
Dutch c.
Oves Cervical C.
ProtectaCap c.
stockinette c.
Universal reducer c.
vault c.
Vimule c.

CAPA
Child and Adolescent Psychiatric
  Assessment

capacitation
sperm c.

capacitive
capacity
alveolar-arterial oxygen diffusing c.
bladder c.
closing c. (CC)
corticosteroid-binding globulin-
  binding c. (CB-GBC)
cystometric c.
diffusing c.
fetal blood oxygen-carrying c.
forced vital c. (FVC)
functional residual c. (FRC)
inspiratory c. (IC)
iron-binding c. (IBC)
lung c. (CL)
maximum breathing c.
oxygen-diffusing c.
plasma iron-binding c.
pulmonary diffusing c.
reduced bladder c.
renal reserve filtration c. (RRFC)
serum bilirubin-binding c.
total iron-binding c. (TIBC)
total lung c. (TLC)
urinary concentrating c.
vital c. (VC)

NOTES

Capasee diagnostic ultrasound system
CAPD
    central auditory processing disorder
    continuous ambulatory peritoneal dialysis
capillariasis
    hepatic c.
capillary
    c. angioma
    c. BLL
    c. blood gas (CBG)
    c. blood gas sampling
    dilated c.
    distended c.
    c. dropout
    c. electrophoresis
    c. electrophoresis/frontal analysis
      (CE/FA)
    c. end loop
    c. erection
    c. filling time
    c. hemangioma
    c. isoelectric focusing technique
    c. leak
    c. leak injury
    c. leak syndrome (CLS)
    nail-fold c.
    c. pattern
    c. refill
    c. refill time
    tortuous c.
capillosus
    Bacteroides c.
capita (*pl. of* caput)
capital femoral epiphysis
capitate bone
capitellar
    c. epiphysis
    c. osteochondritis
capitellum
    displaced c.
    osteochondritis of c.
capitis
    Pediculus humanus var c.
capitis (*gen. of* caput)
caplet
    Advil Cold & Sinus C.'s
    Dristan Sinus C.'s
    Miles Nervine C.'s
    Sinumist-SR C.'s
    TripTone C.'s
Capnocytophaga canimorsus
capnograph
    Microstream c.
capnography
    low-flow sidestream c.
capnometry
Capoten
capped uterus
capreomycin

caproate
    17alpha-hydroxyprogesterone c.
    hydroxyprogesterone c.
    17-hydroxyprogesterone c.
Capronor
Caprosyn monofilament suture
capsaicin
capsicum
Capsin
capsularis
capsular stripping
capsulatum
    Histoplasma c.
capsule
    boric acid c.
    Bowman c.
    contraceptive suppository c.
    Crosby c.
    Crosby-Kugler pediatric c.
    Dexedrine Spansule c.
    Glisson c.
    Heyman c.'s
    joint c.
    Kadian sustained-release
      morphine c.'s
    Norvir c.
    ruptured c.
    Uro-Mag c.
    Virilon c.
    Watson c.
capsulotomy
    posterior knee c.
CAPTA
    Child Abuse Prevention and Treatment
    Act
captopril
capture
    ovum c.
caput, gen. **capitis**, pl. **capita**
    c. medusae
    pediculosis capitis
    c. quadratum
    c. succedaneum
    tinea capitis
Capute scale
Carafate
caramel test
carateum
    Treponema c.
carbachol
carbamazepine (CBZ)
Carbamide
carbamide peroxide
carbamoyl phosphate synthetase (CPS)
carbamoyltransferase
    ornithine c. (OCT)
carbapenem
carbarsone
carbazole

carbenicillin
carbergoline
carbetocin
Carb-HD
    Cal C.-HD
carbimazole
carbinoxamine maleate
carbinoxamine and pseudoephedrine
carbogen
carbohydrate
    c. deficient glycoprotein (CDG)
    c. homeostasis
    c. homeostasis transporter
    c. intolerance
    c. malabsorption
    c. metabolism
    c. overloading
    c. tolerance
carbohydrate-deficient glycoprotein syndrome (type I, II) (CDGS)
carbohydrate-free
    Ross c.-f. (RCF)
Carbolith
carbon
    c. dioxide (CO_2)
    c. dioxide gas
    c. dioxide laser
    c. dioxide laser beam conization
    c. dioxide retention
    c. monoxide (CO)
    c. monoxide poisoning
    c. monoxide toxicity
    c. tetrachloride
carbon-13 urea breath test
carbon-14 test
carbonaceous sputum
carbonate
    calcium c.
    lithium c.
carbonic
    c. acid
    c. anhydrase inhibitor
carbonyl iron
carboplatin
carboplatin/docetaxel
carboprost tromethamine
carboxamide
    dimethyl-triazeno-imidazole c. (DTIC)
carboxyhemoglobin (COHb)
carboxykinase
    phosphoenolpyruvate c. (PEPCK)

carboxylase
    acetyl-CoA c.
    alpha-methylcrotonyl-coenzyme A c.
    c. deficiency
    deficiency of pyruvate c.
carboxylation
carboxyl terminal peptide (CTP)
carboxypeptidase E
carboxyterminal
    c. propeptide
    c. propeptide of type 1 procollagen (PICP)
carbuncle
Carcassonne ligament
carcinoembryonic
    c. antigen (CEA)
    c. antigen 125 (CEA 125)
carcinogen
    chemical c.
carcinogenesis
    pediatric thyroid c.
    radiation c.
carcinogenic
carcinoid
    nonappendiceal c.
    c. syndrome
    c. tumor
carcinoma, pl. **carcinomas, carcinomata (CA)**
    acinic cell c.
    adenocystic c.
    adenoid cystic c.
    adenosquamous c.
    adrenal cortical c.
    advanced c.
    anaplastic c.
    androgen-dependent c.
    c. antigen
    Bartholin gland c.
    basal cell c.
    borderline epithelial ovarian c.
    breast c.
    bulky c.
    cecal c.
    cervical c.
    c. of cervix
    childhood thyroid c.
    choroid plexus c. (CPC)
    clear cell endometrial c.
    colloid c.
    colon c.
    contralateral synchronous c.

C

NOTES

carcinoma *(continued)*
    ductal c.
    embryonal cell c.
    endometrial c.
    endometrioid c.
    epithelial cell ovarian c.
    estrogen-dependent endometrial c.
    estrogen-independent endometrial c.
    FAB staging of c.
    fallopian tube c.
    fibrolamellar hepatocellular c.
    focal lobular c.
    gastric c.
    glassy cell c.
    gynecologic c.
    hepatocellular c. (HCC)
    infantile embryonal c.
    infiltrating ductal c. (IDC)
    infiltrating lobular c. (ILC)
    infiltrating small-cell lobular c.
    inflammatory c.
    intracystic papillary c.
    intraductal papillary c.
    invasive duct c.
    juvenile c.
    keratinizing nasopharyngeal c.
    lobular c.
    lung c.
    medullary thyroid c.
    Merkel cell c.
    mesometanephric c.
    mesonephric c.
    mesonephroid clear-cell c.
    metaplastic c.
    metastatic c.
    microinvasive c. (MICA)
    mucinous c.
    mucoepidermoid c.
    multicentric c.
    multiple nevoid-basal cell c.
      (MNBCC)
    nasopharyngeal c.
    nevoid basal cell c. (NBCC)
    oat cell c.
    ovarian small-cell c.
    papillary endometrial c.
    papillary serous cervical c.
    peritoneal serous papillary c.
    preclinical c.
    primary hepatocellular c. (PHC)
    primary peritoneal c. (PPC)
    rectosigmoid c.
    recurrent c.
    renal cell c.
    renal medullary c.
    scirrhous c.
    secretory c.
    serous c.
    signet ring cell c.
    c. in situ (CIS)
    small cell c.
    sporadic nonfamilial clear cell c.
    squamous cell c.
    thyroid c.
    tubular c.
    uterine corpus c.
    uterine papillary serous c. (UPSC)
    vaginal c.
    verrucous c.
    vulvar adenosquamous c.
    vulvovaginal c.
    well-circumscribed c.
    wolffian duct c.
    yolk sac c.

carcinomatosis
    meningeal c.

carcinosarcoma
    uterine c.

card
    Allen Kindergarten Picture C.'s
    Guthrie c.
    neonatal Guthrie c.
    Peabody Developmental Motor
      Activity C.'s
    Sheridan-Gardiner visual acuity c.'s
    Sonksen-Silver visual acuity c.
    Sonogram fetal ultrasound image c.

cardiac
    c., abnormal facies, thymic
      hypoplasia, cleft palate,
      hypocalcemia syndrome
    c. abnormality
    c. abnormality, abnormal facies,
      thymic hypoplasia, cleft palate,
      hypocalcemia (CATCH 22)
    c. abnormality, T-cell deficit,
      clefting, hypocalcemia
    c. abnormality, T-cell deficit,
      clefting, hypocalcemia phenotype
    c. anomaly
    c. arrest
    c. arrhythmia
    c. asthma
    c. autonomic modulation
    c. catheter
    c. catheterization
    c. compression
    c. cyanosis
    c. dysrhythmia
    c. ejection fraction
    c. event monitor
    c. failure
    c. flow
    c. function
    c. glycoside
    c. hemangioma
    c. hemolytic anemia
    c. lesion

c. looping
c. malformation
c. malposition
c. massage
c. monitoring
c. murmur
c. output
c. rhabdomyoma
c. rhythm disorder
c. rupture
c. septal defect
c. septation
c. silhouette
c. size
c. standstill
c. stun
c. syncope
c. tamponade
c. transplantation
c. trauma
c. troponin T
c. twinning
c. width
cardiac-apnea (CA)
    c.-a. monitor
cardiac-limb syndrome
Cardiff
    C. Count-to-Ten chart
    C. resuscitation bag
Cardilate
cardinal
    c. ligament
    c. movement
    c. point
    c. vein
cardinal-uterosacral
    c.-u. ligament
    c.-u. ligament complex
Cardiobacterium
cardiocranial syndrome
cardioesophageal junction
cardiofacial syndrome
cardiofaciocutaneous (CFC)
cardiogenesis
cardiogenic shock
cardiogenital syndrome
cardiogram
    impedance c.
cardiologist
cardiology
cardiomegaly
cardiomyocyte

cardiomyopathy
    chronic chagasic c.
    diabetic c.
    dilated c.
    fetal c.
    histiocytoid c.
    hypertrophic c.
    idiopathic dilated c.
    ipecac c.
    maternally inherited myopathy
      and c. (MIMyCA)
    neonatal c.
    peripartum c.
    postpartum c.
    restrictive c. (RCM)
    Sengers c.
    subaortic hypertrophic c.
    X-linked c. (XLCM)
    X-linked dilated c. (XLCM)
cardioplegia
    cold potassium c.
cardioplegic solution
cardiopneumograph
cardioprotective effect
cardiopulmonary
    c. bypass
    c. collapse
    c. dysfunction
    c. resuscitation (CPR)
cardiorespiratory
    c. function
    c. homeostasis
    c. monitor
    c. syndrome of obesity in child
cardiorespirogram (CR-gram)
CardioSeal device
cardioskeletal
    c. myopathy
    c. neutropenia
cardiospasm
cardiotachometer
cardiothoracic ratio
cardiothymic shadow
cardiotocogram
    terminal c.
cardiotocograph
cardiotocography (CTG)
    fetal c.
    intrapartum c.
cardiotoxicity
cardiovascular (CV)
    c. calcification

C

NOTES

cardiovascular *(continued)*
    c. collapse
    c. complication
    c. depression
    c. development
    c. effect
    c. malformation (CVM)
    c. manifestation
    c. pertubation
    c. sequela
    c. shock
    c. stabilization
    c. system
cardiovascular/central nervous system syndrome
cardioversion
    synchronized DC c.
cardiovertebral syndrome
carditis
    acute rheumatic c.
    indolent c.
    rheumatic c.
Cardizem
    C. CD
    C. Injectable
    C. SR
care
    ambulatory obstetric c.
    antepartum c.
    antepartum home c.
    breast c.
    custodial c.
    followup c.
    foster c.
    hospice c.
    in-hospital postpartum c.
    Kangaroo C.
    maternal c.
    monitored anesthesia c.
    newborn intensive c. (NBIC)
    obstetric c.
    obstetric-gynecologic c.
    outpatient postpartum c.
    pediatric neurocritical c.
    postoperative c.
    postpartum c.
    preconception c.
    prenatal c.
    prepregnancy c.
    respite c.
    specialized prenatal c.
    substitute c.
    supportive c.
    well-child c. (WCC)
caregiver
    primary c.
caregiver-child interaction
caretaker
    primary c.

Carey-Fineman-Ziter syndrome
Carey Temperament Scale
caries
    dental c.
    early childhood c. (ECC)
CARIFS
    Canadian Acute Respiratory Illness and Flu Scale
carina, pl. **carinae**
carinatum
    pectus c.
carinii
    Pneumocystis c.
C-arm
Carmault clamp
carmine
    indigo c.
Carmi syndrome
Carmol
Carmol-HC Topical
carmustine
Carnation
    C. Follow-Up
    C. Follow-Up soy formula
    C. Good Start formula
Carnegie stage
carneous
    c. degeneration
    c. mole
Carnevale syndrome
Carney syndrome
carnitine
    c. acylcarnitine translocase deficiency
    c. palmitoyltransferase (CPT)
    c. palmitoyltransferase I (CPT I)
    c. palmitoyltransferase II (CPT II)
    c. transferase enzyme disorder
Carnitor
carnivore
Carnoy fixative
carob
    c. gum
    c. seed flour
Caroli
    C. disease
    C. syndrome
Carolina Curriculum for Infants and Toddlers with Special Needs
carotid
    c. artery
    c. artery-cavernous sinus fistula
    c. artery dissection
    c. blood flow (CaBF)
    c. bruit
    left common c.
    right common c.
    c. sinus pressure
carotid-cavernous fistula

carotin
carpal navicular
carpectomy
    proximal row c.
Carpenter syndrome
carphenazine maleate
carpi (*pl. of* carpus)
carp-like mouth
carp mouth
carpopedal spasm
carpus, pl. **carpi**
Carrasyn Hydrogel dressing
carrier
    embryo c.
    Endo-Assist endoscopic ligature c.
    factor V Leiden c.
    fragile X c.
    gene c.
    gestational c.
    heterozygous c.
    latent c.
    linear in-line ligature c.
    Miya hook ligature c.
    obligate c.
    c. protein
    Raz double-prong ligature c.
    c. screening
    silent c.
    c. testing
    translocation c.
CARS
    Childhood Autism Rating Scale
car sickness
cart
    Sensorimedics Horizon
        Metabolic C.
Carter Tubal Assistant
cartilage
    costal c.
    fetal c.
    c. interposition
    c. oligomeric matrix protein
        (COMP)
    c. piercing
cartilage-hair hypoplasia (CHH)
cartilaginous coalition
cartridge
    serum pregnancy assay c.
Cartwright blood group
caruncle
    amniotic c.
    c. of labia

myrtiform c.
urethral c.
caruncula, pl. **carunculae**
    c. hymenalis
    c. myrtiformis
Carus
    C. circle
    C. curve
Carvajal formula
CAS
    central anticholinergic syndrome
    child assessment schedule
CASA
    Child and Adolescent Services
        Assessment
    computer-assisted semen analysis
    computer-assisted semen analyzer
Casal necklace
casanthranol
    docusate and c.
cascade
    coagulation c.
    cytokine c.
    inflammatory c.
    toxic c.
cascara sagrada
case
    index c.
    c. manager
caseating necrosis
caseation
Casec
    C. formula
    C. powder
casein
    c. hydrolysate
    c. hydrolysate formula
    powdered c.
caseosa
    vernix c.
caseous node
caseum
CASG
    Collaborative Antiviral Study Group
CASH
    cancer and steroid hormone
    classic abdominal Semm hysterectomy
    cortical androgen-stimulating hormone
        CASH study
Casodex
cassava bean

NOTES

casseliflavus
>*Enterococcus c.*

Casser fontanelle
casserian fontanelle
CAST
> childhood accidental spiral tibial
> Children of Alcoholics Screening Test

cast
> abduction c.
> bivalved c.
> c. boot brace
> bronchial mucous c.
> cellular c.
> clubfoot c.
> cylinder c.
> decidual c.
> dense c.
> Hexalite c.
> hip spica c.
> hyaline c.
> hypereosinophilic mucoid c.
> long leg c.
> Petri c.
> polysiloxane c.
> red blood cell c.
> Risser localizer c.
> short leg walking c.
> spica c.
> thumb spica c.
> urinary c.
> uterine c.

Castaneda procedure
castellani
> *Acanthamoeba c.*

casting
> Cerrobend c.
> inhibitive c.
> serial c.

Castleman disease
castor
> c. bean
> c. bean poisoning
> c. oil

castrated
castration
Castroviejo fixation forceps
Cast syndrome
CAT
> Clinical Adaptive Test
> computed axial tomography
>> CAT scanning

cat
> c. bite
> c. dander
> c. eye syndrome (CES)

catabolism
> tissue c.
> unregulated c.

catadidymus

Cataflam
catalase negative
catalytic
catamenia
catamenial
> c. hemoptysis
> c. pneumothorax

catamenogenic
Catania type acrofacial dysostosis
cataplectic attack
cataplexy
Catapres Oral
Catapres-TTS Transdermal
cataract
> c., ataxia, deafness, retardation
>   syndrome
> cerulean c.
> congenital bilateral c.
> developmental c.
> c. formation
> c., hypertrichosis, mental retardation
>   (CAHMR)
> infantile c.
> juvenile c.
> lenticular c.
> c., mental retardation,
>   hypogonadism syndrome
> c., microcephaly, arthrogryposis,
>   kyphosis (CAMAK)
> c., microcephaly, failure to thrive,
>   kyphoscoliosis (CAMFAK)
> c., motor system disorder, short
>   stature, learning difficulty, skeletal
>   abnormalities syndrome
> sunflower c.
> zonular c.

cataract-dental syndrome
cataractogenic
cataract-oligophrenia syndrome
catarrhalis
> *Branhamella c.*
> *Moraxella c.*

catarrhal jaundice
catastrophic
> c. bleeding
> c. hemorrhage
> c. injury

catatonic
> c. behavior
> c. syndrome

CATCH 22
> cardiac abnormality, abnormal facies,
>   thymic hypoplasia, cleft palate,
>   hypocalcemia
> conotruncal cardiac defect, abnormal
>   face, thymic hypoplasia, cleft palate
>> CATCH 22 phenotype
>> CATCH 22 syndrome

catch
midstream c.
catch-up growth
CAT/CLAMS
Clinical Adaptive Test/Clinical Linguistic
and Auditory Milestone Scale
catechol
c. estrogen
c. oxidase
catecholamine
endogenous c.
categorical placement
category
bilineal c.
Catel-Manzke syndrome
catenulatum
Bifidobacterium c.
catgut suture
cathartic
c. colon
magnesium-containing c.
saline c.
cathepsin D
catheter
Alzate c.
Amplatz c.
Angiocath c.
c. angiography
Argyle arterial c.
Arrow c.
arterial c.
AutoGuard c.
balloon septostomy c.
balloon-tipped c.
bile duct c.
Bi-Set c.
bladder c.
Bonnano c.
Bozeman-Fritsch c.
c. breakage
Brevi-Kath epidural c.
Broviac c.
cardiac c.
Caud-A-Kath epidural c.
central venous c. (CVC)
central venous pressure c.
Chemo-Port c.
ChronoFlex c.
CliniCath peripherally inserted c.
Conceptus Soft Torque uterine c.
Conceptus VS c.
Cook c.

Corcath c.
coudé c.
Cystocath c.
Dacron sleeve c.
Davis bladder c.
DeLee suction c.
de Pezzer c.
Dobbhoff c.
Dorros infusion and probing c.
double-balloon c.
double-lumen c.
Drew-Smythe c.
Du Pen epidural c.
c. dysfunction
EASI c.
EchoMark salpingography c.
Ehrlich c.
elastomer c.
c. embolization
Embryon GIFT c.
Embryon HSG c.
Evert-O-Cath drug delivery c.
FAE c.
femoral artery c.
flexible Teflon c.
Fogarty arterial embolectomy c.
Fogarty atrioseptostomy c.
Foley c.
French Gesco c.
Gesco c.
Groshong c.
Haas intrauterine insemination c.
Hohn c.
HUMI c.
Hurwitz c.
hysterosalpingography c.
indwelling c.
indwelling arterial c. (IAC)
indwelling venous c. (IVC)
Infuse-A-Port c.
c. insertion
intrauterine pressure c. (IUPC)
Johnson transtracheal oxygen c.
Judkins c.
jugular bulb c.
KDF-2.3 intrauterine c.
Kendall double-lumen c.
Kish urethral illuminating c.
Koala intrauterine pressure c.
Labcath c.
Labotect c.
Landmark c.

NOTES

C

catheter *(continued)*
    large-bore c.
    L-Cath peripherally inserted
      neonatal c.
    Leonard c.
    LeRoy ventricular c.
    Malecot c.
    malpositioned c.
    MediPort c.
    Mentor c.
    microendoscopic optical c.
    Microtip c.
    Micro-Transducer c.
    Millar microtransducer urethral c.
    Neo-Sert umbilical vessel c.
    On-Command c.
    Opti-Flow c.
    over-the-needle c.
    percutaneous central venous c.
      (PCVC)
    percutaneous femoral venous c.
    percutaneously inserted central
      line c. (PICC)
    percutaneous nephrostomy c.
    peripheral arterial c.
    peripheral intravenous c.
    peripherally inserted c. (PIC)
    peripherally inserted central c.
      (PICC)
    peritoneal c.
    PermCath c.
    Per-Q-Cath c.
    Pezzer c.
    pigtail c.
    PIV c.
    Pleur-evac chest c.
    polyethylene c.
    polyurethane c.
    Port-A-Cath c.
    PRO infusion c.
    c. pullback
    pulmonary thermodilution c.
    Quinton dual-lumen c.
    Raaf c.
    radial arterial c.
    radial artery c.
    Raimondi c.
    red rubber c.
    Release c.
    Reliance urinary control insert c.
    Replogle suction c.
    c. reservoir
    scalp vein c.
    c. sepsis
    c. septostomy
    shearing of c.
    Silastic c.
    silicone c.
    silicon rubber c.
    Soft-Cell c.
    soft seal c.
    Soft Torque uterine c.
    Sones c.
    Soules intrauterine insemination c.
    c. specimen
    Spectranetics c.
    split sheath c.
    Stamey c.
    Stamey-Malecot c.
    Stargate falloposcopy c.
    suction c.
    support c.
    suprapubic c.
    Swan-Ganz c.
    Tenckhoff c.
    tethered c.
    TFX c. stylet
    c. tip placement
    c. toes
    tracheal c.
    transcervical Foley c.
    transcervical tubal access c. (T-
      TAC)
    transducer-tipped c.
    transtracheal c.
    transurethral c.
    triple-lumen c.
    Tygon c.
    umbilical artery c. (UAC)
    umbilical vein c. (UVC)
    umbilical venous c. (UVC)
    umbilical vessel c.
    urinary c.
    uterine cornual access c. (UCAC)
    uterine ostial access c. (UOAC)
    Vabra c.
    Vas-Cath c.
    V-Cath c.
    venous c.
    ventricular c.
    Wallace c.
    water-perfused manometry c.
    whistle-tip c.
    Wholey balloon occlusion c.
    c.-within-a-catheter
    Word Bartholin gland c.
    Word bladder c.
    Yankauer c.
    Zynergy Zolution c.
catheter-associated bacteremia
catheter-in-a-catheter technique
catheterization
    bladder c.
    cardiac c.
    central venous c.
    clean intermittent c. (CIC)
    femoral artery c.
    fetal bladder c.

intraoperative ureteral c.
jugular bulb c.
percutaneous central venous c.
peripheral venous c.
pulmonary artery c.
radial artery c.
scalp vein c.
transvaginal tubal c.
umbilical artery c.
umbilical vein c.
urethral c.
urinary c.
catheter-over-needle technique
catheter-over-wire technique
cathode ray oscilloscope (CRO)
cati
   Toxocara c.
CATS
   Child Abuse Trauma Scale
cat's
c. cry
c. cry syndrome
c. eye pupil
c. eye reflex
c. eye syndrome (CES)
c. urine syndrome
cat-scratch
c.-s. disease (CSD)
c.-s. fever
CatsEye digital camera system
Cattell
C. Infant Intelligence Scale
C. Infant Intelligence Test
Catterall classification (grade 1–4)
cauda
c. equina
c. equina syndrome
caudad
Caud-A-Kath epidural catheter
caudal
c. agenesis
c. analgesia
c. anesthesia
c. appendage, short terminal phalanges, deafness, cryptorchidism, mental retardation syndrome
c. chordamesoderm
c. direction
c. duplication
c. dysplasia
c. dysplasia syndrome

c. neuropore
c. pole
c. regression syndrome (CRS)
caudate
c. hypometabolism
c. nucleus
caudocranial
Cauer forceps
caul
causal
c. embryology
c. independence
c. inference
causalgia
causation
cause
acute cerebellar ataxia of unknown c.
cause-and-effect activity
caustic
c. aspiration
c. ingestion
c. injury
cauterization
Bovie c.
nasal c.
cauterizing ball
cautery
BICAP c.
bipolar c.
Bovie c.
c. conization
Endoclip c.
endoscopic c.
laparoscopic c.
L-shaped c.
monopolar c.
ovarian c.
Oxycel c.
cava, pl. **cavae**
azygos continuation of inferior vena c.
inferior vena c. (IVC)
superior vena c. (SVC)
vena c.
CAVD
congenital absence of vas deferens
cave
Meckel c.
Caverject
cavernosa
corpora c.

NOTES

143

cavernosal
 c. artery thrombosis
 c. fibrosis
 c. infarction
cavernosum
 corpus c.
cavernous
 c. hemangioma
 c. lymphangioma
 c. plexus
 c. sinus
 c. sinusitis
 c. sinus syndrome
 c. sinus thrombosis
 c. venous angioma
CAVH
 continuous arteriovenous hemofiltration
caviae
 Nocardia c.
cavitary
 c. lung disease
 c. tuberculosis
 c. white-matter lesion
cavitation
Cavitron ultrasonic surgical aspirator (CUSA)
cavity
 abdominal c.
 abscess c.
 amniotic c.
 Baer c.
 celomic c.
 chorionic c.
 endometrial c.
 exocelomic c.
 intrauterine c.
 oral c.
 pelvic c.
 peritoneal c.
 pseudomonoamniotic c.
 syringomyelic c.
 thoracic c.
 uterine c.
 ventricles to peritoneal c. (VP)
CAVM
 cerebral arteriovenous malformation
cavovalgus
 talipes c.
cavovarus
 c. deformity
 c. foot
cavum
 c. septum pellucidum
 c. septum pellucidum, cavum vergae, macrocephaly, seizures, mental retardation syndrome
 c. vergae
cavus
 c. foot

 pathological c.
 pes c.
 physiologic c.
 talipes c.
cayetanensis
 Cyclospora c.
Cayler cardiofacial syndrome
CBC
 complete blood count
CBCL
 Child Behavior Checklist
CBF
 cerebral blood flow
CBFV
 cerebral blood flow velocity
CBG
 capillary blood gas
 cord blood gas
 corticosteroid-binding globulin
CB-GBC
 corticosteroid-binding globulin-binding capacity
CBR
 cord blood registry
CBRF
 child behavior rating form
CBS
 child behavioral study
 cystathionine beta-synthase
  CBS deficiency
CBT
 cognitive behavioral therapy
 cord blood transplantation
CBV
 cerebral blood volume
CBZ
 carbamazepine
CC
 clomiphene citrate
 closing capacity
  Adalat CC
  hemoglobin CC
cc
 cubic centimeter
CCA
 congenital contractural arachnodactyly
CCAI
 Clinical Colitis Activity Index
CCAM
 congenital cystic adenomatoid malformation
 cystic congenital adenomatoid malformation
  CCAM (type 1–3)
CCC
 craniocerebellocardiac
  CCC dysplasia
  CCC syndrome

CCCT
   clomiphene citrate challenge test
CCD Spirette
CCG
   Children's Cancer Group
CCH
   chronic cryptogenic hepatitis
CCHB
   congenital complete heart block
CCHD
   cyanotic congenital heart disease
cc/hr
   cubic centimeter per hour
CCHS
   congenital central hypoventilation
      syndrome
CCK
   cholecystokinin
cc/kg/day, cc/kg day
   cubic centimeter per kilogram per day
CCLO
   child-centered literary orientation
CCM
   cerebrocostomandibular
CCMS
   cerebrocostomandibular syndrome
CCNU
   cyclohexylchloroethylnitrosurea
CCPD
   continuous cyclic peritoneal dialysis
CCR
   cumulative conception rate
CCS
   Crippled Children's Services
CCSC
   Children's Coping Strategies Checklist
CCSG
   Children's Cancer Study Group
CCUP
   colpocystourethropexy
CCVM
   congenital cardiovascular malformation
CD
   celiac disease
   conduct disorder
      Cardizem CD
      Ceclor CD
CD4+
      CD4+ cell
      CD4+ level

CD4
      CD4 cell count
      CD4 T cell
CD8
      CD8 cell count
      CD8 T cell
CD34 hematopoietic progenitor cell
CD4:CD8 ratio
CDA
   congenital dyserythropoietic anemia
CDAC
   Clostridium difficile-associated diarrhea
CDAP
   continuous distending airway pressure
CDC
   Centers for Disease Control and
      Prevention
   Communicable Disease Center
CDD
   childhood disintegrative disorder
CDE
   color Doppler energy
      CDE blood group system
CDFI
   color Doppler flow imaging
CDG
   carbohydrate deficient glycoprotein
CDGS
   carbohydrate-deficient glycoprotein
      syndrome (type I, II)
CDH
   congenital diaphragmatic hernia
   congenital dislocated hip
   congenital dislocation of hip
      CDH repair
CDH-ECMO
   congenital diaphragmatic hernia-
      extracorporeal membrane oxygenation
CDHNF
   Children's Digestive Health and Nutrition
      Foundation
CDI
   Children's Depression Inventory
   Cotrel-Dubousset instrumentation
cDICA
   Computerized Diagnostic Interview for
      Children and Adolescents
CDIS
   continuous distention irrigation system
CDL
   Cornelia de Lange

NOTES

C

145

CDLS
 Cornelia de Lange syndrome
cDNA
 complementary deoxyribonucleic acid
 complementary DNA
  cDNA library
CDP
 continuous distending pressure
CDRS-R
 Children's Depression Rating Scale-
  Revised
CDS
 color Doppler sonography
CE
 conductive education
CEA
 carcinoembryonic antigen
CEA 125
 carcinoembryonic antigen 125
ceasmic
cebocephalus
cebocephaly
CECA
 cisplatin, etoposide, Cytoxan, Adriamycin
cecal
  c. carcinoma
  c. pouch
Ceclor CD
cecocolic intussusception
Cecon
cecostomy
cecum
  exstrophic c.
CED
 cranioectodermal dysplasia
Cedax
Cedilanid
Cedocard-SR
CEE
 conjugated equine estrogen
CEEA
 circular end-to-end anastomosis
CeeNU
CEF
 Cytoxan, epirubicin, fluorouracil
CE/FA
 capillary electrophoresis/frontal analysis
cefaclor
cefadroxil monohydrate
Cefadyl
cefamandole
cefazolin sodium
cefdinir
cefepime HCl
cefixime
Cefizox
cefmetazole
Cefobid
cefonicid

cefoperazone sodium
ceforanide
Cefotan
cefotaxime sodium
cefotetan disodium
cefoxitin sodium
cefpodoxime proxetil
cefprozil
ceftazidime
ceftibuten
Ceftin Oral
ceftizoxime
ceftriaxone sodium
cefuroxime
  c. axetil (CAE)
  c. sodium
Cefzil
ceiling
Celera
celery stalking
Celestoderm-EV/2
Celestoderm-V
Celestone
  C. Oral
  C. Phosphate Injection
  C. Soluspan
celiac
  c. antibody
  c. artery
  c. axis
  c. disease (CD)
  c. infantilism
  c. sprue
  c. syndrome
celibacy
celibate
celiohysterectomy
celiohysterotomy
celiomyomectomy
celiomyomotomy
celioparacentesis
celiosalpingectomy
celiosalpingotomy
celioscopy
celiotomy
  exploratory c.
  vaginal c.
cell
  absolute nucleated red blood c.
   (ANRBC)
  activated T c.
  c. adhesion factor (CAF)
  c. adhesion molecule (CAM)
  Alzheimer II c.
  amniogenic c.
  antibody-secreting c. (ASC)
  antigen-presenting c. (APC)
  antigen-sensitive c.
  Askanazy c.

atypical c.
atypical squamous c. (ASC)
B c.
back-selected T c.
band c.
basket c.
Betz c.
BeWo c.
Birbeck granule-positive c.
bite c.
blastomere c.
blister c.
c. block analysis
bone marrow stem c.
Burkitt tumor c.
CD4+ c.
CD34 hematopoietic progenitor c.
CD4 T c.
CD8 T c.
cell-salvaged packed c.
choroid plexus c.
ciliated c.
circulating fetal c.
clue c.
c. collector
committed c.
corona radiata c.
crenated red blood c.
crypt c.
CTL c.
c. culture
cumulus c.
c. cycle
c. cycle-nonspecific drug
c. cycle-specific drug
c. cycling in chemotherapy
cytotoxic memory T c.
daughter c.
decidual c.
dendritic c.
desquamated epithelial c.
c. determination
diploid spermatogonial stem c.
c. division
dome c.
donor T c.
double c.
dysplastic c.
early embryonic c.
effector c.
egg c.

embryonic renomedullary
  interstitial c.
embryonic stem c.
encephalitogenic c.
endodermal c.
endothelial c.
enterochromaffin c.
epithelial c.
epithelioid c.
erythroid progenitor c.
eukaryotic c.
exfoliated squamous c.
extragonadal germ c.
fetal red blood c.
fetouterine c.
c. and flare
foam c.
frozen red blood c.'s
ganglion c.
Gaucher c.
c. generation time
germ c.
giant c.
glandular c.
granulosa lutein c.
c. growth inhibitor
Haller c.
haploid c.
HeLa c.'s
helper T c.
hematopoietic stem c. (HSC)
HLA-identical haploidentical bone
  marrow stem c.
hobnail c.
Hofbauer c.
human endothelial c. (HEC)
Hürthle c.
hyperplasia of beta c.
immunocompetent c.
inclusion c.
c. interaction gene
interstitial c.
Ito c.
K c.
c. kill
killer c.
c. kinetics
koilocytotic c.
Kupffer c.
lack of natural killer c.'s
Langerhans c.
Langhans giant c.

NOTES

147

cell *(continued)*
  leukemic c.
  Leydig c.'s
  lipid c.
  luteal c.
  lutein c.
  lymphoblastoid c.
  lymphoid c.
  lymphokine-activated killer c. (LAK)
  c. lysate
  mast c.
  mastoid air c.
  maturation of c.
  MCF-7 breast cancer c.
  memory c.
  Merkel c.
  mesenchymal c.
  metamyelocyte c.
  monster c.
  multinucleated giant c.
  mutant c.
  myeloblast c.
  myelocyte c.
  myoepithelial c.
  natural killer c. (NK)
  natural killer T c.
  neural crest c.
  neuroblastoma c.
  neuroid c.
  Niemann-Pick c.
  NK c.
  nonencephalitogenic c.
  normoblast c.
  nuclear factor of activated T c. (NFAT)
  nucleated red blood c.
  Opalski c.
  osteoblast-like c.
  owl's eye c.
  packed red blood c.'s (PRBC)
  pancreatic islet c.
  parabasal c.
  peripheral blood mononuclear c. (PBMC)
  peripheral blood stem c. (PBSC)
  pituitary c.
  placental giant c.
  plasma c.
  pneumatic c.
  c. precursor
  pregnancy c.
  pregranulosa c.
  primary embryonic c.
  primordial germ c.
  primordial pluripotent stem c.
  promyelocyte c.
  pronormoblast c.
  Purkinje c.'s
  pyknotic c.
  Raji c.
  C. Recovery System (CRS)
  red blood c. (RBC)
  Reed-Sternberg c.
  renal tubular epithelial c.
  reticuloendothelial c.
  Rh null c.
  C. Saver
  Schwann c.
  senescent red c.
  Sertoli c.
  Sertoli-Leydig c.
  sex c.
  sickle c.
  silver c.
  somatic c.
  c. sorting
  spherocytic red blood c.
  spiculated red blood c.
  spindle c.
  squamous c.
  stellate c.
  stem c.
  steroid c.
  stromal c.
  suppressor T c.
  c. surface antigen
  syncytial c.
  syncytiotrophoblastic tumor giant c.
  syngeneic stem c.
  T c.
  target c.
  T-cell-depleted haploidentical bone marrow stem c.
  technetium-labeled red blood c.
  thecal interstitial c.
  theca lutein c.
  T-helper c.
  totipotent c.
  totipotential c.
  triphasic pattern blastemal c.
  trophoblastic c.
  tuboendometrial c.
  vaginal smear intermediate c.
  vaginal smear parabasal c.
  vaginal smear superficial c.
  Vero c.
  viable endometrial c.
  Vignal c.'s
  white blood c. (WBC)
  WI-38 c.
  WISH c.
  yolk c.
CellCept
cell-extracellular matrix adhesion
cell-mediated immunity (CMI)
Cellolite patty
cell-salvaged packed cell

cellular
- c. blue nevus
- c. cast
- c. cytotoxic mechanism
- c. debris
- c. desmoplastic stroma
- c. division
- c. edema
- c. hypoxia
- c. immunity
- c. immunodeficiency
- c. infiltrate
- c. migration
- c. and molecular regulation of lung development
- c. proteolysis
- c. regulation
- c. viral

cellulicidal

cellulitic phlegmasia

cellulitis
- anaerobic c.
- buccal c.
- cuff c.
- *Haemophilus influenzae* c.
- orbital c.
- pelvic c.
- periorbital skin c.
- peritonsillar c.
- pneumococcal facial c.
- postoperative cuff c.
- preseptal c.
- retropharyngeal c.
- streptococcal c.

cellulosae
- *Cysticercus c.*

cellulose acetate (CA)

Cell-VU disposable semen analysis chamber

celom, coelom

celomic, coelomic
- c. cavity
- c. epithelium
- c. metaplasia

Celontin

celosomia

celosomy

Cel-U-Jec Injection

CEM
- cytosine arabinoside, etoposide, methotrexate

cementum
- dental c.

Cemill

cenadelphus

Cenafed Plus

Cena-K

Cenani-Lenz syndactyly

Cenestin
- C. synthetic conjugated estrogens
- C. tablet

Centany ointment

center
- American Association of Poison Control C.'s (AAPCC)
- arousal c.
- birth care c.
- Children's National Medical C.
- Communicable Disease C. (CDC)
- C.'s for Disease Control and Prevention (CDC)
- c. edge angle
- c. edge angle of Wiberg
- electrophilic c.
- C. for Epidemiological Studies Depression Scale for Children
- epiphyseal ossification c.
- germinal c.
- hotline c.
- lower limb ossification c.
- malleolar ossification c.
- pneumotaxic c.
- Poison Control C. (PCC)
- regional perinatal intensive care c. (RPICC)
- school-based health c. (SBHC)
- tertiary care c.
- X inactivation c. (XIC)

centigray (cGy)

centimeter
- cubic c. (cc)
- c. of water (cmH_2O)

centimorgan (cM)

Centocor CA 125 radioimmunoassay kit

central
- c. alveolar hypoventilation
- c. anticholinergic syndrome (CAS)
- c. atrophy
- c. auditory processing disorder (CAPD)
- c. axis depth dose
- c. cord lesion
- c. cord syndrome

NOTES

149

central *(continued)*
    c. core disease
    c. cyanosis
    c. defect
    c. diabetes insipidus
    c. dogma
    c. fat distribution pattern
    c. gliotic tuft
    c. hepatic hematoma
    c. hyperalimentation
    c. hypothyroidism
    c. hypoventilation syndrome
    c. incisor
    c. jaundice
    c. nervous system (CNS)
    c. nervous system/cardiovascular
      syndrome
    c. nervous system differentiation
    c. nervous system disease
    c. nervous system lymphoma
    c. nervous system trauma
    c. neuroblastoma
    c. neurogenic hyperventilation
    c. placenta previa
    c. pontine myelinolysis
    c. porencephaly
    c. precocious puberty (CPP)
    c. primitive neuroectodermal tumor
      (cPNET)
    c. Recklinghausen disease (type II)
    c. respiratory drive
    c. retinal artery
    c. serotonergic hyperactivity
    c. serotonin abnormality
    c. shunt
    c. sleep apnea
    c. syndrome of rostrocaudal
      deterioration
    c. tendon of perineum
    c. type neurofibromatosis
    c. venous access device (CVAD)
    c. venous catheter (CVC)
    c. venous catheterization
    c. venous catheter placement
    c. venous line (CVL)
    c. venous nutrition (CVN)
    c. venous pressure (CVP)
    c. venous pressure catheter
    c. visual field
central-anterior
centralis
    neurinomatosis c.
    placenta previa c.
centralization
    fetal circulatory c.
centralopathic epilepsy
centrencephalic
    c. epilepsy
    c. system

centric fusion translocation
centrifugation
    Ficoll-Hypaque c.
centrifuge
centrifugum
    leukoderma acquisitum c.
centrilobular necrosis
centripetal spread
centrizonal
    c. hypoxia
    c. sinusoidal distention
centromere interference
centromeric
    c. banding
    c. instability-immunodeficiency
      syndrome
    c. region of chromosome
    c. signal
centronuclear myopathy (CNM)
centrotemporal
    c. epilepsy
    c. spike
Ceo-Two
CEP
    congenital erythropoietic porphyria
cepacia
    Burkholderia c.
    Pseudomonas c.
Cepacol Anesthetic Troche
CEPH
    CEPH family
    CEPH pedigree
cephalad
cephalexin
cephalhematoma, cephalohematoma
    bilateral c.'s
    c. deformans
cephalhydrocele
cephalic
    c. cry
    c. delivery
    c. forceps
    c. pole
    c. presentation
    c. prominence
    c. replacement
    c. tetanus
    c. vein
    c. version
cephalization
    primordial c.
cephalocaudal
    c. film-screen mammogram
    c. sequence
    c. sequence of development
cephalocele
cephalocentesis
cephalodactyly
    Vogt c.

cephalodiprosopus
cephalohematoma (*var. of*
  cephalhematoma)
cephalomelus
cephalometric radiograph
cephalometry
  ultrasonic c.
cephalonia
cephalopagus
cephalopelvic disproportion (CPD)
cephalopelvimetry
cephalopolysyndactyly syndrome
cephalosporin
  first-generation c.
cephalosporin-resistant pneumococcus
cephalostat
cephalothin sodium
cephalothoracopagus
cephalotome
cephalotomy
cephalotribe
cephapirin
cephazolin
cephradine
Ceporacin
Ceporex
Ceptaz
CeraLyte drink mix
ceramidase activity
ceramide
  c. trihexose
  c. trihexoside alpha galactosidase
ceramidosis
c-*erb*
  c-*erb* B-2 oncogene
  c-*erb* B-2 oncoprotein
  c-*erb* B-2 protooncogene
cercaria, pl. **cercariae**
cercarial
  c. dermatitis
  c. skin penetration
cerclage
  Barnes c.
  cervical c.
  Mann isthmic c.
  McDonald cervical c.
  c. placement
  prophylactic c.
  rescue cervical c.
  Shirodkar cervical c.
  transabdominal cervicoisthmic c.
  web c.

cerebella (*pl. of* cerebellum)
cerebellar
  c. asynergia
  c. ataxia
  c. cerebral palsy
  c. degeneration
  c. dysfunction
  c. dysplasia
  c. encephalitis
  c. folia
  c. hemangioblastoma
  c. hematoma
  c. hemisphere compression
  c. hemorrhage
  c. hypertrophy
  c. mutism
  c. neoplasm
  c. nucleus
  c. tonsils
  c. tumor
  c. vermis
  c. vermis agenesis
  c. vermis aplasia
  c. vermis hypogenesis
  c. vermis hypoplasia
  c. vermis hypoplasia, oligophrenia,
    congenital ataxia, ocular
    coloboma, hepatic fibrosis
    (COACH)
cerebellar-vestibular system
cerebelli
  folia c.
  vermis c.
cerebellitis
  acute c.
  postinfectious c.
  viral c.
cerebelloparenchymal disorder (I–IV)
  (CPD)
cerebellotrigeminal and focal dermal
  dysplasia
cerebellum, pl. **cerebella**
  absent c.
  dysplastic gangliocytoma of c.
  inverse c.
cerebral
  c. amebiasis
  c. angiography
  c. angioma
  c. anoxia
  c. arteriovenous malformation
    (CAVM)

NOTES

cerebral *(continued)*
    c. artery aneurysm
    c. artery occlusion
    c. aspergillosis
    c. atrophy
    c. blood flow (CBF)
    c. blood flow velocity (CBFV)
    c. blood volume (CBV)
    c. compression
    c. contusion
    c. cortex
    c. cortical necrosis
    c. dysfunction
    c. dysfunction syndrome
    c. dysgenesis
    c. edema
    c. embolism
    c. falx
    c. function monitor (CFM)
    c. gigantism
    c. glucose metabolism
    c. GM1 gangliosidosis
    c. hematoma
    c. hemisphere
    c. herniation
    c. holosphere
    c. hypoperfusion
    c. hypothermia
    c. infarction
    c. injury
    c. ischemia
    c. laceration
    c. lactic alkalosis
    c. leukodystrophy
    c. leukomalacia
    c. malaria
    c. malformations, seizures, hypertrichosis, overlapping fingers syndrome
    c. metabolic rate
    c., ocular, dental, auricular, skeletal (CODAS)
    c. oximetry
    c. oxygen consumption
    c. palsy (CP)
    c. palsy antecedent
    c. palsy, hypotonic seizures, megalocornea syndrome
    c. paragonimiasis
    c. peduncle
    c. perfusion pressure (CPP)
    c. resuscitation
    c. salt wasting (CSW)
    c. schistosomiasis
    c. swelling
    c. syncope
    c. thrombosis
    c. trypanosomiasis
    c. vasospasm
    c. ventriculomegaly

cerebrale
    cranium c.

cerebral-placental ratio

cerebri
    pseudotumor c.

cerebriform

cerebritis
    lupus c.

cerebroarthrodigital syndrome

cerebroatrophic hyperammonemia

cerebrocostomandibular (CCM)
    c. syndrome (CCMS)

cerebrocutaneous angiomatosis

cerebrofacioarticular (CFA)

cerebrofaciothoracic syndrome or dysplasia

cerebrohepatorenal syndrome (CHRS)

cerebromacular degeneration

cerebroocular
    c. dentoauriculoskeletal (CODAS)
    c. dysgenesis (COD)
    c. dysgenesis-muscular dystrophy (COD-MD)
    c. dysplasia-muscular dystrophy
    c. muscular dystrophy

cerebrooculofacial-skeletal (COFS)

cerebrooculomuscular syndrome (COMS)

cerebrooculonasal syndrome

cerebroosteonephrodysplasia (COND)
    Hutterite c.

cerebroosteonephrosis syndrome

cerebroprotective mechanism

cerebroside lipidosis

cerebrospinal
    c. fluid (CSF)
    c. fluid leak
    c. fluid procalcitonin
    c. fluid sampling

cerebrotendinous xanthomatosis

cerebrovascular
    c. accident (CVA)
    c. disease

cerebrovasculosa

cerebrum

Cerebyx

Ceredase

cereus
    Bacillus c.

cerevisiae
    Saccharomyces c.

Cerezyme

ceroid lipofuscinosis

Cerose-DM

Cerrobend
    C. block
    C. casting

certificate
>birth c.

certified
>c. nurse-midwife (CNM)
>c. registered nurse anesthetist

Certiva vaccine
Cerubidine
cerulea
>macula c.

cerulean cataract
ceruloplasmin
>c. deficiency
>c. level

cerumen
Cerumenex Otic
Cervagem
Cervex-Brush cervical cell sampler
cervical
>c. abnormality
>c. adenitis
>c. adenopathy
>c. agenesis
>c. amputation
>c. anomaly
>c. artery
>c. atresia
>c. atypia
>c. block kit
>c. canal
>c. cannula
>c. cap
>c. carcinoma
>c. carcinoma stimulation
>c. cerclage
>c. clamp
>c. clear cell adenocarcinoma
>c. cockscomb
>c. collar
>c. combing
>c. competence
>c. condyloma
>c. cone biopsy
>c. conization
>c. cord tumor
>c. culture
>c. cytology
>c. dilation
>c. disc space calcification
>c. dysplasia
>c. dystocia
>c. ectopic pregnancy
>c. ectopy

c. ectropion
c. effacement
c. epithelial neoplasia
c. epithelium
c. erosion
c. esophagostomy
c. esophagus
c. eversion
c. examination
c. factor
c. funneling
c. GIFT
c. herpes
c. incision
c. incompetence (CI)
c. incompetence prevention randomized cerclage trial (CIPRACT)
c. infection
c. insemination
c. intraepithelial neoplasia (CIN)
c. isthmus
c. laceration
c. leiomyoma
c. length
c. lesion
c. lymphadenitis
c. lymphadenopathy
c. mass
c. motion tenderness (CMT)
c. mucorrhea
c. mucosa
c. mucus
c. myoma
c. os
c. polyp
c. position
c. priming
c. prolapse
c. rib
c. ripening
c. sarcoma
c. score
c. sinus
c. smear
c. spinal cord injury
c. spine immobilization
c. spine injury
c. spine subluxation
c. stenosis
c. stenosis obstruction
c. stroma

NOTES

cervical *(continued)*
    c. stump
    c. stump cancer
    c. stump tumor
    c. tenaculum
    c. teratoma
    c. tissue impedance range
    topographic c.
    c. transformation zone
    c. venous hum
    c. vertebral fusion
cervical-priming agent
cervicectomy
cervices (*pl. of* cervix)
cervicitis
    chlamydial c.
    chronic c.
    gonorrheal c.
    mucopurulent c.
    nongonococcal c.
cervicofacial actinomycosis
cervicography
cervicomedullary
    c. brainstem glioma
    c. compression
    c. junction
cervicoplasty
cervicotomy
cervicovaginal
    c. fetal fibronectin
    c. fistula
    c. infection
    c. junction
    c. ridge
    c. secretion
Cervidil vaginal insert
Cer-View lateral vaginal retractor
cervigram
Cervilaxin
Cerviprost gel
CerviSoft cytology collection device
cervix, pl. **cervices**
    anterior lip of the c.
    atretic c.
    barrel c.
    barrel-shaped c.
    bifid c.
    carcinoma of c.
    cockscomb c.
    collared c.
    cone biopsy of c.
    congenital atresia of uterine c.
    conization of c.
    dilation of c.
    effacement of c.
    fishmouth c.
    friable c.
    incompetent c.

    international classification of cancer of c.
    malignant tumor of c.
    multiple c.
    c. neoplasm
    short c.
    shortened c.
    strawberry c.
    unfavorable c.
CES
    cat eye syndrome
    cat's eye syndrome
    cranial electrical stimulation
cesarean, cesarean section
    c. delivery
    extraperitoneal c.
    c. hysterectomy
    Kerr c.
    Latzko c.
    low cervical c.
    lower segment c. (LSCS)
    low transverse c. (LTC)
    c. operation
    salvage c.
    c. section (C-section)
    transperitoneal c.
    vaginal birth after c. (VBAC)
CESD
    cholesterol ester storage disease
cesium
    c. candle
    c. cylinder
    c. implant
    c. iodide (CsI)
    c. irradiation
    c. source
cesium-137 (^{137}Cs)
cesium iodide (CsI)
cessation of progress
Cetacaine
Cetacort Topical
Cetamide
Cetaphil
cetirizine hydrochloride
Cetrorelix for injection
Cetrotide
cetyl alcohol
cetylpyridinium
Cevi-Bid
Ce-Vi-Sol
ceylanicum
    Ancylostoma c.
CF
    clavicular fracture
    clubfoot
    cystic fibrosis
    CF test
^{252}Cf
    californium-252

CFA
 cerebrofacioarticular
  CFA syndrome
CFC
 cardiofaciocutaneous
  CFC syndrome
CFL
 calcaneofibular ligament
 cisplatin, 5-fluorouracil, leucovorin
  calcium
CFM
 cerebral function monitor
c-fms protooncogene
CFND
 craniofrontonasal dysplasia
CFR
 coronary flow reserve
CFS
 chronic fatigue syndrome
CFTR
 cystic fibrosis transmembrane regulator
CFU
 colony-forming unit
CFUC
 colony-forming unit in culture
CFU-E
 colony-forming unit erythroid
CG
 chorionic gonadotropin
CGAS
 Children's Global Assessment Scale
CGD
 chronic granulomatous disease
 continuous gastric drip
CGH
 comparative genomic hybridization
CGI
 Clinical Global Impressions
 clinical global index
  CGI scale
cGMP
 cyclic guanosine monophosphate
cGMP-specific
  cGMP-s. phosphodiesterase
  cGMP-s. phosphodiesterase 5
cGy
 centigray
CH
 congenital hypothyroidism
CH$_{50}$
 hemolytic complement
  CH$_{50}$ assay

CHADD
 children and adults with attention deficit
  disorder
Chadwick sign
chaffeensis
  Ehrlichia c.
Chagas disease
chagasic encephalitis
chagoma
chain
 beta c.
 c. cystourethrography
 globin c.
 heavy c.
 kappa c.
 light c.
 c. reaction
 sympathetic c.
chain-breaking antioxidant
chaining
 backward c.
 forward c.
chair
 adaptive c.
 birthing c.
 child's c.
 corner c.
 Midmark 413 power female
  procedure c.
chalasia
chalazion, pl. **chalazia**
challenge
 acrosome reaction with
  ionophore c. (ARIC)
 bee sting c.
 blinded c.
 bronchial provocation c.
 caloric c.
 cow's milk c.
 diuretic c.
 exercise bronchial c.
 gluten c.
 intravenous glucose c.
 methacholine c.
 progestational c.
chamber
 anterior c.
 Cell-VU disposable semen
  analysis c.
 Enhanced Metabolic Testing
  Activity C. (EMTAC)
 face c.

NOTES

C

chamber *(continued)*
    holding c.
    hyperbaric c.
    infundibular c.
    Makler reusable semen analysis c.
    Neubauer c.
    respiratory c.
    vitreous c.
Chamberlain line
Chamberlen forceps
chameleon tongue
chamomile
Champetier de Ribes bag
Chanarin-Dorfman syndrome
Chance fracture
chancre
    hunterian c.
    trypanosomal c.
    tuberculous c.
chancroidal bubo
chancroid ulcer
chandelier sign
change
    atrophic c.
    benign cellular c.'s (BCC)
    breast c.
    concomitant c.
    dietary c.
    failed physiologic c.
    fibrocystic breast c.
    focal c.
    glomerular c.
    harlequin color c.
    hematological c.
    hormonal balance c.
    hormone-stimulated endometrial c.
    hydatidiform c.
    immunohistochemical c.
    immunologic c.
    libidinal c.
    c. of life
    lumbosacral skin pigment c.
    nonproliferative fibrocystic c.
    ovarian cycle c.
    papulosquamous skin c.
    personality c.
    polyneuropathy, organomegaly,
      endocrinopathy, M protein,
      skin c.'s (POEMS)
    postasphyxial c.
    postpartum hemodynamic c.
    proliferative c.
    pupillary c.
    rachitic c.
    retinal c.
    sensorineural c.
    ST c.
    structural airway c.
    visual c.
    wave c.
change-point regression
channel
    common c.
    exposed large venous c.
    sinusoidal c.
    surface epithelium vascular c.
    vascular c.
    voltage-dependent calcium c.
channelopathy
    chloride c.
    sodium c.
2-channel pneumogram
CHAOS
    congenital high airway obstruction
      syndrome
chaotic
    c. atrial tachycardia
    c. eye movement
Chapple syndrome
character
    classifiable c.
    denumerable c.
    discrete c.
    Y-linked c.
characteristic
    c. electroencephalogram pattern
    c. emotional response
    epidemiologic c.
    c. face, hypogenitalism, hypotonia,
      pachygyria syndrome
    isosexual sexual c.
    morphological c.
    organoleptic c.
    receiver operating c. (ROC)
    secondary sex c.
characterization
    immunohistochemical stromal
      leukocyte c.
charcoal
    activated c.
    c. agar
    multidose activated c. (MDAC)
    c. polyp
charcoal-blood medium
Charcot
    C. disease
    C. joint
    C. triad
Charcot-Leyden crystal
Charcot-Marie-Tooth (CMT)
    C.-M.-T. disease
    C.-M.-T. disorder
    C.-M.-T. syndrome (CMTS)
    C.-M.-T. syndrome X-linked
      recessive type II

C.-M.-T. syndrome, X-linked type
II with deafness and mental
retardation
Charcot-Marie-Tooth-Hoffmann
syndrome
CHARGE
coloboma, heart disease, atresia choanae,
retarded growth and development, CNS
anomalies, genital hypoplasia, ear
anomalies and/or deafness
CHARGE association
CHARGE syndrome
Charing Cross experience
Charleston brace
Charlevois-Saguenay syndrome
Charlevoix disease
Charlson comorbidity index
Char syndrome
chart
Allen c.
Babson c.
Ballard c.
BBT c.
Broselow c.
Cardiff Count-to-Ten c.
Denver Developmental c.
Down syndrome growth c.
Genentech growth c.
letter c.
Liley three-zone c.
pedigree c.
picture c.
Ross growth c.
seca-230 Promard wall growth c.
sex-specific CDC growth c.
Snellen acuity c.
star c.
Swedish national growth c.
tumbling E c.
Walker c.
Welch Allyn SureSight eye c.
chartarum
Stachybotrys c.
chaser
Scot-Tussin DM Dough C.'s
Chassar
C. Moir-Sims procedure
C. Moir sling procedure
chaste
chasteberry
chastity

chat
cri du c.
chatter
cocktail c.
CHD
congenital heart disease
congenital hip dislocation
congenital hip dysplasia
congestive heart disease
Cheadle
C. disease
C. syndrome
Chealamide
ChEAT
Children's Eating Attitudes Test
check
developmental c.
c. valve obstruction
checklist
Achenbach Child Behavior C.
asthma symptom c. (ASC)
bed rest c.
Child Behavior C. (CBCL)
Children's Coping Strategies C.
(CCSC)
Developmental Behaviour C.
Hopkins symptom c.
life events c. (LEC)
Pediatric Symptom C. (PSC)
Self-Injury and Self-Restraint c.
(SISRC)
Wing Autistic Disorder
Interview C. (WADIC)
Checklist-Revised
Noncommunicating Children's
Pain C.-R. (NCCPC-R)
Chédiak-Higashi
C.-H. anomaly
C.-H. deficiency
C.-H. syndrome
cheek
chipmunk c.'s
cheese-wiring
cheesy
c. discharge
c. exudate
cheilitis
angular c.
cheilognathopalatoschisis
cheilognathoprosoposchisis
cheilognathoschisis
cheilognathouranoschisis

NOTES

157

cheiloschisis
cheilosis
    angular c.
cheiroarthropathy
    diabetic c.
chelated gadolinium
chelation
    iron c.
    c. therapy
chelator
    iron c.
Chelex bead
chelonae
    Mycobacterium c.
Chemet
chemical
    c. carcinogen
    c. conjunctivitis
    c. dependency
    c. diabetes
    c. peritonitis
    c. pleurodesis
    c. pneumonia
    c. pneumonitis
    c. pregnancy
    c. sampling
    c. shift imaging (CSI)
    c. vaginitis
    c. vulvovaginitis
chemically
    c. exposed
    c. exposed child
chemiluminescence
chemiluminescent
    c. illumination
    c. immunoassay (CIA)
Chemke syndrome
chemoattractant
chemoembolization
C-hemoglobinopathy
chemoimmunotherapy
chemokine
Chemo-Port catheter
chemoprevention
    hormone c.
chemoprophylactic
chemoprophylaxis
    intrapartum c.
    selective intrapartum c. (SIC)
chemoradiation
chemoreceptor
    c. sensitivity
    c. trigger zone (CTZ)
chemoreflex
    laryngeal c.
chemosis
chemotactic
    c. agent
    c. factor

chemotaxis
chemotherapeutic
    c. agent
    c. retroconversion
chemotherapy
    adjuvant c.
    alkylating c.
    antituberculosis c.
    cancer c.
    cell cycling in c.
    CHOP c.
    combination c.
    cyclophosphamide, hydroxydaunorubicin, methotrexate, prednisone c.
    high-dose c.
    intraarterial c.
    intraperitoneal c.
    marrow-ablative c.
    metabolism in intraperitoneal c.
    multidrug c.
    near-myeloablative c.
    neoadjuvant c.
    c. phase trial
    postoperative c.
    prophylactic c.
    c. protocol
    salvage c.
    second-line c.
    VAMP c.
chemotherapy-related neutropenia
Chemstrip
    C. bG
    Micral C.
    C. 4 The OB
    C. 10 with SG
Cheney syndrome
Cheracol D
Cherney incision
cherry-red
    c.-r. macular spot
    c.-r. macule
    c.-r. spot myoclonus syndrome
cherubism, gingival fibromatosis, epilepsy, mental deficiency syndrome
cherub sign
Chesapeake
    hemoglobin C.
Cheshire cat smile
chessboard pattern
chest
    barrel c.
    barrel-shaped c.
    c. compression
    c. examination
    flail c.
    funnel c.
    keel c.
    c. mount

c. pain
c. percussion
c. percussion and auscultation
c. physical therapy (CPT)
c. physiotherapy (CPT)
c. radiograph
c. radiography
c. roentgenography
shield-shaped c.
c. suctioning
c. syndrome
c. trauma
c. tube
c. tube drainage
c. wall motion
c. wall radiation therapy
c. wall rigidity
c. wall weight
c. width
c. x-ray (CXR)

chewable
E.E.S. C.
chewing
rotary c.
Cheyne-Stokes respiration
CHF
congestive heart failure
CHH
cartilage-hair hypoplasia
CHI
closed head injury
Chiari
C. anomaly
C. crisis
C. deformity
C. malformation (type I–IV)
C. net
C. procedure
Chiari-Arnold syndrome
Chiari-Frommel syndrome
chiasma, pl. **chiasmata**
c. formation
c. interference
optic c.
chiasmal glioma
chiasmatic
c. cistern
c. pilocytic astrocytoma
chiasmatic-hypothalamic glioma
Chiba needle
CHIC
Coping Health Inventory for Children

Chicago classification
Chicco breast pump
chicken ovalbumin upstream promoter transcription factor II (COUP)
chickenpox
gestational c.
c. pneumonia
c. vaccine
c. virus
Chid breast pump
chigger bite
Chiggertox
chikungunya virus
Chilaiditi syndrome
chilblain
CHILD
congenital hemidysplasia with ichthyosiform erythroderma and limb defects
CHILD syndrome
child
c. abuse (CA)
c. abuse dwarfism
c. abuse and neglect
C. Abuse Prevention and Treatment Act (CAPTA)
C. Abuse Trauma Scale (CATS)
c. and adolescent burden assessment (CABA)
c., adolescent, and family mental health service (CAFMHS)
c. and adolescent forensic psychiatry
C. and Adolescent Functional Assessment Scale (CAFAS)
C. and Adolescent Psychiatric Assessment (CAPA)
c. and adolescent psychiatrist
C. and Adolescent Services Assessment (CASA)
c. of alcoholic (COA)
c. assessment schedule (CAS)
atopic c.
c. behavioral study (CBS)
C. Behavior Checklist (CBCL)
c. behavior rating form (CBRF)
cardiorespiratory syndrome of obesity in c.
chemically exposed c.
CMV-shedding c.
Down syndrome c. (DSC)
C. Find

NOTES

child *(continued)*
  C. Health and Illness Profile, Adolescent Edition (CHIP-AE)
  c. health questionnaire (CHQ)
  immunocompromised c.
  parent c.
  c. physical abuse (CPA)
  c. protective agency
  C. Protective Services (CPS)
  c. restraint
  c. sexual abuse (CSA)
  C. Sexual Behavior Inventory (CSBI)
  c. of substance abuser (COSA)
  term birth, living c. (TBLC)
  unborn c.
  C. Version of the Retrospective Diagnostic Interview for Borderlines
  very low birth weight c.

child-adult mist (CAM)
childbearing age
childbed fever
childbirth
  Bradley method of prepared c.
  Gamper method of c.
  Grantley Dick-Read method of c.
  Kitzinger method of c.
  natural c.
  physiologic c.

childbirth-related
  c.-r. medical condition
  c.-r. morbidity

child-centered literary orientation (CCLO)
child-directed instruction
childhood
  c. absence epilepsy
  c. accidental spiral tibial (CAST)
  alternating hemiplegia of c.
  c. anxiety
  C. Asthma Management Program (CAMP)
  C. Autism Rating Scale (CARS)
  benign epilepsy of c.
  c. breast
  C. Cancer Survivor Study
  chronic benign neutropenia of c.
  chronic bullous dermatosis of c.
  chronic bullous disease of c.
  chronic idiopathic arthritides of c. (CIAC)
  c. cicatricial pemphigoid
  c. conjunctivitis
  c. disintegrative disorder (CDD)
  c. epileptic encephalopathy
  erythroblastic anemia of c.
  c. fibromyalgia
  c. genital trauma

c. idiopathic thrombocytopenic purpura
irritable colon of c.
limb pain of c.
localized vulvar pemphigoid of c. (LVPC)
overanxious disorder of c.
papular acrodermatitis of c. (PAC)
progressive bulbar paralysis of c.
progressive muscular dystrophy of c.
c. progressive systemic sclerosis
c. pseudohypertrophic muscular dystrophy
reactive attachment disorder of infancy or early c.
recurring digital fibroma of c. (RDFC)
c. schizophrenia
c. severity of psychiatric illness (CSPI)
small round blue cell tumor of c.
c. thyroid carcinoma
transient erythroblastopenia of c. (TEC)
c. trauma questionnaire (CTQ)
universal nose of c.
unstable bladder of c.
vasculitis of c.

childhood-onset schizophrenia (COS)
childlessness
children
  c. and adults with attention deficit disorder (CHADD)
  Aid to Families with Dependent C. (AFDC)
  c. of alcoholic (COA)
  C. of Alcoholics Screening Test (CAST)
  Anxiety Disorder Interview for C.
  anxiety rating for c. (ARC)
  Behavioral Assessment Scale for C. (BASC)
  burden of care interview for c.
  Center for Epidemiological Studies Depression Scale for C.
  Coping Health Inventory for C. (CHIC)
  Developmental Programming for Infants and Young C.
  Diagnostic Interview Schedule for C. (DISC)
  Diagnostic Interview Schedule for C.-Revised (DISC-R)
  emergency medical services for c. (EMS-C)
  Functional Independence Measure for C. (WeeFIM)

HIV Classification for C. (P0, P1,
P2)
Hospital for Sick C. (HSC)
human immunodeficiency virus
infected c.
immune-competent c.
Kaufman Assessment Battery
for C. (KABC)
living c. (LC)
Lower Anchorages and Tethers
for c. (LATCH)
Neurological Examination for C.
(NEC)
Personality Inventory for C. (PIC)
puppet c.
Schedule for Affective Disorders
and Schizophrenia for School-
Age C. (K-SADS)
Silverman and Nelles Anxiety
Disorders Interview Schedule
for C.
Social Support Scale for C.
(SSSC)
Stanford-Binet Intelligence Scale
for C.
State-Trait Anxiety Inventory
for C.
St. Joseph Aspirin-Free Cold
Tablets for C.
term infants, premature infants,
abortions, living c. (TPAL)
Trauma Symptom Checklist for C.
(TSCC)
traumatic aortic injuries in c.
treatment and education of autistic
and related communications
handicapped c. (TEACCH)
Tylenol Cold, C.'s
Wechsler Intelligence Scale for C.
(WISC)
Wechsler Intelligence Scale for C.
III
Wechsler Intelligence Scale for C.-
Revised (WISC-R)
C. with Special Health Care Needs
(CWSN)
women, infants, children (WIC)
children's
C. Cancer Group (CCG)
C. Cancer Study Group (CCSG)
C. Coping Strategies Checklist
(CCSC)

C. Depression Inventory (CDI)
C. Depression Inventory test
C. Depression Rating Scale-Revised
(CDRS-R)
C. Depression Scale
C. Digestive Health and Nutrition
Foundation (CDHNF)
C. Eating Attitudes Test (ChEAT)
C. Global Assessment Scale
(CGAS)
C. Health Insurance Program
(CHIP)
C. Interview for Psychiatric
Disorders (ChIPS)
C. Manifest Anxiety Scale
C. Motrin
C. Motrin Suspension
C. National Medical Center
c. service
C. Silfedrine
child's chair
chills
fevers and c. (F&C)
CHIME
Collaborative Home Infant Monitoring
Evaluation
coloboma, heart defects, ichthyosiform
dermatosis, mental retardation, ear
defects
CHIME syndrome
chimera
chimeric
c. gene
c. protein
chimerism
blood c.
chin
cleft c.
c. dimple
galoche c.
c. lift
c. position
c. quivering
underdeveloped c.
Chinese
C. medicine
C. restaurant syndrome
CHIP
Children's Health Insurance Program
Coping Health Inventory for Parents
chip
gene c.

NOTES

CHIP-AE
  Child Health and Illness Profile,
    Adolescent Edition
chipmunk cheeks
ChIPS
  Children's Interview for Psychiatric
    Disorders
Chiron branched DNA assay
chiropractic
CHL
  crown-heel length
Chlamydia
  C. pecorum
  C. pneumoniae
  C. psittaci
  C. sepsis
  C. trachomatis (CT)
  C. trachomatis ligase chain
    reaction
  C. trachomatis pneumonia
  C. trachomatis tubal infertility
chlamydia
chlamydial
  c. cervicitis
  c. conjunctivitis
  c. infection
  c. pneumonia
  c. urethritis
  c. vaginitis
Chlamydiazyme
  C. immunoassay
  C. test
chloasma
Chlor-100
chloracne
chloral
  c. hydrate
  c. hydrate sedation
chlorambucil
chloramphenicol
chloramphenicol-resistant isolate
chlorcyclizine hydrochloride
chlordecone
chlordiazepoxide
chlorhexidine
  c. gluconate
  c. solution
chloride
  acetylcholine c.
  Adrenalin C.
  aluminum c.
  ammonium c.
  Anectine C.
  bethanechol c.
  calcium c.
  c. channelopathy
  doxacurium c.
  ethyl c.
  ferrous c.

Gebauer ethyl c.
isotonic sodium c.
magnesium c.
mercuric c.
methylbenzethonium c.
obidoxime c.
oxybutynin c.
polyvinyl c.
potassium c. (KCl)
pralidoxime c.
sodium c. (NaCl)
sweat c.
tubocurarine c.
vinyl c.
chloride-losing diarrhea
chloridometer
chloridorrhea
  congenital c.
chlormethiazole
Chlor-Niramine
Chlorohist-LA
chloroma
Chloromycetin Injection
chlorophyllin copper complex
chloroplast DNA
chloroquine phosphate
chloroquine-resistant
  c.-r. malaria
  c.-r. *Plasmodium falciparum*
chloroquine-sensitive *Plasmodium*
  falciparum
chlorosis
chlorothiazide
chlorotrianisene
chlorpheniramine
Chlorpromanyl
chlorpromazine
chlorpropamide
chlorprothixene
Chlortab
chlortetracycline fluorescence test
chlorthalidone
Chlor-Trimeton
  C.-T. Injection
  C.-T. Oral
Chlor-Tripolon
chlorzoxazone
CHN
  congenital hypomyelinating neuropathy
choanae
  atresia c.
choanal
  c. atresia
  c. stenosis
chocolate
  c. agar
  c. agar plate
  c. cyst

choice
    forced c.
choked disc
choke mark
Cholac
cholangiogram
    T-tube c.
cholangiography
    breath-hold MR c.
    magnetic resonance c. (MRC)
    non-breathhold MR c.
    percutaneous c.
    single-film c.
cholangiopancreatography
    endoscopic retrograde c. (ERCP)
    magnetic resonance c. (MRCP)
cholangiopathy
    ascending c.
    infantile obstructive c.
    progressive obliterative c.
cholangitis
    ascending c.
    primary sclerosing c.
    recurrent c.
    sclerosing c.
    suppurative c.
Cholebrine
cholecalciferol
    deficient hydroxylation of c.
cholecystectomy
    laparoscopic c. (LC)
cholecystitis
    acalculous c.
    acute acalculous c.
    hydrops-like c.
cholecystokinin (CCK)
    fasting plasma c.
    postprandial plasma c.
choledochal
    c. cyst
    c. cyst-induced pancreatitis
choledochojejunostomy
    Roux-en-Y c.
choledocholithiasis
choledochus
    ductus c.
    terminal c.
cholelithiasis
    cholesterol c.
cholera
    c. infantum
    c. vaccine

cholerae
    Vibrio c.
choleraesuis
    Salmonella c.
cholestasis
    benign familial recurrent c.
    familial intrahepatic c.
    hyperalimentation-associated c.
    intrahepatic c.
    maternal c.
    neonatal c.
    c., pigmentary retinopathy, cleft
      palate syndrome
    progressive familial intrahepatic c.
      (PFIC)
    total parenteral nutrition-
      associated c.
cholestasis-peripheral pulmonary stenosis
cholestatic
    c. hepatosis of pregnancy
    c. jaundice
    c. liver disease
    c. syndrome
cholesteatoma
    congenital c.
cholesterol
    c. cholelithiasis
    c. 20,22 desmolase
    c. ester
    c. ester storage disease (CESD)
    c. gallstone
    c. granuloma
    LDL c.
    c. oxidase
    plasma c.
    c. stone
    c. synthesis
cholesterolemia
    familial c.
cholestyramine resin
choline
    free c.
    c. magnesium trisalicylate
    c. salicylate
    c. theophyllinate
cholinergic
    c. agonist
    c. crisis
    c. drug
    c. sympathetic function
    c. urticaria
cholinesterase inhibitor

NOTES

C

chondrification
chondroblastic osteosarcoma
chondroblastoma
chondrocyte
chondrodysplasia
    giant cell c.
    Grebe c.
    hereditary c.
    Jansen metaphyseal c.
    c. punctata
    rhizomelic c.
chondrodysplasia-pseudohermaphrodism
  syndrome
chondrodystrophia
    c. calcificans congenita
    c. congenita punctata
    c. congenita tarda
    c. fetalis calcificans
    c. myotonica
chondrodystrophica
    myotonia c.
chondrodystrophic myotonia
chondrodystrophy
    asphyxiating thoracic c.
    atypical c.
    hereditary deforming c.
    myotonic c.
    primary c.
chondroectodermal
    c. dysplasia
    c. dysplasia-like syndrome
chondroitin sulfate
chondrolysis
chondromalacia
    c. fetalis
    c. patella
chondromere
chondromyxoid fibroma
chondroosteodystrophy
chondroplastic dwarfism
chondrosarcoma
    uterine c.
chondrosome
Chooz
CHOP
    cyclophosphamide, hydroxydaunorubicin,
    methotrexate, prednisone
      CHOP chemotherapy
choramphenicol
chorda, pl. **chordae**
    chordae tendinea
    c. tympani
    c. umbilicalis
chordablastoma
chordamesoderm
    caudal c.
chordate
chordee
    c. correction

    dorsal c.
    penile c.
chordoid sarcoma
chordoma
chorea
    benign nonprogressive familial c.
    c. gravidarum
    hereditary benign c.
    Huntington c.
    c. magna
    c. minor
    Sydenham c.
chorea-acanthocytosis
choreic
    c. hand
    c. movement
choreiform movement
choreoathetoid
    c. cerebral palsy
    c. movement
choreoathetosis
    bilateral c.
    familial inverted c.
    paroxysmal kinesigenic c.
choreoathetotic
    c. movement
    c. movement disorder
Chorex
chorioadenoma destruens
chorioallantoic
    c. membrane (CAM)
    c. placenta
    c. vessel
chorioamnionic, chorioamniotic
    c. band
    c. infection
    c. placenta
chorioamnion infection
chorioamnionitis (CA)
    Gardnerella vaginalis c.
    histologic c.
chorioangioma
chorioangiomatosis
chorioangiopagi parasiticus
chorioangiopagus placental vessel
chorioangiosis
chorioblastoma
choriocarcinoma
    nongestational c.
choriodecidua
choriodecidual tissue
chorioembryonic antigen
chorioepithelioma
choriogenesis
choriogonadotropin
    c. alfa
    c. alfa for injection

choriomeningitis
>   experimental lymphocytic c.
>   lymphocytic c.

chorion
>   c. frondosum
>   c. laeve
>   outer c.
>   c. sampling
>   smooth c.
>   villous c.

chorionic
>   c. adrenocorticotropin
>   c. cavity
>   c. cyst
>   c. gonadotropic hormone
>   c. gonadotropin (CG)
>   c. growth hormone
>   c. human recombinant gonadotropin
>   c. plate
>   c. sac
>   c. somamammotropin
>   c. thyrotropin
>   c. vascularization
>   c. vesicle
>   c. vessel thrombus
>   c. villi
>   c. villus biopsy (CVB)
>   c. villus haplotype analysis
>   c. villus infarction
>   c. villus ischemia
>   c. villus sampling (CVS)

chorionicity
chorioretinal anomalies, corpus callosum agenesis, infantile spasms syndrome
chorioretinitis
>   toxoplasmic c.

choriovitelline placenta
choroid
>   c. plexus
>   c. plexus carcinoma (CPC)
>   c. plexus cell
>   c. plexus cyst (CPC)
>   c. plexus papillocarcinoma
>   c. plexus papilloma (CPP)
>   c. plexus primordia
>   c. plexus pulse effect
>   c. tubercle

choroiditis
Chotzen syndrome
CHQ
>   child health questionnaire

Christchurch chromosome

Christian-Andrews-Conneally-Muller syndrome
Christian-Opitz syndrome
Christian syndrome (1, 2)
Christmas
>   C. disease
>   C. factor
>   C. tree bladder
>   C. tree distribution
>   C. tree distribution eruption
>   C. tree pattern

Christ-Siemens-Touraine syndrome
chromaffinoma
Chromagen FA, OB
Chroma-Pak
chromatid
>   sister c.

chromatin
>   sex c.
>   X c.
>   Y c.

chromatofocusing pH range
chromatography
>   amino acid c.
>   denaturing high-performance liquid c.
>   gas c.
>   high-performance liquid c. (HPLC)
>   high-power liquid c. (HPLC)
>   high-pressure liquid c. (HPLC)
>   thin-layer c. (TLC)

chromatolysis
chromatophore nevus of Naegeli
chromhidrosis
>   apocrine c.

chromic
>   #1 c.
>   c. gut pelviscopic loop ligature
>   c. phosphate

chromium
chromogen
chromogene
chromohydrotubation
chromomere
chromoneme
chromopertubation
chromophobe
chromophobic adenoma
chromophore
chromosomal
>   c. aberration
>   c. analysis

NOTES

chromosomal *(continued)*
- c. anomaly
- c. banding
- c. breakage-immunodeficiency syndrome
- c. defect
- c. deletion
- c. disorder
- c. dysfunction
- c. inversion
- c. karyotype
- c. marker
- c. mosaicism
- c. nondisjunction
- c. pattern
- c. segment
- c. sex
- c. structural abnormality
- c. study
- c. translocation

chromosome
- c. 1–23
- c. aberration
- accessory c.
- acentric c.
- acrocentric c.
- c. analysis
- arm of c.
- artificial c.
- B c.
- bacterial artificial c. (BAC)
- c. banding
- bivalent c.
- c. breakage
- c. breakage test
- centromeric region of c.
- Christchurch c.
- c. complement
- contiguous gene syndrome of c. 13
- daughter c.
- c. deletion
- deletion of c.
- derivative c.
- dicentric c.
- c. diploid/tetraploid mixoploidy syndrome
- expansion of c.
- founder c.
- fractured c.
- fragile X c.
- gametic c.
- giant c.
- c. GI deletion syndrome
- heterotropic c.
- heterotypical c.
- homologous c.
- human artificial c. (HAC)
- inactivated X c.
- insertion of c.
- inversion of c.'s
- c. 9 inversion syndrome
- c. 15 inverted duplication
- inverted X c.
- iso-X c.
- c. jumping
- c. knob
- lampbrush c.
- late replicating c.
- long arm of c. (q)
- long arm of Y c.
- c. map
- c. mapping
- marker X c.
- metacentric c.
- metaphase c.
- c. microdeletion
- mitochondrial c.
- mitotic c.
- c. 1–22 monosomy syndrome
- c. 17 mutation
- nonhomologous c.
- nucleolar c.
- odd c.
- 4p+ c.
- c. paint
- c. pair
- c. pairing
- c. 9p disorder
- Philadelphia c. (Ph1)
- c. 8p mosaic tetrasomy
- polytene c.
- c. 1p–22p deletion syndrome
- c. 1p–22p monosomy
- c. 1p–22p trisomy
- c. 1q–22q deletion syndrome
- c. 1q–22q duplication syndrome
- c. 1q–22q monosomy
- c. 1q–22q tetrasomy syndrome
- c. 1q–22q triplication syndrome
- c. 1q–22q trisomy
- c. 8 recombinant syndrome
- c. reduction
- c. 1–22 ring syndrome
- c. sequencing
- sex c.
- sex-linked c.
- short arm of c. (p)
- small c.
- somatic c.
- submetacentric c.
- supernumerary c.
- supernumerary marker c. (SMC)
- c. 22 supernumerary marker (SMG22)
- telocentric c.
- c. tetraploidy syndrome
- c. triploidy syndrome

c. 1–22 trisomy
c. 1–22 trisomy syndrome
Turner syndrome in female with
  X c.
c. 14 uniparental disomy syndrome
unpaired c.
W c.
c. walking
X c.
c. XA
c. X autosome translocation
  syndrome
c. X fragility syndrome
c. X inversion syndrome
XO c.
c. XO syndrome
c. Xp21 deletion syndrome
c. Xp22 deletion syndrome
c. X pentasomy
c. Xp21 monosomy
c. Xq deletion syndrome
c. Xq duplication syndrome
c. Xq monosomy
c. Xq trisomy
XX c.
c. XXX syndrome
c. 47,XXX syndrome
c. XXXXX syndrome
c. XXXXY syndrome
c. XXY syndrome
Y c.
yeast artificial c. (YAC)
c. Y;18 translocation syndrome
chromospermism
chromotubation
chronic
c. active hepatitis
c. adhesive arachnoiditis
c. adrenal insufficiency
c. anovulation
c. aspiration
c. aspiration syndrome
c. asthma
c. atrophic vulvitis
c. behavior problem
c. benign neutropenia
c. benign neutropenia of childhood
c. biopsychosocial syndrome
c. bullous dermatitis
c. bullous dermatosis of childhood
c. bullous disease of childhood
c. cervicitis

c. chagasic cardiomyopathy
c. compartment syndrome
c. conjunctival infection
c. constipation
c. cryptogenic hepatitis (CCH)
c. cyanide toxicity
c. cystic mastitis
c. eczematoid dermatitis
c. fatigue syndrome (CFS)
c. focal encephalitis
c. Gaucher disease
c. glomerulonephritis
c. granulomatous amebic
  encephalitis
c. granulomatous disease (CGD)
c. headache
c. hydrocephalus
c. hyperreninemia
c. hypertension
c. hypertransfusion program
c. hypertrophic gastritis
c. hypertrophic vulvitis
c. hypervitaminosis A
c. idiopathic arthritides of
  childhood (CIAC)
c. idiopathic intestinal
  pseudoobstruction (CIIP)
c. idiopathic neutropenia
c. idiopathic urticaria
c. illness
c. inflammatory demyelinating
  polyneuropathy (CIDP)
c. inflammatory demyelinating
  polyradiculoneuropathy (CIDP)
c. interstitial fibrosis
c. interstitial salpingitis
c. intertrigo
c. intestinal pseudoobstruction
c. intravascular hemolysis
c. iridocyclitis
c. ITP
c. juvenile arthritis
c. lung disease (CLD)
c. lung disease of maturity
c. lymphocytic leukemia (CLL)
c. lymphocytic meningitis
c. lymphocytic thyroiditis
c. mastoiditis
c. meningococcemia
c. meningoradiculomyelitis
c. mitral insufficiency
c. motor tic disorder

C

NOTES

chronic *(continued)*
  c. mucocutaneous candidiasis
  c. mumps encephalitis
  c. myelocytic leukemia
  c. myelogenous leukemia (CML)
  c. neuromuscular disease (CNMD)
  c. neuronopathic Gaucher disease
  c. non-A-E hepatitis
  c. nonspecific diarrhea
  c. nonspecific diarrhea of infancy
  c. nonspherocytic hemolytic anemia
  c. obstructive bronchitis
  c. osteomyelitis
  c. otitis media (COM)
  c. pancreatitis
  c. papilledema
  c. parvoviral infection
  c. pelvic infection
  c. pelvic pain (CPP)
  c. peripheral neuropathy
  c. pneumonitis of infancy (CPI)
  c. progressive ataxia
  c. progressive encephalitis
  c. progressive external
    ophthalmoplegia (CPEO)
  c. pulmonary disease
  c. pulmonary histoplasmosis
  c. pulmonary insufficiency
  c. pupillary syndrome
  c. pyogenic lymphadenitis
  c. recurrent multifocal osteomyelitis
    (CRMO)
  c. rejection
  c. relapsing polyradiculoneuropathy
  c. renal failure (CRF)
  c. renal insufficiency
  c. respiratory acidosis
  c. rhinosinusitis
  c. SCFE
  c. schistosomiasis
  c. scrotal hypothermia
  c. sickle cell lung disease
  c. sinusitis
  c. spongiform encephalopathy
  c. subglottic stenosis
  c. suppurative otitis media (CSOM)
  c. synovial inflammation
  c. syphilitic meningitis
  c. tic
  c. tic disorder (CTD)
  c. tonsillar herniation
  c. unremitting
    polyradiculoneuropathy
  c. vascular disease
  c. vitamin A intoxication
chronica
    pityriasis lichenoides c. (PLC)
chronicus
    lichen simplex c. (LSC)

ChronoFlex catheter
chronograph
chronological age
chronotherapy
    phase delay c.
chronotropic
    c. effect
    c. response
chronotropy
CHRS
    cerebrohepatorenal syndrome
Chryseobacterium
Chrysosporium
CHT
    closed head trauma
    combined hormone therapy
    contralateral head turning
CHTN
    Cooperative Human Tissue Network
Chudley-Lowry-Hoar syndrome
Chudley syndrome (1, 2)
Churg-Strauss
    C.-S. syndrome
    C.-S. vasculitis
Chvostek sign
chyle
chyliform
chylomicron
    c. formation
    c. retention disease
chylomicronemia syndrome
chylopericardium
chylothorax
    congenital c.
chylous
    c. ascites
    c. liquid
    c. pleural effusion
chyluria
chymopapain
CI
    cervical incompetence
    cord insertion
C.I.
    Colour Index
Ci
    curie
CIA
    chemiluminescent immunoassay
CIAC
    chronic idiopathic arthritides of
    childhood
Cianchetti syndrome
CIC
    clean intermittent catheterization
cicatricial
    c. alopecia
    c. lesion
    c. retinal disease

cicatrix
ciclopirox
CID
  combined immunodeficiency
  cytomegalic inclusion disease
cidal level
Cidex soak
cidofovir topical gel
Cidomycin
CIDP
  chronic inflammatory demyelinating
    polyneuropathy
  chronic inflammatory demyelinating
    polyradiculoneuropathy
CIE
  counterimmunoelectrophoresis
Ciel
  Kay C.
ciguatera
  c. fish poisoning
  c. intoxication
CIIP
  chronic idiopathic intestinal
    pseudoobstruction
cilastatin
  imipenem and c.
cilia (*pl. of* cilium)
  immotile c.
ciliaris
  tylosis c.
ciliary
  c. biopsy
  c. blush
  c. dyskinesia
  c. dysmotility
  c. flush
  c. function
  c. function study
  c. muscle
  c. nerve
  c. neurotrophic factor (CNTF)
  c. paralysis
  c. spasm
ciliated
  c. cell
  c. cell endometrial adenocarcinoma
  c. metaplasia
cilium, pl. **cilia**
  immotile cilia
Ciloxan
cimetidine

CIN
  cervical intraepithelial neoplasia
cineangiocardiography
  biplane c.
cineangiogram
  continuous c.
cineangiography
  biplane c.
  radionuclide c.
cinedefecography
  anal sphincter c.
Cineloop
  C. image review ultrasound system
  C. Ultrasound
cine loop
cine-MRI
cineradiography
cingulate gyrus
cinnarizine
Cinobac
cinoxacin
Cin-Quin
CIPRACT
  cervical incompetence prevention
    randomized cerclage trial
Cipro
  C. HC Otic
  C. Injection
  C. Oral
Ciprodex otic suspension
ciprofloxacin hydrochloride
circadian
  c. cycle
  c. rhythm
  c. rhythm dyssomnia
circinate balanitis
circle
  Baudelocque uterine c.
  Carus c.
  Huguier c.
  c. of Willis
  c. of Willis aneurysm
circling disease
Circon-ACMI
  C.-ACMI cannula
  C.-ACMI hysteroscope
  C.-ACMI trocar
CircPlus compression wrap/dressing
circuit
  failed Fontan c.

NOTES

circular
    c. end-to-end anastomosis (CEEA)
    c. reaction
circulating
    c. anticoagulant
    c. estrogen
    c. fetal cell
    c. hormone
    c. neutrophils
    c. platelet antibody
    c. testosterone
circulation
    airway, breathing, c. (ABC)
    collateral c.
    duct-dependent pulmonary c.
    duct-dependent systemic c.
    extracorporeal c. (ECC)
    fetal cardiovascular c.
    fetal-placental c.
    fetal pulmonary c.
    fetoplacental c.
    hypophysial portal c.
    hypothalamic-hypophysial portal c.
    parallel c.
    persistence of fetal c.
    persistent fetal c. (PFC)
    pituitary-hypothalamic c.
    c. time
    umbilical cardiovascular c.
    uteroovarian c.
    uteroplacental c.
circulation-cavopulmonary connection
circulatory
    c. arrest
    c. collapse
    c. crossover
    c. system
circumcise
circumcision
    c. clamp
    Mogen c.
    pharaonic c.
    c. status
    Sunna c.
circumduction
    c. gait
    c. movement
circumference
    abdominal c. (AC)
    arm c.
    fetal abdominal c.
    head c. (HC)
    mean arm muscle c. (MAMC)
    midarm c. (MAC)
    midarm muscle c. (MAMC)
    occipitofrontal c. (OFC)
    sonographic abdominal c.
circumferential
    c. burn

    c. eversion
    c. eversion of urethral epithelium
    c. examination
    c. ringed creases of limbs
    c. skin crease of limb
    c. skin creases-psychomotor retardation syndrome
circumflexa
    ichthyosis linearis c.
circumflex artery
circummarginate placenta
circumoral pallor
circumscribed
    c. mass
    c. neurodermatitis
    well-c.
circumscripta
    myositis ossificans c.
circumscriptum
    angiokeratoma c.
    lymphangioma c.
circumscriptus
    albinismus c.
Circumstraint
circumvallata
    placenta c.
circumvallate placenta
cirrhonosus
cirrhosis
    biliary c.
    compensated c.
    cryptogenic c.
    decompensated c.
    endemic Tyrolean infantile c.
    end-stage c.
    hepatic c.
    hypertrophic c.
    Indian childhood c. (ICC)
    liver c.
    c. of liver
    macronodular c.
    micronodular liver c.
    postnecrotic c.
    primary biliary c. (PBC)
    progressive biliary c.
    pseudolobular c.
cirsoid aneurysm
cirsomphalos
CIS
    carcinoma in situ
cisapride
cis-**atracurium**
CISCA
    cisplatin, Cytoxan, Adriamycin
cisplatin
    c., Ara-C, caffeine (CAC)
    bleomycin, etoposide, c. (BEP)
    c., Cytoxan, Adriamycin (CISCA)

c., etoposide, Cytoxan, Adriamycin
(CECA)
c., 5-fluorouracil, leucovorin
calcium (CFL)
intraperitoneal c.
c., methotrexate, vinblastine (CMV)
vinblastine, bleomycin, c. (VBP)

9-cis-retinoic acid
cistern
    basal c.
    chiasmatic c.
    prominent quadrigeminal plate c.
cisternal puncture
cisterna magna
cisternography
    isotope c.
    radioisotope c.
cistron
citalopram
citizen
    Association for Retarded C.'s
    (ARC)
Citracal
citrate
    c. blood sample
    caffeine c.
    calcium c.
    c. and citric acid
    clomiphene c. (CC)
    cyclofenil c.
    diphenhydramine c.
    fentanyl c.
    lithium c.
    magnesium c.
    oral transmucosal fentanyl c.
    (OTFC)
    potassium c.
    sufentanil c.
    tamoxifen c.
    toremifene c.
    c. toxicity
citrated caffeine
citric acid cycle
Citrobacter
    C. amalonaticus
    C. braakii
    C. diversus
    C. farmeri
    C. freundii
    C. koseri
    C. sedlakii

    C. werkmanii
    C. youngae
citrovorum factor
citrulline
    plasma c.
citrullinemia
citrullinuria
citta
cittosis
C-IV
    Pemoline C-IV
CJD
    Creutzfeldt-Jakob disease
    iatrogenic CJD
    new variant CJD
CK
    creatine kinase
CKC
    cold knife conization
CK-MB
    myocardial muscle creatine kinase
    isoenzyme
CL
    cleft lip
    lung capacity
    lung compliance
CLA
    conjugated linoleic acid
    X-linked cerebellar ataxia
clade
Clado anastomosis
cladogenesis
Cladosporium herbarum
cladribine
Claforan
clamp
    Allis c.
    Babcock c.
    back c.
    Backhaus c.
    Ballantine c.
    Buxton c.
    Carmault c.
    cervical c.
    circumcision c.
    DeBakey aortic c.
    extracutaneous vas fixation c.
    Gomco circumcision c.
    Heaney c.
    Hoffmann c.
    hysterectomy c.
    ICSI Massachusetts c.

C

NOTES

clamp *(continued)*
    Kelly c.
    Kocher c.
    Lahey c.
    Lem-Blay circumcision c.
    Mogen c.
    Péan c.
    pediatric bulldog c.
    pediatric vascular c.
    pedicle c.
    Pennington c.
    thoracic c.
    thyroid Lahey c.
    umbilical c.
    vulsellum c.
    Willett c.
    Winston cervical c.
    Yellen c.
    Zeppelin c.
clamped down
clamping
    cord c.
CLAMS
    Clinical Linguistic and Auditory Milestone Scale
clamshell-type catheter occlusion device
Clara cell 16 protein
Clarion hearing implant
Claripex
clarithromycin
Claritin
    C. RediTab
    C. syrup
Claritin-D 24-Hour
Clark
    C. classification of vulvar melanoma
    C. mechanistic classification
    C. microstaging system
Clarke
    C. column
    C. ligator scissor forceps
Clarke-Hadfield syndrome
Clarus model 5169 peristaltic pump
CLAS
    congenital localized absence of skin
clasped thumbs-mental retardation syndrome
clasp-knife
    c.-k. phenomenon
    c.-k. response
classic
    c. abdominal Semm hysterectomy (CASH)
    c. celiac disease
    c. medulloblastoma
    c. migraine
    c. migraine headache
    c. plaque psoriasis
    c. X-linked recessive muscular dystrophy
classical
    c. cesarean section
    c. galactosemia
    c. genetics
    c. incision extension
    c. lissencephaly
    c. migraine
    c. transverse incision
    c. uterine incision
classifiable character
classification
    Abramson c.
    Acosta c.
    AFUD c.
    American Foundation of Urologic Diseases c.
    Angle c.
    Astler-Coller modification of Dukes c.
    Barbero-Marcial c.
    Bethesda 2001 cervical cytology c.
    Bethesda System Pap smear c.
    Blaustein c.
    Caldwell-Moloy c.
    Catterall c. (grade 1–4)
    Chicago c.
    Clark mechanistic c.
    Cori c.
    de la Cruz c.
    Delbet fracture c. (type I–IV)
    Denver c.
    Dripps-American Society of Anesthesiologists c.
    Dukes c.
    EULAR c.
    FAB c.
    histologic c.
    HIV c.
    ILAR peripheral arthritis c.
    Jansky c.
    Jewett c.
    Kajava c.
    King c.
    microinvasive carcinoma c.
    Moss c.
    PAAS c.
    Pulec and Freedman c.
    Reese-Ellsworth c.
    Risser c.
    Rye c.
    Salter-Harris c.
    Schuknecht c.
    Sillence c. of osteogenesis imperfecta (type I, IA, IB, II, III, IV, IVA, IVB)
    Tanner c. (1–5)
    TNM c.

Wassel c.
White c.
Wolfe c. of breast cancer
Zero to Three children's mental
    health diagnostic c.

clastic lesion
clastogenic stress
clathrin
clavicle
congenital pseudoarthrosis of the c.
clavicular
c. fracture (CF)
c. injury
c. pseudarthrosis
c. shaft
claviculectomy
distal c.
clavulanate
c. potassium
ticarcillin c.
clavulanic acid
Clavulin
clawfoot
clawhand
c. deformity
c. deformity repair
clawing
clay
green c.
CLD
chronic lung disease
cytoplasmic lipid droplet
clean
c. intermittent catheterization (CIC)
c. intermittent self-catheterization
clean-catch
c.-c. midstream urine sample
c.-c. technique
c.-c. urinalysis
c.-c. urine specimen
cleaner
Sklar aseptic germicidal c.
clean-out
bowel c.-o.
cleanser
Dey-Wash skin wound c.
clear
c. cell adenocarcinoma
c. cell endometrial carcinoma
c. cell hidradenoma
c. cell sarcoma
c. cell tumor

c. cell vaginal cancer
C. Eyes
c. mucoid sputum
clearance
creatinine c.
c. of fetal product
immune c.
mucociliary c.
ultrafiltration virus c.
urate c.
urea c.
virus c.
xenon c.
Clearblue
C. Easy
C. Improved
clearing
throat c.
ClearPlan
C. Easy
C. Easy fertility monitor
C. Easy ovulation predictor
ClearSite hydrogauze dressing
Clearview hCG pregnancy test
ClearView uterine manipulator
cleavage
embryonic c.
manual c.
c. plan
c. stage
c. syndrome
cleaved
c. amplified polymorphic sequence
c. embryo
cleft
bilateral schizencephalic c.
branchial c.
c. chin
complete c.
c. face
genital c.
c. hand
hyobranchial c.
incomplete c.
intergluteal c.
c. jaw
Lanterman c.
laryngeal c.
laryngotracheoesophageal c.
c. lip (CL)
c. lip, cleft palate, lobster claw
    deformity syndrome

C

NOTES

cleft *(continued)*
  c. lip-nasal reconstruction
  c. lip and palate (CLP)
  nasal alar cartilage c.
  c. nasal deformity correction
  natal c.
  orofacial c.
  oroorbital c.
  c. palate (CP)
  c. palate, diaphragmatic hernia, coarse facies, acral hypoplasia syndrome
  c. palate-lateral synechia (CPLS)
  c. palate, microcephaly, large ears, short stature syndrome
  c. palate repair
  postalveolar c.
  c. premaxillary process
  c. spine
  Stillman c.
  submucous c.
  syndromic c.
  c. vertebrae
  visceral c.
clefting
  ankyloblepharon, ectodermal dysplasia, c. (AEC)
  ectrodactyly, ectodermal dysplasia, c. (EEC)
  hypertelorism, microtia, c. (HMC)
  c., ocular anterior chamber defect, lid anomalies syndrome
cleidocranial
  c. digital dysostosis
  c. dysplasia
  c. dysplasia syndrome
cleidocranialis
  dysostosis c.
  dysplasia c.
cleidocraniodigitalis
  dysostosis c.
cleidocraniopelvina
  dysostosis c.
cleidofacialis
  dysplasia c.
cleidorhizomelic syndrome
cleidorrhexis
cleidotomy
cleidotripsy
clemastine
clenched
  c. fist injury
  c. fist and pleural effusion
  c. fists
Cleocin
  C. HCl
  C. HCl Oral
  C. Pediatric Oral
  C. Phosphate

  C. T
  C. vaginal cream
  C. Vaginal Ovules
Clevedon positive pressure respirator
click
  aortic ejection c.
  ejection c.
  hip c.
  midsystolic c.
  Ortolani c.
  pulmonary ejection c.
  c. stimulus
clidinium
clidoic
Clifford syndrome
climacteric
  grand c.
  c. history
  c. psychosis
  c. syndrome
climacterium
Climara
  C. estradiol transdermal system
  C. estradiol transdermal system patch
climatic bubo
clinch knot
clindamycin
  c. phosphate
  c. phosphate topical solution
Clindoxyl
clinic
  National Fertility C.
  Teen-Tot C.
clinical
  C. Adaptive Test (CAT)
  C. Adaptive Test/Clinical Linguistic and Auditory Milestone Scale (CAT/CLAMS)
  c. assessment in neuropsychology
  c. cohort study
  C. Colitis Activity Index (CCAI)
  c. crib
  c. dating
  C. Evaluation of Language Fundamentals-Preschool
  C. Evaluation of Language Fundamentals, 3rd Edition
  c. finding
  C. Global Impressions (CGI)
  c. global index (CGI)
  c. grouping
  C. Linguistic and Auditory Milestone Scale (CLAMS)
  c. pelvimetry
  c. pregnancy
  c. prognosis
  c. response
  c. risk assessment (CRA)

C. Risk Index for Babies (CRIB)
c. staging
c. type
clinically significant arrhythmia (CSA)
CliniCath peripherally inserted catheter
clinicopathologic
clinicopathological analysis
Clinistix
Clinitek 50 urine chemistry analyzer
Clinitest assay
clinocephaly
clinodactyly
fifth finger c.
clinometacarpy
Clinoril
clioquinol
clip
Bleier c.
fentendo c.
Filshie c.
Hulka c.
Hulka-Clemens c.
c. technique
towel c.
clitoral
c. engorgement
c. hood
c. hypertrophy
c. ischemia
c. length
c. nerve
c. neurofibroma
c. sensitivity
c. strangulation
c. therapy device (CTD)
clitoridectomy
clitoriditis, clitoritis
clitoris, gen. **clitoridis,** pl. **clitorides**
bifid c.
c. crisis
c. enlargement
fascia clitoridis
glans c.
phimosis clitoridis
c. tourniquet syndrome (CTS)
clitorism
clitoritis (*var. of* clitoriditis)
clitoromegaly
clitoroplasty
clivus, pl. **clivi**
inferior c.

CLL
chronic lymphocytic leukemia
CLN
neuronal ceroid lipofuscinosis
CLO
congenital lobar overinflation
cloaca
congenital c.
cloacae
Enterobacter c.
cloacal
c. duct
c. exstrophy
c. extrophy
c. malformation
c. membrane
c. plate anomaly
cloaking
periosteal c.
clobetasol propionate
Clocort Maximum Strength
clocortolone
Cloderm Topical
clodronate
clofazimine
clofibrate
Clomid
clomiphene
c. citrate (CC)
c. citrate challenge test (CCCT, C3T)
c. fetal malformation
clomiphene-resistant polycystic ovary syndrome
clomipramine hydrochloride
clomocycline
clonality
clonal selection theory
clonazepam
clone
c. bank
DNA c.
molecular c.
overlapping c.'s
recombinant c.
clonic
c. movement
c. seizure
clonidine hydrochloride
cloning
DNA c.
embryo c.

NOTES

cloning *(continued)*
    functional c.
    gene c.
    positional c.
    c. vector
clonogenic
    c. assay
    c. technique
clonorchiasis
Clonorchis sinensis
clonus
    ankle c.
    sustained c.
clopamide
Cloquet node
clorazepate
closed
    c. bite
    c. chest massage
    c. comedo
    c. drainage
    c. endotracheal tube suctioning
    c. fist injury
    c. head injury (CHI)
    c. head trauma (CHT)
    c. neural tube defect
    c. thoracotomy
closed-circuit video recording
closed-loop
    c.-l. obstruction
    c.-l. system passing electrode
closing
    c. capacity (CC)
    c. coagulum
    c. ring of Winkler-Waldeyer
clostridia (*pl. of* clostridium)
clostridial
    c. bacteremia
    c. myonecrosis
    c. otitis media
    c. toxin
Clostridium
    C. botulinum
    C. botulinum type A toxin
    C. botulism
    C. difficile
    C. difficile-associated diarrhea (CDAC)
    C. freundii
    C. perfringens
    C. ramosum
    C. septicum
    C. spiroforme
    C. tetani
clostridium, pl. **clostridia**
    clostridia septicemia
closure
    anterior neural tube c.
    bilabial c.

    delayed primary c.
    ductus c.
    early midsystolic c.
    epiphyseal c.
    Gestalt c.
    hysterical glottic c.
    incision c.
    laryngeal c.
    lip c.
    neural tube c.
    neurosurgical c.
    nonlocking c.
    palatal fistula c.
    percutaneous patent ductus arteriosus c.
    physial c.
    posterior neural tube c.
    premature airway c.
    premature ductus arteriosus c.
    primary c.
    secondary c.
    Steri-Strip skin c.
    tertiary c.
    Tom Jones c.
    transcatheter c. (TCC)
    ventricular septal defect patch c.
clot
    c. formation
    friable c.
    intraluminal c.
    c. resolution
    c. sectioning
Clotrimaderm
clotrimazole
    c. troche
    c. vaginal cream 2%
clouding
    corneal c.
    infantile corneal c.
    mental c.
    c. of sensorium
cloudy
    c. cornea
    c. mastoid
    c. sputum
Clouston syndrome
cloven spine
cloverleaf
    c. skull
    c. skull deformity
    c. skull syndrome
cloxacillin
clozapine
CLP
    cleft lip and palate
CLS
    capillary leak syndrome
CLSE
    calf lung surfactant extract

CLTM
    continuous long-term monitoring
clubbing
        digital c.
        c. of fingers and toes
        hereditary c.
        c. of nails
clubfoot, club foot (CF)
        adductus c.
        arthrogrypotic c.
        c. cast
        congenital c.
        c. deformity
        c. dysplasia
        equinus c.
        idiopathic c.
        medial rotation c.
        neurogenic c.
        positional c.
        rigid c.
        c. splint
        Turco posteromedial release of c.
        varus c.
clubhand, club hand
        radial c.
        ulnar c.
clue cell
clumsiness
clumsy child syndrome
clunk
        hip c.
cluster
        c. B disorder
        DAZ gene c.
        c. headache
cluster-stratified sampling method
cluttering
Clutton joints
cM
    centimorgan
CMA
    cow's milk allergy
CMD
    congenital muscular dystrophy
        Fukuyama CMD
CMF
    cyclophosphamide, methotrexate, 5-fluorouracil
CMFP
    cyclophosphamide, methotrexate, 5-fluorouracil, and prednisone

Cytoxan, methotrexate, fluorouracil, prednisone
CMFPT
    Cytoxan, methotrexate, fluorouracil, prednisone, tamoxifen
CMFTD
    congenital muscle fiber-type disproportion
CMFVP
    cyclophosphamide, methotrexate, 5-fluorouracil, vincristine, and prednisone
    Cytoxan, methotrexate, fluorouracil, vincristine, prednisone
cmH$_2$O
    centimeter of water
CMI
    cell-mediated immunity
        CMI vacuum extractor
CMI-Mityvac cup
CMI-O'Neil cup
CML
    chronic myelogenous leukemia
CMP
    cow's milk protein
CMT
    cervical motion tenderness
    Charcot-Marie-Tooth
CMTS
    Charcot-Marie-Tooth syndrome
CMV
    cisplatin, methotrexate, vinblastine
    controlled mechanical ventilation
    cytomegalovirus
        disseminated CMV
        CMV enteritis
        CMV retinitis
CMVF
    cytomegalovirus
CMVIG
    cytomegalovirus immune globulin
    cytomegalovirus immunoglobulin
CMV-IGIV
    cytomegalovirus immune globulin intravenous
CMV-seronegative transplant patient
CMV-shedding child
c-*myc* oncogene
CN
    calcaneonavicular
CNAP
    continuous negative airway pressure

NOTES

C

CNB
core needle biopsy
CNBr
cyanogen bromide
CNBr activated Sepharose
CNEP
continuous negative extrathoracic
pressure
CNF
congenital nephrotic syndrome, Finnish
CNFS
craniofrontonasal syndrome
CNLDO
congenital nasolacrimal duct obstruction
CNM
centronuclear myopathy
certified nurse-midwife
CNMD
chronic neuromuscular disease
CNPAS
congenital nasal pyriform aperture
stenosis
CNS
central nervous system
CNS aneurysm
CNS development
CNS dysfunction
CNS hemorrhage
CNS infarction
CNS leukemia
CNS malignancy
primary angiitis of CNS (PACNS)
CNS tumor
CNTF
ciliary neurotrophic factor
CO
carbon monoxide
end-tidal CO
CO_2
carbon dioxide
end-tidal CO_2
CO_2 laser
pressure of CO_2
^{60}Co
cobalt-60
COA
child of alcoholic
children of alcoholic
CoA
aortic arch coarctation
coenzyme A
COACH
cerebellar vermis hypoplasia,
oligophrenia, congenital ataxia, ocular
coloboma, hepatic fibrosis
COACH syndrome
coach's finger
coactivated antagonists
coadministration

coagulase
coagulase-negative
c.-n. bacteremia
c.-n. *Staphylococcus*
coagulase-positive *Staphylococcus*
coagulation
c. abnormality
argon beam c.
bipolar diathermy c.
c. cascade
cold c.
c. defect
c. disorder
disseminated intravascular c. (DIC)
c. disturbance
c. factor
c. factor zymogen
c. profile
c. study
c. test
coagulative myocytolysis
coagulator
argon beam c. (ABC)
cold c.
Elmed BC 50 M/M digital
bipolar c.
Malis CMC-II bipolar c.
coagulopathy
consumption c.
consumptive c.
disseminated intravascular c. (DIC)
hereditary c.
heritable c.
incipient c.
inherited c.
maternal c.
coagulum
closing c.
necrotic c.
coalescent mastoiditis
coalition
calcaneonavicular c.
cartilaginous c.
congenital tarsal c.
fibrinous c.
osseous c.
tarsal c.
coal tar
coaptation
c. bipolar forceps
urethral c.
coarctation
abdominal c.
c. of aorta
aortic c.
aortic arch c. (CoA)
complex c.
juxtaductal aortic c.
postductal c.

preductal c.
recurrent c.
residual c.
simple c.
coarse
c. calcification
c. facial features
c. rale
c. tremor
coast
c. of California café au lait spots
c. of Maine café au lait spots
coat
buffy c.
lipopolysaccharide c.
Coat-A-Count
C.-A.-C. assay
C.-A.-C. neonatal 17
hydroxyprogesterone kit
coated Vicryl Rapide suture
Coats disease
coaxial
c. flow
c. position
c. sheath cut-biopsy needle
cobalamin
c. adenosyltransferase
c. reductase deficiency
cobalt
c. megavoltage machine
c. poisoning
radioactive c.
cobalt-60 (^{60}Co)
c.-60 moving strip technique
Coban dressing
Cobas fast centrifugal analyzer
Cobb
C. measurement technique
C. method
C. syndrome
cobblestone
c. appearance
c. sessile polyp
cobblestoning of conjunctiva
Cobb-Ragde needle
co-bedding
Coblation-Channeling surgical procedure
COC
combined oral contraceptive
coca
Erythroxylum c.

cocaine
c. addiction
c. baby
crack c.
freebase c.
c. hydrochloride powder
liquified powder c.
c. test
tetracaine, adrenaline, c. (TAC)
tetracaine, epinephrine, c.
cocci (*pl. of* coccus)
coccidioidal
c. granuloma
c. placentitis
Coccidioides immitis
coccidioidin reaction
coccidioidomycosis
disseminated c.
c. meningitis
coccobacillary
c. bacteria
c. form
coccobacillus
HACEK c.
coccus, pl. **cocci**
gram-negative cocci
gram-positive cocci
coccygeal
c. fracture
c. muscle
coccygeus muscle
coccygodynia
coccyx, pl. **coccyges**
cochlea
cochlear
c. aqueduct
c. implant
cochleopalpebral reflex
cochleosaccular degeneration
cochleovestibular paresis
Cochrane Pregnancy and Childbirth Database
Cockayne syndrome (A, B)
Cockayne-Touraine variant of dominant dystrophic epidermolysis bullosa
cock-robin
c.-r. position
c.-r. sign
cockscomb
cervical c.
c. cervix

NOTES

cocktail
c. chatter
GI c.
lytic c.
c. party patter
c. party syndrome
pediatric c.
COD
cerebroocular dysgenesis
CODAS
cerebral, ocular, dental, auricular, skeletal
cerebroocular dentoauriculoskeletal
CODAS syndrome
code
genetic c.
codeine
Fioricet With C.
guaifenesin and c.
Guiatussin With C.
Mallergan-VC With C.
promethazine, phenylephrine, c.
Tylenol With C. No. 2, 3, 4
codfish vertebra
coding
phonological c.
cod liver oil
Codman
C. Accu-Flow shunt
C. triangle
COD-MD
cerebroocular dysgenesis-muscular
dystrophy
COD-MD syndrome
codominance
codominant
c. gene
c. inheritance
codon
stop c.
termination c.
Codoxy
coefficient
bone attenuation c.
c. of fat absorption
c. of inbreeding
inbreeding c.
intraclass correlation c.
kappa c.
c. of parentage
coelom (*var. of* celom)
coelomic (*var. of* celomic)
coenzyme A (CoA)
coenzyme Q10
coercive feeding
coeur en sabot
coexistent fetus
coexisting fracture
cofactor
c. deficiency

heparin c. II (HCII)
molybdenum c.
ristocetin c.
tetrahydrobiopterin c. (BH$_4$)
COF/COM
Cytoxan, Oncovin, fluorouracil plus
Cytoxan, Oncovin, methotrexate
coffee-grounds
c.-g. drainage
c.-g. emesis
c.-g. hematemesis
c.-g. material
Coffey suspension
Coffin-Lowry syndrome
Coffin-Siris
C.-S. defect
C.-S. syndrome
Coffin-Siris-Wegienka syndrome
Coffin syndrome (1, 2)
COFS
cerebrooculofacial-skeletal
COFS syndrome
Cogan
congenital ocular motor apraxia
(type C.) (COMA)
C. syndrome
Cogentin
Co-Gesic
cognition
spatial c.
cognitive
c. ability
c. behavior
c. behavioral therapy (CBT)
c. deficiency
c. delay
c. developmental milestone
c. disability
c. domain
c. impairment
c. therapy
c. toxicity
cognitive-behavioral psychotherapy
cognitive-diathesis model
cognitive-stress diathesis
CO$_2$Guard
COH
controlled ovarian hyperstimulation
cohabitation
COHb
carboxyhemoglobin
Cohen
C. criteria
C. procedure
C. syndrome
C. transtrigonal technique
C. uterine cannula

cohesion
    lexical c.
    referential c.
cohort
    Dunedin birth c.
    c. study
coil
    Dacron fiber-coated c.
    DuctOcclud c.
    Margulies c.
    metal c.
    MRCP using HASTE with a
        phased array c.
    c. occlusion
    c. spring diaphragm
coiled artery
coiling
coin
    c. biopsy
    esophageal c.
    c. ingestion
    c. lesion
coincident pregnancy
coinfection
    beta-hemolytic streptococcal c.
coining
coital
    c. age
    c. contact
    c. dependence
    c. factor
    c. position
    c. timing
coitarche
coition
coitus
    c. incompletus
    c. interruptus
    c. la vache
    c. reservatus
Coke-colored urine
COL7A1 gene
Colace
cola-colored
    c.-c. neonate
    c.-c. urine
Colaris genetic susceptibility test
colarium
Co-Lav
Colax
**Colcher-Sussman x-ray pelvimetry
    technique**

colchicine
cold
    c. abscess
    c. agglutinin
    c. agglutinin disease
    c. anaphylaxis
    c. antibody
    c. biopsy forceps
    c. coagulation
    c. coagulator
    common c.
    c. cup biopsy
    c. hemagglutinin disease
    c. intolerance
    c. knife biopsy
    c. knife cervical conization
    c. knife cone
    c. knife cone biopsy
    c. knife conization (CKC)
    c. knife method
    c. nodule
    c. panniculitis
    c. potassium cardioplegia
    c. stress
    c. urticaria
    c. water near drowning
cold-adapted
    c.-a. influenza vaccine (CAIV)
    c.-a. intranasal influenza vaccine
Cold-Eeze
cold-induced myotonia
Cole
    C. endotracheal tube
    C. intubation procedure
    C. orotracheal tube
    C. syndrome
Cole-Carpenter syndrome
colectomy
**Cole-Hughes macrocephaly-mental
    retardation syndrome**
coleocele
coleotomy
Cole-Rauschkolb-Toomey syndrome
colfosceril palmitate
coli
    ampicillin-resistant *Escherichia c.*
    Balantidium c.
    Campylobacter c.
    enterohemorrhagic *Escherichia c.*
        (EHEC)
    enteropathogenic *Escherichia c.*
        (EPEC)

NOTES

C

coli (continued)
>> enterotoxigenic *Escherichia c.* (ETEC)
>> *Escherichia c.*
>> familial adenomatous polyposis c.
>> hemorrhagic *Escherichia c.*
>> Shiga toxin-producing *Escherichia c.* (STEC)

Colibri forceps
colic
>> c. artery
>> biliary c.
>> infantile c.
>> c. intussusception
>> meconial c.
>> menstrual c.
>> Monday morning c.
>> non-Wessel c.
>> ovarian c.
>> renal c.
>> tubal c.
>> uterine c.
>> Wessel c.

colicky abdominal pain
coliform
>> c. bacteria
>> c. organism

colistimethate sodium
colistin
colitis
>> acute fulminant c.
>> acute infectious c.
>> allergic c.
>> amebic c.
>> antibiotic-associated c.
>> Crohn c.
>> eosinophilic allergic c.
>> fulminant ulcerative c.
>> granulomatous c.
>> hemorrhagic c.
>> Hirschsprung c.
>> infectious c.
>> inflammatory c.
>> lymphoplasmacytic c.
>> mild ulcerative c.
>> moderate ulcerative c.
>> necrotizing c.
>> protein-induced eosinophilic c. (PEC)
>> pseudomembranous c.
>> steroid-dependent c.
>> tuberculous c.
>> ulcerative c.

colla (*pl. of* collum)
Collaborative
>> C. Antiviral Study Group (CASG)
>> C. Group on Hormonal Factors in Breast Cancer
>> C. Home Infant Monitoring Evaluation (CHIME)
>> C. Perinatal Study (CPS)

CollaCote dressing
collagen
>> bovine dermal c.
>> C-terminal propeptide of type I c.
>> GAX c.
>> c. I, III, IV, V, X
>> microfibrillar c.
>> c. vascular disease
>> c. vascular disorder
>> c. weakness

collagenase
>> human neutrophil c.

collagenization
collagenosis
>> mediastinal c.
>> perforating c.
>> reactive perforating c. (RPC)

collapse
>> acute circulatory c.
>> cardiopulmonary c.
>> cardiovascular c.
>> circulatory c.

collapse-consolidation lesion
collapsed subpectoral implant
collar
>> cervical c.
>> c. of pearls
>> Philadelphia c.
>> sebaceous c.
>> venereal c.
>> c. of Venus

collared cervix
collarette of rash
Collastat
collateral
>> c. blood flow
>> c. circulation
>> c. ligament stability
>> systemic venous c. (SSVC)
>> venous c.

collateralization
>> coronary c.

collection
>> breath-by-breath method of gas c.
>> extravascular fluid c.
>> first-morning urine c.
>> 72-hour stool c.
>> 24-hour urine c.
>> oocyte c.
>> subphrenic gas c.

collector
>> cell c.
>> Cytobrush cell c.
>> Cytobrush-Plus cell c.
>> Cytopick endocervical and uterovaginal cell c.

Endocell endometrial cell c.
Flexi-Seal fecal c.
Leukotrap red cell c.
Papette cervical c.
Uterobrush endometrial sample c.
Wallach-Papette disposable cervical
cell c.

Colles
C. fascia
C. fracture
colli (*gen. of* collum)
colliculus, pl. **colliculi**
inferior c.
collimation
pinhole c.
collimator
collinearity
Collins
C. law
C. test
collodion
c. baby
c. skin
colloid
c. carcinoma
c. cyst
c. infusion
c. oncotic pressure
c. osmotic pressure (COP)
radioactive c.
c. solution
collum, gen. **colli**, pl. **colla**
pterygium colli
Collyrium Fresh Ophthalmic
coloboma
c., clefting, mental retardation
syndrome
c. cleft lip/palate-mental retardation
syndrome
congenital iris c.
c., heart defects, ichthyosiform
dermatosis, mental retardation, ear
defects (CHIME)
c., heart disease, atresia choanae,
retarded growth and development,
CNS anomalies, genital
hypoplasia, ear anomalies and/or
deafness (CHARGE)
c., mental retardation,
hypogonadism, obesity syndrome

c., microphthalmos, hearing loss,
hematuria, cleft lip/palate
syndrome
c., obesity, hypogenitalism, mental
retardation syndrome
ocular c.
coloboma-anal atresia syndrome
coloboma-hepatic fibrosis
colobomatous defect
colocecal bladder augmentation
colocolic intussusception
colocolponeopoiesis
colocolpopoiesis
colon
aganglionic c.
ascending c.
c. carcinoma
cathartic c.
descending c.
giant c.
nervous c.
c. pouch
rectosigmoid c.
sigmoid c.
spastic c.
transverse c.
colonic
c. aganglionosis
c. B-cell lymphoma
c. conduit diversion
c. dysmotility
c. interposition
c. obstruction
c. plug
c. polyp
c. polyposis
c. stasis
c. stricture
colonization
candida c.
oropharyngeal c.
stool c.
vaginal c.
colonopathy
fibrosing c.
colonoscopic release
colonoscopy
surveillance c.
colony count
colony-forming
c.-f. unit (CFU)

NOTES

colony-forming *(continued)*
    c.-f. unit in culture (CFUC)
    c.-f. unit erythroid (CFU-E)
colony-stimulating
    c.-s. activity (CSA)
    c.-s. factor (CSF)
color
    c. analog scale
    c. Doppler energy (CDE)
    c. Doppler flow imaging (CDFI)
    c. Doppler sonography (CDS)
    c. Doppler ultrasonography
    c. echocardiogram
    flight of c.
    C. Power Angio imaging
    C. Trails Test
    c. vision
Colorado tick fever
color-coded duplex Doppler
colorectal
    c. anastomosis
    c. cancer
    c. disease
    c. tumor
color-flow Doppler
colorimetric reverse dot blot hybridization
3-color immunofluorescence
ColorMate TLc BiliTest System
ColorpHast Indicator Strips
coloscope
    ZM-1 c.
colostomy
    diverting c.
    double-barrel c.
    fecal diversion c.
    c. formation
    protective c.
    temporary diverting c.
    transverse loop c.
colostration
colostric
colostrorrhea
colostrous
colostrum
Colour Index (C.I.)
Colovage
colovaginal fistula
colpatresia
colpectasis, colpectasia
colpectomy
    partial c.
    skinning c.
    total c.
colpitis mycotica
colpocele
colpocleisis
    Latzko c.
    Le Fort partial c.

colpocystitis
colpocystocele
colpocystoplasty
colpocystotomy
colpocystoureterotomy
colpocystourethropexy (CCUP)
colpodynia
colpohyperplasia
    c. cystica
    c. emphysematosa
colpohysterectomy
colpohysteropexy
colpohysterotomy
colpomicroscopy
colpomycosis
colpomyomectomy
colpopathy
colpoperineopexy
    abdominal sacral c.
colpoperineoplasty
colpoperineorrhaphy
    posterior c.
colpopexy
    abdominal sacral c.
    sacral c.
    sacrospinous c.
    transvaginal sacrospinous c.
colpoplasty
colpopoiesis
colpoptosis, colpoptosia
colporectopexy
colporrhagia
colporrhaphy
    anterior c.
    anteroposterior c.
    Goffe c.
    posterior c.
colporrhexis
colposcope
    CooperSurgical overhead c.
    Leisegang c.
    Zeiss c.
    Zoomscope c.
colposcopic
    c. diagnosis
    c. examination
    c. grading of cervical dysplasia
    c. screening
colposcopically directed brushing
colposcopist
colposcopy
    digital imaging c.
    endocervical canal c.
    estrogen-assisted c.
    vulvar c.
colposcopy-trained
colpospasm

colpostat
    afterload c.
    Henschke c.
colpostenosis
colpostenotomy
colposuspension
    abdominal sacrospinous ligament c.
    Burch c.
    laparoscopic retropubic c.
colpotomy incision
colpoureterotomy
colpourethrocystopexy
    retropubic c.
colpourethropexy
    Burch c.
    modified Burch c.
colpoxerosis
Columbia Impairment Scale
column
    Clarke c.
    spinal c.
    vertebral c.
columnar
    c. epithelium
    c. epithelium papilla
Coly-Mycin
    C.-M. M
    C.-M. S Otic drop
Colyte-Flavored Combitube
COM
    chronic otitis media
COMA
    congenital ocular motor apraxia
    congenital ocular motor apraxia (type
      Cogan)
    cyclophosphamide, Oncovin,
      methotrexate, arabinosylcytosine
coma
    diabetic c.
    hepatic c.
    hyperammonemic hepatic c.
    hyperosmolar nonketotic c.
    myxedema c.
    nonketotic hyperosmolar c.
    pentobarbital c.
comatose
combat crawl
Combidex MRI contrast agent
combination
    apnea-hypopnea c.
    c. chemotherapy
    consonant-vowel c.

    c. estrogen-progestin contraceptive
    estrogen-progestogen c.
    norgestrel/ethinyl estradiol c.
    c. oral contraceptive
    xanthan/guar c.
combined
    c. birth control pill
    c. hormone therapy (CHT)
    c. immunodeficiency (CID)
    c. injectable contraceptive
    c. nevus
    c. oral contraceptive (COC)
    c. pregnancy
    c. spinal-epidural (CSE)
    c. version
combing
    cervical c.
CombiPatch
Combitube
Combivir
comedo, pl. **comedos, comedones**
    closed c.
    c. extractor
    open c.
comedocarcinoma
comedomastitis
comedones (*pl. of* comedo)
comedonicus
    nevus c.
comedos (*pl. of* comedo)
Comfort personal lubricant gel
Comhist LA
comitant strabismus
commando crawl
comma-shaped organism
commensal flora
comminuted fracture
commission
    physician payment review c.
      (PPRC)
commissioning couple
commissural
    c. lip pit
    c. separation
commissure
    anterior c.
    labial c.
    posterior c.
commissurotomy
    mitral c.
committed cell

NOTES

committee
    National Vaccine Advisory C.
      (NVAC)
common
    c. atrium
    c. blue nevus
    c. channel
    c. cold
    c. hepatic duct
    c. migraine
    c. migraine headache
    c. sheath reimplant
    c. variable hypogammaglobulinemia
    c. variable immunodeficiency (CVI,
      CVID)
    c. wart
common-inlet single right ventricle
commotio
    c. cordis
    c. retinae
communal traumatic experiences
  inventory (CTEI)
communicable
    c. disease
    C. Disease Center (CDC)
    c. illness
communicating
    c. hydrocephalus
    c. uterus
communication
    c. aid
    augmentative and alternative c.
      (AAC)
    autocrine c.
    c. board
    c. book
    c. disorder
    c. domain
    facilitated c. (F/C)
    fetal-maternal c.
    fistulous vascular c.
    interatrial c. (IAC)
    nonverbal c.
    paracrine c.
    total c.
    vascular c.
communicative development inventory
communis
    macula c.
    truncus arteriosus c.
community-acquired (CA)
    c.-a. methicillin-resistant
      Staphylococcus aureus (CAMRSA)
community medicine
comorbid anxiety disorder
comorbidity
    psychological c.
COMP
    cartilage oligomeric matrix protein

    cyclophosphamide, Oncovin,
      methotrexate, prednisone
    COMP drug regimen
compacta
Companion 318 Nasal CPAP System
comparative
    c. embryology
    c. genomic hybridization (CGH)
    c. mapping
comparison view
compartment
    adductor interosseous c.
    calcaneal c.
    extracellular fluid c.
    lateral c.
    medial c.
    superficial c.
    c. syndrome
compartmentalization
compassionate use
compatibility
    maternal-fetal HLA c.
Compazine
compensated
    c. cirrhosis
    c. hydrocephalus
    c. shock
compensatory
    c. antiinflammatory syndrome
    c. articulation
    c. erythropoiesis
    c. gliosis
    c. hyperinsulinemia
    c. movement
    c. scoliosis
competence
    cervical c.
    cultural c.
competing anion
complaint
    psychosomatic c.
    somatic c.
Compleat
    C. Modified formula
    C. Pediatric formula
complement
    c. chemotactic factor
    chromosome c.
    c. C3 level
    c. deficiency
    c. deficiency disorder
    c. deposition
    c. fixation
    c. fixation test
    hemolytic c. (CH_{50})
    c. receptor
    serum c.
    c. test

total hemolytic c.
c. value
complemental inheritance
complementary
c. and alternative medicine (CAM)
c. deoxyribonucleic acid (cDNA)
c. DNA (cDNA)
c. gene
c. RNA
c. sequence
complementation test
complement-fixing serum antibody
complete
c. abortion
c. androgen insensitivity syndrome (CAIS)
c. androgen resistance syndrome
c. atrioventricular block
c. atrioventricular canal
c. blood count (CBC)
c. breech presentation
c. cerebellar aplasia
c. cleft
c. cord transection
c. DiGeorge syndrome
c. feminizing testes syndrome
c. fetal heart block
c. fracture
c. hernia
c. hydatidiform mole
c. isosexual precocity
c. linkage
c. placenta previa
c. precocious puberty
c. radial aplasia
c. rectal prolapse
c. remission
c. subtalar release (CSTR)
c. suppression pattern
c. testicular feminization
c. transposition
c. transposition of great arteries
c. transposition of great vessels
c. vulvar duplication
complete/complete/+ station
complex
Adam c.
c. adnexal endometrioma
AIDS dementia c. (ADC)
AIDS-related c. (ARC)
amphotericin B cholesteryl sulfate c.

amphotericin B lipid c.
amyotrophic lateral sclerosis-Parkinson-dementia c.
antigen-antibody c.
antiinhibitor coagulant c.
axial mesodermal dysplasia c.
blepharophimosis, ptosis, epicanthus inversus, telecanthus c.
blocked premature atrial c.
cardinal-uterosacral ligament c.
chlorophyllin copper c.
c. coarctation
c. congenital heart disease
C. 15 cream
del 11/aniridia c.
Diana c.
disseminated *Mycobacterium avium* c. (DMAC)
early amnion vascular disruption c.
Eisenmenger c.
Electra c.
c. enteral feeding
epispadias-exstrophy c.
facioauriculovertebral malformation c.
Fallot c.
c. febrile seizure
gene c.
generalized bilaterally synchronous sharp-wave and slow-wave c.'s
Ghon c.
Gollop-Wolfgang c.
c. heart defect
human factor IX c.
c. hyperplasia
immune c. (IC)
iron dextran c.
Jocasta c.
lap-belt c.
lateral collateral ligament c.
Lear c.
limb-body wall c. (LBWC)
major histocompatibility c. (MHC)
c. mass
membrane attack c.
c. motor tic
Mycobacterium avium c. (MAC)
Mycobacterium avium-intracellulare c. (MAC)
Mycobacterium fortuitum c.
c. myoclonic epilepsy
nipple-areola c.

C

NOTES

complex *(continued)*
  Oedipus c.
  ostiomeatal c.
  c. partial epilepsy
  c. partial seizure (CPS)
  c. partial status epilepticus
  Phaedra c.
  pyruvate dehydrogenase c. (PDHC deficiency)
  QS c.
  c. regional pain syndrome (CRPS)
  Rh c.
  sicca c.
  spermatic venous c.
  spike and wave c.
  synaptonemal c.
  c. syndactyly
  triangular fibrocartilaginous c. (TFCC)
  tuberous sclerosis c. (TSC)
  tuboovarian c. (TOC)
  c. unroofed coronary sinus (CUCS)
  uterosacral c.
  VATER c.
  vitamin B c.
  c. vocal tic
  von Meyenburg c.

complexion
  florid c.
  pallid c.

compliance
  lung c. (CL)
  pulmonary c.
  tympanic membrane c.

complicated
  c. gastroesophageal reflux
  c. meconium ileus
  c. migraine
  c. migraine headache

complication
  abortion c.
  antenatal c.
  antepartum c.
  cardiovascular c.
  end-organ c.
  intraoperative c.
  intrapartum c.
  late c.
  microvascular c.
  neurodevelopmental c.
  neurologic c.
  obstetric c.
  operative site c.
  postoperative c.
  pregnancy c.
  pulmonary c.
  respiratory c.
  thromboembolic c.
  vascular c.

component
  blood c.
  buffy coat c.
  diastolic c.
  extensive intraductal c. (EIC)
  extracellular matrix c.
  systolic c.
  terminal complement c.

composite allograft
composition
  body c.

compound
  artificial lung-expanding compound (ALEC)
  c. heterozygote
  c. nevus
  nitroimidazole c.
  c. pregnancy
  c. presentation
  progestational c.
  pteridine ring c.
  C. W

Compoz
  C. Gel Caps
  C. Nighttime Sleep Aid

Comprecin
compressed air-driven nebulizer
compressibility
compression
  brainstem c.
  cardiac c.
  cerebellar hemisphere c.
  cerebral c.
  cervicomedullary c.
  chest c.
  cord c.
  esophageal c.
  external pneumatic calf c. (EPC)
  c. force
  c. fracture
  head c.
  c. injury
  intermittent pneumatic c.
  intrauterine c.
  joint c.
  mechanical c.
  c. myelopathy
  pneumatic c.
  spinal cord c.
  spot c.
  thorax c.
  tracheal c.
  tracheobronchial c.
  c. ultrasonography
  uterine c.
  vein c.
  vertebral artery c.
compression-rarefaction strain
compressive dressing

compressor
Pari Proneb Turbo c.
c. urethra
compressus
fetus c.
compromise
airway c.
angiitic luminal c.
fetal c.
microcirculatory c.
neurovascular c.
respiratory c.
severe respiratory c.
compromised fetus
Compton effect
compulsion
compulsive
c. echolalia
c. self-mutilation
computed
c. axial tomography (CAT)
c. tomography (CT)
c. tomography laser mammography (CTLM)
computer-aided diagnosis (CAD)
computer-assisted
c.-a. semen analysis (CASA)
c.-a. semen analyzer (CASA)
computerized
C. Diagnostic Interview for Children and Adolescents (cDICA)
c. tomographic (CT)
COMS
cerebrooculomuscular syndrome
Comtrex Cough Formula
Comvax vaccine
conal muscle
concave temporalis muscle
concavity
concealed
c. hemorrhage
c. penis
c. rectal prolapse
conceive
C. Ovulation Predictor
PreCare C.
concentrate
factor c.
platelet c.
protein C c.

concentrated
c. oral sucrose
c. urine
concentration
alpha-tocopherol c.
ambient oxygen c.
anti-HBsAg c.
bicarbonate c.
blood alcohol c. (BAC)
cord blood leptin c.
cortisol c.
elevated sweat chloride c.
fetal leptin c.
fetal steroid c.
fetal thrombopoietin c.
glucose c.
hemoglobin c.
hepatic iron c. (HIC)
hydrogen in c. (pH)
inhibin c.
intracellular hydrogen ion c. (pHi)
lipoprotein c.
maternal steroid c.
mean cell hemoglobin c. (MCHC)
mean corpuscular hemoglobin c. (MCHC)
mean hemoglobin c.
mean plasma iron c.
minimal bacterial c. (MBC)
minimal inhibitory c. (MIC)
minimum inhibitory c. (MIC)
plasma amino acid c.
plasma bilirubin c. (PBC)
plasma histamine c.
plasma iron c.
plasma phosphate c.
plasma retinol c.
plasma theophylline c.
plasma vitamin A c.
platelet c.
pulmonary tissue c. (PTC)
serum albumin c.
serum amino acid c.
serum ferritin c.
serum lactate dehydrogenase c.
serum lithium c.
serum melatonin c.
serum protein c.
steroid c.
sweat chloride c.
concentrica
encephalitis periaxialis c.

NOTES

concentric sclerosis
concept
concepti (*pl. of* conceptus)
conception
    c. age
    assisted c.
    estimated date of c. (EDC)
    evacuation of retained products
      of c. (ERPC)
    natural c.
    products of c. (POC)
    retained products of c. (RPC)
    wrongful c.
Conceptrol
conceptus, pl. **concepti**
    C. fallopian tube catheterization
      system
    C. Soft Torque uterine catheter
    C. VS catheter
Concerta
concha bullosa
Concise Plus hCG urine test
concisus
    Campylobacter c.
concomitant change
concordance
concordant twins
concrete pelvis
concussion
    labyrinthine c.
    spinal c.
    c. syndrome
COND
    cerebroosteonephrodysplasia
condition
    childbirth-related medical c.
    fetal c.
    intersex c.
    local ovarian c.
    maternal systemic c.
    neonatal c.
    nonangiitic vasculopathic c.
    nonvertiginous c.
    orthopaedic c.
    preexisting maternal medical c.
    Questionnaire for Identifying
      Children with Chronic C.'s
      (QuICCC)
    vertiginous c.
    X-linked dominant c.
    X-linked recessive c.
conditional probability
conditioned
    c. orientation reflex (COR)
    c. play audiometry
conditioning regimen
condom
    female c.
    intravaginal c.

    male c.
    Ramses C.
    Reality C.
    The Female C.
    vaginal c.
    Women's Choice c.
conductance
    airway c.
conduct disorder (CD)
conduction
    c. analgesia
    c. anesthesia
    antidromic c.
    c. defect
    orthodromic c.
conductive
    c. education (CE)
    c. hearing impairment
    c. hearing loss
    c. tissue
conductivity
conduit
    fetal vascular c.
    homograft c.
    ileal c.
    intestinal c.
    urinary c.
conduplicato corpore
condyle
    lateral c.
    medial c.
condyloma
    c. acuminatum
    anal c.
    cervical c.
    c. latum
    recalcitrant c.
    resistant c.
    vulvar c.
condylomatous
Condylox solution
cone
    c. biopsy
    c. biopsy of cervix
    cold knife c.
    ectoplacental c.
    transvaginal c.
    vaginal c.
confetti lesion
Confide HIV test kit
configuration
    brachycephalic c.
    hourglass c.
    villoglandular c.
confinement
    estimated date of c. (EDC)
    expected date of c. (EDC)
    postpartum c.

confirmation
> microscopic c.
> tissue c.

conflict

confluent
> c. eyebrows
> c. plaque

Conformant dressing

confusion
> postictal c.

confusional
> c. arousal
> c. migraine

congenita
> adrenal hypoplasia c.
> aglossia c.
> alacrima c.
> alopecia totalis c.
> amaurosis c.
> amyoplasia c.
> amyotonia c.
> aplasia axialis extracorticalis c.
> aplasia cutis c.
> arthrochalasis multiplex c.
> arthrogryposis multiplex c. (AMC)
> bitemporal aplasia cutis c.
> chondrodystrophia calcificans c.
> cutis marmorata telangiectatica c.
> dyskeratosis c.
> erythropoietic porphyria c.
> hypertrichosis universalis c.
> ichthyosis c.
> macrosomia adiposa c.
> myotonia c.
> pachyonychia c.
> paramyotonia c.
> pseudoglioma c.
> pterygoarthromyodysplasia c.
> spondyloepiphyseal dysplasia c.
> syngnathia c.
> Thomsen myotonia c.
> X-linked dyskeratosis c.

congenital
> c. abducens facial paralysis
> c. absence
> c. absence of iron-binding protein
> c. absence of lactase
> c. absence of vas deferens
>   (CAVD)
> c. acromicria syndrome
> c. adrenal hyperplasia (CAH)
> c. adrenal hypoplasia

> c. adrenal lipoid hyperplasia
> c. afibrinogenemia
> c. aganglionic megacolon
> c. agranulocytosis
> c. aleukia
> c. alveolar dysplasia
> c. alveolar proteinosis
> c. amaurosis of retinal origin
> c. amblyogenic stimulus
> c. AME
> c. amegakaryocytic
>   thrombocytopenia
> c. amputation
> c. analgesia
> c. anemia of newborn
> c. anemia syndrome
> c. anomaly
> c. anosmia
> c. anosmia-hypogonadotropic
>   hypogonadism syndrome
> c. anterolateral tibial angulation
> c. aortic stenosis
> c. aplastic anemia
> c. arthromyodysplastic syndrome
> c. articular rigidity
> c. asplenia
> c. ataxia
> c. atelectasis
> c. athetosis
> c. atransferrinemia
> c. atresia of bile duct
> c. atresia of uterine cervix
> c. aural atresia
> c. bilateral cataract
> c. bone marrow failure syndrome
> c. bronchiectasis
> c. bronchopulmonary malformation
> c. bullous urticaria pigmentosa
> c. candidiasis
> c. carbohydrate malabsorption
> c. cardiac defect
> c. cardiac disease
> c. cardiovascular malformation
>   (CCVM)
> c. cataracts, sensorineural deafness,
>   Down syndrome facial appearance,
>   short stature, mental retardation
>   syndrome
> c. central hypoventilation
> c. central hypoventilation syndrome
>   (CCHS)
> c. cerebral aneurysm

C

NOTES

congenital *(continued)*

- c. chloridorrhea
- c. choledochal dilation
- c. cholesteatoma
- c. chylothorax
- c. clasped thumbs
- c. clasped thumbs-mental retardation syndrome
- c. cloaca
- c. clubfoot
- c. complete AV block
- c. complete heart block (CCHB)
- c. condylar deformity
- c. contractural arachnodactyly (CCA)
- c. contracture of extremity
- c. cutaneous candidosis
- c. cutis aplasia
- c. cystic adenomatoid malformation (CCAM)
- c. cystic adenomatoid malfunction
- c. cytomegalovirus
- c. defect of phosphofructokinase
- c. dermal melanocytosis
- c. diaphragmatic hernia (CDH)
- c. diaphragmatic hernia of Bochdalek
- c. diaphragmatic hernia-extracorporeal membrane oxygenation (CDH-ECMO)
- c. dislocated hip (CDH)
- c. dislocation
- c. dislocation of hip (CDH)
- c. dislocation of patella
- c. diverticulum
- c. double pylorus
- c. duodenal atresia
- c. dyserythropoietic anemia (CDA)
- c. dyskeratosis
- c. ectodermal dysplasia of face
- c. ectodermic scalp defect
- c. ectropion
- c. elephantiasis
- c. elevation of the scapula
- c. emphysema, cryptorchidism, penoscrotal web, deafness, mental retardation syndrome
- c. enamel abnormality
- c. encephalo-ophthalmic dysplasia
- c. endothelial corneal dystrophy
- c. epulis
- c. epulis of the newborn
- c. erythropoietic porphyria (CEP)
- c. esophageal stenosis
- c. esotropia
- c. eventration
- c. extremity lymphedema
- c. facial diplegia

- c. familial lymphedema with ocular findings
- c. fibrosarcoma
- c. fibular hemimelia
- c. folate malabsorption
- c. generalized lipodystrophy
- c. generalized phlebectasia
- c. glaucoma
- c. glenoid dysplasia
- c. goitrous hypothyroidism
- c. granulocytopenia
- c. growth hormone deficiency
- c. Guillain-Barré syndrome
- c. hairy nevus
- c. hearing loss
- c. heart block
- c. heart defect
- c. heart defect syndrome
- c. heart disease (CHD)
- c. Heinz body anemia
- c. hemidysplasia with ichthyosiform erythroderma and limb defects (CHILD)
- c. hemiparesis
- c. hemiplegia
- c. hemolytic anemia with aplastic crisis
- c. hemolytic jaundice
- c. hepatic fibrosis
- c. hereditary hematuria
- c. hereditary retinoschisis
- c. herpes
- c. heterochromia
- c. high airway obstruction syndrome (CHAOS)
- c. hip disease
- c. hip dislocation (CHD)
- c. hip disorder
- c. hip dysplasia (CHD)
- c. hydantoin syndrome
- c. hydronephrosis
- c. hypertrichosis-osteochondrodysplasia-cardiomegaly syndrome
- c. hypertrophic pyloric stenosis
- c. hypoaldosteronism
- c. hypocupremia syndrome
- c. hypofibrinogenemia
- c. hypogammaglobulinemia
- c. hypogonadotropic hypogonadism
- c. hypomagnesemia
- c. hypomyelinating neuropathy (CHN)
- c. hypomyelination
- c. hypopituitarism
- c. hypoplastic anemia
- c. hypothalamic hamartoblastoma
- c. hypothyroidism (CH)
- c. hypothyroidism syndrome

c. hypotonia
c. ichthyosiform
c. ichthyosiform erythroderma
c. ichthyosis
c. ichthyosis-mental retardation-spasticity syndrome
c. ichthyosis-trichodystrophy syndrome
c. infection
c. injury
c. insensitivity
c. insensitivity to pain
c. intestinal aganglionosis
c. intestinal band
c. intrinsic factor deficiency
c. iris coloboma
c. jerky nystagmus
c. kyphosis
c. lacrimal duct obstruction
c. lactase deficiency
c. lactic acidosis
c. laryngeal stridor
c. laxity of ligament
c. LCMV syndrome
c. lesion
c. lethal hypophosphatasia
c. leukemia
c. lipase/colipase deficiency
c. lipoatrophic diabetes
c. lip pit
c. listeriosis
c. lobar emphysema
c. lobar overinflation (CLO)
c. localized absence of skin (CLAS)
c. longitudinal deficiency
c. longitudinal deficiency of fibula
c. longitudinal deficiency of tibia
c. long QT syndrome
c. lung malformation
c. macular degeneration
c. manifestation
c. megakaryocytic hypoplasia
c. melanocytic nevus
c. mesoblastic nephroma
c. metatarsus adductus
c. metatarsus varus
c. microcephaly, hiatus hernia, nephrotic syndrome
c. microvillus atrophy
c. miosis
c. multiple myofibromatosis

c. muscle fiber-type disproportion (CMFTD)
c. muscular dystrophy (CMD)
c. muscular dystrophy with central nervous system involvement
c. muscular hypertrophy-cerebral syndrome
c. muscular torticollis
c. myasthenia
c. myasthenia gravis
c. mydriasis
c. myopathy
c. myotonic dystrophy
c. nasal pyriform aperture stenosis (CNPAS)
c. nasolacrimal duct obstruction (CNLDO)
c. neonatal ascites
c. nephrosis
c. nephrotic syndrome
c. nephrotic syndrome, Finnish (CNF)
c. nerve deafness
c. neutropenia
c. nevomelanocytic nevus
c. nevus
c. nonhemolytic jaundice
c. nonhemolytic unconjugated hyperbilirubinemia
c. nonregenerative anemia
c. nonspherocytic hemolytic anemia
c. obliterative jaundice
c. obstruction of nasolacrimal duct
c. obstructive müllerian malformation
c. ocular motor apraxia (COMA)
c. ocular motor apraxia (type Cogan) (COMA)
c. oculofacial paralysis
c. osteopetrosis
c. palatopharyngeal incompetence (CPI)
c. paretic neurosyphilis
c. paroxysmal atrial tachycardia
c. pendular nystagmus
c. perilymphatic fistula
c. peritoneal band
c. pernicious anemia
c. photosensitive porphyria
c. pigmental nevus
c. pneumonia
c. portosystemic venous shunt

NOTES

193

congenital *(continued)*
- c. posteromedial bowing
- c. posteromedial tibial angulation
- c. postural deformity
- c. progressive muscular dystrophy with mental retardation
- c. progressive oculoacousticocerebral degeneration
- c. pseudarthrosis
- c. pseudoarthrosis
- c. pseudoarthrosis of the clavicle
- c. pseudoarthrosis of tibia
- c. pseudohydrocephalic progeroid syndrome
- c. pterygium
- c. ptosis
- c. pulmonary lymphangiectasia
- c. RBC aplasia
- c. retinitis blindness (CRB)
- c. retinitis pigmentosa
- c. rocker-bottom foot
- c. rubella
- c. rubella infection
- c. rubella syndrome (CRS)
- c. sensory neuropathy
- c. sideroblastic anemia
- c. skin aplasia
- c. sodium diarrhea
- c. spastic paraplegia
- c. spherocytosis
- c. stationary night blindness
- c. stippled epiphysis
- c. STORCH infection
- c. structural defect
- c. suprabulbar paresis
- c. supraspinous fossa
- c. syphilis
- c. syphilitic infection
- c. tarsal coalition
- c. TC II deficiency
- c. tendo Achillis contracture
- c. tertiary neurosyphilis
- c. 6th nerve palsy
- c. thoracic scoliosis
- c. thrombocytopenia, Robin sequence, agenesis of corpus callosum, distinctive facies, developmental delay syndrome
- c. thyroid deficiency
- c. thyroid deficiency with muscular hypertrophy
- c. tibial hemimelia
- c. toxoplasmosis
- c. tracheal stenosis
- c. transport defect
- c. trypsinogen deficiency
- c. tuberculosis
- c. tubular stenosis
- c. unilateral lower lip paralysis
- c. universal muscular hypoplasia
- c. upper airway malformation
- c. urinary tract obstruction
- c. vaginal adenosis
- c. vaginal aplasia
- c. varicella syndrome
- c. vertical talus
- c. warfarin syndrome

congenitale
- poikiloderma c.

congenitalis
- alopecia c.
- heredoretinopathia c.

Congest

congestion
- passive venous c.
- pelvic vein c.
- pulmonary vascular c.
- vascular c.

congestive
- c. cardiomyopathy-hypergonadotropic hypogonadism syndrome
- c. gastropathy
- c. heart disease (CHD)
- c. heart failure (CHF)

conglobata
- acne c.

conglutination

Congo virus

conical teeth

conidial forest

conidium, pl. **conidia**

coning of brain

conization
- carbon dioxide laser beam c.
- cautery c.
- cervical c.
- c. of cervix
- cold knife c. (CKC)
- cold knife cervical c.
- hot knife c.
- laser cervical c.
- laser excisional c.
- loop diathermy cervical c.

conjoined
- c. tendon
- c. twins

conjugata
- c. anatomic pelvis
- c. diagonalis pelvis
- c. externa pelvis
- c. vera pelvis

conjugate
- anatomic c.
- c. axis
- diagonal c.
- c. diameter of the pelvic inlet
- effective c.
- external c.

false c.
c. of inlet
internal c.
meningococcal c.
obstetric c.
obstetric c. of outlet
c. of pelvic outlet
c. pneumococcal vaccine
c. pupil
true c.
c. upward gaze
urinary steroid c.

conjugated
c. antichlamydial monoclonal
  antibody
c. bilirubin
c. equine estrogen (CEE)
c. estrogen and meprobamate
c. estrogens
c. hyperbilirubinemia
c. linoleic acid (CLA)

conjugation activity
conjunctiva, pl. **conjunctivae**
bulbar c.
cobblestoning of c.
palpebral c.
xerosis c.

conjunctival
c. hyperemia
c. infection
c. injection
c. nevus
c. scraping
c. suffusion
c. telangiectasis

conjunctivitis
acquired c.
acute epidemic c.
acute hemorrhagic c.
acute perinatal c.
acute purulent c.
allergic c.
bacterial c.
bilateral c.
chemical c.
childhood c.
chlamydial c.
exudative c.
follicular c.
gonococcal c.
herpes simplex viral c.
inclusion body of chlamydial c.

infantile purulent c.
membranous c.
neonatal c.
palpebral c.
pediatric gonococcal c.
pseudomembranous c.
purulent c.
shipyard c.
silver nitrate c.
trachoma inclusion c. (TRIC)
vernal c.
viral c.

conjunctivitis-otitis syndrome
Conmed electrosurgical pencil
connatal form
connection
anomalous pulmonary venous c.
circulation-cavopulmonary c.
decidua-macrophage c.
total anomalous pulmonary
  venous c. (TAPVC)
total cavopulmonary c.

connective
c. tissue
c. tissue disease
c. tissue disorder
c. tissue nevus

connector
domino c.
T c.
tube c.
Y c.

Conners
C. Abbreviated Parent Questionnaire
C. Hyperactivity indices
C. Rating Scale (CRS)
C. Scale

connexin
Conn syndrome
conorii
  Rickettsia c.
conotruncal
c. abnormality
c. anomaly face syndrome (CTAF)
c. cardiac defect, abnormal face,
  thymic hypoplasia, cleft palate
  (CATCH 22)
c. cardiac malformation
c. facial anomaly
c. facial syndrome
c. heart defects
c. septum

NOTES

195

conotruncus
Conradi
    C. disease
    C. syndrome
Conradi-Hünermann syndrome
consanguineous
    c. mating
    c. parents
consanguinity
    parental c.
CoNS bacteremia
conscious
    body c.
    c. sedation
consciousness
    altered state of c. (ASC)
    level of c. (LOC)
    loss of c.
consecutive loss
consensus sequence
consent
    informed c.
    written c.
conservation
    breast c.
conservative
    c. drug use
    c. management
    c. surgery
    c. therapy
conserved
    evolutionarily c.
    c. sequence
consideration
    adrenal morphologic c.
consolability
    face, legs, activity, cry, c.
     (FLACC)
consolidation
    alveolar c.
    basilar c.
    lobar c.
    lung c.
    pneumonic c.
consonant
    glide c.
    nasal c.
consonant-vowel combination
constancy
    object c.
constant
    association c.
    dissociation c.
    c. exotropia
    c. flow end-inspiratory airway
     occlusion
    Michaelis-Menten dissociation c.
    c. positive airway pressure

    pulmonary time c.
    c. strabismus
    c. tidal volume
constellates
    Streptococcus c.
Constilac
constipation
    chronic c.
    functional c.
    idiopathic c.
constituent
constitution
    genetic c.
constitutional
    c. delay of puberty
    c. dwarfism
    c. growth delay
    c. hirsutism
    c. precocious puberty
    c. short stature
constraint-induced movement therapy
constriction
    c. band syndrome
    fetal ductus arteriosus c.
    ring c.
    c. ring
constrictive
    c. pericarditis
    c. pericarditis-dwarfism syndrome
construct
    solid rod segmental c.
construction
    Abbe vaginal c.
    Davydov vagina c.
    Frank vaginal c.
Constulose
consultant
    PID c.
consumption
    cerebral oxygen c.
    c. coagulopathy
    maternal alcohol c.
    oxygen c.
    oxygen c. per minute (Vo_2)
consumptive
    c. coagulopathy
    c. thrombocytopenia
contact
    c. allergen
    coital c.
    c. dermatitis
    c. factor
    heater probe thermal c.
    kangaroo c.
    c. sensitization
    sexual c.
    sperm-cervical mucus c. (SCMC)
    c. vulvovaginitis

contagion
    c. factor
    symptom c.
contagiosa
    impetigo c.
contagiosum
    molluscum c.
contagious
containment
    surgical c.
contaminant
contaminate
contamination
    bacterial c.
content
    aortic oxygen c.
    aspiration of gastric c.'s
    bone mineral c. (BMC)
    evacuation of uterine c.'s
    fatty acid c.
    mixed venous oxygen c.
    poverty of c.
    pulmonary arterial oxygen c.
    pulmonary venous oxygen c.
    quantitative analysis of fat c.
    total body iron c.
Contigen
    C. Bard collagen implant
    C. glutaraldehyde cross-linked
      collagen implant
contig map
contiguous
    c. gene deletion syndrome
    c. gene syndrome of chromosome
    13
    c. pigmentation
Contin
    MS C.
continence ring
continent
    c. ileostomy
    c. supravesical bowel urinary
      diversion
    c. urinary pouch
contingency table
contingent reinforcement
continua
    epilepsia partialis c.
continuant
continuous
    c. ambulatory peritoneal dialysis
      (CAPD)

    c. arteriovenous hemofiltration
      (CAVH)
    c. blood gas monitoring
    c. cineangiogram
    c. cyclic peritoneal dialysis
      (CCPD)
    c. distending airway pressure
      (CDAP)
    c. distending pressure (CDP)
    c. distention irrigation system
      (CDIS)
    c. epidural analgesia
    c. fetal heart monitoring
    c. gastric drip (CGD)
    c. glucose infusion
    c. intravenous oxytocin drip
    c. long-term monitoring (CLTM)
    c. milk infusion
    c. negative airway pressure
      (CNAP)
    c. negative extrathoracic pressure
      (CNEP)
    C. Performance Task
    c. performance test (CPT)
    c. positive airway pressure (CPAP)
    c. running monofilament suture
    c. shunt murmur
    c. subcutaneous infusion (CSQI)
    c. subcutaneous insulin infusion
    c. subcutaneous insulin injection
    c. tracheal gas insufflation
    c. tube feeding
    c. variation
    c. venovenous hemodialysis
      (CVVHD)
    c. venovenous hemofiltration
      (CVVH)
    c. wave Doppler
    c. wave Doppler interrogation
continuous/combined treatment
continuous-dose combined oral
    contraceptive
continuous-wave ultrasound imaging
continuum
    infantile Refsum disease c.
contour
    cranial c.
contoured tilting compression
    mammography
Contour Profile anatomically shaped
    silicone breast

NOTES

contraception
    barrier method of c.
    emergency c. (EC)
    hormonal emergency c.
    lactational amenorrhea method
      of c.
    long-acting c.
    morning-after c.
    oral c.
    postcoital c. (PCC)
    rhythm method of c.
    vaginal ring c.
    Yuzpe regimen of combined oral
      contraceptives for emergency c.

contraceptive
    all-progestin c.
    barrier c.
    combination estrogen-progestin c.
    combination oral c.
    combined injectable c.
    combined oral c. (COC)
    continuous-dose combined oral c.
    c. device
    c. diaphragm
    c. effectiveness
    estrogen-progestin c.
    estrophasic oral c.
    Estrostep oral c.
    c. failure
    c. failure rate
    c. film
    c. foam
    c. history
    hormonal c.
    c. implant
    implantable hormonal c.
    injectable hormonal c.
    intrauterine c. device (IUCD)
    intravaginal c.
    c. jelly
    Lea's shield female barrier c.
    long-acting c.
    low-dose oral c.
    low steroid content combined
      oral c.
    c. method
    monophasic oral c.
    oral c. (OC)
    oral steroid c.
    ParaGard T380A intrauterine
      copper c.
    progestin-only injectable c.
    progestin-only oral c.
    progestin oral c.
    c. ring
    Seasonale oral c.
    sequential oral c.
    c. sponge
    steroid c.

    c. suppository capsule
    c. technique
    triphasic oral c.
    vaginal c.

contract
    behavior c.

contracted pelvis

contractile

contractility
    LV c.
    uterine c.

contraction
    atrial c.
    atrial premature c. (APC)
    Braxton Hicks c.
    myometrial c.
    pelvic c.
    premature atrial c.
    premature ventricular c. (PVC)
    smooth muscle c.
    c. stress test (CST)
    tetanic uterine c.'s
    uterine c.
    ventricular premature c. (VPC)
    volume c.
    Z degree of c.'s
    Z' degree of c.'s
    Z'' degree of c.'s

contractural
    c. arachnodactyly disease
    c. arachnodactyly syndrome

contracture
    congenital tendo Achillis c.
    flaccid c.
    flexion c.
    gastrocnemius c.
    general triceps c.
    heel-cord c.
    joint c. (JC)
    multiple articular c.
    c., muscle atrophy, oculomotor
      apraxia syndrome
    Volkmann ischemic c.

contraindication

contralateral
    c. head turning (CHT)
    c. hernia
    c. hypertrophy
    c. hypertrophy of testes
    c. ovary
    c. ovulation
    c. reflux
    c. synchronous carcinoma

contrasexual precocity

contrast
    barium c.
    Echovist c.
    c. esophagogram
    c. venography

contrecoup injury
control
    airway c.
    birth c.
    bladder c.
    glycemic c.
    head c.
    motor c.
    poor head c.
    seizure c.
    trunk c.
    waitlist c.
controlled
    c. ileal release budesonide
    c. intubation
    c. mechanical ventilation (CMV)
    c. ovarian hyperstimulation (COH)
    c. vaginal delivery
controller
    Pepcid AC Acid C.
controversial
controversy
    transfusion c.
contused tissue
contusion
    cerebral c.
    iliac crest c.
    myocardial c.
    pulmonary c.
conundrum
conus, pl. **coni**
    c. medullaris syndrome
    subaortic c.
convalescent
    c. sera
    c. serum
convection-warmed incubator
convergence
    poor c.
convergent
    c. nystagmus
    c. sidewalls
    c. squint
    c. strabismus
conversion
    c. disorder
    extraglandular c.
    c. reaction
    skin test c.
convex probe
convoluted tubule
convolution

convulsion
    afebrile c.
    B_6-dependent c.
    benign familial neonatal c. (BFNC)
    benign idiopathic neonatal c.
    benign infantile familial c.'s (BIFC)
    epileptic c.
    febrile c.
    focal c.
    gelastic c.
    generalized c.
    multifocal clonic c.
    myoclonic c.
    neonatal c.
    puerperal c.
    salaam c.
    tonic-clonic c.
convulsive
    c. seizure
    c. status epilepticus
cooing
Cook
    C. aspirator
    C. catheter
Cooke-Medley Hostility Scale
Cookie Insert
Cooks syndrome
Cooley anemia
cooling blanket
cool-mist
    c.-m. humidifier
    c.-m. vaporizer
cool shock
Coombs
    C. antibody
    C. positive
    C. test
Coombs-negative autoimmune hemolytic anemia
Coombs-positive isoimmune hemolytic anemia
Cooper
    C. fascia
    C. irritable breast
    suspensory ligaments of C.
    C. syndrome
cooperative
    C. Human Tissue Network (CHTN)
    c. study of sickle cell disease (CSSCD)

NOTES

cooperativity
 theca-granulosa cell c.
Coopernail sign
CooperSurgical
 C. overhead colposcope
coordination
 eye-hand c.
 hand-eye c.
 poor c.
 visual-motor c.
coordinator
 service c.
cooximeter analyzer
COP
 colloid osmotic pressure
Copaxone
Copeland
 C. fetal scalp electrode
 C. Symptom Checklist for
 Attention Deficit Disorders
coping
 C. Health Inventory for Children
 (CHIC)
 C. Health Inventory for Parents
 (CHIP)
 c. self-statement
copious
 c. antibiotic irrigation
 c. discharge
copper
 c. deficiency
 c. deficiency anemia
 c. deposition
 hepatic c.
 c. homeostasis
 c. metabolism
 serum c.
 c. sulfate ingestion
 c. T–380A IUD
 C. T intrauterine device
 c. toxicosis
 c. transport disease
 urinary c.
copper-histidine
copper-induced rhabdomyolysis
copper-wire appearance
coprolalia
coproporphyria
 hereditary c. (HCP)
coproporphyrin
 c. excretion
 urinary c.
 urinary c. I
copropraxia
copulation plug
copy
 DNA c.
 large single c.
 small single c.

COR
 conditioned orientation reflex
cor
 c. biloculare
 c. pulmonale
 c. triatriatum
 c. triatriatum dexter
 c. triloculare biatriatum
coracoclavicular ligament
Corcath catheter
cord
 c. abnormality
 c. accident
 bifid spinal c.
 c. blood
 c. blood acidosis
 c. blood bank
 c. blood bilirubin
 c. blood erythropoietin level
 c. blood gas (CBG)
 c. blood hemoglobin
 c. blood leptin concentration
 c. blood registry (CBR)
 c. blood sample
 c. blood transplantation (CBT)
 body coils of c.
 c. clamping
 c. compression
 c. entanglement
 false vocal c.
 furcate insertion of c.
 genital c.
 heel c.
 hemisection of c.
 c. IgG level
 c. insertion (CI)
 kinked c.
 c. lipoma
 medullary c.
 milking of umbilical c.
 nephrogenic c.
 noncoiled c.
 nuchal c.
 omphalomesenteric c.
 palpable c.
 c. plasma leptin
 presentation of c.
 c. prolapse
 prolapsed c.
 prolapse of umbilical c.
 rete c.'s
 c. serum level
 sex c.
 spermatic c.
 spinal c.
 c. stem cell marrow transplantation
 tethered spinal c.
 three-vessel c.
 tight heel c.

c. torsion
c. transection
two-vessel c.
umbilical c.
velamentous insertion of c.
c. vessel identification
vitelline c.
vocal c.
Cordarone
cordate pelvis
Cordguard
  C. II
  C. umbilical cord sampler
cordiform
  c. pelvis
  c. uterus
cordis
  accretio c.
  bulbus c.
  commotio c.
  ectopia c.
  thoracoabdominal ectopia c.
Cordis-Hakim shunt
cordocentesis
cordotomy
Cordran SP
core
  c. biopsy
  C. Dynamics disposable cannula
  C. Dynamics disposable trocar
  c. needle biopsy (CNB)
  c. temperature
corectopia
Corey ovum forceps
Corgard
Cori
  C. classification
  C. disease
  C. enzyme deficiency
Coricidin-D Tablets
Coricidin Tablets
Cori-Forbes disease
coring
  c. biopsy gun
  intramyometrial c.
  myometrial c.
  uterine c.
corkscrew
  c. appearance
  c. conjunctival blood vessel
  c. maneuver

Cormax Ointment
cornea, gen. **corneae**
  arcus corneae
  cloudy c.
  macula corneae
  c. verticillata
  wetting defect of c.
  xerosis c.
corneal
  c. abrasion
  c. clouding
  c. damage
  c. dystrophy
  c. edema
  c. enlargement
  c. haze
  c. hypoesthesia
  c. leukoma
  c. light reflection
  c. light reflex test
  c. opacification
  c. opacity
  c. scarring
  c. staining
  c. stippling
  c. trauma
  c. ulcer
  c. ulceration
Cornelia
  C. de Lange (CDL)
  C. de Lange syndrome (CDLS)
corneocyte
corneoscleral angle
corner
  c. chair
  c. fracture
Corner-Allen test
corneum
  stratum c.
cornification
cornified
Corning method
Cornoy solution
cornu, pl. **cornua**
  c. uteri
  uterine c.
cornual
  c. anastomosis
  c. gestation
  c. pregnancy
  c. resection

C

NOTES

Corometrics
- C. fetal monitor
- C. Gold Quik Connect Spiral electrode tip
- C. 118 maternal/fetal monitor
- C. Model 900SC in-office mammography

corona
- c. of penis
- c. radiata
- c. radiata cell

coronal
- c. craniosynostosis
- c. sulcus
- c. suture
- c. suture line of skull
- c. synostosis

coronary
- c. aneurysm
- c. arteriovenous fistula
- c. artery aneurysm (CAA)
- c. artery disease
- c. artery fistula (CAF)
- c. artery lesion (CAL)
- c. collateralization
- c. flow reserve (CFR)
- c. heart disease
- c. sinus
- c. sinusoid
- c. thrombosis
- c. vasospasm

coronary-cameral fistula
coronavirus
corpora (*pl. of* corpus)
corporal
- c. cavernosal patch
- c. punishment

corporis
- pediculosis c.
- *Pediculus humanus c.*
- tinea c.

corpus, pl. corpora
- c. albicans cyst
- c. callosum
- c. callosum agenesis, chorioretinal abnormality syndrome
- c. callosum agenesis, chorioretinopathy, infantile spasms syndrome
- c. callosum agenesis, facial anomalies, salaam seizures syndrome
- c. callosum hypoplasia, retardation, adducted thumbs, spastic paraparesis, hydrocephalus (CRASH)
- c. callosum partial agenesis
- corporas cavernosa
- corpora cavernosa

- c. cavernosum
- c. fibrosum
- c. hemorrhagicum
- corpora lutea
- c. luteum
- c. luteum cyst
- c. luteum deficiency syndrome
- c. luteum dysfunction
- c. luteum function
- c. luteum insufficiency
- c. luteum size
- c. luteum spurium
- c. luteum verum
- pediculosis c.
- corpora quadrigemina
- c. spongiosum
- c. subthalamicum
- tinea c.
- uterine c.
- c. of uterus

corpuscle
- Bennett small c.'s
- genital c.
- Hassall c.
- meconium c.
- Nunn engorged c.'s

corpus-to-cervix ratio
correctable lesion
corrected gestational age
correction
- chordee c.
- cleft nasal deformity c.
- Dwyer c.
- endoscopic c.
- loss of c.
- spectacle c.
- surgical c.

corrective surgery
Correct-Revised
- Percentage of Consonants C.-R. (PCC-R)

correlate
Corrigan sign
corrodens
- *Bacteroides c.*
- *Eikenella c.*

CorrTest method
corrupting
Corsi block tapping test
Corson myoma grasping forceps
CortaGel Topical
Cortaid
- C. Maximum Strength Topical
- C. with Aloe Topical

Cortamed
Cortate
Cort-Dome
- C.-D. High Potency Suppository
- C.-D. Topical

Cortef
C. Feminine Itch Topical
C. Oral
Cortenema enema
cortex, pl. **cortices**
adrenal c.
cerebral c.
double c.
fetal zone of adrenal c.
frontoparietal sensorimotor c.
irregular c.
mastoid c.
metaphysial c.
motor c.
nociferous c.
ovarian c.
renal c.
visual c.
cortical
c. agenesis
c. androgen-stimulating hormone (CASH)
c. architecture
c. atrophy
c. blindness
c. bone
c. dysgenesis
c. dysplasia
c. granule
c. granule exocytosis
c. gyral abnormality
c. hemorrhage
c. hyperostosis
c. implantation
c. mantle
c. mass
c. necrosis
c. nephron
c. reaction
c. reflex myoclonus
c. scintigraphy
c. spreading depression
c. supremacy stage
c. thrombophlebitis
c. thumbing
c. tuber
c. vision
c. visual impairment (CVI)
corticalis
agenesia c.
cortices (*pl. of* cortex)
corticography

corticoid
corticomedullary
c. differentiation
c. junction
corticospinal tract dysfunction
corticosteroid
antenatal c.
fluorinated c.
inhaled c. (ICS)
c. therapy
c. treatment
corticosteroid-binding
c.-b. globulin (CBG)
c.-b. globulin-binding capacity (CB-GBC)
corticosteroid-induced
c.-i. atrophy
c.-i. osteoporosis
corticosterone
corticostriatal
corticotrope
corticotropin
corticotropin-like intermediate lobe peptide
corticotropin-releasing
c.-r. factor
c.-r. hormone (CRH)
c.-r. inhibitor
Corticreme
Cortiment
cortin
double c.
cortisol
c. concentration
24-hour urinary free c.
c. level
plasma c.
c. response
salivary c.
urinary free c.
cortisol-binding globulin
cortisol-cortisone shuttle
cortisone
Cortisporin
C. Ophthalmic Suspension
C. Otic
C. Otic Suspension
Cortisporin-TC
C.-TC otic
C.-TC Otic Suspension
Cortizone-5, -10 Topical
Cortoderm

NOTES

cortol
Cortone Acetate
Cortrosyn stimulation test
corynebacteria
Corynebacterium
    C. diphtheriae
    C. haemolyticum
    C. minutissimum
    C. parvum
    C. vaginalis
    C. vaginitis
coryza
    allergic c.
COS
    childhood-onset schizophrenia
COSA
    child of substance abuser
co-segregation
co-sleeping
Cosmegen
cosmetic acne
cost
    response c.
costal
    c. cartilage
    c. cartilage interposition
    c. margin
CO-stat end tidal breath analyzer
Costello syndrome
costochondral junction
costochondritis
costovertebral
    c. angle (CVA)
    c. angle tenderness (CVAT)
    c. angle tenderness to percussion
    c. dysplasia
cosyntropin stimulation test
cot
    finger c.
Cotazym
Cotazym-S
cotinine level
co-transporter-1
    sodium/glucose c.-t.-1
Cotrel-Dubousset instrumentation (CDI)
cotrimoxazole trimethoprim
Cotte operation
Cottle-Neivert retractor
cotton
    c. pledget
    c. swab method
    c. swab test
cotton-ball exudate
cotton-tipped
    c.-t. applicator
    c.-t. swab
cotton-wool spot (CWS)
co-twin
    death of c.

cotyledon
    fetal c.
    maternal c.
    c. perfusion system
    placental c.
cotyledonary placenta
coudé catheter
cough
    barking c.
    brassy c.
    bronchospastic c.
    croupy c.
    Diphen C.
    habit c.
    harassing c.
    Pedituss C.
    psychogenic c.
    c. receptor
    rhonchorous c.
    seal-like c.
    Silphen C.
    staccato c.
    staccato-like c.
    c. syncope
    c. test
    c. tic
    uterine c.
    whooping c.
Cough-Cold
    PediaCare C.-C.
coughing
    paroxysmal c.
    voluntary c.
cough-pressure transmission ratio
Cough-X lozenge
Coulter
    C. Channelyser cell analyzer
    C. counter
Coumadin
coumadinization
coumarin
    c. derivative
    c. syndrome
council
    Interagency Coordinating C. (ICC)
counseling
    genetic c.
    nondirective c.
    preconception c.
    prenatal genetic c.
Counsellor-Davis artificial vagina operation
Counsellor-Flor modification of McIndoe technique
Counsellor vaginal mold
counselor
    genetic c.
count
    absolute band c. (ABC)

absolute CD4 c.
absolute lymphocyte c.
absolute neutrophil c.
amniotic fluid white blood cell c.
bacterial c.
blood c.
CD4 cell c.
CD8 cell c.
colony c.
complete blood c. (CBC)
differential cell c.
erythrocyte c.
fetal kick c.
fetal movement c.
granulocyte c.
Guthrie c.
hemolysis, elevated liver enzymes, low platelet c. (HELLP)
kick c.
lamellar body c. (LBC)
lap c.
leukocyte c.
platelet c.
reticulocyte c.
sperm c.
white blood cell c.
counter
Coulter c.
c. stab wound incision
Sysmex NE8000 cell c.
counterimmunoelectrophoresis (CIE)
counterpulsation
intraaortic balloon c.
counterregulatory hormone release
counterrotation
counting
fetal movement c.
COUP
chicken ovalbumin upstream promoter transcription factor II
coup injury
couple
commissioning c.
c. testing
coupler
couplet
coupling
c. defect
receptor c.
course
aberrant c.
long c.

short c.
ureteral c.
court-ordered obstetrical intervention
couvade
Couvelaire uterus
cover
Bili mask phototherapy eye c.
Sheathes ultrasound probe c.
c. test
coverage
polymicrobial c.
Covera-HS
covering
epidermal c.
Coverlet dressing
Covermark
Cover-Roll gauze
Cover-Strip wound closure strip
covert loss
cover-uncover eye test
Cowchock-Fischbeck syndrome
Cowchock syndrome
Cowden
C. disease
C. syndrome
Cowdry types A, B inclusion body
cowlick
Cowper gland
cowperian duct
cow's
c. milk allergy (CMA)
c. milk challenge
c. milk intolerance
c. milk protein (CMP)
c. milk protein allergy
COX
cyclooxygenase
COX pathway
COX-1
cyclooxygenase-1
COX-2
cyclooxygenase-2
COX-2 inhibitor
Cox
C. proportional hazard
C. proportional hazard model
coxa, pl. coxae
c. magna
c. plana
c. valga
c. vara
c. vara deformity

NOTES

coxarthrosis
Coxiella burnetii
coxoauricular syndrome
Coxsackie
coxsackievirus
      c. A (1-22,24)
      C. A16 infection
      c. B (1-6)
      C. B enterovirus infection
CP
   cerebral palsy
   cleft palate
CPA
   child physical abuse
C-palmitic acid
CPAP
   continuous positive airway pressure
      CPAP machine
      nasal CPAP
      CPAP ventilator
CPC
   choroid plexus carcinoma
   choroid plexus cyst
CPD
   cephalopelvic disproportion
   cerebelloparenchymal disorder (I–IV)
CPE
   cytopathic effect
CPEO
   chronic progressive external
     ophthalmoplegia
C-peptide level
CPI
   chronic pneumonitis of infancy
   congenital palatopharyngeal
     incompetence
CPK
   creatine phosphokinase
CPLS
   cleft palate-lateral synechia
      CPLS syndrome
cPNET
   central primitive neuroectodermal tumor
CPP
   central precocious puberty
   cerebral perfusion pressure
   choroid plexus papilloma
   chronic pelvic pain
CPR
   cardiopulmonary resuscitation
CPS
   carbamoyl phosphate synthetase
   Child Protective Services
   Collaborative Perinatal Study
   complex partial seizure
      CPS deficiency
      CPS ID chromogenic medium
cps
   cycle per second

CPT
   carnitine palmitoyltransferase
   chest physical therapy
   chest physiotherapy
   continuous performance test
      CPT I, II deficiency
CPT I
   carnitine palmitoyltransferase I
CPT II
   carnitine palmitoyltransferase II
cPVL
   cystic periventricular leukomalacia
C1q
      C1q assay
      C1q binding
      deficiency of C1q
C-R
      Bicillin C.-R.
CR
      Norpace CR
CRA
   clinical risk assessment
crab louse
crack
      c. baby
      c. cocaine
cracked
      c. mucous membrane
      c. pot sound
cracked-pot
      c.-p. head
      c.-p. sign
      c.-p. sound
crackle
      bubbly c.
      fine inspiratory c.
crackling rale
cradle
      auditory response c.
      c. cap
      Criss Cross C.
cradleboard
cramp
      leg c.
      menstrual c.
      menstrual-like c.
      nocturnal leg c.
      writer's c.
cramping
      uterine c.
cranberry
Crandall ectodermal dysplasia syndrome
Crane-Heise syndrome
crania (*pl. of* cranium)
cranial
      c. bruit
      c. contour
      c. duplication
      c. echoencephalography

c. electrical stimulation (CES)
c. encephalocele
c. epidural abscess
c. fasciitis
c. hypothermia
c. meningocele
c. molding helmet
c. nerve defect
c. nerve (II–XII)
c. nerve nucleus
c. nerve palsy
c. nerve testing
c. neuritis
c. orthosis
c. sclerosis, osteopathia striata, macrocephaly syndrome
c. sclerosis with striated bone disease
c. sign
c. space
c. suture
c. synostosis
c. ultrasonography
c. ultrasound
craniectomy
endoscopic strip c.
suboccipital c.
cranioacrofacial syndrome
craniobasal bone
CranioCap cranial orthosis
craniocarpotarsal
c. dystrophy
c. syndrome
craniocaudal view
craniocerebellocardiac (3C, CCC)
c. syndrome
craniocerebral trauma
craniocervical
c. dystonia
c. junction
c. myelopathy
cranioclasia, cranioclasis
cranioclast
craniocleidodysostosis
craniodiaphyseal, craniodiaphysial
c. dysplasia
craniodidymus
cranioectodermal dysplasia (CED)
craniofacial
c. anomalies, polysyndactyly syndrome
c. anomaly

c., deafness, hand syndrome
c. disproportion
c. dissociation
c. dysmorphism, absent corpus callosum, iris colobomas, connective tissue dysplasia syndrome
c. dysmorphism-polysyndactyly syndrome
c. dysmorphology
c. dysostosis
c. tumor
craniofacies
craniofenestria
craniofrontal dysplasia
craniofrontonasal
c. dysostosis
c. dysplasia (CFND)
c. syndrome (CNFS)
craniolacunia
craniomalacia
craniomeningocele
craniometaphyseal, craniometaphysial
c. dysplasia
craniooculofrontonasal malformation
cranioorodigital syndrome
craniopagus
craniopathy
craniopharyngioma
cranioplasty
craniorachischisis
craniorhiny
cranioschisis
cranioskeletal dysplasia with acroosteolysis
craniospinal rachischisis
craniostenosis
craniostosis
craniosynostosis
c., arachnodactyly, abdominal hernia syndrome
c., arthrogryposis, cleft palate syndrome
c., ataxia, trigeminal anesthesia, parietal anesthesia and pons, vermis fusion syndrome
Boston-type c.
coronal c.
metopic c.
primary c.
sagittal c.
secondary c.

NOTES

207

craniosynostosis *(continued)*
    single-suture c.
    syndromic c.
craniosynostosis-lid anomalies syndrome
craniosynostosis-marfanoid habitus
craniosynostosis-radial aplasia syndrome
craniosynostotic syndrome
craniotabes
craniothoracopagus syncephalus
craniotome
craniotomy
craniotubular
    c. dysplasia
    c. dysplasia, growth retardation,
      mental retardation, ectodermal
      dysplasia, loose skin
cranium, pl. **crania**
    c. bifidum
    c. bifidum cysticum
    c. bifidum occultum
    c. cerebrale
    visceral c.
    c. viscerale
crankshaft phenomenon
Cranley Maternal-Fetal Attachment
  Scale
CRASH
    corpus callosum hypoplasia, retardation,
      adducted thumbs, spastic paraparesis,
      hydrocephalus
      CRASH syndrome
craving
    dietary c.
    food c.
    pica c.
    salt c.
crawl
    belly c.
    combat c.
    commando c.
crawling aid
CRB
    congenital retinitis blindness
CRCT
    creamatocrit
    volume percent of cream in milk
C-reactive protein (CRP)
cream, creme
    Acticin C.
    Aldara c.
    Amino-Cerv pH 5.5 cervical C.
    AVC C.
    Bactroban c.
    Balmex c.
    butoconazole 2% c.
    Cleocin vaginal c.
    clotrimazole vaginal c. 2%
    Complex 15 c.
    Cutivate c.

    Decadron Phosphate C.
    dihydrotestosterone c.
    Elimite C.
    EMLA c.
    emollient c.
    Estrace vaginal c.
    estradiol vaginal c.
    Eucerin Plus C.
    Exact C.
    Fungoid C.
    gentamicin c.
    Gynazole-1 vaginal c.
    imiquimod c.
    intravaginal c.
    Lamisil C.
    LCD c.
    lidocaine-prilocaine c.
    Masse Breast C.
    miconazole nitrate vaginal c.
    Monistat 3 vaginal c.
    Mother2Be breast nourishing c.
    Mother2Be nipple restoration c.
    Neosporin C.
    Nivea c.
    Nupercainal c.
    Nutraderm c.
    nystatin and triamcinolone c.
    penciclovir c.
    Pen Kera moisturizing c.
    permethrin 5% c.
    Preparation-H hydrocortisone c.
    Purpose c.
    RVPaque c.
    silver sulfadiazine c.
    Sklar c.
    SSD C.
    stearin-lanolin c.
    Sulfamylon c.
    Sween C.
    Terazol 3, 7 vaginal c.
    Topicort c.
    triple sulfa c.
    Trivagizole 3 vaginal c.
    U-Cort c.
    vaginal c.
    vasodilator c.
    Vite E C.
    Zonalon Topical C.
creamatocrit (CRCT)
creamy vulvitis
crease
    allergic c.
    earlobe c.
    flexural c.
    palmar c.
    plantar c.
    simian c.
    single transverse palmar c.
    sole c.

Sydney c.
transversal nasal c.
crease/pit
ear c.
creatine
c. deficiency
c. kinase (CK)
c. kinase MB
c. phosphokinase (CPK)
creatinine
c. clearance
c. phosphokinase
Credé
C. maneuver
C. maneuver of eyes
C. maneuver of uterus
C. prophylaxis
creep
creeping eruption
Cre/loxP system
cremasteric
c. fascia
c. reflex
c. response
creme (*var. of* cream)
cremnocele
crenated red blood cell
crenation sign
Creola body
Creon 10, 20
Creo-Terpin
crepitant rale
crepitation
crepitus
crescendo murmur
crescent
c. cell anemia
c. formation
crescentic
c. fashion
c. glomerulonephritis
c. lesion
Crescent pillow
Crescormon
CREST
calcinosis, Raynaud phenomenon,
esophageal dysmotility, sclerodactyly,
telangiectasia
CREST syndrome
crest
iliac c.
neural c.

posterior iliac c.
superior iliac c.
Cresylate
creta
placenta c.
placenta previa c.
cretin dwarfism
cretinism
athyrotic c.
endemic c.
c. idiocy
cretinism-muscular hypertrophy syndrome
cretinoid dysplasia
Creutzfeldt-Jakob
C.-J. disease (CJD)
C.-J. syndrome
CRF
chronic renal failure
anemia of CRF
CR-gram
cardiorespirogram
CRH
corticotropin-releasing hormone
cri
c. du chat
CRIB
Clinical Risk Index for Babies
CRIB score
crib
clinical c.
c. death
open c.
tongue c.
Crib-O-Gram
cribriform
c. fracture
c. hymen
c. plate
cribrosa
lamina c.
macula c.
cricoarytenoid
c. articulation
c. joint
cricoid
c. pressure
c. split
c. split procedure
cricopharyngeal incoordination of infancy
cricothyroidectomy

NOTES

cricothyroid membrane
cricothyroidotomy
    needle c.
cricothyrotomy
    needle c.
    surgical c.
cri-du-chat syndrome
CRIES
    crying, requires oxygen, increased vital
    signs, expression, sleepless
    CRIES postoperative pain scale
Crigler-Najjar
    C.-N. disease (type I, II)
    C.-N. syndrome (type I, II)
Crile
    C. forceps
    C. hemostat
Crile-Wood needle holder
Crimean-Congo hemorrhagic fever
criminal abortion
criminology
Crinone bioadhesive progesterone gel
Crippled Children's Services (CCS)
crisis, pl. **crises**
    abdominal c.
    acute adrenal c.
    acute splenic sequestration c.
    addisonian c.
    adrenal c.
    aplastic c.
    autonomic c.
    blast c.
    Chiari c.
    cholinergic c.
    clitoris c.
    congenital hemolytic anemia with
     aplastic c.
    developmental c.
    encephalopathic c.
    Fabry c.
    hemolytic c.
    hepatic c.
    hypercalcemic c.
    hypertensive c.
    c. intervention
    intrahepatic vasoocclusive c.
    lupus c.
    megaloblastic c.
    oculogyric c.
    pain c.
    scleroderma renal c.
    sequestration c.
    sickle cell c.
    sickling c.
    splenic sequestration c.
    thyroid c.
    thyrotoxic c.
    transient aplastic c. (TAC)
    vasoocclusive c.

Crisponi syndrome
Criss Cross Cradle
crisscross heart
crista
    c. dividens
    c. supraventricularis
criteria, sing. **criterion**
    Amsel c.
    Beighton c.
    Bell staging c.
    Berne c.
    Cohen c.
    family history research
     diagnostic c. (FH-RDC)
    GOS c.
    ICSD c.
    Jones rheumatic fever diagnostic c.
    Joshi c.
    Kass c.
    Lorber c.
    modified Beighton c.
    Norris-Carroll c.
    Nugent c.
    criterion overlap
    Oxford diagnostic c.
    Ranson c.
    revised Jones c.
    Rochester c.
    Rome c.
    Shimada c.
    Spiegel c.
    Spiegelberg c.
    Sydenham chorea c.
criterion-referenced test
critical
    c. aortic stenosis
    c. body weight
    c. care monitoring
    c. illness neuromuscular disease
    c. pulmonic stenosis
    c. temperature
    c. weight hypothesis
Criticare H formula
Crixivan
CRL
    crown-rump length
CRMO
    chronic recurrent multifocal osteomyelitis
CRO
    cathode ray oscilloscope
crocodile
    c. skin
    c. tongue
Crohn
    C. colitis
    C. disease
Crolom
Crome syndrome

cromoglycate
> disodium c.
> PMS-Sodium C.
> sodium c.

cromolyn
> atropine c.
> c. sodium
> c. sodium inhalation aerosol

Cronkhite-Canada syndrome
crooked fingers syndrome
crop
> c. of macules
> c. of papules
> rash c.

Crosby capsule
Crosby-Kugler pediatric capsule
cross
> c. breeding
> bridging c.
> dihybrid c.
> monohybrid c.
> reciprocal c.
> C. syndrome
> c. table

crossbite
cross-brain oxygen extraction
crossed
> c. adductor reflex
> c. extension reflex
> c. fused ectopia
> c. polysyndactyly

cross-eye
crossing over
crosslink
> TSRH c.

cross-link
> N-telopeptide c.-l.'s (NTx)

cross-linking
Cross-McKusick-Breen syndrome
cross-modal fluency
crossover
> circulatory c.

cross-reaction
cross-sectional
cross-table lateral film
crotamiton
crouch gait
croup
> diphtheritic c.
> membranous c.
> C. score
> spasmodic c.

croupette
croupy cough
Crouzon
> C. craniofacial dysostosis
> C. disease
> C. syndrome

crowded teeth
crowding
> dental c.
> fetal c.
> c. theory

Crowe sign
crown-heel length (CHL)
crowning
crown-rump length (CRL)
crow's nest
CRP
> C-reactive protein

CRPS
> complex regional pain syndrome

CRS
> caudal regression syndrome
> Cell Recovery System
> congenital rubella syndrome
> Conners Rating Scale

CRST
> calcinosis, Raynaud phenomenon,
> sclerodactyly, telangiectasia
> CRST syndrome

cruces (*pl. of* crux)
cruciferous vegetable
crude risk ratio
Cruex Topical
Cruiser hip abduction brace
cruising
crunch
> mediastinal c.

crus, gen. **cruris,** pl. **crura**
> paired crura
> tinea cruris

crush injury
crusta lactea
crusted
> c. lesion
> c. scabies

crusting telangiectasia keratosis
crutches
> Lofstrand c.

crux, pl. **cruces**
cruzi
> *Trypanosoma c.*

Cruz trypanosomiasis

NOTES

211

cry
> cat's c.
> cephalic c.
> high-pitched c.
> hoarse c.
> uterine c.
> voiceless c.
> weak c.

cryaerophilia
> *Campylobacter c.*

crying
> c. cat syndrome
> c., requires oxygen, increased vital signs, expression, sleepless (CRIES)

CRYOcare cryoablation system
cryocauterization
cryocautery
cryoconization
cryofibrinogenemia
cryoglobulin
> polyclonal c.

cryoglobulinemia
Cryogun
> Wallach LL100 cryosurgical C.

cryoinjury
Cryomedics
> C. disposable LLETZ electrode
> C. electrosurgery system

cryomyolysis
cryoprecipitate transfusion
cryopreservation
> oocyte c.

cryopreserved
> c. embryo
> c. valved allograft

cryoprotectant
cryosurgery
cryothalamectomy
cryotherapy
Cryovial
crypt
> c. abscess
> c. cell
> c. cell mitosis
> c. depth
> c. hyperplasia
> c. hypoplasia
> c.'s of Lieberkühn

cryptic
> c. hemangioma
> c. hyperandrogenism
> c. tuber

cryptoazoospermia
cryptocephalus
cryptococcal
> c. antigen
> c. meningitis

cryptococcosis
> cutaneous c.
> extrapulmonary c.
> pulmonary c.

Cryptococcus neoformans **var.**
> *neoformans*

cryptodidymus
cryptogenic
> c. cirrhosis
> c. fibrosing alveolitis
> c. hepatitis
> c. infantile spasm

cryptomenorrhea
cryptomerorachischisis
cryptomicrotia-brachydactyly syndrome
cryptophthalmos, cryptophthalmia
> c. syndrome

cryptophthalmos-syndactyly syndrome
cryptorchidism
> bilateral c.
> unilateral c.

cryptorchid testis
cryptosporidiosis
Cryptosporidium parvum
cryptotia
crypt-villus architecture
Cryselle tablet
crystal
> calcium c.
> Charcot-Leyden c.
> indinavir c.
> urate c.
> c. violet

CrystalEyes endoscopic video system
crystallina miliaria
crystalline lens
crystallization
> fern leaf c.

crystalloid
> miliaria c.
> Reinke c.'s
> c.'s of Reinke
> c. solution

crystalluria
> renal tubular c.

Crystapen
C&S
> culture and sensitivity

^{137}Cs
> cesium-137
> ^{137}Cs level

CS-5 cryosurgical system
CSA
> child sexual abuse
> clinically significant arrhythmia
> colony-stimulating activity

CsA
> cyclosporin A

Csaba stain

Csapo abortion
CSBI
  Child Sexual Behavior Inventory
CSD
  cat-scratch disease
CSE
  combined spinal-epidural
    CSE anesthesia
C-section
  cesarean section
    LUST C-section
CSF
  cerebrospinal fluid
  colony-stimulating factor
    bloody CSF
    CSF glycine
    CSF lymphocytic pleocytosis
    CSF otorrhea
    CSF rhinorrhea
    CSF VDRL
    xanthochromic CSF
C-shaped curve
CSI
  chemical shift imaging
CsI
  cesium iodide
Csillag disease
C-Solve-2
CSOM
  chronic suppurative otitis media
CSPI
  childhood severity of psychiatric illness
CSQI
  continuous subcutaneous infusion
CSSCD
  cooperative study of sickle cell disease
CST
  contraction stress test
    antepartum fetal CST
    fetal CST
C$_{19}$-steroid
CSTR
  complete subtalar release
CSW
  cerebral salt wasting
    CSW syndrome
CT
  Chlamydia trachomatis
  computed tomography
  computerized tomographic
    CT guidance
    CT laser mammography
    CT pelvimetry
    CT scan
    CT scanning
C3T
  clomiphene citrate challenge test
CTAF
  conotruncal anomaly face syndrome
CTD
  chronic tic disorder
  clitoral therapy device
CTEI
  communal traumatic experiences inventory
C-telopeptide
  type I collagen C.-t.
C-terminal propeptide of type I collagen
CTG
  cardiotocography
C-thalassemia
CTL
  cytotoxic T lymphocyte
    CTL cell
    CTL response
CTLM
  computed tomography laser mammography
CTNS
  cystinosis, nephropathic (cytinosin)
    CTNS gene
CTP
  carboxyl terminal peptide
CTQ
  childhood trauma questionnaire
CTS
  clitoris tourniquet syndrome
CTX
  cyclophosphamide
CTZ
  chemoreceptor trigger zone
Cu-7 intrauterine device
cube pessary
cubic
  c. centimeter (cc)
  c. centimeter per hour (cc/hr)
  c. centimeter per kilogram per day (cc/kg/day, cc/kg day)
cubitus
  c. valgus
  c. valgus deformity
  c. varus
cuboid

NOTES

CUCS
    complex unroofed coronary sinus
Cue Fertility Monitor
cued speech
cuff
    c. cellulitis
    Ethox c.
    muscular c.
    neonatal c.
    posterior vaginal c.
    vaginal c.
cuffed
    c. endotracheal tube
    c. ET tube
cuffing
    pericapillary inflammatory c.
cuirass respirator
culbertsoni
    Acanthamoeba c.
culdeplasty
cul-de-sac
    c.-d.-s. biopsy
    Douglas c.-d.-s.
    c.-d.-s. of Douglas
    c.-d.-s. obliteration
    posterior c.-d.-s.
    rectouterine c.-d.-s.
culdocentesis
    equivocal c.
    nondiagnostic c.
culdoplasty
    Halban c.
    high McCall c.
    Marion-Moschcowitz c.
    Mayo c.
    McCall c.
    prophylactic c.
    Torpin-Waters-McCall c.
culdoscope
culdoscopy
culdotomy
Culex
    C. nigripalpus
    C. pipiens
    C. quinquefasciatus
    C. tarsalis
Culiseta melanura
Cullen sign
cultivable virus
cultural
    c. artifact
    c. competence
cultural artifact
culture
    amniotic fluid cell c.
    blood c.
    broth c.
    cell c.
    cervical c.

    colony-forming unit in c. (CFUC)
    epiglottic surface c.
    extended c.
    c. fertilization
    fibroblast c.
    gastric aspirate c.
    GBS screening c.
    gonorrhea c.
    nasal swab c.
    oocyte c.
    purified chick embryo cell c.
     (PCEC)
    screening c.
    c. and sensitivity (C&S)
    shell vial c.
    sputum c.
    test-of-cure c.
    tracheal-aspirate c.
    Ureaplasma c.
    Uricult c.
    urine c.
    in vitro human intestinal organ c.
cultured skin fibroblast
culture-negative
    c.-n. cytomegalovirus infection
    c.-n. neutrocytic ascites
culture-specific determinant
culturing
    viral c.
cumulative
    c. conception rate (CCR)
    c. gene
    c. parental dysfunction
cumulus
    c. cell
    c. oophorus
    c. ovaricus
cuneiform bone
cup
    Bird OP c.
    CMI-Mityvac c.
    CMI-O'Neil c.
    cut-away c.
    cut-out c.
    c. ear
    c. feeding
    heel c.
    c. insemination
    Instead feminine protection c.
    Malmstrom c.
    Milex cervical c.
    Mityvac obstetric vacuum
     extractor c.
    Mityvac Super M c.
    O'Neil c.
    Tender-Touch vacuum birthing c.
    vacuum c.
    zinc-free plastic specimen c.

Cupid's
    C. bow
    C. bow curve
    C. bow upper lip
cupped metaphysis
cupping
    optic nerve c.
    c. of optic nerve head
Cuprimine
cupriuria
cuprophane hemodialyzer membrane
cuproprotein
Curaderm dressing
Curafil dressing
curage
Curagel Hydrogel dressing
curare
Curasorb calcium alginate dressing
curative
curdy discharge
C-urea
    C-u. breath test
    C-u. serology
curet (*var. of* curette)
curetment
curetment (*var. of* curettement)
curettage
    blunt c.
    dilation and c. (D&C)
    endocervical c. (ECC)
    endometrial c. (EMC)
    fractional dilation and c.
    radial c.
    repeat c.
    sharp c.
    suction and c. (S&C)
    suction, dilation, and c.
    vacuum c.
    vaginal interruption of pregnancy
      with dilatation and c. (VIP-DAC)
curette, curet
    Accurette endometrial suction c.
    banjo c.
    Berkeley suction c.
    Bumm c.
    Duncan c.
    Green uterine c.
    Heaney c.
    Helix endocervical c.
    Helix uterine biopsy c.
    Kelly-Gray c.
    Kevorkian c.

    Kevorkian-Younge c.
    Mi-Mark disposable endocervical c.
    Novak c.
    optical aspirating c. (OAC)
    Pipelle endometrial suction c.
    Pipet C.
    Randall suction c.
    Shapleigh c.
    Sims c.
    St. Clair-Thompson c.
    suction c.
    Thomas c.
    Townsend endocervical biopsy c.
    uterine c.
    Vabra suction c.
    Yankauer c.
    Z-Sampler endometrial suction c.
curettement, curetment
curetting
    endocervical c.
curie (Ci)
curly toe
Curosurf
    C. intratracheal suspension
    C. poractant alpha
Curran syndrome
currant jelly stool
Currarino triad
currens
    larva c.
current
    diathermy c.
Curretab Oral
Curry-Jones syndrome
Curschmann spiral
curse
    Ondine c.
Curtis syndrome
curtsey sign
curvature
    abnormal penile c.
    dorsal penile c.
    excessive penile c.
    lateral c.
    penile c.
    c. of spine
    thoracolumbar kyphotic c.
curve
    Barnes c.
    biologic satiation c.
    Carus c.
    C-shaped c.

C

NOTES

215

curve *(continued)*
- Cupid's bow c.
- flow-volume c.
- Friedman labor c.
- growth c.
- hemoglobin-oxygen dissociation c.
- isodose c.
- Kaplan-Meier survival c.
- Liley c.
- lumbar c.
- oxygen dissociation c.
- Risser c.
- saddleback temperature c.
- sexual response c.
- c. of Spee
- S-shaped c.
- standard c.

curved
- c. finger
- c. hemostat
- c. Mayo scissors

Curvularia lunata

curvus
- *Campylobacter c.*

CUSA
- Cavitron ultrasonic surgical aspirator

CUSALap accessory needle

Cusco speculum

Cushing
- C. disease
- C. effect
- C. forceps
- C. syndrome
- C. triad

cushingoid
- c. appearance
- c. body habitus
- c. facies
- c. syndrome

cushion
- birth c.
- c. defect of heart
- endocardial c.
- scintimammography prone breast c.
- sucking c.

cusp

cuspid

custodial care

cutaneocerebral angioma

cutaneomeningospinal angiomatosis

cutaneous
- c. albinism
- c. angioma
- c. anthrax
- c. atrophy
- c. blanching
- c. candidiasis
- c. cryptococcosis
- c. dimple
- c. diphtheria
- c. ectoderm
- c. fetal blood flow
- c. fibrosis
- c. hemangioma
- c. hepatic porphyria
- c. larva migrans
- c. leishmaniasis
- c. lesion
- c. mastocytosis
- c. melanoma
- c. melanosis
- c. mucormycosis
- c. nevus
- c. nodule
- c. pressure pulse
- c. pyelostomy
- c. shunt
- c. sporotrichosis
- c. tag
- c. telangiectasis
- c. tuberculosis
- c. ureterostomy
- c. urticaria
- c. vasculitis
- c. vesicostomy

cutaneous mastocytosis

cut-away cup

cutdown
- greater saphenous vein c.
- c. method

cut-down liver

cutis
- aplasia c.
- c. aplasia of scalp
- c. elastica
- c. hyperelastica
- c. laxa
- c. marmorata
- c. marmorata alba
- c. marmorata telangiectatica
- c. marmorata telangiectatica congenita
- tuberculosis verrucosa c.
- c. verticis gyrata
- c. verticis gyrata, thyroid aplasia, mental retardation syndrome
- xanthosis c.

Cutivate cream

cutoff sign

cut-out cup

cut section

cutter
- Endopath ETS-Flex endoscopic articulating linear c.
- Endopath EZ35 endoscopic linear c.
- endoscopic linear c.
- Polaris reusable c.'s

cutting
>>c., annoyance, guilt, eye-opener (CAGE)
>>c. loop

Cuvier
>>duct of C.

CV
>cardiovascular

CVA
>cerebrovascular accident
>costovertebral angle
>>CVA tenderness

CVAD
>central venous access device

CVAT
>costovertebral angle tenderness

CVB
>chorionic villus biopsy

CVC
>central venous catheter

CVI
>common variable immunodeficiency
>cortical visual impairment

CVID
>common variable immunodeficiency

CVL
>central venous line
>>tunneled CVL

CVM
>cardiovascular malformation

CVN
>central venous nutrition

CVP
>central venous pressure
>>CVP line

CVS
>chorionic villus sampling

CVVH
>continuous venovenous hemofiltration

CVVHD
>continuous venovenous hemodialysis

CWS
>cotton-wool spot

CWSN
>Children with Special Health Care Needs

CXR
>chest x-ray

CY 2010

cyanide toxicity

cyanocobalamin

cyanogen bromide (CNBr)

cyanosis
>acral c.
>cardiac c.
>central c.
>differential c.
>nail bed c.
>oral mucosa c.
>perioral c.
>peripheral c.
>pulmonary c.
>slate-gray c.

cyanotic
>c. breathholding spell
>c. congenital heart disease (CCHD)
>c. congenital heart lesion
>c. flush
>c. heart disease
>c. newborn

cyclacillin

cyclamate
>calcium c.
>sodium c.

cyclandelate

cyclase
>adenylate c.

cyclazocine

cycle
>battering c.
>cell c.
>circadian c.
>citric acid c.
>ectopic P-P c.
>endometrial c.
>estrogen-progestin artificial c.
>female reproductive c.
>fertility c.
>futile c.'s
>genesial c.
>glutamate c.
>initiated c.
>intrauterine pressure c.
>itch-scratch c.
>Krebs c.
>c. length
>menstrual ovarian c.
>ovarian c.
>ovulatory menstrual c.
>periodic breathing c. (PBC)
>c. per second (cps)
>reproductive c.
>respiratory c.
>sexual response c.

NOTES

cycle *(continued)*
>spontaneous menstrual c.
>urea c.

CycleBeads fertility device
cycle-monitoring detail
cyclencephalus
cycle-nonspecific agent
cycle-specific agent
Cyclessa tablet
cyclic
>c. adenosine monophosphate (cAMP)
>c. adenosine monophosphate test
>c. antidepressant poisoning
>c. guanosine monophosphate (cGMP)
>c. hormone production
>c. mastalgia
>c. neutropenia
>c. proliferative endometrium
>c. sloughing
>c. uterine bleeding
>c. vomiting
>c. vomiting syndrome
>c. vulvitis
>c. vulvodynia
>c. vulvovaginitis

cyclicity
>postmenarchal c.

cycling
cyclizine lactate
Cyclocort Topical
cyclocryotherapy
cyclodestructive procedure
Cyclofem
cyclofenil citrate
Cyclogyl
cycloheximide
cyclohexylchloroethylnitrosurea (CCNU)
cyclohydrolase
>guanosine triphosphate c.

Cyclomen
cyclomethycaine
Cyclomydril
cyclooxygenase (COX)
>c.-1 (COX-1)
>c.-2 (COX-2)
>platelet c.

cyclooxygenase-2-derived prostanoid
cyclopentanoperhydrophenanthrene
cyclopenthiazide
cyclopentolate hydrochloride
cyclophosphamide (CTX)
>c., Adriamycin, cisplatin (CAP)
>c., doxorubicin (Adriamycin), Oncovin (vincristine), prednisone
>c., doxorubicin, cisplatin
>c., doxorubicin, and 5-fluorouracil (CAF)

c., hydroxydaunorubicin, methotrexate, prednisone (CHOP)
>c., methotrexate, 5-fluorouracil (CMF)
>c., methotrexate, 5-fluorouracil, and prednisone (CMFP)
>c., methotrexate, 5-fluorouracil, vincristine, and prednisone (CMFVP)
>c., Oncovin, methotrexate, arabinosylcytosine (COMA)
>c., Oncovin, methotrexate, prednisone (COMP)
>vincristine, actinomycin D, c. (VAC)

cyclopia
cyclopism
cycloplegic
cyclopropane
Cyclo-Provera
cyclops
>c. hypognathus
>C. procedure

cycloserine
Cyclospora cayetanensis
cyclosporiasis
cyclosporin A (CsA)
cyclosporine
cyclosporine-induced gingival overgrowth
cyclothiazide
cyclothymia
cyclothymic disorder
cycrimine hydrochloride
cyesis
Cyklokapron
Cylert
Cylex
Cylexin
cylinder
>c. cast
>cesium c.
>Delclos c.
>muscle c.

cylindrical embryo
cyllosoma
cymbocephaly
Cynapin
CYP11B1 gene
CYP11B2 gene
CYP21A gene
CYP21B gene
CYP21 genotyping
cypionate
>estradiol c.
>hydrocortisone c.
>testosterone c.

Cypress facial neuromusculoskeletal syndrome

cyproheptadine
    c. hydrochloride
    c. receptor blocker
cyproterone acetate
cyst
    acne c.
    adnexal c.
    allantoic c.
    alveolar c.
    aneurysmal bone c.
    apocrine c.
    arachnoid c.
    c. aspiration
    autonomous ovarian follicular c.
    Baker c.
    Bartholin gland c.
    benign pineal c.
    bilateral choroid plexus c.
    blue dome c.
    branchial cleft c.
    breast c.
    bronchogenic c.
    calcified outline of c.
    chocolate c.
    choledochal c.
    chorionic c.
    choroid plexus c. (CPC)
    colloid c.
    corpus albicans c.
    corpus luteum c.
    Dandy-Walker c.
    dental lamina c.
    dentigerous c.
    dermoid c.
    dermoid c. of ovary
    duplication c.
    dysontogenetic c.
    echinococcal c.
    Echinococcus granulosus hydatid c.
    endometrial c.
    enterogenous c.
    epidermal inclusion c.
    epidermoid c.
    epithelial inclusion c.
    eruptive vellus hair c.
    esophageal duplication c.
    extraaxial arachnoid c.
    fetal ovarian c.
    follicular c.
    functional ovarian c.
    Gartner duct c.
    gartnerian c.

    germinal inclusion c.
    gingival c.
    glioependymal c.
    hydatid c.
    inclusion c.
    intraabdominal c.
    involution c.
    keratin c.
    keratinized c.
    keratinous c.
    lacteal c.
    leptomeningeal c.
    luteal ovarian c.
    massive ovarian c.
    mesonephric c.
    milk c.
    mucous retention c.
    müllerian c.
    multilocular c.
    multilocular thymic c. (MTC)
    multiloculated c.
    multiple c.
    Naboth c.
    nabothian c.
    neoplastic c.
    neurenteric c.
    noncommunicating c.
    oil c.
    omental c.
    omphalomesenteric c.
    oophoritic c.
    ovarian c.
    paraovarian c.
    paratubal c.
    paraurethral c.
    parenchymal c.
    pericardial c.
    pilar c.
    pilonidal c.
    pineal c.
    popliteal c.
    porencephalic c.
    posterior fossa arachnoid c.
    pseudoporencephalic c.
    renal cortex c.
    rete c. of ovary
    retrocerebellar arachnoidal c.
    Sampson c.
    sebaceous c.
    second branchial cleft c.
    siderophagic c.
    simple c.

C

NOTES

cyst *(continued)*
 skin c.
 solitary bone c.
 sperm-containing c.
 subcapsular c.
 subepidermal keratin c.
 suprasellar arachnoid c.
 tarry c.
 tension c.
 theca lutein c.
 thyroglossal duct c.
 trichilemmal c.
 umbilical c.
 unicameral bone c.
 unilocular ovarian c.
 urachal c.
 vaginal dysontogenetic c.
 vaginal embryonic c.
 vaginal inclusion c.
 vestibular c.
 vitelline duct c.
 vitellointestinal c.
 vulvar inclusion c.
 wolffian remnant c.
Cystadane
cystadenocarcinoma
 mucinous c.
 ovarian c.
 papillary serous c.
 serous c.
cystadenofibroma
cystadenoma
 apocrine c.
 benign mucinous c.
 mucinous c.
 ovarian proliferative c.
 serous c.
 vulvar apocrine c.
Cystagon
cystathionine
 c. beta-synthase (CBS)
 c. synthase
 c. synthase deficiency
cystathioninemia
cystathioninuria
cystatin C
cysteamine
cystectomy
 Bartholin c.
 ovarian c.
 vulvovaginal c.
cysteine hydrochloride
cystencephalus
cystic
 c. adenomatoid malformation
 (CAM)
 c. adenomatoid malformation of
 lung

 c. adenomatous malformation
 (CAM)
 c. adnexal mass
 c. brainstem glioma
 c. cerebellar neoplasm
 c. congenital adenomatoid
 malformation (CCAM)
 c. dilation
 c. dilation of intrahepatic bile duct
 c. disease of the breast
 c. encephalomalacia
 c. endometrial hyperplasia
 c. fibrosis (CF)
 c. fibrosis transmembrane regulator
 (CFTR)
 c. glandular hyperplasia
 c. hydatid disease
 c. hygroma
 c. hyperplasia of the breast
 c. kidney
 c. lesion
 c. leukomalacia
 c. lymphangioma
 c. medial necrosis
 c. mole
 c. myoma degeneration
 c. nephroma
 c. ovarian mass
 c. periventricular leukomalacia
 (cPVL)
 c. PVL
 c. renal disease
 c. sac
 c. teratoma
 c. teratoma of ovary
 c. wall
 c. Walthard rest
cystica
 osteitis fibrosis c.
 osteogenesis imperfecta c.
 spina bifida c.
cysticercosis
 parenchymatous cerebral c.
Cysticercus cellulosae
cysticum
 cranium bifidum c.
 epithelioma adenoides c.
 lymphangioma c.
cyst-induced pancreatitis
cystine
 c. deposition
 c. stone
cystinosis
 infantile neuropathic c.
 c., nephropathic (cytinosin) (CTNS)
 neuropathic c.
 ocular nonnephropathic c.
cystinuria
 transient neonatal c.

cystitis
    acute c.
    bacterial c.
    eosinophilic c.
    hemorrhagic c.
    honeymoon c.
    Hunner interstitial c.
    interstitial c.
    irradiation c.
    postoperative c.
    postradiation c.
    radiation c.
cystoblast
Cystocath catheter
cystocele
    paravaginal c.
    c. repair
cystoduodenostomy
cystogastrostomy
cystogram
    sleep c.
cystography
    indirect c.
    radionuclide voiding c. (RVC)
    voiding c.
cystojejunostomy
cystometer
    Lewis recording c.
cystometric capacity
cystometrics
    office c.
cystometrogram
    eyeball c.
    multichannel c.
cystometrography
cystometry
cystoperitoneal shunt
cystopexy
cystoplasty
    augmentation c.
cystosarcoma phyllodes
cystoscopic transurethral tumor resection
cystoscopy
    rigid c.
    c. table
Cystospaz
Cystospaz-M
cystostomy
    suprapubic c.
cystotomy
    suprapubic c.

cystourethrocele
cystourethrogram
    voiding c. (VCUG)
cystourethrograph
    voiding c. (VCUG)
cystourethrography
    chain c.
    metallic bead-chain c.
    voiding c. (VCUG)
cystourethropexy
    needle c.
    retropubic c.
    vaginal c.
cystourethroscopy
Cytadren
cytarabine
cytidine
    c. diphosphate-choline
    c. diphosphate-diacylglycerol
    c. monophosphate
cytinosin
    cystinosis, nephropathic (c.) (CTNS)
cytoarchitectonic
cytoarchitectural development
cytoarchitecture
Cytobrush
    C. cell collector
    C. Plus endocervical cell sampler
    C. Plus GT
    C. spatula
    Zelsmyr C.
Cytobrush-Plus cell collector
cytochalasin
cytochrome
    c. *b*
    c. *b* system
    c. *c* oxidase deficiency
    c. *c* oxidative enzyme
    c. oxidase test
    P450 c.
    c. P450scc
CytoGam
cytogenetic
    c. analysis
    bone marrow c.'s
    c. line
    c. map
    c. study
cytoid body
cytokine
    c. cascade
    c. granulocyte

NOTES

cytokine *(continued)*
    c. modulator
    pleiotropic c.
    proinflammatory c.
cytokinemia
    fetal c.
    maternal c.
cytokine-related dysmotility
cytologic
    c. analysis
    c. atypia
    c. screening
    c. smear
    c. study
    c. washing
cytological
    c. band
    c. map
cytology
    aspiration biopsy c. (ABC)
    bland c.
    brush c.
    c. brush
    cervical c.
    peritoneal c.
    scrape c.
    sputum c.
    urine c.
    vaginal c.
cytolysis
cytolytic vaginitis
cytomegalic inclusion disease (CID)
cytomegalovirus (CMV, CMVF)
    congenital c.
    c. disease
    c. immune globulin (CMVIG)
    c. immune globulin intravenous (CMV-IGIV)
    c. immunoglobulin (CMVIG)
    c. infection
    prenatal c.
    c. seropositive
    c. total immunoglobulin assay
    transfusion-associated c.
cytomegalovirus-specific immunoglobulin
cytomegaly syndrome
Cytomel Oral
cytometer
    Epics XL flow c.
cytometry
    flow c.
cytopathic effect (CPE)
cytopathogenesis
cytopathologic evaluation
cytopathy
    mitochondrial c.
cytopenia
    autoimmune c.
    intermittent hematologic c.

cytophagocytosis
cytophilic antibody
Cytopick endocervical and uterovaginal cell collector
cytopipette
cytoplasm
    bubble gum c.
cytoplasmic
    c. inheritance
    c. lipid droplet (CLD)
    c. membrane
    c. trait
cytoreduction
cytoreductive surgery
CytoRich process
Cytosar-U
cytosine
    c. arabinoside
    c. arabinoside, etoposide, methotrexate (CEM)
    c. nucleotide
cytoskeleton
cytosol
cytosolic tyrosine transaminase deficiency
Cytospray
cytotechnician
Cytotec induction
cytotoxic
    c. agent
    c. edema
    c. effect
    c. factor
    c. lymphocyte response
    c. memory T cell
    c. T lymphocyte (CTL)
cytotoxicity
    antibody-dependent cell-mediated c. (ADCC)
cytotoxin
    vero c.
cytotrophoblast
    malignant c.
Cytovene
Cytoxan
    C., Adriamycin, fluorouracil (CAF)
    C., Adriamycin, fluorouracil, tamoxifen, Halotestin (CAFTH)
    C., Adriamycin, leucovorin, calcium, fluorouracil (CALF)
    C., Adriamycin, leucovorin, calcium, fluorouracil, ethinyl estradiol (CALF-E)
    C., epirubicin, fluorouracil (CEF)
    fluorouracil, epirubicin, C. (FEC)
    C., methotrexate, fluorouracil, prednisone (CMFP)
    C., methotrexate, fluorouracil, prednisone, tamoxifen (CMFPT)

C., methotrexate, fluorouracil, vincristine, prednisone (CMFVP)

C., Oncovin, fluorouracil plus Cytoxan, Oncovin, methotrexate (COF/COM)

Czerny anemia

NOTES

C

δ (*var. of* delta)
2D
    2D Doppler
    2D echocardiogram
D₄
    leukotriene D_4 (LTD_4)
D₂
    prostaglandin D_2
D920
    Audio Doppler D920
DA
   developmental age
   dextroamphetamine
   ductus arteriosus
DAA
   digital auditory aerobics
   double aortic arch
dacarbazine
    Adriamycin (doxorubicin),
      bleomycin, vinblastine, d. (ABVD)
    mesna, Adriamycin, Ifosfamide, D.
      (MAID)
dacliximab
daclizumab
Dacron
    D. fiber
    D. fiber-coated coil
    D. patch
    D. sleeve catheter
dacryoadenitis
dacryocystitis
    acute d.
dacryocystorhinostomy
dacryocystostenosis
dacryostenosis
dactinomycin
dactylitis
    blistering distal d.
    sickle cell d.
    tuberculous d.
dactylomegaly
DA-DAPI, DA/DAPI
    distamycin A/4-6-diamidino-2-
      phenylindole
    DA-DAPI stain
DAG
    diacylglycerol
Dagenan
DAI
    diffuse axonal injury
daily
    d. activity
    d. fetal movement record
    d. routine
Dakin antibacterial solution

Dalacin C
Dale
    D. abdominal binder
    D. Foley catheter holder
dalfopristin
Dalkon shield
Dall-Miles cable grip procedure
Dalmane
Dalrymple sign
damage
    brain d.
    corneal d.
    hepatocellular d.
    macromolecular d.
    minimal brain d.
    neuronal d.
    obstetric d.
    obturator nerve d.
    parenchymal d.
    pelvic floor d.
    placental d.
    tubal d.
    tubal inflammatory d. (TID)
    vestibular d.
    virus-induced epithelial d.
    white matter d. (WMD)
D-amino acid
DAMP
    deficits in attention, motor control,
    perception
dAMP
    deoxyadenylic acid
D-amphetamine
Damus-Kaye-Stansel
    D.-K.-S. anastomosis
    D.-K.-S. operation
    D.-K.-S. procedure
danazol
    low-dose d.
dance
    hilar d.
    D. sign
    St. Vitus d.
dancer's ankle
dancing
    d. eye
    d. eye movement
    d. eyes/dancing feet disorder
    d. eye syndrome
    d. feet
dander
    animal d.
    cat d.
Dandy-Walker
    D.-W. cyst

D

Dandy-Walker *(continued)*
D.-W. deformity
D.-W. formation
D.-W. malformation
D.-W. malformation-basal ganglia
    disease-seizures syndrome
D.-W. syndrome (DWS)
Dandy-Walker-like syndrome
Dane particle
Danforth sign
danger
radiation d.
dangerousness
Danlos
D. disease
D. syndrome
Danocrine
danthron
D-antigen isoimmunization
Dantrium
dantrolene sodium
Danus-Fontan procedure
Danus-Stanzel repair
DAP
diastolic arterial pressure
direct agglutination pregnancy
    DAP test
Dapa
dapsone
Daranide
Daraprim
Darier
D. disease
D. sign
Darier-White disease
darifenacin
darkened reflex
dark-field
d.-f. examination
d.-f. microscopy
dark urine
Darrow-Gamble syndrome
darting tongue
Dartos fascia
Darvocet
Darvocet-N 100
Darvon
Darwin
D. ear
D. theory of evolution
darwinian
d. evolution
d. fitness
d. reflex
dashboard perineum
DAT
dementia of the Alzheimer type
direct antiglobulin test

data
Fibroid Registry for Outcomes D.
    (FIBROID)
hemodynamic d.
morphologic d.
mortality d.
oximetric d.
sociodemographic d.
database
automatic karyotype system d.
Cochrane Pregnancy and
    Childbirth D.
OSSUM d.
POSSUM d.
Vermont-Oxford Neonatal D.
datalink
Vaccine Safety D. (VSD)
date
d. of birth (DOB)
post d.'s
small for d.'s
dating
biopsy d.
clinical d.
endometrial d.
pregnancy d.
daughter
d. cell
d. chromosome
DES d.
daunomycin
daunorubicin
DAV
dibromodulcitol with Adriamycin and
    vincristine
Davidenkow syndrome
David-O'Callaghan syndrome
Davis
D. bladder catheter
D. & Geck (DG)
Davydov
D. procedure
D. vagina construction
dawn phenomenon
Dawson
D. disease
D. encephalitis
DAX1 gene
day
Acutrim Late D.
calorie per kilogram per d.
    (cal/kg/day, cal/kg day)
cubic centimeter per kilogram
    per d. (cc/kg/day, cc/kg day)
d. of life (DOL)
daycare
DAZ
deleted in azoospermia
    DAZ gene cluster

daze
DAZL1 autosomal homolog
dazzle reflex
dB
  decibel
DBA
  Diamond-Blackfan anemia
DBCP
  dibromochloropropane
d-Biotin
DBS
  diffuse brain swelling
D&C
  dilation and curettage
DCA
  directional coronary atherectomy
DCCT
  diabetes control and complications trial
DCD
  developmental coordination disorder
DCFS
  Department of Children and Family
    Services
DCIS
  ductal carcinoma in situ
DCL
  diffuse cutaneous leishmaniasis
dCMP
  deoxycytidylic acid
DCS
  Department of Children's Services
DD
  developmental disability
DDAVP nasal spray
ddC
  zalcitabine
2D, 3D echocardiography
DDH
  developmental displacement of hip
  developmental dysplasia of hip
DDI
  decision-to-delivery interval
ddI
  didanosine
D-dimer
DDP
  cis-diamminedichloroplatinum
DDST
  Denver Developmental Screening Test
DE
  diatomaceous earth
    DE slurry

D&E
  dilation and evacuation
de
  De Crecchio syndrome
  de Grouchy syndrome 1, 2
  de la Chapelle dysplasia
  de la Cruz classification
  de la Cruz classification of
    congenital aural atresia
  de Lange syndrome
  de Lange syndrome 1, 2
  de Morsier-Gauthier syndrome
  de Morsier syndrome
  de novo
  de novo balanced chromosome
    rearrangement
  de novo balanced translocation
  de novo deletion
  de Pezzer catheter
  De Sanctis-Cacchione syndrome
  de Toni-Fanconi-Debré acute
    syndrome
  de Toni-Fanconi syndrome
  De Vaal disease
  De Vaal syndrome
  De Vega tricuspid annuloplasty
dead
  d. fetus syndrome
  full term, born d. (FTBD)
  d. space
  d. space technique
DEAE
  diethylaminoethyl
  DEAE beads
deaf-blindness
deafness
  adventitious d.
  coloboma, heart disease, atresia
    choanae, retarded growth and
    development, CNS anomalies,
    genital hypoplasia, ear anomalies
    and/or d. (CHARGE)
  congenital nerve d.
  diabetes insipidus and mellitus with
    optic atrophy and d.
    (DIDMOAD)
  eighth nerve d.
  d., femoral epiphyseal dysplasia,
    short stature, developmental delay
  goitrous hypothyroidism with d.
  hereditary progressive bulbar
    paralysis with d.

D

NOTES

deafness *(continued)*
 d., hypogonadism, hypertrichosis, short stature
 ichthyosiform erythroderma, corneal involvement, d.
 d., imperforate anus, hypoplastic thumbs
 keratitis, ichthyosis, d. (KID)
 lentigines (multiple), electrocardiographic abnormalities, ocular hypertelorism, pulmonary stenosis, abnormalities of genitalia, retardation of growth, and d. (sensorineural) (LEOPARD)
 maturity onset d.
 neurosensory d.
 d., onychoosteodystrophy, mental retardation (DOOR)
 pontobulbar palsy with neurosensory d.
 prelingual d.
 progressive bulbar palsy with perceptive d.
 retardation of growth and d.
 sensorineural d.
deafness-causing allele variant
deafness-craniofacial syndrome
deafness-nephritis syndrome
Deal syndrome
deaminase
 adenosine d. (ADA)
 polyethylene glycol-modified adenosine d. (PEG-ADA)
death
 apoptotic cell d.
 brain d.
 d. by calcium
 d. of co-twin
 crib d.
 early embryonic d.
 false-negative d.
 fetal brain d.
 infant d.
 injury-related maternal d.
 intrapartum d.
 intrauterine d. (IUD)
 intrauterine fetal d.
 maternal d.
 neonatal d.
 nonmaternal d.
 perinatal d.
 postoperative sudden d.
 single intrauterine d.
 sudden infant d. (SID)
 sudden intrauterine unexplained d.
 sudden unexpected d. (SUD)
Deaver retractor

DEB
 diepoxybutane
DeBakey
 D. aortic clamp
 D. tissue forceps
debrancher enzyme deficiency
debranching enzyme deficiency
Debré-Sémélaigne syndrome
débridement
 broad d.
 thoracoscopic pleural d.
debriefing
debris
 amniotic d.
 cellular d.
 fetal d.
 keratinous d.
 keratotic d.
 nuclear d.
 stone d.
Debrox Otic
debt
 sleep d.
debulking
 optimal d.
 ovarian carcinoma d.
 surgical d.
 tumor d.
 d. of tumor
debut
 sexual d.
Decadron
 D. Oral
 D. Phosphate Cream
 D. Phosphate Injection
 D. Respihaler
 D. Turbinaire
Decadron-LA Injection
Deca-Durabolin
Decaject Injection
Decaject-LA Injection
decalvans
 keratosis follicularis spinulosa d.
decamethonium bromide
decancellation
 talar d.
decannulate
Decanoate
 Hybolin D.
decanoate
 Haldol D.
decapeptide
decapitate
decapitation
decarboxy
decarboxylase
 glutamic acid d. (GAD)
 ornithine d.
 pyruvate d.

decarboxylation
decay
    bottle tooth d.
    tooth d.
decay-accelerating factor
deceleration
    abnormal d.
    early d.'s
    fetal heart rate d.
    d. injury
    late d.
    d. phase
    U-shaped d.
    variable d.
decerebrate
    d. posturing
    d. rigidity
decerebration
decibel (dB)
decidua
    d. basalis
    d. capsularis
    d. compacta
    ectopic d.
    d. menstrualis
    d. parietalis
    d. polyposa
    tuberous subchorial hematoma of
      the d.
    d. vera
decidual
    d. arteriolar atherosis
    d. arteriolopathy
    d. cast
    d. cell
    d. endometritis
    d. fibrinoid necrosis
    d. fibrin thrombosis
    d. floor
    d. lumen
    d. mural thickening
    d. prolactin synthesis
    d. reaction
decidualization
decidualized endometrium
decidua-macrophage connection
deciduas tuberosa papulosa
deciduate placenta
deciduation
deciduitis
deciduoma
    Loeb d.

deciduous teeth
decision-to-delivery interval (DDI)
decline
declining ovarian function
Declomycin
decoding stage
Decofed Syrup
decompensated
    d. cirrhosis
    d. shock
decompensation
decomposition
decompression
    gastric d.
    nasogastric d.
    silo d.
    small intestine d.
    uterine d.
    vaginal d.
Decon
decondensation
    sperm chromatin d.
decondensed spermhead injection
decongestant
    Balminil D.
    nasal d.
decontamination
    gastrointestinal d.
decorticate posturing
decortication
    pleural d.
decreased
    d. anal tone
    d. appetite
    d. attending skill
    d. biparietal diameter
    d. breath sound
    d. commissural separation
    d. gastrointestinal motility
    d. libido
    d. mucosal surface
    d. propulsion
    d. red blood cell survival
    d. sphincter tone
    d. talocalcaneal angle
    d. urine output
decrescendo diastolic murmur
decubitus
    d. film
    d. position
    d. ulcer
decussation

D

NOTES

dedicated Doppler probe
deep
- d. circumflex iliac artery
- d. dyspareunia
- d. hypothermia and total circulatory arrest (DHCA)
- d. hypothermic circulatory arrest
- d. partial-thickness burn
- d. set eyes
- d. sleep
- d. systemic hypothermia
- d. tendon reflex (DTR)
- d. tendon reflex delayed relaxation phase
- d. transverse arrest
- d. vein thrombophlebitis
- d. vein thrombosis (DVT)
- d. venous thrombosis (DVT)

deep-knee bend
deer tick
DEET
- diethyltoluamide
- n,n-diethyl-m-toluamide

defasciculation
defecating proctogram
defecation
defecography
defect
- absence d.
- acyanotic congenital cardiac d.
- amino acid transport d.
- anatomic support d.
- androgen synthesis d.
- anterior apical vault d.
- anterior neural tube d.
- aorticopulmonary window d.
- arteriovenous canal d.
- atrial septal d. (ASD)
- atrioventricular canal d.
- atrioventricular septal d.
- biochemical d.
- biosynthetic d.
- birth d.
- cardiac septal d.
- central d.
- chromosomal d.
- closed neural tube d.
- coagulation d.
- Coffin-Siris d.
- coloboma, heart defects, ichthyosiform dermatosis, mental retardation, ear d.'s (CHIME)
- colobomatous d.
- complex heart d.
- conduction d.
- congenital cardiac d.
- congenital ectodermic scalp d.
- congenital heart d.

- congenital hemidysplasia with ichthyosiform erythroderma and limb d.'s (CHILD)
- congenital d. of phosphofructokinase
- congenital structural d.
- congenital transport d.
- conotruncal heart d.'s
- coupling d.
- cranial nerve d.
- dehalogenase d.
- dental d.
- diaphragmatic d.
- distal sacral d.
- early constraint d.
- endocardial cushion d. (ECD)
- enzyme d.
- erythrocyte acquired d.
- eustachian tube d.
- fetal structural d.
- fibrocortical d.
- fibrous cortical d.
- genetic d.
- genitourinary d.
- Hartnup d.
- heart d.
- hydroxylase enzyme d.
- intercalary d.
- intracardiac d.
- intrauterine filling d.
- intrauterine positional d.
- iodide trap d.
- laterality d.
- lobulation d.
- luteal phase d. (LPD)
- metaphysial fibrous d.
- microphthalmia with linear skin d.'s (MLS)
- midline facial d.
- mitochondrial respiratory chain d.
- müllerian fusion d.
- nail d.
- neural tube d. (NTD)
- nonneural congenital d.
- open neural tube d.
- opsonin d.
- ovulatory d.
- paraumbilical d.
- paravaginal d.
- pelvic support d.
- perineal d.
- peroxidase d.
- Pi type ZZ gene d.
- pleiotropic functional d.
- radial ray d.
- recessive disorder d.
- red blood cell membrane d.
- relative afferent d.
- sacral neural tube d.

septal d.
single gene d.
sinus venosus d.
skeletal d.
skin d.
spinal column closure d.
structural brain d.
structural heart d.
subclavian artery d.
supracristal ventricular septal d.
T-cell activation d.
terminal transverse acheiria d.
terminal transverse limb d.
testis migration d.
third-degree d.
unbalanced AV canal d.
unrestrictive ventricular septal d.
urea cycle enzyme d.
urinary concentrating d.
uterine lateral fusion d.
ventral wall d.
ventricular septal d. (VSD)
ventriculoseptal d. (VSD)
vertebral arch d.
vertebral column d.
visual field d.
X-linked uric aciduria enzyme d.

defectiva
Abiotrophia d.
defective
d. abdominal wall syndrome
d. eye abduction
d. primary platelet aggregation
d. purine metabolism
d. tryptophan absorption
defect-specific repair
defeminization
defensins
vaginal fluid neutrophil d.
defensiveness
oral tactile d.
tactile d.
defensive obstetrics
deferens
bilateral congenital absence of
vas d. (BCAVD)
congenital absence of vas d.
(CAVD)
vas d.
deferiprone

deferoxamine
d. challenge test
d. mesylate
defervesced
defervescence
defiant behavior
defibrillation
defibrillator
Lifepak d.
deficiency
abdominal muscle d.
abdominal muscular d.
acid ceramidase d.
acid maltase d. (AMD)
acquired antithrombin III d.
acquired C1 INH d.
acquired growth hormone d.
acquired protein C, S d.
ACTH d.
adenosine deaminase d.
adenylosuccinate d.
adenylosuccinate lyase d. (ASLD)
adrenocorticotropic hormone d.
AGA d.
aldosterone d.
alpha-antilysin d.
alpha-1 antitrypsin d.
alpha-glucosidase d.
alpha-lipoprotein d.
alpha-N-acetylgalactosaminidase d.
alpha-reductase d.
15 alpha-reductase d.
American Association on
Mental D. (AAMD)
Andersen d.
antibody d.
antiplasmin d.
antithrombin III d.
apoenzyme d.
arginase d.
argininosuccinic acid synthetase d.
arylsulfatase-activator d.
ascorbic acid d.
ataxia with isolated vitamin E d.
AT3 d. (types I, II)
B_6 d.
3beta-dehydrogenase d.
beta-galactosidase-1 d.
11-beta-HSD2 d.
11-beta-hydroxysteroid
dehydrogenase type 2 d.
biotinidase d.

D

NOTES

deficiency *(continued)*
brancher d.
branching enzyme d.
calcium d.
carboxylase d.
carnitine acylcarnitine translocase d.
d. of C4-binding protein
CBS d.
C2–C9 d.
ceruloplasmin d.
C1 esterase inhibitor d.
Chédiak-Higashi d.
cobalamin reductase d.
cofactor d.
cognitive d.
complement d.
congenital growth hormone d.
congenital intrinsic factor d.
congenital lactase d.
congenital lipase/colipase d.
congenital longitudinal d.
congenital TC II d.
congenital thyroid d.
congenital trypsinogen d.
copper d.
Cori enzyme d.
CPS d.
CPT I, II d.
C1r d.
creatine d.
cystathionine-beta-synthase d.
cystathionine synthase d.
cytochrome *c* oxidase d.
cytosolic tyrosine transaminase d.
debrancher enzyme d.
debranching enzyme d.
dense body d.
developmental d.
dihydropteridine reductase d.
dihydrotestosterone receptor d.
  (DHTR)
disaccharidase d.
EFA d.
enterokinase d.
enzyme d.
epinephrine d.
erythrocyte enzyme d.
erythrocyte glutathione
  peroxidase d.
erythrocyte phosphoglycerate
  kinase d.
erythrocyte pyruvate kinase d.
d. of factor B, D
factor D, H d.
factor I–XIII d.
familial APOA-I d.
familial lecithin:cholesterol
  acyltransferase d.
femoral d.

fibrinogen d.
folate folic acid d.
folic acid d.
formiminotransferase d.
fructose galactokinase d.
FUCA d.
GABA transaminase d.
galactokinase d.
galactosylceramide beta-
  galactosidase d.
GALC d.
GALE d.
GALT d.
genetic isolated CD59 d.
glucoamylase d.
glucocorticoid d.
glucosamine-6-sulfate d.
glucuronyl transferase d.
glutamate formiminotransferase d.
glutathione synthetase d.
glycerol kinase d. (GKD)
glycogen synthetase d.
GnRH d.
gonadotropic d.
G6PD d.
granule d.
growth hormone d. (GHD)
growth hormone receptor d.
  (GHRD)
GUSB d.
HCS d.
heparin cofactor II d.
hepatic lipase d.
hereditary xanthinuria d.
hexosaminidase A d.
HGPRT d.
HMWK d.
holocarboxylase synthetase d.
homozygous glucose-6-phosphate
  dehydrogenase d.
hormone d.
humoral antibody d.
11-hydroxylase d.
17-hydroxylase d.
21-hydroxylase d.
hyperammonemia due to ornithine
  transcarbamoylase d.
IDA d.
idiopathic growth hormone d.
IDS d.
IDUA d.
IgA d.
IgE d.
IgG2 d.
IgG4 d.
IgM d.
immune d.
immunoglobulin G subclass d.
insulin d.

interleukin d.
intrinsic sphincter d. (IDS, ISD)
iron d.
isolated gonadotropin d.
isolated growth hormone d.
  (IGHD)
lactase d.
lactose d.
LCAD d.
LCAD/MCAD d.
LCAD/VLCAD d.
LCHAD d.
LDH d.
leukocyte adhesion d. (LAD)
liver phosphorylase d.
longitudinal d.
LPL d.
luteal phase d.
magnesium d.
MCAD d.
mental d.
merosin d.
methionine synthase d.
MHC class I antigen d.
micronutrient d.
molybdenum cofactor d. (MCD)
monoamine oxidase A d.
MPO d.
multiple acyl-coenzyme A
  dehydrogenase d. (MADD)
multiple carboxylase d.
multiple pituitary hormone d.
  (MPHD)
multiple sulfatase d. (MSD)
muscle adenosine monophosphate
  deaminase d.
muscle carnitine
  palmityltransferase d.
muscle phosphofructokinase d.
myeloperoxidase d.
myophosphorylase d.
N-acetylgalactosamine-4-sulfatase d.
N-acetylglutamate synthetase d.
neuraminidase d.
neutrophil actin d.
neutrophil chemotactic d.
neutrophil G6PD d.
nonclassic 21-hydroxylase d.
OCT d.
d. of C1q
ornithine-ketoacid
  aminotransferase d.

ornithine transcarbamylase d.
  (OTCD)
5-oxoprolinase d.
PAI d.
pancreatic exocrine d.
PDHC d.
PEPCK d.
peroxisomal d.
PFK d.
PGK d.
phosphofructokinase d.
phosphorylase kinase d.
PK d.
placental progesterone d.
placental sulfatase d.
plasminogen activator inhibitor d.
PNP d.
postinfectious secondary lactase d.
prekallikrein d.
primary carnitine d.
primary immune d. (PID)
primary neuraminidase d.
prolactin d.
prolidase d.
properdin d.
propionyl CoA carboxylase d.
prostacyclin d.
protein C, S d.
proximal femoral focal d.
pseudocholinesterase d.
pyridoxine d.
d. of pyruvate carboxylase
RAG d.
red blood cell enzyme d.
red blood cell phosphoglycerate
  kinase d.
riboflavin d.
SCAD d.
SCOT d.
secondary carnitine d.
selective IgA d.
serotonin d.
skeletal calcium d.
sphincter d.
sphingolipid activator protein d.
steroid sulfatase d.
STS d.
sucrase-isomaltase d.
sulfite oxidase d.
sulfoiduronate sulfatase d. (SIDS)
surfactant protein d.
systemic carnitine d.

D

NOTES

deficiency *(continued)*
    systemic fatty acid d.
    TBG d.
    terminal complement component d.
    tetany of vitamin D d.
    tetrahydrobiopterin d.
    thiamin d.
    thymic-dependent d.
    thyroid d.
    thyroid-binding globulin d.
    thyrotropin d.
    thyroxine-binding globulin d.
    tocopherol d.
    TPI d.
    TPMT d.
    transcobalamin (I, II) d. (TC)
    transglutaminase d.
    trifunctional protein d. (TFP)
    triose phosphate isomerase d.
    type I, II AT3 d.
    tyrosine aminotransferase d.
     (TATD)
    tyrosine transaminase d.
    upper limb d.
    urocanase d.
    vitamin A d. (VAD)
    vitamin B_{12} d.
    vitamin C d.
    vitamin D d.
    vitamin E d.
    vitamin K d.
    xanthine oxidase d.
    X-linked congenital glycerol
     kinase d.
    X-linked monoamine oxidase d.
    xylulose dehydrogenase d.
    y-cystathionase d.
    zinc d.
deficiency-1
    leukocyte adhesion d.-1 (LAD-1)
deficiency-2
    leukocyte adhesion d.-2 (LAD-2)
deficient hydroxylation of cholecalciferol
deficit
    attention d.
    d.'s in attention, motor control,
     perception (DAMP)
    base d.
    dichotic listening d.
    fluid d.
    focal neurologic d.
    hemisensory d.
    lexical-syntactic d.
    naming speed d.
    neurodevelopmental d.
    posterior column sensory d.
    pragmatic and semantic-
     pragmatic d.'s
    sensory d.

    spinothalamic sensory d.
    d. therapy
definitive surgery
Definity suspension for IV injection
deflazacortum
deflection
deflexion abnormality
defloration
defoaming
deformans
    cephalhematoma d.
    dystonia musculorum d. (DMD)
    myodysplasia fetalis d.
    myodystrophia fetalis d.
    osteochondrodystrophia d.
deformation
    plastic d.
    shear-strain d.
deformational occipital plagiocephaly
deformity
    adduction d.
    angular d.
    antimongoloid d.
    Arnold-Chiari d.
    back-knee d.
    barrel chest d.
    bell-clapper d.
    bend d.
    bowing d.
    bunionette d.
    calcaneovalgus d.
    cavovarus d.
    Chiari d.
    clawhand d.
    cloverleaf skull d.
    clubfoot d.
    congenital condylar d.
    congenital postural d.
    coxa vara d.
    cubitus valgus d.
    Dandy-Walker d.
    equinovarus pes d.
    equinus d.
    fixed flexion d.
    foot d.
    forefoot d.
    genu varum d.
    gibbous d.
    gooseneck d.
    gunstock d.
    habit tic d.
    hindfoot valgus d.
    hip d.
    hyperextension d.
    inversion d.
    Jaccoud d.
    jaw d.
    joint d.
    kleeblattschädel d.

limb reduction d. (LRD)
lobster-claw d.
lordotic d.
Madelung d.
Michel d.
mitten hand d.
neurogenic equinus d.
pes cavus d.
ping-pong ball d.
postural d.
protuberant step d.
pseudo-Hurler d.
rachitic bone d.
recurvatum d.
rigid supination d.
round back d.
saber shin d.
saddle-nose d.
sandle gap foot d.
shepherd's crook d.
silver fork d.
spinning-top d.
split-foot d.
Sprengel d.
static d.
supratip nasal tip d.
talipes equinovarus d.
thumb in palm d.
torsional d.
Volkmann d.
windswept d.
wryneck d.
defunctionalized bladder
degenerate
d. consensus primer
d. oligonucleotide primer (DOP)
degenerated fibroadenolipoma
degenerating myoma
degeneration
anterior horn cell d.
axonal d.
carneous d.
cerebellar d.
cerebromacular d.
cochleosaccular d.
congenital macular d.
congenital progressive
oculoacousticocerebral d.
cystic myoma d.
dominant Dovne honeycomb
retinal d.
dying-back axonal d.

familial striatal d.
hepatolenticular d.
hereditary oligophrenic
cerebellolental d.
hyaline myoma d.
hypobetalipoproteinemia,
acanthocytosis, retinitis
pigmentosa, and pallidal d.
(HARP)
infantile neuronal d.
infantile striatonigral d.
joint d.
Leber congenital tapetoretinal d.
malignant d.
molar d.
mucoid myoma d.
myocardial fiber d.
nuclear d.
oligodendroglial d.
olivopontocerebellar d.
pallidal d.
pulpal d.
red d.
retinal pigmentary d.
sarcomatous myoma d.
spinocerebellar d.
spongy d.
subacute combined d.
tapetoretinal d.
uterine fibroid carneous d.
uterine fibroid red d.
vitelliform d.
wallerian d.
white matter d.
degenerativa
melanosis corii d.
degenerative
d. arthritis
d. osteoarthritis
degloving injury
deglutition
degradable starch microsphere (DSM)
degradation
fibrin d.
ganglioside d.
glycoprotein d.
degranulation
degree of kindred
30-degree lens
70-degree lens
45-degree skin traction
dehalogenase defect

NOTES

dehiscence
  asymptomatic d.
  episiotomy d.
  uterine scar d.
  wound d.
dehydrated
dehydration
  d. fever
  hemorrhagic d.
  hypernatremia d.
  hypernatremic d.
  hyperosmolar d.
  hypertonic d.
  hyponatremic d.
  hypotonic d.
  hypovolemic d.
  isonatremic d.
  isotonic d.
  mild d.
  moderate d.
  d., poisoning, trauma (DPT)
  severe d.
dehydrocholate (DHC)
7-dehydrocholesterol
dehydroepiandrosterone (DHEA)
  d. sulfate (DHEAS)
  d. sulfate loading test
dehydrogenase
  acetyl-CoA d.
  20alpha-dihydroprogestin d.
  17beta-estradiol d.
  3beta-hydroxysteroid d. (3betaHSD)
  electron transfer flavoprotein d.
    (ETF-DH)
  glucose-6-phosphate d. (G6PD)
  15-hydroxyprostaglandin d.
  18-hydroxysteroid d.
  hydroxysteroid d. type 2 (HSD2)
  isovaleryl-CoA d.
  lactate d. (LDH)
  lactic acid d. (LDH)
  long-chain acyl-CoA d. (LCAD)
  long-chain 3-hydroxyacyl-CoA d.
    (LCHAD)
  long-chain hydroxyacyl-coenzyme
    A d. (LCHAD)
  long- and medium-chain acyl-
    CoA d. (LCAD/MCAD)
  long- and very-long-chain acyl-
    CoA d. (LCAD/VLCAD)
  medium-chain acyl-CoA d.
    (MCAD)
  pyruvate d.
  short-chain acyl coenzyme A d.
    (SCAD)
  short-chain hydroxyacyl-coenzyme
    A d. (SCHAD)
  succinate d.

  very long chain acyl-CoA d.
    (VLCAD)
dehydrogenation
  pyruvate d.
dehydroisoandrosterone sulfate
dehydroxylase
  phenylalanine d.
déjà vu
Dejerine disease
Dejerine-Klumpke syndrome
Dejerine-Sottas
  D.-S. atrophy
  D.-S. disease
  D.-S. syndrome
DeJuan forceps
Dekasol Injection
Dekasol-L.A. Inject
del
  deletion
    del 11/aniridia complex
    Del Aqua-5, -10 Gel
    del Castillo syndrome
Delalutin
Delaprem
Delatestryl Injection
delavirdine
Delaxin
delay
  adaptive d.
  atrioventricular conduction d.
  benign maturation d.
  cognitive d.
  constitutional growth d.
  deafness, femoral epiphyseal
    dysplasia, short stature,
    developmental d.
  developmental d.
  global developmental d.
  growth d.
  language d.
  neurodevelopmental d.
  physiologic d.
  puberal d.
  radial-femoral d.
  short stature, hyperextensibility of
    joints and/or inguinal hernia,
    ocular depression, Rieger
    anomaly, teething d. (SHORT)
  speech d.
  d. syndrome
delayed
  d. bone age
  d. deep tendon reflex
  d. fertilization
  d. first stage
  d. gastric emptying
  d. hypersensitivity
  d. implantation
  d. menarche

d. menstruation
d. motor development
d. myelopathy
d. neuropsychological sequela (DNS)
d. orthostatic intolerance
d. primary closure
d. puberty
d. relaxation phase
d. repair
d. sexual maturation
d. sleep phase syndrome (DSPS)
d. thyrotropin elevation
d. tooth eruption
d. transfusion reaction
d. union

delayed-phase computed tomography
delayed-type hypersensitivity (DTH)
Delbet fracture classification (type I–IV)
Delclos
D. cylinder
D. ovoid

Delcort Topical
DeLee
D. forceps
D. instrumentation
D. maneuver
D. suction catheter
D. suction device
D. suctioning
D. Universal retractor

Delestrogen
deleted in azoospermia (DAZ)
deletion (del)
autosomal d.
chromosomal d.
chromosome d.
d. of chromosome
de novo d.
elastin gene d.
gene d.
interstitial d.
d. 1p–22p syndrome
d. 1q–22q syndrome
d. 1–22 syndrome
terminal d.
Xp d.
d. Xp21 syndrome
d. Xp22 syndrome
d. Xq syndrome

Delfen
delinquency

delinquent
delirium, pl. **deliria**
d., infection, atrophic urethritis/vaginitis, pharmaceuticals, psychological, excess urine
d., infection, pharmacology, psychology, endocrinopathy, restricted mobility, stool impaction (DIAPPERS)

delivered
pregnancy, uterine, not d. (PUND)

Deliver formula
delivery
abdominal d.
d. area
assisted breech d.
assisted cephalic d.
assisted spontaneous vaginal d.
asynchronous multifetal d.
breech vaginal d.
cephalic d.
cesarean d.
controlled vaginal d.
Duncan mechanism of placental d.
elective cesarean d.
en caul d.
expected date of d. (EDD)
failed forceps d.
fear of d.
fear-causing d.
fearless first d.
forceps d. (FD)
high forceps d.
instrumental d.
labor and d. (L&D)
low forceps d.
midforceps d.
d. mode
natural d.
near-term d.
normal spontaneous vaginal d. (NSVD)
normal vaginal d.
operative vaginal d.
outlet forceps d.
oxygen d.
perimortem d.
postmortem d.
precipitate labor and d.
precipitous d.
premature d.
preterm d.

D

NOTES

delivery *(continued)*
 d. record
 d. room
 rotational d.
 route of d.
 sequential d.
 soft cup vacuum d.
 spontaneous cephalic d.
 spontaneous preterm d.
 spontaneous vaginal d. (SVD)
 sterile, spontaneous, controlled
  vaginal d. (SSCVD)
 sterile, spontaneous vaginal d.
  (SSVD)
 sunny-side up d.
 term d.
 traumatic d.
 twin d.
 underwater d.
 vacuum-assisted d.
 vacuum extraction d.
 vacuum extractor d.
 vaginal breech d.
 vertex d.
Delleman syndrome
Dellepiane hysterectomy
Delorme procedure
Delsym
delta, δ
 d. agent
 d. hepatitis
 d. OD$_{450}$
 d. phalanx
 D. shunt
 d. sleep
 d. wave
Delta-Cortef Oral
delta-F508 cystic fibrosis
Deltasone
Deltatrac II indirect calorimeter
deltoid
 d. insertion
 d. muscle
 d. paralysis
delusion
 grandiose d.
Demadex
 D. Injection
 D. Oral
demand
 d. effect
 d. feeding
demander
 entitled d.
demarcated
demecarium
demeclocycline

dementia
 d. of the Alzheimer type (DAT)
 Heller d.
Demerol
demineralization
 acral d.
 bone d.
demise
 fetal d.
 intrapartum d.
 intrauterine fetal d.
 single fetal d.
 single-twin d.
 spontaneous preterm labor with
  intrapartum d.
 twin d.
Demodex
 D. brevis
 D. folliculorum
 D. phylloides
demographic
Demons-Meigs syndrome
Demser
Demulen
 D. 1/35
 D. 1/50
demyelinating encephalopathy
demyelination
 inflammatory d.
 symmetric d.
demyelinative
demyelinogenic leukodystrophy
denature
denaturing
 d. gradient gel electrophoresis
 d. high-performance liquid
  chromatography
Denavir
dendritic
 d. arborization
 d. cell
 d. cell-related disorder
 d. keratitis
denervation
dengue
 d. hemorrhagic fever
 d. shock syndrome
 d. virus
Denhardt solution
denial stage
denidation
Denis
 D. Browne bar
 D. Browne clubfoot splint
 D. Browne night splint
 D. Browne pouch
Denman spontaneous evolution
Dennen forceps
Dennett diet

Dennie
> D. line
> D. lines of lower eyelids

Dennie-Marfan syndrome

Dennie-Morgan
> D.-M. fold
> D.-M. line

Dennyson-Fulford extraarticular subtalar arthrodesis

Denonvilliers fascia

Denorex

de novo

dens
> hypoplastic d.

densa
> sublamina d.

dense
> d. adhesion
> d. band
> d. body
> d. body deficiency
> d. cast
> d. striation

densitometer
> DXA d.
> Expert bone d.
> Hologic 1000 QDR d.
> OsteoAnalyzer d.
> PIXI bone d.
> QDR-1500 bone d.

densitometry
> bone d.
> dynamic spiral CT lung d.

density
> areal bone mineral d. (aBMD)
> arterial linear d.
> bone d.
> bone mineral d. (BMD)
> fat d.
> d. gradient
> hip bone d.
> hypoechoic d.
> increased bone d.
> lamellar body number d.
> optical d.
> soft-tissue d.
> d. spectral array
> volumetric bone d.
> volumetric bone mineral d. (vBMD)

dental
> d. abscess
> d. avulsion
> d. caries
> d. cementum
> d. crowding
> d. defect
> d. enamel hypoplasia
> d. extrusion
> d. extrusion/lateral luxation
> d. intrusion
> d. lamina cyst
> d. speech appliance
> d. trauma

dentate
> d. line
> d. nucleus

dentatorubral atrophy

dentatorubral-pallidoluysian atrophy (DRPLA)

dentia praecox

denticulate hymen

dentigerous cyst

dentin dysplasia

dentinogenesis imperfecta

dentition
> permanent d.
> primary d.

dentoalveolar unit

dentoauriculoskeletal
> cerebroocular d. (CODAS)

dentooculoosseous dysplasia

denuded surface

denumerable character

Denver
> D. classification
> D. Developmental chart
> D. Developmental Screening Test (DDST)
> D. Developmental Screening Test II
> D. Home Screening Questionnaire
> D. hydrocephalus shunt
> D. II screening

Denys-Drash syndrome

deodorant artifact

deossification

deoxyadenosine

deoxyadenosylcobalamin

deoxyadenylic acid (dAMP)

deoxy ATP

NOTES

239

deoxycholate
    amphotericin B d. (AmBd)
deoxycorticosterone (DOC)
deoxycytidylic acid (dCMP)
deoxy-D-glucose
deoxyguanylic acid (dGMP)
deoxyhemoglobin
deoxynucleotide triphosphate
deoxypyridinoline (Dpd)
deoxyribonuclease (DNAse, DNase)
deoxyribonucleic
    d. acid (DNA)
    d. acid analysis
    d. acid index
deoxyribonucleotide
15-deoxyspergualin
deoxythymidylic acid (dTMP)
Depacon
Depakene
Depakote sprinkle
department
    D. of Children and Family
        Services (DCFS)
    D. of Children's Services (DCS)
    D. of Children and Youth Services
    pediatric emergency d. (PED)
    D. of Public Social Services
        (DPSS)
Depen
dependence
    coital d.
    vitamin D d.
dependency
    chemical d.
    pyridoxine d.
dependent
    d. edema
    d. pooling
depersonalization
depigmentation
    d. disorder
    postinflammatory d.
depigmented nevus
depigmentosus
    nevus d.
depilation
depleted
    lymphocyte d.
depletion
    germ-cell d.
    intravascular volume d.
    juvenile spermatogonial d.
    T-cell d.
Depo-Estradiol Injection
Depogen Injection
depolarization
    atrial premature d.
    ectopic ventricular d.
    ventricular premature d.

Depo-Medrol Injection
depo-medroxyprogesterone
**depomedroxyprogesterone acetate
    (DMPA)**
depo-MPA
Deponit
Depopred Injection
Depo-Provera Injection
deposit
    electron-dense subepithelial d.
    granular osmiophilic d.
    macrocephaly with feeblemindedness
        and encephalopathy with
        peculiar d.'s
deposition
    complement d.
    copper d.
    cystine d.
    diffuse perivillous fibrinoid d.
    fat d.
    fibrin d.
    hemosiderin d.
    IgA mesangial d.
    immunoglobulin d.
    neonatal elastin d.
depot
    Androcur D.
    fat d.
    Lupron D.
    Lupron D.-3 Month
    Lupron D.-4 Month
    d. medroxyprogesterone
    d. medroxyprogesterone acetate
        (DMPA)
    Sandostatin LAR D.
Depo-Testadiol
Depo-Testosterone Injection
Depot-Ped
    Lupron D.-P.
depressed
    d. fontanelle
    d. scar
    d. sensorium
    d. skull fracture
depression
    agitated d.
    anaclitic d.
    anxiety d.
    atypical d.
    bipolar d.
    bright white light therapy for
        postpartum d.
    cardiovascular d.
    cortical spreading d.
    double d.
    fetal skull d.
    inbreeding d.
    intimate partner d.
    melancholic d.

narcotic d.
neonatal respiratory d.
paternal postnatal d.
ping-pong ball d.
posteromedial articular d.
postictal d.
postnatal d. (PND)
postpartum d.
prepuberal d.
psychotic d.
d. rating scale
respiratory d.
d. screening
D. Self-Rating Scale
d. stage
treatment-refractory d.
unipolar d.

depressive
d. disorder
d. symptom

depressor
d. anguli oris
d. anguli oris muscle
d. anguli oris muscle hypoplasia
  syndrome
tongue d.
torque d.

deprivation
d. amblyopia
antagonist-induced gonadotropin d.
estrogen d.
idiocy by d.
oxygen d.
social d.

depth
crypt d.
d. dose
d. perception
d. relationship
vertical pocket d.

derangement
internal d.
physiologic d.

Dercum disease
derealization
derecruitment
derepressed gene
derivation
sexual d.

derivative
acetoxyprogesterone d.
17-α-acetoxyprogesterone d.

d. chromosome
coumarin d.
19-nortestosterone d.
purified protein d. (PPD)

Dermablend
Dermabond
dermabrasion
Dermacentor
  D. andersoni
  D. variabilis
Dermacort Topical
dermal
d. erythropoiesis
d. melanocytosis
d. nevus
d. sinus
d. sinus tract
d. vasculitis
d. vitiligo

Dermarest Dricort Topical
Derma-Smoothe/FS Topical
Dermasone
dermatan
d. sulfate
d. sulfate accumulation

dermatitic
dermatitidis
  Blastomyces d.
dermatitis, pl. **dermatitides**
allergic contact d.
atopic d.
brawny d.
burnlike d.
Candida diaper d.
candidal diaper d.
cercarial d.
chronic bullous d.
chronic eczematoid d.
contact d.
diaper d.
eczematoid d.
d. enteropathica
exfoliative d.
follicular d.
friction d.
d. gangrenosa infantum
d. herpetiformis (DH)
d. herpetiformis-associated gluten-
  sensitive enteropathy
infectious eczematoid d.
infective d.
irradiation d.

D

NOTES

dermatitis *(continued)*
  irritant contact d.
  irritant diaper d.
  isolated vulvar seborrheic d.
  Jacquet erosive diaper d.
  juvenile plantar d.
  mask of atopic d.
  monilial diaper d.
  neonatal bullous d.
  nickel d.
  nummular d.
  occlusion d.
  papular d. of pregnancy (PDP)
  perianal d.
  periorificial d.
  photosensitive d.
  progesterone d.
  psoriatic d.
  rebound d.
  rhus d.
  scalp seborrheic d.
  scaly d.
  seborrheic d.
  shoe contact d.
  tide mark d.
  d. venenata
  vulvar seborrheic d.
  weeping d.
dermatofibroma
dermatofibrosarcoma protuberans
dermatofibrosis lenticularis disseminata
dermatoglyphic
  d. abnormality
  d. finding
  d. pattern
dermatoglyphics
dermatoleukodystrophy
dermatology
  neonatal d.
  pediatric d.
dermatomal distribution
dermatomegaly
dermatomyositis (DM)
  amyopathic juvenile d.
  juvenile d. (JDM, JDMS)
  primary idiopathic d.
dermatomyositis/polymyositis (DMPM)
dermatoosteolysis
  Kirghizian d.
Dermatop
dermatophyte
  d. infection
  d. lesion
  d. test medium (DTM)
dermatophytid reaction
dermatophytosis
dermatosis, pl. **dermatoses**
  acute febrile neurophilic d.
  bullous d.

  dermolytic bullous d.
  ichthyosiform d.
  idiopathic d.
  juvenile plantar d.
  d. of kwashiorkor
  linear IgA d.
  plantar d.
  Siemens-Bloch pigmented d.
  vulvar d.
dermis
  papillary d.
  reticular d.
  thinned d.
dermocyma
dermoepidermal junction
dermographism
  white d.
dermoid
  d. cyst
  d. cyst of ovary
  epibulbar d.
  d. sinus
  d. sinus tract
Dermolate Topical
dermolipoma
dermolysis bullosa
dermolytic bullous dermatosis
dermopathy
  nephrogenic fibrosing d.
  restrictive d.
Dermoplast
dermotrichic syndrome
Dermovate
Dermtex HC with Aloe Topical
Derogatis Brief Symptom Inventory
Deronil
derotation femoral osteotomy
Derry syndrome
DES
  diethylstilbestrol
  Dissociative Experience Scale
  dysequilibrium syndrome
  DES daughter
  DES exposure
25-desacetyl rifapentine
DESAD
  National Collaborative Diethylstilbestrol
  Adenosis Project
desalination
desaturate
desaturation
  red d.
Desbuquois syndrome
Descemet membrane
descending
  d. aorta
  d. aorta anastomosis
  d. colon
  left anterior d. (LAD)

descensus uteri
descent
    aberrant course of testicular d.
    fetal d.
    rapid d.
    rotation and d.
    second-degree d.
    spontaneous d.
    testicular d.
    third-degree d.
Deschamps ligature
descriptive embryology
Desenex
    Prescription Strength D.
desensitization
    imaginal d.
    pituitary d.
desert rheumatism
Desferal Mesylate
desferrioxamine
    d. mesylate
    d. therapy
desflurane
desiccate
design
    family-based d.
designated donor blood
designation
    eligibility d.
designed
    Dortmund Nutritional and
        Anthropometrical Longitudinally D.
        (DONALD)
designer
    Pharsight Trial D.
desipramine
desire
    hypoactive sexual d.
    inhibited sexual d.
    sexual d.
Desitin
deslanoside
deslorelin
Desmarres
    D. forceps
    D. retractor
desmethylimipramine
desmins
desmiognathus
desmocranium
desmoid tumor

desmolase
    cholesterol 20,22 d.
Desmons syndrome
desmoplasia
    intratumoral d.
desmoplastic
    d. medulloblastoma
    d. small round cell tumor
        (DSRCT)
desmopressin
    d. acetate nasal spray
    desmopressin acetate
    intranasal d.
desmosome
Desocort
Desogen
desogestrel
    ethinyl estradiol and d.
    d. and ethinyl estradiol
desonide
DesOwen Topical
desoximetasone
desoxycholate amphotericin B
desoxycorticosterone (DOC)
Desoxyn
desquamated epithelial cell
desquamation
    follicular d.
    perineal d.
    periungual d.
desquamative
    d. inflammatory vaginitis
    d. interstitial pneumonia (DIP)
    d. interstitial pneumonitis (DIP)
desquamativum
    erythroderma d.
Desquam-E Gel
Desquam-X Gel
destruction
    hypothalamic-hypophysial d.
    iatrogenic d.
    physial d.
    postirradiation d.
destruens
    chorioadenoma d.
    molar d.
desultory labor
Desyrel
detachment
    exudative retinal d.
    retinal d.
    rhegmatogenous d.

D

NOTES

detachment *(continued)*
    serous retinal d.
    tractional retinal d.
    urethral d.
detail
    cycle-monitoring d.
Detect HIV-1 assay
detection
    mammographic d.
    prenatal d.
    d. rate
detector
    Pedi-cap d.
detergens
    liquor carbonis d.
deterioration
    central syndrome of rostrocaudal d.
    fetal d.
determinant
    antigen d.
    culture-specific d.
    d. group
    sialyl Lewis X d.
determination
    blood gas d.
    bone age d.
    cell d.
    emesis pH d.
    fetal sex d.
    gender d.
    hematocrit d.
    hemoglobin A1c d.
    parentage d.
    prenatal sex d.
    scalp pH d.
    selective renal vein renin d.
    sex d.
    sweat chloride d.
    testis d.
    ultrasonographic d.
detorsion
    manual d.
detoxification
Detroit Test of Learning Aptitude 2
detrusor
    d. hyperreflexia
    d. instability
    d. muscle
    d. overactivity
    d. pressure
    d. sphincter dyssynergia
    d. tone
detrusorrhaphy
detumescence
devascularization
development
    abnormal fetal d.
    adaptive d.
    alveolar stage of lung d.

    arrested d.
    Assessment in Infancy Ordinal Scales of Psychological D.
    axillary hair d.
    Bayley Scales of Infant D. (BSID)
    Bayley Scales of Infant D.-II (BSID-II)
    breast d.
    Brigance Diagnostic Inventory of Early D.
    canalicular stage of lung d.
    cardiovascular d.
    cellular and molecular regulation of lung d.
    cephalocaudal sequence of d.
    CNS d.
    cytoarchitectural d.
    delayed motor d.
    dissociated motor d.
    early follicular d.
    embryonic d.
    emotional d.
    endometrial d.
    Erikson stages of growth and d.
    excretory system d.
    expressive language d.
    fetal d.
    fetal lung d.
    fine motor d.
    genital d.
    goiter d.
    Griffith Scale of Mental D.
    gross d.
    gross motor d.
    hearing d.
    infant d.
    language d.
    lung growth and d.
    male genital duct d.
    mental d.
    National Institute of Child Health and Human D. (NICHD)
    neurologic d.
    normal fetal d.
    Ordinal Scales of Intellectual D.
    phonological d.
    pseudoglandular stage of lung d.
    psychosocial d.
    pulmonary vascular d.
    receptive language d.
    reproductive system d.
    saccular stage of lung d.
    social d.
    d. specialist
    speech d.
    stromal d.
    Tanner stages of d. (1–5)
    Tanner staging of genital d. (1–5)

trilineage d.
visual d.
developmental
    d. age (DA)
    d. area
    d. assessment
    d. assessment score
    D. Behaviour Checklist
    d. cataract
    d. check
    d. coordination disorder (DCD)
    d. crisis
    d. deficiency
    d. delay
    d. delay-multiple strawberry nevi
      syndrome
    d. diapause
    d. disability (DD)
    d. disorder
    d. displacement of hip (DDH)
    d. dysfluency
    d. dyslexia
    d. dysphasia
    d. dysplasia of hip (DDH)
    d. flatfoot
    d. genu varum
    d. hip disease
    d. hip dysplasia
    d. issue
    d. language disorder (DLD)
    d. level
    d. milestone
    d. motor quotient (DMQ)
    d. pattern
    d. pattern disorder
    D. Profile-II (DP-II)
    D. Programming for Infants and
      Young Children
    d. quotient (DQ)
    d. screening
    d. stage
    d. surveillance
    D. Test of Visual-Motor Integration
Deventer pelvis
deviant volitional movement
deviated septum
deviation
    axis d.
    eye d.
    jaw d.
    left axis d.
    right axis d.

septal d.
sexual d.
standard d. (SD)
Devic disease
device
    AcuTrainer d.
    AeroChamber spacer d.
    alternative communication d.
    Amplatzer d.
    antisiphon d.
    aspiration-tulip d.
    Atad Ripener d.
    augmentative communication d.
    AutoPap automated screening d.
    autostapling d.
    barium-impregnated plastic
      intrauterine d.
    BVM d.
    Cameco syringe pistol aspiration d.
    CardioSeal d.
    central venous access d. (CVAD)
    CerviSoft cytology collection d.
    clamshell-type catheter occlusion d.
    clitoral therapy d. (CTD)
    contraceptive d.
    Copper T intrauterine d.
    Cu-7 intrauterine d.
    CycleBeads fertility d.
    DeLee suction d.
    Diva laparoscopic morcellator d.
    Donnez d.
    double-balloon d.
    double-umbrella d.
    dynamic orthotic cranioplasty d.
    Eder cord blood collection d.
    electric suction d.
    Endo Stitch laparoscopic
      suturing d.
    Eros-CTD eroscillator d.
    evacuation d.
    ExacTech glucose measuring d.
    external urethral barrier d.
    FemCap barrier contraceptive d.
    Femcept d.
    Finapres d.
    flutter d.
    FNA-21 fine-needle aspiration d.
    Gianturco-Grifka vascular
      occlusion d.
    GynoSampler endometrial
      sampling d.
    handheld flutter d.

D

NOTES

device *(continued)*
    HemoCue AB hemoglobin measurement d.
    Hollister collecting d.
    Ilizarov d.
    intrauterine d. (IUD)
    intrauterine contraception d. (IUCD)
    intrauterine contraceptive device (IUCD)
    knee height measuring d.
    left ventricular assist d. (LVAD)
    Lippes-type intrauterine d.
    Macroplastique implantable d.
    Makler insemination d.
    McMaster Family Assessment D.
    M-cup vacuum extraction d.
    Medilog 9000 polysomnography d.
    Model 5315 sequential compression d.
    Mucat cervical sampling d.
    Multiload Cu-375 intrauterine d.
    Multispatula cervical sampling d.
    Niplette d.
    One Step Button gastrostomy d.
    OraSure d.
    OsteoView d.
    Papette d.
    Poly CS d.
    Progestasert intrauterine d.
    progesterone-releasing T-shaped d.
    Protocult stool sampling d.
    ReliefBand d.
    Scopette d.
    Seitzinger d.
    Shug male contraceptive d.
    STARFlex d.
    STOP nonsurgical permanent contraception d.
    umbrella d.
    Uterine Explora Curette endometrial sampling d.
    vacuum clitoral therapy d.
    Venodyne pneumatic compressive d.
    ventricular assist d.
    Wallach Endocell collection d.
    Z sampler endometrial sampling d.
DeWeese axis traction forceps
Dewey obstetrical forceps
deworm
DEXA
    dual-energy x-ray absorptiometry
    DEXA scan
Dexacidin Ophthalmic
Dexacort
    D. Phosphate Respihaler Oral Inhaler
    D. Phosphate Turbinaire
    D. Phosphate Turbinaire Intranasal Aerosol

Dex-A-Diet
dexamethasone
    methotrexate, bleomycin, doxorubicin, cyclophosphamide, Oncovin, d. (m-BACOD)
    d., neomycin and polymyxin B
    pulse d.
    d. suppression test
    d. suppression testing (DST)
    d. therapy
    vincristine and d.
Dexameth Oral
Dexasone L.A. Injection
Dexasporin Ophthalmic
Dexatrim
dexbrompheniramine
dexchlorpheniramine
Dexedrine Spansule capsule
dexfenfluramine
Dexide
    D. disposable cannula
    D. disposable trocar
Dexon
    D. II suture
    D. mesh
    D. Plus suture
Dexone
    D. LA
    D. LA Injection
    D. Tablet
dexpanthenol
dexrazoxane
dexter
    cor triatriatum d.
dextran (DX)
    d. 40
    HMW d.
    iron d.
    LMW d.
    low molecular weight d. (LMWD)
    d. sulfate
dextran-70 barrier material
dextrans
    limit d.
dextrin
    d. sulfate
    d. sulfate gel
dextrinosis
    limit d.
dextroamphetamine (DA)
    d. saccharate
    d. sulfate
dextrocardia
    mirror-image d.
dextrocardia/situs inversus syndrome
dextro formula
dextromethorphan
    guaifenesin and d.

dextroposition
anomalous right pulmonary vein d.
d. of heart
dextrose in water
Dextrostix (D-stix)
D. reagent strip
dextrosuria
dextrothyroxine
dextrotransposition (D-transposition)
dextroversion
Dey-Drop Ophthalmic Solution
Dey-Wash skin wound cleanser
DF
diabetic fetopathy
DFA
direct fluorescent antibody
direct fluorescent antigen
DFA stain
DFA staining
DFA test
D-fenfluramine
DFFRY gene
DFMO
difluoromethyl ornithine
DFNA3
autosomal dominant nonsyndromic
hearing loss
DFNB1
autosomal recessive nonsyndromic
hearing loss
DFS
disease-free survival
DG
Davis & Geck
DG Softgut suture
D-galactose
dGMP
deoxyguanylic acid
DGSX
X-linked dysplasia-gigantism syndrome
DH
dermatitis herpetiformis
DHA
docosahexaenoic acid
DHC
dehydrocholate
DHCA
deep hypothermia and total circulatory
arrest
DHE
dihydroergotamine

DHEA
dehydroepiandrosterone
DHEA sulfate
DHEAS
dehydroepiandrosterone sulfate
DHS Tar
DHT
dihydrotestosterone
DHTR
dihydrotestosterone receptor deficiency
DI
diabetes insipidus
donor insemination
DIA
dot immunobinding assay
DiaBeta
diabetes
borderline d.
brittle d.
bronze d.
chemical d.
congenital lipoatrophic d.
d. control and complications trial
(DCCT)
drug-induced d.
D. in Early Pregnancy Study
gestational d.
d. insipidus (DI)
d. insipidus, diabetes mellitus, optic
atrophy (DIDMO)
d. insipidus and mellitus with
optic atrophy and deafness
(DIDMOAD)
insulin-dependent d.
insulin-dependent d. mellitus
(IDDM)
juvenile d.
juvenile-onset d.
ketosis-prone d.
ketosis-resistant d.
latent d.
lipoatrophic d.
maternal d.
maturity-onset d.
d. mellitus, mental retardation,
lipodystrophy, dysmorphic traits
syndrome
d. mellitus (type 1, 2) (DM)
d. neonatorum
non-insulin-dependent d.
non-insulin-dependent d. mellitus
(NIDDM)

D

NOTES

247

diabetes *(continued)*
>   overt insulin-dependent d. mellitus
>   pregestational d.
>   D. Prevention Trial
>   streptozocin-induced d.
>   sugar d.
>   transient neonatal d. (TND)

diabetes-deafness syndrome
diabetes-related congenital malformation
Diabetic
>   D. Tussin DM
>   D. Tussin EX

diabetic
>   d. acidosis
>   d. cardiomyopathy
>   d. cheiroarthropathy
>   d. coma
>   d. embryopathy
>   d. fetopathy (DF)
>   insulin-dependent d.
>   d. ketoacidosis (DKA)
>   d. mother
>   d. nephropathy
>   non-insulin-dependent d.
>   pregnant d.
>   d. retinopathy

diabeticorum
>   necrobiosis lipoidica d. (NLD)

diabetogenic effect of pregnancy
Diabinese
diacetate
>   diflorasone d.
>   ethinyl estradiol and ethynodiol d.
>   ethynodiol d.
>   propylene glycol d.

diacylglycerol (DAG)
diadochokinesis
diagnosis, pl. **diagnoses**
>   antenatal d.
>   colposcopic d.
>   computer-aided d. (CAD)
>   established medical d.
>   fetal d.
>   genetic d.
>   histologic d.
>   histopathological d.
>   neonatal d.
>   preimplantation d.
>   preimplantation genetic d. (PGD)
>   prenatal genetic d.
>   ultrasonographic d.
>   ultrasound d.

diagnostic
>   d. accuracy
>   d. hysteroscope
>   d. imaging
>   D. Interview for Genetic Study (DIGS)
>   D. Interview Schedule for Children (DISC)
>   D. Interview Schedule for Children-Revised (DISC-R)
>   d. mammography
>   d. maneuver
>   d. overshadowing
>   d. peritoneal lavage (DPL)
>   d. procedure
>   d. radiation
>   D. and Statistical Manual of Mental Disorders - 4th Edition (DSM-IV)
>   d. ultrasonography

diagnostics
>   Amplicor PCR d.
>   DNA d.
>   Roche D.
>   Vivigen d.

diagonal conjugate
diakinesis
>   d. stage
>   d. stage of oocyte meiosis

dialectical
dialysate protein loss
dialysis, pl. **dialyses**
>   continuous ambulatory peritoneal d. (CAPD)
>   continuous cyclic peritoneal d. (CCPD)
>   kidney d.
>   peritoneal d. (PD)

dialytic parabiosis
diameter
>   anteroposterior d. of the pelvic inlet
>   aortic root d.
>   AP d.
>   Baudelocque d.
>   biischial d.
>   biparietal d. (BPD)
>   bitemporal d.
>   conjugate d. of the pelvic inlet
>   decreased biparietal d.
>   fetal biparietal d.
>   gestational sac mean d.
>   increased anteroposterior chest d.
>   internal d.
>   intertuberous d.
>   Loehlein d.
>   d. mediana
>   narrow bifrontal d.
>   d. obliqua
>   oblique d.
>   obstetric conjugate d.
>   occipitofrontal d.
>   occipitomental d.
>   plane of greatest d.
>   plane of least d.

posterior sagittal d.
suboccipitobregmatic d.
trachelobregmatic d.
d. transversa
transverse d.
2-diameter pocket technique
Diamine T.D.
3,3′ diaminobenzidine
diaminobenzidine
3,3′ d.
***cis*-diamminedichloroplatinum (DDP)**
c.-d. II
diamniotic
d. dichorionic placenta
d. twins
Diamond-Blackfan
D.-B. anemia (DBA)
D.-B. congenital hypoplastic anemia
D.-B. juvenile pernicious anemia
D.-B. syndrome
diamond-shaped murmur
Diamox Sequels
Diana
D. complex
D. Project
Dianabol
Dianeal dialysis solution
Diaparene
diapause
developmental d.
embryonic d.
diapedetic leukocyte
diaper
d. dermatitis
double d.'s
d. rash
d. syndrome
triple d.'s
zinc-free plastic-lined d.
diaphanography
diaphoresis
diaphoretic
diaphragm
arcing spring d.
coil spring d.
contraceptive d.
duodenal d.
eventration of d.
everted d.
flat spring d.
hinged spring d.
intrauterine d.

Ortho All-Flex d.
d. palsy
d. paralysis
pelvic d.
d. pessary
plication of d.
urogenital d.
diaphragmatic
d. agenesis
d. atony
d. defect
d. eventration
d. hernia
d. hernia, abnormal face, distal limb anomalies syndrome
d. hernia, distal digital hypoplasia syndrome
d. hernia, exophthalmos, hypertelorism syndrome
d. hernia, myopia, deafness syndrome
d. hiatus
d. injury
d. plication
d. trauma
diaphysial, diaphyseal
d. aclasis
d. dysplasia
d. fibular osteotomy
d. fracture
d. osteomyelitis
diaphysis, pl. **diaphyses**
Diapid
DIAPPERS
delirium, infection, pharmacology, psychology, endocrinopathy, restricted mobility, stool impaction
diarrhea
antibiotic-associated d. (AAD)
bloody d.
chloride-losing d.
chronic nonspecific d.
Clostridium difficile-associated d. (CDAC)
congenital sodium d.
explosive watery d.
infantile d.
nosocomial d.
osmotic d.
pediatric viral d.
protracted d.
secretory d.

NOTES

diarrhea *(continued)*
    toddler's d.
    traveler's d. (TD)
    watery d.
diarrhea-associated hemolytic uremic syndrome
diarrheal
    d. dehydration illness
    d. shellfish poisoning
diarrhea-malnutrition syndrome
diarrheic
diarthrodial
    d. joint
    d. muscle
diary
    baby's day d.
    food d.
    headache d.
    retraining d.
    urinary d.
    voiding d.
DiaScreen reagent strip
Diasorb
diastasis
    d. recti
    symphysis pubis d.
diastatic fracture
Diastat Rectal Delivery System
diastematomyelia
diastole
diastolic
    d. arterial pressure (DAP)
    d. blood pressure
    d. component
    d. gradient
    d. murmur
    d. overload
    d. overload pattern
    d. thrill
diastomyelia
diastrophic
    d. dwarf
    d. dwarfism
    d. dysplasia
diathermy
    d. current
    electrocoagulation d.
    excision d.
    laparoscopic ovarian d.
    d. loop excision
diathesis, pl. **diatheses**
    bleeding d.
    cognitive-stress d.
    familial d.
    gouty d.
    hemorrhagic d.
diatomaceous earth (DE)
diatrizoate
    meglumine d.

Diazemuls Injection
Diazepam Intensol
diazo reaction
diazoxide
dibasic
    d. amino acid
    d. aminoaciduria
Dibbell
    D. cleft lip-nasal reconstruction
    D. cleft lip-nasal revision
Dibenzyline
dibrachia
dibromochloropropane (DBCP)
dibromodulcitol with Adriamycin and vincristine (DAV)
dibucaine
DIC
    disseminated intravascular coagulation
    disseminated intravascular coagulopathy
dicentric chromosome
dicephalic twins
dicephalus
dicheilia
dicheiria
dichloroacetic acid
dichlorphenamide
dichorionic, dichorial
    d. placenta
    d. placentation
    d. twins
dichorionic-diamniotic (di-di)
    d.-d. placenta
    d.-d. twins
dichotic
    d. listening
    d. listening deficit
dichotomous
dichotomy
Dickinson syndrome
Dick test
diclofenac
    d. potassium
    d. sodium
dicloxacillin sodium
DICOM
    digital imaging and communication in medicine
dictyate
    d. stage
    d. stage of oocyte meiosis
dicumarol resistance
dicyclomine hydrochloride
didactic material
didanosine (ddI)
didelphic
didelphys
    uterus d.
di-di
    dichorionic-diamniotic

DIDMO
diabetes insipidus, diabetes mellitus,
optic atrophy
DIDMO syndrome
DIDMOAD
diabetes insipidus and mellitus with optic
atrophy and deafness
DIDMOAD syndrome
Didronel
didymus
Dieckmann intraosseous needle
diembryony
diencephalic
d. syndrome (DS)
d. syndrome of infancy
d. system n
diencephalon
Dienestrol Vaginal
Dientamoeba fragilis
diepoxybutane (DEB).
diet
ADA d.
ad libitum d.
AHA Step One D.
American Diabetes Association d.
American Heart Association Step
One D.
Atkins d.
BRAT d.
BRATT d.
Dennett d.
elemental d.
elimination d.
fluid d.
galactose-free d.
glutamine-supplemented d.
gluten-free d. (GFD)
glycemic index d.
high-calorie d.
high-fiber d.
high-phosphate d.
K d.
K+2 d.
ketogenic d.
lactose-free d.
Lorenzo's oil d.
low-branched-chain amino acid d.
low-cholesterol d.
low-fat d.
low-phenylalanine d.
low-protein d.
low-residue d.

low-salt d.
low-sodium d.
migraine d.
Moro-Heisler d.
non-casein-based d.
d. and nutrition
polymeric d.
PSMF d.
Pulmocare d.
pureed d.
d. recommendation
semifluid d.
Sippy d.
traffic-light d.
vegetarian d.
dietary
d. amenorrhea
d. change
d. craving
d. fat
d. fiber
d. habit
d. problem
d. protein enterocolitis
d. supplement
Dieter forceps
Dieterle stain
diethylamide
lysergic acid d. (LSD)
diethylaminoethyl (DEAE)
diethylcarbamazine
diethyldithiocarbamate
diethylenetriaminepentaacetic acid (DTPA)
diethylpropion
diethylstilbestrol (DES)
d.-exposed
diethyltoluamide (DEET)
diet-induced hypochloremic metabolic alkalosis
dietitian
Dieulafoy gastric lesion
DIF
direct immunofluorescence
DIF test
DiFerrante syndrome
difference
arteriovenous oxygen d.
gender d.
intrapair birth weight d.
racial d.

NOTES

251

differential
>d. agglutination test
>d. cell count
>d. cyanosis
>d. detection hypothesis
>d. effect
>manual d.
>d. temperature sensor (DTS)
>d. treatment hypothesis
>d. vascular resistance

differentiation
>alveolar myofibroblast d.
>central nervous system d.
>corticomedullary d.
>embryonic d.
>extraembryonic d.
>fetal sexual d.
>ganglionic d.
>genital d.
>hematopoietic d.
>lymphopoietic d.
>male sex d.
>schwannian d.
>sexual d.
>somatic d.
>terminal lung d.
>testicular d.

Differin gel

difficile
>*Clostridium d.*

difficulty
>attentional d.
>feeding d.
>d. sleeping
>swallowing d.

diffusa
>neurospongioblastosis d.

diffuse
>d. astrocytoma
>d. axonal injury (DAI)
>d. brain swelling (DBS)
>d. cortical thrombophlebitis
>d. cutaneous leishmaniasis (DCL)
>d. cutaneous mastocytosis
>d. cystic polycystic kidney disease
>d. esophageal spasm
>d. fasciitis
>d. fibrocystic disease
>d. globoid body sclerosis
>d. globoid cell cerebral sclerosis
>d. glomerular sclerosis
>d. hyperpigmentation
>d. intestinal polyp
>d. mesangial sclerosis (DMS)
>d. mesangial sclerosis-ocular abnormalities syndrome
>d. mixed lymphocytic plasmacytic disease
>d. morbilliform rash

>d. neonatal hemangiomatosis
>d. nonmalignant lymphadenopathy
>d. periaxial encephalitis
>d. perivillous fibrinoid deposition
>d. proliferative glomerulonephritis
>d. proliferative lupus nephritis
>d. small cell cleaved lymphoma
>d. tensor brain MRI

diffusing
>d. capacity
>d. capacity of lung for carbon monoxide (DL$_{co}$)

diffusion

diffusion-weighted
>d.-w. imaging (DWI)
>d.-w. magnetic resonance imaging

diffusum
>angiokeratoma corporis d.

diflorasone diacetate

Diflucan

diflunisal

difluoromethyl ornithine (DFMO)

Digene
>D. HPV Assay
>D. Hybrid Capture II HPV Test

DiGeorge
>D. anomaly
>D. malformation sequence
>D. microdeletion syndrome

digestion

digestive system

Dighton-Adair syndrome

Digibind

Digilab FTS 40A spectrometer

digit
>bambooing of d.
>hypoplastic d.
>rudimentary-type d.
>sausage d.
>D. Span Subtest
>supernumerary d.
>d. syndactyly
>trigger d.

digital
>d. anomalies, short palpebral fissures, atresia of esophagus or duodenum syndrome
>d. auditory aerobics (DAA)
>d. clubbing
>d. fibroma
>d. imaging colposcopy
>d. imaging and communication in medicine (DICOM)
>d. mammographic imaging screening trial (DMIST)
>d. mammography
>d. mammography system
>d. pitting
>d. pulp

d. radiography
d. subtraction angiography
d. tuft
d. ulceration
d. ultrasound
digitalis effect
digitalis-induced arrhythmia
digitata
    Laminaria d.
digitoorofacial syndrome (I–V)
digitooropalatal syndrome
digitorenocerebral syndrome (DRC)
digitotalar dysmorphism
digitoxin
Digitrapper portable pH recorder
dignathus
digoxigenin-labeled deoxyuridine triphosphate
digoxin
    d. immune fab
    d. monotherapy
digoxin-like immunoreactive factor (DLIF)
DIGS
    Diagnostic Interview for Genetic Study
digyny
dihybrid cross
dihydoprogesterone
dihydralazine
dihydrate
    azithromycin d.
dihydrochloride
    quinine d.
    triethylene tetramine d.
dihydrocodeine bitartrate
dihydrocodeinone
dihydroergotamine (DHE)
    d. mesylate
dihydrofolate
    d. reductase
    d. reductase inhibitor
dihydromorphinone hydrochloride
dihydropteridine
    d. reductase
    d. reductase deficiency
dihydrotachysterol
5-dihydrotachysterol
dihydrotestosterone (DHT)
    d. cream
    d. receptor deficiency (DHTR)

1,25-dihydroxycholecalciferol
dihydroxyphenylalanine (dopa, DOPA, Dopa)
dihydroxyprogesterone acetophenide
9-13-dihydroxypropoxymethyl guanine
1,25-dihydroxyvitamin D$_3$
diiodohydroxyquin
diiodohydroxyquinoline
diiodothyronine (T2)
    d. test
diiodotyrosine (DIT)
diisopropyl
    d. fluorophosphate
    d. iminodiacetic acid (DISIDA)
Dilacor XR
Dilantin syndrome
Dilapan hygroscopic cervical dilator
dilatation (*var. of* dilation)
dilated
    d. bowel loop resection
    d. capillary
    d. cardiomyopathy
    d. cisterna magna
    d. collateral vein
    fingertip d.
    d. intestinal loop
    d. optic vessel
    d. posterior urethra
    d. renal pelvis
    d. vein
dilating reflux
dilation, dilatation
    aorta d.
    cervical d.
    d. of cervix
    congenital choledochal d.
    d. and curettage (D&C)
    cystic d.
    esophageal d.
    d. and evacuation (D&E)
    Frank technique of d.
    fusiform d.
    gastric d.
    lumen d.
    persistent ventricular d.
    pneumatic d.
    posthemorrhagic ventricular d. (PHVD)
    premature cervical d.
    saccular d.
    urinary tract d.
    d. of ventricle

NOTES

253

dilator
#10 d.
bougie d.
Dilapan hygroscopic cervical d.
Goodell d.
Hanks d.
Hegar d.
hygroscopic d.
iris d.
laminaria cervical d.
Lucite d.
mechanical cervical d.
osmotic d.
Pharmaseal disposable cervical d.
Pratt d.
retained hygroscopic cervical d.
rocket d.
Soehendra d.
vaginal d.
Walther d.
Dilaudid
D. Injection
D. Oral
D. Suppository
Dilaudid-HP Injection
dildo, dildoe
dilemma
diltiazem
dilute
d. Surfaxin
d. urine
diluted formula
dilutional anemia
dimeglumine
gadopentetate d.
dimelia
dimenhydrinate
dimension
hyperactive/impulsive d.
inattention d.
left ventricular end-diastolic d.
left ventricular end-systolic d.
dimer
metalloprotein d.
dimercaprol
dimercaptosuccinic acid
dimeric
d. inhibin A level
d. protein
Dimetane Extentabs
dimethindene maleate
dimethothiazine mesylate
dimethyl
d. phthalate
d. sulfoxide (DMSO)
dimethyl-triazeno-imidazole carboxamide (DTIC)
dimethylxanthine
dimetria

dimidiate
diminazene
diminished fremitus
Dimitri disease
dimorphism
sexual d.
dimorphous leprosy
dimple
acromial d.
anal d.
chin d.
cutaneous d.
lumbosacral d.
pilonidal d.
pretibial skin d.
sacral d.
vaginal d.
Dinamap blood pressure monitor
dinitrate
isosorbide d. (ISDN)
dinitrochlorobenzene (DNCB)
d. therapy
dinitrofluorobenzene
dinitrophenylhydrazine
dinoprostone cervical gel
dinoprost tromethamine
dinucleotide
flavin adenine d. (FAD)
Diochloram
Diocto
Diocto-C
diode
argon d.
light-emitting d.
Diodoquin
dioecious
Dioeze
Diomycin
DIOS
distal intestinal obstruction syndrome
diosgenin
Diosuccin
Diovan
diovular twins
dioxide
carbon d. (CO_2)
end-tidal carbon d. (E_TCO_2)
fraction of alveolar carbon d. ($FACO_2$)
fraction in expired gas of carbon d. ($FECO_2$)
partial pressure of arterial carbon d. ($PaCO_2$)
partial pressure carbon d. (PCO_2)
pressure of carbon d.
sulfur d.
dioxin
dioxyline

DIP
  desquamative interstitial pneumonia
  desquamative interstitial pneumonitis
dipalmitoyl phosphatidylcholine (DPPC)
Dipentum
diphallus
diphasic
diphemanil methylsulfate
diphenadione
Diphenadryl
Diphenatol
Diphen Cough
diphencyprone
Diphenhist
diphenhydramine citrate
diphenoxylate and atropine
diphenylhydantoin
diphenyl tetrazolium bromide
diphenylthiourea
diphosphate
  galactose uridine d.
  menadiol sodium d.
  uridine d. (UDP)
diphosphate-choline
  cytidine d.-c.
diphosphate-diacylglycerol
  cytidine d.-d.
diphosphoglycerate
diphtheria
  d. antitoxin
  cutaneous d.
  laryngeal d.
  nasal d.
  d., pertussis, tetanus (DPT)
  pharyngeal d.
  tetanus and d. (Td)
  d., tetanus, acellular pertussis
    vaccine (DTPa)
  d., tetanus-pertussis immunization
  d., tetanus, pertussis vaccine (DTP)
  tetanus toxoid and d.
  d., tetanus toxoid, acellular
    pertussis vaccine
  d., tetanus toxoid, pertussis (DTP)
  d., tetanus toxoids, whole-cell
    pertussis vaccine
  d., tetanus toxoid, whole-cell
    pertussis (DTPw)
  d. toxin (DT)
  d. toxoids-acellular pertussis
  d. toxoid with pertussis

diphtheriae
  Corynebacterium d.
diphtheritic
  d. croup
  d. membrane
  d. toxic myocarditis
diphtheroid
diphthong
diphyllobothriasis
Diphyllobothrium latum
DIPI
  direct intraperitoneal injection
  direct intraperitoneal insemination
dipivefrin
dipivoxil
  adefovir d.
diplegia
  atonic astatic d.
  congenital facial d.
  facial d.
  faciolingual-masticatory d.
  infantile d.
  spastic d.
diplococcus, pl. **diplococci**
  gram-positive d.
Diplococcus pneumoniae
diplogenesis
diploid
  d. distribution
  d. merogony
  d. spermatogonial stem cell
diploid/tetraploid mixoploidy
diploid/triploid mixoploidy
diploidy
diplomyelia
diplopagus
diplopia
  monocular d.
diplosomatia
diplosome
diplotene phase of meiosis
diploteratology
dipodia
dipole
Diprivan Injection
Diprolene
  D. AF Topical
  D. Glycol
dipropionate
  beclomethasone d.
  betamethasone d.
Diprosone Topical

NOTES

255

dipstick
    leukocyte esterase d.
    d. test
    urine d.
dipus
dipygus parasiticus
dipyridamole
    d. myocardial scintigraphy
    d. stress integrated backscatter
dipyrone
direct
    d. agglutination pregnancy (DAP)
    d. antiglobulin test (DAT)
    d. bilirubin
    d. Coombs test
    d. egg injection
    d. extension
    d. fluorescent antibody (DFA)
    d. fluorescent antigen (DFA)
    d. hyperbilirubinemia
    d. immunofluorescence (DIF)
    d. immunofluorescent staining
    d. immunohistochemical staining
    d. intraperitoneal injection (DIPI)
    d. intraperitoneal insemination
      (DIPI)
    d. laryngoscopy
    d. microscopy
    d. oocyte sperm transfer (DOST)
    d. oocyte transfer (DOT)
    d. ophthalmoscope
    d. orbital floor fracture
    d. stimulation
    d. stimulation of pancreas
    d. suicide risk (DSR)
    d. vision internal urethrotomy
      (DVIU)
    d. wet mount
directed
    d. amplification of minisatellite
      region DNA
    d. donor
Directigen Flu A
direction
    caudal d.
    pelvic d.
    rostral d.
directional coronary atherectomy (DCA)
directive
    advance d.
directly observed therapy (DOT)
direct-reacting bilirubin
dirithromycin
Dirofilaria
    D. immitis
    D. tenuis
dirty background
disability
    cognitive d.

    developmental d. (DD)
    intellectual d.
    language-based learning d.
    learning d. (LD)
    mobility d.
    motor d.
    National Joint Committee on
      Learning D.'s (NJCLD)
    neurodevelopmental d.
    neurologic d.
    nonverbal learning d. (NVLD)
    reading d.
    selective reading d.
    social-emotional learning d.
    specific reading d.
disabled
    orthopedically d.
disaccharidase deficiency
disaccharide intolerance
DiSala syndrome
Disalcid
disappearance
    fetal d.
disarray
    myofiber d.
    panlobar d.
disassociation
disaturated
    d. lecithin
    d. phosphatidylcholine
DISC
    Diagnostic Interview Schedule for
      Children
disc, disk
    choked d.
    dragged d.
    embryonic d.
    EMLA anesthetic d.
    glandular d.
    herniated d.
    d. herniation
    intervertebral d. (IVD)
    juvenile intervertebral d.
    Merkel tactile d.
    neovascularization of d. (NVD)
    optic d.
    placental d.
    tilted d.
    trilaminar embryonic d.
discernment
    gustatory d.
discharge
    adherent vaginal d.
    cheesy d.
    copious d.
    curdy d.
    epileptiform d.
    foul-smelling d.
    frothy d.

generalized epileptogenic d.
gleety d.
hypersynchronous d.
hypersynchrony of neural d.'s
interictal d.
leukorrheal d.
mucous d.
neural d.
newborn rehospitalization after
  early d.
nipple d.
partial epileptogenic d.
pathologic d.
physiologic d.
polyspike d.
pulsatile d.
purulent nasal d.
sharp-wave d.
urethral d.
vaginal d.

DisCide disinfecting towel
disciform keratitis
discitis (*var. of* diskitis)
discoid
d. eczema
d. lateral meniscus
d. lesion
d. lupus
d. rash

discoloration
heliotropic d.
prominent skin d.
skin d.

discomfort
internal d.
suprapubic d.

discontinuity
ossicular d.

discontinuous lesion
discoordinated uterine action
discoplacenta
discordance
atrioventricular d.
birth weight d.
twin birth weight d.

discordancy
growth d.

discordant
d. artery flow velocity waveform
d. twin growth
d. twins
d. umbilical arteries

DISC-R
Diagnostic Interview Schedule for
  Children-Revised
discrepancy
leg length d. (LLD)
size-date d.
discrepant
discrete
d. character
d. subaortic stenosis (DSS)
discrete-trial learning
discrimination
auditory d.
right-left d.
tactile d.
two-point d.
DISCUS
Dyskinesia Identification System:
  Condensed User Scale
discus
Advair D.
d. proligerus
Serevent D.
disease (*See also* syndrome)
ABO hemolytic d.
ABO hemolytic d. of the newborn
acid lipase deficiency d.
acid peptic d.
acquired heart d.
acute fulminant d.
acute graft versus host d.
  (AGVHD, aGVHD)
acute neuronopathic Gaucher d.
acute respiratory d. (ARD)
acyanotic congenital heart d.
Addison d.
adhesive d.
adult-onset polycystic kidney d.
adult polycystic d.
adult Refsum d.
advanced-stage d.
Albers-Schönberg d.
Albright d.
Alexander d.
allergic bowel d.
allogenic d.
alloimmune d.
Alpers d.
alpha-1 antitrypsin d.
Alzheimer d.
American Foundation of
  Urologic D.'s (AFUD)

D

NOTES

disease *(continued)*

Andersen d.
Anderson d.
Anderson-Fabry d.
anterior horn cell d.
antiglomerular basement membrane antibody d.
Antopol d.
aortic valve d.
Apert d.
Apert-Crouzon d.
Aran-Duchenne d.
arterial occlusive d.
arterial vascular d.
atypical Kawasaki d.
autoimmune d.
autosomal dominant medullary cystic kidney d. (ADMCKD)
autosomal dominant polycystic d.
autosomal dominant polycystic kidney d. (ADPKD)
autosomal recessive polycystic kidney d. (ARPKD)
Azorean d.
Baló d.
Barlow d.
Bassen-Kornzweig d.
Batten d.
Batten-Mayou d.
Beck d.
Becker d.
Béguez César d.
Behçet d.
Behr d.
benign breast d.
Berger renal d.
Best d.
Bielschowsky-Jansky d.
blistering d.
Bloodgood d.
Blount d.
Bornholm d.
Bourneville d.
Bourneville-Brissaud d.
Brailsford d.
breast d.
Brill d.
Brill-Zinsser d.
brittle-bone d.
bronze Schilder d.
Brown-Symmers d.
Bruton d.
bubble boy d.
Buhl d.
Byler d.
Caffey d.
Caffey-Kenny d.
Caisson d.
Calvé-Perthes d.

Canavan d.
Canavan-van Bogaert-Bertrand d.
Caroli d.
Castleman d.
cat-scratch d. (CSD)
cavitary lung d.
celiac d. (CD)
central core d.
central nervous system d.
central Recklinghausen d. (type II)
cerebrovascular d.
Chagas d.
Charcot d.
Charcot-Marie-Tooth d.
Charlevoix d.
Cheadle d.
cholestatic liver d.
cholesterol ester storage d. (CESD)
Christmas d.
chronic Gaucher d.
chronic granulomatous d. (CGD)
chronic lung d. (CLD)
chronic neuromuscular d. (CNMD)
chronic neuronopathic Gaucher d.
chronic pulmonary d.
chronic sickle cell lung d.
chronic vascular d.
chylomicron retention d.
cicatricial retinal d.
circling d.
classic celiac d.
Coats d.
cold agglutinin d.
cold hemagglutinin d.
collagen vascular d.
colorectal d.
communicable d.
complex congenital heart d.
congenital cardiac d.
congenital heart d. (CHD)
congenital hip d.
congestive heart d. (CHD)
connective tissue d.
Conradi d.
contractural arachnodactyly d.
cooperative study of sickle cell d. (CSSCD)
copper transport d.
Cori d.
Cori-Forbes d.
coronary artery d.
coronary heart d.
Cowden d.
cranial sclerosis with striated bone d.
Creutzfeldt-Jakob d. (CJD)
Crigler-Najjar d. (type I, II)
critical illness neuromuscular d.
Crohn d.

Crouzon d.
Csillag d.
Cushing d.
cyanotic congenital heart d.
  (CCHD)
cyanotic heart d.
cystic d. of the breast
cystic hydatid d.
cystic renal d.
cytomegalic inclusion d. (CID)
cytomegalovirus d.
Danlos d.
Darier d.
Darier-White d.
Dawson d.
Dejerine d.
Dejerine-Sottas d.
Dercum d.
De Vaal d.
developmental hip d.
Devic d.
diffuse cystic polycystic kidney d.
diffuse fibrocystic d.
diffuse mixed lymphocytic
  plasmacytic d.
Dimitri d.
disseminated adenovirus d.
distal tubal d.
diverticular d.
Dorfman-Chanarin d.
duct-dependent heart d.
Dukes d.
Duncan d.
Duroziez d.
early-onset d.
end-stage kidney d.
end-stage liver d.
end-stage renal d. (ESRD)
Erb-Goldflam d.
Erdheim d.
ethanolaminosis in glycogen-
  storage d.
Eulenburg d.
exanthematous d.
exertional reactive airway d.
extraabdominal organ system d.
extramammary Paget d.
Fabry d.
Fahr d.
Fairbank d.
familial Alzheimer d. (FAD)
familial Creutzfeldt-Jakob d.

Farber d.
Fazio-Londe d.
Feer d.
fetal heart d.
fibrocystic d.
fifth venereal d.
FIGO (stage I–IV) d.
Filatov-Dukes d.
first d.
Folling d.
Fong d.
Forbes d.
Fordyce d.
fourth venereal d.
Fox-Fordyce d.
free neuraminic acid storage d.
free sialic acid storage d.
Freiberg d.
Fukuyama d.
fulminant d.
gallbladder d.
Gambian d.
ganglioside storage d.
gastroesophageal reflux d. (GERD)
Gaucher d. (perinatal lethal type)
Gaucher d. (type 1–3)
gay bowel d.
Gee d.
Gee-Herter d.
Gee-Herter-Heubner d.
genetic d.
genetotrophic d.
genital ulcer d. (GUD)
gestational trophoblastic d. (GTD)
Gianotti d.
Gierke d.
Gilbert d.
Gitelman d.
glandular d.
Glanzmann d.
Glenárd d.
glomerular renal d.
glomerulocystic d.
glycogen storage d. (type Ia–Id,
  II–VII) (GSD)
Goldstein d.
graft versus host d. (GVHD)
granulomatous d.
Graves d.
Greenfield d.
group B streptococcus d.
Günther d.

D

NOTES

259

disease *(continued)*
  Hailey-Hailey d.
  Hallervorden-Spatz d.
  hand-foot-and-mouth d. (HFMD)
  Hand-Schüller-Christian d.
  Hansen d.
  Hartnup d.
  HbH d.
  heart d.
  Heller-Döhle d.
  helminthic d.
  hemoglobin C, M, S, SC, SD d.
  hemolytic d.
  hemorrhagic d.
  Henoch d.
  hepatic glycogen storage d.
  hepatobiliary d.
  hepatocellular d.
  hereditary d.
  heredoconstitutional d.
  heredodegenerative d.
  Hers d.
  Hirschsprung d.
  Hodgkin d.
  homologous d.
  hookworm d.
  horn cell d.
  Hünermann d.
  Huntington d. (HD)
  Hurler d.
  Hutinel d.
  hyaline membrane d. (HMD)
  hydatid d.
  hydrocephaloid d.
  hypophosphatemic bone d.
  hypothalamic d.
  iatrogenic Creutzfeldt-Jakob d.
  I-cell d.
  idiopathic peptic ulcer d.
  immune complex d.
  immunoproliferative small
    intestinal d.
  inclusion cell d.
  infantile Alexander d.
  infantile celiac d.
  infantile Gaucher d.
  infantile motor neuron d.
  infantile polycystic d.
  infantile polycystic kidney d.
    (IPKD)
  infantile Refsum d.
  infectious d.
  inflammatory bowel d. (IBD)
  International Classification of D.'s
    (ICD)
  International Society for the Study
    of Vulvar D. (ISSVD)
  interstitial lung d. (ILD)
  intranuclear hyaline inclusion d.
  intraperitoneal endometrial
    metastatic d.
  ischemic heart d. (IHD)
  isoimmune hemolytic d.
  Jaksch d.
  Jansky-Bielschowsky d.
  Jeune d.
  Joseph d.
  juvenile Alexander d.
  juvenile hereditary motor neuron d.
  juvenile neuronopathic Gaucher d.
  juvenile-onset inflammatory
    bowel d.
  juvenile-onset multisystem
    inflammatory d. (JOMID)
  juvenile Paget d.
  juvenile Parkinson d.
  juvenile rheumatic d.
  Kashin-Bek d.
  Kawasaki d. (KD)
  Keshan d.
  kidney d.
  Kienböck d.
  Kikuchi d.
  Kimmelstiel-Wilson d. (KW)
  kinky-hair d. (KHD)
  Kirner d.
  kissing d.
  Köhler bone d.
  Kok d.
  Kostmann d.
  Kozlowski d.
  Krabbe d. (KD)
  Kramer d.
  Krause d.
  Kufs d.
  Kugelberg-Welander d.
  kuru d.
  KW d.
  kwashiorkor d.
  Kyasanur Forest d.
  kyphoscoliotic heart d.
  Lafora body d.
  Langdon Down d.
  late hemorrhagic d.
  latent celiac d.
  Leber d.
  Legg-Calvé-Perthes d. (LCPD)
  Legg-Perthes d.
  Legionnaires d.
  Leigh d.
  Leiner d.
  Lesch-Nyhan d.
  Letterer-Siwe d.
  Lhermitte-Duclos d.
  Libman-Sacks d.
  linear IgA d.
  lipid storage d.
  Little d.

liver d.
Lobstein d.
Lou Gehrig d.
lower airway d.
Luft d.
Lyell d.
Lyme d.
lymphocyte-depleted Hodgkin d.
lymphocyte-predominant Hodgkin d.
lymphohematogenous d.
lymphoproliferative d.
lymphoproliferative/myeloproliferative d.
lysosomal storage d.
Machado-Joseph d.
mad cow d.
Maher d.
maple syrup urine d. (MSUD)
marble bone d.
Marburg d.
Marion d.
Maroteaux-Lamy d.
mast cell d.
maternal cyanotic heart d.
McArdle d.
MEB d.
medullary cystic d.
Melnick-Needles d.
Menetrier d.
Ménière d.
Merzbacher-Pelizaeus d.
metabolic bone d.
metastatic Crohn d. (MCD)
microvillus inclusion d. (MID)
Miege d.
Mikulicz d.
milk precipitin d.
Milroy d.
Minamata d.
minimal change d.
Minot d.
mitochondrial d.
mitral valve d.
mixed cellularity Hodgkin d.
mixed connective tissue d. (MCTD)
Moeller-Barlow d.
Mondor d.
Morquio d.
Morquio-Brailsford d.
Morquio-Ullrich d.
motor neuron d.

moyamoya d.
Mucha-Habermann d.
mucopolysaccharide storage d. (I–VIII)
multicentric Castleman d.
multicystic kidney d.
Münchausen d.
mycobacterial d.
N-acetylneuraminic acid storage d. (NSD)
nemaline rod d.
neonatal chest d.
neonatal cyanotic congenital heart d.
neonatal gonococcal d.
neonatal iron-storage d. (NISD)
neoplastic trophoblastic d.
neurodevelopmental d.
neurogenic hip d.
neurologic demyelinating d.
neuromuscular d.
neutral lipid storage d.
new variant Creutzfeldt-Jakob d. (nvCJD)
Nicolas-Favre d.
Niemann-Pick d. type A (NPA)
Niemann-Pick d. type B (NPB)
Niemann-Pick d. type C (NPC)
Niemann-Pick d. type D (NPD)
Niemann-Pick d. (type I, II)
nodular sclerosing Hodgkin d.
nodular thyroid d.
noncirrhotic ascitic d.
noncyanotic congenital heart d.
nonmetastatic gestational trophoblastic d. (NMGTD)
non-Rh D/non-ABO hemolytic d.
Norrbottnian Gaucher d.
Norrie d.
NYHA classification of heart d.
oasthouse urine d.
obliterative coronary artery d.
obstructive lung d.
obstructive respiratory d.
occlusive vascular d.
Oguchi d.
oligoarticular d.
Ollier d.
Oppenheim d.
optic nerve d.
oral Crohn d.
organic brain d.

D

NOTES

261

disease *(continued)*
organic heart d.
Osgood-Schlatter d. (OSD)
Osler-Weber-Rendu d. (OWRD)
Owren d.
OXPHOS d.
oxygen toxicity lung d.
Paas d.
Paget d.
Panner d.
parathyroid d.
parenchymal lung d.
Parkinson d.
pediatric infectious d. (PID)
pediatric spectrum of d. (PSD)
Pelizaeus-Merzbacher d. (PMD)
pelvic adhesive d. (PAD)
pelvic Castleman d.
pelvic inflammatory d. (PID)
peptic ulcer d. (PUD)
periodontal d.
peripheral arterial d.
peroxisomal d.
Perthes d.
Peyronie d.
Phocas d.
phytanic acid storage d.
ping-pong spread of d.
pink d.
Pityrosporum d.
placental site gestational
  trophoblastic d.
platelet-type von Willebrand d.
PNAC liver d.
polycystic kidney d. (PKD)
polycystic ovarian d. (PCOD)
polycystic ovary d. (PCOD, POD)
polycystic renal d.
polyglandular autoimmune d. (type
  I, II)
Pompe glycogen storage d. (type I,
  II)
Portuguese d.
postabortal pelvic inflammatory d.
postpartum pleuropulmonary and
  cardiac d.
postrheumatic valve d.
posttransplant lymphoproliferative d.
  (PTLD)
Pott d.
Potter d.
preinvasive cervical d.
premalignant d.
Pringle d.
prion d.
pseudo-Crouzon d.
pseudo-von Willebrand d.
psychosomatic d.
puff-of-smoke d.

pulmonary parenchymal d.
pulmonary valve d.
pulmonary venoocclusive d.
pulseless d.
Pyle d.
pyramidal tract d.
radiation-induced heart d. (RIHD)
Ramstedt d.
Raynaud d.
reactive airways d. (RAD)
Recklinghausen d. (type I, II)
Reclus d.
refractory Crohn d.
Refsum d.
rehabilitation among women with
  coronary artery d. (REACH)
renal cystic d.
Rendu-Osler-Weber d.
restrictive lung d.
restrictive respiratory d.
retroviral d.
Rh D d.
rheumatic heart d.
rheumatic valvular heart d.
Rh hemolytic d.
Rh isoimmune hemolytic d.
Rh d. of newborn
Ribbing d.
rickettsial d.
Riga-Fede d.
rippling muscle d.
Ritter d.
Rosai-Dorfman d.
Rotor d.
Roussy-Lévy d.
runt d.
Salla d.
Sandhoff d.
Sanfilippo d. A, B, C, D
Santavuori d.
Saunders d.
SC d.
Scheuermann d.
Schilder d.
Schimmelbusch d.
Schindler d.
Scholz d.
Schwartz-Jampel d.
sclerocystic d. of the ovary
sclerotic skin d.
SD d.
secondary moyamoya d.
secretory d.
Seitelberger d.
Sever d.
sexually transmitted d. (STD)
sialic acid storage d.
sickle cell d. (SCD)
sickle cell-hemoglobin C, D d.

sickle cell-thalassemia d.
silent celiac d.
silent pelvic inflammatory d.
silo filler's d.
Simmonds d.
sixth d.
skin d.
skin-eye-mouth d.
slapped cheek d.
Sly d.
sphingolipid storage d.
Spielmeyer-Vogt d.
spinocerebellar degenerative d.
sporadic Creutzfeldt-Jakob d.
Stargardt d.
startle d.
Steinert d.
Sticker d.
Still d.
storage d.
stress-related peptic ulcer d.
Strumpell-Lorrain d.
Sturge-Weber d.
subacute neuronopathic Gaucher d.
Swift d.
Takayasu d.
Tangier d.
Tarui d.
Taussig-Bing d.
Tay-Sachs d.
T-cell-mediated d.
Terson d.
Thiemann d.
thin basement membrane d.
  (TBMD)
third d.
Thomsen d.
thromboembolic d. (TED)
thrombohemolytic d.
thyroid d.
Tillaux d.
Tourette d.
transplant coronary artery d.
Trevor d.
triglyceride storage d.
trophoblastic neoplastic d.
tubulointerstitial d.
ulceroglandular d.
Ullrich d.
underlying d.
Underwood d.
Unverricht d.

Unverricht-Lundborg d.
upper motor neuron d.
Urbach-Wiethe d.
urea cycle d.
uveomeningitic d.
valvular heart d.
van Bogaert d.
vascular d.
venereal d. (VD)
venoocclusive d. (VOD)
Vogt-Spielmeyer d.
Volkmann d.
Voltolini d.
von Gierke glycogen storage d.
von Hippel-Lindau d.
von Recklinghausen d.
von Willebrand d. (type IIB, III)
Vrolik d.
Waldenström d.
Waldmann d.
Wegner d.
Weil d. (leptospirosis)
Weill d. (polyosteochondritis)
Werdnig-Hoffmann d. (type I–III)
Werlhof d.
Wernicke d.
wet lung d.
Whipple d.
Wilkie d.
Wilkins d.
Williams d.
Wilson d.
Winckel d.
Wolman d.
woolly hair d.
X-linked chronic granulomatous d.
X-linked dominant d.
X-linked recessive d.
Zellweger d.
Zinsser d.
Zuska d.
disease-free survival (DFS)
**disease-modifying antirheumatic drug
  (DMARD)**
disengagement
disequilibrium
    linkage d.
    d. syndrome
    test of linkage d.
    transmission d.
disfigurement
disgerminoma

NOTES

dish
- d. face
- insemination d.
- Uri-Two petri d.

DISIDA
- diisopropyl iminodiacetic acid

disiens
- *Prevotella d.*

disinfectant
- Sklar aseptic germicidal d.

disinfection
- vaginal d.

disinhibited

disinhibition

disintegrate

disintegration

disintegrin

Disipal

disk (*var. of* disc)

Diskhaler metered-dose inhaler

diskitis, discitis
- intervertebral d.

Diskus inhaler

dislocated
- d. elbow, bowed tibiae, scoliosis, deafness, cataract, microcephaly, mental retardation syndrome
- d. hip
- d. mandible
- d. patella
- d. testis

dislocating patella

dislocation
- atlantoaxial d.
- atlantooccipital d.
- C1 to C2 d.
- congenital d.
- congenital hip d. (CHD)
- elbow d.
- facet d.
- femoral head d.
- Galeazzi fracture d.
- habitual shoulder d.
- lens d.
- mandibular d.
- metacarpophalangeal d.
- Monteggia fracture d.
- multiple d.'s
- peroneal d.
- radial head d.
- subluxation d.
- teratologic d.
- testicular d.

dislodged tube

dismissing attachment

dismutase
- extracellular superoxide d.
- recombinant human superoxide d. (rhSOD)

dismutase-1
- superoxide d.-1

disodium
- cefotetan d.
- d. cromoglycate
- edetate calcium d.
- etidronate d.
- intermittent cyclical etidronate d.
- moxalactam d.
- ticarcillin d.

D isoimmunization

disomus

disomy
- uniparental d. (UPD)

disopyramide

disorder
- acid-base d.
- acquired platelet d.
- acute stress d. (ASD)
- adjustment d.
- affective d.
- aggressive conduct d.
- alcohol-related neurodevelopmental d. (ARND)
- alpha-chain d.
- amniotic fluid volume d.
- androgen excess d.
- anterior pituitary d.
- antisocial personality d. (ASPD)
- anxiety d.
- arousal d.
- arrest d.
- articulation d.
- Asperger d.
- athetotic movement d.
- attachment d.
- attention deficit d. (ADD)
- attention deficit hyperactivity d. (ADHD)
- autism spectrum d. (ASD)
- autistic d.
- autistic spectrum d. (ASD)
- autosomal chromosome d.
- autosomal dominant genetic d.
- autosomal recessive d.
- avoidant d.
- basal ganglia d.
- behavioral, anxiety, mood, and other types of d.'s (BAMO)
- binge eating d. (BED)
- bipolar d. (type 1, 2) (BPD)
- body dysmorphic d. (BDD)
- borderline personality d.
- brain d.
- breathing-related sleep d.
- cardiac rhythm d.
- carnitine transferase enzyme d.
- central auditory processing d. (CAPD)

cerebelloparenchymal d. (I–IV)
  (CPD)
Charcot-Marie-Tooth d.
childhood disintegrative d. (CDD)
children and adults with attention
  deficit d. (CHADD)
Children's Interview for
  Psychiatric D.'s (ChIPS)
choreoathetotic movement d.
chromosomal d.
chromosome 9p d.
chronic motor tic d.
chronic tic d. (CTD)
cluster B d.
coagulation d.
collagen vascular d.
communication d.
comorbid anxiety d.
complement deficiency d.
conduct d. (CD)
congenital hip d.
connective tissue d.
conversion d.
Copeland Symptom Checklist for
  Attention Deficit D.'s
cyclothymic d.
dancing eyes/dancing feet d.
dendritic cell-related d.
depigmentation d.
depressive d.
developmental d.
developmental coordination d.
  (DCD)
developmental language d. (DLD)
developmental pattern d.
Diagnostic and Statistical Manual
  of Mental D.'s - 4th Edition
  (DSM-IV)
disruptive behavior d.
dissociative d.
dominant d.
dysthymic d.
dystonic dyskinetic d.
eating d.
embryogenic induction d.
emotional d.
endocrine d.
epithelial d.
expressive language d.
factitious d.
familial bipolar mood d.
FAO d.

fetal iodine deficiency d. (FIDD)
food avoidance emotion d. (FAED)
fragile X d.
full-syndrome eating d.
functional gastrointestinal d.
gamma-chain d.
gamma-loop d.
gastrointestinal d.
gender identity d. (GID)
generalized anxiety d. (GAD)
genetic d.
glomerular d.
glycogen storage d.
GSH pathway d.
Hartnup d.
hematologic d.
hematopoietic d.
heme metabolism d.
hepatic parenchymal d.
heredodegenerative d.
histiocytic d.
human leukocyte antigen-
  associated d.
hyperkinetic d.
hypoactive sexual desire d.
hypothalamic-pituitary d.
impulse spectrum d.
infantile sialic acid storage d.
  (ISSD)
inherited bleeding d.
International Classification of
  Sleep D.'s (ICSD)
intersex d.
intestinal d.
kifafa seizure d.
lactation d.
language d.
late luteal phase dysphoric d.
  (LLPDD)
laterality d.
learning d.
leukorrheal d.
lipid metabolism d.
lipid storage d.
lower respiratory tract d.
lymphoproliferative d.
lysosomal enzyme d.
lysosomal storage d.
major depressive d. (MDD)
manic-depressive d.
mendelian genetic d.
metabolic d.

NOTES

disorder *(continued)*

metal metabolism d.
Methods for Epidemiology of
    Child and Adolescent Mental D.'s
    (MECA)
migrational d.
mixed receptive-expressive
    language d. (MRELD)
monogenic d.
mood d.
motility d.
multifactorial d.
multigenic d.
multiple complex developmental d.
    (MCDD)
muscle glycogen storage d.
musculoskeletal d.
myeloproliferative d.
myoneural junction d.
National Organization for
    Rare D.'s (NORD)
neural tube d.
neurocutaneous d.
neurologic d.
neurological d.
neuromuscular d.
neuronal migration d.
neuropsychiatric d.
nonmendelian d.
nonneoplastic epithelial d.
nonspecific esophageal motility d.
    (NEMD)
nonverbal perceptual-organization-
    output d.
obsessive-compulsive d. (OCD)
obsessive-compulsive personality d.
    (OCPD)
oppositional d.
oppositional defiant d. (ODD)
opsoclonus d.
orgasmic d.
ovarian d.
overanxious d. (OAD)
oxidation d.
pain d.
panic d.
paranoid personality d.
parathyroid d.
parkinsonian movement d.
partial-syndrome eating d.
periodic movement d.
peripheral auditory d.
peroxisomal congenital d.
peroxisome import d.
personality d. (PD)
pervasive developmental d. (PDD)
petit mal-like seizure d.
phonological d.
phytanic acid oxidation d.

pituitary d.
platelet d.
polygenic d.
polygenic/multifactorial d.
porphyrin metabolism d.
posterior pituitary d.
posttransplant lymphoproliferative d.
    (PTLD)
posttraumatic stress d. (PTSD)
Practice Parameters for the
    Assessment and Treatment of
    Anxiety D.'s
premenstrual dysphoric d. (PMDD)
primary bullous d.
Primary Care Evaluation of
    Mental D.'s (PRIME-MD)
primary immunodeficiency d.
protraction d.
pulmonary d.
purine metabolism d.
qualitative d.
quantitative d.
recessive d.
recurrent affective d.
REM sleep behavior d.
reproductive d.
Rett d.
rheumatologic d.
rhythmic movement d.
rumination d.
schizoaffective d.
schizoid personality d.
schizophreniform d.
Screen for Child Anxiety-Related
    Emotional D.'s (SCARED)
seasonal affective d. (SAD)
seizure d.
semantic-pragmatic d.
separation anxiety d. (SAD)
sex-linked d.
sexual arousal d.
sexual aversion d.
sexual pain d.
sickling d.
single-gene d.
sleep terror d.
sleep-wake transition d.
sleepwalking d.
social anxiety d.
somatization d.
somatoform d.
speech d.
stereotypical movement d.
storage d.
substance-induced psychotic d.
substance use d. (SUD)
symptomatic primary
    immunodeficiency d.

test of variables of attention
  deficit d.
thought d.
tic d.
Tourette d. (TD)
transient myeloproliferative d.
  (TMD)
transient tic d.
transport d.
triad of head tilt d.
unifactorial d.
urea cycle d.
urinary tract d.
vesicobullous d.
voice d.
vulvovaginal d.
Werdnig-Hoffmann d.
within-the-infant depressive d.
X-linked dominant d.
X-linked recessive d.
year 7 conduct d.
disordered renal acidification
disorganized
  d. behavior
  d. brainstem nuclei
Disotate
dispar
  Entamoeba d.
  Veillonella d.
dispenser
  Baxa oral d.
  Exacta-Med oral d.
DisperDose
DisperMox oral suspension
dispermy
disperse placenta
dispersion
  Taylor d.
displaced
  d. capitellum
  d. pinna
  d. supracondylar fracture
displacement
  d. implantation
  inner canthus d.
  lateral head d. (LHD)
  lateral sperm head d.
  rotatory d.
  uterine d.
display
  M-mode d.

disposable
  d. bottle
  d. 23-gauge butterfly needle
  d. wipe
disproportion
  cephalopelvic d. (CPD)
  congenital muscle fiber-type d.
    (CMFTD)
  craniofacial d.
  fetopelvic d.
  fiber-type d.
  limb d.
disproportionate dwarfism
disputed maternity
disruption
  anal sphincter d.
  bilateral corticobulbar d.
  inferior vena cava d.
  ossicular d.
  perineal sphincter d.
  surgical d.
  synchondrosis d.
  traumatic aortic d.
  tubular d.
disruptive
  d. behavior disorder
  D. Behavior Disorder Scale
  d. proboscis
dissecans
  osteochondritis d. (OCD)
dissecting aortic aneurysm
dissection
  aortic d.
  axillary node d.
  blunt and sharp d.
  carotid artery d.
  gauze d.
  groin d.
  inguinal-femoral node d.
  inverted-Y detrusor d.
  partial zona d. (PZD)
  pelvic node d.
  retroperitoneal d.
  selective inguinal node d.
  sharp d.
  traumatic d.
dissector
  Endo-Assist cutting d.
  Kittner d.
  Maryland d.
  plasma d.

NOTES

D

dissector *(continued)*
    Polaris reusable d.
    spud d.
disseminata
    dermatofibrosis lenticularis d.
disseminated
    d. adenovirus disease
    d. candidiasis
    d. CMV
    d. coccidioidomycosis
    d. gonococcal infection
    d. gonorrhea
    d. granuloma
    d. granulomatous vasculitis
    d. hemangiomatosis
    d. herpes infection
    d. histoplasmosis
    d. intravascular coagulation (DIC)
    d. intravascular coagulation state
    d. intravascular coagulopathy (DIC)
    d. lupus erythematosus
    d. *Mycobacterium avium complex* (DMAC)
    d. sclerosis
    d. tuberculosis
    d. varicella
dissemination
    iatrogenic d.
    peritoneal d.
disseminatus
    lupus erythematosus d.
dissimilar twins
dissociate
dissociated
    d. motor development
    d. movement
dissociation
    albuminocytologic d.
    atrioventricular d.
    d. constant
    craniofacial d.
    electroclinical d.
    electromechanical d. (EMD)
    hemoglobin-oxygen d.
    immune complex d. (ICD)
dissociative
    d. disorder
    D. Experience Scale (DES)
    d. phenomenon
    d. symptom
dissolution of clot formation
dissymmetry
distal
    d. arthrogryposis, hypopituitarism, mental retardation, facial anomalies syndrome
    d. arthrogryposis, mental retardation, characteristic facies syndrome

    d. arthrogryposis (type I, II)
    d. claviclectomy
    d. collecting duct
    d. dilated bowel segment resection
    d. esophageal atresia
    d. esophageal pH monitoring
    d. femoral skeletal traction
    d. humeral physial fracture
    d. ileum
    d. intestinal obstruction
    d. intestinal obstruction syndrome (DIOS)
    d. jejunum
    d. limb deficiency-mental retardation syndrome
    d. occlusion
    d. onycholysis
    d. RTA
    d. sacral defect
    d. shaft hypospadias
    d. splenorenal shunt
    d. symmetric sensorimotor neuropathy
    d. tongue bud
    d. transverse limb defects, mental retardation, spasticity syndrome
    d. trichorrhexis nodosa
    d. triradius
    d. tubal disease
    d. tubal microsurgery
    d. tubal obstruction
    d. tuft
    d. vagina
distamycin A/4-6-diamidino-2-phenylindole (DA-DAPI, DA/DAPI)
distance
    genetic d.
    intercapillary d.
    (Mustardé ratio) inner canthal distance/interpupillary d. (ICD/IPD)
    source-to-axis d. (SAD)
    source-to-skin d. (SSD)
    d. vision
distasonis
    Bacteroides d.
distemper
    canine d.
distended
    d. abdomen
    d. capillary
distending pressure
distensae
    striae cutis d.
distention, distension
    abdominal d.
    centrizonal sinusoidal d.
    gaseous d.
    jugulovenous d. (JVD)
    lacrimal sac d.

distichiasis
distigmine bromide
distortion
    body-image d.
    lobular d.
    segregation d.
    tubal d.
distractibility
distractible
    hyperactive d.
distraction
distress
    fetal d.
    iatrogenic fetal d.
    neonatal d.
    psychological d.
    respiratory d.
    transient fetal d.
distribution
    butterfly d.
    Christmas tree d.
    dermatomal d.
    diploid d.
    gaussian d.
    malar d.
    d. pattern
    tetraploid d.
    trigeminal nerve d.
    watershed d.
distributive shock
disturbance
    architectural d.
    d. of attachment
    behavioral d.
    coagulation d.
    electrolyte d.
    feeding d.
    growth d.
    immunologic d.
    menstrual d.
    mental d.
    ovulatory d.
    serious emotional d. (SED)
    sleep d.
    thought d.
    visual d.
disturbed
    emotionally d.
    d. equilibrium syndrome
disulfiduria
    mercaptolactate-cysteine d. (MCDU)
disulfiram

disuse
    d. amblyopia
    d. muscular atrophy
    d. syndrome
DIT
    diiodotyrosine
dithiothreitol
Ditropan XL
Diuchlor H
Diulo
Diurese-R
diuresis
    alkaline d.
    glycosuric d.
    osmotic d.
    solute d.
diuretic
    d. challenge
    loop d.
    mercurial d.
    potassium-sparing d.
    d. renography
    thiazide d.
Diuril
diurnal
    d. enuresis
    d. micturition
    d. rhythm
diurnus
    pavor d.
Diva
    D. laparoscopic morcellator
    D. laparoscopic morcellator device
divalproex sodium
divergens
    Babesia d.
divergent
    d. fetal growth
    d. rectus muscle
    d. strabismus
diversion
    bilateral ureteral d.
    biliopancreatic d.
    colonic conduit d.
    continent supravesical bowel urinary d.
    ileal loop d.
    ileocecal conduit d.
    Koch pouch d.
    loop d.
    Mainz pouch d.

NOTES

D

diversion *(continued)*
    partial external biliary d. (PEBD)
    urinary d.
diversity
    genetic d.
diversus
    Citrobacter d.
diverticula (*pl. of* diverticulum)
diverticular disease
diverticulectomy
    urethral d.
diverticulitis
    suburethral d.
diverticulosis
diverticulum, pl. **diverticula**
    bladder d.
    congenital d.
    Hutch d.
    Meckel d.
    Nuck d.
    pharyngeal d.
    porencephalic d.
    tubal d.
    urethral d.
    urinary d.
diverting
    d. colostomy
    d. colostomy with pull-through
      procedure
    d. enterostomy
diving reflex
division
    cell d.
    cellular d.
    equatorial d.
    meiotic d.
    miotic d.
    d. of pancreatic ring
    premature centromere d.
    transcervical d.
    urethral plate d.
divisum
    pancreas d.
divorce
Dix-Hallpike maneuver
dizygotic twin
dizygous
dizziness
    orthostatic d.
DKA
    diabetic ketoacidosis
DL$_{co}$
    diffusing capacity of lung for carbon
      monoxide
DLD
    developmental language disorder
DLIF
    digoxin-like immunoreactive factor

DM
    dermatomyositis
    diabetes mellitus (type 1, 2)
      Diabetic Tussin DM
      Fenesin DM
      Genatuss DM
      Guiatuss DM
      Halotussin DM
      Hold DM
      Koffex DM
      Mytussin DM
      Poly-Histine DM
      Silphen DM
      Siltussin DM
      Tolu-Sed DM
DMAC
    disseminated *Mycobacterium avium*
      complex
DMARD
    disease-modifying antirheumatic drug
DMD
    Duchenne de Boulogne muscular
      dystrophy
    Duchenne muscular dystrophy
    dystonia musculorum deformans
DMD/BMD
    Duchenne de Boulogne muscular
      dystrophy/Becker muscular dystrophy
    Duchenne muscular dystrophy/Becker
      muscular dystrophy
      DMD/BMD gene
DMIST
    digital mammographic imaging screening
      trial
D-mosaic blood type
DMP-266
DMPA
    depomedroxyprogesterone acetate
    depot medroxyprogesterone acetate
DMPM
    dermatomyositis/polymyositis
DMQ
    developmental motor quotient
      fine motor total DMQ
      gross motor total DMQ
DMS
    diffuse mesangial sclerosis
DMSO
    dimethyl sulfoxide
DNA
    deoxyribonucleic acid
      DNA amplification
      DNA amplification fingerprinting
      DNA analysis
      branched DNA
      chloroplast DNA
      DNA clone
      DNA cloning
      complementary DNA (cDNA)

DNA copy
DNA diagnostics
directed amplification of
  minisatellite region DNA
DNA dual color probe
exogenous DNA
genomic DNA
heterochromatic DNA
heteroduplex DNA
homoduplex DNA
DNA hybridization
DNA hybridization assay
DNA index
kinetoplast DNA
DNA library
DNA ligase
DNA marker
mitochondrial DNA (mtDNA)
DNA nucleotidylexotransferase
DNA nucleotidyltransferase
plasmid DNA
DNA ploidy
DNA polymerase
DNA probe test
randomly amplified polymorphic
  DNA
recombinant DNA
repetitive DNA
DNA replication
satellite DNA
DNA sequence
synthetic DNA
DNA testing
DNA typing
DNA-based testing
DNA-directed RNA polymerase
DNAse, DNase
  deoxyribonuclease
  DNAse B factor
  human recombinant DNase
DNCB
  dinitrochlorobenzene
  DNCB therapy
DNS
  delayed neuropsychological sequela
Doan's
  Extra Strength D.
  Original D.
DOB
  date of birth

Dobbhoff
  D. catheter
  D. nasogastric feeding tube
DOBI
  dynamic optical breast imaging system
Dobrava virus
dobutamine hydrochloride
Dobutrex
DOC
  deoxycorticosterone
  desoxycorticosterone
docetaxel
docosahexaenoic acid (DHA)
docosapentaenoic acid
doctor
  medical d. (MD)
  d. of medicine
docusate
  d. calcium
  d. and casanthranol
  sodium d.
  d. sodium
Döderlein
  D. bacillus
  D. hysterectomy technique
  D. method
  D. method of vaginal hysterectomy
  D. roll-flap operation
dog
  d. bite
  d. tick
dogma
  central d.
Döhle body
DOL
  day of life
Dolacet
dolasetron
dolichocephalic
dolichocephaly
dolichopellic, dolichopelvic
dolichostenomelia
doll's
  d. eye maneuver
  d. eye phenomenon
  d. eye reflex
  d. eye response
  d. eyes
  d. head maneuver
Dolobid
Dolophine

D

NOTES

Dolphin

D. hysteroscopic fluid management system

D. instrument

domain

adaptive d.

cognitive d.

communication d.

fine motor d.

gross motor d.

hyperactivity/impulsivity d.

inattention d.

language d.

perceptual d.

Revised Gesell Language D.

self-help d.

shedding d.

social-emotional d.

Domeboro

Otic D.

D. solution

dome cell

domestic

d. abuse

d. violence

d. violence evaluation

d. violence treatment

domesticum

Pyronema d.

domiciliary monitoring

dominance

eye d.

incomplete d.

thromboxane d.

d. variance

dominant

autosomal d.

d. choroidal sclerosis

d. disorder

d. Dovne honeycomb retinal degeneration

d. dystrophic epidermolysis bullosa

d. follicle

d. gene

d. hand

d. inheritance

d. lethal trait

d. recurrent ataxia

X-linked d. (XLD)

dominantly

d. hyperactive

d. hyperactive impulsive type

Dominic-R questionnaire

domino connector

domperidone

Donahue syndrome

DONALD

Dortmund Nutritional and Anthropometrical Longitudinally Designed

DONALD study

Donald-Fothergill operation

Donald procedure

Donath-Landsteiner cold hemolysin

donation

autologous blood d.

egg d.

embryo d.

oocyte d.

ovum d.

sperm d.

Done nomogram

dong quai

Donnagel

Donnan equilibrium

Donna-Sed

Donnatal

Donnez device

Donohue syndrome

donor

artificial insemination d. (AID)

artificial insemination by d. (AID)

cadaveric d.

directed d.

egg d.

d. egg

embryo d.

d. insemination (DI)

intrafamilial genoidentical d.

oocyte d.

d. oocyte

d. oocyte transfer

sperm d.

d. sperm

d. T cell

d. twin

d. venous graft

donor-specific blood

Donovan body

donovanosis

DOOR

deafness, onychoosteodystrophy, mental retardation

DOOR syndrome

DOP

degenerate oligonucleotide primer

dopa, DOPA, Dopa

dihydroxyphenylalanine

L-dopa

levodopa

Dopamet

dopamine

d. hydrochloride

d. receptor agonist

dopaminergic
>   d. agonist
>   d. system

dopa-responsive dystonia (DRD)

Dopcord recorder

Doppler
>   Acuson color D.
>   color-coded duplex D.
>   color-flow D.
>   continuous wave D.
>   2D D.
>   D. echocardiography
>   D. effect
>   D. evaluation
>   FetalPulse Plus fetal D.
>   D. flow
>   D. flow study
>   D. flow-velocity waveform
>   Imex Pocket-Dop OB D.
>   D. myocardial performance index
>   D. principle
>   D. probe
>   pulsed wave D.
>   range-gated D. (RGD)
>   D. scanning
>   D. shift
>   D. shift spectra
>   spectral D.
>   transcranial D. (TCD)
>   D. ultrasonography
>   D. ultrasound
>   D. velocimetry

Doppler-guided ligation

Dopplex

Dopram

Doptone fetal stethoscope

d'orange
>   peau d.

Dorcol

Dorfman-Chanarin disease

dormant basket cell hypothesis

Dormin Oral

dornase alfa

Dorros infusion and probing catheter

dorsal
>   d. birthing position
>   d. bunion
>   d. chordee
>   d. extension splint
>   d. hood
>   d. kyphosis
>   d. lithotomy position

>   d. myeloschisis
>   d. penile curvature
>   d. penile nerve block (DPNB)
>   d. radiculitis
>   d. rhizotomy
>   d. supine position

dorsalis
>   d. pedis
>   d. pedis pulse
>   tabes d.

dorsiflexion

dorsogluteal

dorsum, pl. **dorsa**
>   d. linguae

Dortmund Nutritional and Anthropometrical Longitudinally Designed (DONALD)

DORV
>   double-outlet right ventricle

Doryx

DOS
>   dysosteosclerosis
>   DOS Softgel

dosage
>   antepartum d.

dosage-sensitive sex reversal (DSS)

dose, dosage
>   average radiation d.
>   bolus d.
>   cancericidal d.
>   central axis depth d.
>   depth d.
>   gene d.
>   maximal permissible d.
>   minimal effective d. (MED)
>   minimum lethal d. (MLD)
>   physiologic replacement d.
>   priming d.
>   radiation d.
>   radiation absorbed d. (rad)
>   rescue d.

dosing
>   extended internal d.

DOST
>   direct oocyte sperm transfer

Dostinex

DOT
>   directly observed therapy
>   direct oocyte transfer

dot
>   black d.
>   d. ELISA test

NOTES

dot (*continued*)
    glistening d.
    d. immunobinding assay (DIA)
    Mittendorf d.
    Schüffner d.
dot-blot
    d.-b. HPV hybridization test
    d.-b. hybridization
    d.-b. procedure
    d.-b. technique
dothiepin
double
    d. aortic arch (DAA)
    d. breech presentation
    d. cell
    d. collecting system
    d. cortex
    d. cortex syndrome
    d. cortin
    d. depression
    d. diapers
    d. diaper treatment
    d. elevator palsy
    d. epiphyses
    d. footling presentation
    d. gloving
    d. helix
    d. hemiplegia
    d. hump sign of an enterocele
    d. intussusception
    d. lip
    d. pylorus
    d. ring
    d. setup examination
    d. strength (XX)
    d. thyroid ectopia
    d. ureter
    d. uterus
    d. vacuolization
double-balloon
    d.-b. catheter
    d.-b. device
double-bank
    d.-b. bili lights
    d.-b. phototherapy
double-barrel colostomy
double-blanket phototherapy
double-bleb sign
double-blind study
double-bubble
    d.-b. flushing reservoir
    d.-b. gas shadow
    d.-b. isolette
    d.-b. sign
    d.-b. ventriculoperitoneal shunt
double-catheter technique
double-contrast CT scan
Doublecortin
double-focus tube

double-freeze technique
double-inlet
    d.-i. left ventricle
    d.-i. right ventricle
double-insulated incubator
double-J stent
double-lumen
    d.-l. airway
    d.-l. catheter
    d.-l. venovenous ECMO
double-lung transplantation
double-mouthed uterus
double-onlay preputial flap
double-orifice mitral valve
double-outlet
    d.-o. right ventricle (DORV)
    d.-o. ventricle
double-sandwich ELISA
double-switch procedure
double-tooth tenaculum
double-tract sign
double-umbrella device
double-volume exchange transfusion
double-walled
    d.-w. bubble Isolette
    d.-w. incubator
doubling time
douche
    fan d.
    Fritsch d.
    iodine d.
    Massengill d.
    maternal d.
    povidone-iodine d.
    vaginal d.
    yogurt d.
douching
    postcoital d.
    vinegar d.
doughnut pessary
doughnut-shaped mass
doughy
    d. mass
    d. skin
Douglas
    D. abscess
    D. bag
    cul-de-sac of D.
    D. cul-de-sac
    D. mechanism
    D. method
    D. pouch
    semilunar fold of D.
    D. spontaneous evolution
douglascele
doula
dovetail sign
dowager's hump

Dowling-Meara epidermolysis bullosa simplex
down
    clamped d.
    morbus D.
    D. stigmata
    strain d.
    D. syndrome
    D. syndrome child (DSC)
    D. syndrome growth chart
    testes d.
downbeat nystagmus
Downes score
downgaze
    tonic d.
downregulate
downregulation regimen
down slant
downslanting
    d. eyes
    d. palpebral fissure
downsloping palpebral fissure
downstream
downturned mouth
downward gaze
doxacurium chloride
doxapram hydrochloride
doxazosin
doxepin
Doxil
doxorubicin hydrochloride
Doxy-100
Doxycin
doxycycline
    d. hyclate
    d. monohydrate
doxylamine
Doxy Oral
Doxytec
Doyen vaginal hysterectomy
doylei
    Campylobacter jejuni subspecies *d.*
Doyle operation
Dpd
    deoxypyridinoline
D-penicillamine
DPI
    dry powder inhaler
    dynamic pulmonary imaging
DP-II
    Developmental Profile-II

DPL
    diagnostic peritoneal lavage
DPNB
    dorsal penile nerve block
DPPC
    dipalmitoyl phosphatidylcholine
DPSS
    Department of Public Social Services
DPT
    dehydration, poisoning, trauma
    diphtheria, pertussis, tetanus
DQ
    developmental quotient
DR
    human lymphocyte antigen-locus DR
dracunculiasis
Dracunculus medinensis
Dräger thermal gel mattress
dragged disc
dragging of retina
dragon
    d. pyelogram
    d. sign
drain
    butterfly d.
    fluted d.
    Freyer suprapubic d.
    Jackson-Pratt d.
    Penrose d.
    peritoneal d.
    retroperitoneal d.
    Shirley wound d.
drainage
    anomalous pulmonary venous d.
    chest tube d.
    closed d.
    coffee-grounds d.
    felon d.
    hematoma d.
    incision and d. (I&D)
    intercostal d.
    d., irrigation, fibrinolytic therapy (DRIFT)
    lymphatic d.
    lymph node d.
    mastoid d.
    mediastinal air d.
    nasogastric d.
    open flap d.
    open pericardial d.
    percutaneous catheter d.

D

NOTES

drainage *(continued)*
    postural d. (PD)
    primary peritoneal d. (PPD)
    d. procedure
    pulmonary venous d.
    suction d.
    syringopleural d.
    syringosubarachnoid d.
    d. system
    thoracic duct d.
    in utero d.
    vaginal d.
    waterseal d.
draining otitis media
drain-pipe urethra
Dramamine II
Drapanas mesocaval shunt
drape
    barrier laparoscopy d.
    Ioban d.
    iodophor-impregnated adhesive d.
Drash syndrome
draught
    Black D.
Draw-a-Person Test
drawing
    human figure d.
    line d.
DRC
    digitorenocerebral syndrome
DRD
    dopa-responsive dystonia
    dystrophia retinae pigmentosa-dysostosis
    DRD syndrome
Drenison
dressing
    alginate wound d.
    AlgiSite d.
    Algosteril d.
    Allevyn d.
    Aquacel d.
    Aquasorb d.
    Biobrane/HF d.
    Biopatch d.
    BlisterFilm d.
    BreakAway d.
    Carrasyn Hydrogel d.
    ClearSite hydrogauze d.
    Coban d.
    CollaCote d.
    compressive d.
    Conformant d.
    Coverlet d.
    Curaderm d.
    Curafil d.
    Curagel Hydrogel d.
    Curasorb calcium alginate d.
    Exuderm d.
    d. forceps

    Fuller shield rectal d.
    FyBron calcium alginate d.
    hydrogel d.
    Iodosorb absorptive d.
    Kalginate d.
    Nu Gauze d.
    Nu-Gel d.
    occlusive d.
    PanoPlex d.
    PolyMem d.
    polyurethane d.
    SignaDRESS d.
    Silon wound d.
    StrataSorb d.
    SurePress d.
    SureSite d.
    THINsite d.
    Transorbent d.
    Veingard d.
    Viasorb d.
Drews forceps
Drew-Smythe catheter
Dri-Dot
    Monosticon D.-D.
    Prognosticon D.-D.
drier
    Savant Speed-Vac d.
DRIFT
    drainage, irrigation, fibrinolytic therapy
drift
    genetic d.
    pure random d.
drill
    bladder retraining d.
drilling
    zona d. (ZD)
drink
    Boost nutritional d.
Drinker respirator
drinking
    binge d.
    social d.
drip
    continuous gastric d. (CGD)
    continuous intravenous oxytocin d.
    intravenous d. (IVD)
    postnasal d.
    sterile water gastric d. (SWGD)
dripping
    candle d.
Dripps-American Society of Anesthesiologists classification
Drisdol
Dristan Sinus Caplets
drive
    central respiratory d.
    respiratory d.
    d. for thinness
    ventilatory d.

driver
    Laurus ND-260 needle d.
driving
    Mothers Against Drunk D.
    (MADD)
Drize
droloxifene
dromedary hump
dronabinol
drooling
drooping
    d. lily appearance
    d. lily appearance of lower
    collecting system
drop
    d. attack
    Auro Ear D.'s
    Ayr saline d.'s
    Coly-Mycin S Otic D.
    E-R-O Ear D.'s
    foot d.
    head d.
    Mallazine Eye D.
    methylcellulose d.'s
    Murine Ear D.'s
    Mylicon d.'s
    parasympathomimetic d.
    Phazyme infant d.'s
    Polytrim eye d.'s
    Robitussin-DM infant d.'s
    Rondec D.'s
    saline nose d.'s
    d. seizure
    silver nitrate d.'s
    sympatholytic d.
    Triaminic Oral Infant D.'s
    vitamin C d.'s
droperidol and fentanyl
droplet
    cytoplasmic lipid d. (CLD)
    d. infection
dropout
    capillary d.
    d. of capillary end loop
    echo d.
dropped beat
dropsy
    d. of the fetus
    iatrogenic preterm birth maternal d.
Drosophila
    D. melanogaster diaphanous gene
    D. mutation

drospirenone/ethinyl estradiol
Drotic Otic
drowning
    cold water near d.
    dry d.
    freshwater near d.
    near d.
    saltwater near d.
    very cold water near d.
    warm water near d.
    wet d.
drowsiness
Droxia Hydrea
DRPLA
    dentatorubral-pallidoluysian atrophy
    hereditary DRPLA
DRSP
    drug-resistant *Streptococcus pneumoniae*
drug
    acetylcysteine d.
    d. addiction
    adrenergic d.
    alcohol and other d.'s (AOD)
    alcohol, tobacco, and other d.'s
    (ATOD)
    anthelminthic d.
    antianxiety d.
    antibacterial d.
    antibiotic d.
    anticholinergic d.
    anticonvulsant d.
    antidepressant d.
    antiepileptic d. (AED)
    antifungal d.
    antihistamine d.
    antihypertensive d.
    antimalarial d.
    antineoplastic d.
    antipsychotic d.
    antispastic d.
    antithyroid d.
    anxiolytic d.
    d. baby
    bactericidal d.
    bacteriostatic d.
    beta-adrenergic d.
    beta-lactamase-stable d.
    bronchodilator d.
    cell cycle-nonspecific d.
    cell cycle-specific d.
    cholinergic d.

D

NOTES

drug *(continued)*
    disease-modifying antirheumatic d. (DMARD)
    d. fever
    gateway d.
    d. holiday
    illicit d.
    immunosuppressive d.
    d. ingestion
    intramuscular d.
    intranasal d.
    intravenous d.
    narcotic d.
    neuroleptic d.
    nonestrogen d.
    nonsteroidal antiinflammatory d. (NSAID)
    orphan d.
    ototoxic d.
    over-the-counter d.
    ovulation-inducing d.
    parasympatholytic d.
    prenatally exposed to d.'s (PED)
    prescription d.
    d. prophylaxis
    psychedelic d.
    psychiatric d.
    psychoactive d.
    psychotropic d. (PTD)
    d. reaction pruritus
    recreational d.
    d. resistant
    social d.
    stimulant d.
    tocolytic d.
    tranquilizer d.
drug-depressed infant
drug-induced
    d.-i. acne
    d.-i. diabetes
    d.-i. dystonia
    d.-i. gynecomastia
    d.-i. hematuria
    d.-i. hemolytic anemia
    d.-i. hirsutism
    d.-i. neonatal goiter
    d.-i. neutropenia
    d.-i. pancreatitis
    d.-i. rash
    d.-i. systemic lupus erythematosus
drug-related
    d.-r. anaphylaxis
    d.-r. purpura
drug-resistant
    d.-r. *Streptococcus pneumoniae* (DRSP)
    d.-r. tuberculosis
drunk
drusen

dry
    d. birth
    d. chemical burn
    d. drowning
    d. eye
    d. eye syndrome
    d. labor
    d. mucous membrane
    d. pericarditis
    d. pleurisy
    d. powder inhaler (DPI)
    d. skin
    d. socket
    d. vagina
    d. weight
Drysol
DS
    diencephalic syndrome
        Bactrim DS
        Septra DS
        Sulfatrim DS
        Tolectin DS
        WinRho DS
DSC
    Down syndrome child
        Parafon Forte DSC
DSM
    degradable starch microsphere
DSM-IV
    Diagnostic and Statistical Manual of Mental Disorders - 4th Edition
1D sodium dodecyl sulfate gel
DSPS
    delayed sleep phase syndrome
DSR
    direct suicide risk
DSRCT
    desmoplastic small round cell tumor
D-S-S
DSS
    discrete subaortic stenosis
    dosage-sensitive sex reversal
DST
    dexamethasone suppression testing
D-stix
    Dextrostix
DT
    diphtheria toxin
D-Tach removal needle
D-TGA
    D-transposition of great arteries
DTH
    delayed-type hypersensitivity
DTIC
    dimethyl-triazeno-imidazole carboxamide
        DTIC-Dome
DTIC-Dome
DTM
    dermatophyte test medium

dTMP
deoxythymidylic acid
DTP
diphtheria, tetanus, pertussis vaccine
diphtheria, tetanus toxoid, pertussis
DTP vaccine
DTPA
diethylenetriaminepentaacetic acid
DTPA radionuclide scan
DTPa
diphtheria, tetanus, acellular pertussis
vaccine
DTPw
diphtheria, tetanus toxoid, whole-cell
pertussis
DTR
deep tendon reflex
D-transposition
dextrotransposition
D-transposition of great arteries
(D-TGA)
DTS
differential temperature sensor
Du
blood group D variant equivalent to Rh-
negative
Du Pen epidural catheter
Du variant blood type
Duac topical gel
dual-energy
d.-e. photon absorptiometry
d.-e. x-ray
d.-e. x-ray absorptiometry (DEXA,
DXA)
d.-e. x-ray absorptiometry scan
dual nucleoside analog reverse
transcriptase inhibitor
Dual-Pak
Monistat D.-P.
dual-photon absorptiometry
Duane
D. anomaly
D. retraction syndrome
Duarte variant galactosemia
DUB
dysfunctional uterine bleeding
Dubin-Johnson syndrome
dublin
Salmonella d.
dubliniensis
Candida d.
Dubois abscess

Dubowitz
D. evaluation
D. examination
neonatal maturity classification
of D.
D. Neurological Assessment
D. Scale for Infant Maturity
D. score
D. syndrome
Dubowitz/Ballard Exam for Gestational
Age
Duchenne
D. de Boulogne muscular
dystrophy (DMD)
D. de Boulogne muscular
dystrophy/Becker muscular
dystrophy (DMD/BMD)
D. muscular dystrophy (DMD)
D. muscular dystrophy/Becker
muscular dystrophy (DMD/BMD)
D. myodystrophy
D. palsy
D. paralysis
D. syndrome
D. type pseudohypertrophic
progressive muscular dystrophy
Duchenne-Griesinger syndrome
duckbill speculum
Duckett
D. procedure
D. transverse preputial island flap
duckfoot, pl. **duckfeet**
Ducrey bacillus
ducreyi
Haemophilus d.
duct
allantoic d.
apocrine d.
Bartholin d.
bile d.
blocked d.
branchial d.'s
cloacal d.
common hepatic d.
congenital atresia of bile d.
congenital obstruction of
nasolacrimal d.
cowperian d.
d. of Cuvier
cystic dilation of intrahepatic
bile d.
distal collecting d.

NOTES

D

duct *(continued)*
    eccrine sweat d.
    d. ectasia
    ejaculatory d.
    focally dilated d.
    follicular d.
    Gartner d.
    gartnerian d.
    genital d.
    gland d.
    greater vestibular gland d.
    imperforate nasolacrimal d.
    inspissated d.
    intrahepatic bile d.
    lacrimal d.
    lactiferous d.
    male genital d.
    mesonephric d.
    metanephric d.
    minor vestibular gland d.
    müllerian d.
    nasolacrimal d.
    omphalomesenteric d.
    paramesonephric d.
    paraurethral d.
    patent omphalomesenteric d.
    paucity of interlobular bile d.
    (PILBD)
    pilosebaceous d.
    Reichel cloacal d.
    sebaceous d.
    Skene d.
    solitary dilated d.
    stenotic nasolacrimal d.
    Stensen d.
    sweat d.
    thyroglossal d.
    vanishing bile d.
    vestibular d.
    vitelline d.
    vitellointestinal d.
    wolffian d.
ductal
    d. adenoma
    d. carcinoma
    d. carcinoma in situ (DCIS)
    d. ectasia
    d. hyperplasia
    d. inflammation
    d. obstruction
    d. papilloma
    d. plate malformation
    d. shunt
    d. shunting
ductal-dependent
    d.-d. lesion
    d.-d. pulmonary blood flow
duct-dependent
    d.-d. heart disease

    d.-d. pulmonary blood flow
    d.-d. pulmonary circulation
    d.-d. systemic circulation
DuctOcclud coil
ductule
    bile d.
ductuli efferentia
ductus, pl. **ductus**
    d. arteriosus (DA)
    d. arteriosus persistens
    bilateral d.
    d. choledochus
    d. closure
    d. venosus
Duffy
    D. antigen
    D. system
Dufourmentel transpostion flap technique
Duhamel procedure
Dührssen incision
Dukes
    D. classification
    D. disease
Dulbecco
    D. medium
    D. phosphate buffered saline
Dulcolax
Dull-C
dullness
    absolute cardiac d.
    area of cardiac d. (ACD)
    flank d.
    d. to percussion
    shifting d.
    span of liver d.
3D ultrasound
dumbbell tumor
dummy
    d. source
    d. spacer
Dumontpallier pessary
dumping syndrome
Duncan
    D. curette
    D. disease
    D. folds
    D. knot
    D. mechanism
    D. mechanism of placental delivery
    D. placenta
    D. position
    D. presentation
    D. slipknot
    D. syndrome
    D. test
Dunedin
    D. birth cohort
    D. longitudinal study

duodenal
>d. atresia
>d. diaphragm
>d. duplication
>d. fluid
>d. ileus
>d. obstruction
>d. resection
>d. stenosis
>d. ulcer
>d. vacuolization

duodenale
>*Ancylostoma d.*

duodenitis
duodenum
>Z-shaped d.

DuoFilm
Duosol
Duotrate
dup
>duplication
>dup (10p)/del (10q) syndrome
>dup (1p)–(22p) syndrome
>dup (9q)/del(9p) syndrome
>dup (1q)–(22q) syndrome
>dup (Xq) syndrome

duplex
>d. kidney
>d. scanning
>d. ultrasound
>d. uterus

duplicated
>d. elastic lamina
>d. ureter
>d. vagina

duplicate uterus
duplication (dup)
>d. anomaly
>bowel d.
>caudal d.
>chromosome 15 inverted d.
>complete vulvar d.
>cranial d.
>d. cyst
>duodenal d.
>enteric d.
>fetal d.
>foregut d.
>d. of gallbladder
>gastric d.
>gastrointestinal d.
>gene d.

>d. of ileum
>intestinal d.
>intrachromosomal d.
>mirror d.
>penile d.
>d. 1p–22p syndrome
>d. 1q–22q syndrome
>renal d.
>ureteral d.
>urethral d.
>d. Xq syndrome

duplication-deficiency syndrome
duplicitas
>d. anterior
>d. symmetros

Du-positive mother
dura
>d. mater
>d. mater allograft

durable power of attorney
Durabolin
Duracillin AS
Duraclon Injection
Dura-Estrin
Duragen
Duragesic Transdermal
dural
>d. arteriovenous malformation
>d. ectasia
>d. sinus thrombosis
>d. spinal angioma
>d. venous thrombosis

Duralon-UV nylon membrane
Duralutin
Duramist Plus
Duramorph Injection
DuraNeb portable nebulizer
DuraPrep surgical solution
Duraquin
Dura-Tabs
>Quinaglute D.-T.

Duratears
duration
>D. Nasal Solution
>d. of symptoms

Duratuss-G
Duretic
Duricef
Duroziez disease
duskiness
dusky skin

NOTES

dust
>   d. mite
>   nuclear d.

Dutch
>   D. cap
>   D. pessary

Duval forceps

Duverney gland

DVIU
>   direct vision internal urethrotomy

DVSS
>   dysfunctional voiding scoring system

DVT
>   deep vein thrombosis
>   deep venous thrombosis
>   silent DVT

dwarf
>   diastrophic d.
>   d. pelvis
>   Russell d.
>   d. syndrome

dwarfism
>   achondroplastic d.
>   acromesomelic d.
>   alopecia, contracture, d. (ACD)
>   Amsterdam d.
>   asexual d.
>   ateliotic d.
>   bird-headed d.
>   Brissaud d.
>   camptomelic d.
>   d., cerebral atrophy, keratosis
>   follicularis
>   child abuse d.
>   chondroplastic d.
>   d., congenital medullary stenosis
>   syndrome
>   constitutional d.
>   d. and cortical thickening of
>   tubular bones
>   d., cortical thickening of tubular
>   bones, transient hypocalcemia
>   cretin d.
>   diastrophic d.
>   disproportionate d.
>   d., eczema, peculiar facies
>   familial bird-headed d.
>   geleophysic d.
>   genital d.
>   hypophysial d.
>   hypothyroid d.
>   d., ichthyosiform erythroderma,
>   mental deficiency syndrome
>   infantile d.
>   Kniest d.
>   Langer mesomelic d.
>   Laron d.
>   lean spastic d.
>   Lenz-Majewski hyperostotic d.

lethal neonatal d.
Lorain-Lévi d.
metatropic d.
microcephalic primordial d. 1
micromelic d.
mulibrey nanism or d.
nanocephalic d.
d., onychodysplasia syndrome
osteodysplastic primordial d.
osteoglophonic d.
ovarian d.
parastremmatic d.
d., pericarditis syndrome
pituitary d.
d., polydactyly, dysplastic nails
    syndrome
polydystrophic d.
primordial d.
psychosocial d.
rhizomelic d.
Robinow d.
Russell-Silver d.
Saldino-Noonan d.
Seckel d.
sexual d.
short-limb d.
short-rib d.
Silver d.
Silver-Russell d.
six-fingered d.
Smith-McCort d.
thanatophoric d.
Walt Disney d.

DWI
>   diffusion-weighted imaging

DWS
>   Dandy-Walker syndrome

Dwyer
>   D. correction
>   D. correction of scoliosis

DX
>   dextran

DXA
>   dual-energy x-ray absorptiometry
>   DXA densitometer

d-xylose

dyadic

Dyadic Adjustment Scale

Dyazide

Dyban oocyte fixation technique

Dyclone

dyclonine

dydrogesterone

dye
>   aniline d.
>   azo d.
>   Berwick d.
>   d. decolorization test
>   d. disappearance test

Evans blue d.
formazan d.
indigo carmine d.
iodinated d.
methylene blue d.
triple d.
Dyggve-Melchior-Clausen syndrome
dying-back axonal degeneration
Dyke-Davidoff syndrome
Dynabac
Dynacin Oral
Dyna-Hex
dynamic
d. exercise testing
d. graciloplasty
d. image on ultrasound
d. mutation
d. optical breast imaging system (DOBI)
d. orthotic cranioplasty device
d. pes varus
d. posturography
d. pulmonary imaging (DPI)
d. spiral CT lung densitometry
d. splint
dynamics
androgen d.
family d.
flow velocity d.
toxic d.
Dynamite mattress system
Dynapen
dynein
left/right d.
dynorphin
dyphylline
Dyrenium
dysacousia, dysacusis
dysadrenalism
dysarthria
dysarthritic speech
dysautonomia
familial d.
dysbetalipoproteinemia
dyscalculia
dyscephalia
Francois d.
Hallermann-Streiff d.
d. mandibulooculofacialis
dyscephaly
d., congenital cataract, hypotrichosis syndrome

mandibulo-oculofacial d.
oculomandibular d.
dyschezia
dyschondroplasia
Voorhoeve d.
dyscontrol
episodic d.
dyscoria
dyscrasia
blood d.
sonography blood d.
dysdiadochokinesis
dysembryoma
dysembryoplasia
dysencephalia splanchnocystica
dysenteriae
Shigella d. (type 1)
dysentery
amebic d.
bacillary d.
Shigella d.
dysequilibrium syndrome (DES)
dyserythropoiesis
dysesthetic vulvodynia
dysfibrinogenemia
dysfibronectinemic Ehlers-Danlos syndrome
dysfluency
abnormal d.
developmental d.
dysfluent speech
dysfunction
adrenal axis d.
arm d.
auditory d.
autonomic nervous system d. (ANSD)
AV node d.
B-cell d.
bilirubin-induced neurologic d. (BIND)
bladder d.
bone marrow d.
brain d.
cardiopulmonary d.
catheter d.
cerebellar d.
cerebral d.
chromosomal d.
CNS d.
corpus luteum d.
corticospinal tract d.

NOTES

dysfunction *(continued)*
   cumulative parental d.
   endocrine pancreatic d.
   endothelial d.
   erectile d.
   eustachian tube d.
   exocrine pancreatic d.
   familial vocal cord d.
   family d.
   female sexual d.
   gait d.
   generalized autonomic d.
   global neurologic d.
   gonadal d.
   HPA d.
   hypertonic uterine d.
   hypothalamic d.
   hypothalamic-pituitary d.
   hypotonic uterine d.
   left ventricular d. (LVD)
   LV d.
   lymphocyte d.
   metabolic disorder with hepatic d.
   metabolic disorder with
     neurologic d.
   microcirculatory d.
   minimal brain d. (MBD)
   minimal cerebral d.
   minor cerebral d.
   motor perception d.
   neurogenic bladder d.
   neuromotor d.
   neutrophil actin d.
   oculomotor d.
   oral-motor d.
   ovarian axis d.
   palatorespiratory d.
   pancreatic d.
   papillary muscle d.
   placental d.
   postoperative bladder d.
   postoperative voiding d.
   psychosexual d.
   renal d.
   sacroiliac d.
   serotonergic d.
   sexual d.
   sinus node d. (SND)
   social-occupational d.
   spinal cord d.
   sudomotor d.
   T-cell d.
   temporomandibular joint d.
   testicular d.
   thyroid d.
   thyroid gland d.
   transient pharyngeal muscle d.
   urinary bladder d.
   uterine d.
   vocal cord d. (VCD)
   voiding d.
dysfunctional
   d. family
   d. labor pattern
   d. uterine bleeding (DUB)
   d. voiding
   d. voiding scoring system (DVSS)
dysgammaglobulinemia
dysgenesis, dysgenesia
   autosomal congenital tubular d.
   cerebral d.
   cerebroocular d. (COD)
   cortical d.
   familial pure gonadal d.
   gonadal d.
   iridocorneal mesodermal d.
   d. mesostromalis anterior
   mixed gonadal d. (MGD)
   müllerian d.
   d. neuroepithelialis retinae
   ovarian d.
   partial gonadal d.
   penile d.
   pure gonadal d.
   renal d.
   reticular d.
   seminiferous tubule d.
   d. syndrome
   testicular d.
   tubular d.
   X-linked recessive d.
   XX-type gonadal d.
   XY gonadal d.
dysgenetic
   d. gonad
   d. ovotestis
   d. testis
dysgenic
dysgenitalism
dysgerminoma
   ovarian d.
dysgeusia
dyshepatia
   lipogenic d.
dyshidrosis
dyshidrotic eczema
dyshormonogenesis
dyskaryosis
dyskeratoma
   warty d.
dyskeratosis
   d. congenita
   congenital d.
dyskinesia, dyskinesis
   ciliary d.
   exertion-induced d.
   D. Identification System: Condensed
     User Scale (DISCUS)

kinesigenic paroxysmal d.
orofacial d.
primary ciliary d. (PCD)
sleep-induced d.
tardive d.
withdrawal d.
dyskinetic cerebral palsy
dyslexia
developmental d.
dyslexic
dyslipidemia
dysmaturative myopathy
dysmature
d. infant
d. neonate
dysmaturity syndrome
dysmegakaryocytopoiesis
dysmenorrhea
acupuncture for d.
essential d.
functional d.
intrinsic d.
mechanical d.
membranous d.
obstructive d.
ovarian d.
primary d.
secondary d.
spasmodic d.
tubal d.
ureteral d.
uterine d.
vaginal d.
dysmenorrheal membrane
dysmetria
ocular motor d.
dysmorphic
d. erythrocyte
d. face
d. facial feature
d. facies
d. syndrome
dysmorphism
digitotalar d.
facial d.
major d.
mandibulo-oculofacial d.
minor d.
dysmorphogenesis
otomandibular facial d.
dysmorphologist

dysmorphology
craniofacial d.
d. examination
dysmotile cilia syndrome
dysmotility
ciliary d.
colonic d.
cytokine-related d.
gastric d.
gastrointestinal d.
small bowel d.
d. syndrome
dysmotility-sclerodactyly-telangiectasia
dysmyelinatus
status d.
dysmyelinogenic
dysmyelopoiesis
dysnomia
dysontogenesis
dysontogenetic cyst
dysorganoplasia
dysosmia
dysosteogenesis
dysosteosclerosis (DOS)
dysostosis, pl. **dysostoses**
acrocraniofacial d.
acrofacial d.
Catania type acrofacial d.
cleidocranial digital d.
d. cleidocranialis
d. cleidocraniodigitalis
d. cleidocraniopelvina
craniofacial d.
d. craniofacialis with hypertelorism
craniofrontonasal d.
Crouzon craniofacial d.
dystrophia retinae pigmentosa-d.
 (DRD)
d. enchondralis metaepiphysaria
epiphyseal d.
frontofacionasal d.
Genée-Wiedemann acrofacial d.
 (GWAFD)
d. generalisata
hereditary polytopic enchondral d.
hypomandibular faciocranial d.
mandibulofacial d. (MFD)
d. mandibulofacials
maxillofacial d.
metaphysial d.
d. multiplex
mutational d.

D

NOTES

dysostosis *(continued)*
    Nager type acrofacial d.
    orodigitofacial d.
    otofacial d.
    otomandibular d.
    pelvicocleidocranial d.
    preaxial acrofacial d.
    preaxial mandibulofacial d.
    Rodriguez lethal acrofacial d.
    Treacher Collins mandibulofacial d.
    unilateral mandibulofacial d.
dysostotic idiocy, gargoylism, lipochondrodystrophy syndrome
dyspareunia
    deep d.
    Friedrich criteria for d.
    insertional d.
    secondary vestibular d.
    vestibular d.
dyspepsia
    functional d.
    nonulcer d.
dysphagia
    motility-related d.
    nonneurogenic d.
dysphasia
    developmental d.
dysphonia
    spasmodic d.
    spastic d.
dysphoria
    premenstrual d.
dysphoric
    d. mood
    d. reaction
dyspigmentation
dysplasia
    acetabular d.
    acromelic frontonasal d.
    acromesomelic d.
    acromicric d.
    acropectorovertebral d.
    agyria-pachygyria cortical d.
    alveolar capillary d.
    anal sphincter d.
    angel-shaped phalangoepiphyseal d. (ASPED)
    anhidrotic ectodermal d.
    anhydrotic ectodermal d.
    arrhythmogenic right ventricular d. (ARVD)
    arteriohepatic d. (AHD)
    asphyxiating thoracic d.
    atriodigital d.
    azoospermia, renal anomaly, cervicothoracic spine d. (ARCS)
    bone d.
    bony d.
    boomerang d.

BOR d.
bronchopulmonary d. (BPD)
3C d.
camptomelic d.
caudal d.
CCC d.
cerebellar d.
cerebellotrigeminal and focal dermal d.
cerebrofaciothoracic syndrome or d.
cervical d.
chondroectodermal d.
cleidocranial d.
d. cleidocranialis
d. cleidofacialis
clubfoot d.
colposcopic grading of cervical d.
congenital alveolar d.
congenital encephalo-ophthalmic d.
congenital glenoid d.
congenital hip d. (CHD)
cortical d.
costovertebral d.
craniodiaphyseal d.
cranioectodermal d. (CED)
craniofrontal d.
craniofrontonasal d. (CFND)
craniometaphyseal d.
craniotubular d.
cretinoid d.
de la Chapelle d.
dentin d.
dentooculoosseous d.
developmental hip d.
diaphysial d.
diastrophic d.
dyssegmental d.
ectodermal d.
endocervical glandular d.
epiphyseal d.
d. epiphysealis hemimelia
d. epiphysealis hemimelica
d. epiphysealis punctata
facial ectodermal d.
faciocardiomelic d.
faciogenital d.
familial focal facial dermal d.
Fanconi d.
fetal skeletal d.
fibromuscular d.
fibrous d.
focal cortical d.
focal facial dermal d. (type I, II)
focal facial ectodermal d.
frontofacionasal d.
frontometaphysial d.
frontonasal d. (FND)
geleophysic d.
glenoid d.

Goldenhar oculauricular vertebral d.
gonadal d.
gracile bone d.
Grebe d.
hereditary bone d.
hereditary ectodermal d.
hereditary expansile polyostotic
  osteolytic d.
hereditary retinal d.
hidrotic ectodermal d.
high-grade cervical d.
hip d.
Holt-Oram atriodigital d.
hydrocephalus, agyria, retinal d.
  (HARD)
hypohidrotic ectodermal d.
immunoosseous d.
intestinal neuronal d.
intraepithelial cervical d.
iridodental d.
ischiopatellar d.
Kniest d.
Kniest-like d.
Kozlowski spondylometaphysial d.
kyphomelic d.
Langer mesomelic d.
lateral facial d. (LFD)
Lenz d.
lethal bone d.
d. linguofacialis
low-grade d. (LGD)
lymphatic d.
mammary d.
mandibular-acral d.
mandibuloacral d.
Margarita Island type ectodermal d.
d. marginalis posterior
maxillonasal d.
medullary d.
mesectodermal d.
mesomelic d.
metaphoric d.
metaphysial d.
metatropic d.
Mexican cardiomelic d.
microglandular d.
mild acetabular d.
müllerian duct aplasia, renal
  agenesis/ectopia, cervical
  somite d. (MURCS)
multicystic renal d.
multiple epiphyseal d.

myxoid d.
necrotic facial d.
neonatal osseous d.
nerve d.
neurogenic hip d.
neuronal d.
oculoauricular d.
oculoauriculovertebral d.
oculodentodigital d.
d. oculodentodigitalis
oculodentoosseous d. (ODOD)
odontoonychodermal d.
OFD with tibial d.
olfacto-ethmoidohypothalamic d.
olfactogenital d.
ophthalmomandibulomelic d.
optic nerve d.
osseous-oculodental d.
OSSUM database of skeletal d.'s
osteodental d. (ODD)
osteofibrous d.
osteoglophonic d.
otospondylomegaepliphyseal d.
pelvis capsular d.
pelvis-shoulder d.
polycystic fibrous d.
polyostotic fibrous d.
porencephaly cortical d.
posterior urethral valves, unilateral
  reflux, renal d. (VURD)
pseudoachondroplastic d.
pseudodiastrophic d.
ptosis of eyelids, diastasis recti,
  hip d.
pulmonary d.
punctate epiphyseal d.
radial d.
radiation d.
Rapp-Hodgkin ectodermal d.
renal medullary d.
retinal d.
right ventricular d.
Robinow mesomelic d.
Schimke immunoosseous d.
Schmid metaphyseal d.
Schneckenbecken d.
septooptic-pituitary d.
Silverman-Handmaker
  dyssegmental d.
skeletal d.
sphenoid d.

D

NOTES

dysplasia *(continued)*
  split hand-cleft lip/palate and
    ectodermal d. (SCE)
  sponastrime d.
  spondyloepimetaphyseal d. (SEMD)
  spondyloepiphyseal d. (SED)
  spondylometaphyseal d.
  spondyloperipheral d.
  spondylothoracic d.
  squamous d.
  Stickler d.
  Streeter d.
  d. syndrome
  thanatophoric d.
  thymic d.
  trichorhinophalangeal multiple
    exostosis d.
  trichorino-auriculophalangeal multiple
    exostoses d.
  urinary tract d.
  ventricular d.
  vertebral (defects), (imperforate)
    anus, tracheoesophageal (fistula),
    radial and renal (d.) (VATER)
dysplastic
  d. cell
  d. cortical architecture
  d. gangliocytoma
  d. gangliocytoma of cerebellum
  d. kidney
  d. nevus
  d. nevus syndrome
dyspnea
  paroxysmal nocturnal d. (PND)
  d. of pregnancy
dyspraxia
dysproteinemia
dysprothrombinemia
dysraphia
  olfacto-ethmoidohypothalamic d.
  d. of spine
  tectocerebellar d.
dysraphism
  occult spinal d.
  spinal d.
dysregulated
  d. behavior
  d. insulin secretion
dysregulation
  autonomic d.
  hypothalamic-pituitary-adrenal
    axis d.
  immune d.
  temperature d.
dysrhythmia
  cardiac d.
  gastric d.
  ventricular d.
dyssegmental dysplasia

dyssomnia
  circadian rhythm d.
  extrinsic d.
  infant d.
  intrinsic d.
dysspermia
dyssynergia
  detrusor sphincter d.
dystasia
  hereditary areflexic d.
dystaxia cerebralis infantilis
dysthymia
dysthymic disorder
dysthyroidal infantilism
dystocia
  abdominal d.
  all-fours maneuver for shoulder d.
  cervical d.
  fetal d.
  maternal d.
  placental d.
  shoulder d.
  vaginal soft tissue d.
dystocia-dystrophia syndrome
dystonia
  buccomandibular d.
  craniocervical d.
  dopa-responsive d. (DRD)
  drug-induced d.
  early-onset d.
  focal d.
  generalized d.
  idiopathic torsion d.
  d. musculorum deformans (DMD)
  myoclonic d.
  oromandibular d.
  paroxysmal d.
  primary d.
  progressive d.
  secondary d.
  segmental d.
  symptomatic d.
  tardive d.
  torsion d.
  transient d.
dystonia-deafness syndrome
dystonia-parkinsonism
dystonic
  d. cerebral palsy
  d. dyskinetic disorder
  d. hyperextension
  d. posturing
  d. reaction
dystopia canthorum
dystrophia
  d. bullosa hereditaria, typus
    maculosus
  d. retinae-dysacousis syndrome

d. retinae pigmentosa-dysostosis (DRD)

dystrophic
d. calcification
d. epidermolysis bullosa
d. myopathy
d. nail
d. tooth

dystrophica
epidermis bullosa d.

dystrophin gene
dystrophinopathy
dystrophy
adult pseudohypertrophic muscular d.
Aran-Duchenne muscular d.
asphyxiating thoracic d. (ATD)
autoimmune polyendocrinopathy, candidiasis, ectodermal d. (APECED)
autosomal recessive muscular d.
Becker-Kiener muscular d.
Becker muscular d. (BMD)
Becker pseudohypertrophic muscular d.
Becker type progressive muscular d.
benign X-linked recessive muscular d.
cerebroocular dysgenesis-muscular d. (COD-MD)
cerebroocular dysplasia-muscular d.
cerebroocular muscular d.
childhood pseudohypertrophic muscular d.
classic X-linked recessive muscular d.
congenital endothelial corneal d.
congenital muscular d. (CMD)
congenital myotonic d.
corneal d.
craniocarpotarsal d.
Duchenne de Boulogne muscular d. (DMD)
Duchenne de Boulogne muscular dystrophy/Becker muscular d. (DMD/BMD)
Duchenne muscular d. (DMD)
Duchenne muscular dystrophy/Becker muscular d. (DMD/BMD)

Duchenne type pseudohypertrophic progressive muscular d.
early corneal d.
Emery-Dreifuss muscular d.
endothelial d.
Erb juvenile muscular d.
facioscapulohumeral muscular d. (FSHD)
familial osseous d.
FSH muscular d.
Fukuyama congenital muscular d. (FCMD)
giant neuroaxonal d.
gingival fibromatosis-corneal d.
hereditary bullous d.
humeroperoneal muscular d.
infantile neuroaxonal d.
infantile thoracic d.
Jeune thoracic d.
juvenile epithelial corneal d.
juvenile muscular d.
juvenile myotonic d.
Landouzy d.
Landouzy-Dejerine muscular d.
Leyden-Möbius muscular d.
limb girdle muscular d.
macular d.
Meesmann corneal d.
micropolygyria with muscular d.
mild X-linked recessive muscular d.
muscular d. (MD)
myotonic d. (MD)
myotonic muscular d.
nail d.
neuroaxonal d.
neurovascular d.
ocular muscular d.
oculocerebral d.
oculocerebrorenal d.
oculopharyngeal muscular d.
osteochondromuscular d.
peroneal muscular d.
pseudohypertrophic adult muscular d.
pseudohypertrophic progressive muscular d.
reflex sympathetic d. (RSD)
scapulohumeral muscular d.
scapuloperoneal d.
Schnyder crystalline corneal d. (SCCD)

NOTES

dystrophy *(continued)*
  scleroatonic muscular d.
  secondary nail d.
  severe childhood autosomal
   recessive muscular d. (SCARMD)
  short-limb d.
  spinal muscular d.
  Steinert myotonic d.
  thoracic asphyxiant d.
  thoracic-pelvic-phalangeal d.
  twenty-nail d.
  vulvar d.
  X-linked recessive muscular d.
dysuria
dysuria-pyuria syndrome
dysuria-sterile pyuria syndrome
dyszoospermia

E

E antigen
E autoantibody
E Pam
E sign

E_1

estrone
prostaglandin E_1 (PGE_1)
synthetic prostaglandin E_1

E_2

estradiol
eutopic endometrium prostaglandin E_2
prostaglandin E_2 (PGE_2)

E3

unconjugated estriol

E_3

estriol

E_4

leukotriene E_4 (LTE_4)

17beta-E2 transdermal drug-delivery system

E6-E7 gene

EA

early amniocentesis
esophageal atresia

EAA

excitotoxic amino acid

EABT

estrogen add-back therapy

EACA

epsilon-aminocaproic acid

EAE

experimental allergic encephalomyelitis

Eagle-Barrett syndrome

Eagle test

EAR

early asthmatic response

ear

e. anomaly
Aztec e.
bat e.
e. canal
e. crease/pit
cup e.
Darwin e.
external e.
glue e.
inner e.
laser office ventilation of e.'s (LOVE)
left e.
lop e.
low-set e.'s
malformed e.

middle e.
Morel e.
Mozart e.
Otocalm E.
outer e.
e., patella, short stature (EPS)
prominent e.
satyr e.
scroll e.
e. speculum
swimmer's e.
tugging at e.'s
e. ventilation tube
Wildermuth e.

EarCheck

ear-cough reflex

eardrum

perforated e.
e. perforation

Earle

E. balanced salt solution
E. culture medium

earlobe

bifid e.
e. crease

early

e. adolescence
e. amniocentesis (EA)
e. amnion vascular disruption complex
e. asthmatic reaction
e. asthmatic response (EAR)
e. cardiac motion
e. childhood caries (ECC)
E. Childhood Special Education Program
e. congenital syphilis
e. constraint defect
e. corneal dystrophy
e. deceleration
e. educator
e. embryonic cell
e. embryonic death
e. embryonic loss
e. enteral feeding
e. follicular development
e. infantile autism
e. infantile epileptic encephalopathy
e. intervention
e. interventionist
e. intervention program (EIP)
E. Language Milestone (ELM)
E. Language Milestone scale
e. mature
e. midsystolic closure

E

early *(continued)*
    e. morning irritability
    E. Neonatal Neurobehavioral Scale
    e. neonate
    E. and Periodic Screening,
        Diagnosis, and Treatment
        (EPSDT)
    e. pregnancy factor
    e. pregnancy loss
    e. pregnancy test (EPT)
    e. pregnancy wastage
    e. proliferative phase
    e. satiety
    e. stromal invasion
early-discharge program
early-onset
    e.-o. diabetes mellitus-epiphyseal
        dysplasia syndrome
    e.-o. disease
    e.-o. dystonia
    e.-o. Parkinsonism-mental retardation
        syndrome
    e.-o. preeclampsia
    e.-o. schizophrenia (EOS)
    e.-o. sepsis
earth
    diatomaceous e. (DE)
EAS
    Emotionality Activity Sociability Scale
EASI
    extraamniotic saline infusion
    EASI catheter
Easprin
Eastern
    E. blot
    E. blot test
    E. equine encephalitis (EEE)
Eastman-Bixler syndrome
easy
    e. bruisabilty
    Clearblue E.
    ClearPlan E.
    e. fatigability
eater
    picky e.
eating
    E. Attitudes Test
    binge e.
    e. disorder
    e. disorder not otherwise specified
        (EDNOS)
    e. disorders examination (EDE)
    E. Disorders Inventory
    E. Disorders Inventory Score for
        Interoceptive Awareness Affect
    e. habit
Eaton-Lambert myasthenic syndrome
EB
    epidermolysis bullosa

EBCT
    electron-beam computed tomography
EBLL
    elevation of blood lead level
EBM
    epidermolysis bullosa, macular type
EBNA
    Epstein-Barr nuclear antigen
EBNS
    endoscopic bladder neck suspension
Ebola hemorrhagic fever
Ebstein
    E. anomaly
    E. malformation
EBV
    Epstein-Barr virus
EBV-related B-cell lymphoma
EC
    emergency contraception
E-cadherin protein
ECBI
    Eyberg Child Behavior Inventory
ecbolic
ECC
    early childhood caries
    endocervical curettage
    extracorporeal circulation
eccentric
    e. exercise
    e. gaze
    e. orifice
eccentrochondrodysplasia
eccentrochondroplasia
eccentroosteochondrodysplasia
ecchymosis
    periorbital e.
    postauricular e.
    trocar site e.
ecchymotic Ehlers-Danlos syndrome
ECCL
    encephalocraniocutaneous lipomatosis
Eccocee ultrasound system
eccrine
    e. bromhidrosis
    e. sweat duct
    e. sweat gland
    e. sweating
eccyesis
ECD
    endocardial cushion defect
ECF
    executive cognitive functioning
    extracellular fluid
ECG *(var. of* EKG)
echinococcal cyst
echinococcosis
    alveolar e.
Echinococcus
    E. granulosus

E. *granulosus* hydatid cyst
E. *multilocularis*
echinocyte
Echistatin
ECHO
    enteric cytopathogenic human orphan
    enterocytopathogenic human orphan
echo, pl. **echoes**
    echocardiogram
    echocardiograph
    echoencephalogram
      echo Doppler gradient
      echo dropout
      echo formation
      scattered echo
      single shot fast spin echo (SSFSE)
      specular echo
echocardiogram (echo, echoes)
    color e.
    2D e.
    fetal e.
    M-mode e.
    two-dimensional e.
echocardiograph (echo, echoes)
echocardiography
    abdominal fetal e.
    A-mode e.
    2D, 3D e.
    Doppler e.
    fetal e.
    M-mode e.
    real-time e.
    transesophageal e. (TEE)
    transpericardial e.
    transthoracic e.
EchoCheck
echodensity
echoencephalogram (echo, echoes)
echoencephalography
    cranial e.
echo-free zone
echogenic
    e. cardiac focus
    e. fetal bowel
    e. tissue
echogenicity
echogram
    M-mode e.
echo-guided balloon atrial septostomy
echolalia
    compulsive e.

echolucency
    periventricular e. (PVEL)
echolucent area
EchoMark salpingography catheter
echoplanar functional magnetic
  resonance imaging
echopraxia
Echo-Screen
echothiophate iodide
Echotip
    E. Norfolk aspiration needle
    E. percutaneous entry needle
echoviral meningitis
echovirus, ECHO virus
    e. 9 meningitis
Echovist contrast
eclampsia
    e. nutans
    puerperal e.
    superimposed e.
eclamptic
    e. idiocy
    e. retinopathy
    e. seizure
eclamptogenic, eclamptogenous
ECLS
    extracorporeal life support
ECLT
    euglobulin clot lysis time
ECM
    erythema chronicum migrans
      ECM rash
ECMO
    extracorporeal membrane oxygenation
      double-lumen venovenous ECMO
      venovenous ECMO
E_TCO_2
    end-tidal carbon dioxide
ECochG, ECoG
    electrocochleography
E-Complex-600
econazole
Econopred Plus Ophthalmic
ECOR
    extracorporeal CO_2 removal
Ecostatin
Ecotrin
Ecowarm gel warmer
ECP
    emergency contraception pill
    emergency contraceptive pill
    eosinophilic cationic protein

NOTES

ECR
   endocervical resection
ecstasy
ECT
   electroconvulsive therapy
ectasia, ectasis
   annuloaortic e.
   arterial e.
   duct e.
   ductal e.
   dural e.
   familial aortic e.
   mammary duct e.
   scoliosis with dural e.
ecthyma gangrenosum
ectocervical lesion
ectocervix
   friable e.
ectoderm
   cutaneous e.
ectodermal
   e. dysplasia
   e. dysplasia, cleft lip and palate, hand and foot deformity, mental retardation syndrome
   e. dysplasia, cleft lip and palate, mental retardation, syndactyly syndrome (I, II)
   e. dysplasia of face
   e. dysplasia, mental retardation, syndactyly syndrome
   e. ridge
ectoendocervical junction
ectolecithal
ectomere
ectomesoblast
ectoneurodermal hamartoma
ectopagus
ectoparasite
ectopia
   e. cordis
   crossed fused e.
   double thyroid e.
   infrahyoid e.
   e. lentis
   e. lentis et pupillae
   renal e.
   ureteral e.
ectopic
   e. anus
   e. atrial tachycardia
   e. decidua
   e. endometrial tissue
   e. endometrium
   e. gastric mucosa
   e. implant
   e. implantation
   e. ovarian tissue
   e. pancreatic rest
   e. pinealoma
   e. P-P cycle
   e. pregnancy (EP)
   e. testis
   e. thyroid
   e. ureter
   e. ureterocele
   e. ventricular depolarization
ectoplacental cone
ectopy
   cervical e.
Ectosone
ectrodactyly
   e., ectodermal dysplasia, clefting (EEC)
   e., ectodermal dysplasia and cleft lip/palate syndrome
   e., mandibulofacial dysostosis syndrome
   e., spastic paraplegia, mental retardation syndrome
ectrodactyly-cleft lip/palate syndrome
ectromelia
ectrometacarpia
ectrometatarsia
ectrophalangia
ectropion
   cervical e.
   congenital e.
ectrosyndactyly
ECV
   external cephalic version
   extracellular volume
eczema
   asteatotic e.
   atopic e.
   discoid e.
   dyshidrotic e.
   e. herpeticum
   infantile e.
   e. marginatum
   e. neonatorum
   nipple e.
   nummular e.
   plaque of nummular e.
   seborrheic e.
   e. vaccinatum
eczematization
eczematoid
   e. dermatitis
   e. lesion
   e. skin rash
eczematous
   e. candida
   e. halo nevus
   e. rash
   e. skin lesion
EDAS
   encephaloduroarteriosynangios

EDC
    estimated date of conception
    estimated date of confinement
    expected date of confinement
EDD
    expected date of delivery
Eddowes syndrome
EDE
    eating disorders examination
Edecrin
    E. Oral
    E. Sodium Injection
edema
    angioneurotic e.
    benign transient optic disc e.
    Berlin e.
    brain e.
    brawny e.
    cellular e.
    cerebral e.
    corneal e.
    cytotoxic e.
    dependent e.
    focal cerebral e.
    gestational e.
    hereditary e.
    high-altitude cerebral e. (HACE)
    high-altitude pulmonary e. (HAPE)
    idiopathic scrotal e.
    indurative e.
    intercellular e.
    interstitial e.
    ischemic e.
    labial e.
    laryngeal e.
    leg e.
    lung e.
    malignant brain e.
    menstrual e.
    e. neonatorum
    neurogenic pulmonary e.
    noncardiac pulmonary e.
    optic nerve e.
    periorbital e.
    peritonsillar e.
    pitting e.
    placental e.
    postasphyxial cerebral e.
    postthoracotomy pulmonary e.
    premenstrual e.
    presternal e.
    pulmonary e.
    rebound e.
    retinal e.
    scrotal e.
    segmental e.
    subglottic e.
    suborbital e.
    tonsillar e.
    vasogenic e.
    villous e.
    vulvar e.
edematous papilla
Eden-Lawson hysterectomy
EdenTec 2000W in-home cardiorespiratory monitor
Eder cord blood collection device
edetate calcium disodium
Edex
edge effect
EDIN behavioral score
edinburgensis
    typus e.
Edinburgh
    E. malformation syndrome
    E. Postnatal Depression Scale (EPDS)
Edinger-Westphal nucleus
edition
    Bayley Scales of Infant Development-Motor, 2nd E.
    Child Health and Illness Profile, Adolescent E. (CHIP-AE)
    Clinical Evaluation of Language Fundamentals, 3rd E.
    Receptive-Expressive Emergent Language Scale, 2nd E. (REEL-2)
    Stanford-Binet Intelligence Scale, 4th E.
    Stanford-Binet Memory Scale, 4th E.
    Wechsler Adult Intelligence Scale, 3rd E.
    Wechsler Intelligence Scale, 3rd E.
Edmonston-Zagreb measles vaccine
EDNOS
    eating disorder not otherwise specified
EDRF
    endothelium-derived relaxing factor
edrophonium
    e. chloride
    e. test
EDS
    Ehlers-Danlos syndrome

NOTES

E

EDTA
ethylenediaminetetraacetic acid
EDTA-anticoagulated Vacutainer
EDTA-Vacutainer
educable
education
E. for All Handicapped Children
Act
American College of Graduate
Medical E. (ACGME)
Bradley childbirth e.
conductive e. (CE)
E. of the Handicapped
Amendments of 1986
Lamaze childbirth e.
special e.
educator
early e.
infant e.
EDV
end-diastolic velocity
end-diastolic volume
umbilical arterial EDV
Edwards-Gale syndrome
Edwardsiella tarda
Edwards syndrome
E$_{dyn}$
respiratory system elastance
EE
electrosurgical excision
ethinyl estradiol
EEA stapler
EEC
ectrodactyly, ectodermal dysplasia,
clefting
EEC syndrome
EECS
extraembryonic celomic space
EEE
Eastern equine encephalitis
EEG
electroencephalogram
electroencephalography
amplitude-integrated EEG
interictal EEG
EEG/polygraphic/video monitoring
EELV
end-expiratory lung volume
eelworm
EENT
eyes, ears, nose, throat
EEP
end-expiratory phase
end-expiratory pressure
EER
extraesophageal reflux
EES
erythromycin ethylsuccinate
expandable esophageal stent

E.E.S.
E. 200, 400
E. Chewable
E. Granules
EFA
essential fatty acid
EFA deficiency
EFAS
embryofetal alcohol syndrome
EFE
endocardial fibroelastosis
primary EFE
efface
effacement
cervical e.
e. of cervix
effect
Accutane e.
adiabatic e.
adverse maternal e.
anemic e.
antiendometriotic e.
antiestrogen e.
antiestrogenic e.
antiinflammatory e.
Arias-Stella e.
ball-valve e.
Bohr e.
brain-sparing e.
bystander e.
cardioprotective e.
cardiovascular e.
choroid plexus pulse e.
chronotropic e.
Compton e.
Cushing e.
cytopathic e. (CPE)
cytotoxic e.
demand e.
differential e.
digitalis e.
Doppler e.
edge e.
Eisenmenger e.
estrogen e.
estrogen-agonist uterine e.
estrogenic e.
fetal e.
fetal alcohol e.'s (FAE)
first-pass e.
founder e.
halo e.
Hawthorne e.
hormonal e.
hypnotic e.
iatrogenic e.
inotropic e.
jet cooling e.
Mach band e.

marijuana e.
mass e.
maternal e.
mitogenic e.
muscarinic e.
neurologic adverse e.
perinatal e.
pituitary gonadotropin e.
Posiero e.
progestational e.
psychological e.
returning-soldier e.
salutary e.
sedative e.
side e.
siphon e.
social factor e.
star e.
systemic side e.
teratogenic e.
waterhammer e.
white coat e.
Yom Kippur e.

effective
   e. conjugate
   e. refractory period

effectiveness
   contraceptive e.

effector cell

efferentia
   ductuli e.

efferent limb

Effexor

efficacious

efficacy
   oral contraceptive e.
   in vitro e.

efficiency
   female fertility e.
   sleep e.

effluvium, pl. **effluvia**
   anagen e.
   telogen e.

efflux

effortless regurgitation

effusion
   bilateral otitis media with e.
    (BOME)
   boggy synovial e.
   chylous pleural e.
   clenched fist and pleural e.
   hemorrhagic pleural e.

lingular e.
malignant pleural e.
middle ear e. (MEE)
otitis media with e. (OME)
otitis media without e.
parapneumonic pleural e.
pericardial e.
pleural e.
subdural e.
transudative pleural e.
tuberculous pleural e.

Efidac/24

EFM
   electronic fetal monitoring
   external fetal monitoring

EFNEP
   expanded food nutrition education
    program

EFS
   event-free survival

Efudex Topical

EFW
   estimated fetal weight

EGA
   estimated gestational age

Egan mammography

EG/BUS
   external genitalia/Bartholin, urethral, and
    Skene glands

EGD
   esophagogastroduodenoscopy

EGF
   epidermal growth factor

EGFR
   epidermal growth factor receptor

egg
   e. activation
   e. cell
   e. donation
   e. donor
   donor e.
   frozen e.
   e. membrane
   e. on a string
   e. phospholipid
   e. retrieval
   e. transport
   e. yolk extender

eggbeater running pattern

EGNB
   enteric gram-negative bacillary

E

NOTES

Egnell
- E. breast pump
- E. vacuum

egodystonic
ego-oriented individual therapy (EOIT)
egophony
egosyntonic
egress
- neutrophil e.

EH
- endometrial hyperplasia

EHEC
- enterohemorrhagic *Escherichia coli*

Ehlers-Danlos
- E.-D. syndrome (EDS)

EHM
- embryonic heart motion

Ehrlich catheter
Ehrlichia
- E. *chaffeensis*
- E. *phagocytophilia*
- E. *sennetsu*

ehrlichiosis
- granulocytic e.
- human granulocytic e. (HGE)
- human monocytic e. (HME)

EIA
- enzyme immunoassay
- enzyme immunosorbent assay
- exercise-induced asthma

EIB
- erythema induration of Bazin
- exercise-induced bronchospasm

EIC
- extensive intraductal component

eicosanoid
eicosapentaenoic acid
EIFT
- embryo intrafallopian transfer

eight-ball hyphema
eight-cell embryo
eight-drugs-in-one-day treatment series
eighth nerve deafness
Eikenella corrodens
EIM
- extraintestinal manifestation

EI/MV
- endotracheal intubation and mechanical ventilation

EIN
- endometrial intraepithelial neoplasia

Einstein
- E. Neonatal Neurobehavioral Assessment Scale (ENNAS)
- E. screening test

Einthoven triangle
EIP
- early intervention program

eIPV
- enhanced inactivated polio vaccine

Eisenmenger
- E. complex
- E. effect
- E. physiology
- E. syndrome

EITB
- enzyme-linked immunotransfer blot

ejaculate
- sperm-free e.

ejaculation
- e. failure
- premature e.
- retrograde e.

ejaculatory duct
ejecta
- laser e.

ejection
- e. click
- milk e.
- e. murmur
- e. reflex

EKC
- epidemic keratoconjunctivitis

EKG, ECG
- electrocardiogram
- electrocardiography
- pediatric EKG

Eklund
- E. mammography technique
- E. positioning system

ektacytometer
elastance
- respiratory system e. (E_{dyn})
- static e. (E_{st})

elastase
- fecal pancreatic e.

elastic
- e. bandaging
- e. canal
- e. lamina
- e. recoil of the bronchus
- e. stocking
- e. tissue hyperplasia

elastica
- cutis e.

elasticity
- blood vessel e.

elasticum
- pseudoxanthoma e.

elastin (ELN)
- e. gene deletion

elastography
- magnetic resonance e. (MRE)

elastolysis
- generalized e.

elastomer catheter
elastosis perforans serpiginosa

Elavil
elbow
    e. dislocation
    e. fracture
    Little League e.
    nursemaid's e.
    pitcher's e.
    prone on e.'s (POE)
    pulled e.
    tennis e.
ELBW
    extremely low birth weight
        ELBW infant
ELBWI
    extremely low birth weight infant
Eldecort Topical
elderly primigravida
EleCare
    E. formula
    E. nutritional supplement
Elecsys 1010 analyzer
elective
    e. abortion
    e. abortion material
    e. cesarean delivery
    e. cesarean section
    e. termination
Electra complex
electric
    e. breast pump
    e. suction device
    e. vacuum aspiration
    e. vacuum aspirator
electrical
    e. accustimulation
    e. alternans
    e. burn
    e. stimulation
electrocardiogram (EKG, ECG)
    fetal e.
electrocardiography (EKG, ECG)
    abdominal fetal e.
    fetal e.
electrocautery
    AmpErase e.
    bipolar e.
    Endoclip monopolar e.
    laparoscopic e.
    transurethral e.
electroclinical dissociation

electrocoagulation diathermy
electrocochleography (ECochG, ECoG)
    round window e. (RWECochG)
electroconvulsive therapy (ECT)
electrocortical silence
electrode
    Aspen laparoscopy e.
    ball e.
    e. balloon
    bipolar e.
    Bugbee e.
    closed-loop system passing e.
    Copeland fetal scalp e.
    Cryomedics disposable LLETZ e.
    fetal scalp e. (FSE)
    Kontron e.
    Littmann ECG e.
    LLETZ-LEEP active loop e.
    loop e.
    Medi-Trace e.
    REM PolyHesive II patient
     return e.
    rollerball e.
    RollerBar e.
    roller-barrel e.
    RollerLoop vaporizing loop e.
    scalp e.
    spiral e.
    unipolar e.
    Valleylab ball e.
    Valleylab loop e.
electrodesiccation
electrodialyzed whey formula
electroejaculation
electroencephalogram (EEG)
    amplitude-integrated e. (aEEG)
electroencephalographic sleep study
electroencephalography (EEG)
    quantitative e. (qEEG)
    video e.
electrogastrography
Electro-Gel conductivity gel
electrographic background abnormality
electrohysterograph
electrohysterography
electrolysis
electrolyte
    e. balance
    e. disturbance
    e. imbalance
    e. loss
    e. therapy

NOTES

E

electromagnetic
    e. radiation
    e. spectrum
electromechanical
    e. dissociation (EMD)
    e. morcellation
electromembrane
    therapeutic e. (TEM)
electrometrogram
electromyelogram (EMG)
electromyogram (EMG)
    surface e. (SEMG)
electromyography (EMG)
    anal sphincter e.
    surface e. (SEMG)
    transabdominal uterine e.
electron
    e. microscopy
    e. microscopy of stool
    e. transfer flavoprotein (ETF)
    e. transfer flavoprotein
      dehydrogenase (ETF-DH)
    e. volt (eV)
electron-beam computed tomography (EBCT)
electron-dense subepithelial deposit
electronic
    e. communication aid
    e. fetal heart rate monitoring
    e. fetal monitoring (EFM)
    e. scale
electronystagmography (ENG)
electrooculogram
electrooculography
electrophilic center
electrophoresis
    capillary e.
    denaturing gradient gel e.
    fluorophore-assisted carbohydrate e. (FACE)
    e. gel
    hemoglobin e.
    high-performance capillary e. (HPCE)
    Laurell (rocket) immune e.
    polyacrylamide gel e.
    pulsed field gel e. (PFGE)
    RNA e.
    thermal gel gradient e.
electrophoretic mobility shift assay (EMSA)
electrophrenic stimulation
electroporation
electroretinal abnormality
electroretinogram (ERG)
electroretinography (ERG)
Electroscope disposable scissors
electroshield monitoring system

electroshock
    maximal e. (MES)
    e. therapy
electrospray ionization mass spectrometry (ESIMS)
electrosurgery
electrosurgical
    e. excision (EE)
    e. loop excision
    e. plume
    e. wire
elegance
    sartorial e.
elegans
    Abiotrophia e.
Elejalde syndrome
Elek test
Elema angiocardiogram
element
    immature neural e.
    IS e.
    transposable e.
elemental
    e. diet
    e. iron
elephant
    e. man
    e. pelvis
elephantiasis
    congenital e.
    genital e.
    e. vulvae
elevate
    rest, ice, compression e. (RICE)
elevated
    e. bile acid
    e. cardiac output
    e. conjugated bilirubin
    e. enzyme activity
    e. fetal hemoglobin
    e. intracranial pressure
    e. liver enzymes
    e. obstetric risk
    e. renin
    e. sweat chloride concentration
    e. transaminase
elevation
    alpha-fetoprotein e.
    e. of blood lead level (EBLL)
    delayed thyrotropin e.
    fetus growth e.
    periosteal e.
    posterior pharyngeal wall e.
    rest, ice, compression, e. (RICE)
    ST-segment e.
elevator
    Boyle uterine e.
    lemon-squeezer obstetrical e.
    Somer uterine e.

U e.
uterine e.
Wadia e.

ELF
epithelial lining fluid
pulmonary ELF
elfin facies hypercalcemia syndrome
elfinlike facies
ELIFA
enzyme-linked immunofiltration assay
eligibility designation
eligible
elimination diet
Elimite Cream
ELISA
enzyme-linked immunosorbent assay
double-sandwich ELISA
Lyme ELISA
ELISA test
ELISpot
solid-phase enzyme-linked immunospot
ELISpot assay
ELISpot test
Elixicon
elixir
Brofed E.
Bromaline E.
Bromanate E.
Lortab E.
Tylenol and Codeine E.
Elixophyllin
Elliot forceps
ellipsis
elliptical uterine incision
elliptocyte
elliptocytic anemia
elliptocytosis
hereditary e. (HE)
spherocytic hereditary e.
Ellis-Sheldon syndrome
Ellis-van Creveld syndrome
ELM
Early Language Milestone
ELM scale
Elmed
E. BC 50 M/M digital bipolar
coagulator
E. peristaltic irrigation pump
Elmiron
ELN
elastin
Elocon

elongation
rete ridge e.
urethral e.
ELP
exogenous lipoid pneumonia
ElSahy-Waters syndrome
Elscint ESI-3000 ultrasound
Elspar
ELT
euglobulin lysis time
Eltor
Eltroxin
elucidation
EM
erythema multiforme
EMA
endomysium antibody
epithelial membrane antigen
E-Mac
English MacIntosh
E-Mac laryngoscope blade
emaciated
Emadine
emancipated minor
EMB
ethambutol
embarrassment
respiratory e.
Embden-Meyerhof pathway
embolectomy
Fogarty arterial e. (FAE)
Embolex
emboli (*pl. of* embolus)
embolic abscess
embolism (*See also* embolus)
air e.
amniotic fluid e. (AFE)
cerebral e.
fat e.
pulmonary e. (PE)
pulmonary fat e.
embolization
angiographic e.
aortopulmonary collateral coil e.
arterial e.
catheter e.
fibroid e.
patent ductus arteriosis coil e.
pelvic arterial e.
e. therapy
transcatheter coil e.
transcatheter uterine artery e.

E

NOTES

embolization *(continued)*
    transvenous coil e.
    uterine artery e. (UAE)
    uterine fibroid e. (UFE)
embolus, pl. **emboli** *(See also* embolism)
    air e.
    amniotic fluid e.
    gas e.
    massive pulmonary e.
    occluding spring e.
    pulmonary e.
    septic e.
    trophoblastic e.
Embosphere microsphere
embrace reflex
embroscopy
embryatrics
embryectomy
embryo
    abnormal e.
    e. biopsy
    e. carrier
    cleaved e.
    e. cloning
    cryopreserved e.
    cylindrical e.
    e. donation
    e. donor
    eight-cell e.
    e. encapsulation
    endometrial e.
    four-cell e.
    frozen e.
    gastrulating e.
    e. intrafallopian transfer (EIFT)
    Janosik e.
    multicelled e.
    nodular e.
    preimplantation e. (PIE)
    presomite e.
    previllous e.
    pronuclear e.
    e. reduction
    somite e.
    Spee e.
    e. splitting
    stunted e.
    tetraploid e.
    e. thawing
    e. thawing with transfer
    e. transfer (ET)
    triploid e.
    two-cell e.
embryoblast
embryocardia
embryocide
embryoctony
embryofetal alcohol syndrome (EFAS)

embryofetoscopy
    transabdominal thin-gauge e.
    (TGEF)
embryogenesis
embryogenic induction disorder
embryography
embryoid
embryologic malformation
embryology
    breast e.
    causal e.
    comparative e.
    descriptive e.
    experimental e.
    genital tract e.
    Leydig cell e.
    reproductive tract e.
embryoma
embryomorphous
Embryon
    E. GIFT catheter
    E. GIFT transfer catheter set
    E. HSG catheter
embryonal
    e. cell carcinoma
    e. RMS
    e. sarcoma
    e. tumor
embryonate
embryonic
    e. anideus
    e. axis
    e. blastoderm
    e. branchial system
    e. cleavage
    e. development
    e. diapause
    e. differentiation
    e. disc
    e. esophagus
    e. genome activation
    e. heart motion (EHM)
    e. hemoglobin
    e. loss
    e. neural retina
    e. neural tube
    e. noxae
    e. organ culture study
    e. period
    e. renomedullary interstitial cell
    e. sac
    e. stem cell
    e. testicular regression syndrome
    e. tissue
embryoniform
embryonization
embryonum
    smegma e.
embryony

embryopathology
embryopathy
    alcoholic e.
    e. alcoholica
    diabetic e.
    heparin e.
    isotretinoin e.
    retinoic acid e.
    rubella e.
    thalidomide e.
    trimethadione e.
    valproic acid e.
    warfarin e.
embryoplastic
embryoscope
embryoscopy
embryotome
embryotomy
embryotoxic
embryotoxon
    posterior e.
embryotrophy
EMC
    endometrial curettage
Emcyt
EMD
    electromechanical dissociation
emedastine
emergency
    e. cesarean section
    e. contraception (EC)
    e. contraception pill (ECP)
    e. contraceptive pill (ECP)
    hypertensive e.
    e. medical services for children
      (EMS-C)
    e. medicine
    e. surgery
    surgical e.
emergent injury
Emerson respirator
Emery-Dreifuss
    E.-D. muscular dystrophy
    E.-D. syndrome
emesis
    bile-stained e.
    bilious e.
    coffee-grounds e.
    intractable e.
    e. pH determination
    posttussive e.

    salivation, lacrimation, urination,
      defecation, gastrointestinal distress,
      and e. (SLUDGE)
emetic agent
EMG
    electromyelogram
    electromyogram
    electromyography
    exomphalos, macroglossia, gigantism
      MyoTrac EMG
      EMG syndrome
Emgel
eminence
    malar e.
    median e.
emission
    evoked otoacoustic e. (EOAE)
    nasal air e.
    otoacoustic e. (OAE)
    transient evoked otoacoustic e.
      (TEOAE)
EMIT
    enzyme-multiplication immunoassay
      technique
    enzyme-multiplied immunoassay
      technique
Emko
EMLA
    eutectic mixture of local anesthetics
      EMLA anesthetic disc
      EMLA cream
      EMLA disc topical anesthetic
        adhesive system
      EMLA patch
emmenagogic
emmenagogue
emmenia
emmenic
emmeniopathy
emmenology
Emmet operation
emmetropia
Emmett cervical tenaculum
Emmett-Gellhorn pessary
Emo-Cort
emollient cream
emotional
    e. abuse
    e. amenorrhea
    e. development
    e. disorder
    e. lability

E

NOTES

emotional *(continued)*
> e. milestone
> e. response
> e. state

Emotionality Activity Sociability Scale (EAS)
emotionally
> e. disturbed
> e. impaired

empathy
emphysema
> congenital lobar e.
> lobar e.
> perivascular e.
> pulmonary interstitial e. (PIE)
> subcutaneous e.

empiric
> e. therapy
> e. treatment

empirical
empirically
Empirin
Empirynol Plus contraceptive gel
emprosthotonos
empty
> e. scrotum syndrome
> e. sella syndrome

emptying
> abnormal gastric e.
> bladder e.
> delayed gastric e.
> gastric e.

empyema
> encapsulated e.
> epidural e.
> intracranial e.
> e. necessitatis
> subdural e.
> symptomatic chronic e.

EMR
> endomyometrial resection

EMRN
> encephalomyeloradiculoneuropathy

EMS
> encephalomyosynangiosis

EMSA
> electrophoretic mobility shift assay

EMS-C
> emergency medical services for children

EMTAC
> Enhanced Metabolic Testing Activity Chamber

EM/TEN
> erythema multiforme/toxic epidermal necrolysis

emulsion
> fat e.
> Soyacal IV fat e.
> Travamulsion IV fat e.

Emulsoil
en
> en bloc
> en bloc resection
> en caul delivery
> en face position

EnAbl thermal ablation system
enalapril
enalaprilat
enamel
> e. hypoplasia
> mottled e.

enamelogenesis
enanthate
> estradiol e.
> norethindrone e. (NET-EN)
> testosterone e.

enanthem
> hemorrhagic e.
> oral e.

Enbrel
encainide
Encap
> Novo-Rythro E.

encapsulated empyema
encapsulation
> embryo e.

Encare
enceinte
encelitis, enceliitis
encephalitide
encephalitis, pl. **encephalitides**
> acute chagasic e.
> acute influenza A e.
> allergic e.
> arboviral e.
> brainstem e.
> California e.
> cerebellar e.
> chagasic e.
> chronic focal e.
> chronic granulomatous amebic e.
> chronic mumps e.
> chronic progressive e.
> Dawson e.
> diffuse periaxial e.
> Eastern equine e. (EEE)
> enterovirus e.
> epidemic e.
> equine e.
> focal postviral e.
> giant cell e.
> hemorrhagic e.
> herpes simplex e. (HSE)
> herpes simplex virus e.
> herpesvirus e.
> influenza A e.
> Japanese e.
> La Crosse e.

e. lethargica
Marie-Strümpell e.
measles inclusion body e. (MIBE)
multinucleated cell e.
mumps e.
neonatal HSV-1, -2 e.
periaxial e.
e. periaxialis concentrica
postinfectious e.
postinfluenza vaccination e.
postmeasles e.
postviral e.
Powassan e.
progressive e.
psychoses cum encephalatides
Rasmussen e.
Russian spring-summer e.
Schilder e.
septic e.
St. Louis e. (SLE)
subacute e.
tick-borne e. (TBE)
Toxoplasma e.
toxoplasmic e.
varicella e.
Venezuelan equine e. (VEE)
viral e.
Western equine e. (WEE)
encephalitogenic cell
encephaloarteriosynangiosis
encephalocele
cranial e.
frontal e.
hydrocephalus, agyria, retinal
  dysplasia with or without e.
  (HARD+/-E)
nasal e.
parietal e.
transalar sphenoidal e.
encephaloclastic
encephalocraniocutaneous lipomatosis
  (ECCL)
encephalocraniofacial
e. angiomatosis
e. neuroangiomatosis
encephaloduroarterial synangiosis
encephaloduroarteriosynangios (EDAS)
encephalofacial angiomatosis
encephalofacialis
angiomatosis e.
neuroangiomatosis e.

encephalomalacia
cystic e.
multicystic e.
periventricular e.
polycystic e.
encephalomeningocele
encephalomere
encephalomyelitis
acute disseminated e. (ADEM)
allergic e.
experimental allergic e. (EAE)
fatal e.
immune-mediated disseminated e.
inflammatory demyelinating e.
postinfectious e. (PIE)
postrabies vaccine e.
varicella-zoster e.
encephalomyelocele
encephalomyelopathy
Leigh necrotizing e.
mitochondrial e.
encephalomyeloradiculoneuropathy
  (EMRN)
encephalomyopathy
e. of Leigh
mitochondrial e.
subacute necrotizing e.
encephalomyosynangiosis (EMS)
encephalopathic crisis
encephalopathy
AIDS e.
anoxic-ischemic e.
bilirubin e.
bovine spongiform e. (BSE)
Brett epileptogenic e.
burn e.
childhood epileptic e.
chronic spongiform e.
demyelinating e.
early infantile epileptic e.
epileptic e.
epileptogenic e.
fatal neonatal hyperammonemic e.
hepatic e. (HE)
human immunodeficiency virus e.
hypertensive e.
hypoxic e.
hypoxic-ischemic e. (HIE)
infantile epileptic e.
infantile subacute necrotizing e.
late radiation e.
lead e.

E

NOTES

encephalopathy *(continued)*
    Leigh subacute necrotizing e.
    metabolic e.
    mitochondrial e.
    myoclonic e.
    necrotizing e.
    neonatal e. (NE)
    neonatal hypoxic-ischemic e.
    nonspecific e.
    overt bilirubin e.
    phenytoin e.
    plateau e.
    postasphyxial e.
    postvaccinal e.
    progressive e.
    radiation e.
    Reye hepatic e.
    Sarnat e.
    spongiform e.
    static e.
    subacute necrotizing e.
    transient bilirubin e.
    transmissible spongiform e. (TSE)
    uremic e.
    Wernicke e. (WE)
    e. with prolinemia
encephalotomy
encephalotrigeminal
    e. angiomatosis
    e. syndrome
enchondral ossification
enchondroma, pl. **enchondromata**
    multiple bone enchondromata
enchondromatosis
encode
encoding
encopresis
encranius
encu method
encyesis
end
    e. bud
    e. ileostomy
    E. Lice Liquid
endadelphos
Endantadine
endarterectomy
endarteritis
    infective e.
    obliterative e.
Endcaps
    Glucolet E.
end-diastolic
    e.-d. velocity (EDV)
    e.-d. volume (EDV)
endemic
    e. Burkitt lymphoma
    e. cretinism
    malaria e.

    e. syphilis
    e. Tyrolean infantile cirrhosis
endemicity
Endermologie LPG system
Enders Edmonston measles strain
end-expiratory
    e.-e. lung volume (EELV)
    e.-e. phase (EEP)
    e.-e. pressure (EEP)
end-inspiratory airway occlusion
endoanal
    e. ultrasonography
    e. ultrasound
Endo-Assist
    E.-A. cutting dissector
    E.-A. endoscopic forceps
    E.-A. endoscopic knot pusher
    E.-A. endoscopic ligature carrier
    E.-A. endoscopic needle holder
    E.-A. retractable blade
    E.-A. retractable scalpel
    E.-A. sponge aspirator
Endo-Avitene
    E.-A. hemostatic material
    E.-A. microfibrillar collagen
    hemostat
endobronchial tuberculosis
endocarcinoma
endocardial
    e. cushion
    e. cushion defect (ECD)
    e. fibroelastosis (EFE)
    e. fibrosis
    e. sclerosis
    e. thrombus
endocarditis
    acute bacterial e.
    bacterial e.
    enterococcal e.
    fetal e.
    fungal e.
    infectious e. (IE)
    infective e. (IE)
    Libman-Sacks e.
    marantic e.
    nonbacterial thrombotic e.
    subacute bacterial e. (SBE)
    thrombotic e.
    verrucous e.
endocardium
    mural e.
endocavitary radiation therapy
Endocell endometrial cell collector
endocervical
    e. aspirator
    e. canal
    e. canal colposcopy
    e. curettage (ECC)
    e. curetting

e. glandular dysplasia
e. mucosa
e. polyp
e. resection (ECR)
e. sample
e. sampling
e. sampling brush
e. sinus tumor
endocervicitis
endocervix
endochondral ossification
endochondroma
endochorion
Endoclip
E. cautery
E. monopolar electrocautery
endocolpitis
endocrine
e. disorder
e. factor
e. gland
e. manifestation
e. nonfunctional testis
e. pancreatic dysfunction
e. system
endocrinologic sex
endocrinologist
endocrinology
pediatric e. (PdE)
reproductive e.
endocrinology-infertility
reproductive e.-i.
endocrinopathy
endocytosis
receptor-mediated e.
endoderm
endodermal
e. cell
e. sinus
e. sinus tumor (EST)
endodermatosis
endoesophageal pH
endogenicity/melancholia
endogenous
e. catecholamine
e. estrogen
e. estrogenic stimulation
e. fat
e. gonadotropin
e. gonadotropin activity suppression
e. hormonal production
e. hormone

e. opiate
e. opiate receptor
e. opioid
e. opioid peptide
e. pyrogen
e. steroid
Endo GIA 30 suture stapler
endoglin
endograsper
roticulating e.
EndoLive 3-D stereo video endoscope
Endoloop suture
endoluminal
e. stent
e. stenting
endomesenchymal tract
endometria (*pl. of* endometrium)
endometrial
e. ablation
e. ablator
e. adenoacanthoma
e. adhesion
e. aspirator
e. atrophy
e. biopsy
e. breakdown
e. cancer
e. cannula
e. carcinoma
e. cavity
e. clear cell adenocarcinoma
e. curettage (EMC)
e. cycle
e. cycling activity
e. cyst
e. dating
e. development
e. embryo
e. histology
e. hyperplasia (EH)
e. implant
e. intraepithelial neoplasia (EIN)
e. involvement
e. metastasizing leiomyoma
e. milieu
e. morphology
e. neoplasia
e. neoplasm
e. polyp
e. proliferation
e. protein
e. receptor

NOTES

endometrial *(continued)*
- e. resection
- e. resection and ablation (ERA)
- e. sampling
- e. sarcoma
- e. secretory adenocarcinoma
- e. shedding
- e. spiral artery
- e. stimulation
- e. stripe
- e. stroma
- e. stromal sarcoma (ESS)
- e. thickness
- e. tuberculosis
- e. tumor
- e. vaporization

endometrioid
- e. carcinoma
- e. epithelial cell tumor

endometrioma
- complex adnexal e.
- large e.
- ovarian e.

endometriosis
- adhesive e.
- AFS Revised Classification of E.
- asymptomatic mild e.
- extrapelvic e.
- e. interna
- internal e.
- nonpigmented e.
- ovarian e.
- pelvic e.
- pulmonary e.
- rectosigmoid colon e.
- retroperitoneal e.
- small bowel e.
- stromal e.
- tubal e.
- urinary tract e.
- vulvar e.

endometriosis-associated infertility

endometriotic
- e. focus
- e. implant
- e. lesion
- e. tissue

endometritis
- bacteriotoxic e.
- decidual e.
- e. dissecans
- nonpuerperal e.
- postpartum e.
- puerperal e.

endometrium, pl. **endometria**
- atrophic e.
- cyclic proliferative e.
- decidualized e.
- ectopic e.
- eutopic e.
- hyperechoic e.
- hypersecretory e.
- inactive e.
- menstrual e.
- nonpregnant e.
- proliferative e.
- quiescent e.
- secretory e.
- Swiss cheese e.
- tubal e.

endometropic

endomyocardial
- e. biopsy
- e. fibrosis

endomyometria (*pl. of* endomyometrium)

endomyometrial resection (EMR)

endomyometritis
- postpartum e.

endomyometrium, pl. **endomyometria**

endomysial staining

endomysium antibody (EMA)

endoneurial fibrosis

endonuclease
- e. analysis
- restriction e.

endoparametritis

Endopath
- E. bladeless trocar
- E. endoscopic articulating stapler
- E. ETS-Flex endoscopic articulating linear cutter
- E. EZ35 endoscopic linear cutter
- E. needle tip electrosurgery probe
- E. Optiview optical surgical obturator
- E. TriStar trocar
- E. Ultra Veress needle

endopelvic fascia

endopeptidase

endoperoxide

endophthalmitis
- nematode e.

endophytic

endoplasm

endoplasmic reticulum (ER)

Endopouch Pro specimen-retrieval bag

endorectal
- e. flap
- e. pull-through

endoreduplication

end-organ complication

endorphin, dopamine, and prostaglandin theory

endosalpinges (*pl. of* endosalpinx)

endosalpingiosis
- atypical e.

endosalpingitis

endosalpingoblastosis
endosalpinx, pl. **endosalpinges**
endoscope
EndoLive 3-D stereo video e.
MicroLap e.
mother and baby e.
Olympus GIF-XP10 video e.
Pentax EG-2430 video e.
Pentax FG 24-x video e.
rigid open-tube e.
Storz e.
endoscopic
e. bladder neck suspension (EBNS)
e. cautery
e. choroid plexus extirpation
e. correction
e. elastic band ligation
e. ethmoidectomy
fetal e.
e. incision
e. incision with flap
e. linear cutter
e. microsurgery
e. retrograde
cholangiopancreatography (ERCP)
e. sclerotherapy
e. sinus surgery
e. strip craniectomy
e. unroofing
e. variceal ligation (EVL)
e. variceal sclerotherapy (EVS)
endoscopy
flexible fiberoptic e.
Endoshears
endosonography
Endosound endoscopic ultrasound
endosperm
Endo Stitch laparoscopic suturing device
Endotek
E. OM-3 Urodata monitor
E. UDS-1000 monitor
E. urodynamics system
endothelia (*pl. of* endothelium)
endothelial
e. cell
e. cell activation
e. cell lysate
e. dysfunction
e. dystrophy
e. nitric oxide synthetase

endothelin
e. plasma level
e. receptor-B gene
endothelin-1 (ET-1)
endothelin-2 (ET-2)
endothelin-3 (ET-3)
e. gene
endotheliochorial placenta
endothelio-endothelial placenta
endotheliosis
glomerular capillary e.
endothelium, pl. **endothelia**
fenestrated vascular e.
vascular e.
endothelium-derived relaxing factor (EDRF)
endotoxemia
endotoxic shock
endotoxin
gram-negative e.
lipopolysaccharide e.
meningococcal e.
endotracheal (ET)
e. intubation (ETI)
e. intubation and mechanical ventilation (EI/MV)
e. tube
endotrachelitis
endovaginal
e. finding
e. imaging
multiplane e. (MEVA)
e. probe
e. sonography
e. transducer
e. ultrasonography
e. ultrasound (EVUS)
endovascular hemolytic-uremic syndrome
endovasculitis
hemorrhagic e.
end-point dilution method
Endrate
Endrin
end-stage
e.-s. cirrhosis
e.-s. heart failure
e.-s. kidney disease
e.-s. liver disease
e.-s. renal disease (ESRD)
end-systolic
e.-s. stress (ESS)

NOTES

end-systolic *(continued)*
    e.-s. volume (ESV)
    e.-s. wall stress
end-tidal
    e.-t. breath carbon monoxide
    e.-t. carbon dioxide (E_TCO_2)
    e.-t. CO
    e.-t. CO_2
    e.-t. CO_2 monitoring
    e.-t. CO_2 tension
end-to-side
    e.-t.-s. anastomosis
    e.-t.-s. portocaval shunt
Enduron
enema
    air e.
    air-contrast barium e.
    antegrade continence e. (ACE)
    barium e.
    Cortenema e.
    Fleet Mineral Oil E.
    Gastrografin e.
    hydrogen peroxide e.
    lactulose e.
    oil e.
    phosphate e.
    e. procedure
    rectocolonic saline e.
    retention e.
    Rowasa e.
    soapsuds e.
    water e.
    water-soluble contrast e.
Ener-B
energy
    color Doppler e. (CDE)
    e. expenditure
    e. healing
    e. metabolism
EnfaCare LIPIL formula
Enfamil
    E. A.R. LIPIL formula
    E. Human Milk Fortifier
    E. Human Milk Fortifier formula
    E. LactoFree LIPIL formula
    E. LIPIL Low iron formula
    E. LIPIL with iron formula
    E. Next Step ProSobee LIPIL
      formula
    E. Nutramigen LIPIL formula
    E. Pregestimil formula
    E. Premature LIPIL formula
    E. ProSobee LIPIL formula
enflurane
ENG
    electronystagmography
engaged head
engagement

Engerix-B
    E.-B hepatitis B vaccine
    E.-B immunization
engineering
    genetic e.
Englert forceps
English
    E. lock
    E. MacIntosh (E-Mac)
    manual E.
    E. position
    signed E. (SE)
    signed exact E. (SEE)
    E. yew
Engman syndrome
engorged
    e. breast
    e. vessel
engorgement
    breast e.
    clitoral e.
    e. of intussusceptum
    vascular e.
    venous e.
engraftment
    fetal e.
Engstrom respirator
enhanced
    e. inactivated polio vaccine (eIPV)
    E. Metabolic Testing Activity
      Chamber (EMTAC)
    e. urinalysis
enhanced-potency MAb
enhancement
    acoustic e.
    e. factor
    immunologic e.
    rapid acquisition with resolution e.
      (RARE)
enhancer
    surfactant-associated protein C e.
enigmatic fever
enjoyment
    sexual e.
enkephalin
enlarged
    e. cavum septum
    e. cavum septum pellucidum
    e. liver
    e. posterior fossa
enlargement
    abdominal e.
    areolar e.
    bony e.
    breast e.
    clitoris e.
    corneal e.
    lymph node e.
    muscle e.

parotid e.
pelvis e.
sellar e.
uterine e.
Enlon
enmeshment
ENNAS
Einstein Neonatal Neurobehavioral
Assessment Scale
enolase
neuron-specific e. (NSE)
enophthalmos
enoxacin
enoxaparin
Enpresse tablet
Enseals
potassium iodide E.
ensu method
Ensure
E. High Protein formula
E. Plus HN formula
E. with Fiber formula
EN-tabs
Azulfidine EN-t.
Entamoeba
E. dispar
E. gingivalis
E. histolytica
entanglement
cord e.
fetal e.
ENTec coblator plasma system
enteral feeding
enteric
e. adenovirus
e. cytopathogenic human orphan
(ECHO)
e. duplication
e. feeding
e. fever
e. gentamicin
e. gram-negative bacillary (EGNB)
e. hyperoxaluria
e. infection
e. neuropeptide
enteritidis
Salmonella e.
enteritis
bacterial e.
Campylobacter e.
CMV e.
inflammatory bacterial e.

regional e.
rotavirus e.
tuberculous e.
viral e.
Enterobacter
E. cloacae
E. pneumonia
Enterobacteriaceae
enterobiasis
Enterobius vermicularis
enterocele
anterior e.
double hump sign of an e.
pulsion e.
e. repair
traction e.
enterochromaffin
e. cell
e. cell stimulation
enterococcal endocarditis
Enterococcus
E. casseliflavus
E. faecalis
E. faecium
enterococcus, pl. enterococci
glycopeptide-resistant e. (GRE)
vancomycin-resistant e. (VRE)
viridans e.
enterocolic fistula
enterocolitica
Yersinia e.
enterocolitis
allergic e.
autistic e.
dietary protein e.
Hirschsprung e.
necrotizing e. (NEC)
pseudomembranous e.
e. syndrome
enterocutaneous fistula
enterocyte
enterocytopathogenic human orphan
(ECHO)
Enterocytozoon
E. bieneusi
E. intestinalis
enteroenteric fistula
enterogenous cyst
enteroglucagon
enterohemorrhagic *Escherichia coli*
(EHEC)

E

NOTES

enterohepatic
> e. recirculation
> e. shunt
> e. shunting

enterokinase deficiency
enteromenia
enteropathica
> acrodermatitis e.
> dermatitis e.

enteropathogenic *Escherichia coli* **(EPEC)**
enteropathy
> autoimmune e. (AIE)
> dermatitis herpetiformis-associated gluten-sensitive e.
> gluten e.
> gluten-induced e.
> gluten-sensitive e.
> protein-losing e.

enteroscopy
> small bowel e.

enterostomal therapy
enterostomy
> diverting e.
> proximal e.
> Santulli e.

Entero-Test
enterotoxigenic *Escherichia coli* **(ETEC)**
enterotoxin
> e. F
> sporulation e.

enterovaginal fistula
enterovesical fistula
enteroviral
> e. infection
> e. meningitis
> e. meningoencephalitis
> e. myocarditis

enterovirus
> e. 71
> e. encephalitis
> nonpolio e.

Entex LA
enthesis
> tender e.

enthesitis
enthesopathy
entitled demander
Entocort
entrapment
> head e.
> intrapartum head e.
> penile zipper e.
> saphenous nerve e.

entrapped temporal horn
Entree
> E. II trocar and cannula system
> E. Plus trocar and cannula system

EntriStar
> E. Gastrostomy System
> E. Skin Level Tube
> E. Skin Level Tube for gastrostomy

entropy
enucleation
> surgical e.

Enulose
enunciate
enuresis
> diurnal e.
> head banding e.
> nocturnal e.
> pad and bell technique for e.
> primary nocturnal e.
> secondary e.

enuretic episode
envelope
> lipid e.
> peritoneal e.

envenomation
> arachnid e.
> snakebite e.

environment
> Home Observation for the Measurement of the E. (HOME)
> hormonal e.
> least restrictive e. (LRE)
> natural e.
> thermal neutral e.

environmental
> e. risk
> e. teratogen
> e. tobacco smoke (ETS)
> e. toxin
> e. trigger
> e. variance

Envision endocavity probe
Enzone
enzygotic twin
enzymatic block
enzyme
> e. activity
> angiotensin-converting e. (ACE)
> antioxidant e.
> e. assay
> cytochrome *c* oxidative e.
> e. defect
> e. deficiency
> elevated liver e.'s
> exogenous pancreatic e.
> human recombinant antioxidant e.
> e. immunoassay (EIA)
> e. immunosorbent assay (EIA)
> inosinate pyrophoshorylase e.
> major detoxificating e.
> peroxidative e.
> proteolytic e.

rare-cutter e.
recombinant e.
e. replacement therapy
restriction e.
e. supplement
Taq I e.
TNF-alpha converting e.
zinc-dependent e.
enzyme-linked
e.-l. antiglobulin test
e.-l. immunofiltration assay (ELIFA)
e.-l. immunosorbent assay (ELISA)
e.-l. immunotransfer blot (EITB)
enzyme-multiplication immunoassay technique (EMIT)
enzyme-multiplied immunoassay technique (EMIT)
enzymic acid hydrolysis
enzymopathy
EOAE
evoked otoacoustic emission
EOIT
ego-oriented individual therapy
EOM
equal ocular movement
extraocular movement
EOS
early-onset schizophrenia
eosin
hematoxylin and e. (H&E)
e. stain
eosin-4 stain
eosinopenia
eosinophilia
nonallergenic rhinitis with e.
peripheral e.
pulmonary e.
pulmonary infiltrate with e. (PIE)
sputum e.
eosinophilia-myalgia syndrome
eosinophilic
e. adenoma
e. allergic colitis
e. ascites
e. cationic protein (ECP)
e. cystitis
e. esophagitis
e. fasciitis
e. gastroenteritis
e. gastroenteropathy
e. granuloma

e. infiltrate
e. leukemia
e. meningitis
e. meningoencephalitis
e. myocarditis
e. myositis
e. nonallergic rhinitis
e. pleocytosis
e. pneumonia
e. pustular folliculitis (EPF)
eosinophil peroxidase
EP
ectopic pregnancy
etoposide
EPC
external pneumatic calf compression
EPDS
Edinburgh Postnatal Depression Scale
EPEC
enteropathogenic *Escherichia coli*
ependyma
ependymitis
granular e.
ependymoblastoma
ependymoma
posterior fossa anaplastic e.
supratentorial anaplastic e.
eperezolid
EPF
eosinophilic pustular folliculitis
ephaptic interaction
ephebiatrics
ephebic
ephebogenesis
ephebogenic
ephebology
ephedrine
racemic e.
e. sulfate
ephelis, pl. **ephelides**
ephemeral
e. fever
e. temperature
EPI
extremely premature infant
Epi
E. E-Z Pen
E. E-Z Pen-Jr
epiblast
epiblepharon
epibulbar dermoid
epicanthal fold

NOTES

epicanthus inversus
epicardial pacing
epicardium
epicomus syndrome
epicondyle
    traction apophysitis of medial e.
epicondylitis
    lateral e.
epicranial aponeurosis
Epics XL flow cytometer
epicutaneous test
epidemic
    e. capillary bronchitis
    e. encephalitis
    e. keratoconjunctivitis (EKC)
    e. keratoconjunctivitis adenovirus
    e. motor polyradiculoneuritis
    e. parotitis
    e. pleurodynia
    e. relapsing fever
    e. vertigo
epidemica
    myalgia cruris e.
epidemiologic, epidemiological
    E. Catchment Program
    e. characteristic
    e. feature
    e. genetics
    e. study
epidemiology
epidermal
    e. covering
    e. growth factor (EGF)
    e. growth factor receptor (EGFR)
    e. hyperkeratosis
    e. inclusion cyst
    e. melanocyte
    e. nevus
    e. nevus syndrome
epidermidis
    Staphylococcus e.
epidermis, pl. epidermides
    e. bullosa dystrophica
epidermodysplasia verruciformis
epidermoid cyst
epidermolysis
    e. bullosa (EB)
    e. bullosa acquisita
    e. bullosa letalis
    e. bullosa, macular type (EBM)
    e. bullosa simplex
    e. bullosa simplex of feet
    e. bullosa simplex of hands
epidermolytic
    e. hyperkeratosis
    e. toxin
Epidermophyton floccosum
epidermophytosis

epididymal
    e. sperm
    e. sperm aspiration
    e. vessel vasculitis
epididymis, pl. epididymides
    appendix e.
epididymitis
    postoperative congestive e.
epididymoorchitis
epididymovasostomy
epidural
    e. abscess
    e. analgesia
    e. anesthesia
    e. empyema
    e. hemangioma
    e. hematoma
    e. hemorrhage
    e. morphine
    e. opioid
Epifoam
Epifrin
epigastric
    e. artery
    e. hernia
    e. pain
    e. tenderness
epigastrium
epigastrius
epigenesis
epigenetic event
epiglottal blockage
epiglottic surface culture
epiglottis
    omega-shaped e.
epiglottitis
    acute e.
epignathus
epilepsia partialis continua
epilepsy
    abdominal e.
    absence e.
    benign childhood e.
    benign focal e.
    benign myoclonic e.
    benign neonatal e.
    benign partial e.
    benign rolandic e. (BRE)
    centralopathic e.
    centrencephalic e.
    centrotemporal e.
    childhood absence e.
    complex myoclonic e.
    complex partial e.
    extratemporal e.
    fictitious e.
    focal e.
    E. Foundation
    grand mal e.

idiopathic e.
infantile e.
International League Against E.
  (ILAE)
jacksonian e.
juvenile absence e.
juvenile myoclonic e.
e. management
midtemporal e.
myoclonic e.
myoclonic e. with ragged red
  fibers (MERRF)
myoclonus e.
nocturnal e.
partial complex e.
petit mal e.
photosensitive e.
posttraumatic e.
primary generalized e.
progressive bulbar palsy with e.
progressive myoclonic e.
psychomotor e.
reactive e.
reflex e.
rolandic e.
secondary e.
e. seizure
severe myoclonic e.
startle e.
sylvian e.
symptomatic e.
television e.
temporal lobe e.
typical absence e.
vestibulogenic e.
video game e.
visual reflex e.

epileptic
e. aura
e. convulsion
e. encephalopathy
e. idiocy
e. myoclonus
e. seizure
e. syndrome

epilepticus
absence status e.
complex partial status e.
convulsive status e.
febrile status e.
idiopathic status e.
limbic status e.

nonconvulsive status e. (NCSE)
partial status e.
refractory status e. (RSE)
status e. (SE)
symptomatic status e.

epileptiform
e. activity
e. discharge

epileptogenesis
epileptogenic
e. encephalopathy
e. lesion

epileptogenicity
epileptologist
epileptology
epiloia
epimenorrhagia
epimenorrhea
epimyoepithelial island
Epinal
epinephrine
aerosolized racemic e.
e. deficiency
higher-dose therapy with e. (HDE)
lidocaine and e.
Marcaine with e.
e. provocation
racemic e.
self-injectable e.
Xylocaine With E.

epineurium
EpiPen
E. Jr.
E. Sr.

epipericardial connective tissue
epiphora
epiphyseal, epiphysial
e. closure
e. dysostosis
e. dysplasia
e. dysplasia, microcephaly,
  nystagmus syndrome
e. dysplasia, short stature,
  microcephaly, nystagmus syndrome
e. growth
e. growth plate
e. ossification center
e. plate injury
e. stapling
e. syndrome

epiphyses (*pl. of* epiphysis)
epiphysiodesis

NOTES

E

315

epiphysiolysis
epiphysis, pl. **epiphyses**
    capital femoral e.
    capitellar e.
    congenital stippled e.
    double epiphyses
    femoral e.
    intraarticular e.
    proximal femoral e.
    proximal tibial e.
    radial e.
    slipped e.
    slipped capital femoral e. (SCFE)
    slipped upper femoral e. (SUFE)
    stippled e.
    stippling of epiphyses
    tibial e.
    upper humeral e.
epiplocele
epiploia
epipodophyllotoxin
epipygus
epirubicin
episcleritis
episioperineoplasty
episioperineorrhaphy
episioplasty
episiorrhaphy
episiostenosis
episiotomy
    bilateral mediolateral e.'s
    e. dehiscence
    first-degree e.
    fourth-degree e.
    median e.
    mediolateral e.
    midline e.
    prophylactic e.
    e. repair
    ruptured e.
    second-degree e.
    e. site
    third-degree e.
Episkopi blindness
episode
    enuretic e.
    hyperammonemic e.
    hypomanic e.
    hypotonic-hyporesponsive e.'s
     (HHEs)
    mitochondrial encephalomyelopathy,
     lactic acidosis, strokelike e.'s
    mitochondrial encephalomyopathy,
     lactic acidosis, strokelike e.'s
     (MELAS)
    mitochondrial myopathy,
     encephalopathy, lactic acidosis,
     strokelike e.'s
    nonprimary first e.

    present e.
    protracted depressive e.
    Schedule for Affective Disorders
     and Schizophrenia for School-Age
     Children-Present E. (K-SADS-P)
    strokelike e.
    syncopal e.
    vasoocclusive e.
episodic
    e. angioedema
    e. ataxia (1, 2)
    e. blanching
    e. dyscontrol
    e. dyscontrol syndrome
    e. flushing
    e. hypoglycemia
    e. memory
episome
epispadias
    female e.
    simple e.
epispadias-exstrophy complex
epistasis
epistatic
epistaxis
    recurrent e.
    refractory e.
epistemology
episthotonos
epitarsus
epitaxy
17-epitestosterone
epithelial
    e. atrophy
    e. autoantibody localization
    e. bud
    e. cancer
    e. cell
    e. cell abnormality
    e. cell ovarian carcinoma
    e. cell proliferation
    e. disorder
    e. hyperplasia
    e. inclusion cyst
    e. keratitis
    e. lining fluid (ELF)
    e. liver tumor
    e. membrane antigen (EMA)
    e. ovarian cancer (stage I–IV)
    e. pearl
    e. plug
    e. serous tumor
    e. stromal ovarian neoplasm
    e. stromal tumor
    e. tuft
epithelialization
epithelial-mesenchymal interaction
epitheliochorial placenta

epithelioid
e. cell
e. cell nevus
e. leiomyosarcoma
epithelioma
e. adenoides cysticum
basal cell e.
calcifying e.
epithelium, pl. **epithelia**
acetowhite e.
airway e.
artificial vaginal e.
atypical e.
celomic e.
cervical e.
circumferential eversion of
urethral e.
columnar e.
germinal e.
infarction of oral e.
luminal e.
native squamous e.
oral e.
ovarian germinal e.
papilla of columnar e.
respiratory e.
retinal pigment e. (RPE)
squamous e.
stratified squamous e.
surface e.
urethral e.
urogenital e.
uterine e.
white e.
Epitol
epitope
epitopic
epituberculosis
epitympanic recess
Epivir-HBV
EPO
erythropoietin
evening primrose oil
Epo
erythropoietin
epoch
growth e.
sleep e.
epoetin alfa
Epogen
epoophorectomy
epoophoron

EPP
erythropoietic protoporphyria
Eppendorfer
E. biopsy forceps
E. biopsy punch
Eppy/N
Eprolin
EPS
ear, patella, short stature
EPS syndrome
EPSDT
Early and Periodic Screening, Diagnosis,
and Treatment
EPSDT program
epsilon-aminocaproic acid (EACA)
epsilon toxin
Epstein-Barr
E.-B. nuclear antigen (EBNA)
E.-B. virus (EBV)
Epstein pearls
EPT
early pregnancy test
epulis
congenital e.
e. gravidarum
e. of newborn
e. of pregnancy
Equagesic
equal
e. conjoined twins
e. ocular movement (EOM)
equalization
pressure e. (PE)
equation
Hadlock e.
Harris-Benedict basal energy
expenditure e.
Henderson-Hasselbalch e.
Schofield weight- and height-based
resting energy expenditure
prediction e.
Starling e.
equatorial
e. division
e. plane
equi
Rhodococcus e.
equilibration
equilibrium
acid-base e.
Donnan e.
genetic e.

NOTES

equilibrium (*continued*)
- Hardy-Weinberg e.
- linkage e.
- e. phase
- e. reaction
- Starling e.

equina
- cauda e.

equine
- e. antitoxin
- e. encephalitis
- e. estrogen

equinovalgus
- talipes e.

equinovarus
- fetal talipes e.
- idiopathic talipes e.
- neurogenic talipes e.
- pes e.
- e. pes deformity
- talipes e. (TEV)

equinus
- ankle e.
- e. clubfoot
- e. deformity
- e. gait
- e. position
- talipes e.

equivalent
- genome e. (GE)
- lethal e.
- meconium ileus e.

equivocal culdocentesis

ER
- endoplasmic reticulum
- estrogen receptor

ERA
- endometrial resection and ablation
- evoked response audiometry
- ERA resectoscope sheath

eradication therapy

Er alpha
- estrogen receptor alpha

Erb
- E. juvenile muscular dystrophy
- E. palsy
- E. syndrome

Erb-Charcot syndrome

Erb-Duchenne
- E.-D. palsy
- E.-D. paralysis

Erbe
- E. electrical coagulation instrument
- E. electrical cutting instrument

Er beta
- estrogen receptor beta

Erb-Goldflam
- E.-G. disease
- E.-G. syndrome

Erb-Klumpke palsy

ERCP
- endoscopic retrograde cholangiopancreatography

Erdheim disease

erectile
- e. dysfunction
- e. structure
- e. tissue

erection
- artificial e.
- capillary e.
- penile e.

erethism

ERG
- electroretinogram
- electroretinography

ergocalciferol

ergogenic

ergometer
- bicycle e.

ergonovine maleate

ergosterol

ergot

ergotamine tartrate

Ergotrate

Erhardt
- E. developmental prehension assessment
- E. forceps

erigentes
- nervi e.

Erikson stages of growth and development

Erlacher-Blount syndrome

Erlenmeyer flask appearance

E-R-O Ear Drops

Eronen syndrome

Eros-CTD
- E.-CTD eroscillator device

E-rosette receptor

erosion
- bony e.
- cervical e.
- mesh e.
- subglottic e.

erosive
- e. adenomatosis of nipple
- e. esophagitis
- e. rhinitis
- e. vulvitis

ERP
- event-related potential

ERPC
- evacuation of retained products of conception

erratic
- e. blood pressure
- e. temperature

error
>alpha e.
>beta e.
>Garrodian inborn e.
>inborn e.
>metabolic e.
>refractive e.

ERT
>estrogen replacement therapy

ertapenem sodium
erucic acid
eructation
eruption
>bullous drug e.
>Christmas tree distribution e.
>creeping e.
>delayed tooth e.
>Kaposi varicelliform e.
>maculopapular e.
>monomorphous papular e.
>morbilliform e.
>papular e.
>papulosquamous e.
>polymorphous light e.
>pruritic vesiculopapular e.
>purpuric light e.
>scarlatiniform e.
>seabather's e.
>vesicobullous e.
>vesiculopapular e.
>violaceous e.

eruptive
>e. fever
>e. hidradenoma
>e. lichen planus
>e. nevus
>e. syringoma
>e. temperature
>e. vellus hair cyst
>e. xanthoma

ERV
>expiratory reserve volume

Er:YAG laser
Erybid
Eryc
Erycette
EryDerm
Erygel
Erymax
EryPed

erysipelas
>e. internum
>necrotizing e.

Erysipelothrix rhusiopathiae
Ery-Tab
erythema
>e. chronicum migrans (ECM)
>fixed e.
>gingival e.
>heliotropic e.
>e. induration of Bazin (EIB)
>e. infectiosum
>Jacquet e.
>linear gingival e.
>e. marginatum
>e. migrans
>e. multiforme (EM)
>e. multiforme exudativum
>e. multiforme/toxic epidermal necrolysis (EM/TEN)
>e. neonatorum toxicum
>e. nodosum
>e. nodosum leprosum
>ocular e.
>palmar e.
>periorbital violaceous e.
>periungual e.
>scarlatiniform e.
>toxic e.
>e. toxicum neonatorum
>vasculitic e.
>violaceous e.
>vulvovaginal e.

erythematosus
>disseminated lupus e.
>drug-induced systemic lupus e.
>lupus e. (LE)
>neonatal lupus e. (NLE)
>systemic lupus e. (SLE)

erythematous
>e. blush
>e. confluent plaque
>e. cutaneous plaque
>e. halo
>e. macule
>e. papule
>e. rash
>e. satellite lesion

erythrasma of vulva
erythredema polyneuropathy
erythrityl tetranitrate
Erythro-Base

NOTES

319

erythroblastic
    e. anemia
    e. anemia of childhood
erythroblastopenia
    transient e.
erythroblastosis
    ABO e.
    fetal e. (FE)
    e. fetalis
    e. neonatorum
Erythrocin
erythrocyte
    e. acquired defect
    burr-shaped e.
    e. count
    dysmorphic e.
    e. enzyme deficiency
    e. glutathione peroxidase deficiency
    e. membrane
    e. mosaicism
    packed e.
    e. phosphoglycerate kinase
      deficiency
    e. pyruvate kinase deficiency
    e. sedimentation rate (ESR)
    e. transfusion
erythrocytopoiesis
erythrocytosis
    familial e.
    stress e.
erythroderma
    atopic e.
    bullous congenital ichthyosiform e.
    congenital ichthyosiform e.
    e. desquamativum
    exfoliative e.
    generalized e.
    ichthyosiform e.
    nonbullous congenital
      ichthyosiform e.
erythrodermic
erythrohepatic
    e. porphyria
    e. protoporphyria
erythroid
    colony-forming unit e. (CFU-E)
    e. hyperplasia
    e. hypoplasia
    mature burst-forming unit e. (M-
      BFU-E)
    e. progenitor
    e. progenitor cell
erythrokeratodermia
    symmetric progressive e.
    e. variabilis
erythroleukoblastosis
erythromelalgia
Erythromid

erythromycin
    e. estolate
    e. ethylsuccinate (EES)
    e. lactobionate
erythron
erythrophagocytic lymphohistiocytosis
erythroplasia
    Queyrat e.
    Zoon e.
erythropoiesis
    compensatory e.
    dermal e.
    e. failure
    megaloblastic e.
    stress e.
erythropoietic
    e. porphyria
    e. porphyria congenita
    e. protoporphyria (EPP)
erythropoietin (EPO, Epo)
    human e.
    recombinant human e. (r-EPO,
      rHuEPO, rHuEpo)
    serum e.
Erythroxylum coca
Eryzole
ES
    Pertussin ES
    Vicodin ES
ESA Coulochem multi-electrode
Escalante syndrome
escape
    e. beats
    e. rhythm
escharotomy
Escherichia
    E. coli
    E. coli sepsis
    E. coli vaccine
Esclim
    E. estradiol transdermal system
    E. patch
    E. Transdermal
    E. transderm system
Escobar syndrome
escutcheon
E-selectin
Eserine
ESIMS
    electrospray ionization mass spectrometry
Eskalith
esmolol hydrochloride
esodeviation
esophageal
    e. anastomosis
    e. atresia (EA)
    e. candidiasis
    e. coin
    e. compression

e. dilation
e. duplication cyst
e. foreign body
e. hiatus
e. manometry
e. perforation
e. pressure
e. reflux
e. replacement
e. rupture
e. spasm
e. sphincter
e. stenosis
e. stricture
e. transection
e. ulceration
e. web
esophagectomy
esophagitis
allergic e.
eosinophilic e.
erosive e.
infectious e.
monilial e.
peptic e.
reflux e.
tetracycline-induced e.
viral e.
esophago-deglutition response
esophagoduodenostomy
esophagogastroduodenoscopy (EGD)
esophagogram
barium e.
contrast e.
esophagography
barium e.
esophagoscope
Holinger infant e.
esophagoscopy
esophagostomy
cervical e.
esophagotracheal primordium
esophago-UES-contractile reflex
esophagram
barium e.
Gastrografin e.
esophagus, pl. **esophagi**
Barrett e.
cervical e.
embryonic e.
nutcracker e.
stenosis of e.

EsopHogram software
esophoria
esotropia
accommodative e.
congenital e.
espundia
ESR
erythrocyte sedimentation rate
ESRD
end-stage renal disease
ESS
endometrial stromal sarcoma
end-systolic stress
essential
e. amino acid
e. benign pentosuria
e. dysmenorrhea
e. fatty acid (EFA)
e. fructosuria
e. hypertension
e. myoclonus
e. thrombocythemia (ET)
e. tremor
e. vulvodynia
Essiac
EST
endodermal sinus tumor
E$_{st}$
static elastance
established
e. medical diagnosis
e. risk
Estalis
Estar
ester
cholesterol e.
L-valine e.
phorbol e.
tosylarginine methyl e. (TAME)
esterase
tosylarginine methyl ester e.
esterified estrogen
Estes
E. operation
E. procedure
estetrol
esthesioneuroblastoma
esthiomene
estimated
e. date of conception (EDC)
e. date of confinement (EDC)

NOTES

estimated *(continued)*
  e. fetal weight (EFW)
  e. gestational age (EGA)
estimation
  gestational age e.
  e. of gestational age
estimator
  maximum likelihood e.
Estinyl
estolate
  erythromycin e.
Estrace
  E. Oral
  E. vaginal cream
Estra-D
Estraderm
  E. Transdermal
  E. transdermal system
  E. TTS
estradiol (E_2)
  17beta-e.
  e. assay
  bound e.
  e. cypionate
  e. cypionate and
    medroxyprogesterone acetate
  Cytoxan, Adriamycin, leucovorin,
    calcium, fluorouracil, ethinyl e.
    (CALF-E)
  desogestrel and ethinyl e.
  drospirenone/ethinyl e.
  e. enanthate
  ethinyl e. (EE)
  ethynodiol diacetate and e.
  exogenous e.
  free e.
  e. level
  levonorgestrel and ethinyl e.
  micronized 17beta e.
  norethindrone acetate and ethinyl e.
  norgestimate and ethinyl e.
  pre-hCG e.
  e. receptor
  e. suppression
  e. transdermal system
  e. vaginal cream
  e. valerate
estradiol/levonorgestrel
estradiol/norethindrone acetate
estradiol/norgestimate
estradiol-releasing silicone vaginal ring
estramustine phosphate sodium
estrane
Estrasorb
Estratab
Estratest
  E. HS
  E. Oral
Estren-Dameshek subtype

Estring estradiol vaginal ring
estriol (E_3)
  e. level
  salivary e.
  unconjugated e. (E3, uE3)
estrogen
  e. add-back therapy (EABT)
  e. agonist
  e. antagonist
  e. breakthrough bleeding
  catechol e.
  Cenestin synthetic conjugated e.'s
  circulating e.
  conjugated e.'s
  conjugated equine e. (CEE)
  e. deprivation
  e. effect
  endogenous e.
  equine e.
  esterified e.
  e. excess
  fetal e.
  health, osteoporosis, progestin, e.
    (HOPE)
  e. level
  e. loss
  e. metabolism
  oral conjugated e.
  orally administered e.
  postcoital e.
  prevent postmenopausal Alzheimer
    with replacement e.'s (PREPARE)
  e. receptor (ER)
  e. receptor alpha (Er alpha)
  e. receptor beta (Er beta)
  e. receptor localization
  e. replacement
  e. replacement therapy (ERT)
  serum e.
  e. sulfotransferase
  e. surge
  e. synthesis
  synthetic conjugated e.
  transdermal e.
  uninterrupted e.
  unopposed e.
  e. window etiologic hypothesis
  e. withdrawal
  e. withdrawal bleeding
  e.'s with methyltestosterone
  women's angiographic vitamins
    and e. (WAVE)
estrogen-agonist uterine effect
estrogen-assisted colposcopy
estrogen-dependent
  e.-d. endometrial carcinoma
  e.-d. neoplasia
estrogenic effect

estrogen-independent endometrial
 carcinoma
estrogen-induced prolactinoma
estrogenization
 introital e.
estrogenized mucosa
estrogen-only HRT
estrogen/progesterone ratio
estrogen-progesterone withdrawal
 bleeding
estrogen-progestin
 e.-p. artificial cycle
 e.-p. contraceptive
 e.-p. replacement therapy
 e.-p. test
estrogen-progestogen combination
estrone (E$_1$)
 oral e.
 e. sulfate
estrophasic oral contraceptive
estropipate
Estrostep
 E. Fe
 E. oral contraceptive
Estroven
estrus
ESV
 end-systolic volume
ET
 embryo transfer
 endotracheal
 essential thrombocythemia
 K+ Care ET
 ET tube
ET-1
 endothelin-1
ET-2
 endothelin-2
ET-3
 endothelin-3
etanercept
ETEC
 enterotoxigenic *Escherichia coli*
E-tegrity test
E-test
ETF
 electron transfer flavoprotein
ETF-DH
 electron transfer flavoprotein
 dehydrogenase
ETH
 ethionamide

ethacrynic acid
ethambutol (EMB)
Ethamide
ethane
 exhaled e.
ethanol (EtOH)
 blood e.
 e. poisoning
ethanolaminosis in glycogen-storage
 disease
ethchlorvynol
ether
Ethibond polybutilate-coated polyester
 suture
Ethicon
 E. disposable cannula
 E. disposable trocar
Ethiguard needle
ethinamate
ethinyl
 e. estradiol (EE)
 e. estradiol and desogestrel
 e. estradiol and ethynodiol
 diacetate
 e. estradiol and levonorgestrel
 e. estradiol and norethindrone
 e. estradiol and norgestimate
 e. estradiol and norgestrel
 e. testosterone
ethiodized oil
Ethiodol
ethionamide (ETH)
ethisterone
ethmocephaly, ethmocephalus
 e. syndrome
ethmoid
 e. bone
 e. sinus
ethmoidectomy
 endoscopic e.
ethnic heritage
ethnicity
ethoheptazine citrate
ethologic
ethopropazine hydrochloride
ethosuximide
ethotoin
Ethox cuff
ethoxzolamide
Ethrane
ethyl
 e. alcohol (EtOH)

NOTES

ethyl *(continued)*
 e. biscoumacetate
 e. chloride
ethylenediamine
ethylenediaminetetraacetic acid (EDTA)
ethylene glycol
ethylester
 tryptophan e.
ethylmalonic-adipic aciduria
ethylnorepinephrine
ethylphenylephrine
ethylsuccinate
 erythromycin e. (EES)
ethynodiol
 e. diacetate
 e. diacetate and estradiol
Ethyol
ETI
 endotracheal intubation
etidronate
 e. disodium
 sodium e.
etiocholanolone
etiologic fraction of tubal infertility
etiology
 fever of unknown e. (FUE)
 opsoclonus-myoclonus e.
etiopathogenesis
etiopathogeny
etoglucid
EtOH
 ethanol
 ethyl alcohol
etomidate
Etopophos
etoposide (EP)
 Adriamycin, Oncovin,
  prednisone, e. (AOPE)
 Ara-C, Platinol, e. (APE)
 e. phosphate
etoricoxib
etretinate
ETS
 environmental tobacco smoke
EUB-405
 E. ultrasound scanner
 E. ultrasound system
Eubacterium
eucalcemia
eucapnia
Eucerin Plus Cream
euchromatin
Eudermic surgical glove
eugenics
euglobulin
 e. clot lysis time (ECLT)
 e. lysis time (ELT)
euglycemia
 newborn e.

eugonadal amenorrhea
eugonadism
eugonadotropic
 e. amenorrhea
 e. hypogonadism
 e. oligospermia
eukaryote
eukaryotic cell
EULAR
 European League Against Rheumatism
 EULAR classification
Eulenburg disease
Euler and Byrne score
eumelanin
eumenorrheic woman
eunuch
eunuchoid
 e. gigantism
 e. habitus
eunuchoidism
 female e.
 hypergonadotropic e.
 hypogonadotropic e.
euphoria
euphoriant
euploid
 e. abortion
 e. pregnancy
euploidy
eupnea
eupneic
euprolactinemic woman
Eurax Topical
Euro-Med FNA-21 aspiration needle
European League Against Rheumatism
 (EULAR)
europium
eustachian
 e. tube
 e. tube defect
 e. tube dysfunction
eutectic mixture of local anesthetics
 (EMLA)
euthymic
euthyroid sick syndrome
Eutonyl
eutopic
 e. congenital hypothyroidism
 e. endometrium
 e. endometrium prostaglandin E_2
eV
 electron volt
evacuation
 air e.
 e. device
 dilation and e. (D&E)
 fimbrial e.
 molar e.
 e. proctography

e. of retained products of
conception (ERPC)
surgical e.
e. of uterine contents
evacuator
smoke e.
uterine e.
evaluation
Acute Physiology and Chronic
Health E. (APACHE)
audiometric e.
Collaborative Home Infant
Monitoring E. (CHIME)
cytopathologic e.
domestic violence e.
Doppler e.
Dubowitz e.
fluoro-urodynamic e.
genetic e.
infertility e.
intrapartum e.
longitudinal interval followup e.
(LIFE)
mental status e.
midtrimester ultrasonographic e.
physical capacity e. (PCE)
postpartum e.
posttreatment e.
psychomotor e.
rape crisis e.
sonographic e.
urological e.
uterine e.
women's ischemia syndrome e.
(WISE)
evanescent maculopapular rash
Evans
E. blue dye
E. calcaneal lengthening
E. syndrome
Evans-Steptoe procedure
evaporated
e. milk
e. milk formula
evaporation
evening primrose oil (EPO)
event
acute life-threatening e. (ALTE)
apneic e.
apparent life-threatening e. (ALTE)
asphyxial e.
epigenetic e.

iatrogenic e.
idiopathic apparent life-
threatening e.
inciting e.
intracellular e.
life e.
e. monitor
thromboembolic e. (TE)
unexplained apparent life-
threatening e. (UALTE)
event-free survival (EFS)
eventration
congenital e.
e. of diaphragm
diaphragmatic e.
event-related potential (ERP)
Everard Williams procedure
Everone
Evershears
E. bipolar laparoscopic forceps
E. bipolar laparoscopic scissors
eversion
cervical e.
circumferential e.
e. injury
vaginal e.
everted diaphragm
Evert-O-Cath drug delivery catheter
evidence
e. of anticipation
laparoscopic e.
rape e.
sexual assault forensic e. (SAFE)
evisceration
vaginal e.
Evista
E-Vitamin
EVL
endoscopic variceal ligation
EVLW
extravascular lung water
evoked
e. otoacoustic emission (EOAE)
e. potential
e. potential technique
e. response
e. response audiometry (ERA)
evolution
darwinian e.
Darwin theory of e.
Denman spontaneous e.

NOTES

325

evolution *(continued)*
    Douglas spontaneous e.
    spontaneous e.
evolutionarily conserved
Evra
    Ortho E.
EVS
    endoscopic variceal sclerotherapy
EVUS
    endovaginal ultrasound
Ewing
    E. sarcoma
    E. sarcoma gene
    E. tumor
EX
    Diabetic Tussin EX
ex
    ex lap
    Touro Ex
    ex utero intrapartum technique
     (EXIT)
    ex utero intrapartum tracheloplasty
     (EXIT)
    ex utero intrapartum treatment
     (EXIT)
    ex vivo
    ex vivo fertilization
    ex vivo liver-directed gene therapy
exacerbation
    asthma e.
Exacta-Med oral dispenser
Exact Cream
ExacTech glucose measuring device
Exact-Touch Saccomanno Pap smear
  collection system
exaggerated craniocaudal view
Exami-Gown gown
examination, exam
    abdominal e.
    Allen and Capute neonatal
     neurodevelopmental e.
    audiometric e.
    Ballard e.
    benign breast e.
    bimanual pelvic e.
    buffy coat e.
    cervical e.
    chest e.
    circumferential e.
    colposcopic e.
    dark-field e.
    double setup e.
    Dubowitz e.
    dysmorphology e.
    eating disorders e. (EDE)
    eye e.
    manipulative e.
    neonate e.
    neurologic e.

    newborn e.
    obstetric ultrasound e.
    Pediatric Early Elemental E.
     (PEEX)
    pelvic e.
    peripubertal e.
    personality disorder e. (PDE)
    preparticipation sports e. (PSE)
    prepuberal e.
    radiological e.
    rectal e.
    rectoabdominal e.
    rectovaginal e.
    roentgenographic e.
    routine screening cervical e.
    self-breast e. (SBE)
    serial digital e.'s
    serial neurologic e.
    slit-lamp e.
    speculum e.
    sterile speculum e.
    sterile vaginal e. (SVE)
    stool e.
    swab e.
    targeted ultrasonographic e.
    vaginal e.
    VCU e.
exanthem
    bacterial e.
    Boston e.
    laterothoracic e.
    maculopapular e.
    measles e.
    papular e.
    pediatric e.
    polymorphous e.
    scarlet fever e.
    toxin-induced scarlet fever e.
    unilateral laterothoracic e. (ULE)
    vesicular e.
    viral e.
exanthema
    e. multiforme exudativum
    rheumatic e.
exanthematous disease
excavator
excavatum
    pectus e.
eXcel-DR Glasser laparoscopic needle
excess
    adrenal e.
    androgen e.
    e. androgen
    apparent mineralocorticoid e.
     (AME)
    base e.
    estrogen e.
    glucocorticoid e.
    hyponatremia of water e.

iatrogenic androgen e.
sodium e.
soluble antigen e.
TBG e.
excessive
e. acid secretion
e. amniotic fluid
e. blood loss
e. hoarseness
e. insulin action
e. insulin secretion
e. penile curvature
e. pulmonary arterial flow
e. QT prolongation
e. sleeping
e. sweating
e. villous maturation
exchange
fetal-maternal e.
perfluorocarbon-assisted gas e.
plasma e.
regional gas e. (R_{AW})
sister chromatid e.
Starling law of transcapillary e.
e. transfusion (EXT)
excision
atrial septum e.
e. diathermy
diathermy loop e.
electrosurgical e. (EE)
electrosurgical loop e.
laparoscopic cornual e.
large loop e.
laser e.
local e.
needle e.
radical e.
radical local e.
repeat-loop e.
thyroglossal duct cyst e.
wide e.
excisional biopsy
excitation
excitement
sexual e.
excitotoxic
e. amino acid (EAA)
e. injury
e. mechanism
e. necrosis
excitotoxicity
exclamation-mark hair

exclusion
allelic e.
excoriation
excrescence
internal e.
ovarian e.
excreta
excrete
excretion
coproporphyrin e.
fractional e.
glucose e.
sodium e.
urinary e.
urobilinogen e.
water e.
excretory
e. system development
e. urogram
excursion
thoracic wall e.
excyst
metacercaria e.
executive
e. cognitive functioning (ECF)
e. function
Exelderm Topical
exemestane
exencephalia
bifid e.
exencephaly
exenteration
anterior e.
anterior pelvic e.
pelvic e.
posterior e.
posterior pelvic e.
pyelonephritis in e.
stress reaction in e.
total pelvic e.
exercise
bladder-stretching e.
e. bronchial challenge
eccentric e.
e. intolerance
isometric quadriceps e.
Kegel e.'s
maternal e.
pelvic muscle e.
pelvic muscle-strengthening e.
e. recommendation
visual training e.

NOTES

exercise-induced
  e.-i. amenorrhea
  e.-i. asthma (EIA)
  e.-i. bronchospasm (EIB)
  e.-i. hematuria
  e.-i. incontinence
exertional reactive airway disease
exertion-induced dyskinesia
exfoliated squamous cell
exfoliation
  e. failure
  lamellar e.
exfoliative
  e. dermatitis
  e. erythroderma
exhaled
  e. ethane
  e. pentane
exhaustion
  maternal e.
  ovarian follicle e.
exhibitionism
EXIT
  ex utero intrapartum technique
  ex utero intrapartum tracheloplasty
  ex utero intrapartum treatment
  EXIT procedure
exit plan
Exna
exocelomic
  e. cavity
  e. membrane
exocervical sample
exocervix
exocrine
  e. pancreatic dysfunction
  e. pancreatic hypoplasia
  e. pancreatic insufficiency
exocytosis
  cortical granule e.
exodeviation
exogastric lesion
exogenous
  e. DNA
  e. estradiol
  e. estrogen administration
  e. estrogenic stimulation
  e. gonadotropin
  e. gonadotropin stimulation
  e. hormone
  e. lipoid pneumonia (ELP)
  e. medication
  e. obesity
  e. pancreatic enzyme
  e. steroid
  e. surfactant

  e. surfactant therapy
  e. thyroxine treatment
exomphalos, macroglossia, gigantism (EMG)
exon
exonuclease
Exophiala werneckii
exophoria
exophthalmos
  apparent e.
  pulsating e.
exophytic
  e. lesion
  e. mass
  e. wart
exostosis, pl. **exostoses**
  calcified e.
  multiple cartilaginous exostoses
  pelvic e.
  subungual e.
  trichorhinophalangeal multiple e. (TRAMPE)
Exosurf Neonatal
exotoxemia
exotoxin
  e. C
  Pseudomonas e.
exotoxin-A
  streptococcal e.-A (SPEA)
exotropia
  constant e.
  intermittent e.
expandable esophageal stent (EES)
expanded food nutrition education program (EFNEP)
expander
  AccuSpan tissue e.
  Becker tissue e.
  tissue e.
  volume e.
expansion
  e. of chromosome
  GAA trinucleotide e.
  palatal e.
  plasma volume e.
  volume e.
expectancy
  life e.
expectant management
expected
  e. date of confinement (EDC)
  e. date of delivery (EDD)
expectorant
  Benylin E.
expectorate
expenditure
  energy e.
  nonresting energy e. (NREE)
  resting energy e. (REE)

total daily energy e. (TDEE)
total energy e.

experience
  appropriate learning e.
  Charing Cross e.
  Positive Reinforcement in the
    Menopausal E. (PRIME)
  separation-reunion e.

experimental
  e. allergic encephalomyelitis (EAE)
  e. embryology
  e. lymphocytic choriomeningitis
  e. obesity
  e. pneumococcal meningitis

Expert bone densitometer
expiration
expiratory
  e. apnea
  e. flow volume
  e. grunting
  e. to inspiratory ratio
  e. noise
  e. reserve volume (ERV)
  e. scan
  e. stridor

expire
explanted
exploration
  oral e.

exploratory
  e. celiotomy
  e. laparotomy

explosive watery diarrhea
exponential
exposed
  chemically e.
  e. large venous channel

exposure
  airway, breathing, circulation and
    control bleeding, disability, e.
    (ABCDE)
  anesthetic gas e.
  DES e.
  fetal androgen e.
  intrauterine e.
  lead e.
  maternal mercury e.
  methamphetamine e.
  needlestick e.
  prenatal diethylstilbestrol e.
  radiation e.
  teratogen e.

teratogenic e.
toxin e.
in utero e.
in utero drug e. (IUDE)

expressed sequence tag
expression
  abnormal gene e.
  facial e.
  gene e.
  Human Gene E. (HuGE)
  Human Genome E. (HuGE)
  oncogene e.

expressionless face
expressive
  e. aphasia
  e. language
  e. language development
  e. language disorder
  E. One-Word Picture Vocabulary
    Test

expressivity
expulsion
expulsive
  e. force
  e. pains

exsanguination
  fetal e.

Exsel shampoo
exstrophic
  e. cecum
  e. vagina

exstrophy
  bladder e.
  e. of the bladder
  cloacal e.

EXT
  exchange transfusion

Extencaps
  Micro-K 10 E.

extended
  e. culture
  e. end-to-end anastomosis
  e. family
  e. field irradiation therapy
  e. internal dosing
  e. radical hysterectomy
  e. radical mastectomy
  e. rubella syndrome

extended-release methylphenidate
extended-spectrum penicillin
extender
  egg yolk e.

NOTES

E

329

extension
classical incision e.
direct e.
J e.
medial hip rotation in e.
midline vertical uterine e.
paracervical e.
parametrial e.
protective e.
Score for Neonatal Acute
  Physiology-Perinatal E. (SNAP-PE)
T e.
vaginal e.
extensive
e. alveolar exudate
e. intraductal component (EIC)
e. support
extensor
e. fit
e. hypertonus
e. leg posture
e. thrust pattern
Extentabs
Dimetane E.
Quinidex E.
exteriorization
uterine e.
externa
malignant otitis e.
otitis e. (OE)
external
e. anal sphincter
e. anal thrombosis
e. auditory canal
e. auditory meatus
e. beam irradiation
e. beam radiation therapy
e. branchial sinus
e. cephalic version (ECV)
e. cephalic version and spontaneous
  vertex
e. conjugate
e. ear
e. femoral torsion
e. fetal monitoring (EFM)
e. genitalia/Bartholin, urethral, and
  Skene glands (EG/BUS)
e. hemorrhage
e. hordeolum
e. hydrocephalus
e. iliac artery
e. jugular vein catheter placement
e. jugular venipuncture
e. male genitalia
e. oblique muscle
e. ophthalmoplegia
e. os
e. otitis

e. pneumatic calf compression
  (EPC)
e. radiation therapy
e. rotation
e. sphincter muscle
e. surface
e. tibial torsion
e. urethral barrier device
e. urethral meatus
e. version
e. virilization
e. x-ray therapy
externalizing
e. behavior
E. Behavior Scale
e. score
exterogestate
extinction
extirpation
Amreich vaginal e.
endoscopic choroid plexus e.
extirpative surgery
extra
e. ossification
E. Strength Doan's
extraabdominal organ system disease
extraamniotic
e. pregnancy
e. saline infusion (EASI)
extraaxial
e. arachnoid cyst
e. fluid
extracapsular growth
extracardiac
e. abnormality
e. anomaly
e. conduit cavopulmonary
  anastomosis
e. malformation
e. shunt
extracellular
e. fluid (ECF)
e. fluid compartment
e. matrix
e. matrix component
e. matrix signal
e. plasma potassium
e. superoxide dismutase
e. volume (ECV)
extrachorial pregnancy
extrachromosomal inheritance
extracorporeal
e. circulation (ECC)
e. CO_2 removal (ECOR)
e. life support (ECLS)
e. membrane oxygenation (ECMO)
e. rewarming
extracortical axial aplasia
extracranial foreign body

extract
    calf lung surfactant e. (CLSE)
    malt soup e.
    modified bovine surfactant e.
    pyrethrum e.
extraction
    breech e.
    cross-brain oxygen e.
    internal podalic version and
      breech e.
    Marshall-Taylor vacuum e.
    menstrual e.
    partial breech e.
    peripheral fractional oxygen e.
      (PFOE)
    podalic e.
    spontaneous breech e.
    testicular sperm e. (TESE)
    total breech e.
    vacuum e.
extractor
    Bird vacuum e.
    CMI vacuum e.
    comedo e.
    Kobayashi vacuum e.
    Malmstrom vacuum e.
    Mityvac vacuum e.
    M-type e.
    mucus e.
    Murless head e.
    Murless vacuum e.
    O'Neil vacuum e.
    plastic cup vacuum e.
    Silastic cup e.
    Silc e.
    soft-cup e.
    Tender-Touch e.
    TRIzol RNA e.
    vacuum e.
extracutaneous
    e. sporotrichosis
    e. vas fixation clamp
extradural
    e. abscess
    e. anesthesia
    e. block
    e. hematoma
extraembryonic
    e. bleed
    e. celomic space (EECS)
    e. differentiation
    e. fetal membrane

    e. location
    e. mesoderm
extraesophageal reflux (EER)
extrafamily offender
extrafascial total abdominal
  hysterectomy
extraglandular
    e. conversion
    e. testosterone production
extraglomerular
extragonadal
    e. germ cell
    e. germ cell tumor
extrahepatic
    e. bile duct resection
    e. biliary atresia
    e. biliary tract
    e. biliary tree
    e. portal vein obstruction
    e. presinusoidal obstruction
extraintestinal manifestation (EIM)
extralobar sequestration
extraluminal
    e. fluid
    e. gas bubble
extramammary Paget disease
extramedullary hematopoiesis
extramembranous pregnancy
extramural upper airway obstruction
extranodal
    e. marginal zone
    e. marginal zone B-cell lymphoma
    e. tumor
extranumerary nipple
extraocular
    e. movement (EOM)
    e. muscle
    e. muscle surgery
extraordinary urinary frequency
  syndrome
extraosseous Ewing sarcoma
extraovular placement
extrapelvic
    e. endometriosis
    e. malignancy
    e. solid tumor
extraperitoneal
    e. cesarean
    e. insufflation
extraplacental membrane
extrapolate
extrapolation

E

NOTES

extrapulmonary
    e. cryptococcosis
    e. extravasation
    e. extravasation of air
    e. tuberculosis
extrapyramidal
    e. cerebral palsy
    e. lesion
    e. manifestation
    e. movement
    e. nervous system
    e. sign
    e. tract
extrapyramidal-pyramidal syndrome
extrarenal
    e. pheochromocytoma
    e. rhabdoid tumor
    e. saline
extrasystole
extratemporal epilepsy
extrathoracic
    e. obstruction
    e. tuberculosis
    e. ventilator
extrauterine
    e. life
    e. pregnancy
extravasation
    blood e.
    extrapulmonary e.
    e. injury
extravascular
    e. fluid collection
    e. lung water (EVLW)
extraventricular
extravesical
    e. mass
    e. ureteral reimplantation
extravillous trophoblast
extreme
    e. benign hyperbilirubinemia
    e. leukocytosis
extremely
    e. low birth weight (ELBW)
    e. low birth weight infant
      (ELBWI)
    e. premature infant (EPI)
extremis
    in e.
extremity
    congenital contracture of e.
    flaccid e.
    long thin e.
    lower e. (LE)
    e. lymphedema
    upper e. (UE)
extrinsic
    e. alveolar alveolitis
    e. compression of airway

    e. dyssomnia
    e. extravesical mass
    e. pathway inhibitor
extrophy
    cloacal e.
extrusion
    dental e.
    oocyte e.
    placental e.
    e. reflex
extrusion/lateral luxation
extrusive luxation
extubate
extubation
exuberant callus
exudate
    alveolar fibrinous e.
    cheesy e.
    cotton-ball e.
    extensive alveolar e.
    fibrinopurulent e.
    fibrinous e.
    inflammatory e.
    opaque white e.
    peritoneal e.
    subretinal e.
    tonsillar e.
    tonsillopharyngeal e.
exudative
    e. ascites
    e. conjunctivitis
    e. meningitis
    e. pharyngitis
    e. retinal detachment
    e. tonsillitis
exudativum
    erythema multiforme e.
    exanthema multiforme e.
Exuderm dressing
Eyberg Child Behavior Inventory
   (ECBI)
eye
    amblyopic e.
    Clear E.'s
    Credé maneuver of e.'s
    dancing e.
    deep set e.'s
    e. defects-diffuse renal mesangial
      sclerosis syndrome
    e. deviation
    doll's e.'s
    e. dominance
    downslanting e.'s
    dry e.
    e.'s, ears, nose, throat (EENT)
    e. examination
    e. inflammation
    lazy e.
    e. movement

muscle, liver, brain, e. (mulibrey)
nonfixing e.
ox's e.
e. popping
raccoon e.'s
e. retraction with adduction
e. salvage therapy
e. slant
sunset e.'s
sunsetting e.'s
widely spaced e.'s
eyeball cystometrogram
eyebrow
confluent e.'s
ichthyosis, cheek, e. (ICE)
eyeground
eye-hand coordination
eyelash trichomegaly
eyelid
Dennie lines of lower e.'s

fusion of e.'s
heliotrope e.
e. muscle
e. squeezing
e. tumor
eye-of-the-tiger sign
eye-opener
cutting, annoyance, guilt, e.-o. (CAGE)
Eyesine Ophthalmic
EZ-EM
EZ-EM Bio-Gun automated biopsy system
EZ-EM PercuSet amniocentesis tray
E-Z Heat hot pack
Ezide
E-Z-On Vest

NOTES

E

$F_{2\ alpha}$
  prostaglandin $F_{2\ alpha}$ (PGF2 alpha)
FA
  Fanconi anemia
  femoral anteversion
    Nestabs FA
    FA screening
F.A.
  Mission Prenatal F.A.
FAA
  febrile antigen agglutination
    FAA gene
FAB
  French-American-British
    FAB classification
    FAB staging of carcinoma
fab
  digoxin immune f.
FABP
  finger arterial blood pressure
fabric
  Solumbra 30+ SPF f.
Fabricius
  bursa of F.
Fabry
    F. crisis
    F. disease
FACE
  fluorophore-assisted carbohydrate
    electrophoresis
    FACE kit
face (*See also* facies)
  abnormal f.
  asymmetry of f.
  bovine f.
  f. chamber
  cleft f.
  congenital ectodermal dysplasia
    of f.
  dish f.
  dysmorphic f.
  ectodermal dysplasia of f.
  expressionless f.
  fetal f.
  f., legs, activity, cry, consolability
    (FLACC)
  f. mask
  f. presentation
  round moon f.
  f. tent
  f. underdevelopment
face/chin presentation
face-near-straight-down (FNSD)
face-out, whole-body plethysmograph

FACES
  Family Adaptability and Cohesion
    Evaluation Scale
FACES-III
  Family Adaptability and Cohesion Scale-
    III
face-straight-down (FSD)
facet
  f. dislocation
  jumped f.
  locked f.
  medial talocalcaneal f.
  subtalar f.
  f. syndrome
face-to-pubes position
face-to-side (FTS)
facial
  f. affect recognition
  f. angioma
  f. anomaly
  f. asymmetry
  f. buttress
  f. clefting syndrome, Gypsy type
  f. diplegia
  f. dysmorphia syndrome
  f. dysmorphism
  f. dysplasia, hyperextensibility of
    joints, clinodactyly, growth
    retardation, mental retardation
    syndrome
  f. ectodermal dysplasia
  f. expression
  f. expression and sleeplessness
  f. nerve
  f. nerve injury (FNI)
  f. nerve palsy
  f. nerve paralysis
  f. pain
  f. vein insertion
facial-digital-genital syndrome
facialis
  herpes f.
faciei
  lupus miliaris disseminatum f.
facies (*See also* face)
  abnormal f.
  asymmetric crying f. (ACF)
  birdlike f.
  f. bovina
  bovine f.
  Campbell Soup kid f.
  cushingoid f.
  dwarfism, eczema, peculiar f.
  elfinlike f.
  flat f.

F

facies *(continued)*
    moon f.
    moon-shaped f.
    peculiar f.
    Potter f.
    progeroid f.
    seborrheic-like f.
    soup kid f.
    thalassemia f.
    triangular f.
facilitated communication (F/C)
facility
    intermediate care f. (ICF)
facioauriculovertebral (FAV)
    f. anomalad
    f. malformation complex
    f. spectrum (FAVS)
faciocardiomelic dysplasia
faciocardiorenal syndrome
faciocerebroskeletocardiac syndrome
faciocutaneoskeletal (FCS)
faciodigitogenital syndrome
faciogenital
    f. dysplasia
    f. syndrome
faciolingual-masticatory diplegia
faciooculoacousticorenal (FOAR)
faciopalatoosseous (FPO)
facioscapulohumeral (FSH)
    f. muscular dystrophy (FSHD)
    f. syndrome of Landouzy-Dejerine
faciotelencephalic malformation
faciotelencephalopathy
Facit polyp forceps
$FACO_2$
    fraction of alveolar carbon dioxide
FACS
    fluorescence-activated cell sorter
FACT
    Functional Assessment of Cancer
    Therapy
Fact
    F. Plus
    F. Plus Pro pregnancy test
factitial panniculitis
factitious
    f. disorder
    f. disorder by proxy (FDP)
    f. precocious puberty
factor
    acidic fibroblast growth f. (FGFa)
    activated clotting f. X
    alloimmune f.
    angiogenic growth f.
    antihemophilic f. (AHF)
    atrial natriuretic f. (ANF)
    autocrine-acting growth f.
    autocrine motility f. (AMF)
    autocrine/paracrine-acting growth f.

    autoimmune f.
    azoospermia f. (AZF)
    basic fibroblast growth f. (bFGF)
    bifidus f.
    binding protein-2 insulinlike
      growth f.
    binding protein-3 insulinlike
      growth f.
    biomedical f.
    biotin f.
    blocking f.
    brain-derived neurotrophic f.
      (BDNF)
    cell adhesion f. (CAF)
    cervical f.
    chemotactic f.
    chicken ovalbumin upstream
      promoter transcription f. II
      (COUP)
    Christmas f.
    ciliary neurotrophic f. (CNTF)
    citrovorum f.
    coagulation f.
    coital f.
    colony-stimulating f. (CSF)
    complement chemotactic f.
    f. concentrate
    contact f.
    contagion f.
    corticotropin-releasing f.
    cytotoxic f.
    decay-accelerating f.
    deficiency of f. B, D
    f. D, H deficiency
    digoxin-like immunoreactive f.
      (DLIF)
    DNAse B f.
    early pregnancy f.
    endocrine f.
    endothelium-derived relaxing f.
      (EDRF)
    enhancement f.
    epidermal growth f. (EGF)
    fecundity f.
    fetal f.
    fibrin stabilizing f.
    fibroblast growth f. (FGF)
    fibroblast pneumocyte f.
    follicular f.
    glass f.
    glial cell line derived
      neurotrophic f. (GDNF)
    gonadotropin-releasing f. (GnRH,
      GRF)
    granulocyte colony-stimulating f.
      (G-CSF)
    granulocyte-macrophage colony-
      stimulating f. (GM-CSF)
    growth f. (GF)

growth control f.
growth-like f.
Hageman f.
helper f.
hepatocyte growth f. (HGF)
hepatocyte nuclear f. (HNF)
hidden rheumatoid f.
highly purified f. IX
HMWK f.
home f.
human antihemophilic f.
human sperm cytosolic f.
humoral f.
hyaluronic acid f.
hyaluronidase f.
f. I, II, IIa, III-VIII, X-XIII
immune f.
immunologic f.
infertility f.
insulinlike growth f. (IGF)
intrauterine f.'s
intrinsic f. (IF)
f. I–XIII deficiency
keratinocyte growth f. (KGF)
kidney-derived growth f.
labile f.
leukemia inhibitory f. (LIG)
lifestyle f.
lymphocyte-activating f.
f. M
macrophage-activating f. (MAF)
macrophage colony-stimulating f.
macrophage-inhibition f.
male f.
maternal f.
maturation-promoting f. (MPF)
menarche f.
microbial f.
migration inhibitory f. (MIF)
mitosis-promoting f. (MPF)
mixed lymphocyte reaction
  blocking f.
mortality risk f.
M-phase-promoting f.
M protein f.
müllerian duct inhibitory f.
müllerian inhibiting f. (MIF)
müllerian inhibitory f. (MIF)
necrotizing f.
nephritic f.
nerve growth f. (NGF)
obstetric risk f.

ovarian f.
paracrine-acting growth f.
paternal f.
perinatal risk f.
perisphincteric f.
PK f.
placental growth f. (PGF)
plasma coagulation f. VIII, IX
plasma thromboplastin antecedent f.
platelet-activating f.
platelet-derived growth f.
postnatal f.
precipitating f.
predisposing f.
pregnancy risk f. (PRF)
prenatal risk f.
primary testis-determining f.
prognostic f.
prolactin inhibiting f. (PIF)
prolactin releasing f. (PRF)
properdin f. B
prostacyclin-stimulating f. (PSF)
proteinase f.
psychosocial f.
purified human f. IX
recombinant antihemophilic f.
recombinant f. VIIa
Rh f.
rhesus f.
rheumatoid f. (RF)
risk f.
Service Utilization and Risk F.'s
  (SURF)
somatic cell-derived growth f.
  (SCF)
specific transcription f.
spreading f.
stable f.
streptokinase f.
Stuart f.
Stuart-Prower f.
testis-determining f. (TDF)
tissue f.
transfer f.
transforming growth f. (TGF)
transforming growth f. 1 (TGF-1)
tubal f.
tumor angiogenesis f. (TAF)
tumor-limiting f.
tumor necrosis f. (TNF)
tumor necrosis f. alpha (TNF-
  alpha)

NOTES

factor *(continued)*
    uterine f.
    f. V^{Leiden}
    vascular endothelial growth f.
      (VEGF)
    vascular permeability f.
    f. VIIa (FVIIa)
    f. VIII:C
    f. VIII hemophilia
    f. VII, VIII inhibitor
    f. V Leiden
    f. V Leiden carrier
    f. V Leiden mutation
    f. V Leiden mutation test
    f. V Leiden thrombophilia
    von Willebrand f. (vWF)
    f. V polypeptide
    work f.
    f. Xa inhibition assay
factor-1
    recombinant human insulin-like
      growth f.-1 (rhIGF-1)
    steroidogenic f.-1 (SF-1)
    thyroid transcription f.-1 (TTF-1)
Factrel
facultative scotoma
FAD
    familial Alzheimer disease
    flavin adenine dinucleotide
Fadhil syndrome
fading
fadir sign
FADS
    fetal akinesia deformation sequence
FAE
    fetal alcohol effects
    Fogarty arterial embolectomy
      FAE catheter
      FAE syndrome
faecalis
    Enterococcus f.
faecium
    Enterococcus f.
FAED
    food avoidance emotion disorder
Fagan Test of Infant Intelligence
FAH
    fumarylacetoacetate hydrolase
Fahr disease
failed
    f. breastfeeding
    f. Fontan circuit
    f. forceps delivery
    f. intrauterine pregnancy
    f. physiologic change
    f. reduction
failure
    acute renal f. (ARF)
    bilateral gonadal f.

    bone marrow f.
    cardiac f.
    chronic renal f. (CRF)
    congestive heart f. (CHF)
    contraceptive f.
    ejaculation f.
    end-stage heart f.
    erythropoiesis f.
    exfoliation f.
    fertility f.
    fimbrial f.
    fulminant hepatic f. (FHF)
    gonadal f.
    growth f.
    heart f.
    high-output f.
    hypothalamic f.
    hypoxic respiratory f.
    impending renal f.
    implantation f.
    kidney f.
    left ventricular f.
    multiorgan system f.
    multiple organ f.
    multiple organ system f. (MOSF)
    neurogenic respiratory f.
    ovarian f.
    premature ovarian f. (POF)
    primary testicular f.
    f. to progress
    progressive central nervous
      system f.
    progressive renal f.
    renal f.
    reproductive f.
    respiratory f.
    right-sided heart f.
    severe growth f.
    f. to thrive (FTT)
    treatment f.
    ventilatory f.
faint
    vasovagal f.
Fairbank
    F. disease
    F. skeletal abnormality
Fairbank-Keats syndrome
falciform hymen
falciparum
    f. malaria
    Plasmodium f.
Falk-Shukuris operation
fall-away response
falling
    f. sickness
    f. of the womb
fallopian
    f. pregnancy
    f. tube

f. tube carcinoma
f. tube mass
f. tube metastasis
f. tube prolapse
f. tube sperm perfusion (FTSP)
falloposcope
falloposcopy
Fallot
acyanotic tetralogy of F.
F. complex
F. pentalogy
pentalogy of F.
pink tetralogy of F.
F. syndrome
tetralogy of F. (tet, TF, TOF)
trilogy of F.
F. trilogy
Falope
F. ring
F. ring applicator
F2 alpha
prostaglandin F2 (PGF2 alpha)
false
f. conjugate
f. fontanelle
f. heteroovular twins
f. knot
f. knot of umbilical cord
f. labor
f. localizing sign
f. mole
f. negative
f. pains
f. pelvis
f. positive
f. pregnancy
f. vocal cord
f. waters
false-negative death
false-positive
falx, pl. **falces**
cerebral f.
f. laceration
f. sign
FAMA
fluorescent antibody against membrane
antigen
fluorescent antimembrane antibody test
FAMA assay
famciclovir
familial
f. achalasia

f. adenomatous polyposis
f. adenomatous polyposis coli
f. alobar holoprosencephaly
f. Alzheimer disease (FAD)
f. aortic ectasia
f. aortic ectasia syndrome
f. APOA-I deficiency
f. ataxia-hypogonadism syndrome
f. atypical multiple mole melanoma
syndrome
f. benign hematuria
f. bipolar mood disorder
f. bird-headed dwarfism
f. cardiac myxoma
f. cardiac myxoma syndrome
f. centrolobal sclerosis
f. cholesterolemia
f. chylomicronemia syndrome
f. combined hyperlipidemia (FCHL)
f. congenital alopecia, mental
retardation, epilepsy, unusual EEG
syndrome
f. congenital fourth cranial nerve
palsy
f. congenital superior oblique
oculomotor palsy
f. congenital trochlear nerve palsy
f. Creutzfeldt-Jakob disease
f. defective apolipoprotein B-100
f. diathesis
f. dominant thrombocytopenia
f. dysautonomia
f. endocrine-neuroectodermal
abnormalities syndrome
f. erythroblastic anemia
f. erythrocytosis
f. erythrophagocytic
lymphohistiocytosis (FEL)
f. exudative vitreoretinopathy (FEV)
f. focal facial dermal dysplasia
f. glomerulonephritis
f. glycinuria
f. granulomatous arteritis
f. hemiplegic migraine (FHM)
f. hemophagocytic
lymphohistiocytosis (FHLH)
f. Hibernian fever
f. hirsutism
f. hypercalcemia
f. hypercalcemia with hypocalciuria
(FHH)
f. hypercholesterolemia

F

NOTES

339

familial *(continued)*
- f. hyperglycerolemia
- f. hyperinsulinemic hypoglycemia
- f. hyperinsulinism of infancy
- f. hyperlipidemia
- f. hyperlysinemia
- f. hyperprolinemia
- f. hypertriglyceridemia (FHTG)
- f. hypoalphalipoproteinemia
- f. hypobetalipoproteinemia
- f. hypocalciuric hypercalcemia (FHH)
- f. hypofibrinogenemia
- f. hypokalemic periodic paralysis
- f. hypomagnesemia
- f. hypophosphatemia (FHR)
- f. hypophosphatemic rickets
- f. iminoglycinuria
- f. infertility
- f. insomnia syndrome
- f. intrahepatic cholestasis
- f. inverted choreoathetosis
- f. juvenile gout
- f. juvenile hyperuricemic nephropathy
- f. juvenile nephrophthisis (FJN)
- f. lecithin:cholesterol acyltransferase deficiency
- f. lipodystrophy
- f. lipoid adrenal hyperplasia
- f. loading
- f. lumbosacral syringomyelia
- f. lymphedema praecox
- f. macrocephaly
- f. macroglossia-omphalocele syndrome
- f. male precocious puberty
- f. Mediterranean fever (FMF)
- f. multiple endocrine adenomatosis
- f. multiple lipomatosis
- f. muscular atrophy
- f. neonatal seizure
- f. neuroblastoma
- f. neurovisceral lipidosis
- f. olivopontocerebellar atrophy
- f. osseous dystrophy
- f. osteochondrodystrophy
- f. ovarian cancer
- f. panhypopituitarism
- f. polysyndactyly-craniofacial anomalies syndrome
- f. protein intolerance
- f. pterygium syndrome
- f. pure gonadal dysgenesis
- f. pyridoxine-dependency syndrome
- f. recurrent hematuria
- f. short stature
- f. spastic paraparesis
- f. spastic paraplegia (FSP)
- f. spinal neurofibromatosis
- f. striatal degeneration
- f. tendency
- f. third and fourth pharyngeal pouch syndrome
- f. thrombophilia
- f. trait
- f. tremor
- f. Turner syndrome
- f. vasopressin-sensitive diabetes insipidus
- f. visceral myopathy
- f. visceral neuropathy
- f. vocal cord dysfunction

familiaris
- osteopathia dysplastica f.

family
- F. Adaptability and Cohesion Evaluation Scale (FACES)
- F. Adaptability and Cohesion Scale-III (FACES-III)
- CEPH f.
- f. dynamics
- f. dysfunction
- dysfunctional f.
- F. Environment Scale (FES)
- extended f.
- gene f.
- f. history
- f. history research diagnostic criteria (FH-RDC)
- F. Inventory of Resources for Management (FIRM)
- F. Medical Leave Act (FMLA)
- f. member presence (FMP)
- f. planning
- *Poxviridae* f.
- f. selection
- f. therapy

family-based
- f.-b. design
- f.-b. test

family-centered
- f.-c. approach
- f.-c. obstetrics

famotidine

Famvir

Fanconi
- F. anemia (FA)
- F. aplastic anemia
- F. dysplasia
- F. pancytopenia
- F. pancytopenia syndrome

Fanconi-Albertini Zellweger syndrome
Fanconi-Bickel syndrome
Fanconi-Petrassi syndrome
Fanconi-Prader syndrome
Fanconi-Schlesinger syndrome
fan douche

fanning
fan-shaped hemorrhagic infarction
Fansidar
fantasy
    revenge f.
fantasy/make-believe world
FAO
    fatty acid oxidation
    FAO disorder
faradism
Farber
    F. disease
    F. lipogranulomatosis
    F. syndrome
    F. test
farcinica
    Nocardia f.
Fareston
farmeri
    Citrobacter f.
farmer's lung
Farre white line
Farr test
farsightedness
FAS
    fetal alcohol syndrome
    Functional Assessment Scale
fascia, pl. fascias, fasciae
    f. adherens
    Camper f.
    f. clitoridis
    Colles f.
    Cooper f.
    cremasteric f.
    Dartos f.
    Denonvilliers f.
    endopelvic f.
    Gerota f.
    inferior f.
    f. lata
    f. lata allograft
    f. lata suburethral sling
    obturator f.
    perirectal f.
    plantar f.
    presacral f.
    pubocervical f.
    Scarpa f.
    Smead-Jones closure of peritoneum and f.
    subserous f.
    superior f.

    tensor fasciae latae (TFL)
    transversalis f.
fascial
    f. flap
    f. necrosis
    f. reconstruction
    f. sling procedure
    f. strip
fascicle
fasciculata
    zona f.
fasciculation
    muscle f.
    tongue f.
fasciculus, pl. fasciculi
    syndrome of median longitudinal f.
fasciitis, fascitis
    cranial f.
    diffuse f.
    eosinophilic f.
    gas gangrene f.
    necrotizing myositis/f.
    nodular f.
    plantar f.
Fasciola hepatica
fascioliasis
fascioscapulohumeral
fascitis (*var. of* fasciitis)
fashion
    crescentic f.
    forward roll f.
    Halban f.
    Moschcowitz f.
FASIAR
    follicle aspiration, sperm injection, and assisted rupture
Faslodex
FAST
    Focused Assessment by Sonography for Trauma
    FAST blood test
fast
    f. channel syndrome
    f. neutron
    protein modified f. (PMF)
    protein-sparing modified f. (PSMF)
fastener
    ROC XS suture f.
FASTER
    first abarelix depot study for treating endometriosis rapidly

NOTES

FASTER *(continued)*
first and second trimester evaluation of risk

fasting
f. blood sugar
f. plasma cholecystokinin
f. plasma glucose (FPG)
f. serum insulin

FAT
female athlete triad

fat
f. absorption
f. analysis
body f.
f. density
f. deposition
f. depot
dietary f.
f. distribution pattern
f. embolism
f. emulsion
endogenous f.
f. flap
f. flexor hallucis longus tendon
f. herniation
f. malabsorption
f. mass (FM)
f. metabolism
microscopic f.
f. necrosis
percent body f. (PBF)
f. plane
preperitoneal f.
unsaturated f.

fatal
f. cutaneous aspergillosis
f. encephalomyelitis
f. familial insomnia
f. infantile myopathy
f. neonatal hyperammonemic encephalopathy

fate mapping
fat-free mass (FFM)
fatigability
easy f.
increased f.

fatigue
f. fracture
f. syndrome

fat-induced infarction
fatty
f. acid
f. acid-coenzyme A
f. acid content
f. acid oxidation (FAO)
f. acid profile
f. halo
f. infiltration

f. liver
f. liver of pregnancy

faun tail nevus
FAV
facioauriculovertebral

fava
f. bean
f. bean ingestion

favism
FAVS
facioauriculovertebral spectrum

Fazio-Londe
F.-L. atrophy
F.-L. disease

FBEP
Fort Bragg evaluation project

FBM
fetal bone marrow
fetal breathing movement

5-FC
5-fluorocytosine

F&C
fevers and chills

F/C
facilitated communication

FCHL
familial combined hyperlipidemia

FCMD
Fukuyama congenital muscular dystrophy

FCS
faciocutaneoskeletal
FCS syndrome

FD
forceps delivery

FDA
Food and Drug Administration

FDIU
fetal death in utero

FDP
factitious disorder by proxy
fibrinogen degradation product

FE
fetal erythroblastosis

Fe
iron
Estrostep Fe
Loestrin Fe
Microgestin Fe 1.5/30
Microgestin Fe 1/29
Norlestrin Fe
Slow Fe

fear
f. of delivery
f. food
pregnancy f.
social-evaluative f.

fear-causing delivery
fearless first delivery
feasible

feature
> coarse facial f.'s
> dysmorphic facial f.
> epidemiologic f.
> grotesque f.'s
> f. matching
> mongoloid f.'s
> mood-congruent psychotic f.
> sharp facial f.'s

febrile
> f. antigen agglutination (FAA)
> f. baby
> f. convulsion
> f. morbidity
> f. myalgia
> f. nonhemolytic transfusion reaction
> f. paroxysm
> f. seizure
> f. status epilepticus
> f. UTI

FEC
> fluorouracil, epirubicin, Cytoxan

fecal
> f. acidity
> f. bolus
> f. calprotectin
> f. diversion colostomy
> f. hoarding
> f. impaction
> f. incontinence
> f. marker
> f. microflora
> f. occult blood testing (FOBT)
> f. pancreatic elastase
> f. shedding
> f. shedding of virus
> f. streptococci
> f. water loss

fecalith
> appendiceal f.
> calcified f.

fecaloma, scatoma
fecal-oral spread
feces
FECO$_2$
> fraction in expired gas of carbon dioxide

fecund
fecundability
fecundate
fecundation
fecundity
> f. factor

> natural f.
> f. selection

fed
> bottle f.
> nipple f.

feed
> bottle f.
> full enteral f.
> full nipple f.
> trophic f.
> tube f.

feedback
> tubuloglomerular f.

feeder
> Brecht f.
> f. layer

feeding
> ad lib f.
> Alimentum f.
> bolus tube f.
> f. bradycardia
> coercive f.
> complex enteral f.
> continuous tube f.
> cup f.
> demand f.
> f. difficulty
> f. disturbance
> early enteral f.
> enteral f.
> enteric f.
> finger f.
> Finkelstein f.
> gastric enteral f.
> gastric tube f.
> f. gastrostomy
> gavage f.
> G-tube f.
> hydrolyzed f.
> f. intolerance
> intragastric f.
> intravenous f.
> liquid f.
> by mouth f.
> nasoduodenal f.
> nasogastric drip f.
> nasogastric tube f.
> nipple f.
> p.o. f.
> poor f.
> f. problem
> f. regimen

NOTES

343

feeding *(continued)*
    scheduled f.
    syringe f.
    transpyloric enteral f.
    transpyloric tube f.
    f. tube
Feelings About Yourself instrument
Feer disease
feet *(pl. of* foot)
FEF
    forced expiratory flow
Feiba VH Immuno
Feilchenfeld forceps
Feingold syndrome
Feinmesser-Zelig syndrome
FEL
    familial erythrophagocytic
      lymphohistiocytosis
felbamate
Felbatol
Feldene
felis
    Afipia f.
    Rickettsia f.
Felix-Weil reaction
felon drainage
Felty syndrome
female
    f. athlete triad (FAT)
    f. condom
    f. epispadias
    f. eunuchoidism
    f. fertility efficiency
    f. fertility inefficiency
    f. genital mutilation (FMG)
    f. genital tract mutilation (FGTM)
    f. karyotype
    phenotypic f.
    f. pseudohermaphroditism
    f. pseudo-Turner syndrome
    f. reproductive cycle
    f. reproductive tract
    F. Sexual Distress Scale (FSDS)
    f. sexual dysfunction
    F. Sexual Function Index (FSFI)
    f. sexual response
    f. sterilization
    f. sterilization procedure
    super f.
    triple-X f.
Femara
FemCap barrier contraceptive device
Femcaps
Femcept device
femhrt
feminine
feminization
    complete testicular f.

    f. syndrome
    testicular f.
feminizing
    f. adrenal tumor
    f. surgery
    f. testes syndrome
Feminone
Femiron
Femizol-M
Femogen Forte
Femogex
femora
    biologically plastic f.
femoral
    f. antetorsion
    f. anteversion (FA)
    f. artery catheter
    f. artery catheterization
    f. bulb
    f. circumflex artery
    f. cutaneous nerve
    f. deficiency
    f. epiphysis
    f. head dislocation
    f. hernia
    f. hypoplasia unusual facies
      (FHUF)
    f. length
    f. lymph node
    f. neck
    f. neuropathy
    f. osteosarcoma
    f. osteotomy
    f. retroversion
    f. shaft fracture
    f. testis
    f. torsion
    f. triangle
femoral-facial syndrome
femoral-tibial angle
femoris
    rectus f.
FemPatch
FemSoft continence insert
Femstat 3
femtomole/milligram (fm/mg)
femur
    f. length (FL)
    metaphysial lesion of distal f.
    NSA of f.
femur-fibula-ulna (FFU)
FEN
    fluids, electrolytes, nutrition
fencing
    f. position
    f. reflex
Fenesin DM
fenestrata
    placenta f.

fenestrated vascular endothelium
fenestration
    Fontan f.
    laparoscopic f.
    third ventricle f.
fenfluramine
fenoterol
fentanyl
    f. citrate
    droperidol and f.
    f. lollipop
    f. patch
    TTS f.
fentendo
    fetal endoscopic tracheal occlusion
    fentendo clip
    fentendo plug
fentomole/milligram
Fenton vaginoplasty
Fe₃O₄
    magnetite
Feosol
Feostat
FEP
    free erythrocyte protoporphyrin
FER
    frozen embryo replacement
Feratab
ferberizing
Ferber method
Fergon
Ferguson reflex
Fer-In-Sol
    F.-I.-S. supplement
    F.-I.-S. vitamins
Fer-Iron
fermentans
    Mycoplasma f.
fermentum
    Lactobacillus f.
fern
    f. leaf crystallization
    f. leaf pattern
    f. leaf tongue
    f. test
ferning
    f. pattern
    f. technique
    vaginal fluid f.
fern-positive Nitrazine
Ferospace
Ferralyn Lanacaps

ferric
    f. chloride reaction
    f. chloride test
    f. hyaluronate adhesion barrier
    f. sulfate
Ferriman-Gallwey
    F.-G. hirsutism score
    F.-G. hirsutism scoring system
Ferris Smith-Sewall retractor
ferritin
    F. IRMA kit
    f. level test
    serum f.
Ferro-Sequels
ferrous
    f. chloride
    f. fumarate
    f. gluconate
    f. sulfate (FeSO₄)
Fertil-A-Chron
fertile
    f. period
    f. phase
fertility
    f. agent
    f. cycle
    f. failure
    f. rate
    subsequent f.
fertilizable life span
fertilization
    f. age
    assisted f.
    culture f.
    delayed f.
    ex vivo f.
    microassisted f.
    minimal-stimulation in vitro f.
    oocyte f.
    in vitro f. (IVF)
    in vivo f.
fertilized
    f. oocyte
    f. ovum
Fertinex
FES
    Family Environment Scale
FeSO₄
    ferrous sulfate
fes **protooncogene**
fetal
    f. abdominal circumference

NOTES

fetal (*continued*)
- f. Accutane syndrome
- f. acid-base balance
- f. acidemia
- f. acidosis
- f. acoustic stimulation test
- f. activity test
- f. adrenal gland
- f. age
- f. akinesia deformation sequence (FADS)
- f. akinesia syndrome
- f. alcohol effects (FAE)
- f. alcohol syndrome (FAS)
- f. aminopterin-like syndrome
- f. aminopterin syndrome
- f. anasarca
- f. androgen exposure
- f. anemia
- f. aneuploidy
- f. anoxia
- f. anticoagulant syndrome
- f. aorta
- f. aortic blood flow
- f. aortic Doppler velocimetry
- f. arrhythmia
- f. arterial oxygen saturation (FS_pO_2)
- f. arterial velocimetry
- f. arthrogryposis
- f. ascites
- f. asphyxia
- f. aspiration syndrome
- f. assessment technique
- f. attitude
- f. biometry
- f. biophysical profile
- f. biparietal diameter
- f. birth injury
- f. bladder catheterization
- f. blood gases
- f. blood glucose
- f. blood oxygen-carrying capacity
- f. blood pH
- f. blood study
- f. blood value
- f. blood volume
- f. body movement
- f. bone marrow (FBM)
- f. BPP
- f. bradycardia
- f. brain
- f. brain death
- f. brain disruption sequence
- f. brain sparing
- f. brain stem auditory evoked potential
- f. breathing
- f. breathing movement (FBM)
- f. capillary branching
- f. cardiac activity
- f. cardiac function
- f. cardiac motion
- f. cardiac rhabdomyoma
- f. cardiomyopathy
- f. cardiotocography
- f. cardiovascular circulation
- f. cartilage
- f. cellular growth
- f. cerebral oxygenation
- f. chromosome abnormality
- f. circulatory centralization
- f. cocaine syndrome
- f. compromise
- f. condition
- f. congenital hyperplasia
- f. cord blood
- f. cortisol infusion
- f. cotyledon
- f. cranial artery
- f. crowding
- f. CST
- f. cystic hygroma
- f. cytokinemia
- f. cytomegalovirus infection
- f. death rate
- f. death in utero (FDIU)
- f. debris
- f. demise
- f. demise in utero
- f. descent
- f. deterioration
- f. development
- f. diabetes insipidus
- f. diagnosis
- f. Dilantin syndrome
- f. disappearance
- f. distress
- f. distress in labor
- f. distress syndrome
- F. Dopplex monitor
- f. dose limit
- f. drug therapy
- f. ductus arteriosus constriction
- f. duplication
- f. dysmaturity syndrome
- f. dystocia
- f. echocardiogram
- f. echocardiography
- f. effect
- f. effects of alcohol
- f. electrocardiogram
- f. electrocardiography
- f. endocarditis
- f. endoscopic
- f. endoscopic tracheal occlusion (fentendo)
- f. engraftment

f. entanglement
f. erythroblastosis (FE)
f. erythroid progenitor
f. estrogen
f. exsanguination
f. face
f. face syndrome
f. facies syndrome
f. factor
f. fibronectin (FFN, fFN)
f. fibronectin assay
f. fibronectin measurement
f. fibronectin test
f. foot length (FFL)
f. fracture
f. gigantism
f. gigantism, renal hamartoma,
  nephroblastomatosis syndrome
f. goiter
f. grasping
f. growth aberration
f. growth measurement
f. growth parameters
f. growth restriction (FGR)
f. growth retardation
f. habitus
f. HC/AC
f. head
f. head position
f. heart
f. heart action
f. heart activity
f. heart disease
f. heart frequency (FHF)
f. heart rate (FHR)
f. heart rate deceleration
f. heart rate monitor
f. heart rate monitoring
f. heart rate pattern
f. heart rate reactivity
f. heart rate variability
f. heart sounds
f. hemoglobin (HbF)
f. hemolysis
f. hemorrhage
f. hiccup
f. histocompatibility antigen
f. hormone
f. hydantoin syndrome (FHS)
f. hydronephrosis
f. hydrops
f. hydrostatic pressure

f. hypercarbia
f. hyperglycemia
f. hyperinsulinism
f. hypotrophy
f. hypoxia
f. imaging
f. inflammatory response
f. inflammatory response syndrome
f. intracranial anatomy
f. iodine deficiency disorder
  (FIDD)
f. isotretinoin syndrome
f. jeopardy
f. karyotype
f. kick count
f. LDL level
f. leptin concentration
f. lie
f. limb
f. liver
f. lobectomy
f. loss
f. LOU
f. lung development
f. lung fluid
f. lung liquid
f. lung maturation
f. lung maturity (FLM)
f. lung readiness
f. maceration
f. macrosomia
f. malformation
f. malnutrition
f. malpresentation
f. maturity testing
f. membrane
f. metabolism
f. methotrexate syndrome
f. monitoring strip
f. morbidity
f. mortality
f. movement assessment
f. movement count
f. movement counting
f. movement profile
f. neck fold thickness
f. nonimmune hydrops
f. NST
f. nuchal translucency thickness
f. number
f. nutrition
f. nutritional deprivation syndrome

F

NOTES

fetal *(continued)*

- f. oculocerebrorenal syndrome of Lowe
- f. organogenesis
- f. outcome
- f. outline
- f. ovarian cyst
- f. overgrowth syndrome
- f. oximetry monitoring
- f. oxygen saturation
- f. paramethadione-trimethadione syndrome
- f. parathyroid suppression
- f. phenytoin syndrome
- f. physiologist
- f. pole
- f. postural abnormality
- f. posture
- f. prematurity
- f. presentation
- f. pulmonary circulation
- f. pulmonary hypoplasia
- f. pulmonary maturity
- f. pulmonary sequestration
- f. pulmonary vascular resistance
- f. pulse oximetry
- f. pyelectasis
- f. red blood cell
- f. reduction
- f. reentrant SVT
- f. rejection
- f. resorption
- f. retention
- f. risk
- f. rubella syndrome
- f. sac
- f. scalp blood pH
- f. scalp blood sampling
- f. scalp electrode (FSE)
- f. scalp monitoring
- f. scalp oxygenation
- f. scalp platelet sampling
- f. scalp stimulation
- f. seizure
- f. serum
- f. sex determination
- f. sexual differentiation
- f. shoulder extraction force
- f. skeletal anomaly
- f. skeletal dysplasia
- f. skin sampling
- f. skull depression
- f. small parts
- f. somatic activity
- f. souffle
- f. spine position
- f. spleen
- f. startle response
- f. station
- f. status
- f. stem cell transplantation
- f. steroid concentration
- f. structural defect
- f. structural malformation
- f. surgery
- f. surgical procedure
- f. surveillance
- f. surveillance technique
- f. surveillance test
- f. surveillance testing
- f. swallowing
- f. tachycardia
- f. talipes equinovarus
- f. thalidomide
- f. thoracic abnormality
- f. thrombocytopenia
- f. thrombopoietin concentration
- f. thrombotic vasculopathy (FTV)
- f. tissue biopsy
- f. tissue implant
- f. tissue transplant
- f. tobacco syndrome
- f. tone
- f. toxoplasmosis
- f. tracheal occlusion
- f. transfusion
- f. transfusion syndrome
- f. trauma
- f. trimethadione syndrome
- f. ultrasound
- f. urination
- f. urine
- f. uropathy
- f. valproate syndrome (FVS)
- f. varicella syndrome (FVS)
- f. vascular anomaly
- f. vascular conduit
- f. vascular impedance
- f. vasculitis
- f. ventriculomegaly
- f. version in utero
- f. viability
- f. warfarin syndrome
- f. wastage
- f. weight
- f. well-being
- f. zone of adrenal cortex

fetalis

chondromalacia f.
erythroblastosis f.
hydrops f.
ichthyosis f.
immune hydrops f.
maternal hydrops f.
maternal parvovirus f.
nonimmune hydrops f. (NIHF)
opisthotonos f.
rachitis f.

fetalism
fetal-maternal
    f.-m. communication
    f.-m. exchange
    f.-m. hemorrhage
    f.-m. medicine
fetal-neonatal transition
fetal-pelvic index
fetal-placental
    f.-p. circulation
    f.-p. insufficiency
    f.-p. steroidogenesis
    f.-p. unit
FetalPulse
    F. Plus fetal Doppler
    F. Plus monitor
fetal-to-neonatal transition
Fetasonde fetal monitor
fetation
feticide
    selective f.
fetid breath
fetoamniotic shunt
fetofetal
    f. transfusion
    f. transfusion syndrome
fetography
fetology
fetomaternal
    f. alloimmune thrombocytopenia
     (FMAIT)
    f. bleed
    f. hemorrhage (FMH)
    f. transfusion (FMT)
    f. transfusion reaction
fetometry
    ultrasonic f.
    ultrasound f.
fetoneonatal estrogen-binding protein
fetopathy
    diabetic f. (DF)
fetopelvic disproportion
fetoplacental
    f. access
    f. anasarca
    f. blood volume
    f. circulation
    f. function
    f. transfusion
fetoprotein
    amniotic fluid alpha f. (AFAFP)
    maternal serum alpha f. (MSAFP)

fetor
    f. hepaticus
    f. oris
fetoscope
    Hillis-DeLee f.
fetoscopic laser occlusion of
   chorioangiopagus vessels (FLOC)
fetoscopy
fetotoxic
fetotoxicity
fetouterine cell
fetu
    fetus in f.
fetus, pl. fetuses
    acardiac f.
    f. acardiacus
    f. acardius
    amorphous f.
    f. amorphus
    asynclitic position of f.
    calcified f.
    Campylobacter f.
    coexistent f.
    f. compressus
    compromised f.
    dropsy of the f.
    f. in fetu
    f. growth elevation
    growth-restricted f.
    growth-retarded f.
    habitus of f.
    harlequin f.
    HLA-compatible f.
    ichthyosis f.
    impacted f.
    just-viable f.
    macerated f.
    mummified f.
    near-viable f.
    nonhydropic f.
    nonstressed f.
    nonvertex f.
    nonviable f.
    nuchal translucency in a f.
    paper-doll f.
    papyraceous f.
    f. papyraceus
    parasitic f.
    postmature f.
    presentation of f.
    previable f.
    retroperitoneal f.

F

NOTES

fetus *(continued)*
 Rh-sensitized f.
 f. sanguinolentis
 singleton f.
 sireniform f.
 sirenomelic f.
 stressed f.
 stunted f.
 triploid f.
 trisomic f.
 vanishing f.
 viable f.
 Vibrio f.
fetus-to-fetus transplant
Feuerstein-Mims syndrome
Feulgen stain
FEV
 familial exudative vitreoretinopathy
 forced expiratory volume
FEV$_1$
 forced expiratory volume in 1 second
fever
 absorption f.
 acute rheumatic f. (ARF)
 African tick bite f.
 Argentine hemorrhagic f.
 arthritis of rheumatic f.
 artificial f.
 aseptic f.
 biphasic f.
 blackwater f.
 f. blister
 Bolivian hemorrhagic f.
 boutonneuse f.
 cat-scratch f.
 childbed f.
 f.'s and chills (F&C)
 Colorado tick f.
 Crimean-Congo hemorrhagic f.
 dehydration f.
 dengue hemorrhagic f.
 drug f.
 Ebola hemorrhagic f.
 enigmatic f.
 enteric f.
 ephemeral f.
 epidemic relapsing f.
 eruptive f.
 familial Hibernian f.
 familial Mediterranean f. (FMF)
 Flinders Island spotted f.
 glandular f.
 Haverhill f.
 hay f.
 hemorrhagic f.
 inanition f.
 intermittent f.
 intrapartum maternal f.
 Katayama f.
 Korean hemorrhagic f.
 Lassa f.
 louse-borne f.
 maternal f.
 Mediterranean f.
 milk f.
 Omsk hemorrhagic f.
 Oriental spotted f.
 Oroya f.
 paratyphoid f.
 parrot f.
 parturient f.
 PediaCare F.
 Pel-Ebstein f.
 periodic f.
 pharyngoconjunctival f.
 phlebotomus f.
 f. phobia
 Pontiac f.
 puerperal f.
 Q f.
 Queensland f.
 query f.
 quotidian f.
 rat-bite f.
 recrudescence of f.
 relapsing f.
 revised Jones criteria for diagnosis
 of acute rheumatic f.
 rheumatic f.
 Rift Valley f.
 Rocky Mountain spotted f. (RMSF)
 saddleback f.
 San Joaquin f.
 scarlet f.
 South African tick f.
 spirillary rat-bite f.
 spotted f.
 staphylococcal scarlet f.
 surgical scarlet f.
 tactile f.
 three-day f.
 tick f.
 tick-borne relapsing f.
 transitory f.
 trench f.
 tsutsugamushi f.
 typhoid f.
 typhus f.
 f. of undetermined origin (FUO)
 undulant f.
 unexplained f.
 f. of unknown etiology (FUE)
 f. of unknown origin (FUO)
 uveoparotid f.
 Valley f.
 West Nile f.
 yellow f.
FeverAll

Fèvre-Languepin syndrome
fexofenadine
FF
    flatfoot
FFL
    fetal foot length
FFM
    fat-free mass
FFN, fFN
    fetal fibronectin
FFP
    fresh frozen plasma
FFU
    femur-fibula-ulna
      FFU syndrome
FGF
    fibroblast growth factor
FGFa
    acidic fibroblast growth factor
FGFR, FGF-R
    fibroblast growth factor receptor
FGFR3
    fibroblast growth factor receptor 3
FGR
    fetal growth restriction
fgr protooncogene
FG syndrome
FGTM
    female genital tract mutilation
FHF
    fetal heart frequency
    fulminant hepatic failure
FHH
    familial hypercalcemia with hypocalciuria
    familial hypocalciuric hypercalcemia
FHLH
    familial hemophagocytic
      lymphohistiocytosis
FHM
    familial hemiplegic migraine
FHR
    familial hypophosphatemia
    fetal heart rate
      FHR acceleration
      FHR baseline
      nonreassuring FHR
FH-RDC
    family history research diagnostic criteria
FHS
    fetal hydantoin syndrome
    Floating-Harbor syndrome

FHTG
    familial hypertriglyceridemia
FHUF
    femoral hypoplasia unusual facies
      FHUF syndrome
FIA
    fluorescent immunoassay
fiber
    f. bone
    Dacron f.
    dietary f.
    myoclonus epilepsy with ragged
      red f.'s (MERRF)
    myometrial f.
    parasympathetic f.
    Perdiem F.
    postsynaptic f.
    Purkinje f.'s
    ragged red f. (RRF)
    Rosenthal f.
Fiberall
    F. Powder
    F. Wafer
FiberCon
fiberglass jacket
fiberoptic
    f. bronchoscopy
    f. headband
    f. phototherapy (FO-PT)
Fibersource HN formula
fiber-type disproportion
fibril
    anchoring f.
fibrillary
    f. astrocytoma
    f. gliosis
fibrillation
    atrial f.
    f. potential
fibrillatory wave
fibrillin
fibrin
    basal perivillous f.
    f. degradation
    f. degradation product
    f. deposition
    f. sheath
    f. split product (FSP)
    f. stabilizing factor
    f. thrombus
Fibrindex test

F

NOTES

351

fibrinogen
- f. abnormality
- f. deficiency
- f. degradation product (FDP)
- plasma f.
- radiolabeled f.
- serial maternal serum f.
- f. split product

fibrinogen-fibrin
- f.-f. degradation product
- fibrinogen-fibrin conversion syndrome

fibrinoid
- f. degeneration of astrocytes
- f. leukodystrophy
- f. necrosis

fibrinolysis
- f. inhibitor
- tissue activator-induced f.

fibrinolytic
- f. agent
- f. and clotting system
- f. therapy

fibrinopurulent exudate

fibrinous
- f. coalition
- f. exudate
- f. pericarditis
- f. polyp

fibroadenolipoma
- degenerated f.

fibroadenoma
- giant f.
- intracanalicular f.
- juvenile f.
- pericanalicular f.

fibroareolar tissue

fibroblast
- f. culture
- cultured skin f.
- genital skin f.
- f. growth factor (FGF)
- f. growth factor-10 null phenotype
- f. growth factor receptor (FGFR, FGF-R)
- f. growth factor receptor 3 (FGFR3)
- human embryo f. (HEF)
- f. pneumocyte factor

fibroblastic osteosarcoma
fibroblastoid synoviocyte
fibrochondrogenesis
fibrocortical defect

fibrocystic
- f. breast
- f. breast change
- f. disease

fibrodysplasia ossificans progressiva (FOP)

fibroelastosis
- endocardial f. (EFE)
- prenatal f.

fibroepithelial polyp
fibrogenesis
FIBROID
- Fibroid Registry for Outcomes Data

fibroid
- calcified uterine f.
- f. embolization
- intramural f.
- lower uterine segment f.
- F. Registry for Outcomes Data (FIBROID)
- submucous f.
- subserous f.
- uterine f.

fibroidectomy
fibrolamellar hepatocellular carcinoma

fibroma
- benign nasopharyngeal f.
- chondromyxoid f.
- digital f.
- histiocytic f.
- infantile digital f.
- f. molle gravidarum
- nasopharyngeal f.
- nonossifying f.
- ossifying f.
- ovarian f.
- periungual f.
- sternocleidomastoid f.
- subungual f.
- vulvar f.

fibromatosis
- gingival f.
- infantile f.
- ovarian f.
- pelvic f.

fibromectomy

fibromuscular
- f. cervical stroma
- f. dysplasia

fibromyalgia
- childhood f.

fibromyoma, pl. **fibromyomata**
- uterine f.

fibromyxoid stroma

fibronectin
- cervicovaginal fetal f.
- fetal f. (FFN, fFN)
- oncofetal f.
- f. receptor

fibroplasia
- retrolental f. (RLF)

fibropurulent

fibrosa
- osteitis f.

fibrosarcoma
congenital f.
fibrosing
f. adenomatosis
f. adenosis
f. colonopathy
f. inflammation
f. mediastinitis
fibrosis
cavernosal f.
cerebellar vermis hypoplasia,
oligophrenia, congenital ataxia,
ocular coloboma, hepatic f.
(COACH)
chronic interstitial f.
coloboma-hepatic f.
congenital hepatic f.
cutaneous f.
cystic f. (CF)
delta-F508 cystic f.
endocardial f.
endomyocardial f.
endoneurial f.
focal f.
focal tubulointerstitial f. (FTIF)
gum f.
hepatic f.
horseshoe f.
idiopathic diffuse interstitial f.
interstitial f.
meningeal f.
neoplastic f.
obstructing periuretal f.
peribronchial f.
peritoneal f.
peritubular f.
portal f.
postradiation periureteral f.
pulmonary interstitial f.
retroperitoneal f.
retropubic f.
f. scoring
tubular interstitial f.
fibrosum
molluscum f.
pedunculated molluscum f.
fibrothecoma
fibrotic ophthalmoplegia
fibrous
f. anlage
f. connective tissue
f. cortical defect

f. dysplasia
f. dysplasia of jaw
fibrovascular
f. tissue
f. tumor
fibroxanthoma
fibula
congenital longitudinal deficiency
of f.
fibular
f. hemimelia
f. osteotomy
f. shaft fracture
Fick
F. method
F. principle
Ficoll-Hypaque centrifugation
fictitious epilepsy
FIDD
fetal iodine deficiency disorder
fiddle-string adhesion
fidget
fidgety
Fiedler myocarditis
field
f. block
central visual f.
high power f. (hpf)
involved f. (IF)
low power f. (lpf)
tangential breast f.
f. of view
f. of vision
visual f.
fifth
f. digit syndrome
f. finger clinodactyly
f. phacomatosis
f. venereal disease
fifth-day fit
fight-and-flight response
fighter
Flimm F.
FIGLU
formiminoglutamic acid
FIGLU-uria
formiminoglutamicaciduria
FIGO
International Federation of Gynecology
and Obstetrics
FIGO nomenclature

F

NOTES

FIGO *(continued)*
    FIGO (stage I–IV) disease
    FIGO staging
figure
    Gesell f.
    Matching Familiar F.'s (MFF)
    mitotic f.
figure-of-eight
    f.-o.-e. apparatus
    f.-o.-e. clavicle strap
    f.-o.-e. harness
    f.-o.-e. strapping
figure-of-four test
figure-of-three sign
filament
    myosin f.
    sarcomeric f.
filamentous hemagglutinin
filariasis
Filatov-Dukes disease
filgrastim
filial generation
filiform
    f. adnatum
    f. papule
    f. plaque
    f. wart
Filippi syndrome
Fillauer night splint
filled and spilled
fillet
filling
    bladder f.
    ventricular f.
film
    contraceptive f.
    cross-table lateral f.
    decubitus f.
    scoliosis f.
    tear f.
    tibial f.
    upright chest f.
    vaginal contraceptive f. (VCF)
Filmtab
    Rondec F.
filmy adhesion
Filshie
    F. clip
    F. clip applicator
filter
    Greenfield f.
    HEPA f.
    leukocyte-depletion f.
    leukocyte-removal f.
    leukodepletion f.
    Millipore f.
    f. paper (FP)
    vena caval f.
filtered specimen trap

filtrate
    glomerular f.
filtration
    f. fraction
    glass-wool f.
    glomerular f.
    rate of fluid f. (Qf)
filum terminale
fimbria, pl. **fimbriae**
    flowering-out of f.
    mushrooming of f.
    f. ovarica
fimbrial
    f. adhesion
    f. ectopic pregnancy
    f. evacuation
    f. failure
    f. obstruction
    f. prolapse
fimbriated end of fallopian tube
fimbriectomy
    Uchida f.
fimbriocele
fimbrioplasty
    Bruhat laser f.
Finapres
    F. blood pressure monitor
    F. device
finasteride
find
    Child F.
finding
    clinical f.
    congenital familial lymphedema
      with ocular f.'s
    dermatoglyphic f.
    endovaginal f.
    histopathological f.
    laboratory f.
    pathologic f.
    sonographic f.
    ultrasonic endovaginal f.
Findley folding pessary
fine
    f. inspiratory crackle
    f. lens opacity
    f. Metzenbaum scissors
    f. motor
    f. motor-adaptive skill
    f. motor development
    f. motor domain
    f. motor index
    f. motor milestone
    f. motor total DMQ
Fine-Lubinsky syndrome
fine Metzenbaum scissors
fine-needle
    f.-n. aspiration (FNA)
    f.-n. aspiration biopsy (FNAB)

finger
  f. agnosia
  f. arterial blood pressure (FABP)
  baseball f.
  bent f.
  boutonnière f.
  coach's f.
  f. cot
  curved f.
  f. feeding
  f. gnosis
  f. grasp
  index f.
  Madonna f.
  mallet f.
  middle f.
  f. opposition
  overriding f.
  f. plethysmography
  pollicization of index f.
  ring f.
  seal f.'s
  spider f.
  webbed f.'s
fingerbreadth
fingernail
finger-nose-finger test
fingerprint
fingerprinting
  DNA amplification f.
  plasmid f.
fingerspelling
fingerstick
finger-tapping test
fingertip
  f. dilated
  f. number writing test
finger-to-nose test
Finkelstein feeding
Finnish
  congenital nephrotic syndrome, F. (CNF)
FIO$_2$, FiO$_2$
  fraction of inspired oxygen
Fioricet With Codeine
fire
  f. ant allergy
  f. setting
  St. Anthony's f.
fire-setting behavior

FIRM
  Family Inventory of Resources for Management
firm hepatomegaly
first
  f. abarelix depot study for treating endometriosis rapidly (FASTER)
  f. bicuspid
  f. degree prolapse
  f. disease
  f. heart sound
  f. Korotkoff sound
  f. parallel pelvic plane
  f. permanent molar
  f. primary molar
  F. Response ovulation predictor
  f. and second branchial arch syndrome
  f. and second trimester evaluation of risk (FASTER)
  f. stage of labor
  f. trimester
  f. trimester screening
  f. trimester termination
first-cycle clinical pregnancy
first-degree
  f.-d. AV block
  f.-d. burn
  f.-d. episiotomy
  f.-d. hypospadias
  f.-d. laceration
first-generation
  f.-g. cephalosporin
  f.-g. progesterone
first-line measure
first-morning urine collection
first-pass effect
FISCA
  Functional Impairment Scale for Children and Adolescents
FISH
  fluorescent in situ hybridization
  FISH analysis
fish
  f. oil
  f. poisoning
  f. skin
Fisher
  infantile choreoathetosis of F.
  F. and Paykel RD1000 resuscitator
fisherman's knot
Fisher-Race Rh system nomenclature

F

NOTES

Fishman syndrome
fishmouth
    f. abnormality
    f. cervix
    f. meatus
    f. vertebra
fish-shaped mouth
fish-tank granuloma
fishy odor
FISS
    Flint Infant Security Scale
fissure
    abnormal palpebral f.
    Ammon f.
    anal f.
    f. in ano
    antimongoloid palpebral f.
    azygos f.
    downslanting palpebral f.
    downsloping palpebral f.
    mild downslant to palpebral f.
    palpebral f.
    rectal f.
    f. of sternum
    superior vesical f.
    upslanting palpebral f.
fissured
    f. lips
    f. tongue
fissuring
fist
    clenched f.'s
fisting
    f. of hands
fistula, pl. **fistulae, fistulas**
    anterior rectoperineal f.
    arterioportal f.
    arteriovenous f.
    branchial cleft f.
    bronchobiliary f.
    bronchoesophageal f.
    bronchopleural f.
    bronchopulmonary f. (BPF)
    carotid artery-cavernous sinus f.
    carotid-cavernous f.
    cervicovaginal f.
    colovaginal f.
    congenital perilymphatic f.
    coronary arteriovenous f.
    coronary artery f. (CAF)
    coronary-cameral f.
    enterocolic f.
    enterocutaneous f.
    enteroenteric f.
    enterovaginal f.
    enterovesical f.
    gastrointestinal f.
    genitourinary f.
    hepatic arteriovenous f.

H-type tracheoesophageal f.
H-type transesophageal f.
intestinal f.
intracranial arteriovenous f.
intrahepatic arterioportal f.
lacteal f.
mammary f.
metroperitoneal f.
microcephaly, mesobrachyphalangy,
    tracheoesophageal f.
palatal f.
perianal f.
perilymphatic f. (PLF)
perineal f.
perineovaginal f.
peripheral arteriovenous f.
persistent gastrocutaneous f.
postradiation f.
rectal-fourchette f.
rectolabial f.
rectourethral f.
rectovaginal f.
rectovestibular f.
rectovulvar f.
renal f.
sinus f.
spit f.
systemic arteriovenous f.
tracheocutaneous f.
tracheoesophageal f. (TEF, TOF)
transesophageal f. (TEF)
tubovaginal f.
umbilical f.
urachal f.
ureter f.
ureterovaginal f.
urethrocutaneous f.
urethrovaginal f.
urinary f.
urogenital f.
uteroperitoneal f.
vesicocutaneous f.
vesicouterine f.
vesicovaginal f.
vesicovaginorectal f.
vestibular f.
vitelline f.
fistulogram
fistulotomy
fistulous vascular communication
fit
    arrest/akinetic f.
    extensor f.
    fifth-day f.
    flexor f.
    mixed flexor/extensor f.
    uncinate f.
fitness
    darwinian f.

Fitz-Hugh-Curtis syndrome
Fitzsimmons syndrome
five-component vaccine
five-hop test
five-hour glucose tolerance test
five-word sentence
fixation
    buttonpexy f.
    complement f.
    flexible intramedullary f.
    iliococcygeal f.
    intramedullary rod f.
    Nichols sacrospinous f.
    f. nystagmus
    percutaneous pin f.
fixative
    Carnoy f.
fixator
    Ilizarov external f.
fixed
    f. allele
    f. erythema
    f. flexion deformity
    f. pulmonary hypertension
    f. stenosis
fixed-deficit ataxia
fixed-wing transport
FJN
    familial juvenile nephrophthisis
FK binding protein
FL
    femur length
FLACC
    face, legs, activity, cry, consolability
    FLACC scale
flaccid
    f. contracture
    f. extremity
    f. lesion
    f. paralysis
    f. paraparesis
    f. paraplegia
    f. paresis
    f. quadriparesis
    f. tetraplegia
    f. tone
flaccidity
    penile f.
flag sign
Flagyl
    F. 375
    F. Oral

flail
    f. chest
    f. foot
    f. mitral leaflet (FML)
FLAIR
    fluid-attenuated inversion recovery
    FLAIR sequence
flaking
    periungual f.
flame burn
flammeus
    nevus f.
flange
    tracheostomy tube f.
flank
    bluish discoloration of f.
    bulging f.
    f. dullness
    f. mass
    f. pain
flanking region
flap
    bladder f.
    Boari f.
    bridging f.
    bulbocavernosus fat f.
    butterfly f.
    Byers f.
    double-onlay preputial f.
    Duckett transverse preputial
     island f.
    endorectal f.
    endoscopic incision with f.
    fascial f.
    fat f.
    foreskin f.
    gluteal free f.
    island f.
    lateral transverse thigh f.
    latissimus dorsi f.
    liver f.
    maple leaf f.
    Martius bulbocavernosus fat f.
    McCraw gracilis myocutaneous f.
    Mustardé cheek f.
    myocutaneous f.
    onlay island f.
    Ponten fasciocutaneous f.
    preputial f.
    Rubens f.
    saddlebag f.
    f. tracheostomy

NOTES

F

flap *(continued)*
    TRAM f.
    TRAMP f.
    vaginal wall f.
    vein f.
    Warren f.
flare
    cell and f.
Flarex
flaring
    f. of ala nasi
    alar f.
    f. and grunting
    grunting and f.
    metaphysial f.
    nasal f.
flash
    hot f.
    f. VEP
flashback
flashlamp-pulsed
    f.-p. dye laser
    f.-p. laser therapy
Flashtab
flat
    f. abdominal radiograph
    f. acetabular roof
    f. affect
    f. back
    f. facies
    f. fontanelle
    f. frontal bone
    f. nasal bridge
    f. nose
    f. pelvis
    f. red-black telangiectasia
    f. spring diaphragm
    f. wart
flatfoot (FF)
    calcaneovalgus f.
    developmental f.
    flexible f.
    hypermobile f.
    peroneal spastic f.
    physiologic f.
flatness to percussion
flattened
    f. occiput
    f. villus
flatulence
Flatulex
flava
    macula f.
flavimaculatus
    fundus f.
flavin adenine dinucleotide (FAD)
Flaviviridae
Flavobacterium

flavoprotein
    electron transfer f. (ETF)
flavus
    Aspergillus f.
flecainide acetate
Fleet
    F. Babylax Rectal
    F. Mineral Oil Enema
    F. Pain Relief
    F. Phospho-Soda
fleeting paralysis
Fleming ovoid
Flents breast comfort pack
flesh-colored papule
fleshy mole
Fletcher-Suit applicator
fleur-de-lis breast reconstruction pattern
flexible
    f. fiberoptic bronchoscopy
    f. fiberoptic endoscopy
    f. flatfoot
    f. hysteroscope
    f. intramedullary fixation
    f. kyphosis
    f. pes planovalgus
    f. Teflon catheter
flexion
    f. contracture
    f. reflex
    f. spasm
flexion-distraction injury
flexion-extension
Flexi-Seal fecal collector
flexneri
    Shigella f.
    Shigella f. (type 2b)
flexor
    f. fit
    f. hallucis longus tendon
    f. tone
flexural
    f. area
    f. crease
flexure
    basicranial f.
    splenic f.
flight
    f. of color
    f. of ideas
Flimm Fighter
Flinders Island spotted fever
Flint Infant Security Scale (FISS)
FLM
    fetal lung maturity
    FLM test
floating
    f. great toe

f. membrane
f. thumb
Floating-Harbor syndrome (FHS)
FLOC
   fetoscopic laser occlusion of
   chorioangiopagus vessels
floccosum
   Epidermophyton f.
flocculation
Flonase
flood
flooding
floor
   decidual f.
   orbital f.
   pelvic f.
Flo-Pack
floppy
   f. infant
   f. infant syndrome
   f. larynx
flora
   commensal f.
   microbial f.
   prepuberal vaginal f.
   skin f.
   uterine f.
   vaginal f.
Florical
florid
   f. complexion
   f. pulmonary valvular incompetence
   f. toxemia
Florida pouch
Florinef Acetate
Florone
flottant
   pouce f.
flour
   carob seed f.
Flovent Rotadisk
flow
   aboral f.
   f. angulation
   blood f. (Q̇)
   bulk f.
   cardiac f.
   carotid blood f. (CaBF)
   cerebral blood f. (CBF)
   coaxial f.
   collateral blood f.
   cutaneous fetal blood f.

f. cytometric analysis
f. cytometry
f. cytometry analysis
Doppler f.
ductal-dependent pulmonary
   blood f.
duct-dependent pulmonary blood f.
excessive pulmonary arterial f.
fetal aortic blood f.
forced expiratory f. (FEF)
gene f.
hyperemic cerebral blood f.
f. karyotyping
menstrual f.
f. murmur
myocardial blood f.
outward menstrual f.
f. pattern
placental blood f.
pulmonary arterial f.
pulmonary blood f. (PBF)
f. rate
renal blood f. (RBF)
renal plasma f.
retrograde axoplasmic f.
retrograde menstrual f.
reversed end-diastolic f.
splanchnic blood f.
systemic f.
to-and-fro f.
torrential pulmonary f.
umbilical blood f.
umbilical venous f.
urine f.
uterine blood f.
uteroplacental blood f.
f. velocity dynamics
f. velocity waveform
venous f.
f. void
volume f.
flowering-out of fimbria
FlowGel barrier material
flowmeter
   laser-Doppler f.
FlowStat
Flowtron DVT prophylaxis unit
flow-volume
   f.-v. curve
   f.-v. loop
Floxin Otic
floxuridine in hepatic metastasis

F

NOTES

flu
　　influenza
Fluanxol
flucloxacillin
fluconazole
fluctuance
fluctuant
fluctuating tone
fluctuation
　　mood f.
flucytosine
5-flucytosine
Fludara
fludarabine
fludrocortisone
fluency
　　cross-modal f.
　　verbal f.
flufenamic acid
fluid
　　amniotic f. (AF)
　　ascitic f.
　　BAL f.
　　Bamberger f.
　　body f.
　　f. bolus
　　bronchoalveolar f.
　　cerebrospinal f. (CSF)
　　f. deficit
　　f. diet
　　duodenal f.
　　f.'s, electrolytes, nutrition (FEN)
　　epithelial lining f. (ELF)
　　excessive amniotic f.
　　extraaxial f.
　　extracellular f. (ECF)
　　extraluminal f.
　　fetal lung f.
　　follicular f.
　　foul-smelling amniotic f.
　　hemorrhagic spinal f.
　　f. homeostasis
　　human oviduct f. (HOF)
　　hydrocele f.
　　hysteroscopy f.
　　interstitial f.
　　intracellular f. (ICF)
　　intravascular f.
　　isotonic f.
　　maintenance f.
　　meconium-stained amniotic f.
　　　(MSAF)
　　middle ear f. (MEF)
　　milky f.
　　negative balance of body f.
　　f. overload
　　peripancreatic f.
　　peritoneal f.
　　proteinaceous subretinal f.

　　pseudochylous milky f.
　　f. replacement
　　f. replacement therapy
　　f. restriction
　　f. resuscitation
　　retained fetal lung f. (RFLF)
　　f. retention
　　seminal f.
　　serosanguineous f.
　　f. sift
　　sperm-counting f.
　　subretinal f.
　　synovial f.
　　third spacing of f.
　　tracheobronchial aspirate f. (TAF)
　　transcapillary f.
　　ventricular f.
　　viscous f.
　　f. wave
　　xanthochromic f.
fluid-attenuated inversion recovery
　　(FLAIR)
fluke
　　lung f.
flulike syndrome
Flumadine Oral
flumazenil
flumecinol
FluMist vaccine
flunisolide
flunitrazepam
fluocinolone acetonide
fluocinonide
Fluoderm
Fluogen
fluorangiography
fluorescein
　　f. fundus angiography
　　f. isothiocyanate
　　f. sodium
　　f. stain
　　f. treponema antibody test
fluorescein-conjugated monoclonal
　　antibody test
fluorescein-labeled milk
fluorescence
　　f. actin staining test
　　f. depolarization analysis
　　f. spot test
fluorescence-activated cell sorter (FACS)
fluorescens
　　Pseudomonas f.
fluorescent
　　f. antibody against membrane
　　　antigen (FAMA)
　　f. antimembrane antibody test
　　　(FAMA)
　　f. immunoassay (FIA)
　　f. polarization

f. polarization immunoassay (FPIA)
f. in situ hybridization (FISH)
f. treponemal antibody (FTA)
f. treponemal antibody absorption
(FTA-ABS)

fluoridation
fluoride
polyvinylidene f. (PVDF)
slow-release sodium f.
sodium f.

Fluorigard
Fluori-Methane
fluorinated corticosteroid
fluorine
Fluorinse
fluorocortisone
5-fluorocytosine (5-FC)
fluorodeoxyuridine (FUDR)
9-fluorohydrocortisone
fluoroimmunoassay
time-resolved f.

fluorometholone (FML)
fluorophore-assisted carbohydrate electrophoresis (FACE)
fluorophosphate
diisopropyl f.

Fluoroplex Topical
fluoroquinolone
fluoroscope
fluoroscopic guidance
fluoroscopy
airway f.
image intensification f.

fluorouracil
Cytoxan, Adriamycin, f. (CAF)
Cytoxan, Adriamycin, leucovorin, calcium, f. (CALF)
Cytoxan, epirubicin, f. (CEF)
f., epirubicin, Cytoxan (FEC)

5-fluorouracil (5-FU)
intraperitoneal 5-f.

fluoro-urodynamic evaluation
Fluothane
fluoxetine
f. HCl
f. hydrochloride

fluoxymesterone
flupentixol, flupenthixol
fluphenazine
flurandrenolide
flurazepam
flurbiprofen

flush
breast f.
ciliary f.
cyanotic f.
heparin-lock f.
hot f.
malar f.
f. method
orgasmic f.
vasomotor f.

flushing
episodic f.

flutamide
fluted drain
fluticasone
f. propionate
f. propionate dry powder inhaler
f. propionate inhalation powder

flutter
atrial f.
f. device
f. isthmus
ocular f.
f. wave

flutter-like oscillation
fluvoxamine maleate
flux
bile acid f.

Fluzone
fly
Spanish f.
tsetse f.

flying squirrel typhus
flying-T pelvis
FM
fat mass

FMAIT
fetomaternal alloimmune thrombocytopenia

FMF
familial Mediterranean fever

FMG
female genital mutilation

FMH
fetomaternal hemorrhage

FML
flail mitral leaflet
fluorometholone
FML Forte

FMLA
Family Medical Leave Act

NOTES

F

fm/mg
femtomole/milligram
FMP
family member presence
FMR1
fragile site mental retardation 1
FMR1 gene
FMR2
fragile site mental retardation 2
fMRI
functional MRI
FMRP
fragile X mental retardation protein
FMT
fetomaternal transfusion
FNA
fine-needle aspiration
FNA-21
F. fine-needle aspiration device
F. needle
FNAB
fine-needle aspiration biopsy
FND
frontonasal dysplasia
FNI
facial nerve injury
FNSD
face-near-straight-down
FO
foot orthosis
foam
Because vaginal f.
f. cell
contraceptive f.
intravaginal f.
f. rubber vaginal form
Sklar f.
F. Stability Index (FSI)
f. stability test (FST)
FoamCare
F. cleansing system
F. double scrub brush
FOAR
faciooculoacousticorenal
FOAR syndrome
FOBT
fecal occult blood testing
focal
f. atrophy
f. axonal swelling
f. brainstem glioma
f. cerebral edema
f. change
f. convulsion
f. cortical dysplasia
f. dermal hypoplasia
f. dermal hypoplasia syndrome
f. dystonia
f. epilepsy

f. facial dermal dysplasia (type I, II)
f. facial ectodermal dysplasia
f. fibrosis
f. glomerulosclerosis
f. hemorrhage
f. heterotopia
f. lobular carcinoma
f. lupus nephritis
f. motor seizure
f. mucopolysaccharidosis
f. neurologic deficit
f. nodular hyperplasia
f. pontine leukoencephalopathy
f. postviral encephalitis
f. scleroderma
f. segmental glomerular sclerosis
f. and segmental glomerular
sclerosis-hyalinosis
f. segmental glomerulosclerosis
(FSGS)
f. segmental lupus
glomerulonephritis
f. segmental proliferative
glomerulonephritis
f. spot size
f. tubulointerstitial fibrosis (FTIF)
f. villitis
f. vulvitis
Focalin tablet
focally dilated duct
focus, pl. **foci**
echogenic cardiac f.
endometriotic f.
hyperechogenic foci
occult f.
Simon f.
focused
F. Assessment by Sonography for
Trauma (FAST)
f. computed tomography
Foerster sponge-holding forceps
Fogarty
F. arterial embolectomy (FAE)
F. arterial embolectomy catheter
F. atrioseptostomy catheter
fogo selvagem
Foille Medicated First Aid
folacin
folate
f. antagonist
f. folic acid deficiency
f. level
fold
absent antihelical f.
antihelical f.
aryepiglottic f.
broad ligament f.
Dennie-Morgan f.

Duncan f.'s
epicanthal f.
genitocrural f.
gluteal f.
head and tail f.
f. of Hoboken
Juvara f.
lateral umbilical f.
median umbilical f.
nuchal f.
Pawlik f.
pleuroperitoneal f.
rectouterine f.
rugal f.
skin f.
splanchnic f.
umbilical f.
urogenital f.
folding frequency
Foley
F. catheter
F. tube
folia (*pl. of* folium)
foliaceus
pemphigus f.
folic
f. acid
f. acid antagonist
f. acid deficiency
folinic acid
folium, pl. **folia**
cerebellar folia
folia cerebelli
folia of cerebellum
folia linguae
folia vermis
folia of vermis
folk medicine
follicle
antral f.
f. aspiration, sperm injection, and
assisted rupture (FASIAR)
f. aspiration tube
atretic f.
dominant f.
graafian f.
luteinized unruptured f.
f. maturation stimulation
Naboth f.
nabothian f.
preantral f.
preovulatory f.

primary f.
primordial f.
f. regulatory protein (FRP)
f. steroidogenesis
f. stimulating hormone
follicle-stimulating hormone (FSH)
follicular
f. atrophoderma, basal cell
carcinoma syndrome
f. atrophoderma, basocellular
proliferation, hypotrichosis
syndrome
f. attrition
f. bronchitis
f. conjunctivitis
f. cyst
f. dermatitis
f. desquamation
f. development arrest
f. duct
f. factor
f. fluid
f. function
f. hematoma
f. hyperplasia
f. maturation
f. ostium
f. phase
f. phase gonadotropin secretion
f. plugging
f. scoring
f. tonsillitis
f. urethritis
f. vulvitis
follicularis
dwarfism, cerebral atrophy,
keratosis f.
keratosis f.
folliculitis
eosinophilic pustular f. (EPF)
fungal f.
hot tub f.
Staphylococcus epidermidis f.
folliculogenesis
folliculorum
Demodex f.
folliculostatin
Folling disease
follistatin
Follistim
Follistim/Antagon kit

NOTES

F

follitropin
    f. alpha
    f. beta
followup, follow-up
    f. care
    Carnation F.'s
    long-term f.
Follow-Up Soy formula
Folvite
folylpolyglutamate
fomepizole
fomite
    hand-to-eye f.
Fong disease
Fontaine syndrome
Fontan
    F. fenestration
    F. operation
    F. principle
    F. procedure
fontanelle, fontanel
    anterior f.
    anterolateral f.
    bulging f.
    Casser f.
    casserian f.
    depressed f.
    false f.
    flat f.
    Gerdy f.
    mastoid f.
    posterior f.
    posterolateral f.
    pulsatile f.
    sagittal f.
    scaphoid f.
    f. sign
    sphenoid f.
    sunken anterior f.
fonticulus, pl. fonticuli
food
    f. allergen
    f. avoidance emotion disorder
    (FAED)
    f. challenge test
    f. craving
    f. diary
    F. and Drug Administration (FDA)
    fear f.
    f. foraging
    F. Guide Pyramid
    f. impaction
    f. insecurity
    f. poisoning
    f. police
    f. seeking
    solid f.
    thermic effect of f. (TEF)
food-antigen sensitization

food-borne illness
food-induced
    f.-i. enterocolitis syndrome
    f.-i. pulmonary hemosiderosis
foot, pl. feet
    athlete's f.
    bilateral club feet
    calcaneovalgus f.
    cavovarus f.
    cavus f.
    club f.
    congenital rocker-bottom f.
    dancing feet
    f. deformity
    f. drop
    epidermolysis bullosa simplex of
    feet
    flail f.
    Friedreich f.
    high arch f.
    hyperdorsiflexed f.
    Madura f.
    Morand f.
    narrow f.
    f. orthosis (FO)
    f. presentation
    pronated f.
    reel f.
    rockerbottom f.
    spatula f.
    Z f.
footballer's migraine
football-shaped vesicle
foot-drop
footling breech presentation
footplate
    astrocyte f.
footprinting
foot-progression angle (FPA)
FOP
    fibrodysplasia ossificans progressiva
FO-PT
    fiberoptic phototherapy
foraging
    food f.
foramen, pl. foramina
    bulboventricular f.
    f. of Luschka
    f. of Magendie
    f. magnum
    f. of Monro
    f. of Morgagni
    f. of Morgagni hernia
    outlet foramina
    f. ovale
    f. ovale persistence
    parietal foramina
    pleuroperitoneal f.
    f. primum

f. secundum
sternomastoid f.
stylomastoid f.
Forane
Forbes-Albright syndrome
Forbes disease
force
    acceleration-deceleration f.
    compression f.
    expulsive f.
    fetal shoulder extraction f.
    oncotic f.
    physician-applied f.
    shearing f.
    Starling f.
    United States Preventive Services
      Task F. (USPSTF)
forcé
forced
    f. bowel training
    f. choice
    f. expiratory flow (FEF)
    f. expiratory volume (FEV)
    f. expiratory volume in 1 second
      (FEV$_1$)
    f. grasping reflex
    f. grasp reflex
    f. vital capacity (FVC)
forced-air blanket
Force GSU argon-enhanced
  electrosurgery system
forceps
    Adson f.
    alligator f.
    Allis f.
    Allis-Abramson breast biopsy f.
    Apple Medical bipolar f.
    Arruga-Nicetic capsule f.
    artery f.
    ASSI bipolar coagulating f.
    atraumatic f.
    axis-traction f.
    Babcock f.
    Bailey-Williamson f.
    Baird f.
    Bakchaus towel f.
    Barton f.
    bayonet f.
    Bellucci alligator f.
    BiCoag f.
    Bierer ovum f.
    Billroth tumor f.

Bill traction handle f.
biopsy f.
bipolar laparoscopic f.
f. birth trauma
Bishop-Harmon f.
Bozeman uterine dressing f.
Brown-Adson tissue f.
Castroviejo fixation f.
Cauer f.
cephalic f.
Chamberlen f.
Clarke ligator scissor f.
coaptation bipolar f.
cold biopsy f.
Colibri f.
Corey ovum f.
Corson myoma grasping f.
Crile f.
Cushing f.
DeBakey tissue f.
DeJuan f.
DeLee f.
f. delivery (FD)
Dennen f.
Desmarres f.
DeWeese axis traction f.
Dewey obstetrical f.
Dieter f.
dressing f.
Drews f.
Duval f.
Elliot f.
Endo-Assist endoscopic f.
Englert f.
Eppendorfer biopsy f.
Erhardt f.
Evershears bipolar laparoscopic f.
Facit polyp f.
Feilchenfeld f.
Foerster sponge-holding f.
Francis f.
Fujinon biopsy f.
Gelhorn f.
Gerald f.
Glassman f.
Greven f.
Haig-Fergusson f.
Halsted mosquito f.
Haugh f.
Hawk-Dennen f.
Heaney-Ballantine f.
Heaney hysterectomy f.

NOTES

forceps *(continued)*
    high f.
    Hildebrandt uterine hemostatic f.
    Hirst placental f.
    Hodge f.
    hot biopsy f.
    Hunt bipolar f.
    Iselin f.
    Jacobson hemostatic f.
    Jaws f.
    jeweler's f.
    Juers f.
    Kelly tissue f.
    Kelly vulsellum f.
    Kevorkian-Younge biopsy f.
    Kjelland f.
    Kjelland-Barton f.
    Kjelland-Luikart f.
    Kleppinger bipolar f.
    Lahey f.
    Lalonde delicate hook f.
    laparoscopic plasma f.
    Laufe-Piper f.
    Laufe polyp f.
    Laurer f.
    Leff f.
    Levret f.
    Livernois-McDonald f.
    Llorente dissecting f.
    low f.
    Luikart f.
    Luikart-Simpson f.
    f. maneuver
    Mazzariello-Caprini f.
    McGee f.
    McGill f.
    McKernan-Adson f.
    McKernan-Potts f.
    McLane f.
    McPherson f.
    Nadler f.
    Nägele f.
    Neville-Barnes f.
    nonfenestrated f.
    obstetric f.
    Ochsner f.
    outlet f.
    ovum f.
    paddle f.
    Palmer ovarian biopsy f.
    Péan f.
    pelvic f.
    Pennington f.
    Perez-Castro f.
    Phaneuf uterine artery f.
    Piper f.
    Pistofidis cervical biopsy f.
    pituitary f.
    Polaris reusable f.

    Pollock f.
    preemie Simpson f.
    punch biopsy f.
    Quinones uterine-grasping f.
    radial jaw biopsy f.
    Randall stone f.
    Reddick-Saye f.
    Reiner-Knight f.
    ring f.
    Rochester-Ochsner f.
    Rochester-Péan f.
    Roger f.
    f. rotation
    Russian tissue f.
    Saenger ovum f.
    Scanzoni f.
    Schroeder tenaculum f.
    Schroeder vulsellum f.
    Schubert uterine biopsy f.
    Seitzinger tripolar cutting f.
    Semken f.
    Shea f.
    Shearer f.
    Shute f.
    Simpson f.
    Singley f.
    Sopher ovum f.
    sponge f.
    sponge-holding f.
    spoon f.
    Stolte f.
    suture grasper f.
    Tabb crura tissue f.
    Tarnier axis-traction f.
    tendon f.
    Therma Jaw hot urologic f.
    Thomas-Gaylor biopsy f.
    Tischler cervical biopsy f.
    Tischler-Morgan uterine biopsy f.
    tissue f.
    trial f.
    Tucker-McLane f.
    Tucker-McLane-Luikart f.
    uterine tenaculum f.
    Utrata f.
    Willett f.
    Winter placental f.
    Yeoman f.
    Z-Clamp hysterectomy f.

Forchheimer spot
Fordyce
    F. disease
    F. granule
    F. spot
forebag
forefoot
    f. abduction
    f. adduction
    f. adductus

f. deformity
f. valgus
f. varus
foregut
f. duplication
f. malformation
forehead
broad f.
foreign
f. body
f. body aspiration
f. body salpingitis
forekidney
forelock
white f.
foremilk
forensic specimen
foreplay
foreskin
f. flap
large f.
forest
conidial f.
forewaters
fork
replication f.
forking
aqueductal f.
form
balsa vaginal f.
child behavior rating f. (CBRF)
coccobacillary f.
connatal f.
foam rubber vaginal f.
Lucite f.
MedWatch f.
parenchymatous f.
phosphorylated drug f.
racemose f.
serous f.
Teacher Rating F. (TRF)
Teacher Report F. (TRF)
Vineland Adaptive Behavior Scales, Survey F.
Ware Short F.-35
formaldehyde
formalin
formation
abscess f.
alveolar saccule f.
blood vessel f.
bone f.

cataract f.
chiasma f.
chylomicron f.
clot f.
colostomy f.
crescent f.
Dandy-Walker f.
dissolution of clot f.
echo f.
kerion f.
macular star f.
neoaorta f.
onion bulb f.
perivascular pseudorosette f.
pneumatocele f.
popcorn f.
primary lung bud f.
recurrent hernia f.
sequestrum f.
somite f.
subcutaneous catheter tunnel f.
terminal blush f.
uterine window f.
formative yolk
Forma water-jacketed incubator
formazan dye
formboard
forme fruste
formic acid
formiminoglutamic acid (FIGLU)
formiminoglutamicaciduria (FIGLU-uria)
formiminotransferase
f. deficiency
f. deficiency syndrome
formula
Accupep HPF enteral f.
Advance f.
Advera f.
AL 110 f.
Alcare f.
Alimentum f.
Alitraq f.
Alsoy 1, 2 f.
Bazett f.
BC Cold Powder Non-Drowsy F.
Brozek body fat percentage f.
20-calorie f.
24-calorie f.
Carnation Follow-Up soy f.
Carnation Good Start f.
Carvajal f.
Casec f.

F

NOTES

formula *(continued)*
 casein hydrolysate f.
 Compleat Modified f.
 Compleat Pediatric f.
 Comtrex Cough F.
 Criticare H f.
 Deliver f.
 dextro f.
 diluted f.
 EleCare f.
 electrodialyzed whey f.
 F. EM oral solution
 EnfaCare LIPIL f.
 Enfamil A.R. LIPIL f.
 Enfamil Human Milk Fortifier f.
 Enfamil LactoFree LIPIL f.
 Enfamil LIPIL Low iron f.
 Enfamil LIPIL with iron f.
 Enfamil Next Step ProSobee
  LIPIL f.
 Enfamil Nutramigen LIPIL f.
 Enfamil Pregestimil f.
 Enfamil Premature LIPIL f.
 Enfamil ProSobee LIPIL f.
 Ensure High Protein f.
 Ensure Plus HN f.
 Ensure with Fiber f.
 evaporated milk f.
 Fibersource HN f.
 Follow-Up Soy f.
 fortified f.
 full-strength f.
 Glucerna f.
 glucose f.
 goat's milk f.
 Gorlin f.
 half-strength f.
 Hardy-Weinberg f.
 high-caloric density f.
 high-calorie f.
 high-fructose f.
 high-glucose f.
 homemade f.
 hydrolysate f.
 hydrolyzed premature f.
 hypercaloric f.
 Infalyte f.
 Intralipid f.
 Isocal HN f.
 Isomil DE f.
 Isosource 1.5 Cal f.
 Isosource HN f.
 Isosource Standard f.
 I-Soyalac f.
 Jevity Plus f.
 Kaopectate Advanced F.
 Kindercal f.
 LactoFree LIPIL f.
 lactose-containing f.

 lactose-free f.
 Liposyn f.
 Lohman-Brozek body fat
  percentage f.
 Lonalac f.
 Lytren f.
 Magnacal f.
 Mall f.
 MCT oil f.
 Mead Johnson f.
 menstrual f.
 Meritene f.
 Microlipid f.
 milk-based f.
 Moducal f.
 Mollifene Ear Wax Removing F.
 Mollison f.
 Neocate One+ f.
 Newtrition Isofiber f.
 Newtrition Isotonic f.
 nucleotide-fortified f.
 Nutramigen f.
 Nutren 1.0, 1,5, 2.0 f.
 Nutren 1.0 with Fiber f.
 Osmolite HN f.
 Oxepa f.
 Parent's Choice f.
 Parkland f.
 Pedialyte f.
 PediaSure with Fiber f.
 Peptamen Jr. f.
 Perative f.
 Polycose liquid f.
 Polycose powder f.
 Portagen f.
 powdered milk f.
 predigested f.
 Pregestimil f.
 preterm f.
 prethickened f.
 Profiber f.
 ProMod f.
 Promote with Fiber f.
 Propac Plus f.
 ProSobee f.
 protein hydrolysate f.
 Pulmocare f.
 quarter-strength f.
 rapid dissolution f. (RDF)
 RCF f.
 Rehydralyte f.
 Resource Just for Kids with
  Fiber f.
 Resource Plus f.
 Resource Standard f.
 Sabbagha f.
 semielemental casein hydrolysate f.
 Similac 2 Advance f.
 Similac Alimentum Advance f.

Similac Human Milk Fortifier f.
Similac Isomil Advance 2 f.
Similac Isomil DF f.
Similac Lactose Free Advance f.
Similac Natural Care Advance f.
Similac NeoSure Advance f.
Similac PM 60/40 f.
Similac Special Care 20, 24, 40 f.
Similac with iron f.
Siri body fat percentage f.
sodium-free f.
soy-based protein isolate f.
Spearman-Brown prediction f.
sucrose-free f.
Sumacal f.
Suplena f.
Sustacal Plus f.
Sustagen f.
three-quarter strength f.
Tolerex f.
TraumaCal f.
Triaminic AM Decongestant F.
TwoCal HN f.
vegetable oil fat-based f.
Vicks F. 44
Vicks F. 440
Vital High Nitrogen f.
Vitaneed f.
Vivonex Pediatric f.
Vivonex Plus f.
Vivonex Ten f.
WHO f.
formula-feeding woman
fornix, pl. **fornices**
posterior f.
posterior vaginal f.
vaginal f.
Forsius-Eriksson type ocular albinism
Forssman
F. antigen
F. titer
Fortaz
Fort Bragg evaluation project (FBEP)
Forte
Biotin F.
FML F.
Robinul F.
Zone-A F.
Fortel ovulation test
fortification spectrum
fortified formula

fortifier
Enfamil Human Milk F.
human milk f. (HMF)
Similac Human Milk F. (SHMF)
Fortovase
fortuitum
Mycobacterium f.
Forvade
forward
f. chaining
f. roll fashion
f. roll method
f. tandem gait
forward-bending test
Fosamax
foscarnet
Foscavir
fosfomycin tromethamine
fosinopril
fosphenytoin
fossa, gen. and pl. **fossae**
congenital supraspinous f.
enlarged posterior f.
iliac f.
ischiorectal f.
f. navicularis
olecranon f.
f. ovalis
posterior cranial f.
shallow acetabular fossae
f. of Waldeyer
foster care
Fostex
F. Bar
F. 10% BPO Gel
Fothergill-Donald operation
Fothergill-Hunter operation
Fothergill operation
Fototar
foul-smelling
f.-s. amniotic fluid
f.-s. discharge
foundation
Children's Digestive Health and
Nutrition F. (CDHNF)
Epilepsy F.
MedicAlert F.
National Osteoporosis F.
founder
f. chromosome
f. effect
Fountain syndrome

F

NOTES

four-cell embryo
four-chamber view
fourchette
    posterior f.
four-day syndrome
four-flap Z-plasty
four-hour rule
Fourier transform infrared
  microspectroscopy
four-leaf clover pattern
Fournier teeth
four-point position
four-quadrant assessment
four-site skinfold test
fourth
    Bartholomew rule of f.'s
    f. heart sound
    f. nerve palsy
    f. parallel pelvic plane
    f. phacomatosis
    f. stage of labor
    f. venereal disease
fourth-degree
    f.-d. burn
    f.-d. episiotomy
    f.-d. laceration
foveal hypoplasia
fowleri
    Naegleria f.
Fowler position
Fowler-Stephens orchiopexy
Fox-Fordyce disease
FP
    filter paper
    FP blood lead testing
FPA
    foot-progression angle
FPG
    fasting plasma glucose
FPIA
    fluorescent polarization immunoassay
FPO
    faciopalatoosseous
    FPO syndrome
FRA, fra
    fragile
    fragile chromosome site
    fragile gene
fraction
    f. of alveolar carbon dioxide
      ($FACO_2$)
    cardiac ejection f.
    f. in expired gas of carbon
      dioxide ($FECO_2$)
    filtration f.
    increased globulin f.
    f. of inspired oxygen (FIO_2, FiO_2)
    left ventricular ejection f. (LVEF)
    plasma f.

    recombination f.
    regurgitant f.
    shortening f.
    S phase f.
fractional
    f. dilation and curettage
    f. excretion
    f. excretion of sodium
    f. shortening
fractionated sterotactic radiotherapy
fractionation
fracture
    avulsion f.
    basal skull f.
    basilar skull f.
    bend f.
    birth f.
    blowout f.
    bowing f.
    boxer's f.
    bucket-handle f.
    buckle f.
    bursting f.
    calcaneal f.
    Chance f.
    clavicular f. (CF)
    coccygeal f.
    coexisting f.
    Colles f.
    comminuted f.
    complete f.
    compression f.
    corner f.
    cribriform f.
    depressed skull f.
    diaphysial f.
    diastatic f.
    direct orbital floor f.
    displaced supracondylar f.
    distal humeral physial f.
    elbow f.
    fatigue f.
    femoral shaft f.
    fetal f.
    fibular shaft f.
    Galeazzi f.
    greenstick f.
    growing f.
    growth plate f.
    hangman's f.
    hindfoot f.
    hip f.
    impacted f.
    indirect orbital floor f.
    intertrochanteric f.
    intrauterine f.
    Jefferson f.
    Jones stress f.
    juvenile Tillaux f.

laryngeal f.
lateral condylar f.
Le Fort f.
linear skull f.
Maisonneuve f.
Malgaigne f.
mastoid bone f.
maternal f.
medial epicondylar f.
metacarpal f.
metaphysial f.
middle third of clavicle f.
Monteggia f.
NOE f.
nonaccidental spiral tibial f.
nondisplaced lateral condylar f.
nonpathologic f.
oblique f.
olecranon f.
open f.
orbital blowout f.
orbital wall f.
osteochondral f.
osteoporotic f.
patellar f.
pathologic f.
f. pattern
pelvic f.
f. of penis
physial f.
ping-pong f.
plastic deformation f.
plate f.
pond f.
proximal humeral stress f.
pubic ramus stress f.
radial head f.
radial neck f.
f. reduction
f. remodeling
rib f.
Salter-Harris classification of f.
Salter-Harris epiphyseal f.
Salter-Harris f. (type I–V)
scapular f.
shear f.
skull f.
sleeve f.
spinal compression f.
spiral tibial f.
sternal f.
stress f.

supracondylar humeral f.
talar dome f.
thoracic spine f.
tibial shaft f.
tibial stress f.
f. of Tillaux
Tillaux f.
toddler's f.
torus f.
transverse f.
triplane f.
ulnar styloid f.
vertebral f.
vertebral compression f.
zygomaticomaxillary f.

fractured
f. chromosome
f. sternum

fragile (FRA, fra)
f. chromosome site (FRA, fra)
f. chromosome site 1 (FRAXE1)
f. chromosome site 2 (FRAX2)
f. chromosome site E (FRAXE)
f. chromosome site F (FRAXF)
f. gene (FRA, fra)
medically f.
f. site mental retardation 1
(FMR1)
f. site mental retardation 2
(FMR2)
f. tissue
f. X analysis
f. X carrier
f. X chromosome
f. X disorder
f. X gene (FRAX)
f. X mental retardation protein
(FMRP)
f. X mental retardation syndrome
f. Xq syndrome
f. X syndrome (FRAX, FXS)
f. X type A

fragilis
Bacteroides f.
Dientamoeba f.

fragilitas ossium
fragment
f. antigen binding
anucleate f.
Okazaki f.
placental f.
restriction f.

NOTES

F

fragment · fremitus

fragment *(continued)*
    retained placental f.
    urinary beta-core f.
fragmentation
    f. of necrotic bone
    uterine f.
fragmented poikilocyte
Fragmin
frame
    open reading f.
    reading f.
frameshift mutation
Franceschetti-Goldenhar syndrome
Franceschetti-Jadassohn syndrome
Franceschetti-Klein syndrome
Franceschetti syndrome
Franceschetti-Zwahlen-Klein syndrome
Franceschetti-Zwahlen syndrome
Francisella
    F. tularensis
    F. tularensis subspecies holarctica
Francis forceps
Francois
    F. dyscephalia
    F. dyscephalic syndrome
frank
    f. ambiguity
    f. breech
    f. breech presentation
    F. nonsurgical perineal autodilation
    F. procedure
    F. technique of dilation
    F. vaginal construction
Frankenhäuser
    F. ganglion
    F. plexus
Franklin-Dukes test
Frank-Starling
    F.-S. mechanism
    F.-S. principle
    F.-S. relationship
Frantz tumor
frappage therapy
Fraser-Francois syndrome
Fraser-like syndrome
Fraser syndrome
FRAST
    Free Running Asthma Test
frataxin
fraternal twins
FRAX
    fragile X gene
    fragile X syndrome
FRAX2
    fragile chromosome site 2
FRAXE
    fragile chromosome site E
FRAXE1
    fragile chromosome site 1

FRAXE2
FRAXE-associated mental retardation
FRAXF
    fragile chromosome site F
FRAXq27 syndrome
FRAX28 syndrome
fra(X) syndrome
Frazier suction tip
FRC
    functional residual capacity
FreAmine
freckling
    axillary f.
    inguinal f.
Fredet-Ramstedt
    F.-R. operation
    F.-R. procedure
free
    F. & Active
    f. androgen index
    F. to Be Me body image program
    f. beta hCG
    Breathe F.
    f. choline
    f. erythrocyte protoporphyrin (FEP)
    f. estradiol
    f. fatty acid
    f. hydroxyl radical
    f. iron
    f. neuraminic acid storage disease
    f. peritoneal air
    f. radial generation
    F. Running Asthma Test (FRAST)
    f. sialic acid storage disease
    f. testosterone
    f. testosterone index
    f. thyroxine
    f. thyroxine index
    f. tongue
    f. tracheal autograft
    f. triiodothyronine
    f. water calculation
freebase cocaine
free-floating loop
free-flow oxygen
Freeman cookie cutter areola marker
Freeman-Sheldon syndrome
freeze-thaw-freeze
freezing process
Freezone Solution
Frei
    F. antibody
    F. test
Freiberg
    F. disease
    F. infraction
Frejka pillow splint
fremitus
    diminished f.

tactile f.
vocal f.
frena (*pl. of* frenum)
French
F. Foley balloon
F. Gesco catheter
F. hysteroscope
F. lock
French-American-British (FAB)
24 French Foley balloon
7 French sheath
frenectomy
frenoplasty
frenotomy
frenulum, pl. **frenula**
f. labiorum pudendi
f. linguae
lingual f.
multiple oral frenula
frenum, pl. **frena**
Frenzel maneuver
frequency
allele f.
f. dysuria syndrome
fetal heart f. (FHF)
folding f.
high f. (HF)
low f. (LF)
Nyquist f.
pulse f.
recombination f.
spectral edge f. (SEF)
urinary f.
fresh frozen plasma (FFP)
fresh-packed RBCs
freshwater near drowning
freudian
Freud theory
Freund
F. adjuvant
F. operation
freundii
Citrobacter f.
Clostridium f.
Freyer suprapubic drain
friable
f. cervix
f. clot
f. ectocervix
f. hair
Fria muscle training device & program
Friberg microsurgical agglutination test

fricative
glottal f.
friction
f. dermatitis
f. diaper rash
f. rub
Friedman
F. labor curve
F. rabbit test
F. Splint brace
Friedman-Lapham test
Friedreich
F. ataxia
F. foot
Friedrich criteria for dyspareunia
Fried syndrome
Friend syndrome
frigid
Frigiderm
frigidity
Fritsch
F. douche
F. syndrome
Fritsch-Asherman syndrome
Froben-SR
frogleg
f. lateral radiograph
f. position
f. posture
f. view
frog-legged
Fröhlich syndrome
frondlike
frontal
f. baldness
f. bones scalloping
f. bossing
f. encephalocele
f. horn
f. plagiocephaly
f. pole area
f. suture
frontoanterior
left f. position (LFA)
f. position
right f. position (RFA)
frontodigital syndrome
frontofacionasal
f. dysostosis
f. dysplasia
frontometaphysial dysplasia
frontonasal dysplasia (FND)

NOTES

frontoparietal sensorimotor cortex
frontoposterior
    left f. position (LFP)
    f. position
    right f. position (RFP)
frontostriatal
frontotemporal cortical atrophy
frontotransverse
    left f. position (LFT)
    f. position
    right f. position (RFT)
front-to-back wiping
frostbite
frothy discharge
frottage
frozen
    f. biopsy
    f. egg
    f. embryo
    f. embryo replacement (FER)
    f. ovum
    f. pelvis
    f. plasma
    f. red blood cells
    f. section
    f. semen
    f. smile puckered lips
    f. sperm
    f. zygote
frozen-thawed embryo transfer
FRP
    follicle regulatory protein
fructokinase
fructose
    f. galactokinase deficiency
    f. intolerance
    f. intolerance test
fructosemia
fructosuria
    benign f.
    essential f.
fruity breath odor
frusemide
fruste
    forme f.
Fryns-Moerman syndrome
Fryns syndrome (1–3)
Fryns-van den Berghe syndrome
FS
    AmpliTaq DNA polymerase F.
FSD
    face-straight-down
FSDS
    Female Sexual Distress Scale
FSE
    fetal scalp electrode
FSFI
    Female Sexual Function Index

FSGS
    focal segmental glomerulosclerosis
FSH
    facioscapulohumeral
    follicle-stimulating hormone
      FSH antagonist
      FSH binding inhibitor
      highly purified FSH
      FSH inhibition
      FSH level
      FSH MAIAclone immunoradiometric assay
      FSH muscular dystrophy
      purified urinary FSH
      FSH secretion
FSHD
    facioscapulohumeral muscular dystrophy
FSI
    Foam Stability Index
FS$_p$O$_2$
    fetal arterial oxygen saturation
FSP
    familial spastic paraplegia
    fibrin split product
FST
    foam stability test
FT
    full term
FTA
    fluorescent treponemal antibody
      FTA test
FTA-ABS
    fluorescent treponemal antibody absorption
FTBD
    full term, born dead
3F thermistor wire
FTIF
    focal tubulointerstitial fibrosis
FTS
    face-to-side
FTSP
    fallopian tube sperm perfusion
FTT
    failure to thrive
      FTT syndrome
FTV
    fetal thrombotic vasculopathy
5-FU
    5-fluorouracil
FUCA
    alpha-L-fucosidase
      FUCA deficiency
Fucidin
fucosidase
fucosidosis
FUDR
    fluorodeoxyuridine

FUE
    fever of unknown etiology
fugax
    amaurosis f.
fugue state
Fuhrmann syndrome
Fuhrman pleural drainage set
Fujinon
    F. biopsy forceps
    F. flexible hysteroscope
Fukuyama
    F. CMD
    F. congenital muscular dystrophy
    (FCMD)
    F. disease
    F. syndrome
FUL
    functional urethral length
fulguration
full
    f. breech presentation
    f. enteral feed
    f. inclusion
    f. lepromatous leprosy
    f. mutation
    f. nipple feed
    f. term (FT)
    f. term, born dead (FTBD)
    f. tuberculoid leprosy
    f. venography
Fuller
    F. Albright syndrome 1
    F. shield
    F. shield rectal dressing
fullness
    periorbital f.
full-strength formula
full-syndrome eating disorder
full-term
    f.-t. infant
    f.-t. newborn
    f.-t. pregnancy
full-thickness
    f.-t. bowel biopsy
    f.-t. burn
    f.-t. intestinal biopsy
    f.-t. necrosis
    f.-t. skin graft
fulminans
    acne f.
    neonatal purpura f.
    purpura f.

fulminant
    f. disease
    f. early-onset neonatal pneumonia
    f. hepatic failure (FHF)
    f. hepatitis
    f. sepsis
    f. ulcerative colitis
fulminating meningitis
fulvestrant
Fulvicin
    F. P/G
    F. U/F
fumarate
    ferrous f.
    quetiapine f.
fumarylacetoacetate hydrolase (FAH)
fumes
fumigatus
    Aspergillus f.
function
    adrenocortical f.
    atrioventricular node f.
    axon-reflex f.
    binocular f.
    bladder f.
    bowel f.
    brain f.
    brainstem f.
    cardiac f.
    cardiorespiratory f.
    cholinergic sympathetic f.
    ciliary f.
    corpus luteum f.
    declining ovarian f.
    executive f.
    fetal cardiac f.
    fetoplacental f.
    follicular f.
    global assessment of f. (GAF)
    hypothalamic-pituitary f.
    impaired cognitive f.
    kidney f.
    leukocyte f.
    luteal f.
    mitochondrial f.
    mucociliary f.
    myocardial f.
    oromotor f.
    ovarian f.
    peroneal nerve f.
    pituitary-adrenal f.
    pituitary gland f.

NOTES

F

function *(continued)*
 pituitary-ovarian f.
 placental f.
 pulmonary f.
 renal tubular f.
 reproductive f.
 serotonergic f.
 sexual f.
 sinus node f.
 sympathetic adrenergic f.
 thyroid f.
 urethral f.
 ventricular f.
functional
 f. abdominal pain
 f. age
 f. alveolus
 f. asplenia
 F. Assessment of Cancer Therapy (FACT)
 F. Assessment Scale (FAS)
 f. behavior
 f. brain activity
 f. brain imaging
 f. cloning
 f. constipation
 f. dysmenorrhea
 f. dyspepsia
 f. electrical stimulation
 f. gastrointestinal disorder
 f. impairment
 F. Impairment Scale for Children and Adolescents (FISCA)
 f. incontinence
 F. Independence Measure for Children (WeeFIM)
 f. MRI (fMRI)
 f. murmur
 f. outlet obstruction
 f. ovarian cyst
 f. posterior rhizotomy
 f. prepuberal castrate syndrome
 f. pulmonary atresia
 f. residual capacity (FRC)
 f. urethral length (FUL)
function-enhancing mutation
functioning
 executive cognitive f. (ECF)
 global level of f. (GLOF)
 f. tumor
fundal
 f. height
 f. height measurement
 f. placentation
 f. plication
 f. pressure
 f. tenderness

Fundamentals-Preschool
 Clinical Evaluation of Language F.-P.
fundectomy
fundi *(pl. of* fundus)
fundic gland polyp
fundoplication
 laparoscopic f. (LF)
 Nissen f.
 Thal f.
fundus, pl. **fundi**
 f. albipunctatus
 f. flavimaculatus
 ghost vessel f.
 incarcerated f.
 optic f.
 red f.
 salt and pepper f.
funduscopic
funduscopy
fundusectomy
fungal
 f. ball
 f. endocarditis
 f. folliculitis
 f. id reaction
 f. infection
 f. meningitis
 f. oil
 f. sepsis
fungating mass
fungemia
fungi *(pl. of* fungus)
fungiform papilla
Fungizone
Fungoid
 F. AF Topical Solution
 F. Cream
fungoides
 mycosis f.
fungus, pl. **fungi**
 f. ball
 lipophilic f.
 umbilical f.
funic
 f. presentation
 f. reduction
 f. souffle
funicular souffle
funiculus, pl. **funiculi**
 f. umbilicalis
funipuncture
funis
funisitis
 necrotizing f.
funnel
 accessory müllerian f.
 f. chest

f. length
f. width
funneling
cervical f.
funnel-shaped pelvis
Funston syndrome
FUO
fever of undetermined origin
fever of unknown origin
Furadantin
Furalan
furan
furazolidone
furcate insertion of cord
furfur
Malassezia f.
furoate
mometasone f.
furosemide
Furoxone
furrow
furrowing
surface f.
furrowlike umbilicus
furuncle
staphylococcal f.
furunculosis
staphylococcal f.
fusaric acid
Fusarium
fused
f. frontal horn
f. raphe
fusiform
f. aneurysm
f. dilation
f. dilation of urethra
f. nerve thickening

fusion
anterior spinal f.
calcaneonavicular f.
cervical vertebral f.
f. of eyelids
f. implantation
incomplete müllerian f.
joint f.
labial f.
labioscrotal f.
müllerian duct f.
postvaginal f.
robertsonian f.
spinal f.
talocalcaneal f.
thought action f.
fusobacteria
Fusobacterium
F. gonidiaformans
F. mortiferum
F. necrophorum
F. nucleatum
fusospirillary gangrenous stomatitis
fusospirochetal gingivitis
futile cycle
FVC
forced vital capacity
FVIIa
factor VIIa
FVS
fetal valproate syndrome
fetal varicella syndrome
FXS
fragile X syndrome
FyBron calcium alginate dressing
fyn protooncogene

NOTES

F

G
  gravida
    G band
    G protein
    G syndrome
G₁
  gap₁
G₂
  gap₂
G₀
  gap₀
g, gm
  gram
GA
  gestational age
GAA
  gossypol acetic acid
    GAA trinucleotide expansion
GABA
  gamma-aminobutyric acid
    GABA transaminase deficiency
gabapentin
GABEB
  generalized atrophic benign
    epidermolysis bullosa
GABHS
  group A beta-hemolytic streptococcus
    GABHS pharyngitis
Gabitril
GAD
  generalized anxiety disorder
  glutamic acid decarboxylase
gadolinium
    chelated g.
gadopentetate dimeglumine
GAF
  global assessment of function
Gaffney joint
GAG
  glycosaminoglycan
Gage sign
gag reflex
Gail breast cancer model
Gaillard syndrome
gain
    absolute length g.
    absolute weight g.
    maternal weight g.
    poor weight g.
    total weight g.
    weight g.
gait
    antalgic g.
    g. apraxia
    g. ataxia

    ataxic g.
    broad-based g.
    circumduction g.
    crouch g.
    g. dysfunction
    equinus g.
    forward tandem g.
    heel-toe g.
    g. laboratory
    lordotic g.
    nonreciprocal g.
    outtoe g.
    reciprocating g.
    shuffling g.
    slapping storklike g.
    teddy-bear g.
    toe-in g.
    toe-out g.
    Trendelenburg g.
    waddling g.
    wide-based shuffling g.
galactacrasia
galactagogue
galactic
galactitol
galactobolic
galactocele
galactocerebrosidase (GALC)
galactogram
    mammary g.
galactography
galactokinase deficiency
galactokinesis
galactolipid
galactometer
galactopoiesis
galactorrhea
galactorrhea-amenorrhea syndrome
galactosamine
galactose
    g. breath test
    g. uridine diphosphate
galactose-free diet
galactosemia
    African American variant g.
    classical g.
    Duarte variant g.
    hereditary g.
    Los Angeles variant g.
    transferase deficient g.
galactose-1-phosphate uridyltransferase
  (GALT)
galactosialidosis
galactosidase
    ceramide trihexoside alpha g.

G

galactosis
galactosuria
galactosylceramide beta-galactosidase
  deficiency
galactosylsphinogosine lipidosis
galactotherapy
Galbiati bilateral fetal ischiopubiotomy
GALC
  galactocerebrosidase
    GALC deficiency
GALE
  UDP-galactose-4-epimerase
    GALE deficiency
galea
Galeazzi
  G. fracture
  G. fracture dislocation
  G. sign
Galen
  aneurysm of vein of G.
  vein of G.
Galileo rigid hysteroscope
Gallant reflex
gallbladder
  atretic g.
  g. disease
  duplication of g.
  hydropic g.
  g. hydrops
  g. resection
  g. stasis
gallinatum
  pectus g.
gallium
  g. scan
  g. scintography
gallium-67
  g. citrate contrast medium
  g. scan
gallop
  protodiastolic g.
  g. rhythm
  summation g.
Galloway-Mowat syndrome
Galloway syndrome
gallstone
  cholesterol g.
  g. pancreatitis
galoche chin
GALT
  galactose-1-phosphate uridyltransferase
  gastrointestinal-associated lymphoid
    tissue
  gut-associated lymphoid tissue
    GALT deficiency
galtonian-Fisher genetics
galtonian trait
Galton law of regression
Gambee suture

Gambian
  G. disease
  G. trypanosomiasis
gamble
  Procter and G. (P&G)
Gamble-Darrow syndrome
gamekeeper's thumb
gametangium
gamete
  aging g.
  g. intrafallopian transfer (GIFT)
  g. manipulation
  g. micromanipulation
  overmature g.
gametic
  g. chromosome
  g. selection
gametogenesis
  ovarian g.
gametokinetic
Gamimune N
gamma
  G. BHC
  g. globulin (GG)
  g. globulin replacement
  g. glutamyl transferase (GGT)
  g. glutamyl transpeptidase
  interferon g. (IFN-gamma)
  g. interferon
  g. knife surgery
  g. ray
gamma-aminobutyric acid (GABA)
gamma-1b
gamma-benzene hexachloride
Gammabulin Immuno
gamma-chain disorder
Gammagard S/D
gamma-irradiated cellular products
  transfusion
gamma-loop disorder
Gammar-IV
Gammar-P IV
Gamper
  G. bowing reflex
  G. method
  G. method of childbirth
gampsodactyly
Gamulin Rh
ganaxolone
ganciclovir
ganglia (*pl. of* ganglion)
gangliocytoma
  dysplastic g.
ganglioglioma
ganglion, pl. **ganglia**
  basal g.
  g. cell
  Frankenhäuser g.
  gasserian g.

herpes zoster of geniculate g.
hypoglossal g.
sympathetic g.
g. trigger theory
volar g.
ganglioneuroblastoma
ganglioneuroma
ganglioneuromatosis
mucosal g.
ganglionic
g. blocker
g. differentiation
ganglioside
g. degradation
g. storage disease
gangliosidosis
adult generalized g.
cerebral GM1 g.
generalized g. GM1 type I
generalized infantile g.
generalized juvenile g.
generalized g. juvenile type
GM2 g.
GM3 g.
g. GM1 juvenile type
g. GM1 late onset without bony
involvement
g. GM1 type II
juvenile GM1 g.
juvenile GM2 g.
neuronal GM1 g.
Sandhoff GM2 g. (type I, II)
gangrene
acute streptococcal g.
gas g.
Meleney synergistic g.
pulmonary g.
spontaneous g. of newborn
streptococcal g.
synergistic g.
gangrenosa
varicella g.
gangrenosum
ecthyma g.
pyoderma g.
gangrenous
g. appendicitis
g. stomatitis
ganirelix
g. acetate
g. acetate injection

GANT
gastrointestinal autonomic nerve tumor
Gantrisin
Azo G.
GAP
gonadotropin-releasing hormone-
associated peptide
gap
anion g.
g. junction
osmotic g.
plasma anion g.
gap$_0$ (G$_0$)
gap$_1$ (G$_1$)
gap$_2$ (G$_2$)
gape
allergic g.
GAPS
Guidelines for Adolescent Preventive
Services
Garamycin
Garatec
Garcia-Lurie syndrome
Gardner
G. Expressive One-Word
Vocabulary Test-Revised
G. syndrome
Gardnerella
G. *vaginalis*
G. *vaginalis* chorioamnionitis
G. vaginitis
Gardner-Silengo-Wachtel syndrome
Gardner-Wells tongs
Gareis-Mason syndrome
gargantuan mastitis
gargoylism
Gariel pessary
garinii
Borrelia g.
Garrodian inborn error
Gartner
G. duct
G. duct cyst
gartnerian
g. cyst
g. duct
gas, pl. **gases**
g. anesthetic
arterial blood g. (ABG)
g. bloat
blood g.
capillary blood g. (CBG)

NOTES

G

gas *(continued)*
    carbon dioxide g.
    g. chromatography
    g. chromatography-mass
      spectrometry (GC-MS)
    g. chromatography-mass
      spectroscopy (GC-MS)
    cord blood g. (CBG)
    g. embolus
    fetal blood gases
    g. gangrene
    g. gangrene fasciitis
    inspired g. (I)
    intervillous blood g.
    intramural g.
    Mylanta G.
    paucity of g.
    sweep g.
    g. transfer
    venous blood g. (VBG)
    volume of expired g. (VE)

GASA
    growth-adjusted sonographic age

gaseous distention

gases *(pl. of* gas)

gas-forming bacteria

Gaskin maneuver

gasless laparoscopy

GasPak jar

gasping respiration

gasseri
        Lactobacillus g.

gasserian ganglion

Gasser syndrome

GAST
    gonadotropin agonist stimulation test

gastric
    g. accommodation
    g. acid hypersecretion
    g. acid hyposecretion
    g. aspirate culture
    g. atony
    g. atrophy
    g. balloon
    g. bubble
    g. bypass
    g. carcinoma
    g. decompression
    g. dilation
    g. duplication
    g. dysmotility
    g. dysrhythmia
    g. emptying
    g. emptying time
    g. enteral feeding
    g. fluid aspiration
    g. inhibitory polypeptide (GIP)
    g. irrigation
    g. lavage

    g. mobilization
    g. mucosa
    g. perforation
    g. peristaltic wave
    g. pull-up
    g. reduction surgery
    g. regurgitation
    g. residual volume (GRV)
    g. residue
    g. stapling
    g. tonometry
    g. tube feeding
    g. tube insertion
    g. visceral hypersensitivity
    g. volvulus
    g. wash
    g. washing
    g. web

gastrinoma

gastritis
    antral g.
    chronic hypertrophic g.
    infectious g.
    lymphocytic g.
    micronodular g.
    nodular g.
    peptic g.

gastroacephalus

gastroamorphus

gastrocnemius
    g. aponeurosis
    g. contracture
    g. muscle

gastrocnemius-semimembranosus bursa

gastrocolic reflex

Gastrocrom

gastrocystoplasty

gastrodidymus

gastroduodenoscopy

gastroenteritis, pl. **gastroenteritides**
    allergic eosinophilic g.
    Campylobacter g.
    eosinophilic g.
    parasitic gastroenteritides
    rotavirus g.
    Salmonella g.
    viral g.

gastroenterologist

gastroenteropathy
    allergic g.
    eosinophilic g.

gastroepiploic artery (GEA)

gastroesophageal (GE)
    g. angle of His
    g. balloon tamponade
    g. incompetence
    g. junction (GEJ)
    g. reflux (GER)

g. reflux disease (GERD)
g. reflux-reflex apnea recording
Gastrografin
G. enema
G. esophagram
gastrointestinal (GI)
g. anaphylaxis
g. anastomosis (GIA)
g. atresia
g. autonomic nerve tumor (GANT)
g. decontamination
g. disorder
g. duplication
g. dysmotility
g. fistula
g. hemorrhage
g. infection
g. loss
g. malignancy
g. manifestation
g. obstruction
g. paraganglioma
g. polyp
g. priming
g. reflux
g. series
g. syndrome
g. tract
g. tube
g. tuberculosis
upper g.
gastrointestinal-associated lymphoid tissue (GALT)
gastrojejunostomy
gastromelus
gastropagus
gastroparesis
gastropathy
AIDS g.
congestive g.
hypertrophic g.
gastrophrenic ligament
gastroplasty
gastroschisis
Silastic silo reduction of g.
gastrostomy
g. button
EntriStar Skin Level Tube for g.
feeding g.
percutaneous endoscopic g. (PEG)
Stamm g.

g. tube
g. tube placement
gastrothoracopagus
gastrula
gastrulating embryo
Gas-X
gate-control
g.-c. hypothesis
g.-c. theory
gated blood pool scanning
gateway drug
Gaucher
G. cell
G. disease (perinatal lethal type)
G. disease (type 1–3)
Gaucher-type histiocyte
21-gauge hypodermic needle
gaussian distribution
Gauss sign
gauze
Aquaphor g.
Cover-Roll g.
g. dissection
iodoform g.
Oxycel g.
Vaseline-impregnated g.
g. wick
gavage feeding
Gaviscon
GAX collagen
gay
g. bowel disease
g., lesbian, bisexual (GLB)
g. relationship
gaze
conjugate upward g.
downward g.
eccentric g.
g. palsy
paralysis of conjugate upward g.
upward g.
gaze-evoked nystagmus
gaze-paretic nystagmus
G-banded
G.-b. cytogenetic aberration
G.-b. karyotype
G-banding
GBM
glomerular basement membrane
GBS
group B streptococcus
Guillain-Barré syndrome

G

NOTES

383

GBS *(continued)*
    GBS meningitis
    GBS screening culture
    GBS (type Ia, Ib, Ic, II, III)
    GBS vaccine
GBV-C
    GB virus C
GB virus C (GBV-C)
GCDAS
    Gesell Child Development Age Scale
GCI
    gestational carbohydrate intolerance
GC-MS
    gas chromatography-mass spectrometry
    gas chromatography-mass spectroscopy
GCPS
    Greig cephalopolysyndactyly syndrome
GCS
    Glasgow Coma Scale
G-CSF
    granulocyte colony-stimulating factor
G-CSF-R
    granulocyte colony-stimulating factor receptor
GDM
    gestational diabetes mellitus
GDNF
    glial cell line derived neurotrophic factor
GDP
    guanyldiphosphate
GDS
    Gesell Developmental Scale
    Gordon diagnostic system
GE
    gastroesophageal
    General Electric
    genome equivalent
    GE RT 3200 Advantage II ultrasound
    GE Senographe 2000D
    GE Senographe 2000D digital mammography system
GEA
    gastroepiploic artery
    GEA graft
Gebauer ethyl chloride
Geck
    Davis & G. (DG)
Gee disease
Gee-Herter disease
Gee-Herter-Heubner disease
Gehrung pessary
GEJ
    gastroesophageal junction
gel
    AccuSite injectable g.
    ACTH g.
    Acthar g.
    Advantage 24 bio-adhesive contraceptive g.
    amethocaine g.
    Ametop g.
    Aquagel lubricating g.
    Aquasonic 100 ultrasound transmission g.
    Benzac AC G.
    BenzaClin topical g.
    Benzac W G.
    Cerviprost g.
    cidofovir topical g.
    Comfort personal lubricant g.
    Crinone bioadhesive progesterone g.
    Del Aqua-5, -10 G.
    Desquam-E G.
    Desquam-X G.
    dextrin sulfate g.
    Differin g.
    dinoprostone cervical g.
    1D sodium dodecyl sulfate g.
    Duac topical g.
    Electro-Gel conductivity g.
    electrophoresis g.
    Empirynol Plus contraceptive g.
    Fostex 10% BPO G.
    H.P. Acthar G.
    Itch-X g.
    keratolytic g.
    MetroGel-Vaginal g.
    metronidazole vaginal g.
    miconazole g.
    Monsel g.
    Multidex g.
    Orabase g.
    Panretin topical g.
    Perfectoderm G.
    povidone-iodine g.
    Prepidil Vaginal G.
    PRO 2000 G.
    PRO/Gel ultrasound transmission g.
    prostaglandin E_2 g.
    Protectaid contraceptive sponge with F-5 g.
    Rid g.
    Scan ultrasound g.
    SonoMix ultrasound g.
    Tisit Blue G.
gelastic
    g. convulsion
    g. seizure
gelatin agglutination test
gelatin-encapsulated microbubble
gelatinosa
    substantia g.
gelatinous
    g. skin
    g. varix

geleophysic
- g. dwarfism
- g. dysplasia

Gelfoam

Gelhorn
- G. forceps
- G. pessary

Gel-Kam

gelling

Gelpi perineal retractor

gel-transfer

gemcitabine

Gemella
- G. *bergeriae*
- G. *haemolysans*
- G. *morbillorum*
- G. *sanguinis*

gemellary pregnancy

gemellipara

gemellology

gemeprost

geminus, pl. **gemini**

gemistocyte

gemmule
- Hoboken g.

Gemonil

Gemzar

Genac

Genahist Oral

Genapap

Genapax

Genaspor

Genatuss DM

Gen-Clobetasol

gender
- g. assignment
- g. determination
- g. difference
- g. dysphoria syndrome
- g. identity disorder (GID)
- g. reversal
- g. role

gene
- g. action
- adhalin g.
- AIRE g.
- allelic g.
- g. amplification
- apoB g.
- autoimmune regulator g.
- autosomal g.
- breast cancer g. 1 (BRCA1, BRCA1 and BRCA2)
- breast cancer g. 2 (BRCA2)
- Bruton/B-cell tyrosine kinase g.
- candidate g.
- g. candidate
- g. carrier
- cell interaction g.
- chimeric g.
- g. chip
- g. cloning
- codominant g.
- COL7A1 g.
- complementary g.
- g. complex
- CTNS g.
- cumulative g.
- CYP21A g.
- CYP11B1 g.
- CYP11B2 g.
- CYP21B g.
- DAX1 g.
- g. deletion
- derepressed g.
- DFFRY g.
- DMD/BMD g.
- dominant g.
- g. dose
- *Drosophila melanogaster* diaphanous g.
- g. duplication
- dystrophin g.
- E6-E7 g.
- endothelin-3 g.
- endothelin receptor-B g.
- Ewing sarcoma g.
- g. expression
- FAA g.
- g. family
- g. flow
- FMR1 g.
- fragile g. (FRA, fra)
- fragile X g. (FRAX)
- GLUT1 g.
- GLUT3 g.
- GUSB g.
- H g.
- hair cortex keratin g. type II
- herpes simplex virus thymidine kinase g.
- histocompatibility g.
- holandric g.

NOTES

G

gene (*continued*)
    homeobox 2 g.
    homeotic g.'s
    housekeeping g.
    HOX A g.
    HPV E7 g.
    human jagged-1 g. (JAG1)
    immune response g.
    immune suppressor g.
    immunoglobulin g.
    imprinted g.
    Ir g.
    Is g.
    jumping g.
    KAL g.
    leaky g.
    lethal g.
    g. library
    g. location
    g. locus
    major capsid protein g.
    g. map
    g. mapping
    marker g.
    MOMP g.
    g. mosaic
    MTHFR g.
    mutant g.
    g. mutation
    NF1 g.
    nonstructural g.
    od g.
    operator g.
    p53 g.
    partner g.
    PAX3 g.
    penetrant g.
    Pi type g.
    Pi type 2 g.
    Pi type 22 g.
    pleiotropic g.
    g. pool
    pRb tumor suppressor g.
    g. probe
    g. product
    PTEN g.
    PTK g.
    p53 tumor suppressor g.
    RBM g.
    recessive g.
    reciprocal g.
    recombinase activating g. (RAG)
    regulator g.
    repressed g.
    repressor g.
    RhCE g.
    RhD g.
    g. sequencing
    sex-conditioned g.

    sex-influenced g.
    sex-limited g.
    sex-linked g.
    SGLT1 g.
    SHOX g.
    silent g.
    sodium/glucose co-transporter g.
    SOX9 g.
    g. splicing
    structural g.
    g. study
    sublethal g.
    suicide g.
    supplementary g.
    suppressor g.
    syntenic g.
    g. targeting
    tdy g.
    g. therapy
    g. transcription
    g. transfer
    transmembrane conductance
      regulator g.
    tumor suppression g.
    tumor suppressor g.
    UBE3A g.
    wild-type g.
    Wilms tumor suppression g.
    X-linked g.
    Y-linked g.

GeneAmp PCR test
Genebs
Genée-Wiedemann
    G.-W. acrofacial dysostosis
      (GWAFD)
    G.-W. syndrome
Genentech
    G. biosynthetic human growth
      hormone
    G. growth chart
genera (*pl. of* genus)
general
    G. Electric (GE)
    g. endotracheal anesthesia
    g. obstetrics
    g. practitioner
    g. reading backwardness (GRB)
    g. triceps contracture
generalisata
    dysostosis g.
    osteitis condensans g.
generalization
generalized
    g. albinism
    g. alopecia
    g. aminoaciduria
    g. anxiety disorder (GAD)
    g. atrophic benign epidermolysis
      bullosa (GABEB)

g. autonomic dysfunction
g. bilaterally synchronous sharp-wave and slow-wave complexes
g. convulsion
g. dystonia
g. elastolysis
g. epileptogenic discharge
g. erythroderma
g. gangliosidosis GM1 adult type
g. gangliosidosis GM1 type I
g. gangliosidosis juvenile type
g. gray matter atrophy
g. hypertrichosis terminalis-gingival hyperplasia syndrome
g. hypotonia, congenital hydronephrosis, characteristic face syndrome
g. infantile gangliosidosis
g. infantile gangliosidosis with bony involvement
g. juvenile gangliosidosis
g. linear interactive modeling (GLIM)
g. lipodystrophy
g. obstructive overinflation
g. phlebectasia
g. pustular psoriasis
g. slowing
g. tetanus
g. tonic-clonic seizure
g. vigilance
g. white matter atrophy

generation
filial g.
free radial g.

generational

generator
migraine g.
Valleylab Force IC electrosurgical g.

genesial cycle

genetic
g. abnormality
g. amniocentesis
g. anomaly
g. bit analysis
g. burden
g. code
g. constitution
g. counseling
g. counselor
g. defect

g. diagnosis
g. disease
g. disorder
g. distance
g. diversity
g. drift
g. engineering
g. engineering technology
g. equilibrium
g. evaluation
g. fine structure
g. heterogeneity
g. history
g. inheritance pattern
g. interference
g. isolated CD59 deficiency
g. line
g. linkage
g. linkage analysis
g. locus
g. map
g. marker
g. material
g. model
g. mutation
g. myopathy
g. polymorphism
g. predisposition
g. screening
g. sex
g. study
g. susceptibility
g. switch
g. syndrome
g. test
g. testing
g. therapy
g. thrombophilia
g. variance

geneticist
medical g.

genetics
behavioral g.
biochemical g.
classical g.
epidemiologic g.
galtonian-Fisher g.
human g.
medical g.
modern g.
multilocal g.

NOTES

G

genetics *(continued)*
    prenatal g.
    reproductive g.
genetotrophic disease
genetous idiocy
Genex
Geneye Ophthalmic
geniculate
    g. herpes
    lateral g.
geniculostriate
genioglossus muscle
genital
    g. actinomycosis
    g. ambiguity
    g. anomaly-cardiomyopathy
      syndrome
    g. aphthous ulcer
    g. cleft
    g. cord
    g. corpuscle
    g. crisis of newborn
    g. development
    g. differentiation
    g. duct
    g. dwarfism
    g. elephantiasis
    g. herpes
    g. infection
    g. lesion
    g. mucosa
    g. mycoplasma
    g. outflow tract
    g. papule
    g. prolapse
    g. prolapse staging
    g. pruritus
    g. ridge
    g. sensation
    g. skin fibroblast
    g. tract embryology
    g. tract integrity
    g. tract malignancy
    g. tract trauma
    g. tract tumor
    g. tubercle
    g. tuberculosis
    g. ulceration
    g. ulcer disease (GUD)
    g. ulcer syndrome
    g. wart
genitalia
    ambiguous external g.
    external male g.
    indifferent g.
    internal g.
    lymphatic drainage of g.
genitalis
    herpes g.

genitalium
    Mycoplasma g.
genitocrural fold
genitofemoral nerve
genitogram with or without IVP
genitopalatocardiac syndrome
genitoplasty
**Genitor mini-intrauterine insemination
  cannula**
genitourinary (GU)
    g. abnormality
    g. atrophy
    g. defect
    g. fistula
    g. sphincter (GUS)
    g. tract
Genoa syndrome
genoblast
genocide
genocopy
genodermatosis, pl. **genodermatoses**
genome
    g. activation
    g. equivalent (GE)
    g. project
genomic
    g. DNA
    g. imprinting
    g. library
    g. in situ hybridization
genomovar
    Burkholderia cepacia g. (III)
    Burkholderia multivorans g. (II)
    g. (I–VI)
Genoptic S.O.P.
Genotropin Injection
genotype
    AA g.
    ACE g.
genotypic assay
genotyping
    CYP21 g.
Genpril
Gen-Probe
    G.-P. amplified CT assay
    G.-P. amplified CT test
Gentacidin
Gent-AK
gentamicin
    g. cream
    enteric g.
    prednisolone and g.
    g. sulfate
gentian violet
GentleLASE Plus
Gentran
Gentrasul
genu
    g. recurvatum

g. valgum
g. varum
g. varum deformity
genucubital position
genuine stress incontinence (GSI)
genupectoral position
genus, pl. **genera**
genus-specific monoclonal antibody
Gen-XENE
Geocillin
geographic tongue
geohelminth
geometric
g. design test
g. mean titer (GMT)
Geopen
geophagia
georgiae
Actinomyces g.
geotaxis
GER
gastroesophageal reflux
Gerald forceps
GERD
gastroesophageal reflux disease
Gerdy fontanelle
Geref
gerencseriae
Actinomyces g.
Gerhardt syndrome
Gerimed
germ
g. cell
g. cell mosaicism
g. cell ovarian neoplasm
g. cell teratoma
g. cell testicular tumor
g. layer
g. line
g. line mosaicism
g. ridge
g. tube test
German
G. lock
G. measles
G. syndrome
germ-cell depletion
germinal
g. cell tumor
g. center
g. epithelium
g. epithelium of Waldeyer

g. inclusion cyst
g. matrix
g. matrix hemorrhage (grade 1–4)
g. membrane
g. pole
g. vesicle
g. vesicle breakdown (GVBD)
g. vesicle stage
g. zone
germinolysis
subependymal g.
germinoma
pineal g.
germ-line mutation
germplasm
Gerota fascia
Gerstmann-Sträussler-Scheinker syndrome
Gerstmann syndrome
Gesco
G. cannula
G. catheter
Gesell
G. Adaptive and Personal Behavior Domain, Revised
G. Child Development Age Scale (GCDAS)
G. Developmental Model
G. Developmental Scale (GDS)
G. Developmental Schedules
G. Developmental Schedules, Revised
G. figure
G. Gross Motor Domain, Revised
G. Infant Scale
G. Preschool Test
G. School Readiness Test
G. test with Knobloch modification
gestagen
gestagenic
Gestalt closure
gestation
anembryonic g.
cornual g.
higher-order g.
monochorionic g.
monochorionic-diamniotic g.
multifetal g.
multiple g.
prolonged g.
stuck twin g.
term g.

NOTES

G

gestation *(continued)*
  tubal g.
  twin g.
  unruptured tubal g.
gestational
  g. abnormality
  g. age (GA)
  g. age assessment
  g. age estimation
  g. carbohydrate intolerance (GCI)
  g. carrier
  g. chickenpox
  g. diabetes
  g. diabetes mellitus (GDM)
  g. edema
  g. growth
  g. hypertension
  g. lupus
  g. mother
  g. proteinuria
  g. psychosis
  g. ring
  g. sac (GS)
  g. sac mean diameter
  g. sac size (GSS)
  g. surrogacy
  g. surrogate
  g. thrombocytopenia
  g. thyrotoxicosis
  g. trophoblastic disease (GTD)
  g. trophoblastic neoplasia (GTN)
  g. trophoblastic tumor (GTT)
gestationis
  herpes g. (HG)
  pemphigoid g.
gestation-specific nomogram
gestator
Gesterol
Gestodene
Gestogen
gestosis, pl. **gestoses**
  second trimester acute g.
Gestrinone
gesturing
GF
  growth factor
GFAP
  glial fibrillary acidic protein
GFD
  gluten-free diet
GFR
  glomerular filtration rate
GG
  gamma globulin
  Lactobacillus rhamnosus strain GG
    (L-GG)
GGT
  gamma glutamyl transferase

GH
  growth hormone
GHBP
  growth hormone-binding protein
GHD
  growth hormone deficiency
GHI
  growth hormone insensitivity
Ghon
  G. complex
  G. tubercle
ghost
  peroxisomal g.
  g. vessel
  g. vessel fundus
GHR
  growth hormone receptor
GHRD
  growth hormone receptor deficiency
GH-RH
  growth hormone-releasing hormone
GHST
  growth hormone stimulation test
GI
  gastrointestinal
  GI bleeding
  GI cocktail
  GI tract venous malformation
GIA
  gastrointestinal anastomosis
  GIA 30
  GIA 60, 80 stapler
  GIA 80 stapler
Gianotti-Crosti syndrome
Gianotti disease
giant
  g. anorectal condyloma acuminatum
  g. axonal neuropathy
  g. baby
  g. cell
  g. cell arteritis
  g. cell chondrodysplasia
  g. cell encephalitis
  g. cell hepatitis
  g. cell myocarditis
  g. cell pneumonia
  g. chromosome
  g. colon
  g. congenital pigmented nevus
  g. coronary artery aneurysm
  g. fibroadenoma
  g. hemangioma
  g. metamyelocyte
  g. neuroaxonal dystrophy
  g. platelet alpha-granule
  g. platelet granulation
  g. platelet syndrome
**Gianturco-Grifka vascular occlusion
  device**

Giardia lamblia
giardiasis
gibbous deformity
gibbus
  lumbar g.
  thoracolumbar g.
Gibco BRL sperm preparation medium
Gibson-Coke method
Gibson murmur
GID
  gender identity disorder
giddiness
Giemsa
  G. banding
  G. stain
Gierke disease
GIFT
  gamete intrafallopian transfer
  granulocyte immunofluorescence test
    cervical GIFT
    intrauterine GIFT
    vaginal GIFT
gigantism
  cerebral g.
  eunuchoid g.
  exomphalos, macroglossia, g.
    (EMG)
  fetal g.
  hyperpituitary g.
  pituitary g.
  Sotos cerebral g.
gigantoblast
gigantocellularis
  nucleus reticularis g.
gigantomastia
giggle incontinence
Gigli
  G. operation
  G. saw
Gilbert
  G. disease
  G. syndrome
Gilbert-Dreyfus syndrome
Gilbert-Lereboullet syndrome
gill
  g. arch skeleton
  G. respirator
Gilles
  G. de la Tourette
  G. de la Tourette syndrome
Gillespie-Numerof Burnout Inventory
Gillespie syndrome

Gillette joint
Gilliam
  G. operation
  G. round ligament
Gilliam-Doleris
  G.-D. operation
  G.-D. uterine suspension
Gilmore Oral Reading Test (GORT)
Gimbernat reflex ligament
gingiva, pl. gingivae
gingival
  g. cyst
  g. cyst of newborn
  g. erythema
  g. fibromatosis
  g. fibromatosis-corneal dystrophy
  g. fibromatosis, hypertrichosis,
    cherubism, mental retardation,
    epilepsy syndrome
  g. fibromatosis, hypertrichosis,
    mental retardation, epilepsy
    syndrome
  g. hyperplasia
  g. hyperplasia, hirsutism,
    convulsions syndrome
  g. hypertrophy-corneal dystrophy
    syndrome
  g. lesion
  g. overgrowth
gingivalis
  Bacteroides g.
  Entamoeba g.
  Porphyromanus g.
gingivitis
  acute necrotizing ulcerative g.
    (ANUG)
  fusospirochetal g.
  herpetic g.
  necrotizing g.
  necrotizing ulcerating g. (NUG)
  pregnancy-associated g.
  Vincent g.
gingivostomatitis
  herpetic g.
  primary herpetic g.
ginkgo biloba
ginseng
Giordano operation
GIP
  gastric inhibitory polypeptide
girdle
  Hitzig g.

G

NOTES

girdle *(continued)*
    limb g. (LG)
    g. weakness
girl
    premenarchal g.
    G.'s, Ritalin LA, and ADHD
      (GRACE)
girth
    abdominal g.
gitalin
Gitelman
    G. disease
    G. syndrome
Gittes
    G. bladder suspension technique
    G. operation
    G. procedure
    G. urethral suspension
GITUP procedure
GK
    glycerol kinase
GKD
    glycerol kinase deficiency
glabella
glabellar response
glabrata
    Candida g.
    Torulopsis g.
gladiatorum
    herpes g.
    tinea g.
gladioli
    Burkholderia g.
gland
    accessory sex g.
    adrenal g.
    apocrine sweat g.
    Bartholin g.
    Brunner g.
    bulbourethral g.
    BUS g.'s
    Cowper g.
    g. duct
    g. duct opening
    Duverney g.
    eccrine sweat g.
    endocrine g.
    external genitalia/Bartholin, urethral,
      and Skene g.'s (EG/BUS)
    fetal adrenal g.
    greater vestibular g.
    holocrine sebaceous g.
    hypoplastic parathyroid g.
    g. infection
    Krause lacrimal accessory g.
    lacrimal g.
    late-onset congenital large
      ectopic g.
    Littre g.

    mammary g.
    meibomian g.
    Méry g.
    Moll g.
    Montgomery g.
    Naboth g.
    nabothian g.
    parathyroid g.
    paraurethral g.
    parotid g.
    periurethral g.
    Philip g.
    pilosebaceous g.
    pineal g.
    pituitary g.
    salivary g.
    sebaceous g.
    Skene g.
    sublingual g.
    submaxillary g.
    sweat g.
    thymus g.
    thyroid g.
    urethral g.
    uterine g.
    vestibular g.
    Wolfring lacrimal accessory g.
glanders
glandular
    g. atypia
    g. atypia lesion
    g. cell
    g. disc
    g. disease
    g. fever
    g. hyperplasia
    g. mastitis
    g. neoplasia
    g. tissue
    g. tularemia
glans
    g. clitoris
    g. penis
glans-cavernosal procedure
glanular
    g. hypospadias
    g. urethral meatus
glanuloplasty
    meatal advancement and g.
    urethral advancement and g.
Glanzmann
    G. disease
    G. syndrome
    G. thrombasthenia
Glanzmann-Riniker syndrome
Glasgow
    G. Coma Scale (GCS)
    G. Meningococcal Septicemia Score
glass factor

Glassman forceps
glass-wool filtration
glassy cell carcinoma
glatiramer acetate
glaucoma
    acute angle closure g.
    congenital g.
    infantile g.
    primary congenital g.
    traumatic g.
Glazunov tumor
GLB
    gay, lesbian, bisexual
    GLB youths
GLB-1
    beta-galactosidase-1
gleet
    vent g.
gleety discharge
Glen Anderson ureteroneocystostomy
Glenárd disease
Glenn
    G. anastomosis
    G. operation
    G. shunt
Glenn-Anderson technique
glenohumeral
    g. instability
    g. joint
glenoid dysplasia
glia
gliadin
glial
    g. cell line derived neurotrophic
      factor (GDNF)
    g. fibrillary acidic protein (GFAP)
glide consonant
gliding movement
gli family zinc-finger transcriptional
  activators
GLIM
    generalized linear interactive modeling
glimepiride
glioblastoma multiforme
glioependymal cyst
glioma
    brainstem g.
    cervicomedullary brainstem g.
    chiasmal g.
    chiasmatic-hypothalamic g.
    cystic brainstem g.
    focal brainstem g.

    optic nerve g.
    g. of optic nerve
    optic pathway g.
    pontine g.
    spinal cord g.
    tectal brainstem g.
gliomatosis peritonei
gliosis
    aqueductal g.
    astrocytic g.
    compensatory g.
    fibrillary g.
    g. uteri
gliotic
    g. reaction
    g. tuft
glipizide
Glisson capsule
glistening dot
global
    g. aphasia
    g. assessment of function (GAF)
    g. brain hypoxia
    g. brain swelling
    g. developmental delay
    g. glomerulosclerosis
    g. hypertonia
    g. hypoplasia
    g. level of functioning (GLOF)
    g. neurologic dysfunction
    g. seasonality score
    G. Severity Index of Brief
      Symptom Inventory (GSI-BSI)
globe
    g. cell anemia
    ruptured g.
globiformis
    Arthrobacter g.
globin chain
globoid
    g. cell cerebral sclerosis
    g. cell leukodystrophy
globoside
globozoospermia
globule
    milk fat g. (MFG)
globulin
    anti-D immune g.
    antilymphocyte g.
    anti-Rh gamma g.
    anti-Rho(D) g.
    antithymocyte g.

G

NOTES

globulin (*continued*)
    botulinum immune g.
    corticosteroid-binding g. (CBG)
    cortisol-binding g.
    cytomegalovirus immune g. (CMVIG)
    gamma g. (GG)
    hepatitis B immune g. (HBIG, H-BIG, HBIg)
    hepatitis immune g.
    human immune g.
    human rabies immune g. (HRIG)
    hyperimmune serum g.
    immune g.
    immune serum g. (ISG)
    intravenous gamma g. (IVGG)
    intravenous immune g. (IVIG, IVIg)
    lymphocyte immune g.
    pregnancy-associated g.
    purified gamma g.
    rabies immune g. (RIG)
    regular immune g.
    respiratory syncytial virus immune g. (RSVIG, RSV-IG)
    respiratory syncytial virus intravenous immune g. (RSV-IGIV, RSV-IVIG)
    Rh immune g. (RhIg)
    Rho(D) immune g.
    sex hormone-binding g. (SHBG)
    specific immune g.
    testosterone-estrogen-binding g.
    tetanus immune g.
    thyroid-binding g. (TBG)
    thyroxine-binding g. (TBG)
    varicella-zoster immune g. (VZIG)
    zoster immune g. (ZIG)

globus
    g. hystericus
    g. pallidus

GLOF
    global level of functioning

glomerular
    g. basement membrane (GBM)
    g. basement membrane antigen
    g. capillary endotheliosis
    g. change
    g. disorder
    g. filtrate
    g. filtration
    g. filtration rate (GFR)
    g. insufficiency
    g. proteinuria
    g. renal disease
    g. sclerosis
    g. sialoglycoprotein
    g. tuft

glomerulation

glomeruli (*pl. of* glomerulus)
glomerulocystic disease
glomerulonephritis
    acute g.
    acute postinfectious g. (APGN)
    acute poststreptococcal g. (APSGN)
    autoimmune g.
    chronic g.
    crescentic g.
    diffuse proliferative g.
    familial g.
    focal segmental lupus g.
    focal segmental proliferative g.
    hemorrhagic cystitis g.
    hypocomplementemic g.
    idiopathic rapidly progressive g.
    immune complex-mediated g.
    membranoproliferative g. (MPGN)
    membranous g.
    mesangial proliferative g.
    mesangiocapillary g. (type I, II) (MPGN)
    necrotizing g.
    pauciimmune g.
    postinfectious g.
    poststreptococcal g.
    proliferative g.
    rapidly progressive g.

glomerulopathy
glomerulosa
    zona g.

glomerulosclerosis
    focal g.
    focal segmental g. (FSGS)
    global g.

glomerulotubular
glomerulus, pl. **glomeruli**
glomus tumor
GLORIA
    gold-labeled optical rapid immunoassay

glossa
glossitis
    benign migratory g.
    candidal g.

glossodynia
glossopalatine ankylosis syndrome
glossopharyngeal nerve
glossoptosis
glottal
    g. fricative
    g. obstruction

glottic
    g. opening
    g. spasm

glottis, pl. **glottides**
glove
    Biogel Reveal g.
    Eudermic surgical g.
    latex g.

Micro-Touch Platex medical g.
Mylar g.
Neolon surgical g.
powder-free g.
SensiCare surgical g.
sheepskin g.
g.'s and socks syndrome
gloving
double g.
glubionate
calcium g.
glucagon
Glucamide
Glucerna formula
glucoamylase deficiency
glucocerebrosidase
macrophage-targeted g.
glucocorticoid
g. deficiency
g. excess
g. insufficiency
glucocorticosteroid therapy
glucogenesis
glucoglycinuria
glucokinase
Glucola screen
Glucolet Endcaps
glucometer
Accu-Chek II g.
G. Elite diabetes care system
Glucostat II g.
G. II
gluconate
calcium g.
chlorhexidine g.
ferrous g.
potassium g.
quinidine g.
gluconeogenesis
hepatic g.
Glucophage
glucosamine
glucosamine-6-sulfate deficiency
glucose
blood g.
g. challenge test
g. concentration
g. excretion
fasting plasma g. (FPG)
fetal blood g.
g. formula
hypertonic g.

g. intolerance
g. meter
g. monitoring
g. oxidase test tape
plasma g.
g. plus insulin
postprandial g.
g. production rate (GPR)
g. reagent stick
serum g.
g. tolerance
g. tolerance test (GTT)
g. transporter (GLUT)
urinary g.
glucose-dependent insulinotropic peptide
glucose-galactose
g.-g. intolerance
g.-g. malabsorption
glucose-intolerant gravida
glucose-6-phosphate dehydrogenase
 (G6PD)
glucosiduronate
Glucostat II glucometer
Glucostix
glucosuria
Glucotrol
glucuronate pregnanediol
glucuronidation
glucuronide
3 alpha-androstanediol g.
androsterone g.
isovaleryl g.
virilizing 3 alpha-androstanediol g.
glucuronosyltransferase
glucuronyl
g. transferase
g. transferase deficiency
g. transferase inactivity
glue
airplane g.
g. ear
glue-sniffing neuropathy
GLUT
glucose transporter
glutamate
arginine g.
g. cycle
g. formiminotransferase deficiency
glutamic
g. acid
g. acid decarboxylase (GAD)
g. acid decarboxylase antibody

NOTES

G

glutamic-oxalacetic
glutamic-pyruvic transaminase
glutamine
glutamine-supplemented diet
glutamyltransferase
glutamyl transpeptidase (GTP)
glutaraldehyde cross-linked collagen
  injection
glutaric
    g. acidemia (type I, II)
    g. aciduria syndrome (type I, II)
    g. aciduria (type I, II)
glutathione (GSH)
    g. peroxidase
    g. S-transferase
    g. S-transferase isoform
    g. synthetase deficiency
glutathionemia
gluteal
    g. fold
    g. free flap
    g. lymph node
    g. muscle
    g. trauma
gluten
    g. allergy
    g. challenge
    g. enteropathy
    g. intolerance
    g. sensitivity
gluten-free diet (GFD)
gluten-induced enteropathy
gluten-sensitive enteropathy
glutethimide
gluteus
    g. maximus muscle
    g. medius limp
    g. medius muscle
    g. minimus muscle
GLUT1 gene
GLUT3 gene
glyburide
glycemia
glycemic
    g. control
    g. index
    g. index diet
glycerin
    g., lanolin and peanut oil
    g. suppository
glycerol
    iodinated g.
    g. kinase (GK)
    g. kinase deficiency (GKD)
glycerophospholipid
glycerophosphorylcholine
glyceryl
    g. guaiacolate
    g. trinitrate (GTN)

glycine
    blood g.
    CSF g.
glycinuria
    familial g.
glycocalyx
glycocorticoid
glycodelin-A
glycogen
    g. accumulation
    g. storage disease (type Ia–Id,
      II–VII) (GSD)
    g. storage disorder
    g. synthetase deficiency
glycogenesis
    hepatic g.
    g. (type I, II)
glycogenosis
    type 7 g.
    von Gierke g.
glycohemoglobin
glycol
    Diprolene G.
    ethylene g.
    polyethylene g.
    propylene g.
glycol-ADA
    polyethylene g.-ADA
glycolic
    Aqua G.
glycolipid metabolism
glycolysis
glycopeptide-resistant enterococcus
  (GRE)
glycophorin C
glycoprotein
    carbohydrate deficient g. (CDG)
    g. degradation
    heterodimeric integral membrane g.
    g. IB/IX
    KL-6 mucinous g.
glycoproteinosis
glycoprotein-producing tumor
glycopyrrolate
glycorrhachia
glycosaminoglycan (GAG)
    g. layer
    urinary g.
glycoside
    cardiac g.
glycosphingolipid
glycosuria
    renal g.
glycosuric diuresis
glycosylated hemoglobin (HgA1c)
glycosylation
Glylorin
Gly-Oxide Oral
Glyset

Glytuss
GM2 gangliosidosis
GM-CSF
    granulocyte-macrophage colony-
        stimulating factor
GMDS
    Griffith Mental Developmental Scale
GM3 gangliosidosis
GMS
    goniodysgenesis, mental retardation, short
        stature
        GMS syndrome
GMT
    geometric mean titer
gnashing
gnathocephalus
Gnathostoma spinigerum
gnathostomiasis
gnosis
        finger g.
GNR
    gram-negative rod
GnRH
    gonadotropin-releasing factor
    gonadotropin-releasing hormone
        GnRH agonist (GNRHa)
        GnRH deficiency
GNRHa
    GnRH agonist
GnRHa
    gonadotropin-releasing hormone agonist
    gonadotropin-releasing hormone analog
GnRH-facilitated
        G.-f. FSH release
        G.-f. LH release
GnRH-independent sexual precocity
goal
        annual g.
goat's milk formula
Goebell-Frangenheim-Stoeckel
    urethrovesical suspension technique
Goebell procedure
Goebell-Stoeckel-Frangenheim procedure
Go-Evac
Goffe colporrhaphy
goiter
        g. development
        drug-induced neonatal g.
        fetal g.
        simple colloid g.
goiter-deafness syndrome
goitrogen ingestion

goitrous
        g. hypothyroidism
        g. hypothyroidism with deafness
Golabi-Ito-Hall syndrome
Golabi-Rosen syndrome (GRS)
gold
        g.-198 (^{198}Au)
        radioactive g.
        g. salt
        g. seed
        g. sodium thiomalate
        g. therapy
Goldberg syndrome
Goldblatt-Vilijoen radial ray hypoplasia
Goldenhar
        G. microphthalmia syndrome
        G. oculauricular vertebral dysplasia
        G. sequence
Goldenhar-Gorlin syndrome
Golden sign of S
Goldie-Coldman hypothesis
gold-labeled optical rapid immunoassay
    (GLORIA)
Goldmann perimeter visual field test
Goldstein disease
Goldston syndrome
Golgi
        G. apparatus
        G. body
        G. stain
Gollop-Wolfgang complex
Goltz
        G. focal dermal hypoplasia
        G. syndrome
Goltz-Gorlin syndrome
Goltz-Peterson-Gorlin-Ravitz syndrome
GoLYTELY
GOMBO
    growth retardation, ocular abnormalities,
        microcephaly, brachydactyly,
        oligophrenia
        GOMBO syndrome
Gomco
        G. bell
        G. circumcision clamp
        G. circumcision technique
Gomez and López-Hernández syndrome
Gomori
        G. methenamine-silver stain
        G. trichrome reaction
        G. trichrome stain
gompertzian growth

NOTES

G

gonad
- dysgenetic g.
- indifferent g.'s
- maternal g.'s
- palpable g.
- streak g.'s
- undifferentiated g.

gonadal
- g. agenesis
- g. agenesis syndrome
- g. aplasia
- g. axis
- g. dysfunction
- g. dysgenesis
- g. dysgenesis syndrome
- g. dysplasia
- g. failure
- g. failure, short stature, mitral valve prolapse, mental retardation syndrome
- g. germ cell neoplasm
- g. hormone treatment
- g. mosaicism
- g. ridge
- g. sex
- g. steroid
- g. steroid suppression
- g. streak
- g. stroma
- g. stromal cell tumor
- g. stromal ovarian tumor

gonadarche
gonadectomy
gonadoblastoma
- ovarian g.

gonadocrinin
gonadoliberin
gonadorelin acetate
gonadostat
gonadotoxin
gonadotrope
gonadotropic deficiency
gonadotropin, gonadotrophin
- g. agonist stimulation test (GAST)
- beta-human chorionic g. (beta-hCG, beta-HCG)
- chorionic g. (CG)
- chorionic human recombinant g.
- endogenous g.
- exogenous g.
- human chorionic g. (hCG, HCG)
- human menopausal g. (hMG)
- g. level
- nicked human chorionic g.
- g. ovulation induction
- pituitary g.
- pulsatile human menopausal g.
- g. regulation
- g. secretion
- g. secretion inhibitor
- urinary chorionic g. (UCG)
- urinary menopausal g.

gonadotropin-dependent precocious puberty
gonadotropin-independent precocious puberty
gonadotropin-induced ovarian hyperstimulation
gonadotropin-releasing
- g.-r. factor (GnRH, GRF)
- g.-r. hormone (GnRH, GRH)
- g.-r. hormone agonist (GnRHa)
- g.-r. hormone analog (GnRHa)
- g.-r. hormone antagonist
- g.-r. hormone-associated peptide (GAP)

gonadotropin-resistant
- g.-r. ovary syndrome
- g.-r. testis

Gonal-F
gonane
gondii
- *Toxoplasma* g.

gonidiaformans
- *Fusobacterium* g.

goniodysgenesis, mental retardation, short stature (GMS)
goniometer
goniometry
gonioscopy
gonoblennorrhea
gonococcal
- g. arthritis
- g. arthritis of newborn
- g. conjunctivitis
- g. infection
- g. ophthalmia
- g. ophthalmia neonatorum
- g. perihepatitis
- g. septicemia
- g. urethritis

gonococcus, pl. **gonococci**
- penicillinase-producing g.

gonorrhea
- g. culture
- disseminated g.
- *Neisseria* g.
- pharyngeal g.

gonorrheal
- g. cervicitis
- g. ophthalmia
- g. salpingitis

gonorrhoica
- macula g.

Gonozyme test
Gonzales blood group

Goodell
>G. dilator
>G. sign

Goodenough-Harris Drawing Test
Goodman syndrome
Goodpasture syndrome
gooseflesh
gooseneck
>g. deformity
>g. deformity of left ventricular outflow tract

Gordofilm Liquid
Gordon
>G. diagnostic system (GDS)
>G. Distractibility Test
>G. reflex
>G. syndrome

Gore-Tex
>G.-T. Soft Tissue Patch
>G.-T. surgical membrane

Gorlin
>G. formula
>G. syndrome (1, 2)

Gorlin-Goltz syndrome
Gorlin-Psaume syndrome
GORT
>Gilmore Oral Reading Test
>Gray Oral Reading Test

GORT-R
>Gray Oral Reading Test-Revised

GOS
>Great Ormond Street
>GOS criteria

goserelin
>g. acetate
>g. acetate implant

gossypiboma
gossypol acetic acid (GAA)
Gott malleable retractor
Gottron
>G. papule
>G. sign

Gougerot-Carteaud syndrome
Goulet retractor
gout
>familial juvenile g.

gouty
>g. arthritis
>g. diathesis

Gower
>hemoglobin G.-1, -2

Gowers
>G. maneuver
>G. sign

gown
>barrier g.
>Exami-Gown g.

gp41
>transmembrane glycoprotein g.

gp120 viral protein
G6PD
>glucose-6-phosphate dehydrogenase
>G6PD deficiency

GPMAL
>gravida, para, multiple births, abortions, live births

GPR
>glucose production rate

G-protein-coupled receptor
graafian
>g. follicle
>g. vesicle

GRACE
>Girls, Ritalin LA, and ADHD

gracile bone dysplasia
gracilis
>*Campylobacter* g.
>g. flap neovagina
>g. flap technique
>g. muscle

graciloplasty
>dynamic g.

grade
>placental g.
>Roenigk g.

graded compression ultrasonography
Gradenigo syndrome
gradient
>A-a g.
>albumin g.
>alveolar-arterial oxygen g.
>alveolar-arterial pressure g.
>arterial-ascitic fluid pH g.
>blood pressure g.
>density g.
>diastolic g.
>echo Doppler g.
>hepatic venous wedge pressure g.
>peak instantaneous g.
>pressure g.
>g. recalled acquisition in the steady state (GRASS)

NOTES

G

gradient *(continued)*
   g. refocused acquisition in steady
      state (GRASS)
   sucrose g.
   transtubular potassium
      concentration g. (TTKG)
   tympanometric g.
grading
   histopathological g.
   Papile g.
   placental g.
   tumor g.
Graefenberg
   G. ring
   G. spot (G-spot)
Graefe-Usher syndrome
graevenitzii
   Actinomyces g.
Grafco breast pump
graft
   allogenic fetal g.
   bilateral myocutaneous g.
   bone g.
   buccal mucosa g.
   donor venous g.
   full-thickness skin g.
   GEA g.
   heterologous g.
   HLA-identical marrow g.
   isogeneic g.
   Martius g.
   oral mucous membrane g.
   polytetrafluoroethylene g.
   sacrocolpopexy g.
   seromuscular intestinal patch g.
   skin g.
   split-thickness g.
   T-cell-depleted g.
   g. versus host disease (GVHD)
   g. versus leukemia (GVL)
Graham
   G. Steell murmur
   G. syndrome
Graham-Rosenblith scale
gram (g, gm)
   oxy-CR g.
   G. stain
grammar
gram-negative
   g.-n. acne
   g.-n. bacilli
   g.-n. bacteria
   g.-n. cocci
   g.-n. endotoxic shock
   g.-n. endotoxin
   g.-n. endotoxin-induced shock
   g.-n. organism
   g.-n. pneumonia

   g.-n. rod (GNR)
   g.-n. ventriculitis
gram-positive
   g.-p. bacilli
   g.-p. bacteria
   g.-p. cocci
   g.-p. diplococcus
   g.-p. organism
   g.-p. rods
Gram-Weigert stain
grand
   g. climacteric
   g. mal
   g. mal attack
   g. mal epilepsy
   g. mal seizure
   g. multipara
   g. multiparity
   g. pregnancy
granddad syndrome
grandiose delusion
grandiosity
grandmother theory
grandmultipara
grandmultiparity
GraNee needle
Granger sign
granisetron
granny knot
Grantley
   G. Dick-Read method
   G. Dick-Read method of childbirth
Grant syndrome
Grant-Ward operation
granular
   g. cell myoblastoma
   g. ependymitis
   g. lung
   g. osmiophilic deposit
   g. urethritis
granulation
   arachnoid g.
   giant platelet g.
   pacchionian g.
   g. tissue
granule
   argyrophilic g.
   Birbeck g.
   Butschli g.
   cortical g.
   g. deficiency
   E.E.S. G.'s
   Fordyce g.
   large lysosome-like g.
   metachromatic cytoplasmic g.
   Nissl g.
   Reilly g.
   sulfur g.

granulocyte
  g. colony-stimulating factor (G-CSF)
  g. colony-stimulating factor receptor (G-CSF-R)
  g. count
  cytokine g.
  g. immunofluorescence test (GIFT)
  g. transfusion
granulocyte-macrophage colony-stimulating factor (GM-CSF)
granulocytic
  g. ehrlichiosis
  g. leukemia
  g. leukocytosis
  g. sarcoma
granulocytopenia
  congenital g.
granulocytopoiesis
granuloma, pl. **granulomata**
  g. annulare
  cholesterol g.
  coccidioidal g.
  disseminated g.
  eosinophilic g.
  fish-tank g.
  g. gluteal infantum
  g. gravidarum
  g. inguinale
  Langhans giant cell g.
  Majocchi g.
  mediastinal g.
  noncaseating sarcoidlike g.
  palisading g.
  progressive g.
  pyogenic g.
  rheumatoid g.
  sperm g.
  swimming pool g.
  telangiectatic g.
  umbilical g.
granulomatis
  Calymmatobacterium g.
granulomatosis
  g. infantiseptica
  juvenile systemic g.
  larval g.
  Wegener g. (WG)
granulomatous
  g. amebic meningoencephalitis
  g. angiitis
  g. calcification

  g. colitis
  g. disease
  g. infection
  g. lymphadenitis
  g. mastitis
  g. myocarditis
  g. perivasculitis
  g. salpingitis
  g. vasculitis
granuloplasty
granulopoiesis
  neutrophil g.
granulosa
  g. cell tumor
  g. lutein cell
  membrane g.
granulosa-stromal cell tumor
granulosa-theca cell tumor
granulosus
  Echinococcus g.
grape mole
graphesthesia
grasp
  finger g.
  inferior pincer g.
  neat pincer g.
  palmar g.
  pincer g.
  plantar g.
  radial digital g.
  radial palmar g.
  g. reflex
  toe g.
  ulnar palmar g.
grasper
  Lion's Claw g.
  MetraGrasp ligament g.
  Polaris reusable g.
grasping
  fetal g.
GRASS
  gradient recalled acquisition in the steady state
  gradient refocused acquisition in steady state
  GRASS MRI
  GRASS MRI technique
grass
  perennial rye g.
  g. pollen
  timothy g.
grating sound

NOTES

G

Graves
> avascular space of G.
> G. bivalve speculum
> G. disease

gravida (G)
> glucose-intolerant g.
> g., para, multiple births, abortions, live births (GPMAL)

gravidarum
> chorea g.
> epulis g.
> granuloma g.
> hydrops g.
> hyperemesis g.
> striae g.

gravidic
> g. retinitis
> g. retinopathy

gravidism
graviditas
> g. examnialis
> g. exochorialis

gravidity
gravid uterus
Gravindex test
gravis
> autoimmune myasthenia g.
> congenital myasthenia g.
> icterus g.
> myasthenia g.
> neonatal myasthenia g.
> transient neonatal myasthenia g.
> g. type Ehlers-Danlos syndrome

Gravlee jet washer
Gravol
gray
> g. baby
> g. baby syndrome
> g. matter
> g. matter heterotopia
> G. Oral Reading Test (GORT)
> G. Oral Reading Test-Revised (GORT-R)
> g. platelet syndrome
> g. scale

gray-scale
> g.-s. imaging
> g.-s. ultrasonography

gray-white junction
GRB
> general reading backwardness

GRE
> glycopeptide-resistant enterococcus

greasy stool
great
> g. arteries
> G. Ormond Street (GOS)
> G. Smoky Mountains Study of Youth (GSMS)

> g. toe
> g. vessel
> g. vessel of thorax

greater
> g. saphenous vein
> g. saphenous vein cutdown
> g. trochanter
> g. trochanteric bursa
> g. vestibular gland
> g. vestibular gland duct

great-grand multipara
Grebe
> G. chondrodysplasia
> G. dysplasia

green
> g. clay
> indocyanine g.
> g. light
> G. uterine curette

Greenfield
> G. disease
> G. filter

greenstick
> g. fracture
> g. injury

greeting spasm
Greig
> G. cephalopolysyndactyly anomaly
> G. cephalopolysyndactyly syndrome (GCPS)
> G. syndrome

grepafloxacin
Greulich
> G. and Pyle bone age
> G. and Pyle radiographic atlas

Greven forceps
Grey Turner sign
GRF
> gonadotropin-releasing factor

GRH
> gonadotropin-releasing hormone
> GRH antagonist

grid
> Self-Injury G. (SIG)

gridiron incision
grief
> anticipatory g.
> perinatal g.

grieving process
Griffith
> G. General Quotient
> G. Mental Developmental Scale (GMDS)
> G. Scale of Mental Development

Grifulvin V
grimace
grimacing
Grimelius stain

grip
milkmaid's g.
g. myotonia
grippotyphosa
Leptospira g.
Grisactin
Griscelli syndrome
Grisel syndrome
griseofulvin microcrystalline
griseus
Streptomyces g.
Grisolle sign
Grisovin
Gris-PEG
groin
g. dissection
g. hernia
g. ringworm
grommet
groove
Blessig g.
Harrison g.
intercondylar g.
intersphincteric g.
neural g.
primitive g.
g. sign
transverse nail g.
vomerian g.
grooved pegboard
Groshong catheter
gross
g. development
g. motor
g. motor development
g. motor domain
g. motor function measure
g. motor index
g. motor milestone
g. motor skill
g. motor total DMQ
grossly bloody stool
grotesque features
ground-glass
g.-g. appearance
g.-g. osteopenia
g.-g. pattern
ground itch
group
g. A beta-hemolytic streptococcal infection

g. A beta-hemolytic streptococcus (GABHS)
Adhesion Scoring G. (ASG)
AIDS Clinical Trials G.
antepartum support g.
g. A streptococcal impetigo
g. A streptococcus
blood g.
g. B streptococcal infection
g. B streptococcal pneumonia
g. B streptococcal sepsis
g. B streptococcus (GBS)
g. B streptococcus disease
Cartwright blood g.
g. C autosome
Children's Cancer G. (CCG)
Children's Cancer Study G. (CCSG)
Collaborative Antiviral Study G. (CASG)
g. C pharyngitis
g. C streptococcus
determinant g.
g. D streptococcus
Gonzales blood g.
g. G streptococcus
Kidd blood g.
Lewis blood g.
linkage g.
Lucarelli bone marrow transplant risk g.
Lutheran blood g.
National Wilms Tumor Study G. (NWTS)
Pediatric Oncology G.
private blood g.
g. problem-solving therapy
Rh blood g.
spotted fever g.
streptococcal g.
support g.
typhus g.
grouping
blood g.
clinical g.
growing fracture
growth
g. arrest
bacterial g.
catch-up g.
g. control factor
g. curve

NOTES

G

growth *(continued)*
    g. delay
    g. discordancy
    discordant twin g.
    g. disturbance
    divergent fetal g.
    epiphyseal g.
    g. epoch
    extracapsular g.
    g. factor (GF)
    g. failure
    g. failure-pericardial constriction
      syndrome
    fetal cellular g.
    gestational g.
    gompertzian g.
    g. hormone (GH)
    g. hormone-binding protein (GHBP)
    g. hormone deficiency (GHD)
    g. hormone immunoassay
    g. hormone insensitivity (GHI)
    g. hormone receptor (GHR)
    g. hormone receptor deficiency
      (GHRD)
    g. hormone release
    g. hormone-releasing hormone (GH-
      RH)
    g. hormone-secreting adenoma
    g. hormone stimulation test
      (GHST)
    g. index
    linear g.
    longitudinal g.
    nonestrogen-regulated g.
    g. parameters
    placental g.
    g. plate
    g. plate fracture
    g. plate injury
    poor linear g.
    g. problem
    puberal g.
    g. rate
    g. retardation
    g. retardation, ocular abnormalities,
      microcephaly, brachydactyly,
      oligophrenia (GOMBO)
    g. retardation, small and puffy
      hands, eczema syndrome
    retarded fetal g.
    skeletal g.
    slow g.
    g. spurt
    g. stunting
    testicular g.
    g. velocity (GV)
    g. zone
growth-adjusted sonographic age
  (GASA)

growth-discordant twins
growth-like factor
growth-remaining method
growth-restricted fetus
growth-retarded fetus
GRS
    Golabi-Rosen syndrome
Grubben syndrome
Gruber syndrome
Grünfelder reflex
grunting
    g. baby syndrome
    expiratory g.
    flaring and g.
    g. and flaring
    g. respiration
GRV
    gastric residual volume
GS
    gestational sac
GSD
    glycogen storage disease (type Ia–Id,
      II–VII)
GSH
    glutathione
      GSH pathway disorder
GSI
    genuine stress incontinence
GSI-BSI
    Global Severity Index of Brief Symptom
      Inventory
GSMS
    Great Smoky Mountains Study of Youth
G-spot
    Graefenberg spot
GSS
    gestational sac size
GT
      Cytobrush Plus GT
GTD
    gestational trophoblastic disease
GTN
    gestational trophoblastic neoplasia
    glyceryl trinitrate
G-to-T transversion mutation
GTP
    glutamyl transpeptidase
    guanosine triphosphate
    guanyltriphosphate
GTT
    gestational trophoblastic tumor
    glucose tolerance test
G-tube feeding
GU
    genitourinary
guaiac-negative stool
guaiacolate
    glyceryl g.
guaiac-positive stool

guaiac test
guaifenesin
  g. and codeine
  g. and dextromethorphan
  g., phenylpropanolamine,
    phenylephrine
Guaifenex DM, LA
guanabenz
guanadrel
guanethidine
guanfacine hydrochloride
guanidine salt
guanidinoacetate
guanine
  9-13-dihydroxypropoxymethyl g.
  g. nucleotide
guanosine
  g. triphosphate (GTP)
  g. triphosphate cyclohydrolase
guanyldiphosphate (GDP)
guanyltriphosphate (GTP)
guard
  high g.
  mouth g.
guardian
  g. ad litem
  G. DNA system
  G. vaginal retractor
gubernacular attachment
gubernaculum
GUD
  genital ulcer disease
Guerin-Stein syndrome
Guiatuss DM
Guiatussin With Codeine
guidance
  CT g.
  fluoroscopic g.
  hand-over-hand g.
  g. officer
  pictorial anticipatory g. (PAG)
  ultrasonographic g.
  ultrasound g.
guide
  Pilot suturing g.
  trocar g.
guidelines
  G. for Adolescent Preventive
    Services (GAPS)
  Bethesda System g.
guidewire

Guillain-Barré-Landry syndrome
Guillain-Barré syndrome (GBS)
guilliermondi
  Candida g.
guilt
  survivor g.
guinea worm infection
gulf
  Lecat g.
gum
  g. arabic rehydration solution
  bean g.
  g. bleeding
  carob g.
  g. fibrosis
  g. hyperplasia
gumma, pl. gummata
  pituitary gland g.
  tuberculous g.
gum-tooth interface
gun
  Bard Biopty g.
  coring biopsy g.
gunstock deformity
Günther disease
gurgling
Gurrieri syndrome
GUS
  genitourinary sphincter
GUSB
  beta-glucuronidase
  GUSB deficiency
  GUSB gene
  GUSB locus
gustatory
  g. discernment
  g. lacrimation
Gustavson syndrome
gut
  g. motility
  g. rest
  g. suture
  g. tonometry
  torsion of g.
  g. vasculitis
gut-associated lymphoid tissue (GALT)
Guthrie
  bacterial inhibition assay method
    of G.
  G. card
  G. count

G

NOTES

Guthrie *(continued)*
    G. muscle
    G. test
guttata
    parapsoriasis g.
    psoriasis g.
guttate
    g. lesion
    g. psoriasis
gutter
    paracolic g.
    pelvic g.
    posterior cul-de-sac g.
GV
    growth velocity
    GV oocytes
GVBD
    germinal vesicle breakdown
GVHD
    graft versus host disease
GVL
    graft versus leukemia
GWAFD
    Genée-Wiedemann acrofacial dysostosis
gym
    jungle g.
gymnastics
gymnast's wrist
GYN
    gynecologic
    gynecological
    gynecologist
    gynecology
gynandroblastoma
gynandromorph
gynatresia
Gynazole-1 vaginal cream
Gynecare Thermachoice uterine balloon therapy system
gynecic
gynecogenic
gynecography
gynecoid
    g. fat distribution pattern
    g. obesity
    g. pelvis
gynecologic, gynecological (GYN)
    g. cancer

    g. cancer patient
    g. carcinoma
    g. history
    g. malignancy
    g. oncology
gynecologist (GYN)
gynecology (GYN)
    adolescent g.
    pediatric g.
gynecomastia
    benign transient g.
    drug-induced g.
    involutional g.
    neonatal g.
    pathological g.
    physiologic g.
    puberal g.
Gynecort Topical
Gyne-Lotrimin Vaginal
Gynemesh PS polypropylene mesh support
Gyne-Sulf
gyniatrics
gyniatry
gynogenetic
Gynol II contraceptive jelly
gynopathy
gynoplasty, gynoplastics
GynoSampler
    G. endometrial aspirator
    G. endometrial sampling device
Gynoscann
gyral
    g. abnormality
    g. anomaly
    g. atrophy
    g. malformation
    g. pattern
gyrata
    cutis verticis g.
gyrate atrophy
Gyrocaps
    Slo-Phyllin G.
gyrus, pl. **gyri**
    cingulate g.
    mushroom g.
    orbitofrontal gyri

H
>H gene
>H and Lewis blood group activity
>H protein

H₂
>histamine 2
>>H₂ blocker

H₁
>histamine 1
>>H₁ receptor

H2O syndrome
H-7000 electron microscope
HA
>hyperalimentation
>hyperandrogenic anovulation
>hypoplastic aorta

Haab stria
HAART
>highly active antiretroviral therapy

Haase rule
Haas intrauterine insemination catheter
HABA
>hydroxybenzoic acid
>>HABA binding test

habenula, pl. **habenulae**
>Haller h.
>h. urethralis

habit
>bladder h.
>bowel h.
>h. cough
>dietary h.
>eating h.
>mentalis h.
>sexual h.
>sleeping h.
>h. tic deformity

HabitEX smoking cessation system
habitual
>h. aborter
>h. abortion
>h. shoulder dislocation
>h. shoulder subluxation
>h. snoring (HS)

habituation
habitus
>body h.
>Buddhalike h.
>craniosynostosis-marfanoid h.
>cushingoid body h.
>eunuchoid h.
>fetal h.
>h. of fetus
>marfanoid h.

HAC
>hexamethylmelamine with doxorubicin and cyclophosphamide
>human artificial chromosome

HACE
>high-altitude cerebral edema

HACEK
>*Haemophilus aphrophilus, Actinobacillus actinomycetemcomitans, Cardiobacterium hominis, Eikenella corrodens, Kingella kingae*
>>HACEK coccobacillus

Hacker hypospadias
Hadlock equation
haematobium
>*Schistosoma h.*

haemolysans
>*Gemella h.*

haemolyticum
>*Arcanobacterium h.*
>*Corynebacterium h.*

Haemophilus
>*H. aphrophilus*
>*H. aphrophilus, Actinobacillus actinomycetemcomitans, Cardiobacterium hominis, Eikenella corrodens, Kingella kingae* (HACEK)
>*H. ducreyi*
>*H. influenzae*
>*H. influenzae* cellulitis
>*H. influenzae* meningitis
>*H. influenzae* type b (HIB)
>*H. influenzae* type b conjugate vaccine
>*H. influenzae* type b immunization
>*H. pertussis* vaccine (HPV)
>*H. vaginalis*
>*H.* vaginitis

Hagedorn
>neutral protamine H. (NPH)

Hageman factor
Haig-Fergusson forceps
Haight baby retractor
Hailey-Hailey disease
hair
>axillary h.
>bamboo h.
>brittle h.
>h. bud
>h. bulb incubation test
>h. cortex keratin gene type II
>h. cotinine analysis
>exclamation-mark h.
>friable h.

H

hair *(continued)*
    h. groomer's syncope
    h. growth phase
    h. loss
    lumbosacral tuft of h.
    Menkes kinky h.
    mental retardation, polydactyly,
      phalangeal hypoplasia, syndactyly,
      unusual face, uncombable h.
    moniliform h.
    h. monster
    h. patch
    pubic h.
    h. pulling
    h. sampling
    sexual h.
    sparse h.
    h. spray
    spun glass h.
    terminal h.
    h. tourniquet
    h. tourniquet injury
    tuft of h.
    twisted h.
    vellus h.
    h. whorl
    wispy h.
HAIR-AN, HAIRAN
    hirsutism, androgen excess, insulin
      resistance, acanthosis nigricans
    hyperandrogenism, insulin resistance,
      acanthosis nigricans
    HAIR-AN syndrome
hairball
hair-brain syndrome
hairless pseudofemale
hairlike tumor
hairline
    low occipital h.
    pubic h.
hair-on-end appearance
hairpin vessel
hairy
    h. leukoplakia
    h. nevus
    h. patch
    h. tongue
Hajdu-Cheney syndrome
Hakim-Adams syndrome
Hakim syndrome
Halban
    H. culdoplasty
    H. fashion
    H. procedure
    H. syndrome
Halbrecht syndrome
halcinonide
Halcion
Haldol Decanoate

Haley's M-O
half-desmosome
half-Fourier acquisition single-shot turbo
    spin-echo (HASTE)
half-kneeling position
half-life
Halfprin
half-strength formula
half-value layer (HVL)
halitosis
Halle
    H. infant nasal speculum
    H. point
Haller
    H. cell
    H. habenula
Hallermann-Streiff
    H.-S. dyscephalia
    H.-S. syndrome
Hallermann-Streiff-François syndrome
Hallermann syndrome
Hallervorden-Spatz
    H.-S. disease
    H.-S. syndrome
Hallopeau-Siemens syndrome
Hall-Pallister syndrome
Hallpike maneuver
Hall-Riggs syndrome
Hall syndrome (1, 2)
hallucal
hallucination
    hypnagogic h.
    olfactory h.
    phobic h.
    tactile h.
    visual phobic h.
hallucinogen
hallucis
    spastic abductor h.
hallux
    purple h.
    h. rigidus
    h. valgus
halo
    h. effect
    erythematous h.
    fatty h.
    h. nevus
    osteopenic h.
    h. sign of hydrops
    H. Sleep System
    h. test
    h. traction
halobetasol
halofantrine
Halog-E
halogen
    h. acne

h. lamp
h. spotlight phototherapy
halogenated hydrocarbon
haloperidol
haloprogin
Halotestin
Cytoxan, Adriamycin, fluorouracil, tamoxifen, H. (CAFTH)
Halotex
halothane
Halotussin DM
Halpern syndrome
Halsted
H. mastectomy
H. mosquito forceps
H. operation
halstedian concept of tumor spread
Haltia-Santavuori neural ceroid lipofuscinosis
Haltran
HAM
human T-cell lymphotrophic virus type I associated myelopathy
hamartin
hamartoblastoma
congenital hypothalamic h.
hypothalamic h.
renal, anus, lung, polydactyly, h. (RALPH)
hamartoma
ectoneurodermal h.
hypothalamic h.
iris h.
mesenchymal h.
neuroectodermal h.
smooth muscle h.
hamartomatosis
hereditary multiple system h.
hamartomatous
h. malformation
h. mass
hamartoneoplastic syndrome
hamartopolydactyly syndrome
HAMD
Hamilton Depression Scale
Hamel syndrome
Ham F10 medium
Hamilton
H. Depression Scale (HAMD)
H. method
Hamman-Rich syndrome

hammer
Quisling h.
h. toe
Hammersmith
hemoglobin H.
hammock
Mersilene gauze h.
Hamou
H. contact microhysteroscope
H. hysteroscope
H. microcolpomicrohysteroscope
H. Micro-Hysteroflator
H. technique
hamster egg penetration assay
hamstring
lengthening of h.
h. lengthening
HAM/TSP
HTLV-I associated myelopathy/tropical spastic paraparesis
hand
ape h.
choreic h.
cleft h.
dominant h.
epidermolysis bullosa simplex of h.'s
fisting of h.'s
h. and head presentation
lobster-claw h.
mechanic's h.
milkmaid's h.
mitten h.
narrow h.
h. preference
vaginal h.
h. ventilation
h. wringing
hand-bagging
handbook
Harriet Lane H.
hand-eye coordination
hand-foot-and-mouth disease (HFMD)
hand-foot-genital syndrome
hand-foot-mouth syndrome
hand-foot syndrome
hand-foot-uterus syndrome
handheld flutter device
handicap
mental h.
neurodevelopmental h.

NOTES

H

handle
    laryngoscope h.
handling
hand-over-hand guidance
handpiece
    PhotoDerm PL h.
Hand-Schüller-Christian
    H.-S.-C. disease
    H.-S.-C. syndrome
hands-feet position
hand-to-eye fomite
hand-to-mouth movement
handwashing
hand-wringing movement
hand-wrist bone age
hanging
    h. panniculus
    h. stirrup
hanging-drop test
hangman's fracture
hangover
Hanhart syndrome
Hanks dilator
Hank's balanced salt solution (HBSS)
Hansel stain
Hansen disease
Hantaan virus
H$_2$-antagonist
hantavirus
    h. cardiopulmonary syndrome
    (HCPS)
    h. immunoglobulin M antibody
    h. pulmonary syndrome
HAODM
    hypoplasia of anguli oris depressor
    muscle
HAPE
    high-altitude pulmonary edema
haplogroup
haploid
    h. cell
    h. set
    h. sperm
    h. spermatozoon
haploidentical bone marrow transplant
haploinsufficiency
haplotype
    maternal HLA h.
    h. relative risk (HRR)
happy
    h. puppet syndrome
    h. wheezer
hapten
hapten-antibody
    hypersensitive h.-a.
haptoglobin
harassing cough

HARD
    hydrocephalus, agyria, retinal dysplasia
    HARD syndrome
HARD+/-E
    hydrocephalus, agyria, retinal dysplasia
    with or without encephalocele
    HARD+/-E syndrome
hard hepatomegaly
Hardikar syndrome
Hardy-Weinberg
    H.-W. equilibrium
    H.-W. formula
    H.-W. law
harelip
harlequin
    h. color change
    h. fetus
    h. ichthyosis
    h. reaction
    h. sign
harmonic
    H. scalpel
    h. tissue imaging
harmony
harness
    figure-of-eight h.
    Kicker Pavlik h.
    Pavlik h.
    Wheaton Pavlik h.
HARP
    hypobetalipoproteinemia, acanthocytosis,
    retinitis pigmentosa, and pallidal
    degeneration
    HARP syndrome
Harpenden
    H. calipers
    H. stadiometer
Harriet Lane Handbook
Harrington
    H. retractor
    H. rod
Harris
    H. growth arrest line
    H. uterine injector (HUI)
    H. view
Harris-Benedict basal energy
  expenditure equation
Harrison
    H. groove
    H. method
    H. sulcus
Harrod syndrome
harsh pansystolic murmur
Hart
    H. line
    H. syndrome
Harter self-esteem questionnaire

Hartmann
>H. sign
>H. solution

Hartnup
>H. defect
>H. disease
>H. disorder

HAS
>hospitalized attempted suicide

Hashimoto thyroiditis

hashish

Hassall corpuscle

Hasson cannula

HASTE
>half-Fourier acquisition single-shot turbo spin-echo
>HASTE sequence

HAstV-1
>human astrovirus type 1

hat
>measuring h.
>silver thermal h.
>thermal h.

Hata phenomenon

hatchet face appearance

hatching
>assisted h. (AH)
>assisted zona h. (AZH)
>blastocyst h.

HATT
>hemagglutination treponemal test

Haugh forceps

Haultain operation

HAV
>hepatitis A vaccine
>hepatitis A virus

Haverhill fever

haversian system

Havrix vaccine

Hawaii
>H. agent
>H. Early Learning Profile (HELP)

Hawk-Dennen forceps

Hawkins
>H. breast localization needle
>H. sign

hawkinsinuria

Haw River syndrome

Hawthorne effect

hay fever

Hayflick
>Wistar Institute Susan H. (WISH)

Hay-Wells syndrome

hazard
>Cox proportional h.

haze
>corneal h.

hazy lung

HB
>hepatitis B
>Recombivax HB

Hb, hgb
>hemoglobin

HbA$_2$
>hemoglobin A$_2$

HBAg
>hepatitis B antigen

HBcAb
>hepatitis B core antibody

HbE
>hemoglobin E
>HbE beta-thalassemia

HBeAb
>hepatitis B early antibody

HbF
>fetal hemoglobin
>hemoglobin F

HbH
>hemoglobin H
>HbH disease
>HbH disease-mental retardation syndrome
>HbH related mental retardation

HBIG, H-BIG, HBIg
>hepatitis B immune globulin

HBIR
>Hering-Breuer inflation reflex

HBL
>hepatoblastoma

HBLP
>hyperbetalipoproteinemia

HbOC
>hepatitis B oligosaccharide-CRM197 vaccine

HbP
>primitive fetal hemoglobin

HBQ
>human health and behavior questionnaire

HbS
>hemoglobin S
>sickle cell hemoglobin

HBsAb
>hepatitis B surface antibody

NOTES

H

411

HBsAg
hepatitis B surface antigen
HbSC
HBS mutation
HBSS
Hank's balanced salt solution
HbSS
homozygosity for hemoglobin S
HbS-Thal
hemoglobin S thalassemia
HBV
hepatitis B vaccine
hepatitis B virus
HC
head circumference
Bancap HC
Prevex HC
HC/AC
head circumference/abdominal
circumference ratio
fetal HC/AC
HC/AC ratio
HCC
hepatocellular carcinoma
H(c)ELISA
hemagglutinin enzyme-linked
immunosorbent assay
HCFA
Health Care Financing Administration
hCG, HCG
human chorionic gonadotropin
free beta hCG
OvuDate hCG
Pro-Step hCG
Tandem Icon II hCG
Test Pack hCG
HCII
heparin cofactor II
HCII coagulation inhibitor
hck protooncogene
HCl
hydrochloride
cefepime HCl
Cleocin HCl
fluoxetine HCl
ondansetron HCl
oxytetracycline HCl
phenazopyridine HCl
ropivacaine HCl
sertraline HCl
valacyclovir HCl
venlafaxine HCl
HCO$_3$
bicarbonate
HCP
hereditary coproporphyria
HCPS
hantavirus cardiopulmonary syndrome

HCRM
home cardiorespiratory monitor
HCS
holocarboxylase
HCS deficiency
hct
hematocrit
HCTZ
hydrochlorothiazide
HCV
hepatitis C virus
HCW
healthcare worker
HD
Huntington disease
HDC-ABMT
high-dose chemotherapy with autologous
bone marrow transplantation
HDCV
human diploid cell rabies vaccine
HDE
higher-dose therapy with epinephrine
HDI 3000 ultrasound
HDL
high-density lipoprotein
HDL cholesterol
HDN
hemolytic disease the newborn
hemolytic disease of newborn
hemorrhagic disease of newborn
HDS
hematuria, dysuria syndrome
HDV
hepatitis D virus
HE
hepatic encephalopathy
hereditary elliptocytosis
spherocytic HE
H&E
hematoxylin and eosin
H&E stain
head
h. banding enuresis
h. banging
h. birth
h. bobbing
h. box
breech h.
h. circumference (HC)
h. circumference/abdominal
circumference ratio (HC/AC)
h. compression
h. control
cracked-pot h.
cupping of optic nerve h.
h. drop
engaged h.
h. entrapment
fetal h.

h. growth velocity
hourglass h.
h. lag
h. louse
malformed radial h.
h. mesoderm
molding of h.
h. pole
h. positioner
h. presentation
H. reflex
h. righting
h. size
H. Start
h. and tail fold
h. tilt
h. titubation
transillumination of h.
h. trauma
h. ultrasound
zygomatic h.

headache
acute h.
analgesic-rebound h.
chronic h.
classic migraine h.
cluster h.
common migraine h.
complicated migraine h.
h. diary
migraine h.
migraine-type h.
migrainous h.
nonmigrainous h.
postdural puncture h.
postlumbar puncture h.
preeclampsia h.
primary h.
recurrent h.
secondary h.
sleep-related h.
spinal h.
tension h.
vascular h.

headband
fiberoptic h.
imaging h.
plagiocephaly h.

headlight
Keeler fiberoptic h.

head-righting
lateral h.-r.

head-sparing intrauterine growth retardation
head-to-head sperm agglutination (H-H)
head-to-tail sperm agglutination (H-T)
head-up tilt (HUT)
healing
energy h.

health
H. Care Financing Administration (HCFA)
h. maintenance organization (HMO)
h. maintenance visit
mental h.
National Institute of Mental H. (NIMH)
National Institutes of H. (NIH)
h., osteoporosis, progestin, estrogen (HOPE)
pediatric public h.
H. Plan Employer Data and Information Set
H. Scan Assess Plus peak flow meter
h. status
World Association for Infant Mental H.

healthcare worker (HCW)
HealthCheck One-Step One Minute pregnancy test
Healthdyne
H. apnea monitor
H. oximeter
H. ventilator

health-related quality of life (HRQOL)
Heaney
H. clamp
H. curette
H. hysterectomy forceps
H. hysterectomy retractor
H. needle holder
H. operation
H. vaginal vault closure technique

Heaney-Ballantine forceps
Heaney-Simon retractor
hearing
h. acuity
h. aid
h. development
h. loss
h. loss, mental deficiency, growth retardation, clubbed digits, EEG abnormalities syndrome

NOTES

H

413

hearing *(continued)*
    residual h.
    h. screening
hearing-loss–nephritis syndrome
heart
    air-filled h.
    h. block
    boot-shaped h.
    crisscross h.
    cushion defect of h.
    h. defect
    h. defect syndrome
    dextroposition of h.
    h. disease
    h. and estrogen/progestin
      replacement study (HERS)
    h. failure
    fetal h.
    hole in h.
    Holmes h.
    hypoplasia of left h. (HLL)
    hypoplastic left h.
    h. lesion
    h. massage
    midline h.
    h. murmur
    h. rate (HR)
    h. rate monitoring
    h. rate power spectral analysis
      (HRSA)
    h. rate variability (HRV)
    h. shadow
    h. sounds
    h. transplant
    h. transplantation
    upstairs-downstairs h.
    h. valve replacement
heartburn
heart-hand syndrome
heart-shaped
    h.-s. pelvis
    h.-s. uterus
heat
    h. loss
    prickly h.
    h. shock protein
    h. transfer mechanism
heater probe thermal contact
heatstroke
Heat-Treated
    Profilnine H.-T.
heave
    apical h.
heavy
    h. chain
    h. metal poisoning
heavy-ion
    h.-i. irradiation
    h.-i. mammography

hebdomadis
    Leptospira interrogans serovar *h.*
hebephrenia
hebephrenic silliness
hebetic
HEC
    human endothelial cell
Hecht pneumonia
hedgehog
    Sonic H.
heel
    h. capillary sampling
    h. cord
    h. cord lengthening
    h. cup
    h. lance (HL)
    h. pain
    h. stick
    h. strike
    Thomas h.
    h. valgus
heel-cord contracture
heel-stick
    h.-s. hematocrit
    h.-s. procedure
heel-to-ear maneuver
heel-toe gait
heel-to-shin test
Heerfordt syndrome
HEF
    human embryo fibroblast
Hegar
    H. dilator
    H. sign
heidelberg
    Salmonella h.
height
    fundal h.
    midparental h.
    minimal acceptable h. (MAH)
    sitting h. (SH)
    symphysis-fundus h.
    h. table
    h. velocity (HV)
    h. velocity Z-score
height-for-age (HFA)
heilmannii
    Helicobacter h.
Heimlich maneuver
Heineke-Mikulicz pyloroplasty
Heiner syndrome
Heinz
    H. body
    H. body hemolytic anemia
Hektoen agar
HeLa
    Henrietta Lacks
    HeLa cells
helcomenia

helical scan
helices (*pl. of* helix)
Helicobacter
    H. heilmannii
    H. pylori
heliotrope
    h. eyelid
    h. pattern
    h. rash
heliotropic
    h. discoloration
    h. erythema
heliox
    helium and oxygen
helium and oxygen (heliox)
helix, pl. helices
    alpha h.
    double h.
    H. endocervical curette
    h. termination peptide
    H. uterine biopsy curette
Helixate
helix-loop-helix transcription
Hellendall sign
Heller
    H. dementia
    H. myotomy
    H. test
Heller-Belsey operation
Heller-Döhle disease
Heller-Nissen operation
Hellin law
Hellin-Zeleny law
HELLP
    hemolysis, elevated liver enzymes, low
      platelet count
      HELLP syndrome
helmet
    cranial molding h.
    plagiocephaly h.
helmet-molding therapy
helminth
helminthic disease
HELP
    Hawaii Early Learning Profile
helper
    h. factor
    T h.
    h. T cell
helplessness
Helpline
    Bed Rest H.

Hemabate
Hemaflex sheath
hemagglutination
    indirect h.
    h. inhibition
    h. inhibition antibody (HIA)
    h. test
    h. treponemal test (HATT)
    Treponema pallidum h. (TPHA)
hemagglutinin
    h. enzyme-linked immunosorbent
      assay (H(c)ELISA)
    filamentous h.
hemagogue
hemangiectasia hypertrophica
hemangiectatic hypertrophy
hemangioblastoma
    cerebellar h.
hemangioendothelioma
    kaposiform h.
hemangioma, pl. hemangiomata
    bone h.
    capillary h.
    cardiac h.
    cavernous h.
    cryptic h.
    cutaneous h.
    epidural h.
    giant h.
    hepatic h.
    infantile hepatic h.
    Kaposi-like form of infantile h.
    lobular capillary h.
    macular h.
    port-wine h.
    proliferating h.
    strawberry h.
    vulvar h.
hemangioma-thrombocytopenia syndrome
hemangiomatosis
    diffuse neonatal h.
    disseminated h.
    pulmonary h.
hemangiomatous branchial clefts/lip
    pseudocleft syndrome
hemangiopericytoma
    infantile h.
hemarthrosis
    acute h.
hematemesis
    coffee-grounds h.

NOTES

Hematest
    H. positive
    H. test
hematobilia
hematocele
    pelvic h.
    pudendal h.
hematocephalus
hematochezia
hematocolpometra
hematocolpos
hematocrit (hct)
    automated h.
    h. determination
    heel-stick h.
    mean menstrual cycle h.
    posttransfusion h.
    spun h.
hematogenous
    h. infection
    h. metastasis
    h. osteomyelitis
    h. primary tuberculosis
    h. seeding
    h. septic arthritis
    h. spread
hematogenously
hematologic
    h. disorder
    h. neoplasia
hematological change
hematology
hematoma
    acute subdural h.
    adrenal h.
    auricular h.
    axillary h.
    central hepatic h.
    cerebellar h.
    cerebral h.
    h. drainage
    epidural h.
    extradural h.
    follicular h.
    hepatic h.
    infected cuff h.
    interhemispheric subdural h.
    interstitial and loculated h.
    intracerebral h.
    intracranial h.
    intraparenchymal h.
    intrauterine h.
    puerperal h.
    retroperitoneal h.
    retroplacental h.
    secondary h.
    subcapsular hepatic h.
    subchorionic h.
    subdural h. (SDH)

    subgaleal h. (SGH)
    sublingual h.
    submental h.
    testicular h.
    traumatic h.
    umbilical cord h.
    uterine h.
    vaginal h.
    vulvar h.
hematometra, hemometra
hematometrocolpos
hematometry
hematomphalocele
hematophagocytic syndrome
hematopoiesis, hemopoiesis
    extramedullary h.
hematopoietic, hemopoietic
    h. differentiation
    h. disorder
    h. stem cell (HSC)
    h. stem cell transplantation
    h. syndrome
    h. system
    h. system stimulator
hematosalpinx, hemosalpinx
hematotrachelos
hematotympanum (*var. of* hemotympanum)
hematoxylin and eosin (H&E)
hematuria
    benign familial h. (BFH)
    benign recurrent h.
    congenital hereditary h.
    drug-induced h.
    h., dysuria syndrome (HDS)
    exercise-induced h.
    familial benign h.
    familial recurrent h.
    macroscopic h.
    h., nephropathy, deafness syndrome
    painless h.
    recurrent gross h. (RGH)
    sickle-cell associated h.
    transient h.
heme
    h. iron
    h. metabolism disorder
    h. oxygenase
    h. oxygenase inhibitor
hemelytrometra
heme-negative stool
heme-positive stool
Hemet Rectal
hemiacardius
hemiacephalus
hemianencephaly
hemianopia, hemianopsia
    bitemporal h.

homonymous h.
transient h.
hemiatrophy
progressive facial h.
hemiatrophy-hemihypertrophy
hemiblock
left anterior h.
hemibody irradiation
hemicardia
hemicephalia
hemicervix
hemichorea
hemicolectomy
hemicord
hemicortectomy
hemicrania
migraine sine h.
hemidesmosome
hemidystonia
hemiepiphysiodesis
hemifacial
h. microsomia (HM)
h. spasm
hemi-Fontan procedure
hemifusion
hemignathia and microtia syndrome
hemihyperplasia
hemihypertrophy
hemihypoplasia
hemihysterectomy
hemimegalencephaly
unilateral h.
hemimelia
congenital fibular h.
congenital tibial h.
dysplasia epiphysealis h.
fibular h.
paraxial fibular h.
paraxial tibial h.
tibial h.
transverse h.
hemimelus
hemin
heminasal
h. aplasia
h. hypoplasia
hemineural plate
hemipagus
hemiparesis
congenital h.
postconvulsive h.
spastic h.

hemiparetic
h. cerebral palsy
h. posture
hemiplegia
acute infantile h.
alternating h.
congenital h.
double h.
infantile h.
postmigrainous stroke h.
spastic h.
syndrome of acute h.
hemiplegic
h. cerebral palsy
h. migraine
hemisection
h. of cord
h. uterine morcellation technique
hemisensory deficit
hemisphere
cerebral h.
hemispherectomy
total h.
hemispheric tumor
hemisyndrome
left h.
hemiuterus
hemivagina
hemivertebra, pl. **hemivertebrae**
hemivulvectomy
hemizona assay (HZA)
hemizygosity
hemizygous
hemobilia
traumatic h.
hemoblastic leukemia
Hemoccult H test
Hemoccult II test
hemochorial placenta
hemochromatosis
hereditary h.
HFE gene for h.
neonatal h. (NH)
hemoconcentration
HemoCue
H. AB hemoglobin measurement
device
H. blood glucose analyzer
H. blood glucose system
H. blood hemoglobin analyzer
H. blood hemoglobin system
H. glucose test

NOTES

H

417

HemoCue *(continued)*
  H. hemoglobin photometer
  H. hemoglobin test
  H. microcurette
hemocystinuria
Hemocyte
hemocytometer
  Neubauer h.
hemodiafiltration
hemodialysis
  continuous venovenous h.
    (CVVHD)
hemodilution
hemodynamic
  h. abnormality
  h. data
  h. instability
  h. monitoring
hemodynamics
  maternal central h.
  uterine h.
Hemofil M
hemofilter
hemofiltration
  continuous arteriovenous h.
    (CAVH)
  continuous venovenous h. (CVVH)
hemoglobin (Hb, hgb)
  h. A
  h. A$_2$ (HbA$_2$)
  h. A1c
  h. A1c determination
  h. Bart
  h. Bart hydrops fetalis syndrome
  h. C
  h. CC
  h. Chesapeake
  h. C, M, S, SC, SD disease
  h. concentration
  cord blood h.
  h. E (HbE)
  h. electrophoresis
  elevated fetal h.
  embryonic h.
  h. F (HbF)
  fetal h. (HbF)
  glycosylated h. (HgA1c)
  h. Gower-1, -2
  h. H (HbH)
  h. Hammersmith
  hereditary persistence of fetal h.
    (HPFH)
  high-affinity h.
  homozygous h. E
  h. Kempsey
  h. Lepore
  h. level
  mean cell h. (MCH)
  mean corpuscular h. (MCH)

  h. M Hyde Park
  h. M Saskatoon
  h. Portland
  primitive fetal h. (HbP)
  reduced h.
  h. S (HbS)
  h. SC
  h. SC, SS phenotype
  h. SD
  serum free h.
  sickle cell h. (HbS)
  h. SS (HbSS)
  h. SS (HbSS)
  h. S solubility test
  h. S thalassemia (HbS-Thal)
  h. S-Thal phenotype
  h. subtype method
  unstable h.
  variant h.
hemoglobinemia
hemoglobinopathy
  sickle cell h.
hemoglobin-oxygen
  h.-o. dissociation
  h.-o. dissociation curve
hemoglobinuria
  march h.
  paroxysmal nocturnal h. (PNH)
hemoglobulinopathy
hemolymphatic stage
hemolysin
  Donath-Landsteiner cold h.
hemolysis
  antibody-mediated h.
  chronic intravascular h.
  h., elevated liver enzymes, low
    platelet count (HELLP)
  fetal h.
  immune h.
  massive intravascular h.
  mechanical h.
  microangiopathic h.
  nonimmune h.
hemolysis-derived black pigment stone
hemolytic
  ABO h. disease of the newborn
  h. anemia
  h. complement (CH$_{50}$)
  h. crisis
  h. disease
  h. disease the newborn (HDN)
  h. uremia syndrome associated with
    pregnancy
  h. uremic syndrome (HUS)
hemolyzed specimen
hemometra *(var. of* hematometra)
Hemonyne
Hemopad

hemopathy
    maternal h.
hemopericardium
hemoperitoneum
    ovulation-associated h.
hemophagocytic
    h. lymphohistiocytosis
    h. syndrome
hemophilia
    h. A, B, C
    acquired h.
    factor VIII h.
hemophiliac
hemophilic arthropathy
hemopneumothorax
hemopoiesis (*var. of* hematopoiesis)
hemopoietic (*var. of* hematopoietic)
hemoptysis
    catamenial h.
HemoQuant assay
hemorrhage
    accidental h.
    adrenal h.
    antepartum h.
    catastrophic h.
    cerebellar h.
    CNS h.
    concealed h.
    cortical h.
    epidural h.
    external h.
    fetal h.
    fetal-maternal h.
    fetomaternal h. (FMH)
    focal h.
    gastrointestinal h.
    germinal matrix h. (grade 1–4)
    idiopathic pulmonary h. (IPH)
    iliopsoas h.
    interhemispheric subarachnoid h.
    intracerebellar h.
    intracranial h. (ICH)
    intraparenchymal h.
    intrapartum h.
    intraretinal h. (IH)
    intraventricular h. (grade 1–4) (IVH)
    maternal-fetal h.
    orbital h.
    perinatal cerebral h.
    periventricular h. (grade 1–4) (PVH)
    periventricular-intraventricular h. (PIVH)
    petechial h.
    pinpoint h.
    placental h.
    postcesarean h.
    posterior fossa h.
    postpartum h. (PPH)
    pulmonary h.
    retinal h.
    retroplacental h.
    scleral h.
    splinter h.
    sternocleidomastoid h.
    subarachnoid h.
    subcapsular hepatic h.
    subchorionic h.
    subconjunctival h.
    subdural h.
    subependymal h. (SEH)
    subependymal germinal matrix h.
    subgaleal h.
    subhyaloid h.
    transplacental h.
    trauma-related acute pelvic h.
    unavoidable h.
    uterine h.
hemorrhagic
    h. colitis
    h. cystitis
    h. cystitis glomerulonephritis
    h. dehydration
    h. diathesis
    h. disease
    h. disease of newborn (HDN)
    h. edema of infancy
    h. enanthem
    h. encephalitis
    h. endovasculitis
    h. *Escherichia coli*
    h. familial nephritis
    h. fever
    h. fever with renal syndrome (HFRS)
    h. hereditary nephritis
    h. pleural effusion
    h. scurvy
    h. shock
    h. shock and encephalopathy syndrome (HSES)
    h. shock syndrome

NOTES

hemorrhagic *(continued)*
  h. spinal fluid
  h. telangiectasia
hemorrhagica
  purpura h.
hemorrhagicum
  corpus h.
hemorrhoid
  Pazo H.
hemorrhoidal
  h. artery
  h. nerve
  h. preparation
hemosalpinx *(var. of* hematosalpinx)
hemosiderin
  h. deposition
  h. laden macrophage
hemosiderinuria
hemosiderosis
  food-induced pulmonary h.
  primary pulmonary h.
  pulmonary h.
  transfusion-induced h.
hemospermia
hemostasis
  intrapartum h.
  surgical h.
hemostat
  Crile h.
  curved h.
  Endo-Avitene microfibrillar
    collagen h.
hemostatic staple line
Hemotene
hemothorax
hemotympanum, hematotympanum
HEMPAS
  hereditary erythroblastic multinuclearity
    with positive acidified serum
    HEMPAS test
Hem-Prep
Hemril-HC Uniserts
Henderson-Hasselbalch equation
Henle
  loop of H.
Hennebert sign
Hennekam lymphangiectasia-lymphedema syndrome
Henoch disease
Henoch-Schönlein purpura (HSP)
Henrietta Lacks (HeLa)
Henschke colpostat
henselae
  Bartonella h.
  Rochalimaea h.
Hensen node
HEP
  hepatoerythropoietic porphyria

HEPA
  high-efficiency particulate air
  HEPA filter
hepadnavirus
Hepalean
heparan
  h. sulfate
  h. sulfate accumulation
  h. sulfate urine test
heparin
  calcium h.
  h. challenge test
  h. cofactor II (HCII)
  h. cofactor II deficiency
  h. cofactor II inhibitor
  h. embryopathy
  h. lock (hep lock)
  low-dose h.
  low molecular weight h. (LMWH)
  minidose h.
  prophylactic h.
  h. sodium
  unfractionated h.
heparin-binding site mutation
heparin–induced thrombocytopenia (HIT)
heparinization
  therapeutic h.
heparinized
  h. lactated Ringer
  h. saline
heparin-lock flush
heparitinuria
hepatectomy
  left h.
  partial h.
  right h.
  total h.
hepatic
  h. amebiasis
  h. arteriovenous fistula
  h. capillariasis
  h. capsular calcification
  h. cirrhosis
  h. coma
  h. copper
  h. copper overload syndrome
  h. crisis
  h. ductular hypoplasia
  h. ductular hypoplasia-multiple
    malformations syndrome
  h. encephalopathy (HE)
  h. fibrosis
  h. focal nodular hyperplasia
  h. gluconeogenesis
  h. glycogenesis
  h. glycogen storage disease
  h. hemangioma
  h. hematoma
  h. infantilism

h. iron concentration (HIC)
h. lipase deficiency
h. lobe
h. metastasis
h. necrosis
h. neoplasm
h. parenchymal disorder
h. porphyria
h. pregnancy
h. rupture
h. sinusoid
h. transaminase
h. transplantation
h. venous wedge pressure gradient
h. wedged venography

hepatica
    Fasciola h.
hepaticojejunostomy
hepaticus
    fetor h.
hepatis
    bacillary peliosis h.
    peliosis h.
    porta h.
hepatitis
    h. A
    h. A, B immunization
    anicteric h.
    autoimmune chronic acute h.
    h. A vaccine (HAV)
    h. A virus (HAV)
    h. B (HB)
    h. B antigen (HBAg)
    h. B arthritis-dermatitis syndrome
    h. B core antibody (HBcAb)
    h. B early antibody (HBeAb)
    biliary neonatal h.
    h. B immune globulin (HBIG, H-BIG, HBIg)
    h. B oligosaccharide-CRM197 vaccine (HbOC)
    h. B surface antibody (HBsAb)
    h. B surface antigen (HBsAg)
    h. B vaccine (HBV)
    h. B virus (HBV)
    h. C
    chronic active h.
    chronic cryptogenic h. (CCH)
    chronic non-A-E h.
    cryptogenic h.
    h. C virus (HCV, HVC)
    h. D

delta h.
h. D virus (HDV)
h. E
h. E virus (HEV)
fulminant h.
h. F virus (HFV)
h. G
giant cell h.
h. G virus (HGV)
herpes h.
hyperalimentation h.
icteric h.
idiopathic neonatal giant-cell h.
h. immune globulin
infectious h.
maternal h.
neonatal cholestatic h.
non-A h.
non-ABCDE h.
non-A, non-B h. (NANBH)
non-B h.
h. screening
serum h.
toxic h.
viral h.

hepatobiliary
    h. disease
    h. scintigraphy
    h. ultrasonography
hepatoblastoma (HBL)
hepatocellular
    h. carcinoma (HCC)
    h. damage
    h. disease
    h. injury
    h. lysome
hepatoclavicular
hepatocyte
    h. growth factor (HGF)
    h. nuclear factor (HNF)
    pleomorphism of h.
hepatoerythropoietic porphyria (HEP)
hepatofacioneurocardiovertebral syndrome
hepatolenticular degeneration
hepatoma
hepatomegaly
    firm h.
    hard h.
hepatopathy
    sickle h.

NOTES

H

hepatoportoenterostomy
hepatopulmonary syndrome (HPS)
hepatorenal
    h. syndrome
    h. tyrosinemia
hepatosplenic candidiasis
hepatosplenomegaly
hepatotoxicity
    nutritional h.
hepatotoxic syndrome
hepatotoxin
hepatotropic virus
HEPES
    N-[2-hydroxyethyl]piperazine N′-[2-
    ethanesulfonic acid]
HEPES-buffered Ham F10 medium
hep lock
    heparin lock
heptavalent
Heptavax-B
Heptest Xa assay
HER
    HIV Epidemiology Research
    HER Study
HER-2/neu protooncogene
herald
    h. bleed
    h. patch
herb
    moxa h.
herbal
    h. medicine
    h. tea
herbarum
    Cladosporium h.
herbicide
Herbst registry
Herceptin
Hercules
    infant H.
hereditaria
    adynamia episodica h.
    alopecia h.
    anemia hypochromica
      sideroachrestica h.
    arthroophthalmopathia h.
    atrophia bulborum h.
    keratitis fugax h.
    porphyria cutanea tarda h.
hereditary
    h. abductor vocal cord paralysis
    h. agenesis of corpus callosum
    h. angioedema (type I)
    h. areflexic dystasia
    h. autonomic neuropathy
    h. benign chorea
    h. benign intraepithelial dyskeratosis
    syndrome

    h. blepharophimosis, ptosis,
    epicanthus inversus syndrome
    h. bone dysplasia
    h. bullous dystrophy
    h. bullous skin dystrophy, macular
    type
    h. chin trembling
    h. chondrodysplasia
    h. clubbing
    h. coagulopathy
    h. coproporphyria (HCP)
    h. cutaneomandibular polyoncosis
    h. deforming chondrodystrophy
    h. disease
    h. DRPLA
    h. dysplastic nevus syndrome
    h. ectodermal dysplasia
    h. ectodermal polydysplasia
    h. edema
    h. elliptocytosis (HE)
    h. epithelial dysplasia of the
    retinae
    h. erythroblastic multinuclearity
    h. erythroblastic multinuclearity
    with positive acidified serum
    (HEMPAS)
    h. expansile polyostotic osteolytic
    dysplasia
    h. familial congenital nephritis
    h. fructose intolerance
    h. galactosemia
    h. hematuria syndrome
    h. hemochromatosis
    h. hemolytic anemia
    h. hemorrhagic telangiectasia (HHT)
    h. interstitial pyelonephritis
    h. lymphedema
    h. macular epidermolysis bullosa
    h. methemoglobinemia
    h. motor-sensory neuropathy (type
    IA, II–VII) (HMSN)
    h. multiple system hamartomatosis
    h. nephritis deafness, abnormal
    thrombogenesis syndrome
    h. neuropathy with liability to
    pressure palsy (HNPP)
    h. nonpolyposis colorectal cancer
    h. nonspherocytic anemia
    h. oligophrenic cerebellolental
    degeneration
    h. optic neuron atrophy
    h. orotic aciduria
    h. osteoarthrophthalmopathy
    h. osteochondrodysplasia
    h. osteodysplasia with acroosteolysis
    h. ovarian cancer
    h. pancreatitis
    h. paroxysmal ataxia

h. persistence of fetal hemoglobin (HPFH)
h. polytopic enchondral dysostosis
h. progressive arthroophthalmopathy
h. progressive bulbar paralysis with deafness
h. pyropoikilocytosis (HPP)
h. renal adysplasia
h. renal agenesis
h. retinal aplasia
h. retinal dysplasia
h. retinoblastoma
h. retinoschisis
h. sensory autonomic neuropathy
h. sensory radicular neuropathy
h. spastic paraplegia
h. spherocytosis
h. spinal muscular atrophy
h. stomatocytosis
h. thrombophilia
h. trait
h. tremor
h. trichodysplasia
h. tyrosinemia
h. urogenital adysplasia
h. xanthinuria deficiency

heredity
autosomal h.
sex-linked h.
X-linked h.

heredoataxia
heredobiologic
heredoconstitutional disease
heredodegeneration
heredodegenerative
h. disease
h. disorder
heredodiathesis
heredofamilial
heredoimmunity
heredolues (*var. of* heredosyphilis)
heredopathia
h. atactica
h. atactica polyneuritiformis
heredoretinopathia congenitalis
heredosyphilis, heredolues
Hering-Breuer inflation reflex (HBIR)
heritability
heritable coagulopathy
heritage
Ashkenazi Jewish h.

ethnic h.
H. Panel genetic screening test
herkogamy
Herlitz epidermolysis bullosa letalis
Hermansky-Pudlak syndrome
hermaphrodite
hermaphroditism
true h.
XX h.
Hernandez syndrome
hernia
abdominal h.
Bochdalek h.
broad ligament h.
complete h.
congenital diaphragmatic h. (CDH)
contralateral h.
diaphragmatic h.
epigastric h.
femoral h.
foramen of Morgagni h.
groin h.
hiatal h.
immunotherapy h.
incarcerated inguinal h.
incisional h.
incomplete h.
indirect inguinal h.
inguinal h.
h. inguinale
internal h.
labial h.
linea alba h.
lung h.
Morgagni h.
ovary in inguinal h.
paraduodenal h.
paraesophageal hiatal h.
peritoneal h.
Petit h.
pleuroperitoneal h.
port site h.
reducible h.
retrocecal h.
retrosternal h.
Richter h.
h. sac
sliding hiatal h.
spigelian h.
strangulated h.
transmesenteric h.
trocar h.

NOTES

H

hernia *(continued)*
    umbilical h.
    uncomplicated h.
    h. uteri inguinale
    ventral h.
herniated
    h. disc
    h. stomach
    h. viscera
herniation
    brain h.
    brainstem h.
    cerebral h.
    chronic tonsillar h.
    disc h.
    fat h.
    midbrain h.
    muscle h.
    syndrome of uncal h.
    transtentorial h.
    uncal h.
herniorrhaphy
herniotomy
    Petit h.
heroin
Her Option uterine cryoablation therapy system
herpangina
Herp-Check test
herpes
    acute neonatal h.
    h. aseptic meningitis
    cervical h.
    congenital h.
    h. facialis
    geniculate h.
    genital h.
    h. genitalis
    h. gestationis (HG)
    h. gladiatorum
    h. hepatitis
    intrauterine h.
    h. keratitis
    neonatal h.
    h. neonatorum
    ophthalmic h.
    orolabial h.
    perinatal h.
    h. simplex (HS)
    h. simplex encephalitis (HSE)
    h. simplex genitalis (HSG)
    h. simplex labialis
    h. simplex pneumonia
    h. simplex viral conjunctivitis
    h. simplex virus (HSV)
    h. simplex virus 1 (HSV1, HSV-1)
    h. simplex virus 2 (HSV2, HSV-2)
    h. simplex virus encephalitis
    h. simplex virus thymidine kinase gene
    h. stomatitis
    toxoplasmosis, other agents, rubella, cytomegalovirus, h.
    h. virus
    h. virus entry mediator (HVEM)
    h. whitlow infection
    h. zoster
    h. zoster of geniculate ganglion
    h. zoster meningitis
    h. zoster ophthalmicus (HZO)
    h. zoster oticus
    h. zoster virus (HZV)
Herpesviridae
herpesvirus
    h. encephalitis
    h. hominis
    human h. 1–8 (HHV1–8)
    Kaposi sarcoma-associated h.
    H. suis
herpetic
    h. corneal infection
    h. gingivitis
    h. gingivostomatitis
    h. keratitis
    h. keratopathy
    h. stomatitis
    h. whitlow
herpeticum
    eczema h.
herpetiform
    h. aphthous ulcer
    h. corneal ulcer
herpetiformis
    dermatitis h. (DH)
    h. epidermolysis bullosa simplex
    impetigo h.
Herplex Liquifilm
Herrick anemia
herringbone pattern
HERS
    heart and estrogen/progestin replacement study
Hers disease
Herson-Todd score
Herter infantilism
Hertig-Rock ovum
Hertoghe sign
hertz (Hz)
hesitancy
Hespan
Hesselbach triangle
hetacillin
hetastarch solution
heteradelphus
heteralius
heterocephalus
heterochromatic DNA

heterochromatin
heterochromia
    congenital h.
    h. of inner canthus
    h. iridis
    h. of iris
heterochromosome
heterocyclic antidepressant
heterodimer
heterodimeric integral membrane glycoprotein
heterodisomy
    maternal uniparental h.
heteroduplex
    h. analysis
    h. DNA
heterodymus
heterogamete
heterogeneity
    allelic h.
    genetic h.
    locus h.
    loss of h. (LOH)
heterogeneous
heterogenic
heterogenicity
heterograft
heteroinoculation
heterokaryon
heterologous
    h. graft
    h. insemination
    h. surfactant
    h. twins
    h. uterine sarcoma
heteromorphous
heteroovular twin
heteropagus
heterophil, heterophile
    h. antibody
    h. antigen
    h. test
heterophilic
heteroplasmy
heteroploid
heteroprosopus
heterosexual
    h. high risk behavior
    h. precocious puberty
    h. relationship
heterosomal aberration
heterosome

heterotaxia syndrome
heterotaxy
    abdominal h.
    h. syndrome
    visceral h.
heterotopia
    band h.
    bilateral periventricular nodular h.
    focal h.
    gray matter h.
    leptomeningeal h.
    mesodermal h.
    neuroglial h.
    neuronal h.
    periventricular nodular gray matter h.
    subcortical band h.
    subcortical laminar h.
    subependymal h.
heterotopic
    h. gray matter
    h. liver transplantation
    h. pregnancy
heterotropic
    h. chromosome
    h. pregnancies
heterotypic
heterotypical chromosome
heterozygosity
heterozygote
    compound h.
    obligate h.
heterozygous
    h. carrier
    h. familial hypercholesterolemia
Heuser membrane
HEV
    hepatitis E virus
hew mutation
Hexa-Betalin
Hexa-CAF
    hexamethylmelamine, cyclophosphamide, doxorubicin, and 5-fluorouracil
hexacetonide
    triamcinolone h.
hexachloride
    gamma-benzene h.
hexachlorocyclohexane
hexachlorophene
    h. bath
    h. wash

NOTES

H

hexadactyly
postaxial h.
preaxial h.
Hexadrol
H. Phosphate Injection
H. Tablet
Hexalen
Hexalite cast
hexamethonium chloride
hexamethyldislazane (HMDS)
hexamethylmelamine
h., cyclophosphamide, doxorubicin, and 5-fluorouracil (Hexa-CAF)
h. with doxorubicin and cyclophosphamide (HAC)
hexamethyl propylene amine oxime (HMPAO)
HMPAO leukocyte scintigraphy
hexamine
hexaploidy
Hexastat
hexenmilch
hexestrol
Hexit
hexocyclium methylsulfate
hexoprenaline sulfate
hexosamine
hexosaminidase
h. A, B
h. A deficiency
serum h. A
hexose
hexylresorcinol
Heyer-Schulte valve
Heyman capsules
Heyman-Herndon clubfoot procedure
Heyns abdominal decompression apparatus
HF
high frequency
HFA
height-for-age
high-functioning autism
Proventil HFA
HFEA
Human Fertilization and Embryology Authority
HFE gene for hemochromatosis
HFFI
high-frequency flow interruption
HFJ
high-frequency jet
HFJ ventilation
HFJ ventilator
HFJV
high-frequency jet ventilation
HFMD
hand-foot-and-mouth disease

HFO
high-frequency oscillation
high-frequency oscillatory
HFO ventilation
HFO ventilator
HFOV
high-frequency oscillatory ventilation
HFPP
high-frequency positive-pressure
HFPP ventilation
HFPP ventilator
HFPPV
high-frequency positive-pressure ventilation
HFRS
hemorrhagic fever with renal syndrome
hFSH
human follicle-stimulating hormone
HFV
hepatitis F virus
high-frequency ventilation
HG
herpes gestationis
HgA1c
glycosylated hemoglobin
hgb (*var. of* Hb)
HGE
human granulocytic ehrlichiosis
HGF
hepatocyte growth factor
HGH, hGH
human growth hormone
HGPRT
hypoxanthine-phosphoribosyltransferase
HGPRT deficiency
HGSIL
high-grade squamous intraepithelial lesion
HGV
hepatitis G virus
H-H
head-to-head sperm agglutination
HHA
hyposmia-hypogonadotropic hypogonadism
HHEs
hypotonic-hyporesponsive episodes
HHH, triple H
hyperornithemia, hyperammonemia, homocitrulinemia
HHH syndrome
HHHO
hypotonia, hypopigmentia, hypogonadism, obesity
HHHO syndrome
HHS
Hoyeraal-Hreidarsson syndrome
HHT
hereditary hemorrhagic telangiectasia

HHV1–8
    human herpesvirus 1–8
HI
    H. antibody
    H. titer
HI-30
    bikinin
HIA
    hemagglutination inhibition antibody
5-HIAA
    5-hydroxyindoleacetic acid
21-HIAA
    21-hydroxyindoleacetic acid
hiatal hernia
hiatus
    diaphragmatic h.
    esophageal h.
    h. hernia, microcephaly, nephrosis syndrome
    h. leukemicus
    urogenital h.
HIB
    Haemophilus influenzae type b
    hypoxia, intussusception, brain mass
Hib
    H. conjugate vaccine
    H. polysaccharide vaccine
Hibiclens
Hibistat
HibTITER
    Acel-Imune H.
    H. vaccine
HIC
    hepatic iron concentration
hiccup, hiccough
    fetal h.
hickey
Hicks version
Hi-Cor-1.0, -2.5 Topical
hidden
    h. penis
    h. rheumatoid factor
    h. testis
hidradenitis suppurativa
hidradenoma
    clear cell h.
    eruptive h.
    papillary h.
hidrotic ectodermal dysplasia
HIE
    hypoxic-ischemic encephalopathy

HIFT
    high-frequency ventilation trial
high
    h. airway obstruction syndrome
    h. altitude perinatal mortality
    h. annular testis
    h. arch foot
    h. bladder pressure
    h. fetal order
    h. forceps
    h. forceps delivery
    h. frequency (HF)
    h. frontal bone
    h. gastrin level
    h. guard
    h. hymenal opening
    h. imperforate anus
    h. intrauterine insemination
    h. McCall culdoplasty
    h. molecular weight (HMW)
    h. molecular weight kininogen (HMWK)
    h. myopia
    h. output
    h. oxygen percentage (HOPE)
    h. oxygen percentage in retinopathy of prematurity (HOPE-ROP)
    h. pain threshold
    h. power field (hpf)
    h. risk
    h. scrotal testis
    h. stirrups
    h. tone
    h. urogenital sinus
    h. uterosacral ligament suspension
high-affinity hemoglobin
high-altitude
    h.-a. cerebral edema (HACE)
    h.-a. pulmonary edema (HAPE)
high-arched palate
high-caloric density formula
high-calorie
    h.-c. diet
    h.-c. formula
high-contrast Bucky imaging
high-density lipoprotein (HDL)
high-dose
    h.-d. chemotherapy
    h.-d. chemotherapy with autologous bone marrow transplantation (HDC-ABMT)
high-efficiency particulate air (HEPA)

NOTES

H

higher-dose
  h.-d. therapy
  h.-d. therapy with epinephrine (HDE)
higher-order
  h.-o. birth
  h.-o. gestation
high-fiber diet
high-flow
  h.-f. nasal cannula
  h.-f. nonrebreather
high-frequency
  h.-f. flow interruption (HFFI)
  h.-f. hearing loss
  h.-f. jet (HFJ)
  h.-f. jet ventilation (HFJV)
  h.-f. oscillation (HFO)
  h.-f. oscillator
  h.-f. oscillatory (HFO)
  h.-f. oscillatory ventilation (HFOV)
  h.-f. positive-pressure (HFPP)
  h.-f. positive-pressure ventilation (HFPPV)
  h.-f. ventilation (HFV)
  h.-f. ventilation trial (HIFT)
  h.-f. ventilator
high-fructose formula
high-functioning autism (HFA)
high-glucose formula
high-grade
  h.-g. cervical dysplasia
  h.-g. squamous intraepithelial lesion (HGSIL, HSIL)
high-intensity click stimulus
highly
  h. active antiretroviral therapy (HAART)
  h. purified factor IX
  h. purified FSH
high-oscillation ventilator
high-output failure
high-performance
  h.-p. capillary electrophoresis (HPCE)
  h.-p. liquid chromatography (HPLC)
high-phosphate diet
high-pitched
  h.-p. bowel sounds
  h.-p. cry
  h.-p. voice
  h.-p. wheeze
high-power liquid chromatography (HPLC)
high-pressure liquid chromatography (HPLC)
high-resolution
  h.-r. banding
  h.-r. chest computed tomography
  h.-r. computed tomography (HRCT)

  h.-r. ultrasonography
  h.-r. ultrasound
high-riding prostate
high-risk
  h.-r. infant
  h.-r. mother
  h.-r. obstetrician
  h.-r. patient
  h.-r. pregnancy
  h.-r. pregnancy assessment
  h.-r. register (HRR)
high-tone hearing loss
high-voltage slow activity (HVSA)
Higoumenakis sign
hilar
  h. cell hyperplasia
  h. cell pathology
  h. cell tumor
  h. dance
  h. lymphadenopathy
  h. region
Hildebrandt uterine hemostatic forceps
Hilgenreiner line
Hillis-DeLee fetoscope
Hillis-Müller maneuver
hilus cell tumor
hindbrain
hindfoot
  h. fracture
  h. valgus
  h. valgus deformity
hindgut
hindwaters
hinge
  knee h.
hinged spring diaphragm
Hinman syndrome
Hinton test
hip
  h. adduction release
  h. bone density
  h. click
  h. clunk
  congenital dislocated h. (CDH)
  congenital dislocation of h. (CDH)
  h. deformity
  developmental displacement of h. (DDH)
  developmental dysplasia of h. (DDH)
  dislocated h.
  h. dysplasia
  h. fracture
  incongruent h.
  irritable h.
  neurogenic dysplasia of h. (NDH)
  nonspherical congruent h.'s
  observation h.
  h. pointer

h. rotation
h. rotation test
snapping h.
spherical congruent h.'s
h. spica cast
subluxed h.
transient marrow edema syndrome
of the h. (TMES)
hip-knee-ankle angle
hip-knee-ankle-foot orthosis (HKAFO)
hippocampal
h. neuron
h. pathologic injury
h. sclerosis
hippocampus
hippocratic nail
hippurate
methenamine h.
hippus
respiratory h.
Hiprex
Hirschberg
H. corneal reflex test
H. light reflex test
hirschfeldii
Salmonella h.
Hirschsprung
H. colitis
H. disease
H. disease, microcephaly, mental
retardation, characteristic facies
syndrome
H. enterocolitis
Hirst placental forceps
hirsute woman
hirsutism
h., androgen excess, insulin
resistance, acanthosis nigricans
(HAIR-AN, HAIRAN)
constitutional h.
drug-induced h.
familial h.
hormonal h.
idiopathic h.
male-pattern h.
moderate h.
postmenopausal h.
h., skeletal dysplasia, mental
retardation syndrome
hirudin
His
angle of H.

bundle of H.
gastroesophageal angle of H.
H. rule
Hispanic
His-Purkinje system
Histadyl
Histalet Forte Tablet
histaminase
histamine
h. 1 (H_1)
h. 2 (H_2)
h. 1 antihistamine
h. fish poisoning
h. interleukin
Histantil
Histatan
histidase
histidine
histidinemia
histidinuria
histiocyte
Gaucher-type h.
sea-blue h.
histiocytic
h. disorder
h. fibroma
h. lymphoma
histiocytoid cardiomyopathy
histiocytoma
malignant fibrous h. (MFH)
histiocytosis
acute disseminated h.
acute disseminated h. X
Langerhans cell h. (LCH)
malignant h.
sinus h.
h. X
histochemical
histocompatibility
h. gene
h. locus antigen
maternal-fetal h.
histocytic necrotizing lymphadenitis
Histofreezer cryosurgical system
histogenesis
histoimmunological origin
histoincompatibility
maternal-fetal h.
histologic
h. abnormality
h. architecture
h. chorioamnionitis

NOTES

H

429

histologic *(continued)*
- h. classification
- h. diagnosis
- h. placental inflammation
- h. sampling

histology
- endometrial h.
- proliferative h.
- Shimada h.
- Shimada-Chatten h.

histolytica
- *Entamoeba h.*

histomorphometry

histone
- h. antigen
- h. H1 kinase

histopathological
- h. diagnosis
- h. finding
- h. grading
- h. study

histopathology

Histoplasma capsulatum

histoplasmosis
- chronic pulmonary h.
- disseminated h.
- infantile disseminated h.
- pulmonary h.

history
- climacteric h.
- contraceptive h.
- family h.
- genetic h.
- gynecologic h.
- menstrual h.
- obstetric h.
- occupational h.
- personal hygiene h.
- prenatal h.
- h. of present illness (HPI)
- reproductive h.
- sexual h.
- sudden infant death unexplained by h.
- urologic h.

histrelin acetate

Histussin NC

HIT
- heparin–induced thrombocytopenia

Hitachi
- H. EUB 420 digital ultrasound
- H. EUB 405 imaging system
- H. UB 420 digital ultrasound system

hitchhiker's thumb

Hitzig girdle

HIV
- human immunodeficiency virus
- HIV classification

HIV Classification for Children (P0, P1, P2)
- HIV Epidemiology Research (HER)
- HIV infected
- HIV infection
- HIV microangiopathy
- HIV test

HIV-1
- human immunodeficiency virus-1
- HIV-1 p24 antigen
- HIV-1 RNA PCR assay

HIVAGEN test

HIV-associated nephropathy

Hi-Vegi-Lip

hives

Hivid

HIVIG
- human immunodeficiency virus immunoglobulin

hiving

HIV-seropositive

HKAFO
- hip-knee-ankle-foot orthosis
- Rochester HKAFO

HL
- heel lance
- humerus length

HLA
- human leukocyte antigen
- HLA-A3
- HLA-B
- HLA-B14,DR1
- HLA-DR
- HLA typing

HLA-A10

HLA-B27 antigen

HLA-B5/B51

HLA-B27-positive

HLA-compatible fetus

HLA-DR7

HLA-DRw11

HLA-DRw53

HLA-identical
- HLA-i. haploidentical bone marrow stem cell
- HLA-i. marrow graft

HLA-matched platelet transfusion

HLA-mismatch

HLHS
- hypoplastic left heart syndrome

HLI
- human leukocyte interferon

HLL
- hypoplasia of left heart

HLP
- hyperlipoproteinemia

HM
- hemifacial microsomia

HMB
    hydroxy beta methylbutyrate
HMC
    hypertelorism, microtia, clefting
        HMC syndrome
HMD
    hyaline membrane disease
        neonatal HMD
HMDS
    hexamethyldislazane
HME
    human monocytic ehrlichiosis
HMF
    human milk fortifier
HMG
        HMG aciduria
hMG
    human menopausal gonadotropin
        HMG aciduria
        hMG/IUI
HMO
    health maintenance organization
HMPAO
    hexamethyl propylene amine oxime
        HMPAO leukocyte scintigraphy
HMS Liquifilm
HMSN
    hereditary motor-sensory neuropathy
        (type IA, II–VII)
HMW
    high molecular weight
        HMW dextran
HMWK
    high molecular weight kininogen
        HMWK deficiency
        HMWK factor
HN
HNF
    hepatocyte nuclear factor
HNPP
    hereditary neuropathy with liability to
        pressure palsy
HNU
    human *neu* unit
HOA
    hypertrophic osteoarthropathy
hoarding
    fecal h.
hoarse
        h. cry
        h. voice

hoarseness
    excessive h.
hobnail cell
Hoboken
        fold of H.
        H. gemmule
        H. nodule
HOBT
    hyperbaric oxygen therapy
hockey stick incision
Hodge
        H. forceps
        H. maneuver
        H. pessary
Hodgkin
        H. disease
        H. lymphoma
Hoehne sign
HOF
    human oviduct fluid
Hofbauer cell
Hoffer procedure
Hoffmann
        H. clamp
        H. reflex
Hogben test
Hogness box
Hohn catheter
HO inhibitor
holandric
        h. gene
        h. inheritance
holarctica
        Francisella tularensis subspecies h.
hold
        H. DM
        h. technique
holder
        Cameco syringe h.
        Dale Foley catheter h.
        needle h.
holding
        breath h.
        h. chamber
hole
        h. in heart
        Murphy h.
holiday
        drug h.
        weekend drug h.
Holinger
        H. infant bougie

NOTES

H

431

Holinger *(continued)*
    H. infant bronchoscope
    H. infant esophageal speculum
    H. infant esophagoscope
    H. infant laryngoscope
Hollingshead 5-factor index
Hollister collecting device
hollow
    h. of sacrum
    h. viscera
Holmes heart
holmium:yttrium-aluminum-garnet
  (Ho:YAG)
holoacardius
holoacranial
holoblastic ovum
holocarboxylase (HCS)
    h. synthetase
    h. synthetase deficiency
holocrine sebaceous gland
hologastroschisis
Hologic
    H. 1000 QDR densitometer
    H. 1000 QDR dual-energy
      absorptiometer
hologynic inheritance
holoprosencephalic proboscis
holoprosencephaly (HPE)
    alobar h.
    h. anomalad
    familial alobar h.
    lobar h.
    semilobar h.
holorachischisis
holosphere
    cerebral h.
holosystolic murmur
holovisceral
Holtain height stadiometer
Holter monitor
Holt-Oram
    H.-O. atriodigital dysplasia
    H.-O. syndrome
Holzgreve syndrome
Homans sign
homatropine
HOME
    Home Observation for the Measurement
    of the Environment
      HOME scale
home
    h. antibiotic infusion therapy
    h. birth
    h. blood glucose monitoring
    h. cardiorespiratory monitor
      (HCRM)
    h. care service
    h. cognitive score
    h. conservative management

    h. factor
    h. management
    H. Observation for the
      Measurement of the Environment
      (HOME)
    h. oxygen
    h. parenteral nutrition (HPN)
    h. pregnancy test
    h. uterine activity monitor
      (HUAM)
    h. uterine activity monitoring
      (HUAM)
    h. uterine monitoring (HUM)
homemade formula
homeobox (HOX)
    h. 2 gene
    short stature h. (SHOX)
homeopathy
homeostasis
    bacterial h.
    body h.
    carbohydrate h.
    cardiorespiratory h.
    copper h.
    fluid h.
    thermal h.
homeostatic lag
homeothermy
    servocontrolled h.
homeotic genes
Homer Wright rosette
homicide
    intimate partner h.
hominis
    Blastocystis h.
    herpesvirus h.
    Mycoplasma h.
    Poliovirus h.
homochronous inheritance
homocitrulinemia
    hyperornithemia,
      hyperammonemia, h. (HHH, triple
      H)
homocitrullinemia
homocysteine loading test
homocystine
homocystinemia
homocystinuria
homoduplex DNA
homogamete
homogeneity
    tissue h.
homogeneous
homogenize
homograft conduit
homokaryon
homolateral weakness
homolog, homologue
    DAZL1 autosomal h.

HomoloGene
homologous
    h. chromosome
    h. disease
    h. insemination
    h. recombination
    h. surfactant
    h. uterine sarcoma
homologue (*var. of* homolog)
homology
homonymous hemianopia
homophilic
homoplasmy
    mutant h.
homosexuality
homothermic
homotropic inheritance
homotypic
homovanillic acid (HVA)
homozygosity for hemoglobin S (HbSS)
homozygote
homozygous
    h. achondroplasia
    h. familial hypercholesterolemia
    h. glucose-6-phosphate
      dehydrogenase deficiency
    h. hemoglobin E
    h. hyperlipidemia (type I, II)
    h. sickle cell anemia
    h. thalassemia
honei
    Rickettsia h.
honeybee allergy
honeycombed appearance
honeycomb lung
honey-crusted plaque
honeymoon cystitis
Honvol
hood
    clitoral h.
    dorsal h.
    h. mist
    h. O$_2$
    h. oxygen
    oxygen h.
    Oxy-Hood oxygen h.
    H. procedure
    Rock-Mulligan h.
    vaginal h.
hook
    Mayo h.

    tenaculum h.
    h. traction technique
hookworm
    h. disease
    h. infection
Hootnick-Holmes syndrome
HOP
    hypothalamic-pituitary-ovarian
    hypothyroxinemia of prematurity
HOPE
    health, osteoporosis, progestin, estrogen
    high oxygen percentage
      Women's HOPE
hopelessness
Hope resuscitation bag
HOPE-ROP
    high oxygen percentage in retinopathy of
      prematurity
      HOPE-ROP study
Hopkins
    H. symptom checklist
    H. syndrome
hopping
    bunny h.
hora somni (at bedtime)
hordeolum, pl. **hordeola**
    external h.
    internal h.
Horizon 2000
horizon
    Streeter h.
horizontal
    h. nystagmus
    h. saccadic gaze paresis
    h. supranuclear gaze palsy
    h. suspension
    h. suspension in newborn
    h. transmission
    h. transmission of virus
Hormodendrum
hormonal
    h. abnormality
    h. antineoplastic therapy
    h. balance change
    h. contraceptive
    h. effect
    h. emergency contraception
    h. environment
    h. hirsutism
    h. implant
    h. level
    h. manipulation

NOTES

H

hormonal *(continued)*
    h. pregnancy test tablet
    h. treatment
hormone
    adrenal androgen-stimulating h. (AASH)
    adrenocortical h.
    adrenocorticotropic h. (ACTH)
    alpha-melanocyte-stimulating h. (alpha-MSH)
    antenatal thyrotropin releasing h.
    anterior pituitary-like h.
    antidiuretic h. (ADH)
    antimüllerian h. (AMH)
    h. assay
    atrial natriuretic h.
    bioactive h.
    calcitropic h.
    cancer and steroid h. (CASH)
    h. chemoprevention
    chorionic gonadotropic h.
    chorionic growth h.
    circulating h.
    h. complex receptor
    cortical androgen-stimulating h. (CASH)
    corticotropin-releasing h. (CRH)
    h. deficiency
    endogenous h.
    exogenous h.
    fetal h.
    follicle stimulating h.
    follicle-stimulating h. (FSH)
    Genentech biosynthetic human growth h.
    gonadotropin-releasing h. (GnRH, GRH)
    growth h. (GH)
    growth h.-releasing hormone (GH-RH)
    human chorionic adrenocorticotropic h.
    human follicle-stimulating h. (hFSH)
    human growth h. (HGH, hGH)
    human urinary follicle-stimulating h. (hu-FSH)
    Humatrope growth h.
    hypothalamic luteinizing hormone-releasing h.
    inappropriate antidiuretic h. (IADH)
    LATS h.
    luteinizing h. (LH)
    luteinizing hormone-releasing h. (LH-RH)
    lutein-stimulating h. (LSH)
    luteotropic h.
    melanocyte-stimulating h.
    müllerian inhibiting h. (MIH)
    ovarian h.
    parathyroid h. (PTH)
    peptide h.
    pituitary h.
    placental h.
    placental growth h. (PGH)
    pregnancy h.
    purified h.
    recombinant follicle stimulating h. (rFSH)
    recombinant human growth h. (rhGH)
    h. replacement therapy (HRT)
    serum parathyroid h.
    sex h.
    Somatrem growth h.
    Somatropin growth h.
    steroid h.
    syndrome of inappropriate secretion of antidiuretic h. (SIADH)
    h. therapy
    thyroid h.
    thyroid-stimulating h. (TSH)
    thyrotropic h.
    thyrotropin releasing h. (TRH)
    tropic h.
    urinary-derived human follicle-stimulating h. (u-hFSH)
    urinary luteinizing h. (uLH)
hormone-producing neoplasm
hormone-receptor complex internalization
hormone-secreting tumor
hormone-stimulated endometrial change
hormonogenesis
hormonotherapy
horn
    h. cell disease
    entrapped temporal h.
    frontal h.
    fused frontal h.
    iliac h.
    noncommunicating uterine h.
    rudimentary uterine h.
    uterine h.
    h. of uterus
Horner syndrome
hornet sting
horse-riding stance
horseshoe
    h. fibrosis
    h. kidney
    h. placenta
HOS
    hypoosmotic swelling
hospice care
hospital
    H. Recliner seat
    H. for Sick Children (HSC)
    h. stabilization

St. Jude Research H.
tertiary referral h.
Texas Scottish Rite H. (TSRH)
hospitalization
antepartum h.
prolonged delivery h.
hospitalized
h. attempted suicide (HAS)
h. bed rest
host
h. defense mechanism
h. response mechanism
hot
h. biopsy
h. biopsy forceps
h. cross bun skull
h. flash
h. flush
h. knife conization
h. nodule
h. potato voice
h. tub folliculitis
hotline center
Hottentot apron
hour
cubic centimeter per h. (cc/hr)
h. of sleep
Sudafed 12 H.
24-hour
Claritin-D 24-H.
24-h. urinary free cortisol
24-h. urine collection
hourglass
h. configuration
h. head
h. uterus
1-hour glucose challenge test
8-hour polysomnography
hour-specific total serum bilirubin
72-hour stool collection
house dust mite
household
housekeeping gene
housemaid's knee
Howell biopsy aspiration needle
Howell-Jolly body
HOX
homeobox
HOX A gene
Hoxa5 null mutant

Ho:YAG
holmium:yttrium-aluminum-garnet
Ho:YAG laser
Hoyeraal-Hreidarsson syndrome (HHS)
HP
Ku-Zyme HP
Profasi HP
H.P.
H.P. Acthar Gel
Mission Prenatal H.P.
HPA
human pancreatic amylase
hypothalamic-pituitary-adrenal
hypothalamic-pituitary axis
HPA axis
HPA dysfunction
HPCE
high-performance capillary
electrophoresis
HPE
holoprosencephaly
hpf
high power field
HPFH
hereditary persistence of fetal
hemoglobin
HPH
hypoxia-induced pulmonary hypertension
HPI
history of present illness
hPL, HPL
human placental lactogen
HPLC
high-performance liquid chromatography
high-power liquid chromatography
high-pressure liquid chromatography
HPN
home parenteral nutrition
HPO
HPO axis
HPP
hereditary pyropoikilocytosis
HPS
hepatopulmonary syndrome
hypertrophic pyloric stenosis
HPV
Haemophilus pertussis vaccine
human papillomavirus
human parvovirus
HPV B19
HPV E7 gene
HPV type 16 capsid antibody

NOTES

435

HPV-associated lesion
HR
    heart rate
H-*ras*
       H-*ras* oncogene
       H-*ras* p21 protein
HRCT
    high-resolution computed tomography
HRHS
    hypoplastic right heart syndrome
HRIG
    human rabies immune globulin
HRQOL
    health-related quality of life
       HRQOL assessment
       HRQOL questionnaire
HRR
    haplotype relative risk
    high-risk register
HRSA
    heart rate power spectral analysis
HRT
    hormone replacement therapy
       estrogen-only HRT
HRV
    heart rate variability
HS
    habitual snoring
    herpes simplex
    hysterosalpingography
       Estratest HS
HSAS
    hydrocephalus due to congenital stenosis
      of aqueduct of Sylvius
HSC
    hematopoietic stem cell
    Hospital for Sick Children
       HSC Scale
HSD2
    hydroxysteroid dehydrogenase type 2
HSE
    herpes simplex encephalitis
H/S Elliptosphere catheter set
HSES
    hemorrhagic shock and encephalopathy
      syndrome
HSG
    herpes simplex genitalis
    hysterosalpingogram
    hysterosalpingography
       HSG tray
HSI
    human seminal (plasma) inhibitor
HSIL
    high-grade squamous intraepithelial
      lesion
HSP
    Henoch-Schönlein purpura
HS-tk gene therapy

HSV
    herpes simplex virus
HSV1, HSV-1
    herpes simplex virus 1
HSV2, HSV-2
    herpes simplex virus 2
       HSV2 proctitis
H-T
    head-to-tail sperm agglutination
HTLV
    human T-cell leukemia virus
HTLV-I
    human T-cell lymphotropic virus type I
       HTLV-I associated
         myelopathy/tropical spastic
         paraparesis (HAM/TSP)
HTLV-II
    human T-cell lymphotropic virus type II
HTP
    hypothalamic, pituitary, thyroid
5-HTT
       serotonin transporter 5-HTT
H-type
       H-t. tracheoesophageal fistula
       H-t. transesophageal fistula
HUAM
    home uterine activity monitor
    home uterine activity monitoring
huang
       ma h.
HuCV
    human calicivirus
Hudson
       H. prongs
       H. T Up-Draft II disposable
       nebulizer
hue
       blue scleral h.
       purple h.
       violaceous h.
       white scleral h.
huffing
Huffman
       H. adolescent speculum
       H. vaginal speculum
       H. vaginoscope
hu-FSH
    human urinary follicle-stimulating
      hormone
HuGE
    Human Gene Expression
    Human Genome Expression
       HuGE index
HuGENET
    Human Genome Epidemiology Network
Hughes syndrome
Huguier circle
Huhner-Sims test
Huhner test

HUI
>Harris uterine injector
>HUI Mini-Flex

Hulka-Clemens clip

Hulka clip

HUM
>home uterine monitoring

hum
>benign venous h.
>cervical venous h.
>venous h.

Humalog
>H. insulin lispro injection
>H. Pen

human
>h. antihemophilic factor
>h. artificial chromosome (HAC)
>h. astrovirus type 1 (HAstV-1)
>h. bite
>h. calicivirus (HuCV)
>h. chorionic adrenocorticotropic hormone
>h. chorionic gonadotropin (hCG, HCG)
>h. chorionic gonadotropin level
>h. diploid cell rabies vaccine (HDCV)
>h. diploid cell vaccine
>h. embryo fibroblast (HEF)
>h. endothelial cell (HEC)
>h. epidermal growth factor-2 oncogene
>h. EP1 receptor
>h. erythropoietin
>h. factor IX complex
>H. Fertilization and Embryology Authority (HFEA)
>h. figure drawing
>H. Figure Drawing Test
>h. follicle-stimulating hormone (hFSH)
>H. Gene Expression (HuGE)
>h. gene therapy
>h. genetics
>H. Genome Epidemiology Network (HuGENET)
>H. Genome Expression (HuGE)
>H. Genome Project
>h. granulocytic ehrlichiosis (HGE)
>h. growth hormone (HGH, hGH)
>h. health and behavior questionnaire (HBQ)

>h. herpesvirus 1–8 (HHV1–8)
>h. immune globulin
>h. immunodeficiency virus (HIV)
>h. immunodeficiency virus-1 (HIV-1)
>h. immunodeficiency virus encephalopathy
>h. immunodeficiency virus immunoglobulin (HIVIG)
>h. immunodeficiency virus infected children
>Insulatard NPH h.
>h. insulin
>h. insulin-induced lipoatrophy
>h. jagged-1 gene (JAG1)
>h. leukocyte antigen (HLA)
>h. leukocyte antigen-associated disorder
>h. leukocyte interferon (HLI)
>h. lymphocyte antigen-locus DR
>h. menopausal gonadotropin (hMG)
>h. milk
>h. milk-fed
>h. milk fortifier (HMF)
>h. monocytic ehrlichiosis (HME)
>Nabi-HB hepatitis B immune globulin h.
>h. neutrophil collagenase
>h. *neu* unit (HNU)
>h. oviduct fluid (HOF)
>h. ovum fertilization test
>h. pancreatic amylase (HPA)
>h. papillomavirus (HPV)
>h. papovavirus BK
>h. parvovirus (HPV)
>h. parvovirus arthropathy
>h. placental lactogen (hPL, HPL)
>h. rabies immune globulin (HRIG)
>h. recombinant antioxidant enzyme
>h. recombinant DNase
>h. scabies
>h. seminal (plasma) inhibitor (HSI)
>h. sperm cytosolic factor
>h. T-cell leukemia virus (HTLV)
>h. T-cell leukemia virus type I, II, III
>h. T-cell lymphotrophic virus type I associated myelopathy (HAM)
>h. T-cell lymphotropic virus 1 tropic meloneuropathy
>h. T-cell lymphotropic virus type I (HTLV-I)

NOTES

H

437

human *(continued)*
    h. T-cell lymphotropic virus type II (HTLV-II)
    h. urinary follicle-stimulating hormone (hu-FSH)
    Velosulin H.
humanus
    Pediculus h.
Humate-P
Humatin
Humatrope
    H. growth hormone
    H. Injection
HumatroPen
Humegon
humeroperoneal muscular dystrophy
humeroradial synostosis
humerus length (HL)
HUMI
    Harris-Kronner uterine manipulator-injector
    HUMI catheter
Humibid L.A.
humidification
    h. therapy
    h. ventilator
humidified
    h. air
    h. isolette
humidifier
    bubbler h.
    cool-mist h.
    Ohio h.
humid stertor
humor
    aqueous h.
    vitreous h.
humoral
    h. antibody
    h. antibody deficiency
    h. factor
    h. immune system
    h. immunity
    h. immunodeficiency
hump
    buffalo h.
    dowager's h.
    dromedary h.
    rib h.
Humulin
    H. 50/50
    H. 70/30
    H. L, N, R, U
    H. Pen
Hünermann disease
Hünermann-Happle syndrome
hunger
    air h.
    unusual h.

Hunner
    H. interstitial cystitis
    H. ulcer
Hunt bipolar forceps
Hunter
    H. canal
    H. syndrome
Hunter-Fraser syndrome
Hunter-Hurler phenotype
hunterian chancre
Hunter-MacMurray syndrome
Hunter-McAlpine craniosynostosis syndrome
Huntington
    H. chorea
    H. disease (HD)
    polyglutamine-expanded H.
Hunt-Reich cannula
Hurler
    H. disease
    H. syndrome
    H. variant
Hurler-like
    H.-l. facial appearance
    H.-l. syndrome
Hurler-Pfaundler syndrome
Hurler-Scheie syndrome
hurry
    intestinal h.
Hurst syndrome
Hürthle cell
Hurwitz catheter
HUS
    hemolytic uremic syndrome
husband
    artificial insemination by h. (AIH)
    therapeutic insemination, h. (THI, TIH)
HUT
    head-up tilt
Hutch diverticulum
Hutchinson
    H. incisor
    H. sign
    H. syndrome
    H. teeth
    H. triad
Hutchinson-Gilford syndrome
hutchinsonian molar
Hutinel disease
Hutterite cerebroosteonephrodysplasia
HUVS
    hypocomplementemic urticarial vasculitis syndrome
Huxley respirator
HV
    height velocity
HVA
    homovanillic acid

HVC
  hepatitis C virus
HVEM
  herpes virus entry mediator
HVL
  half-value layer
HVSA
  high-voltage slow activity
hyaline
  h. body
  h. cast
  h. eosinophilic inclusion
  h. membrane
  h. membrane disease (HMD)
  h. membrane syndrome
  h. myoma degeneration
hyalinosis
  h. cutis et mucosae
  infantile system h.
hyaluronic acid factor
hyaluronidase factor
H-Y antigen
Hyate:C
Hybolin
  H. Decanoate
  H. Improved
hybrid Capture DNA Assay
  somatic h.
hybridization
  allele-specific oligonucleotide h.
  colorimetric reverse dot blot h.
  comparative genomic h. (CGH)
  DNA h.
  dot-blot h.
  fluorescent in situ h. (FISH)
  genomic in situ h.
  multispectral fluorescent in situ h.
    (M-FISH)
  nucleic acid h.
  papillomavirus h.
  polar body in-situ h.
  prenatal interphase fluorescence in
    situ h.
  reverse dot blot h.
  in situ nucleic acid h.
hybridoma technique
hybridus
  Petasites h.
Hybritech
Hycamtin
hyclate
  doxycycline h.

Hycodan
Hycort Topical
HYCX
  hydrocephalus due to congenital stenosis
    of aqueduct of Sylvius
hydantoin syndrome
hydatid
  h. cyst
  h. cyst of Morgagni
  h. disease
  h. mole
  h. polyp
  h. pregnancy
hydatidiform
  h. change
  h. mole
hydatidosis
  alveolar h.
Hyde-Forster syndrome
Hyderm
hydermia
hydradenitis suppurativa
hydralazine
hydramnios, hydramnion
  idiopathic h.
hydranencephaly
hydrate
  chloral h.
hydration
  intravenous h.
  maternal h.
hydraulic UF
hydrazide
  isonicotinic acid h. (INH)
hydrazine sulfate
Hydrea
  Droxia H.
hydremica
hydrencephalocele
hydrencephalomeningocele
hydriodic acid
hydroa
  h. aestivale
  h. gestationis
  h. puerorum
  h. vacciniforme
hydroalcoholic
hydrocarbon
  aliphatic h.
  halogenated h.
  h. pneumonia

NOTES

H

hydrocele
    abdominoscrotal h.
    h. feminae
    h. fluid
    Maunoir h.
    h. muliebris
    Nuck h.
    owl's eyes view of h.
    transitory h.
hydrocelectomy
hydrocephalic
    h. brain swelling
    h. idiocy
    h. lissencephaly
hydrocephalocele
hydrocephaloid disease
hydrocephalus, hydrocephaly
    acquired h.
    acute h.
    h. agyria, retinal dysplasia (HARD)
    h. agyria, retinal dysplasia with or
      without encephalocele (HARD+/-E)
    arrested h.
    benign external h.
    chronic h.
    communicating h.
    compensated h.
    corpus callosum hypoplasia,
      retardation, adducted thumbs,
      spastic paraparesis, h. (CRASH)
    h. due to congenital stenosis of
      aqueduct of Sylvius (HSAS,
      HYCX)
    external h.
    h. ex vacuo
    h. internus
    LICAM gene for X-linked h.
    new-onset h.
    noncommunicating h.
    normal pressure h. (NPH)
    obstructive h.
    otitic h.
    permanent posthemorrhagic h.
    posthemorrhagic h. (PHH)
    shunt-dependent h.
    shunted h.
    h., skeletal anomalies, mental
      disturbances syndrome
    symptomatic progressive h.
    uncompensated h.
    h. with features of VATER
    X-linked h.
hydrocephalus-cerebellar agenesis
  syndrome
Hydrocet
Hydro-chlor
hydrochloride (HCl)
    arginine h.
    Aventyl H.

betaine h.
bupropion h.
buspirone h.
butriptyline h.
cetirizine h.
chlorcyclizine h.
ciprofloxacin h.
clomipramine h.
clonidine h.
cyclopentolate h.
cycrimine h.
cyproheptadine h.
cysteine h.
dicyclomine h.
dihydromorphinone h.
dobutamine h.
dopamine h.
doxapram h.
doxorubicin h.
esmolol h.
ethopropazine h.
fluoxetine h.
guanfacine h.
imipramine h.
isoprenaline h.
levalbuterol h.
loperamide h.
mechlorethamine h.
meclizine h.
mefloquine h.
meperidine h.
mepivacaine h.
methacycline h.
methadone h.
methamphetamine h.
methdilazine h.
methixene h.
methoxamine h.
methylphenidate h.
metoclopramide h.
mitoxantrone h.
Mustargen H.
naftifine h.
naloxone h.
nortriptyline h.
nylidrin h.
olopatadine h.
opipramol h.
OROS methylphenidate h.
paroxetine h.
phenazopyridine h.
piperidolate h.
proguanil h.
promethazine h.
propranolol h.
pseudoephedrine h.
quinacrine h.
ranitidine h.
ritodrine h.

ropivacaine h.
sertraline h.
sulfamethoxazole/phenazopyridine h.
sulfisoxazole/phenazopyridine h.
tetracycline h.
thioridazine h.
thiphenamil h.
tolazoline h.
topotecan h.
trifluoperazine h.
triflupromazine h.
trimethobenzamide h.
tripelennamine h.
triprolidine h.
valacyclovir h.
vancomycin h.
venlafaxine h.
hydrochlorothiazide (HCTZ)
h. and spironolactone
Hydrocil
hydrocodone and acetaminophen
hydrocolloid
hydrocolpocele
hydrocolpos
hydrocortisone
Bactine H.
h. base
h. butyrate
h. cypionate
neomycin (bacitracin), polymyxin
B, h.
h. sodium succinate
h. valerate
Hydrocortone
H. Acetate Injection
H. Oral
H. Phosphate Injection
Hydrocort Topical
hydrocystoma
apocrine h.
vulvar apocrine h.
hydrodensitometry
hydrodissection
HydroDIURIL
hydroflotation
hydroflumethiazide
hydrogel dressing
hydrogen
h. bond
h. breath test
h. in concentration (pH)
h. peroxide

h. peroxide enema
h. peroxide-producing lactobacillus
h. pump inhibitor
Hydrogesic
hydrolase
fumarylacetoacetate h. (FAH)
hydrolethalus syndrome
hydrolysate
casein h.
h. formula
milk protein h. (MPH)
protein h.
hydrolysis
enzymic acid h.
steroid conjugate h.
hydrolysis-resistant
hydrolyzed
h. cow's milk
h. feeding
h. premature formula
h. protein
h. whey
hydroma (*var. of* hygroma)
hydromeningocele
hydrometra
hydrometrocolpos
hydromicrocephaly
hydromorphone
hydromphalus
hydromucocolpos
hydromyelia
hydromyelocele
hydromyelomeningocele
hydronephrocolpos, postaxialpolydactyly, congenital heart disease syndrome
hydronephrosis
congenital h.
fetal h.
intermittent h.
perinatal h.
prenatal h.
progressive h.
unilateral neonatal h.
hydronephrotic kidney
hydroparasalpinx
hydroperoxide
total h. (TH)
hydropertubation
hydrophila
Aeromonas h.
hydrophilic ointment
hydrophobia

NOTES

441

hydrophobic
hydrophthalmia, hydrophthalmos, hydrophthalmus
hydropic
    h. chorionic villus
    h. gallbladder
    h. infant
    h. placental villus
hydrops
    fetal h.
    h. fetalis
    fetal nonimmune h.
    h. folliculi
    gallbladder h.
    h. gravidarum
    immune fetal h.
    intrauterine h.
    Kell h.
    maternal h.
    nonimmune fetal h.
    h. ovarii
    placental h.
    h. tubae profluens
hydrops-like cholecystitis
hydroquinone
    3% h.
hydrorrhea
    h. gravidae
    h. gravidarum
hydrosalpinx
    intermittent h.
hydrostatic
    h. pressure
    h. reduction
hydrosyringomyelia
Hydro-Tex Topical
hydrotherapy
Hydro ThermAblator endometrial ablation system
hydrothorax
    tension h.
hydrotubation
hydroureter
hydroureteronephrosis
hydrovarium
hydroxide
    aluminum h.
    magnesium h.
    potassium h. (KOH)
    sodium h.
hydroxocobalamin
3-hydroxy-3-methylglutaric aciduria
11-hydroxyandrosterone
hydroxybenzoic acid (HABA)
hydroxy beta methylbutyrate (HMB)
hydroxybutyrate
hydroxychloroquine sulfate
25-hydroxycholecalciferol
17-hydroxycorticosteroid

hydroxyeicosatetraenoic acid
11-hydroxyetiocholanolone
5-hydroxyindoleacetic
    5-h. acid (5-HIAA)
    5-h. assay
21-hydroxyindoleacetic acid (21-HIAA)
hydroxyindole-o-methyltransferase
hydroxylase
    17 alpha-h.
    21-h.
    h. enzyme defect
    phenylalanine h. (PAH)
17-hydroxylase
    17-h. deficiency
    17-h. deficiency syndrome
21-hydroxylase
    21-h. deficiency
    21-h. deficiency syndrome
11-hydroxylase deficiency
hydroxylation
    kynurenine h.
hydroxyl radical (OH)
hydroxylysine
3-hydroxy-3-methylglutaryl coenzyme A
hydroxyphenyluria
17-hydroxypregnenolone
hydroxyprogesterone
    h. caproate
    h. and estradiol valerate
17-hydroxyprogesterone (17-OHP)
    17-h. caproate
hydroxyproline
    proline h.
hydroxyprolinemia
15-hydroxyprostaglandin dehydrogenase
hydroxysteroid
    3beta-h. dehydrogenase (3betaHSD)
    h. dehydrogenase type 2 (HSD2)
18-hydroxysteroid dehydrogenase
hydroxyurea
1,25-hydroxyvitamin D
25-hydroxyvitamin-D$_3$
hydroxyzine
hyfrecation
hyfrecator
Hy-Gene seminal fluid collection kit
Hy-Gestrone
hygiene
    perineal h.
    poor dental h.
    sleep h.
hygroma, hydroma
    cystic h.
    fetal cystic h.
    nuchal cystic h.
hygroscopic
    h. dilator
    h. rod
Hylorel

Hylutin
hymen
    h. bifenestratus
    h. biforis
    cribriform h.
    denticulate h.
    falciform h.
    imperforate h.
    infundibuliform h.
    microperforate h.
    redundant h.
    h. sculptatus
    septate h.
    stenotic h.
    h. subseptus
    vertical h.
    virginal h.
hymenal
    h. band
    h. injury
    h. membrane
    h. opening
    h. ring
    h. tag
hymenectomy
hymenitis
Hymenoptera
    H. sign
    H. venom
hymenorrhaphy
hymenotomy
hyobranchial cleft
hyoid
    h. bar
    h. bone
hyointestinalis
    Campylobacter h.
hyoscine
    Isopto H.
    h. methylbromide
hyoscyamine
    h., atropine, scopolamine,
      phenobarbital
    h. sulfate
Hyosophen
hypamnion, hypamnios
Hypan test
Hypaque Meglumine
Hyperab
hyperabduction
    thumb h.

hyperacidity
hyperactive
    h. bowel sounds
    h. distractible
    dominantly h.
    h. impulsivity
hyperactive/impulsive dimension
hyperactivity
    bronchial h.
    central serotonergic h.
    motor h.
hyperactivity/impulsivity domain
hyperacusis
hyperacute
    h. infarction
    h. rejection
hyperadrenalism
hyperaeration
hyperalaninemia
hyperaldosteronism
hyperalimentation (HA)
    central h.
    h. hepatitis
    Intralipid h.
    intravenous h. (IVH)
    Pedtrace-4 h.
    peripheral h.
    TrophAmine h.
hyperalimentation-associated cholestasis
hyperalphalipoproteinemia
hyperammonemia, hyperammoniemia
    cerebroatrophic h.
    h. due to ornithine
      transcarbamoylase deficiency
    h., hyperornithinemia,
      homocitrullinuria
    h., hyperornithinemia,
      homocitrullinuria syndrome
    transient h.
    h. variant
hyperammonemic
    h. episode
    h. hepatic coma
    h. state
    h. syndrome
hyperammoniemia (*var. of*
  hyperammonemia)
hyperamylasemia
hyperandrogenemia
hyperandrogenemic chronic anovulation
  syndrome

NOTES

H

hyperandrogenic
 h. anovulation (HA)
 h. chronic anovulation
hyperandrogenism
 adrenal h.
 cryptic h.
 h. insulin resistance, acanthosis
   nigricans (HAIR-AN, HAIRAN)
 ovarian h.
 h. reversal
hyperargininemia
hyperarousal
hyperbaric
 h. chamber
 h. oxygen
 h. oxygen therapy (HOBT)
 h. oxygen treatment
hyperbetalipoproteinemia (HBLP)
hyperbilirubinemia
 congenital nonhemolytic
   unconjugated h.
 conjugated h.
 direct h.
 extreme benign h.
 idiopathic h.
 indirect h.
 neonatal h.
 prolonged indirect h.
 prolonged unconjugated h.
 transient familial neonatal h.
 unconjugated h.
hyperbilirubinemic
hypercalcemia
 h. elfin-facies syndrome
 familial h.
 familial hypocalciuric h. (FHH)
 hypocalciuric h.
 idiopathic infantile h.
 infantile h.
 h., peculiar facies, supravalvular
   aortic stenosis syndrome
hypercalcemia/Williams-Beuren syndrome
hypercalcemic crisis
hypercalciuria
 absorptive h.
 autosomal recessive renal proximal
   tubulopathy and h. (ARPTH)
 renal h.
hypercaloric formula
hypercapnia
 permissive h.
hypercarbia
 fetal h.
hypercarotenemia
hypercellularity
 mesangial h.
 segmental mesangial h.

hyperchloremia
hyperchloremic
 h. metabolic acidosis
 h. renal acidosis
hypercholesterolemia
 familial h.
 heterozygous familial h.
 homozygous familial h.
hyperchromic acidosis
hypercoagulability
hypercoagulable state
hypercoagulation
hypercortisolism
hypercyanotic spell
hypercyesis, hypercyesia
hyperdactyly
hyperdibasicaminoaciduria
hyperdiploid
hyperdorsiflexed foot
hyperdynamia uteri
hyperdynamic
 h. precordium
 h. ventricle
 h. ventricle with high output
hyperechogenic
 h. foci
 h. material
hyperechogenicity
 renal h.
hyperechoic
 h. bowel
 h. endometrium
 h. mass
hyperekplexia
hyperelastica
 cutis h.
hyperemesis
 h. gravidarum
 h. lactentium
hyperemia
 conjunctival h.
 optic disc h.
 postprandial h.
 posttraumatic h.
hyperemic cerebral blood flow
hyperencephalus
hypereosinophilic
 h. mucoid cast
 h. syndrome
hyperesthesia
hyperestrogenism
hyperexcitability
hyperexpansion
hyperexplexia
hyperextensibility
 knee joint h.
hyperextensible joint
hyperextensile skin

hyperextension
    h. deformity
    dystonic h.
hyperferritinemia
hyperfiltration
hyperfolliculoidism
hyperfractionated
    h. radiation therapy
    h. radiotherapy
hypergalactosis
hypergammaglobulinemia
    polyclonal h.
hypergastrinemia
    infant h.
hypergenitalism
hyperglycemia
    fetal h.
    ketotic h.
    nonketotic h.
    rebound h.
hyperglycemic clamp technique
hyperglycerolemia
    familial h.
hyperglycinemia
    ketotic h.
    nonketotic h. (NKH)
hypergonadism
hypergonadotropic, hypergonadotrophic
    h. amenorrhea
    h. eunuchoidism
    h. hypogonadism
hypergynecosmia
hyperhaploidy
hyperhemolysis
HyperHep
hyperhidrosis
    volar h.
hyperhomocystinemia
hyperhydroxyprolinemia
hyper-IgD syndrome
hyper-IgE syndrome
hyper-IgM syndrome
hyperimmune
    h. Ig
    h. serum globulin
hyperimmunoglobulin
    h. E
    h. E syndrome
hyperimmunoglobulinemia A
hyperinflation
hyperinsulinemia
    compensatory h.

hyperinsulinemic
    h. hypoglycemia
    h. infant
hyperinsulinemic-euglycemic clamp technique
hyperinsulinism
    fetal h.
    h. hyperammonemia syndrome
    h. with hyperammonemia variant
hyperintensity
hyperinvolution
hyperirritable stage
hyperirritant spot
hyperkalemia
hyperkalemic
    h. periodic paralysis
    h. RTA
hyperkeratosis
    epidermal h.
    epidermolytic h.
    palmar and plantar punctate h.
    punctate h.
    striate h.
hyperkeratotic
    h. dry skin
    h. ridge
hyperkinesis
hyperkinetic
    h. behavior pattern
    h. child syndrome
    h. disorder
    h. pulmonary hypertension
hyperkyphosis
hyperlactation
hyperlacticacidemia
hyperlaxity
    joint h.
    skin h.
hyperleukocytosis
hyperlexia
hyperlinearity
    palmar h.
hyperlipidemia
    familial h.
    familial combined h. (FCHL)
    homozygous h. (type I, II)
    mixed h.
    triglyceride h.
hyperlipoproteinemia (HLP)
hyperlordosis
hyperlucency

NOTES

H

hyperlucent
  h. lung
  h. lung syndrome
hyperluteinization
hyperlysinemia
  familial h.
hypermagnesemia
  iatrogenic acute h.
hypermastia
hypermenorrhea
hypermetabolism
hypermethioninemia
hypermetropia
hypermobile
  h. Ehlers-Danlos syndrome
  h. flatfoot
  h. joint
  h. pes planus
hypermobility
  joint h.
  posterior occipitoatlantal h. (POAH)
  h. syndrome
  urethral h.
hypermyelination
hypernasality
hypernasal speech
hypernatremia dehydration
hypernatremic
  h. dehydration
  h. state
hypernitrosopnea
hyperolfaction
hyperopia
  asymmetric h.
hyperornithemia, hyperammonemia, homocitrulinemia (HHH, triple H)
hyperornithinemia
hyperosmolality
hyperosmolar
  h. dehydration
  h. nonketotic coma
  h. state
hyperosmotic agent
hyperostosis
  calvarial h.
  cortical h.
  h. generalisata with striation
  infantile cortical h.
hyperovarianism
hyperoxaluria
  enteric h.
  primary h.
  primary h. type 1 (PH-1)
  secondary h.
hyperoxia test
hyperoxygenation
hyperparasitemia

hyperparathyroidism
  maternal h.
  neonatal h.
hyperperfusion
  ictal h.
hyperphagia
hyperphagic
hyperphenylalaninemia (MHP)
  benign h.
  malignant h.
hyperphosphatemia
hyperphosphaturic syndrome
hyperpigmentation
  brawny h.
  diffuse h.
  periorbital h.
  reticulated h.
  whorled macular h.
hyperpigmented
  h. lesion
  h. lichenified plaque
hyperpipecolic acidemia
hyperpituitary gigantism
hyperplasia
  adenomatous h. (AH)
  adenomatous endometrial h.
  adrenal h.
  adrenocortical h.
  adult-onset congenital adrenal h.
  angiofollicular lymph node h.
  atypical adenomatous h.
  atypical ductal h. (ADH)
  atypical lobular h.
  basal cell h.
  benign lymphoid h.
  h. of beta cell
  complex h.
  congenital adrenal h. (CAH)
  congenital adrenal lipoid h.
  crypt h.
  cystic h. of the breast
  cystic endometrial h.
  cystic glandular h.
  ductal h.
  elastic tissue h.
  endometrial h. (EH)
  epithelial h.
  erythroid h.
  familial lipoid adrenal h.
  fetal congenital h.
  focal nodular h.
  follicular h.
  gingival h.
  glandular h.
  gum h.
  hepatic focal nodular h.
  hilar cell h.
  intimal h.
  Kupffer cell h.

late-onset h.
Leydig cell h.
lipoid adrenal h.
lymphoid h.
lymphonodular h.
microglandular cervical h.
neonatal breast h.
nodular adrenal h.
nodular lymphoid h.
nonclassic adrenal h. (NCAH)
nonclassic congenital adrenal h.
  (NC-CAH)
21-OH nonclassical adrenal h.
parietal cell h.
pigmented nodular adrenal h.
polypoid h.
pseudoepitheliomatous h.
pulmonary lymphoid h. (PLH)
salt-wasting congenital adrenal h.
  (SW-CAH)
sebaceous gland h.
simple h.
simple virilizing congenital
  adrenal h. (SV-CAH)
squamous cell h.
stromal h.
Swiss cheese h.
thymus h.
vulvar squamous h.
hyperplastic
  h. joint
  h. lymphoid tissue
  h. polyp
  h. right heart syndrome
hyperploidy
hyperpnea
hyperpolarization
hyperprogesteronemia
hyperprolactinemia
  nontumoral h.
  tumorous h.
hyperprolactinemia-associated luteal
  phase
hyperprolactinemic amenorrhea
hyperprolinemia
  familial h.
hyperpronate
hyperpronation
hyperprostaglandin E$_2$ syndrome
hyperprostaglandinuric tubular syndrome
hyperpyrexia
  malignant h.

hyperreactio luteinalis
hyperreactivity
hyperreflexia
  detrusor h.
hyperreflexic apnea
hyperrelaxinemia
hyperreninemia
  chronic h.
hyperreninemic hypertension
hyperresonance to percussion
hyperresonant calvarial percussion note
hyperresponsive
hypersecretion
  gastric acid h.
hypersecretory endometrium
hypersegmentation
hypersegmented neutrophil
hypersensitive hapten-antibody
hypersensitivity
  h. angiitis
  delayed h.
  delayed-type h. (DTH)
  gastric visceral h.
  h. pneumonitis
  h. reaction
  h. vasculitis
hypersensitization
hypersensitize
hypersexual behavior
hypersexuality
hypersomnia
  menstrual-associated periodic h.
  primary h.
hypersomnolence
hypersplenism
Hyperstat I.V.
hyperstimulation
  controlled ovarian h. (COH)
  gonadotropin-induced ovarian h.
  ovarian h.
  spontaneous h.
  uterine h.
hypersynchronization
hypersynchronous discharge
hypersynchrony of neural discharges
hypertelorism
  Bixler h.
  dysostosis craniofacialis with h.
  h., microtia, clefting (HMC)
  ocular h.
hypertelorism-hypospadias syndrome

NOTES

H

447

hypertension
  accelerated h.
  benign intracranial h.
  chronic h.
  essential h.
  fixed pulmonary h.
  gestational h.
  hyperkinetic pulmonary h.
  hyperreninemic h.
  hypoxia-induced pulmonary h. (HPH)
  iatrogenic h.
  idiopathic intracranial h. (IIH)
  infantile h.
  intracranial h.
  malignant h.
  maternal h.
  nonproteinuric h.
  pediatric h.
  persistent pulmonary h. (PPH)
  portal h.
  postpartum h.
  pregnancy-associated h.
  pregnancy-induced h. (PIH)
  presinusoidal h.
  primary pulmonary h.
  pulmonary h.
  rebound h.
  renal h.
  renovascular h.
  transient h.
  white coat h.
hypertension-preeclampsia
hypertensive
  h. crisis
  h. emergency
  h. encephalopathy
hyperthecosis
  ovarian stromal h.
  h. ovarii
  stromal h.
hyperthermia
  malignant h. (MH)
  neonatal h.
  h. in newborn
hyperthermic rhabdomyolysis
hyperthyroid
hyperthyroidism
hyperthyrotropinemia
  transient h.
hypertonia
  axial h.
  global h.
hypertonic
  h. dehydration
  h. glucose
  h. saline
  h. saline solution
  h. uterine dysfunction

hypertonicity
hypertonus
  extensor h.
  uterine h.
hypertransaminasemia
hypertransfusion regimen
hypertrichosis
  h., coarse face, brachydactyly, obesity, mental retardation syndrome
  h. lanuginosa
  h. universalis congenita
  vellus h.
hypertrichotic osteochondrodysplasia
hypertriglyceridemia
  familial h. (FHTG)
hypertrophic
  h. bundle
  h. bundle of smooth muscle
  h. cardiomyopathy
  h. cirrhosis
  h. gastropathy
  h. growth zone
  h. interstitial neuropathy of infancy
  h. nail
  h. osteoarthropathy (HOA)
  h. pyloric stenosis (HPS)
  h. scar
  h. stenosis
  h. zone (HZ)
hypertrophica
  hemangiectasia h.
hypertrophied tissue
hypertrophy
  adenoidal h.
  adenotonsillar h.
  atrial h.
  biventricular h.
  cerebellar h.
  clitoral h.
  congenital thyroid deficiency with muscular h.
  contralateral h.
  hemangiectatic h.
  infantile myxedema-muscular h.
  juxtaglomerular apparatus h.
  h. of labia
  labial h.
  left atrial h.
  left ventricular h. (LVH)
  massive breast h.
  myocardial h.
  myocytic h.
  ovarian h.
  pontile h.
  right atrial h.
  right ventricular h. (RVH)
  septal h.
  synovial h.

testicular h.
trigonal h.
ventricular h.
virginal breast h.
hypertropia
ipsilateral h.
hypertrypsinemia
hypertryptophanemia
hypertympany
hypertyrosinemia II
hyperuricemia
X-linked primary h.
hyperuricosuria
hypervalinemia
hyperventilation
central neurogenic h.
h. provocative test
h. syndrome
hypervigilance manifestation
hyperviscosity syndrome
hypervitaminosis
h. A
chronic h. A
hypervolemia
hypesthesia
bilateral stocking h.
hypha, pl. **hyphae**
hyphema
eight-ball h.
traumatic h.
hypnagogic hallucination
hypnotherapeutic
hypnotherapy
hypnotic effect
hypoactive
h. bowel sounds
h. sexual desire
h. sexual desire disorder
hypoactivity
hypoadrenalism neural ceroid lipofuscinosis
hypoalbuminemia
hypoalbuminemic
hypoaldosteronism
congenital h.
hypoallergenic
hypoalphalipoproteinemia
familial h.
primary h.
hypoarousal
sustained autonomic h.

hypobetalipoproteinemia
h., acanthocytosis, retinitis pigmentosa, and pallidal degeneration (HARP)
familial h.
hypocalcemia
cardiac abnormality, abnormal facies, thymic hypoplasia, cleft palate, h. (CATCH 22)
cardiac abnormality, T-cell deficit, clefting, h.
h., dwarfism, cortical thickening syndrome
dwarfism, cortical thickening of tubular bones, transient h.
late neonatal h.
h. and microdeletion 22q11 syndrome
neonatal h.
hypocalcemic
h. seizure
h. tetany
hypocalcification
linear h.
hypocalciuria
familial hypercalcemia with h. (FHH)
hypocalciuric hypercalcemia
hypocalvaria
hypocapnia
hypocarbia
hypocarnitinemia
hypocellularity
hypochloremia
hypochloremic metabolic alkalosis
hypochlorhydria
hypochlorous acid
hypochondriasis
primary h.
secondary h.
hypochondrogenesis
hypochondroplasia syndrome
hypochromic microcytic anemia
hypocitraturia
hypocoagulability
hypocomplementemia
intermittent h.
hypocomplementemic
h. glomerulonephritis
h. urticarial vasculitis syndrome (HUVS)
hypocycloidal tomography

NOTES

449

hypodactyly
hypodense
hypodermoclysis
hypodiploid
hypodontia
hypodysplasia
    renal h.
hypoechogenic area
hypoechoic
    h. density
    h. structure
hypoesthesia
    corneal h.
hypoesthesic skin lesion
hypoestrogenemia
hypoestrogenic woman
hypoestrogenism
hypoferremia
hypofertility
hypofibrinogenemia
    congenital h.
    familial h.
hypofluorescent
hypofolliculogenesis
hypofunction
    adrenal h.
hypogalactia
hypogalactous
hypogammaglobulinemia,
  hypogammaglobinemia
    acquired h.
    adult-onset h.
    common variable h.
    congenital h.
    late-onset h.
    physiologic h.
    transient h.
    X-linked h.
hypoganglionic segment of Aldrich
hypoganglionosis
hypogastric
    h. artery
    h. artery ligation
    h. lymph node
    h. pain
    h. plexus
    h. vein
hypogastropagus
hypogastroschisis
hypogenesis
    cerebellar vermis h.
hypogenital dystrophy with diabetic tendency syndrome
hypogenitalism
hypoglossal
    h. ganglion
    h. nerve
hypoglossia-hypodactyly syndrome

hypoglycemia
    episodic h.
    familial hyperinsulinemic h.
    hyperinsulinemic h.
    hypoketotic h.
    insulin-induced h.
    ketotic h.
    neonatal h.
    nonfamilial hyperinsulinemic h.
    nonhyperinsulinemic h.
    nonketotic h.
    refractory h.
    severe refractory h.
    transient h.
hypoglycemic
    oral h.
    h. seizure
hypoglycin
hypoglycorrhachia
hypoglycosylation
hypognathus
    cyclops h.
hypogonadal woman
hypogonadism
    alopecia, anosmia, deafness, h. (AADH)
    h., alopecia, diabetes mellitus, mental retardation, deafness and ECG abnormalities
    congenital hypogonadotropic h.
    eugonadotropic h.
    hypergonadotropic h.
    hypogonadotropic h.
    hyposmia-hypogonadotropic h. (HHA)
    idiopathic hypothalamic h. (IHH)
    isolated hypogonadotropic h. (IHH)
    primary h.
hypogonadism-anosmia syndrome
hypogonadotropic, hypogonadotrophic
    h. amenorrhea
    h. eunuchoidism
    h. hypogonadism
    h. hypogonadism, anosmia
    h. hypogonadism, mental retardation, microphthalmia syndrome
hypogonadotropism
hypohaploidy
hypohidrotic
    h. ectodermal dysplasia
    h. ectodermal dysplasia, hypothyroidism, agenesis of corpus callosum syndrome
    h. sweating
hypokalemia
hypokalemic
    h. acidosis
    h. alkalosis

h. periodic paralysis
h. salt-losing tubulopathy
hypoketotic hypoglycemia
hypokinesia
hypokinetic
hypokyphosis
hypoleptinemia
hypolordosis
hypomagnesemia
congenital h.
familial h.
ionized h.
neonatal h.
primary h.
hypomagnesemic tetany
hypomandibular faciocranial dysostosis
hypomania
pharmacologically induced h.
hypomanic episode
hypomastia, hypomazia
hypomaturation-hypoplasia
hypomelanosis
Ito h.
h. of Ito
hypomelanotic
hypomelia, hypotrichosis, facial hemangioma syndrome
hypomenorrhea
hypomenorrheic woman
hypomentia
hypometabolic
hypometabolism
caudate h.
hypomyelination
congenital h.
hyponasality
hyponasal speech
hyponatremia of water excess
hyponatremic
h. dehydration
h. seizure
h. state
hypoosmotic swelling (HOS)
hypoovarianism
hypoparathyroidism
idiopathic h.
physiologic transient h.
h., stature, mental retardation, seizures syndrome
hypoperfusion
cerebral h.

interictal h.
splanchnic h.
hypoperistalsis
megacystis, microcolon, intestinal h. (MMIH)
hypopharyngeal-glottal obstruction
hypopharynx
hypophosphatasia
congenital lethal h.
h. tarda
hypophosphatemia
familial h. (FHR)
X-linked h.
hypophosphatemic
h. bone disease
h. rickets
hypophysectomy
hypophysial, hypophyseal
h. amenorrhea
h. dwarfism
h. infantilism
h. portal circulation
hypophysis
hypophysitis
lymphocytic h.
hypopigmentation
perianal h.
vulvar h.
hypopigmented
h. lesion
h. macule
h. mycosis
hypopituitarism
congenital h.
hypopituitary syndrome
hypoplacentosis
hypoplasia
adrenal h.
h. of anguli oris depressor muscle (HAODM)
bilateral lung h.
bilateral optic nerve h.
biliary h.
bone marrow h.
cartilage-hair h. (CHH)
cerebellar vermis h.
congenital adrenal h.
congenital megakaryocytic h.
congenital universal muscular h.
crypt h.
dental enamel h.
enamel h.

NOTES

hypoplasia *(continued)*
    h., endocrine disturbances, tracheostenosis syndrome
    erythroid h.
    exocrine pancreatic h.
    fetal pulmonary h.
    focal dermal h.
    foveal h.
    global h.
    Goldblatt-Vilijoen radial ray h.
    Goltz focal dermal h.
    heminasal h.
    hepatic ductular h.
    ipsilateral lung h.
    iris h.
    laryngeal h.
    h. of left heart (HLL)
    Leydig cell h.
    linear h.
    lipoid adrenal gland h.
    h. of lung
    malar h.
    mandibular h.
    maxillary h.
    midface h.
    midfacial h.
    müllerian h.
    odontoid process h.
    optic nerve h. (ONH)
    orbital bone h.
    oromandibular limb h.
    pancreatic h.
    pontocerebellar h.
    pulmonary h.
    right lung h.
    right ventricular h.
    secondary adrenal h.
    segmental h.
    spondylohumerofemoral h.
    thymic h.
    transient erythroid h.
    transverse arch h.
    tubular h.
    velofacial h.
    h. of vermis
    vermis h.
hypoplasia/hydrocephalus
    X-linked cerebral h.
hypoplastic
    h. anemia
    h. aorta (HA)
    h. congenital anemia syndrome
    h. dens
    h. digit
    h. kidney
    h. labia
    h. left heart
    h. left heart syndrome (HLHS)
    h. left ventricle

    h. lung
    h. mandible
    h. nails
    h. parathyroid gland
    h. patella
    h. penis
    h. philtrum
    h. prostate
    h. pulmonary vascular bed
    h. radius
    h. right heart syndrome (HRHS)
    h. sacrum
    h. superior cerebellar vermis
    h. teeth
    h. thumb
    h. tongue
    h. uterus
    h. zygomatic arch
hypopnea
hypopotassemia
hypoproliferative anemia
hypoproteinemia
    idiopathic h.
hypoprothrombinemia
hypopyon
hyporeflexia
hyposecretion
    gastric acid h.
hyposegmentation
hyposensitization
hyposmia
hyposmia-hypogonadotropic hypogonadism (HHA)
hyposomatotropism
    obesity-related h.
hypospadias
    anterior h.
    balanic h.
    distal shaft h.
    first-degree h.
    glanular h.
    Hacker h.
    middle h.
    midshaft h.
    penoscrotal h.
    perineal h.
    perineoscrotal h.
    posterior h.
    proximal shaft h.
    pseudovaginal perineoscrotal h. (PPSH)
    h. repair
    scrotal h.
    second-degree h.
    subcoronal h.
    third-degree h.
hypospadias-dysphagia syndrome
hypospadias-mental retardation syndrome

hyposplenia
hyposplenism
hypostatic pneumonia
hyposthenuria
hyposulfite
    sodium h.
hypotelorism
    ocular h.
    orbital h.
hypotension
    instantaneous orthostatic h. (INOH)
    maternal h.
    neurally mediated h.
    orthostatic h.
hypotensive anesthesia
hypothalamic
    h. amenorrhea
    h. disease
    h. dysfunction
    h. failure
    h. hamartoblastoma
    h. hamartoblastoma, hypopituitarism, imperforate anus, postaxial polydactyly syndrome
    h. hamartoblastoma syndrome
    h. hamartoma
    h. hypothyroidism
    h. lesion
    h. luteinizing hormone-releasing hormone
    h., pituitary, thyroid (HTP)
    h. set point
    h. tumor
hypothalamic-hypophysial
    h.-h. destruction
    h.-h. portal circulation
hypothalamic-hypophysial-ovarian-endometrial axis
hypothalamic-hypopituitary hypothyroidism
hypothalamic-pituitary
    h.-p. amenorrhea
    h.-p. axis (HPA)
    h.-p. disorder
    h.-p. dysfunction
    h.-p. function
    h.-p. system
hypothalamic-pituitary-adrenal (HPA)
    h.-p.-a. axis dysregulation
hypothalamic-pituitary-gonadal axis
hypothalamic-pituitary-ovarian (HOP)

hypothenar
hypothermia
    cerebral h.
    chronic scrotal h.
    cranial h.
    deep systemic h.
hypothesis, pl. **hypotheses**
    alternative h.
    Barker low birth weight h.
    bayesian h.
    critical weight h.
    differential detection h.
    differential treatment h.
    dormant basket cell h.
    estrogen window etiologic h.
    gate-control h.
    Goldie-Coldman h.
    Knudson two-hit tumorigenesis h.
    Korenman estrogen window h.
    Lyon h.
    school failure h.
    serotonin h.
    susceptibility h.
    two-hit h.
    Wramsby h.
hypothesize
hypothyroid
    h. dwarfism
    h. myopathy
hypothyroidism
    acquired h.
    athyrotic h.
    central h.
    congenital h. (CH)
    congenital goitrous h.
    eutopic congenital h.
    goitrous h.
    hypothalamic h.
    hypothalamic-hypopituitary h.
    maternal thyrotropin receptor blocking antibody-induced congenital h.
    mixed h.
    neonatal nongoitrous h.
    primary h.
    secondary h.
    subclinical h.
    h. syndrome
    tertiary h.
    transient congenital h.
hypothyroid-large muscle syndrome

NOTES

H

453

hypothyroxinemia
    h. of prematurity (HOP)
    transient h.
hypotonia
    benign congenital h.
    benign infantile h.
    bladder h.
    congenital h.
    h., hypopigmentia, hypogonadism,
      obesity (HHHO)
    infantile muscular h.
    muscle h.
    muscular h.
    nonparalytic h.
    h., obesity, hypogonadism, mental
      retardation syndrome
    h., obesity, prominent incisors
      syndrome
    Oppenheim congenital h.
    paralytic h.
    transient h.
    uterine h.
hypotonic
    h. bladder
    h. cerebral palsy
    h. dehydration
    h. myometrium
    h. saline
    h. uterine dysfunction
    h. weakness
hypotonic-hyporesponsive episodes
  (HHEs)
hypotonicity
hypotony
    ocular h.
hypotransferrinemia
hypotrichosis
    Marie-Unna h.
hypotrophy
    fetal h.
hypotropia
hypouricemia
hypovarianism
hypoventilation
    central alveolar h.
    congenital central h.
    h. syndrome
hypovitaminemia
    thiamin h.
hypovitaminosis
hypovolemia
hypovolemic
    h. dehydration
    h. shock
hypoxanthine-phosphoribosyltransferase
  (HGPRT)
hypoxemia
    acute-on-chronic tissue h.
    perinatal h.

hypoxia
    alveolar h.
    cellular h.
    centrizonal h.
    fetal h.
    global brain h.
    intestinal h.
    intrauterine h.
    h., intussusception, brain mass
      (HIB)
    maternal h.
    perinatal h.
    subacute fetal h.
    in utero h.
hypoxia-induced pulmonary hypertension
  (HPH)
hypoxia-ischemia
hypoxic
    h. cell sensitizer
    h. encephalopathy
    h. respiratory failure
    h. spell
    h. vasoconstriction
hypoxic-ischemic
    h.-i. brain injury
    h.-i. cerebral injury
    h.-i. encephalopathy (HIE)
Hyprogest
hypsarrhythmia
hypsarrhythmic pattern
hypsicephaly
Hyrexin
Hyrexin-50 Injection
Hyskon
hysteralgia
hysteratresia
hysterectomized
hysterectomy
    abdominal h.
    abdominovaginal h.
    Bell-Buettner h.
    Bonney abdominal h.
    cesarean h.
    h. clamp
    classic abdominal Semm h.
      (CASH)
    Dellepiane h.
    Döderlein method of vaginal h.
    Doyen vaginal h.
    Eden-Lawson h.
    extended radical h.
    extrafascial total abdominal h.
    laparoscopically assisted radical
      vaginal h.
    laparoscopic-assisted abdominal h.
      (LAAH)
    laparoscopic-assisted vaginal h.
      (LAVH)
    laparoscopic Döderlein h.

laparoscopic supracervical h. (LSH)
Mayo h.
Meigs-Werthein h.
modified radical h.
Munro and Parker classification for
  laparoscopic h.
obstetric h.
paravaginal h.
Pelosi vaginal h.
pelviscopic intrafascial h.
Porro h.
radical h.
Reis-Wertheim vaginal h.
Rutledge classification of
  extended h.
Semm h.
subtotal h.
supracervical h. (SCH)
total abdominal h. (TAH)
vaginal h.
Ward-Mayo vaginal h.
hysteresis
hysteria
hysteric
  h. convulsion
  h. seizure
hysterical
  h. amnesia
  h. glottic closure
  h. mother
  h. paralysis
  h. seizure
  h. syncope
  h. visual loss
hystericus
  globus h.
hysterocele
hysterocleisis
hysterocolposcope
hysterocystopexy
hysterodynia
hysterofiberscope
  Olympus flexible h.
hysterogram
hysterograph
hysterography
hysterolith
hysterolysis
hysterometer
hysteromyoma
hysteromyomectomy
hysteromyotomy

hystero-oophorectomy
hysteropathy
hysteropexy
  abdominal h.
  Alexander-Adams h.
hysterophore
hysteroplasty
hysterorrhaphy
hysterorrhexis
hysterosalpingectomy
hysterosalpingogram (HSG)
hysterosalpingography (HS, HSG)
  h. catheter
hysterosalpingo-oophorectomy
hysterosalpingosonography
hysterosalpingostomy
hysteroscope
  Baggish h.
  Baloser h.
  Circon-ACMI h.
  diagnostic h.
  flexible h.
  French h.
  Fujinon flexible h.
  Galileo rigid h.
  Hamou h.
  Karl Storz 15 French flexible h.
  Liesegang LM-Flex 7 flexible h.
  Olympus h.
  OPERA Star SL h.
  Valle h.
hysteroscopic
  h. approach
  h. endometrial ablation
  h. insufflator
  h. metroplasty
  h. myomectomy
  h. removal
  h. septum resection
  h. surgery
hysteroscopy
  h. fluid
  laparoscopic-assisted vaginal h.
    (LAVH)
hysterosonography
hysterospasm
hysterothermometry
hysterotomy
  abdominal h.
  low transverse h.
  Pelosi h.
  vaginal h.

NOTES

H

hysterotrachelectomy
hysterotracheloplasty
hysterotrachelorrhaphy
hysterotrachelotomy
hysterotubography
hystersonography
hystrix
    ichthyosis h.
Hytakerol
Hytone Topical
Hytuss
Hytuss-2X

Hyzine-50 Injection
HZ
    hypertrophic zone
Hz
    hertz
HZA
    hemizona assay
HZO
    herpes zoster ophthalmicus
HZV
    herpes zoster virus

I

    inspired gas
        I antigen score
        I IFG-binding protein

I-20

    pulse oximeter sensor N-25 and I-20

I_2

    prostaglandin I_2

^{123}I

    iodine-123

^{125}I

    iodine-125

^{127}I

    iodine-127

^{131}I

    iodine-131

^{132}I

    iodine-132

IAA

    ileoanal anastomosis

IAC

    indwelling arterial catheter
    interatrial communication

IADH

    inappropriate antidiuretic hormone
        IADH syndrome

IAHS

    infection-associated hemophagocytic
        syndrome

IAI

    intraabdominal infection
    intraamniotic infection

IALT

    intestine-associated lymphoid tissue

IAP

    intrapartum antibiotic prophylaxis

IASA

    idiopathic acquired sideroblastic anemia

iatrogenic

        i. acute hypermagnesemia
        i. airway injury
        i. androgen excess
        i. anemia
        i. bladder
        i. CJD
        i. complete heart block
        i. Creutzfeldt-Jakob disease
        i. destruction
        i. dissemination
        i. effect
        i. event
        i. fetal distress
        i. hypertension
        i. infertility
        i. menopause
        i. multiple pregnancy (IMP)
        i. pneumothorax
        i. precocious puberty
        i. preterm birth maternal dropsy
        i. pyopneumothorax
        i. ureteral injury
        i. urethral obstruction

IB

    infantile botulism
        Midol IB

ibandronate

IBC

    inflammatory breast cancer
    iron-binding capacity

IBD

    identical by descent
    inflammatory bowel disease

IBDQ

    Inflammatory Bowel Disease
        Questionnaire

IBIDS

    ichthyosis, brittle hair, impaired
        intelligence, decreased fertility, short
        stature
        IBIDS syndrome

IB/IX

        glycoprotein I.
        membrane glycoprotein I.

IBR

    Infant Behavior Record

IBS

    irritable bowel syndrome

IBSN

    infantile bilateral striatal necrosis
        syndrome

IBT

    immunobead test

ibuprofen

Ibuprohm

Ibu-Tab

        I.-T. Junior Strength Motrin

ibutilide

%IBW

    percent of ideal body weight

IC

    immune complex
    inspiratory capacity
    invasive cancer
        Babytherm IC

iC3b receptor

ICA

    islet cell antibody

iCa

    ionized calcium

ICAM1
  intercellular adhesion molecule 1
ICC
  Indian childhood cirrhosis
  Interagency Coordinating Council
ICCR
  International Committee for
    Contraceptive Research
ICD
  immune complex dissociation
  International Classification of Diseases
ICD/IPD
  (Mustardé ratio) inner canthal
    distance/interpupillary distance
ICD-p24 test
ICE
  ichthyosis, cheek, eyebrow
    ICE syndrome
iced
    i. saline
    i. saline submersion
I-cell disease
ICF
  immunodeficiency, centromeric
    instability, facial anomalies
  intermediate care facility
  intracellular fluid
    ICF syndrome
ICFM
  isolated congenital folate malabsorption
ICH
  intracranial hemorrhage
ichthyosiform
    congenital i.
    i. dermatosis
    i. erythroderma
    i. erythroderma, corneal
      involvement, deafness
    i. erythroderma, hair abnormality,
      mental and growth retardation
ichthyosis
    i., alopecia, ectropion, mental
      retardation syndrome
    i., brittle hair, impaired
      intelligence, decreased fertility,
      short stature (IBIDS)
    i., characteristic appearance, mental
      retardation syndrome
    i., cheek, eyebrow (ICE)
    i., cheek, eyebrow syndrome
    i. congenita
    congenital i.
    i. fetalis
    i. fetus
    i., follicularis, atrichia (or
      alopecia), photophobia (IFAP)
    harlequin i.
    i., hypogonadism, mental
      retardation, epilepsy syndrome

    i. hystrix
    lamellar i.
    i. linearis circumflexa
    i., male hypogonadism syndrome
    i., mental retardation, dwarfism,
      renal impairment syndrome
    i., mental retardation, epilepsy,
      hypogonadism syndrome
    i., oligophrenia, epilepsy syndrome
    i., spastic neurologic disorder,
      oligophrenia syndrome
    i. spinosa
    i., split hair, aminoaciduria
      syndrome
    i. uteri
    i. vulgaris
    i. with keratitis and deafness
      syndrome
    X-linked i.
ichthyotic idiocy
ICI
  intracranial injury
ICN
  intensive care nursery
Icon
    I. serum pregnancy test
    I. strep B test
    I. urine pregnancy test
ICP
  intracranial pressure
    ICP monitoring
ICPS
  intrauterine contraceptive progesterone
    system
ICS
  inhaled corticosteroid
  International Continence Society
    ICS bladder prolapse (stage I–III)
ICSD
  International Classification of Sleep
    Disorders
    ICSD criteria
ICSHI
  intracytoplasmic sperm head injection
ICSI
  intracytoplasmic sperm injection
    ICSI Massachusetts clamp
ictal hyperperfusion
icteric
    i. hepatitis
    i. leptospirosis
    i. phase
icterogenic breast milk
icterohaemorrhagiae
    Leptospira i.
icterometer
icterus
    i. gravis
    i. gravis neonatorum

i. neonatorum
physiologic i.
i. praecox
scleral i.

I&D
incision and drainage

IDA
alpha-L-iduronidase
iron deficiency anemia
IDA deficiency

Idaho syndrome
Idamycin PFS
idarubicin
IDC
infiltrating ductal carcinoma
intervertebral disc calcification

IDDM
insulin-dependent diabetes mellitus

IDEA
Individuals with Disabilities Education Act

ideas
flight of i.

ideation
paranoid i.
suicidal i.

identical
i. by descent (IBD)
i. twins

identification
cord vessel i.

identity matrix
ideogram
IDI
intractable diarrhea of infancy

idiocy
amaurotic familial i.
Aztec i.
Batten-Bielschowsky type of late infantile and juvenile amaurotic i.
cretinism i.
i. by deprivation
eclamptic i.
epileptic i.
genetous i.
hydrocephalic i.
ichthyotic i.
inflammatory i.
juvenile amaurotic i.
Kalmuk i.
late infantile amaurotic i.
microcephalic i.

paralytic i.
Spielmeyer-Vogt type of late infantile and juvenile amaurotic i.
traumatic i.
xerodermic i.

idioglossia
idiolalia
idiopathic
i. abortion
i. acquired sideroblastic anemia (IASA)
i. apnea
i. apnea of prematurity
i. apparent life-threatening event
i. cavernous sinusitis
i. cholestasis of pregnancy
i. chronic arthritis
i. clubfoot
i. constipation
i. copper toxicosis
i. dermatosis
i. diffuse interstitial fibrosis
i. diffuse interstitial fibrosis of lung
i. dilated cardiomyopathy
i. epilepsy
i. facial paralysis
i. growth hormone deficiency
i. heel-cord tightness
i. hemolytic uremia syndrome
i. hirsutism
i. hydramnios
i. hyperbilirubinemia
i. hypercalcemia-supravalvular aortic stenosis syndrome
i. hypertrophic subaortic stenosis (IHSS)
i. hypoparathyroidism
i. hypoproteinemia
i. hypothalamic hypogonadism (IHH)
i. infantile hypercalcemia
i. infantile hypercalcemia syndrome
i. infertility
i. intracranial hypertension (IIH)
i. intussusception
i. isosexual precocious puberty
i. juvenile avascular necrosis
i. long Q-T syndrome
i. low molecular weight proteinuria
i. megalencephaly

NOTES

idiopathic *(continued)*
    i. minimal lesion nephrotic syndrome (IMLNS)
    i. neonatal giant-cell hepatitis
    i. nephrotic syndrome (INS)
    i. neutropenia
    i. pancreatitis
    i. peptic ulcer disease
    i. polyserositis
    i. premature adrenarche
    i. premature thelarche
    i. primary renal hematuric proteinuric syndrome
    i. pulmonary hemorrhage (IPH)
    i. rapidly progressive glomerulonephritis
    i. recurrent jaundice of pregnancy
    i. respiratory distress syndrome (IRDS)
    i. scoliosis
    i. scrotal edema
    i. seizure
    i. short stature (ISS)
    i. status epilepticus
    i. steatorrhea
    i. steroid-resistant proteinuria/nephrotic syndrome
    i. talipes equinovarus
    i. thrombocytopenic purpura (ITP)
    i. tibia vara
    i. toe walking (ITW)
    i. torsion dystonia
    i. torticollis
    i. ulcer
    i. urticaria
    i. venous thromboembolism
    i. vulvodynia
idiosome
idiosyncratic marrow aplasia
idiot
    mongolian i.
IDI-Strep B test
IDM
    infant of diabetic mother
    intensive diabetes management
IDMS
    isolated diffuse mesangial sclerosis
idoxifene
idoxuridine
id reaction
IDS
    iduronate sulfatase
    intrinsic sphincter deficiency
    IDS deficiency
IDU
    intravenous drug use
    5-iodo-2′-deoxyuridine

IDUA
    alpha-L-iduronidase
    IDUA deficiency
iduronate sulfatase (IDS)
iduronic acid
IE
    infectious endocarditis
    infective endocarditis
I/E, I:E
    inspiratory to expiratory ratio
IEM
    inborn error of metabolism
IEP
    Individualized Education Program
IES
    Impact of Events Scale
IF
    intrinsic factor
    involved field
    IF radiation
IFA
    immunofluorescent antibody
    immunofluorescent assay
    indirect fluorescent antibody
    IFA test
IFAP
    ichthyosis, follicularis, atrichia (or alopecia), photophobia
    IFAP syndrome
ifenprodil
Ifex
IFI
    intrafollicular insemination
IFN
    interferon
IFN-gamma
    interferon gamma
ifosfamide
IFSP
    Individualized Family Service Plan
Ig
    immunoglobulin
    hyperimmune Ig
IgA
    immunoglobulin A
    IgA AGA test
    IgA antiendomysial
    IgA antiendomysium antibody
    IgA antigliadin
    IgA antireticulin antibody
    IgA deficiency
    IgA HIV antibody test
    IgA mesangial deposition
    secretory IgA
IgA1
    immunoglobulin A subclass 1
IgA2
    immunoglobulin A subclass 2

IgD
>immunoglobulin D
>>IgD antibody

IgE
>immunoglobulin E
>>IgE antibody
>>antistaphylococcal IgE
>>IgE deficiency
>>IgE syndrome

IGF
>insulinlike growth factor
>>IGF-1, -2

IgF
>immunoglobulin F

IGFBP
>insulinlike growth factor-binding protein

IGFBP-3
>insulinlike growth factor-binding protein-3

IgG
>immunoglobulin G
>>IgG antibody
>>IgG antibody titer
>>IgG anti-HAV
>>serovar-specific IgG

IgG2
>immunoglobulin G2
>>IgG2 deficiency

IgG4
>immunoglobulin G4
>>IgG4 deficiency

IgG-IFA test

IGHD
>isolated growth hormone deficiency

IGIV
>immunoglobulin, intravenous

IgM
>immunoglobulin M
>>IgM antibody
>>IgM antibody titer
>>IgM deficiency
>>IgM indirect fluorescent antibody test
>>serovar-specific IgM
>>X-linked immunodeficiency with hyper IgM

IgM-IFA test

ignoring
>active i.

IGT
>impaired glucose tolerance

IH
>intraretinal hemorrhage

IHA
>indirect hemagglutination antibody
>>IHA test

IHD
>ischemic heart disease

IHH
>idiopathic hypothalamic hypogonadism
>isolated hypogonadotropic hypogonadism

IHPS
>infantile hypertrophic pyloric stenosis

IHSS
>idiopathic hypertrophic subaortic stenosis

IIF
>indirect immunofluorescence
>>IIF assay

IIH
>idiopathic intracranial hypertension

IIQ
>Incontinence Impact Questionnaire

IIQ-R
>Incontinence Impact Questionnaire-Revised

IL
>interleukin

ILAE
>International League Against Epilepsy

ILAR
>International League of Associations for Rheumatology
>>ILAR peripheral arthritis classification

ILC
>infiltrating lobular carcinoma

ILD
>interstitial lung disease

ileal
>i. atresia
>i. conduit
>i. interposition
>i. intussusception
>i. limb
>i. loop
>i. loop diversion
>i. perforation
>i. pouch-anal anastomosis (IPAA)
>i. reservoir
>i. stoma
>i. ureter

ileitis
>backwash i.

NOTES

ileitis *(continued)*
    nonspecific i.
    regional i.
    terminal i.
ileoanal
    i. anastomosis (IAA)
    i. pull-through
ileocecal
    i. conduit diversion
    i. intussusception
ileocolic
    i. artery
    i. intussusception
ileocolitis
ileocystoplasty
    Camey i.
ileoentectropy
ileoileal
    i. anastomosis
    i. intussusception
ileoileocolic intussusception
ileostomy
    Bishop-Koop i.
    continent i.
    end i.
ileovesicostomy
    Yang-Monti i.
Iletin
    Lente I. II
    NPH I. I, II
    pork Regular I. II
    Regular I. I, II
ileum
    distal i.
    duplication of i.
    native i.
ileus
    adynamic i.
    complicated meconium i.
    duodenal i.
    meconium i. (MI)
    paralytic i.
    postinfectious i.
    simple meconium i.
    i. subparta
iliac
    i. apophysis maturation index
    i. artery
    i. crest
    i. crest apophysitis
    i. crest contusion
    i. fossa
    i. horn
    i. node
    i. spine
    i. vein
iliococcygeal
    i. fixation
    i. muscle

iliococcygeus
    i. fascia suspension
    i. muscle
iliofemoral artery
ilioneoureterocystotomy
iliopagus
iliopectineal
    i. bursa
    i. line
iliopsoas
    i. hemorrhage
    i. sign
iliothoracopagus
iliotibial
    i. band
    i. band friction syndrome
ilioxiphopagus
ilium
Ilizarov
    I. device
    I. external fixator
    I. limb-lengthening procedure
ill-defined mass
illegal substance
illegitimacy
illegitimate
illicit
    i. drug
    i. drug use
    i. sex
Illinois Test of Psycholinguistic Abilities (IPTA)
illness
    acute i.
    childhood severity of psychiatric i. (CSPI)
    chronic i.
    communicable i.
    diarrheal dehydration i.
    food-borne i.
    history of present i. (HPI)
    Integrated Management of Childhood I. (IMCI)
    leptospiral i.
    lower respiratory i. (LRI)
    manic-depressive i.
    maternal i.
    mental i.
    nonthyroidal i. (NTI)
    present i. (PI)
    prodromal i.
    psychiatric i.
    roseolalike i.
    seroconversion i.
    systemic i.
    upper respiratory i.
    viral lower respiratory i. (VLRI)
illocutionary stage

Illumina
    I. Pro Series CO_2 surgical laser system
    I. Pro Series laparoscopic laser
illuminated vaginal speculum
illumination
    chemiluminescent i.
illuminator
    LightMat surgical i.
Illum syndrome
iLook 15 handheld ultrasound system
iloprost
Ilotycin
IL 2R
ILS17 gene for isolated lissencephaly
ILSX gene for X-linked lissencephaly
IM
    infectious mononucleosis
    intestinal malrotation
    intramuscular
image
    body i.
    i. intensification fluoroscopy
    i. intensifier
    i. recording system
image-degradation amblyopia
image-guided breast biopsy
imager
    peripheral instantaneous X-ray i. (PIXI)
imagery
    traumatic i.
imaginal desensitization
imaging
    chemical shift i. (CSI)
    color Doppler flow i. (CDFI)
    Color Power Angio i.
    continuous-wave ultrasound i.
    diagnostic i.
    diffusion-weighted i. (DWI)
    diffusion-weighted magnetic resonance i.
    dynamic pulmonary i. (DPI)
    echoplanar functional magnetic resonance i.
    endovaginal i.
    fetal i.
    functional brain i.
    gray-scale i.
    harmonic tissue i.
    i. headband
    high-contrast Bucky i.

    magnetic resonance i. (MRI)
    magnetic source i. (MSI)
    mediastinal i.
    medical optimal i. (MOI)
    MIGB i.
    M-mode i.
    neuraxis tumor i.
    OB-View i.
    OPS i.
    phosphorus-31 magnetic resonance i. (^{31}P MRI)
    plantar i.
    prenatal magnetic resonance i.
    radionuclide i.
    rhod-2 i.
    SieScape i.
    thallium i.
    tissue Doppler i. (TDI)
    tissue specific i.
    ultrafast magnetic resonance i.
imbalance
    asymmetric muscle i.
    electrolyte i.
    neuromuscular i.
    ventilation/perfusion i.
imbricated stitch
IMCI
    Integrated Management of Childhood Illness
Imelab vascular diagnostic system
Imerslünd-Grasbeck syndrome
Imerslünd syndrome
Imex
    I. antepartum monitor
    I. Pocket-Dop OB Doppler
Imexlab vascular diagnostic system
imidazole
    topical i.
imidazopyridine
imiglucerase
imino acid
iminoglycinuria
    familial i.
imipemide
imipenem and cilastatin
imipenem-cilastatin sodium
imipramine hydrochloride
imiquimod cream
imitative play
Imitrex Injection
Imlach ring

NOTES

IMLNS
idiopathic minimal lesion nephrotic
 syndrome
immature
i. infant
i. neural element
i. ovarian teratoma
i. placenta
i. social behavior
i. teratoma grade 0–3
immaturity
parathyroid gland i.
pulmonary i.
immediate
i. extrauterine adaptation
i. hypersensitivity reaction
immersion
i. burn
i. oil
static i.
imminent abortion
immitis
Coccidioides i.
Dirofilaria i.
immobile
immobilization
cervical spine i.
Treponema pallidum i. (TPI)
immobilizer
Olympic Neostraint i.
straight-leg i.
immotile
i. cilia
i. cilia syndrome
Immulite
immune
i. clearance
i. complex (IC)
i. complex disease
i. complex dissociation (ICD)
i. complex-mediated
 glomerulonephritis
i. complex-mediated pericarditis
i. complex-mediated vasculitis
i. complex vasculitis
i. deficiency
i. dysregulation
i. factor
i. fetal hydrops
i. globulin
i. hemolysis
i. hydrops fetalis
i. monitoring technique
i. neutropenia
i. phase
i. process
i. response
i. response gene
rubella i.

i. separation technique
i. serum globulin (ISG)
i. suppressor gene
i. surveillance
i. system
i. system anatomy
i. thrombocytopenia
i. thrombocytopenic purpura (ITP)
immune-competent children
immune-mediated
i.-m. abnormality
i.-m. disseminated encephalomyelitis
i.-m. neutropenia
i.-m. thrombocytopenia
immunity
adaptive i.
Burnet acquired i.
cell-mediated i. (CMI)
cellular i.
humoral i.
passive i.
previous maternal i.
immunization
active i.
blood group i.
diphtheria, tetanus-pertussis i.
Engerix-B i.
Haemophilus influenzae type b i.
hepatitis A, B i.
MMR i.
I. Monitoring Program, Active
 (IMPACT)
passive i.
polio i.
preconception i.
prophylactic i.
Recombivax HB i.
Rh i.
tetanus-diphtheria i.
varicella i.
immunizing unit (IU)
Immuno
Feiba VH I.
Gammabulin I.
immunoassay
alpha-fetoprotein enzyme i. (AFP-
 EIA)
BioStar Flu optical i.
chemiluminescent i. (CIA)
Chlamydiazyme i.
enzyme i. (EIA)
fluorescent i. (FIA)
fluorescent polarization i. (FPIA)
gold-labeled optical rapid i.
 (GLORIA)
growth hormone i.
microparticle enzyme i.
nonradioactive i.
nonreactive i.

optical i. (OIA)
Premier Platinum HpSA enzyme i.,
  The
Quantikine human IL-6 I.
radioactive i.
SalEst i.
solid-phase enzyme i.
immunobead test (IBT)
immunobiologic
immunoblastic
  i. lymphoma
  i. sarcoma
immunoblot
  i. assay
  Western i.
immunochemiluminometric insulin assay
immunochemistry
immunochemotherapy
immunocompetence
  maternal i.
immunocompetent cell
immunocompromised child
immunocytochemical
immunocytochemistry
immunodeficiency
  acquired i.
  cellular i.
  i., centromeric heterochromatin
    instability, facial anomalies
    syndrome
  i., centromeric instability, facial
    anomalies (ICF)
  combined i. (CID)
  common variable i. (CVI, CVID)
  humoral i.
  primary i. (PID)
  severe combined i. (SCID)
  X-linked severe combined i. (X-
    SCID)
immunodeficient
immunodiagnosis
immunoelectrophoresis
immunofluorescence
  3-color i.
  direct i. (DIF)
  indirect i. (IIF)
  i. study
immunofluorescent
  i. antibody (IFA)
  i. assay (IFA)
  i. *Chlamydia* test
immunofunctional assay

immunogen
immunogenetics
immunogenic
immunogenicity
immunoglobulin (Ig)
  i. A (IgA)
  i. A nephropathy
  antenatal anti-D i.
  i. antibody
  anti-D i.
  i. A subclass 1 (IgA1)
  i. A subclass 2 (IgA2)
  cytomegalovirus i. (CMVIG)
  cytomegalovirus-specific i.
  i. D (IgD)
  i. deposition
  i. E (IgE)
  i. E level
  i. F (IgF)
  i. G (IgG)
  i. G2 (IgG2)
  i. G4 (IgG4)
  i. gene
  i. G subclass deficiency
  human immunodeficiency virus i.
    (HIVIG)
  i., intravenous (IGIV)
  intravenous i. (IVIG, IVIg)
  intravenous anti-D i.
  i. M (IgM)
  quantitative i.
  respiratory syncytial virus i.
    (RSVIG, RSV-IG)
  respiratory syncytial virus
    intravenous i. (RSV-IGIV, RSV-
    IVIG)
  Rh i.
  RhD i.
  surface i.
  tetanus i. (TIG)
  thyroid-stimulating i.
  varicella-zoster i. (VZIG)
  Venilon human i.
immunohistochemical
  i. change
  i. stromal leukocyte characterization
immunologic
  i. assay
  i. change
  i. disturbance
  i. enhancement
  i. factor

NOTES

immunologic *(continued)*
  i. maladaptation
  i. paralysis
  i. pregnancy test
  i. reaction
  i. screening
  i. study
  i. suppression
  i. surveillance
  i. tolerance
  i. unresponsiveness
immunological infertility
immunology
  maternal i.
  nutritional i.
  placental i.
  transplantation i.
  tumor i.
immunomodulation
immunomodulator
immunomodulatory treatment
immunoosseous dysplasia
immunoperoxidase
  i. stain
  i. technique
immunoproliferative small intestinal disease
immunoprophylaxis
immunoprotein
immunoradiometric assay (IRMA)
immunoreaction
immunoreactive trypsinogen (IRT)
immunoreactivity
immunoresistance
immunosorbent agglutination assay (ISAGA)
immunosuppression
  pharmacologic i.
immunosuppressive
  i. drug
  i. therapy
immunotherapy
  active specific i. (ASI)
  adoptive i.
  allergen i.
  i. hernia
  nonspecific i.
  Pacis BCG i.
  rush i.
  specific i.
  systemic-active nonspecific i.
  tumor i.
Imodium
  I. A-D
  I. Advanced
Imogam
Imovax
IMP
  iatrogenic multiple pregnancy

IMPACT
  Immunization Monitoring Program, Active
impacted
  i. bowel
  i. fetus
  i. fracture
  i. twins
  i. uterus
Impact of Events Scale (IES)
impaction
  delirium, infection, pharmacology, psychology, endocrinopathy, restricted mobility, stool i. (DIAPPERS)
  fecal i.
  food i.
  psychological causes, excessive urine production, restricted mobility, stool i.
  stool i.
impaired
  i. cognitive function
  emotionally i.
  i. glucose tolerance (IGT)
  i. rectal sensation
  i. secretion
  i. taste
  i. vision
impairment
  auditory i.
  bilateral hearing i.
  cognitive i.
  conductive hearing i.
  cortical visual i. (CVI)
  functional i.
  inherited androgen uptake i.
  intrauterine growth i.
  mixed hearing i.
  neurocognitive i.
  neurologic i.
  neurosensory i. (NSI)
  opioidergic control i.
  renal i.
  sensorineural hearing i.
  sensory i.
  somatosensory i.
  unilateral hearing i.
impedance
  acoustic i.
  i. audiometry
  bioelectrical i. (BEI)
  i. cardiogram
  fetal vascular i.
  i. plethysmography
  i. pneumography
  transcephalic i.
  i. tympanometry
impending renal failure

imperfecta
> amelogenesis i.
> dentinogenesis i.
> osteogenesis i. (type I–IV) (OI)
> perinatal lethal osteogenesis i.
> progressive deforming
>   osteogenesis i.
> Sillence classification of
>   osteogenesis i. (type I, IA, IB,
>   II, III, IV, IVA, IVB)

imperforate
> i. anus
> i. anus, hand, and foot anomalies
> i. anus repair
> i. hymen
> i. nasolacrimal duct
> i. urethra
> i. vagina

impervious
> i. sheet
> i. stockinette

impetigo
> Bockhart i.
> bullous i.
> i. contagiosa
> group A streptococcal i.
> i. herpetiformis
> i. neonatorum
> nonbullous i.
> staphylococcal i.
> i. strain

impingement
> i. syndrome
> i. test

Implanon
implant
> benign i.
> Biocell RTV saline-filled breast i.
> breast i.
> cesium i.
> Clarion hearing i.
> cochlear i.
> collapsed subpectoral i.
> Contigen Bard collagen i.
> Contigen glutaraldehyde cross-linked
>   collagen i.
> contraceptive i.
> ectopic i.
> endometrial i.
> endometriotic i.
> fetal tissue i.
> goserelin acetate i.

> hormonal i.
> interstitial i.
> iridium i.
> levonorgestrel i.
> metastatic i.
> Norplant i.
> Organon percutaneous E2 i.
> peritoneal i.
> progestin-only i.
> radioactive i.
> radium i.
> saline i.
> silicone i.
> subdermal i.
> subdermal levonorgestrel i. (SLI)
> subpectoral i.
> transperineal i.
> transvaginal i.
> Zoladex I.

implantable hormonal contraceptive
implantation
> bilateral PC-IOL i.
> blastocyst i.
> i. bleeding
> cortical i.
> delayed i.
> displacement i.
> ectopic i.
> i. failure
> fusion i.
> intrusive i.
> i. phase
> placental i.
> prosthetic graft i.
> i. protein
> radioactive seed i.
> i. theory
> tubouterine i.

impotence
> psychogenic i.

impotent
impregnate
impregnated vaginal packing
impression
> basilar i.
> Clinical Global I.'s (CGI)

Impress Softpatch
imprint
> touch i.

imprinted gene
imprinting
> genomic i.

NOTES

467

improper formula preparation
improved
    Clearblue I.
    Hybolin I.
impulse
    apical i.
    point of maximal i. (PMI)
    point of maximum i. (PMI)
    i. spectrum disorder
impulsive
impulsivity
    hyperactive i.
Imuran
Imuthiol
IMV
    intermittent mandatory ventilation
    intermittent mechanical ventilation
IMx Estradiol Assay
^{111}**In**
    indium-111
in
    rooming in
    in situ
    in situ nucleic acid hybridization
    in situ pinning
    in situ tubularization
    toeing in
    in toto
    in utero (IU)
    in utero drainage
    in utero drainage of fetal bladder
    in utero drug exposure (IUDE)
    in utero exposure
    in utero hypoxia
    in utero percutaneous umbilical
      cord ligation
    in utero reduction
    in utero reduction of herniated
      viscera
    in utero resection
    in utero stem cell therapy
    in utero transplantation
    in vitro
    in vitro antibody production
      (IVAP)
    in vitro efficacy
    in vitro fertilization (IVF)
    in vitro fertilization-embryo transfer
      (IVF-ET)
    in vitro human intestinal organ
      culture
    in vitro maturation
    in vitro resistance
    in vivo
    in vivo fertilization
    in vivo gene therapy
inactivated
    i. poliomyelitis vaccine

    i. polio vaccine
    i. poliovirus
    i. poliovirus vaccine (IPV)
    i. virus vaccine
    i. X chromosome
inactivation
    i. pattern
    random X i.
    X i.
inactive endometrium
inactivity
    alert i.
    glucuronyl transferase i.
inadequacy
    luteal phase i.
inadequate
    i. body awareness
    i. luteal phase
    i. maternal nutrition
inanition fever
inapparent poliomyelitis
inappropriate
    i. antidiuretic hormone (IADH)
    i. antidiuretic hormone secretion
    i. lactation
Inapsine
inattention
    i. dimension
    i. domain
inattention-overactivity with aggression
  (IOWA)
inattentive
inborn
    i. error
    i. error of bile acid biosynthesis
    i. error of bile acid synthesis
    i. error of metabolism (IEM)
inbreeding
    coefficient of i.
    i. coefficient
    i. depression
INCA
    infant nasal cannula assembly
incadronate
incapacitating pain
incarcerated
    i. fundus
    i. gravid uterus
    i. placenta
incarcerated inguinal hernia
incarceration
    uterine i.
Incert bioabsorbable sponge
incessant ovulation
incest
incestuous
incidence
incidentaloma

incipient
    i. abortion
    i. coagulopathy
incision
    abdominal i.
    Bevan i.
    bikini cut i.
    bilateral subcostal i.'s
    boutonnière i.
    buttonhole i.
    cervical i.
    Cherney i.
    classical transverse i.
    classical uterine i.
    i. closure
    colpotomy i.
    counter stab wound i.
    i. and drainage (I&D)
    Dührssen i.
    elliptical uterine i.
    endoscopic i.
    gridiron i.
    hockey stick i.
    infraumbilical i.
    inverted T uterine i.
    Joel-Cohen i.
    Kehr i.
    Lanz i.
    laparoscopic i.
    laparotomy i.
    lazy-S i.
    low-segment transverse i.
    low transverse uterine i.
    low vertical uterine i.
    Maylard i.
    McBurney i.
    midline i.
    paramedian i.
    periumbilical i.
    Pfannenstiel i.
    prior low transverse uterine i.
    prior low vertical uterine i.
    Rockey-Davis i.
    rooftop i.
    saber cut i.
    Sanger i.
    Schuchardt i.
    Sellheim i.
    smiling i.
    subcostal i.
    supraumbilical i.
    transverse skin i.

    uterine i.
    vertical i.
    Y i.
incisional
    i. hernia
    i. neuroma
incisor
    barrel-shaped upper central i.
    central i.
    Hutchinson i.
    intruded i.
    lateral i.
    peg-shaped upper central i.
    prominent maxillary i.
    single central maxillary i. (SCMI)
incisure
    Schmidt-Lantermann i.
inciting event
inclination
    pelvic i.
incline
inclusion
    i. body
    i. body of chlamydial conjunctivitis
    i. cell
    i. cell disease
    i. cyst
    full i.
    hyaline eosinophilic i.
    intracytoplasmic i.
    lipid i.
    Paneth cell i.
    paracrystalline i.
incognito
    tinea i.
incoherence
income
    Supplemental Security I. (SSI)
incomitant strabismus
incompatibility
    ABO i.
    blood group i.
    minor group antigen i.
    platelet-antigen i.
    Rh i.
incompatible blood group antigen
incompetence
    cervical i. (CI)
    congenital palatopharyngeal i. (CPI)
    florid pulmonary valvular i.
    gastroesophageal i.
    organic tricuspid i.

NOTES

incompetence *(continued)*
    palatopharyngeal i.
    pelvic vein i.
    pharyngeal i.
    sphincteric i.
    velopharyngeal i. (VPI)
incompetent
    i. cervix
    i. lower esophageal sphincter
incomplete
    i. abortion
    i. androgen insensitivity
    i. bowel obstruction
    i. breech presentation
    i. cleft
    i. conjoined twins
    i. dominance
    i. foot presentation
    i. hernia
    i. knee presentation
    i. müllerian fusion
    i. precocious puberty
    i. rectal prolapse
incompletus
    coitus i.
incongruent hip
inconsequential occurrence
inconspicuous penis
incontinence
    anal i.
    anorectal i.
    Blaivas classification of urinary i.
    exercise-induced i.
    fecal i.
    functional i.
    genuine stress i. (GSI)
    giggle i.
    I. Impact Questionnaire (IIQ)
    I. Impact Questionnaire-Revised
      (IIQ-R)
    key-in-lock i.
    i. of milk
    mixed i.
    Miyazaki-Bonney test for stress i.
    overflow i.
    paradoxical i.
    passive i.
    postpartum i.
    I. quality-of-life (I-QOL)
    reflex i.
    stress i.
    I. Stress questionnaire (ISQ)
    stress urinary i. (SUI)
    true i.
    urge i.
    urinary exertional i.
    urinary stress i.
incontinentia
    i. pigmenti achromians

    i. pigmenti syndrome
    i. pigmenti (type I, II)
incorporation
    meatal advancement and
      glansplasty i. (MAGPI)
    meatal advancement and
      glanuloplasty i. (MAGPI)
increase
    plasma prorenin i.
increased
    i. anteroposterior chest diameter
    i. bone density
    i. fatigability
    i. femoral anteversion
    i. globulin fraction
    i. intracranial pressure
    i. renin release
    i. vascular resistance
increta
    placenta i.
incubate
incubation period
incubator
    Air Shields i.
    convection-warmed i.
    double-insulated i.
    double-walled i.
    Forma water-jacketed i.
    Ohmeda Care-Plus i.
    single-walled i.
incudiform uterus
incus
indapamide
independence
    causal i.
independent
Inderal LA
indeterminate
    i. leprosy
    i. sleep
indeterminus
    situs inversus i.
index, pl. **indices, indexes**
    acetabular i. (AI)
    age i.
    amniotic fluid i. (AFI)
    anal i. (AI)
    anterior cerebral artery pulsatility i.
      (ACAPI)
    anxiety sensitivity i. (ASI)
    axial acetabular i. (AAI)
    Bailey Physical Development I.
    Bayley Mental Developmental i.
    Bayley Psychomotor
      Developmental I.
    blood cell indices
    body mass i. (BMI)
    borderline amniotic fluid i.
    Broders i.

i. case
Charlson comorbidity i.
Clinical Colitis Activity I. (CCAI)
clinical global i. (CGI)
Colour I. (C.I.)
Conners Hyperactivity indices
deoxyribonucleic acid i.
Doppler myocardial performance i.
Female Sexual Function I. (FSFI)
fetal-pelvic i.
fine motor i.
i. finger
Foam Stability I. (FSI)
free androgen i.
free testosterone i.
free thyroxine i.
glycemic i.
gross motor i.
growth i.
Hollingshead 5-factor i.
HuGE i.
iliac apophysis maturation i.
karyopyknotic i.
Kessner I.
Kruger i.
Kupperman i.
left ventricular stroke work i.
  (LVSWI)
Lloyd-Still i.
McGoon i.
Mengert i.
mental development i. (MDI)
Mentzer i.
migration i. (MI)
mixed obstructive apnea/hypopnea i.
  (MOAHI)
neural i.
nonverbal developmental i.
oxygenation i. (OI)
Parental Stress I. (PSI)
Pearl i.
Pediatric Crohn Disease Activity I.
  (PCDAI)
pelvic i.
pelvic support i. (PSI)
Penetrating Abdominal Trauma I.
  (PATI)
Physiologic Stability I. (PSI)
placental maturity i.
ponderal i. (PI)
Pourcelot i.

Prehospital I. (PHI)
prepregnancy body mass i.
Psychological General Well-Being I.
  (PGWB)
psychomotor development i. (PDI)
pulsatility i. (PI)
quantitative insulin sensitivity
  check i. (QUICKI)
Quetelet body mass i.
radiographic bone strength i.
  (RBSI)
resistance i. (RI)
Rohrer i.
short-increment sensitivity i. (SISI)
Silverman-Anderson i.
State-Trait Anxiety I.-I (STAI-I)
Stuart i.
sun protection behavior i. (SBPI)
testosterone i.
thyroid i.
Tobin i.
total testosterone i.
umbilical coiling i. (UCI)
urinary diagnostic i. (UDI)
weight/height i.
W/H i.
Wintrobe i.
India
  I. ink stain
  I. ink test
  I. rubber skin
Indiana pouch
Indian childhood cirrhosis (ICC)
indican
indicanuria
indications
  maternal i.
indicator
  Bioself fertility i.
  prognostic i.
indices (*pl. of* index)
Indiclor test
indifferent
  i. genitalia
  i. gonadal stage
  i. gonads
indigenous neoplasm
indigo
  i. carmine
  i. carmine dye
indigotin

NOTES

indinavir
- i. calculi
- i. crystal

indirect
- i. bilirubin
- i. calorimetry
- i. Coombs test
- i. cystography
- i. fluorescent antibody (IFA)
- i. hemagglutination
- i. hemagglutination antibody (IHA)
- i. hyperbilirubinemia
- i. immunofluorescence (IIF)
- i. inguinal hernia
- i. laryngoscopy
- i. laser ophthalmoscope
- i. ophthalmoscope
- i. ophthalmoscopy
- i. orbital floor fracture
- i. placentography
- i. visualization

indium-111 (^{111}In)
indium-labeled leukocyte scan
individualized
- I. Education Program (IEP)
- I. Family Service Plan (IFSP)

Individuals with Disabilities Education Act (IDEA)
Indocin
- I. I.V.
- I. I.V. Injection
- I. SR
- I. SR Oral

indocyanine green
indolamine
indolent
- i. carditis
- i. granular CMV retinitis

indomethacin
indrawing
- intercostal i.
- supraclavicular i.

induced
- i. abortion
- i. labor
- i. remission
- i. sputum analysis (ISA)

induction
- Cytotec i.
- gonadotropin ovulation i.
- labor augmentation i.
- menstrual cycle i.
- ovulation i.
- Pitocin i.
- rapid sequence i.
- Spemann i.
- superovulation i.
- i. therapy

induction-to-delivery interval

induration
- nonpitting i.

indurative edema
indusium, pl. **indusia**
- i. griseum

indwelling
- i. arterial catheter (IAC)
- i. cannula
- i. catheter
- i. optode
- i. thumb
- i. venous catheter (IVC)
- i. venous line (IVL)

ineffective myelopoiesis
inefficiency
- female fertility i.

inequality
- limb length i.

inertia
- primary uterine i.
- secondary uterine i.
- true uterine i.
- uterine i.

inertially-induced injury
inevitable abortion
Infalyte formula
infancy
- acropustulosis of i.
- acute hemorrhagic edema of i. (AHEI)
- anaclitic depression of i.
- apnea of i.
- autoimmune neutropenia of i. (ANI)
- benign myoclonus of i.
- benign paroxysmal torticollis of i.
- chronic nonspecific diarrhea of i.
- chronic pneumonitis of i. (CPI)
- cricopharyngeal incoordination of i.
- diencephalic syndrome of i.
- familial hyperinsulinism of i.
- hemorrhagic edema of i.
- hypertrophic interstitial neuropathy of i.
- intractable diarrhea of i. (IDI)
- nonfamilial hyperinsulinism of i.
- normal gastroesophageal reflux of i.
- persistent hyperinsulinemic hypoglycemia of i. (PHHI)
- physiologic anemia of i.
- protracted diarrhea of i.
- severe myoclonic epilepsy in i. (SMEI)
- spongy degeneration of i.
- transient hypogammaglobulinemia of i. (THI)

infancy-onset diabetes mellitus, multiple epiphyseal dysplasia syndrome

Infanrix vaccine
infant
> acid-loaded i.
> aneuploidy i.
> asphyctic i.
> at-risk i.
> I. Behavior Record (IBR)
> i. death
> i. development
> i. development program
> i. development specialist
> i. of diabetic mother (IDM)
> i. dietary supplement
> drug-depressed i.
> dysmature i.
> i. dyssomnia
> i. educator
> ELBW i.
> extremely low birth weight i. (ELBWI)
> extremely premature i. (EPI)
> i. face scale
> floppy i.
> I. Flow nCPAP system
> full-term i.
> i. Hercules
> high-risk i.
> hydropic i.
> i. hypergastrinemia
> hyperinsulinemic i.
> immature i.
> jittery i.
> large-for-dates i.
> LBW i.
> LGA i.
> liveborn i.
> low birth weight i. (LBWI)
> macrosomic i.
> MAS-ECMO i.
> mature i.
> i. morbidity
> i. mortality
> i. mortality rate
> i. nasal cannula assembly (INCA)
> Neurodevelopmental Assessment of Preterm I.'s (NAPI)
> periodic breathing in i.'s
> postmature i.
> postterm i.
> premature i. (PI)
> preterm i.

> i. respiratory distress syndrome (IRDS)
> Rh-positive i.
> SGA i.
> singleton i.
> i. size (IS)
> sleepy i.
> small premature i.
> i. Star high-frequency ventilator
> I. Star 8000 oscillator
> stillborn i.
> i. stimulation program
> i. subdural tap
> i. of substance-abusing mother (ISAM)
> i. suffocation
> i. teacher
> term i.
> very low birth weight i.
> viable i.
> vigorous i.
> VLBW i.
> well-oxygenated i.

infanticide
infantile
> i. achalasia
> i. acquired aphasia
> i. acropustulosis
> i. agranulocytosis
> i. Alexander disease
> i. anorexia
> i. arteriosclerosis
> i. asthma
> i. autism
> i. beriberi
> i. bilateral striatal necrosis syndrome (IBSN)
> i. botulism (IB)
> i. breath-holding response
> i. cataract
> i. celiac disease
> i. cerebellooptic atrophy
> i. cerebral sphingolipidosis
> i. choreoathetosis of Fisher
> i. colic
> i. corneal clouding
> i. cortical hyperostosis
> i. diarrhea
> i. diarrhea rotavirus
> i. digital fibroma
> i. diplegia
> i. disseminated histoplasmosis

NOTES

infantile *(continued)*

- i. dwarfism
- i. eczema
- i. embryonal carcinoma
- i. epilepsy
- i. epileptic encephalopathy
- i. fibromatosis
- i. Gaucher disease
- i. glaucoma
- i. hemangiopericytoma
- i. hemiplegia
- i. hepatic hemangioma
- i. hypercalcemia
- i. hypertension
- i. hypertrophic pyloric stenosis (IHPS)
- i. idiopathic scoliosis
- i. monoclonic seizure
- i. motor neuron disease
- i. muscular hypotonia
- i. muscular torticollis
- i. myoclonic jerk
- i. myoclonic seizure
- i. myofibrillar myopathy
- i. myofibromatosis
- i. myxedema
- i. myxedema-muscular hypertrophy
- i. NCL
- i. neuroaxonal dystrophy
- i. neuronal degeneration
- i. neuropathic cystinosis
- i. obstructive cholangiopathy
- i. onset
- i. optic atrophy-ataxia syndrome
- i. osteopetrosis
- i. paralysis
- i. periarteritis nodosa (IPN)
- i. PKD
- i. poikiloderma
- i. polyarteritis nodosa (IPAN)
- i. polycystic disease
- i. polycystic kidney disease (IPKD)
- i. polyneuritis
- i. progressive spinal muscular atrophy (type I–III)
- i. purulent conjunctivitis
- i. pustulosis
- i. pyknocytosis
- i. Refsum disease
- i. Refsum disease continuum
- i. respiratory distress syndrome
- i. salaam
- i. scurvy
- i. seborrhea
- i. sialic acid storage disorder (ISSD)
- i. sleep apnea
- i. spasm

- i. spasms, hypsarrhythmia, mental retardation syndrome
- i. spasms with mental retardation
- i. spastic paraplegia
- i. spinal muscular atrophy
- i. striatonigral degeneration
- i. subacute necrotizing encephalopathy
- i. syncope
- i. system hyalinosis
- i. tetany
- i. thoracic dystrophy
- i. tibia vara
- i. tremor syndrome

infantile-onset spinocerebellar ataxia

infantilis

- dystaxia cerebralis i.
- poliodystrophia cerebri progressiva i.

infantilism

- Brissaud i.
- cachectic i.
- celiac i.
- dysthyroidal i.
- hepatic i.
- Herter i.
- hypophysial i.
- Lorain-Lévi i.
- muscular i.
- myxedematous i.
- pseudonuchal i.
- regressive i.
- sexual i.

infantis

- *Bifidobacterium i.*

infantiseptica

- granulomatosis i.

infantum

- anemia pseudoleukemica i.
- cholera i.
- dermatitis gangrenosa i.
- granuloma gluteal i.
- *Leishmania i.*
- lichen i.
- roseola i.
- tabes i.

infarction, infarct

- acute myocardial i. (AMI)
- bilirubin i.
- bowel i.
- cavernosal i.
- cerebral i.
- chorionic villus i.
- CNS i.
- fan-shaped hemorrhagic i.
- fat-induced i.
- i. of herniated stomach
- hyperacute i.
- limb i.

maternal floor i.
multiple villous i.'s
myocardial i. (MI)
i. of oral epithelium
parasagittal cortical i.
periventricular i.
placental i.
pulmonary i.
renal i.
i. of skinfold
uric acid i.
white i.

In-Fast bone screw system
Infasurf
I. intratracheal suspension
I. surfactant
Infatab
infected
i. abortion
i. cuff hematoma
HIV i.
vertically i.
infection
acute lower respiratory i. (ALRI)
acute lower respiratory tract i.
(ALRTI)
acute respiratory i. (ARI)
adenovirus i.
adnexal i.
amniotic fluid i.
ascending intrauterine i.
astrovirus i.
asymptomatic i.
asymptomatic urinary tract i.
(AUTI)
bacterial i.
Bartonella henselae i.
benign papillomavirus i.
bloodstream i. (BSI)
bone i.
Calicivirus i.
Campylobacter i.
cervical i.
cervicovaginal i.
chlamydial i.
chorioamnion i.
chorioamnionic i.
chronic conjunctival i.
chronic parvoviral i.
chronic pelvic i.
congenital i.
congenital rubella i.

congenital STORCH i.
congenital syphilitic i.
conjunctival i.
Coxsackievirus A16 i.
Coxsackievirus B enterovirus i.
culture-negative cytomegalovirus i.
cytomegalovirus i.
dermatophyte i.
disseminated gonococcal i.
disseminated herpes i.
droplet i.
enteric i.
enteroviral i.
fetal cytomegalovirus i.
fungal i.
gastrointestinal i.
genital i.
gland i.
gonococcal i.
granulomatous i.
group A beta-hemolytic
streptococcal i.
group B streptococcal i.
guinea worm i.
hematogenous i.
herpes whitlow i.
herpetic corneal i.
HIV i.
hookworm i.
intraabdominal i. (IAI)
intraamniotic i. (IAI)
intraarticular i.
intractable viral i.
intrauterine i. (IUI)
intrauterine parvovirus B19 i.
invasive bacterial i.
IUD-related i.
latent herpes simplex virus i.
lower genital tract i.
lower respiratory i. (LRI)
lower respiratory tract i. (LRTI)
lower urinary tract i.
lytic i.
MAI i.
i. marker
maternal i.
middle ear i.
multiple opportunistic pathogen i.
multiplicity of i. (MOI)
mycotic i.
nail-fold i.
neisserial i.

NOTES

475

infection *(continued)*
    neonatal herpes simplex virus i.
    nonprimary i.
    nontuberculous mycobacterial i.
    nosocomial i.
    nosocomial bacterial i. (NBI)
    opportunistic i.
    overwhelming i.
    papillomavirus i.
    parameningeal i.
    parasitic i.
    paronychial i.
    parvoviral i.
    pediatric gonococcal i.
    pelvic i.
    perinatally acquired HIV i.
    pharyngeal gonococcal i.
    i. point
    polymicrobial pelvic i.
    posthysterectomy i.
    postpartum i.
    prenatal i.
    primary i.
    puerperal i.
    pyogenic i.
    recurrent staphylococcal i.
    respiratory tract i.
    retroperitoneal i.
    rhinocerebral i.
    rickettsial i.
    rubella i.
    SEM i.
    serious bacterial i. (SBI)
    Serratia marcescens i.
    sexually transmitted i. (STI)
    silent congenital CMV i.
    simplex i.
    sinopulmonary tract i.
    skeletal i.
    spirochetal i.
    stage A, B, C, N i.
    staphylococcal i.
    Stenotrophomonas maltophilia i.
    streptococcal i.
    suppurative i.
    surgical i.
    symptomatic i.
    syphilitic i.
    tick-borne i.
    TORCH i.
    transplacental i.
    trichomonal i.
    Trichomonas i.
    upper genital tract i.
    upper respiratory i. (URI)
    upper respiratory tract i. (URTI)
    upper urinary tract i.
    urinary tract i. (UTI)
    uterine i.
    vaginal i.
    varicella i.
    varicella-zoster virus i.
    vertically acquired i.
    Vincent i.
    viral upper respiratory tract i.
    vulvar i.
    vulvovaginal premenarchal i.
    wound i.
    yeast i.
    yersinial i.
    zoonotic i.

infection-associated hemophagocytic syndrome (IAHS)

infectiosum
    erythema i.

infectious
    i. arthritis
    i. colitis
    i. disease
    i. eczematoid dermatitis
    i. endocarditis (IE)
    i. esophagitis
    i. gastritis
    i. hepatitis
    i. lymphocytosis
    i. mononucleosis (IM)
    i. myocarditis
    i. pancreatitis
    i. pericarditis
    i. peritonitis
    i. polyneuritis
    i. pulmonary tuberculosis
    i. rhinitis

infective
    i. dermatitis
    i. endarteritis
    i. endocarditis (IE)
    i. phlebitis

Infectrol Ophthalmic
infecundity
inference
    causal i.
inferior
    i. clivus
    i. colliculus
    i. epigastric artery
    i. fascia
    i. hemorrhoidal nerve
    inferior i.
    i. mesenteric artery
    i. mesenteric vein
    i. olivary nucleus
    i. peduncle
    i. pincer grasp
    i. rectal nerve
    i. straight
    i. turbinate surgery

i. vena cava (IVC)
i. vena cava disruption
infertile
    i. patient
    i. woman
infertility
    i. agent
    anovulatory i.
    asymptomatic i.
    Chlamydia trachomatis tubal i.
    endometriosis-associated i.
    etiologic fraction of tubal i.
    i. evaluation
    i. factor
    familial i.
    iatrogenic i.
    idiopathic i.
    immunological i.
    inherited i.
    i. investigation
    male factor i.
    i. management
    i. perceptions inventory (IPI)
    primary i.
    secondary i.
    i. treatment
    tubal factor i.
    unexplained i.
infestation
    louse i.
    pinworm i.
    threadworm i.
infibulation
infiltrate
    cellular i.
    eosinophilic i.
    inflammatory i.
    interstitial i.
    leukemia i.
    liver i.
    lung i.
    miliary i.
    patchy i.
    perihilar i.
    perivascular eosinophilic i.
    perivascular inflammatory i.
    perivascular polymorphonuclear i.
    plasma cell i.
    pleomorphic cellular i.
    polymorphonuclear i.
    pulmonary i.
    retinal i.

streaky i.
white retinal i.
xanthogranulomatous i.
yellow retinal i.
infiltrating
    i. ductal carcinoma (IDC)
    i. lobular carcinoma (ILC)
    i. small-cell lobular carcinoma
infiltration
    bone marrow i.
    fatty i.
    leukocyte i.
    lidocaine i.
    lymphohistiocytic i.
    lymphomatous i.
    lymphoplasmacytic i.
    nodular i.
    patchy i.
    peribronchial i.
    peribronchiolar i.
    perineal i.
Inflamase
    I. Forte Ophthalmic
    I. Mild Ophthalmic
inflamed
inflammation
    acute renal parenchymal i.
    chronic synovial i.
    ductal i.
    eye i.
    fibrosing i.
    histologic placental i.
    intraamniotic i.
    lymphoplasmacytic i.
    maternal intravascular i.
    orbital i.
    pelvic i.
    portal i.
    transmural i.
    vulvovaginal i.
inflammatory
    i. arteritis
    i. bacterial enteritis
    i. bowel disease (IBD)
    I. Bowel Disease Questionnaire (IBDQ)
    i. bowel malignancy
    i. breast cancer (IBC)
    i. Brown syndrome
    i. carcinoma
    i. cascade
    i. colitis

NOTES

inflammatory *(continued)*
> i. demyelinating encephalomyelitis
> i. demyelination
> i. exudate
> i. idiocy
> i. infiltrate
> i. molecule
> i. myopathy
> i. myositis
> i. polyp
> i. process
> i. pseudotumor (IPT)
> i. response

inflatable ball pessary
inflection
> voice i.

infliximab
influence
> neurobiologic i.

influenza (flu)
> i. A,B,C
> i. A encephalitis
> i. vaccine
> i. virus

influenzae
> *Haemophilus i.*

influenza-like syndrome
influenzal meningitis
informatics
information
> integrate sensory i.
> pediatric dosing i.
> sensory i.

informed
> i. consent
> i. consent disclosure rules

informosome
infraclavicular area
infraction
> Freiberg i.

InfraGuide
infrahyoid ectopia
inframammary
infraorbital nerve
infrapubic ramus
infrared
> i. photocoagulation (IRC)
> i. spectroscopy
> i. thermographic calorimetry (ITC)

infratentorial
> i. tuberculoma
> i. tumor

infraumbilical incision
infravesical obstruction
infundibular
> i. chamber
> i. pulmonic stenosis
> i. stalk

infundibuliform hymen
infundibulopelvic (IP)
> i. ligament
> i. vessel

infundibulum
> i. of fallopian tube
> right ventricular i.

infusate
Infuse-A-Port catheter
infusion
> alkali i.
> apotransferrin i.
> bicarbonate i.
> colloid i.
> continuous glucose i.
> continuous milk i.
> continuous subcutaneous i. (CSQI)
> continuous subcutaneous insulin i.
> extraamniotic saline i. (EASI)
> fetal cortisol i.
> insulin i.
> intraarterial i.
> intralymphatic i.
> intraosseous i. (IOI)
> intravenous i.
> IO i.
> laminaria i.
> i. pump
> vasopressin i.

Ingelman-Sundberg gracilis muscle procedure
ingestion
> accidental caustic i.
> alcohol i.
> caustic i.
> coin i.
> copper sulfate i.
> drug i.
> fava bean i.
> goitrogen i.
> iron i.
> lead i.
> organophosphate i.
> paraquat i.
> toxic i.

Ingram bicycle seat
ingrown toenail
inguinal
> i. adenitis
> i. adenopathy
> i. area
> i. canal
> i. freckling
> i. hernia
> i. ligament
> i. lymphadenectomy
> i. lymphadenitis
> i. lymph node

i. lymph node metastasis
i. triangle
inguinale
granuloma i.
hernia i.
hernia uteri i.
lymphogranuloma i.
inguinal-femoral node dissection
INH
isoniazid
isonicotinic acid hydrazide
inhalation
i. anesthesia
Atrovent Aerosol I.
i. bronchial challenge testing
i. injury
INOmax for i.
intrapulmonary i.
NebuPent I.
nitrogen dioxide i.
i. of nitrous oxide
smoke i.
i. suspension
tobramycin solution for i. (TOBI)
inhaled
i. beta-2 agonist
i. bronchodilator
i. corticosteroid (ICS)
i. nitric oxide (iNO, I-NO)
i. steroid
inhaler
AeroBid-M Oral Aerosol I.
AeroBid Oral Aerosol I.
Azmacort Oral I.
Beconase AQ Nasal I.
Dexacort Phosphate Respihaler
Oral I.
Diskhaler metered-dose i.
Diskus i.
dry powder i. (DPI)
fluticasone propionate dry
powder i.
Nasalide Nasal I.
steroid i.
Vancenase Nasal I.
Vanceril Oral I.
inheritance
amphigonous i.
autosomal dominant i.
autosomal recessive i.
biparental i.
codominant i.

complemental i.
cytoplasmic i.
dominant i.
extrachromosomal i.
holandric i.
hologynic i.
homochronous i.
homotropic i.
maternal i.
matroclinous i.
mendelian i.
mitochondrial i.
monofactorial i.
multifactorial i.
oligogenic i.
polygenic i.
quantitative i.
quasicontinuous i.
recessive i.
sex-linked i.
unit i.
X-linked dominant i.
X-linked recessive i.
Y-linked i.
inherited
i. androgen uptake impairment
i. bleeding disorder
i. coagulopathy
i. hemolytic uremia syndrome
i. infertility
i. thrombophilia in pregnancy
inhibin
i. A, B
i. concentration
i. subunit
i. test
inhibin-A subunit
inhibited sexual desire
inhibiting
inhibition
agglutination i.
behavioral i.
callosal i.
FSH i.
hemagglutination i.
labor i.
luteinization i.
pituitary gonadotropin i.
premature uterine contraction i.
prostaglandin synthesis i.
response i.

NOTES

inhibition *(continued)*
    steroid secretion i.
    vagal i.
inhibitive casting
inhibitor
    ACE i.
    alpha-2 antiplasmin coagulation i.
    alpha-2 antitrypsin i.
    alpha-2AP coagulation i.
    alpha-2AT coagulation i.
    alpha-glucosidase i.
    alpha-2 macroglobulin coagulation i.
    alpha-2M coagulation i.
    alpha-1 protease i.
    alpha-1 proteinase i. (A1PI, a1PI)
    angiotensin-converting enzyme i.
    antithrombin III coagulation i.
    aromatase i.
    AT3 coagulation i.
    calcineurin i.
    CAMP-specific phosphodiesterase i.
    carbonic anhydrase i.
    cell growth i.
    C1 esterase i.
    cholinesterase i.
    C1INH coagulation i.
    corticotropin-releasing i.
    COX-2 i.
    dihydrofolate reductase i.
    dual nucleoside analog reverse transcriptase i.
    extrinsic pathway i.
    factor VII, VIII i.
    fibrinolysis i.
    FSH binding i.
    gonadotropin secretion i.
    HCII coagulation i.
    heme oxygenase i.
    heparin cofactor II i.
    HO i.
    human seminal (plasma) i. (HSI)
    hydrogen pump i.
    leukotriene i.
    lupus i.
    luteinization i.
    luteinizing hormone receptor-binding i.
    M2 i.
    monoamine oxidase i. (MAOI)
    neuraminidase i.
    nonnucleoside reverse transcriptase i. (NNRTI)
    nucleoside reverse transcriptase i. (NRTI)
    oocyte maturation i. (OMI)
    ovum-capture i.
    phosphodiesterase i. (PDI)
    plasminogen activator i. (PAI)
    prostaglandin synthetase i. (PGSI)
    protease i. (PI)
    protein C, S coagulation i.
    proton pump i. (PPI)
    reverse transcriptase i. (RTI)
    secretory leukocyte protease i.
    selective serotonin reuptake i. (SSRI)
    serine protease i. (SERPIN)
    serotonin reuptake i. (SRI)
    serum protease i.
    specific phosphodiesterase i.
    tissue factor pathway i. (TFPI)
    topoisomerase-1 i.
    urinary trypsin i.
inhibitor-1
    plasminogen-activator i.-1 (PAI-1)
inhibitor-2
    plasminogen-activator i.-2 (PAI-2)
in-hospital postpartum care
iniencephaly
iniodymus
iniopagus
iniops
initial apnea
initiated cycle
initiation
    labor i.
    lactation i.
    puberty i.
    sexual i.
inject
    Dekasol-L.A. I.
injectable
    i. bromocriptine
    Cardizem I.
    i. hormonal contraceptive
injection
    adrenaline i.
    Adrucil I.
    A-hydroCort I.
    A-methaPred I.
    Antispas I.
    Apresoline I.
    AquaMEPHYTON I.
    Arfonad I.
    Aristocort Forte I.
    Aristocort Intralesional I.
    Aristospan Intraarticular I.
    Aristospan Intralesional I.
    Astramorph PF I.
    Baci-IM I.
    Benadryl I.
    Bentyl Hydrochloride I.
    bulbar conjunctival i.
    Celestone Phosphate I.
    Cel-U-Jec I.
    Cetrorelix for i.
    Chloromycetin I.
    Chlor-Trimeton I.

choriogonadotropin alfa for i.
Cipro I.
conjunctival i.
continuous subcutaneous insulin i.
Decadron-LA I.
Decadron Phosphate I.
Decaject I.
Decaject-LA I.
decondensed spermhead i.
Definity suspension for IV i.
Dekasol I.
Delatestryl I.
Demadex I.
Depo-Estradiol I.
Depogen I.
Depo-Medrol I.
Depopred I.
Depo-Provera I.
Depo-Testosterone I.
Dexasone L.A. I.
Dexone LA I.
Diazemuls I.
Dilaudid I.
Dilaudid-HP I.
Diprivan I.
direct egg i.
direct intraperitoneal i. (DIPI)
Duraclon I.
Duramorph I.
Edecrin Sodium I.
ganirelix acetate i.
Genotropin I.
glutaraldehyde cross-linked
  collagen i.
Hexadrol Phosphate I.
Humalog insulin lispro i.
Humatrope I.
Hydrocortone Acetate I.
Hydrocortone Phosphate I.
Hyrexin-50 I.
Hyzine-50 I.
Imitrex I.
Indocin I.V. I.
intracardiac i.
intracytoplasmic sperm i. (ICSI)
intracytoplasmic sperm head i.
  (ICSHI)
intraurethral bulk i.
Isuprel I.
Kefurox I.
Kenalog I.
Key-Pred I.

Key-Pred-SP I.
Kytril I.
Lasix I.
Levothroid I.
local methotrexate i.
medroxyprogesterone i.
Minocin IV I.
monotropins for i.
Nebcin I.
Neut I.
nonexudative conjunctival i.
Norditropin I.
Nuromax I.
Nutropin AQ I.
Nydrazid I.
Octocaine I.
Osmitrol I.
paracervical i.
Pentam-300 I.
periurethral collagen i.
pessary i.
Phenergan I.
Prednisol TBA I.
Prorex I.
Protropin I.
Regonol I.
retrograde ureteral dye i.
Romazicon I.
round spermatid nuclei i. (ROSNI)
Saizen I.
i. sclerotherapy
Serostim I.
silicone i.
Solu-Cortef I.
Solu-Medrol I.
Solurex LA I.
Somatropin (rDNA origin) for i.
Sublimaze I.
subtrigonal i.
subureteric Teflon i.
subzonal i. (SUZI)
Sufenta I.
Synthroid I.
Tac-3 I.
Teflon periurethral i.
Terramycin I.M. I.
Ticon I.
Tigan I.
Toposar I.
Toradol I.
transurethral collagen i.
Triam-A I.

NOTES

injection *(continued)*
- Triam Forte I.
- Triostat I.
- urofollitropin for i.
- Valium I.
- Vancocin I.
- Vancoled I.
- Vistaril I.
- Zinacef I.

injector
- Harris-Kronner uterine manipulator-i. (HUMI)
- Harris uterine i. (HUI)
- Injex i.
- MadaJet XL needle-free i.
- Mini-Flex flexible Harris uterine i.

Injex injector

injury
- AAST Organ Injury Scaling of vulva, vagina, bladder, urethral, rectal i. (grade I–V)
- acceleration i.
- accidental fetal i.
- acute i.
- airbag i.
- anoxic-ischemic i.
- asphyxial birth i.
- asphyxial brain i.
- avulsion i.
- axonal i.
- birth i.
- bladder i.
- blowout i.
- blunt cardiac i. (BCI)
- bowel i.
- brachial plexus i. (BPI)
- brain i.
- capillary leak i.
- catastrophic i.
- caustic i.
- cerebral i.
- cervical spinal cord i.
- cervical spine i.
- clavicular i.
- clenched fist i.
- closed fist i.
- closed head i. (CHI)
- compression i.
- congenital i.
- contrecoup i.
- coup i.
- crush i.
- deceleration i.
- degloving i.
- diaphragmatic i.
- diffuse axonal i. (DAI)
- emergent i.
- epiphyseal plate i.
- eversion i.
- excitotoxic i.
- extravasation i.
- facial nerve i. (FNI)
- fetal birth i.
- flexion-distraction i.
- greenstick i.
- growth plate i.
- hair tourniquet i.
- hepatocellular i.
- hippocampal pathologic i.
- hymenal i.
- hypoxic-ischemic brain i.
- hypoxic-ischemic cerebral i.
- iatrogenic airway i.
- iatrogenic ureteral i.
- inertially-induced i.
- inhalation i.
- intracranial i. (ICI)
- intraoperative gastrointestinal i.
- intrapleural i.
- irradiation i.
- ischemic brain i.
- Kehr sign for splenic i.
- large bowel i.
- Lauge-Hansen mechanism of i.
- life-threatening i.
- ligamentous i. (grade I–III)
- lumbosacral plexus i.
- mechanical birth i.
- meniscal i.
- mitochondrial i.
- muscular i.
- musculoskeletal i.
- neonatal brain i.
- neonatal cold i.
- nerve i.
- neurological i.
- neuromuscular i.
- obstetric traction i.
- overuse i.
- oxidative brain i.
- parasagittal cerebral i.
- pelvic nerve i.
- penetrating brain i.
- peripheral nerve i.
- physial i.
- popsicle i.
- i. prevention
- pulmonary i.
- radiation-induced physial i.
- rectal i.
- reperfusion i.
- Salter-Harris classification of epiphyseal plate i.
- scalding i.
- i. severity score (ISS)
- small bowel i.
- spinal cord i.
- splenic i.

I

sports-related i.
straddle i.
stress i.
submersion i.
The I. Prevention Program (TIPP)
thermal i.
tracheobronchial tree i.
traction i.
transfusion-associated lung i.
  (TRALI)
traumatic birth i.
traumatic brain i. (TBI)
ureteral i.
urological i.
vaginal i.
vascular i.
ventilator-induced lung i. (VILI)
ventilatory-associated lung i.
  (VALI)
vessel i.
whiplash i.
injury-related maternal death
inlet
pelvic i.
in-line probe
innate
inner
i. amnion
i. canthus
i. canthus displacement
i. cell mass
i. ear
innervated
innervation
autonomic i.
somatic sensory i.
sympathetic i.
innocent murmur
innocuous
innominate
i. artery
i. bone
i. osteotomy
i. vein
Innova
I. electrotherapy system
I. feminine incontinence treatment
  system
I. pelvic floor stimulator
Innovar
iNO, I-NO
inhaled nitric oxide

inoculata
varicella i.
inoculate
inoculation
inoculum
intranasal i.
INOH
instantaneous orthostatic hypotension
INOmax for inhalation
inorganic mercury salt
inosinate pyrophoshorylase enzyme
inosiplex
inositol trisphosphate
inotropic
i. effect
i. support
i. therapy
inotropy
Inoue-Melnick virus
INOvent delivery system
inpatient
i. management
i. monitoring
InPouch TV subculture kit
input
abnormal cortical visual i.
labyrinthine afferent i.
proprioceptive i.
unequal visual i.
vestibular i.
INR
international normalized ratio
INS
idiopathic nephrotic syndrome
121ins2 mutation
insect
i. bite
i. repellent
i. sting reaction
insecticide
organophosphate i.
insecurity
food i.
insemination
artificial i. (AI)
artificial intravaginal i.
cervical i.
cup i.
direct intraperitoneal i. (DIPI)
i. dish
donor i. (DI)
heterologous i.

NOTES

483

insemination *(continued)*
    high intrauterine i.
    homologous i.
    intrafollicular i. (IFI)
    intraperitoneal i. (IPI)
    intratubal i. (ITI)
    intrauterine i. (IUI)
    intravaginal i. (IVI)
    Makler i.
    subzonal i. (SUZI)
    i. swim-up technique
    therapeutic i.
    therapeutic donor i. (TDI)
    washed intrauterine i.
insensible
    i. fluid loss
    i. water loss (IWL)
insensitive ovary syndrome
insensitivity
    androgen i.
    congenital i.
    growth hormone i. (GHI)
    incomplete androgen i.
    partial (incomplete) androgen i.
      (PAI)
insert
    Cervidil vaginal i.
    Cookie I.
    FemSoft continence i.
    Miconazole 7 vaginal i.
    Monistat 1 Combination Pack
      vaginal i.
insertion
    Achilles tendon i.
    catheter i.
    i. of chromosome
    cord i. (CI)
    deltoid i.
    facial vein i.
    gastric tube i.
    interchromosomal i.
    laminaria tent i.
    marginal cord i.
    i. potential
    saphenous vein catheter i.
    i. sequence
    i. site selection
    subzonal i. (SUZI)
    transpyloric tube i.
    umbilical cord i.
    velamentous cord i.
insertional
    i. dyspareunia
    i. mutagenesis
insipidus
    central diabetes i.
    diabetes i. (DI)
    familial vasopressin-sensitive
      diabetes i.

    fetal diabetes i.
    nephrogenic diabetes i.
    X-linked recessive-type diabetes i.
insomnia
    fatal familial i.
    primary i.
    i. syndrome
insonation
inspiration time (I-time)
inspiratory
    i. capacity (IC)
    i. to expiratory ratio (I/E, I:E)
    i. pressure
    i. reserve volume (IRV)
    i. stridor
    i. time (IT)
    i. whoop
inspire
inspired
    i. gas (I)
    i. oxygen
inspissated
    i. bile
    i. bile syndrome
    i. duct
    i. milk syndrome
    i. mucus
inspissation
    amorphous i.
    mucous i.
INSS
    International Neuroblastoma Staging
      System
instability
    atlantoaxial i.
    bladder i.
    detrusor i.
    glenohumeral i.
    hemodynamic i.
    occipitoatlantal i.
instantaneous orthostatic hypotension
  (INOH)
Instead feminine protection cup
instillation
institute
    National Cancer I. (NCI)
    I. of Personality and Ability
      Testing (IPAT)
institutionalize
instruction
    adult-directed i.
    child-directed i.
instrument
    Dolphin i.
    Erbe electrical coagulation i.
    Erbe electrical cutting i.
    Feelings About Yourself i.
    I-QOL i.

Kevorkian-Younge cervical
  biopsy i.
Keyes biopsy i.
LDS i.
Lusk i.
myoma fixation i.
Newport medical i.
PlasmaKinetic i.
Polaris reusable i.
Welch Allyn AudioPath Platform
  hearing acuity i.

instrumental
  i. delivery
  i. vertex

instrumentation
  anterior spinal i.
  bladder i.
  Cotrel-Dubousset i. (CDI)
  DeLee i.
  Miami Moss i.
  posterior segmental fixation i.
  segmental spinal i.
  TSRH i.

insufficiency
  ACTH i.
  adrenal i.
  adrenocortical i.
  adrenocorticotropic hormone i.
  alacrima, achalasia, adrenal i.
  aortic valve i.
  caloric i.
  chronic adrenal i.
  chronic mitral i.
  chronic pulmonary i.
  chronic renal i.
  corpus luteum i.
  exocrine pancreatic i.
  fetal-placental i.
  glomerular i.
  glucocorticoid i.
  intrapartum uteroplacental i.
  mitral valve i.
  pancreatic exocrine i.
  placental i.
  prerenal i.
  primary adrenal i.
  primary ovarian i.
  pulmonary i.
  renal i.
  respiratory i.
  tricuspid i.
  uterine i.

  uteroplacental i. (UI)
  valvular i.

insufflation
  continuous tracheal gas i.
  extraperitoneal i.
  i. needle
  peritoneal i.
  tubal i.

insufflator
  hysteroscopic i.
  Kidde tubal i.
  laparoscopic i.
  Semm Pelvi-Pneu i.

Insulatard NPH human
insulin
  beef i.
  i. deficiency
  fasting serum i.
  glucose plus i.
  human i.
  i. infusion
  I. Lente L
  i. lipoatrophy
  i. lispro
  maternal i.
  neutral protamine Hagedorn i.
  Novolin i.
  NPH i.
  i. pen
  pork i.
  i. pump
  regular purified pork i.
  i. resistance
  i. response
  I. RIA 100
  i. secretion
  i. sensitivity
  i. sensitivity test
  i. shock
  i. tolerance test

insulinase
insulin-dependent
  i.-d. diabetes
  i.-d. diabetes mellitus (IDDM)
  i.-d. diabetic

insulinemia
insulin-induced hypoglycemia
insulinlike
  i. growth factor (IGF)
  i. growth factor-binding protein
    (IGFBP)

NOTES

insulinlike *(continued)*
    i. growth factor-binding protein-3 (IGFBP-3)
insulinoma
insulinopenia
insulinotropic peptide
insulin-resistant diabetes, acanthosis nigricans, hypogonadism, pigmentary retinopathy, deafness, mental retardation syndrome
insulin-secreting pancreatic tumor
insulitis
insulopenia
Insul-Sheath vaginal speculum sheath
insult
    perinatal i.
insurance
    Social Security Disability I. (SSDI)
InSure
InSync miniform pad
intact membrane
intake
    caloric i.
    maximal oxygen i. (MOI)
    oral i.
    i. and output (I&O, I/O)
    periconceptual i.
    poor caloric i.
    poor oral i.
Intal
Integra
integrate
    i. sensation
    i. sensory information
integrated
    I. Management of Childhood Illness (IMCI)
    i. visual and auditory (IVA)
integration
    Developmental Test of Visual-Motor I.
    sensorimotor i.
    sensory i.
    structural i.
    visual-motor i. (VMI)
    visuomotor i. (VMI)
integrin
    beta-1, -2 i.
integrin-binding
integrity
    genital tract i.
    perineal body i.
intellectual disability
intelligence
    borderline i.
    Fagan Test of Infant I.
    normal i.
    i. quotient (IQ)
    subaverage i.

    i. test
    Wechsler Preschool and Primary Scale of I. (WPPSI)
    Wechsler Preschool and Primary Scale of I.-Revised (WPPSI-R)
intense emotional state
intensifier
    image i.
intensity
intensity/duration ratio (I/T)
intensity/time ratio (I/T)
intensive
    i. care nursery (ICN)
    i. diabetes management (IDM)
    i. phototherapy
    i. special care nursery (ISCN)
    i. special care unit (ISCU)
intensivist
Intensol
    Diazepam I.
intention
    i. myoclonus
    secondary i.
    i. tremor
intentional poisoning
interaction
    actin-myosin i.
    androgen i.
    caregiver-child i.
    ephaptic i.
    epithelial-mesenchymal i.
    Interview Schedule for Social I.
    mother-child i.
    parent-child i.
    poor feeding i.
    sperm-cervical mucus i.
    sperm-mucus i.
    sperm-oocyte i.
    stromal-epithelial i.
interactive play therapy
Interagency Coordinating Council (ICC)
interarticularis
    pars i.
interarytenoid notch
interassay
interatrial communication (IAC)
interbody ankylosis
intercalary
    i. defect
    i. defect of pollical ray
intercalatum
    Schistosoma i.
intercapillary distance
Interceed
    I. barrier material
    I. TC7 absorbable adhesion barrier
intercellular
    i. adhesion molecule 1 (ICAM1)
    i. edema

I

interchange
interchromosomal insertion
intercondylar
    i. groove
    i. notch
    i. radiograph
intercostal
    i. drainage
    i. indrawing
    i. retractions
    i. space
intercourse
    anal i.
    interfemoral i.
    sexual i.
    timed i.
    vulvar i.
intercross
interdigital
    i. candidosis
    i. web
interdigitation
interdisciplinary team
interest
    atypical i.
interface
    gum-tooth i.
    maternal-fetal i.
    placental i.
    tendon-bone i.
interfemoral intercourse
interference
    acoustical i.
    centromere i.
    chiasma i.
    genetic i.
    negative i.
    positive i.
interferon (IFN)
    i. alfa-2a, -2b
    i. alfa-NL
    i. alfa-N1, N2, N3
    alpha i.
    i. alpha
    i. alpha-2a
    i. alpha-2b
    alpha-recombinant i.
    i. beta
    beta i.
    i. beta-1a, -1b
    i. beta-recombinant
    gamma i.

    i. gamma (IFN-gamma)
    i. gamma-1b
    human leukocyte i. (HLI)
    interstitial positive-pressure i. alpha
    leukocyte i.
    lymphoblastoid i.
    i. therapy
interferon-alpha
interfetal membrane
Intergel irrigating solution
intergluteal cleft
interhemispheric
    i. subarachnoid hemorrhage
    i. subdural hematoma
interictal
    i. discharge
    i. EEG
    i. hypoperfusion
    i. myokymia
    i. spike
interkinesis
interleukin (IL)
    i. (1–30)
    i.-1
    i.-1B
    i. deficiency
    histamine i.
interlobar
intermaxillary narrowness
InterMed Bear
intermedia
    thalassemia i.
intermediate
    i. care facility (ICF)
    i. dystonic stage
    i. trophoblast (IT)
intermedius
    Staphylococcus i.
intermenstrual
    i. bleeding
    i. pain
intermittent
    i. cyclical etidronate disodium
    i. exotropia
    i. fever
    i. hematologic cytopenia
    i. hydronephrosis
    i. hydrosalpinx
    i. hypocomplementemia
    i. mandatory ventilation (IMV)
    i. mechanical ventilation (IMV)
    i. pneumatic compression

NOTES

intermittent *(continued)*
    i. porphyria
    i. positive pressure breathing
      (IPPB)
    i. positive pressure ventilation
      (IPPV)
    i. self-catheterization
    i. sterilization
    i. strabismus
    i. support
intermuscular abscess
intern
interna
    endometriosis i.
internal
    i. anal sphincter
    i. branchial sinus
    i. conjugate
    i. derangement
    i. diameter
    i. discomfort
    i. endometriosis
    i. excrescence
    i. femoral torsion
    i. generative organ
    i. genitalia
    i. hernia
    i. hordeolum
    i. iliac artery
    i. jugular vein
    i. jugular vein catheter placement
    i. monitoring
    i. oblique muscle
    i. ophthalmoplegia
    i. os
    i. podalic version
    i. podalic version and breech
      extraction
    i. radiation therapy
    i. representation
    i. respiration
    i. rotation
    i. septation
    i. tibial torsion
internalization
    hormone-receptor complex i.
    receptor i.
internalize
internalizing
    I. Behavior Scale
    i. problem
    i. score
international
    i. classification of cancer of cervix
    I. Classification of Diseases (ICD)
    I. Committee for Contraceptive
      Research (ICCR)
    I. Federation of Gynecology and
      Obstetrics (FIGO)

    I. League Against Epilepsy (ILAE)
    I. League of Associations for
      Rheumatology (ILAR)
    I. Neuroblastoma Staging System
      (INSS)
    i. normalized ratio (INR)
    I. Reference Preparation (IRP)
    I. Society of Gynecologic
      Pathologists (ISGYP)
    I. Society for Gynecologic
      Pathology
    I. Society for Heart Transplantation
      (ISHT)
    I. Society for the Study of Vulvar
      Disease (ISSVD)
    I. Staging System
    I. Union Against Cancer
    I. Unit (IU)
interneuron
    aspiny i.
internist
internuclear ophthalmoplegia
internus
    hydrocephalus i.
    obturator i.
interpeak latency
Interpersonal Support Evaluation List
interphase
interplant
interposition
    antiperistaltic intestinal i.
    cartilage i.
    colonic i.
    costal cartilage i.
    ileal i.
    intestinal i.
    isoperistaltic intestinal i.
interpretation
    mirror image i.
    i. variability
interrogans
    Leptospira i.
interrogation
    continuous wave Doppler i.
interrupted
    i. aortic arch (type A, B)
    i. suture
interruption
    high-frequency flow i. (HFFI)
    vena caval i.
interruptus
    coitus i.
intersex
    i. condition
    i. disorder
    i. problem
intersexuality
inter-simple sequence repeat

intersphincteric
   i. abscess
   i. groove
   i. space
InterStim therapy
interstitial
   i. brachytherapy
   i. cell
   i. cystitis
   i. deletion
   i. edema
   i. fibrosis
   i. fluid
   i. implant
   i. infiltrate
   i. irradiation
   i. keratitis
   i. and loculated hematoma
   i. lung disease (ILD)
   i. mastitis
   i. myocarditis
   i. nephritis
   i. plasma cell pneumonia
   i. pneumonitis
   i. positive-pressure interferon alpha
   i. pregnancy
   i. space
   i. therapy
interstitium
   renal i.
interthreshold zone
intertriginous
   i. area
   i. candidiasis
   i. candidosis
intertrigo
   chronic i.
intertrochanteric fracture
intertuberous diameter
interval
   atlantodens i. (ADI)
   decision-to-delivery i. (DDI)
   induction-to-delivery i.
   PR i.
   prolonged QT i.
   pulse i.
   QT i.
   short PR i.
intervention
   antiinflammatory i.
   behavioral i.
   court-ordered obstetrical i.

crisis i.
early i.
legal i.
mind-body i.
pharmacologic i.
postmenopausal estrogen and
   progestin i. (PEPI)
prenatal smoking i.
psychopharmacological i.
pulsed i.
salvage i.
school-based i.
interventional procedure
interventionist
   early i.
interventricular septum
intervertebral
   i. disc (IVD)
   i. disc calcification (IDC)
   i. diskitis
interview
   Autism Diagnostic I. (ADI)
   Brown and Harris i.
   LEDS i.
   Life Events and Difficulty
      Schedule I.
   prenatal i.
   psychiatric diagnostic i. (PDI)
   I. Schedule for Children and
      Adolescents (ISCA)
   I. Schedule for Social Interaction
Interview-Revised
   Autism Diagnostic I.-R. (ADI-R)
intervillous
   i. blood
   i. blood gas
   i. space
interweaving pattern
intestinal
   i. aganglionosis
   i. atresia
   i. bag
   i. bladder augmentation
   i. bypass procedure
   i. conduit
   i. disorder
   i. duplication
   i. fistula
   i. hurry
   i. hypoxia
   i. interposition
   i. ischemia

NOTES

intestinal *(continued)*
    i. lesion
    i. lymphangiectasia, lymphedema, mental retardation syndrome
    i. malrotation (IM)
    i. mesentery
    i. metaplasia
    i. motility
    i. mucosa
    i. neuronal dysplasia
    i. obstruction
    i. ostomy
    i. parasite
    i. peristalsis
    i. permeability (IP)
    i. polyp
    i. polyposis
    i. pseudoobstruction
    i. telangiectasia
    i. tract
    i. transplantation
    i. villous atrophy
    i. volvulus
intestinalis
    Campylobacter fetus i.
    Enterocytozoon i.
    pneumatosis i.
    pneumatosis cystoides i.
    Septata i.
intestine
    large i.
    small i.
intestine-associated lymphoid tissue (IALT)
intima
intimal
    i. hyperplasia
    i. thickening
intimate
    i. partner
    i. partner depression
    i. partner homicide
intoeing
intolerance
    carbohydrate i.
    cold i.
    cow's milk i.
    delayed orthostatic i.
    disaccharide i.
    exercise i.
    familial protein i.
    feeding i.
    fructose i.
    gestational carbohydrate i. (GCI)
    glucose i.
    glucose-galactose i.
    gluten i.
    hereditary fructose i.
    lactose i.

    lysinuric protein i.
    milk protein i.
    orthostatic i.
    primary lactose i.
    protein i.
    soy protein i.
    transient protein i.
intoxicate
intoxication
    acute scombroid i.
    aluminum i.
    anticonvulsant i.
    barbiturate i.
    botulinus i.
    chronic vitamin A i.
    ciguatera i.
    intrarenal androgenic i.
    lead i.
    manganese i.
    mepivacaine i.
    metal i.
    methylmercury i.
    phenothiazine i.
    salicylate i.
    scombroid i.
    sugar i.
    thallium i.
    vitamin A, D i.
    water i.
intraabdominal
    i. abscess
    i. cyst
    i. infection (IAI)
    i. pressure
    i. streak
    i. surgery
    i. testis
intraamniotic
    i. infection (IAI)
    i. inflammation
intraaortic balloon counterpulsation
intraarterial
    i. chemotherapy
    i. infusion
intraarticular
    i. epiphysis
    i. infection
intraassay
intraatrial
    i. redirection
    i. repair
intrabronchial obstruction
intrabronchiolar obstruction
intracanalicular fibroadenoma
intracardiac
    i. defect
    i. injection
    i. shunt
    i. tunnel

intracavitary
- i. brachytherapy
- i. irradiation
- i. lesion
- i. myoma
- i. radium

intracellular
- i. calcium
- i. event
- i. fluid (ICF)
- i. hydrogen ion concentration (pHi)
- i. mediator
- i. pH (pHi)

intracerebellar hemorrhage
intracerebral
- i. aneurysm
- i. hematoma
- i. seeding of bacteria

intracervical
- i. adhesion
- i. purified porcine relaxin
- i. tent

intrachromosomal duplication
intracisternal therapy
intraclass correlation coefficient
intracoronary ultrasound
intracranial
- i. anatomy
- i. arterial aneurysm
- i. arteriovenous fistula
- i. bleeding
- i. calcification
- i. cystic space
- i. dural vascular anomaly
- i. empyema
- i. foreign body
- i. hematoma
- i. hemorrhage (ICH)
- i. hypertension
- i. injury (ICI)
- i. malformation
- i. pathology
- i. pressure (ICP)
- i. pressure monitoring
- i. suppuration
- i. tumor
- i. venous sinus thrombosis
- i. volume

intractable
- i. diarrhea of infancy (IDI)
- i. emesis
- i. pain

- i. uterine bleeding
- i. viral infection

intracystic papillary carcinoma
intracytoplasmic
- i. inclusion
- i. sperm head injection (ICSHI)
- i. sperm injection (ICSI)

intradermal
- i. nevus
- i. test

IntraDop probe
intraductal
- i. cancer
- i. papillary carcinoma
- i. papilloma

intradural spinal angioma
intraepidermal
- i. blister
- i. spongiosis
- i. vesiculation

intraepithelial
- i. cervical dysplasia
- i. disease progression
- i. dyskeratosis syndrome
- i. endometrial cancer
- i. lesion
- i. neoplasia

intrafallopian transfer
intrafamilial genoidentical donor
intrafamily offender
intrafollicular insemination (IFI)
intragastric
- i. feeding
- i. pH

intrahepatic
- i. arterioportal fistula
- i. bile duct
- i. bile duct paucity
- i. biliary atresia
- i. cholestasis
- i. cholestasis of pregnancy
- i. vasoocclusive crisis

intralesional steroid therapy
intraligamentary ectopic pregnancy
intraligamentous myoma
Intralipid
- I. formula
- I. hyperalimentation

intralobar
- i. pulmonary sequestration
- i. rest

intralobular connective tissue

NOTES

intraluminal
- i. clot
- i. electrical impedance technique
- i. nutrient
- i. plug
- i. pressure
- i. upper airway obstruction
- i. web

intralymphatic infusion

intramammary lymph node

intramedullary
- i. rod
- i. rod fixation
- i. spinal abscess

intramural
- i. fibroid
- i. gas
- i. myoma
- i. pregnancy
- i. thrombus
- i. upper airway obstruction

intramuscular (IM)
- i. block
- i. drug

intramyometrial
- i. coring
- i. mass

intranasal
- i. desmopressin
- i. drug
- i. inoculum
- i. live influenza vaccine
- i. spray

intranatal

intranuclear
- i. hyaline inclusion disease
- i. inclusion body
- i. virion

intraocular
- i. lymphoma
- i. malignancy
- i. optic neuritis
- i. pressure (IOP)
- i. tumor

intraoperative
- i. complication
- i. gastrointestinal injury
- i. lymphatic mapping
- i. radiation
- i. ureteral catheterization

intraosseous (IO)
- i. infusion (IOI)
- i. line placement
- i. needle

intrapair birth weight difference

intraparenchymal
- i. bleed
- i. hematoma
- i. hemorrhage

intrapartum
- i. antibiotic prophylaxis (IAP)
- i. asphyxia
- i. asphyxiation
- i. cardiotocography
- i. chemoprophylaxis
- i. complication
- i. cord prolapse
- i. death
- i. demise
- i. evaluation
- i. fetal heart rate abnormality
- i. fetal monitoring
- i. fetoplacental transfusion
- i. head entrapment
- i. hemorrhage
- i. hemostasis
- i. management
- i. maternal fever
- i. monitor
- i. period
- i. uteroplacental insufficiency

intrapelvic

intraperitoneal
- i. blood transfusion
- i. chemotherapy
- i. cisplatin
- i. endometrial metastatic disease
- i. fetal transfusion
- i. 5-fluorouracil
- i. insemination (IPI)
- i. involvement
- i. pregnancy
- i. radiation therapy

intrapleural injury

intrapsychic phenomenon

intrapulmonary
- i. inhalation
- i. shunt
- i. shunting
- i. shunt ratio (Qs/Qt)
- i. tumor

intrarenal
- i. anastomosis
- i. androgenic intoxication
- i. reflux
- i. venous radical

intraretinal hemorrhage (IH)

intraspinous vascular anomaly

intratesticularly

intrathecal
- i. anti-HIV antibody
- i. medication
- i. methotrexate
- i. narcotic

intrathoracic
- i. airway obstruction
- i. tracheomalacia
- i. tuberculosis

intratonsillar
intratracheal
   i. magnesium (ITMg)
   i. pulmonary ventilation (ITPV)
intratubal insemination (ITI)
intratumoral desmoplasia
intraurethral bulk injection
intrauterine (IU)
   i. acquisition
   i. adhesion
   i. amputation
   i. asphyxia
   i. balloon-type cannula
   i. cavity
   i. cirsoid aneurysm
   i. compression
   i. contraception device (IUCD)
   i. contraceptive device (IUCD)
   i. contraceptive progesterone system (ICPS)
   i. death (IUD)
   i. device (IUD)
   i. diaphragm
   i. exposure
   i. facial necrosis
   i. factors
   i. fetal death
   i. fetal demise
   i. fetal monitoring
   i. filling defect
   i. fracture
   i. GIFT
   i. growth impairment
   i. growth restriction (IUGR)
   i. growth retardation (IUGR)
   i. growth retardation, microcephaly, mental retardation syndrome
   i. hematoma
   i. herpes
   i. hydrops
   i. hypoxia
   i. infection (IUI)
   i. insemination (IUI)
   i. insemination cannula
   i. insemination cannula with mandrel
   i. intraperitoneal fetal transfusion
   i. intussusception
   i. involvement
   i. lymphedema
   i. maternofetal transfusion
   i. parabiotic syndrome

   i. parvovirus B19 infection
   i. pneumonia
   i. position
   i. positional defect
   i. positioning
   i. pregnancy (IUP)
   i. pressure catheter (IUPC)
   i. pressure cycle
   i. pressure measurement
   i. resuscitation
   i. sac
   i. synechia
   i. ureteral obstruction
   i. viral myositis
   i. volume
intravaginal
   i. condom
   i. contraceptive
   i. cream
   i. foam
   i. foreign body use
   i. insemination (IVI)
   i. pouch
   i. prostaglandin
   i. sponge
   i. suppository
   i. testicular torsion
intravasation
intravascular
   i. fluid
   i. oncotic pressure
   i. sickling
   i. transfusion
   i. ultrasonography
   i. ultrasound (IVUS)
   i. volume
   i. volume depletion
intravenous (I.V., IV)
   i. alimentation
   i. anti-D immunoglobulin
   cytomegalovirus immune globulin i. (CMV-IGIV)
   i. drip (IVD)
   i. drug
   i. drug use (IDU)
   i. excretory urography
   i. feeding
   i. fluid therapy
   i. gamma globulin (IVGG)
   i. glucose challenge
   i. hydration
   i. hyperalimentation (IVH)

NOTES

intravenous *(continued)*
    i. immune globulin (IVIG, IVIg)
    i. immunoglobulin (IVIG, IVIg)
    i. infusion
    i. leiomyomatosis
    i. line
    i. line placement
    i. medication
    peripheral i. (PIV)
    i. pyelogram (IVP)
    i. pyelography (IVP)
    scalp i.
    i. urogram (IVU)
    i. urography (IVU)
intraventricular
    i. bleed
    i. fibrinolytic therapy
    i. hemorrhage (grade 1–4) (IVH)
    i. neurocysticercosis
    i. ribavirin
intravesical pressure
intrinsic
    i. asthma
    i. dysmenorrhea
    i. dyssomnia
    i. factor (IF)
    i. flow resistance (R_{int})
    i. PEEP, auto-PEEP
    i. pulsatility
    i. sphincter deficiency (IDS, ISD)
    i. tumor
introducer
    P.D. Access with Peel-Away
      needle i.
introital
    i. estrogenization
    i. papulosis
introitus
    marital i.
    parous i.
    vaginal i.
    virginal i.
Introl bladder neck support prosthesis
intromission
Intron A
intruded incisor
intrusion
    dental i.
    i. symptom
intrusive
    i. implantation
    i. luxation
    i. stress reaction
intubated
intubation
    controlled i.
    endotracheal i. (ETI)
    nasal tube i.
    nasotracheal i.

    neonatal i.
    oral tube i.
    orotracheal i.
    rapid sequence i. (RSI)
    Silastic tube i.
    stenosis post i.
    tracheal i.
intussusception
    apex of i.
    appendiceal i.
    cecocolic i.
    colic i.
    colocolic i.
    double i.
    idiopathic i.
    ileal i.
    ileocecal i.
    ileocolic i.
    ileoileal i.
    ileoileocolic i.
    intrauterine i.
    jejunogastric i.
    prolapsing apex of i.
    retrograde i.
intussusceptum
    engorgement of i.
invaginata
    trichorrhexis i.
invaginated bowel
invagination
    basilar i.
Invanz
invasion
    early stromal i.
    lymphovascular space i. (LVSI)
    myometrial i.
    trophoblastic i.
invasive
    i. bacterial infection
    i. cancer (IC)
    i. candidiasis
    i. cervical cancer
    i. duct carcinoma
    i. hemodynamic monitoring
    i. hydatidiform mole
    i. management
    i. neoplasia
    i. sinusitis
    i. testing
invecta
    Solenopsis i.
inventory
    Battelle Developmental I. (BDI)
    Beck Depression I. (BDI)
    Behavior Problem I. (BPI)
    Children's Depression I. (CDI)
    Child Sexual Behavior I. (CSBI)
    communal traumatic experiences i.
      (CTEI)

communicative development i.
Derogatis Brief Symptom I.
Eating Disorders I.
Eyberg Child Behavior I. (ECBI)
Gillespie-Numerof Burnout I.
Global Severity Index of Brief
    Symptom I. (GSI-BSI)
infertility perceptions i. (IPI)
18-item Birleson Depression I.
Leyton Obsessional I.
Marital Dyadic I.
Maslach Burnout I.
Minnesota Multiphasic
    Personality I. (MMPI)
Neonatal Perception I. (NPI)
Neonatal Withdrawal I. (NWI)
Pediatric Evaluation of Disability I.
    (PEDI)
peer conformity i.
Spielberger State Anxiety I.
standardized reading i.
State-Trait Anxiety I.
Urinary Distress I. (UDI)
Urogenital Distress I. (UDI)
Weinberger Adjustment I. (WAI)
West Haven-Yale Multidimensional
    Pain I.
Inventory-Adolescent
Minnesota Multiphasic
    Personality I.-A. (MMPI-A)
inverse
i. cerebellum
i. polymerase chain reaction
i. ratio ventilation (IRV)
Inversine
inversion
acute uterine i.
appendiceal i.
chromosomal i.
i. of chromosomes
i. deformity
i. duplication (15) chromosome
    syndrome
i. duplication (8p) syndrome
paracentric i.
pericentric i.
puerperal i.
i. stress tilt test
i. 9 syndrome
T-wave i.
uterine i.
i. of the uterus

ventricular i.
i. of viscera
inversion-ligation appendectomy
inversus
blepharophimosis, ptosis,
    epicanthus i. (BPEI)
epicanthus i.
situs i.
visceroatrial situs i.
inverted
i. appendiceal stump
i. duplication of chromosome 15
i. nipple
i. pelvis
i. repeat
i. subcuticular suture
i. T uterine incision
i. X chromosome
inverted-V mouth
inverted-Y detrusor dissection
inverting baseball stitch
invertogram
Investa suture
investigation
infertility i.
Invirase
involucrum, pl. **involucra**
involuntary
i. movement
i. sterilization
involute
involuting nevus
involution
i. cyst
spontaneous i.
spontaneous thymic i.
i. of the uterus
involutional
i. gynecomastia
i. melancholia
i. psychosis
involved field (IF)
involved-field radiation
involvement
adnexal i.
congenital muscular dystrophy with
    central nervous system i.
endometrial i.
gangliosidosis GM1 late onset
    without bony i.
generalized infantile gangliosidosis
    with bony i.

NOTES

involvement *(continued)*
    intraperitoneal i.
    intrauterine i.
    lymph node i.
    lymphovascular space i.
    metastatic axillary i.
    multisite lower genital tract i.
    neurologic i.
    nodal i.
    ocular i.
    pelvic i.
    pleuropulmonary i.
    postponing sexual i. (PSI)
    Tay-Sachs disease with visceral i.
Invos 3100 cerebral oximeter
IO
    intraosseous
        IO infusion
I/O
    intake and output
I&O
    intake and output
Ioban
    I. 2 cesarean sheet
    I. drape
iocetamic acid
iodamide
iodide
    cesium i. (CsI)
    potassium i.
    propidium i.
    saturated solution of potassium i.
      (SSKI)
    sodium i.
    i. therapy
    i. trap defect
iodide-containing medication
iodinated
    i. dye
    i. glycerol
iodine
    i.-123 (^{123}I)
    i.-125 (^{125}I)
    i.-127 (^{127}I)
    i.-131 (^{131}I)
    i.-132 (^{132}I)
    i. douche
    i. 125-labeled fibrinogen scan
    i. povidone solution
    i. stain
    i. supply
    tincture of i.
    urinary i.
iodipamide
5-iodo-2′-deoxyuridine (IDU)
iodoform
    i. gauze
    i. gauze packing
iodomethyl-norcholesterol scanning

Iodopen
iodophor
iodophor-impregnated adhesive drape
iodoquinol
Iodosorb absorptive dressing
iodothyronine level
Iofed PD
iohexol
IOI
    intraosseous infusion
ion
    calcium i.
    i. trapping
Ionamin
Ionasescu syndrome
ionic contrast medium
Ionil-T shampoo
ionization
ionized
    i. calcium (iCa)
    i. hypomagnesemia
    i. magnesium
ionizing radiation
Iontocaine
iontophoresis
    pilocarpine i.
    sweat chloride i.
IOP
    intraocular pressure
iopanoic acid
iothalamate sodium
IOWA
    inattention-overactivity with aggression
Iowa
    I. trumpet
    I. Women's Health Study
IP
    infundibulopelvic
    intestinal permeability
        IP ligament
IPAA
    ileal pouch-anal anastomosis
IPAN
    infantile polyarteritis nodosa
IPAT
    Institute of Personality and Ability
    Testing
        IPAT Depression Scale
ipecac
    i. cardiomyopathy
    syrup of i.
    i. syrup
IPH
    idiopathic pulmonary hemorrhage
IPI
    infertility perceptions inventory
    intraperitoneal insemination
IPKD
    infantile polycystic kidney disease

IPN
infantile periarteritis nodosa
ipodate sodium
IPOL poliovirus vaccine
IPPB
intermittent positive pressure breathing
IPPV
intermittent positive pressure ventilation
ipratropium
i. bromide
i. bromide nasal spray
i. nebulization
iprindole
iproniazid
ipsilateral
i. anhidrosis
i. anisocoria
i. hypertropia
i. lateral rectus muscle
i. lung hypoplasia
i. miosis
ipsilon zone
IPT
inflammatory pseudotumor
IPTA
Illinois Test of Psycholinguistic Abilities
IPV
inactivated poliovirus vaccine
Salk IPV
IPV vaccine
IQ
intelligence quotient
Raven IQ
I-QOL
Incontinence quality of life
I-QOL instrument
^{192}Ir
iridium-192
IRC
infrared photocoagulation
Ircon
IRDS
idiopathic respiratory distress syndrome
infant respiratory distress syndrome
Ir gene
iridectomy
irides (*pl. of* iris)
iridis (*gen. of* iris)
iridium
i.-192 (^{192}Ir)
i. implant
i. wire

iridocorneal mesodermal dysgenesis
iridocyclitis
acute i.
chronic i.
relapsing i.
iridodental dysplasia
iridodonesis
iridogoniodysgenesis with somatic anomalies
irinotecan
iris, gen. **iridis**, pl. **irides**
i., coloboma, ptosis, hypertelorism, mental retardation syndrome
i. dilator
i. hamartoma
heterochromia iridis
heterochromia of i.
i. hypoplasia
i. lesion
i. Lisch nodule
speckled irides
stellate i.
i. vessel
iritis
i. catamenialis
photophobic i.
IRMA
immunoradiometric assay
Iromin-G
iron (Fe)
carbonyl i.
i. chelation
i. chelator
i. deficiency
i. deficiency anemia (IDA)
i. dextran
i. dextran complex
elemental i.
free i.
heme i.
i. ingestion
I. Intern retractor
MicroIron II carbonyl i.
nonheme i.
i. overload
Pedicran with I.
plasma-free i.
i. poisoning
i. requirement
serum i.
i. supplement
total body i.

NOTES

iron *(continued)*
    i. toxicity
    i. turnover
    unbound i.
iron-binding
    i.-b. capacity (IBC)
    i.-b. protein
iron-catalyzed pseudoperoxidation
Irospan
IRP
    International Reference Preparation
irradiated
irradiation
    abdominal i.
    abdominopelvic i.
    axillary i.
    cesium i.
    i. cystitis
    i. dermatitis
    external beam i.
    heavy-ion i.
    hemibody i.
    i. injury
    interstitial i.
    intracavitary i.
    local i.
    low-dose involved-field i.
    low-dose splenic i.
    ovarian-sparing i.
    paraaortic node i.
    pelvic i.
    surface i.
    total body i. (TBI)
    whole-abdomen i.
    whole-body i.
    whole-pelvis i.
irrational
irregular
    i. cortex
    i. menses
    i. rhythm
    i. stereotyped movement
    i. stereotyped vocalization
    i. tooth placement
irregularity
    menstrual i.
irrigant
    Neosporin G.U. I.
irrigation
    bowel i.
    copious antibiotic i.
    gastric i.
    whole-bowel i. (WBI)
irritability
    early morning i.
    reflex i.
irritable
    i. bowel syndrome (IBS)
    i. breast

    i. colon of childhood
    i. hip
irritant
    i. contact dermatitis
    i. diaper dermatitis
    i. receptor
irritation
    i. diaper rash
    meningeal i.
    perineal i.
irritative vulvovaginitis
IRT
    immunoreactive trypsinogen
IRV
    inspiratory reserve volume
    inverse ratio ventilation
Irving
    I. method
    I. tubal ligation
IS
    infant size
    IS element
ISA
    induced sputum analysis
Isaac syndrome
ISAGA
    immunosorbent agglutination assay
ISAM
    infant of substance-abusing mother
ISCA
    Interview Schedule for Children and
      Adolescents
ischemia
    cerebral i.
    chorionic villus i.
    clitoral i.
    intestinal i.
    myocardial i.
    penile i.
ischemic
    i. brain injury
    i. decidual necrosis
    i. edema
    i. exercise test
    i. heart disease (IHD)
ischia (*pl. of* ischium)
ischiadelphus
ischiocavernosus muscle
ischiocavernous
ischiodidymus
ischiomelus
ischiopagus
    i. tripus separation
    i. tripus twins
ischiopatellar dysplasia
ischiopubica
    osteochondritis i.
ischiopubic ramus
ischiopubiotomy

ischiorectal
    i. abscess
    i. fossa
ischiothoracopagus
ischium, pl. **ischia**
ISCN
    intensive special care nursery
ISCU
    intensive special care unit
ISD
    intrinsic sphincter deficiency
ISDN
    isosorbide dinitrate
Iselin forceps
isethionate
    pentamidine i.
ISG
    immune serum globulin
Is gene
ISGYP
    International Society of Gynecologic
    Pathologists
Ishihara
    POU theory of I.
ISHT
    International Society for Heart
    Transplantation
island
    epimyoepithelial i.
    i. flap
    Langerhans i.'s
    Pander i.'s
islander
    Pacific I.
islet
    i. cell adenoma
    i. cell adenomatosis
    i. cell antibody (ICA)
    i. cell tumor
    i.'s of Langerhans
Ismelin
isoametropic amblyopia
isoamylase
isoantibody
isoantigen
Iso-Bid
isobutyric acid
Isocal HN formula
isocarboxazid
isochromatic
isochromosome
    i. 10p syndrome

    i. 12p syndrome
    i. Xq
isodense lesion
isodisomy
    paternal uniparenteral i.
isodose curve
isoechoic
isoenzyme
    MB i.
    myocardial muscle creatine
    kinase i. (CK-MB)
isoetharine
isofluorphate
isoflurane
isoform
    glutathione S-transferase i.
isogeneic graft
isograft
isohemagglutinin
    anti-A, anti-B i.
isoimmune
    i. anemia
    i. fetal thrombocytopenia
    i. hemolytic disease
isoimmunization
    antepartum Rh i.
    blood group i.
    D i.
    D-antigen i.
    Kell i.
    i. in pregnancy
    Rh i.
    rhesus i.
isointense
Isojima test
isolate
    chloramphenicol-resistant i.
isolated
    i. autosomal dominant syndrome
    i. cleft palate
    i. congenital folate malabsorption
    (ICFM)
    i. diffuse mesangial sclerosis
    (IDMS)
    i. double outlet right ventricle
    i. gonadotropin deficiency
    i. growth hormone deficiency
    (IGHD)
    i. hypogonadotropic hypogonadism
    (IHH)
    i. premature menarche

NOTES

isolated *(continued)*
    i. TGA
    i. vulvar seborrheic dermatitis
isolating
isolation
    social i.
Isolette
    Airshields I.
    bubble I.
    double-bubble I.
    double-walled bubble I.
    humidified I.
    temperature-controlled I.
isoleucine
isologous neoplasm
isomer
isomerase
    triose phosphate i. (TPI)
isomerism
isometric quadriceps exercise
Isomil DE formula
isomorphic presentation
isonatremia
isonatremic dehydration
isoniazid (INH)
    prophylactic i.
isonicotinic acid hydrazide (INH)
Isopaque
isoperistaltic intestinal interposition
isoprenaline hydrochloride
Isoprinosine
isopropamide iodide
isopropanol
isopropyl alcohol
isoproterenol
Isoptin SR
Isopto
    I. Atropine Ophthalmic
    I. Carbachol
    I. Carpine
    I. Carpine Ophthalmic
    I. Cetamide
    I. Eserine
    I. Frin
    I. Hyoscine
Isordil
isosexual
    i. idiopathic precocious puberty
    i. precocity
    i. sexual characteristic
isosorbide dinitrate (ISDN)
Isosource
    I. 1.5 Cal formula
    I. HN formula
    I. Standard formula
Isospora belli
isosporiasis
isosthenuria

Isotamine
isothiocyanate
    fluorescein i.
isotonic
    i. bolus
    i. dehydration
    i. electrolyte solution
    i. fluid
    i. PBS
    i. saline
    i. sodium chloride
isotope
    i. cisternography
    radioactive i.
    i. scanning
Isotrate
isotretinoin
    i. dysmorphic syndrome
    i. embryopathy
    i. teratogenic syndrome
Isotrex
isovaleric
    i. acid
    i. aciduria
isovaleryl-CoA dehydrogenase
isovaleryl glucuronide
isovolumic relaxation time (IVRT)
iso-X chromosome
isoxsuprine
I-Soyalac formula
isozyme
ISQ
    Incontinence Stress questionnaire
israelii
    Actinomyces i.
ISS
    idiopathic short stature
    injury severity score
ISSD
    infantile sialic acid storage disorder
issue
    developmental i.
    legal i.
    sexual i.
    social i.
ISSVD
    International Society for the Study of
    Vulvar Disease
isthmi (*pl. of* isthmus)
isthmica nodosa
isthmic occlusion
isthmointerstitial anastomosis
isthmorrhaphy
isthmus, pl. **isthmuses, isthmi**
    cervical i.
    flutter i.
I-Sulfacet
Isuprel Injection

IT
inspiratory time
intermediate trophoblast
I/T
intensity/duration ratio
intensity/time ratio
ITC
infrared thermographic calorimetry
itch
ground i.
swimmer's i.
itchiness
itching
perineal i.
vulvovaginal i.
itch-scratch cycle
Itch-X
I.-X gel
I.-X spray
18-item Birleson Depression Inventory
itersonii
Aquaspirillum i.
ITI
intratubal insemination
I-time
inspiration time
ITMg
intratracheal magnesium
Ito
I. cell
hypomelanosis of I.
I. hypomelanosis
I. method
nevus of I.
I. nevus
I. syndrome
ITP
idiopathic thrombocytopenic purpura
immune thrombocytopenic purpura
acute childhood ITP
chronic ITP
recurrent ITP
ITPV
intratracheal pulmonary ventilation
itraconazole
ITW
idiopathic toe walking
IU
immunizing unit
International Unit
intrauterine
in utero

IUCD
intrauterine contraception device
intrauterine contraceptive device
IUD
intrauterine death
intrauterine device
copper T–380A IUD
ParaGard T380 copper IUD
Saf-T-Coil IUD
IUDE
in utero drug exposure
IUD-related infection
IUGR
intrauterine growth restriction
intrauterine growth retardation
asymmetric IUGR
symmetric IUGR
IUI
intrauterine infection
intrauterine insemination
IUI disposable cannula
IUP
intrauterine pregnancy
IUPC
intrauterine pressure catheter
I.V., IV
intravenous
I.V. anti-D therapy
Hyperstat I.V.
Indocin I.V.
Merrem I.V.
Metro I.V.
Monistat I.V.
scalp I.V.
Vasotec I.V.
IVA
integrated visual and auditory
IVA visual consistency test
IVAP
in vitro antibody production
IVAP assay
IVC
indwelling venous catheter
inferior vena cava
IVD
intervertebral disc
intravenous drip
Quantikine IVD
Iveegam
Ivemark syndrome
ivermectin

NOTES

IVF
    in vitro fertilization
IVF-ET
    in vitro fertilization-embryo transfer
IVF-induced abdominal pregnancy
IVGG
    intravenous gamma globulin
IVH
    intravenous hyperalimentation
    intraventricular hemorrhage (grade 1–4)
IVI
    intravaginal insemination
IVIG, IVIg
    intravenous immune globulin
    intravenous immunoglobulin
IVL
    indwelling venous line
ivory bones
IVP
    intravenous pyelogram

intravenous pyelography
    genitogram with or without IVP
IVRT
    isovolumic relaxation time
IVU
    intravenous urogram
    intravenous urography
IVUS
    intravascular ultrasound
Ivy bleeding time
IWL
    insensible water loss
Ixodes
    I. pacificus
    I. persulcatus
    I. ricinus
    I. scapularis

J
joule
J extension
J needle
J pulmonary receptor
J tracking
JA
juvenile arthritis
jabbering
Jaboulay amputation
Jabs syndrome
Jaccoud deformity
jacket
body j.
fiberglass j.
Orthoplast j.
yellow j.
jackknife
j. position
j. seizure
j. spasm
Jackson
J. membrane
J. right-angle retractor
jacksonian
j. epilepsy
j. march
j. seizure
Jackson-Pratt drain
Jackson-Weiss syndrome (JWS)
Jacobs
J. cannula
J. tenaculum
Jacobsen-Brodwall syndrome
Jacobsen syndrome
Jacobson hemostatic forceps
Jacob syndrome
Jacquemier sign
Jacquet
J. erosive diaper dermatitis
J. erythema
Jadassohn
nevus of J.
J. nevus phakomatosis (JNP)
nevus sebaceus of J. (SNJ)
J. test
Jadassohn-Lewandowski syndrome
Jadassohn-Tieche nevus
Jaeken syndrome
Jaffe-Campanacci syndrome
Jaffe-Lichtenstein syndrome
JAG1
human jagged-1 gene

Jahnke syndrome
Jakob-Creutzfeldt (JC)
J.-C. syndrome
Jaksch
J. anemia
J. disease
J. syndrome
Jamaican vomiting sickness
jamais vu
James syndrome
Jancar syndrome
Janeway lesion
janiceps
j. asymmetrus
j. parasiticus
j. twins
Janosik embryo
Jansen
J. metaphyseal chondrodysplasia
J. syndrome
Jansky-Bielschowsky
J.-B. disease
J.-B. neural ceroid lipofuscinosis
J.-B. syndrome
Jansky classification
Janus
J. report
J. syndrome
Janz syndrome
Japanese
J. B encephalitis virus
J. encephalitis
japonica
Laminaria j.
Rickettsia j.
japonicum
Schistosoma j.
jar
GasPak j.
Jarcho-Levin syndrome
jargon
Jarisch-Herxheimer reaction
Jarit
J. disposable cannula
J. disposable trocar
JAS
juvenile ankylosing spondylitis
Jatene
J. arterial switch procedure
J. operation
J. valve
jaundice
benign j.
black j.
breast-feeding j.

J

jaundice *(continued)*
    breast milk j.
    catarrhal j.
    central j.
    cholestatic j.
    congenital hemolytic j.
    congenital nonhemolytic j.
    congenital obliterative j.
    neonatal cholestatic j.
    j. of newborn
    nuclear j.
    obstructive j.
    peripheral j.
    physiologic j.
    prolonged j.
    Schmorl j.
    unexplained j.
javanica
    Rhus j.
jaw
    bird-beak j.
    cleft j.
    j. cysts, basal cell tumors, skeletal anomalies syndrome
    j. deformity
    j. deviation
    fibrous dysplasia of j.
    j. jerk
    lumpy j.
    j. myoclonus
    parrot j.
    small j.
    j. thrust
    j. thrust-spine stabilization maneuver
Jaws forceps
JC
    Jakob-Creutzfeldt
    joint contracture
    polyomavirus JC
    JC syndrome
    JC virus
JDM
    juvenile dermatomyositis
    juvenile diabetes mellitus
    juvenile-onset diabetes mellitus
    amyopathic JDM
    new-onset JDM
JDMS
    juvenile dermatomyositis
Jefferson fracture
Jehovah's Witness
jejunal
    j. atresia
    j. biopsy
    j. ulcer
jejunal-ileal atresia

jejuni
    Campylobacter j.
    Campylobacter fetus j.
jejunitis
    necrotizing j.
jejunogastric intussusception
jejunoileal
    j. atresia
    j. bypass
jejunojejunal anastomosis
jejunostomy
jejunum
    distal j.
    proximal j.
    villous atrophy of j.
jelly
    Aci-Jel vaginal j.
    j. bean
    contraceptive j.
    Gynol II contraceptive j.
    K-Y lubricating j.
    petroleum j.
    Wharton j.
    Xylocaine j.
Jenamicin
Jenest-28
Jensen syndrome
jeopardy
    fetal j.
jerk
    infantile myoclonic j.
    jaw j.
    myoclonic j.
    j. nystagmus
Jervell and Lange-Nielsen long QT syndrome
Jeryl Lynn mumps strain
Jessner-Cole syndrome
JET
    junctional ectopic tachycardia
jet
    j. cooling effect
    high-frequency j. (HFJ)
    j. nebulizer
    pulsatile air j.
    ureteral j.
    j. ventilation
    j. ventilator
Jeune
    J. disease
    J. syndrome
    J. thoracic dystrophy
Jevity Plus formula
Jew
    Ashkenazi J.
    Sephardic J.
jeweler's forceps
Jewett classification

JGCT
juvenile granulosa cell tumor
juxtaglomerular cell tumor
JGCT of ovary
JIA
juvenile idiopathic arthritis
Jirasek gestation stage
jitteriness
jitters
jittery
j. baby
j. infant
JMML
juvenile myelomonocytic leukemia
JMS
Juberg-Marsidi syndrome
JNP
Jadassohn nevus phakomatosis
Jo-1 antibody
Job syndrome
Jocasta complex
JODM
juvenile-onset diabetes mellitus
Joel-Cohen incision
jogger's
j. amenorrhea
j. ankle
Johanson-Blizzard syndrome
Johnson
J. method
J. neuroectodermal syndrome
J. score 1–10
J. transtracheal oxygen catheter
Johnson-McMillin syndrome
joint
AC j.
j. attention
j. bleed
j. capsule
Charcot j.
Clutton j.'s
j. compression
j. contracture (JC)
cricoarytenoid j.
j. deformity
j. degeneration
diarthrodial j.
j. fusion
Gaffney j.
Gillette j.
glenohumeral j.
hyperextensible j.

j. hyperlaxity
hypermobile j.
j. hypermobility
hyperplastic j.
lax j.
j. laxity
j. line tenderness
metacarpophalangeal j.
metatarsophalangeal j.
naviculocuneiform j.
neural arch j.
Oklahoma ankle j.
painful j.
pelvic j.
j. probability
sacroiliac j.
Select j.
septic j.
j. stability
j. suppuration
swollen j.
synovial j.
temporomandibular j. (TMJ)
JOMID
juvenile-onset multisystem inflammatory disease
Jones
J. and Jones wedge technique
J. procedure
J. rheumatic fever diagnostic criteria
J. stress fracture
J. wedge metroplasty
Jorgenson scissors
Joseph
J. disease
J. syndrome
Josephs-Diamond-Blackfan syndrome
Joshi criteria
Joubert syndrome
Joubert-Boltshauser syndrome
joule (J)
J-pouch
JR
Aerolate JR
Jr.
EpiPen Jr.
Peptamen Jr.
JRA
juvenile rheumatoid arthritis (type I, II)
pauciarticular JRA

NOTES

JRA (*continued*)
    pauciarticular-onset JRA
    polyarticular JRA
J-shaped sella
Juberg-Hayward syndrome
Juberg-Holt syndrome
Juberg-Marsidi syndrome (JMS)
Judkins catheter
Juers forceps
jug handle view
jugular
    j. bulb catheter
    j. bulb catheterization
    j. bulb monitoring
    j. occlusion plethysmography
    j. shunt
    j. vein
    j. vein thrombosis
    j. venous A wave
    j. venous cannulation
    j. venous pressure (JVP)
    j. venous pulse
jugulovenous distention (JVD)
juice
    j. baby
    white grape j.
Juliusberg pustulosis
jumped facet
jumper's knee
jumping
    chromosome j.
    j. Frenchmen of Maine syndrome
    j. gene
    j. translocation
junction
    cervicomedullary j.
    cervicovaginal j.
    corticomedullary j.
    costochondral j.
    craniocervical j.
    dermoepidermal j.
    ectoendocervical j.
    gap j.
    gastroesophageal j. (GEJ)
    gray-white j.
    lumbosacral j.
    mesencephalic-diencephalic j.
    mucocutaneous j.
    neuromuscular j. (NMJ)
    pontomedullary j.
    squamocolumnar j. (SCJ)
    sternochondral j.
    striatothalamic j.
    ureteropelvic j. (UPJ)
    ureterovesical j. (UVJ)
    uterotubal j. (UTJ)
junctional
    j. ectopic tachycardia (JET)
    j. epidermolysis bullosa

    j. nevus
    j. rhythm
    j. tachycardia
jungle gym
Junin virus
Junior Strength Motrin
Junius-Kuhnt syndrome
junky lung
justifiable abortion
just-viable fetus
JustVision diagnostic ultrasound system
Juvara fold
juvenile
    j. absence epilepsy
    j. aldosteronism
    j. Alexander disease
    j. amaurotic idiocy
    j. amyotrophic lateral sclerosis
    j. ankylosing spondylitis (JAS)
    j. arthritis (JA)
    j. avascular necrosis
    j. carcinoma
    j. cataract
    j. cataract, cerebellar atrophy, mental retardation, myopathy syndrome
    j. chronic arthritis
    j. colonic polyp
    j. dermatomyositis (JDM, JDMS)
    j. diabetes
    j. diabetes mellitus (JDM)
    j. dystonic lipidosis
    j. epithelial corneal dystrophy
    j. fibroadenoma
    j. GM1 gangliosidosis
    j. GM2 gangliosidosis
    j. granulosa cell tumor (JGCT)
    j. hereditary motor neuron disease
    j. hyperuricemia syndrome
    j. idiopathic arthritis (JIA)
    j. idiopathic polyarticular arthritis
    j. idiopathic scoliosis
    j. intervertebral disc
    j. kyphosis
    j. melanoma
    j. MLD
    j. muscular dystrophy
    j. muscular torticollis
    j. myasthenia
    j. myelomonocytic leukemia (JMML)
    j. myoclonic epilepsy
    j. myotonic dystrophy
    j. nasopharyngeal angiofibroma
    j. NCL
    j. neuronopathic Gaucher disease
    j. onset
    j. osteomalacia
    j. osteoporosis

j. Paget disease
j. papillomatosis
j. Parkinson disease
j. pelvis
j. periodontitis
j. pernicious anemia
j. pilocytic astrocytoma
j. plantar dermatitis
j. plantar dermatosis
j. polyarthritis
j. polymyositis
j. psoriatic arthritis
j. rheumatic disease
j. rheumatoid arthritis (type I, II) (JRA)
j. spermatogonial depletion
j. spinal muscular atrophy
j. spondyloarthropathy
j. sulfatidosis
j. systemic granulomatosis
j. tabes
j. tibia vara
j. Tillaux fracture
J. Wellness and Health Survey (JWHS)
j. xanthogranuloma (JXG)
j. X-linked retinoschisis

juvenile-onset
j.-o. diabetes
j.-o. diabetes mellitus (JDM, JODM)
j.-o. inflammatory bowel disease
j.-o. multisystem inflammatory disease (JOMID)

juvenilis
arcus j.
kyphoscoliosis dorsalis j.
kyphosis dorsalis j.
osteochondritis deformans j.
osteodystrophia j.

juxtaarticular osteopenia
juxtacardiac
juxtaductal aortic coarctation
juxtaglomerular
j. apparatus hypertrophy
j. cell tumor (JGCT)
j. hyperplasia syndrome

juxtamedullary
juxtapleural inflammatory lesion
juxtapose
juxtaposition
Juzo-Hostess two-way stretch compression stocking
JVD
jugulovenous distention
JVP
jugular venous pressure
JWHS
Juvenile Wellness and Health Survey
J-wire placement
JWS
Jackson-Weiss syndrome
JXG
juvenile xanthogranuloma

NOTES

K
> potassium
>> K cell
>> K diet

K+ 8

K+ 10

K+2 diet

KABC
> Kaufman Assessment Battery for Children

Kabuki
>> K. makeup syndrome (KMS)
>> K. syndrome (KS)

Kadian sustained-release morphine capsules

KAFO
> knee-ankle-foot orthosis

Kagan staging system

Kahn
>> K. approach
>> K. cannula
>> K. test

Kajava classification

KAL
>> KAL gene
>> KAL protein

kala azar

Kalginate dressing

Kalischer syndrome

Kaliscinski ureteral procedure

kaliuresis

kallikrein

kallikrein-kinin system

Kallmann-de Morsier syndrome

Kallmann syndrome

Kalmuk idiocy

Kaltostat packing

kaluresis

kanamycin

Kanana Banana

kangaroo
>> k.'s Care
>> k. contact
>> K. enteral feeding pump
>> K. infusion pump
>> k. pouch

kangarooing

Kanner syndrome

kansasii
>> Mycobacterium k.

Kantor sign

Kantrex

Kaochlor

Kao Lectrolyte

kaolin
>> k. clotting time
>> k. and pectin

Kaon
>> S-F K.

Kaopectate
>> K. Advanced Formula
>> K. II
>> K. Maximum Strength

Kao-Spen

Kapectolin

Kapeller-Adler test

Kaplan-Meier
>> K.-M. method
>> K.-M. survival curve

Kaplan syndrome

Kaposi
>> K. sarcoma (KS)
>> K. sarcoma-associated herpesvirus
>> K. varicelliform eruption
>> K. varicelliform sarcoma

kaposiform hemangioendothelioma

Kaposi-like form of infantile hemangioma

kappa
>> k. chain
>> k. coefficient

Kapur-Toriello syndrome

karaya

Karl
>> K. Storz flexible ureteropyeloscope
>> K. Storz 15 French flexible hysteroscope

Karman cannula

Karnofsky performance status

Karo syrup

Kartagener syndrome

karyogenesis

karyokinesis

karyopyknosis

karyopyknotic index

karyorrhexis

karyosome

karyotheca

karyotype
>> abnormal k.
>> k. analysis
>> atypical k.
>> chromosomal k.
>> female k.
>> fetal k.
>> G-banded k.
>> male k.
>> maternal k.
>> parental k.

karyotype *(continued)*
    paternal k.
    spectral k. (SKY)
    Turner phenotype with normal k.
    45,X k.
    XO k.
    XX k.
    46,XX k.
    47,XX k.
    XXX k.
    XXY k.
    47,XXY k.
    XY k.
    46,XY k.
    47,XY k.
    46,XY/47,XY k.
karyotyping
    flow k.
    spectral k. (SKY)
Kasabach-Merritt
    K.-M. phenomenon
    K.-M. syndrome
Kasai
    K. operation
    K. peritoneal venous shunt
    K. portoenterostomy
    K. procedure
Kashin-Bek disease
Kasof
Kass criteria
katadidymus
Katayama fever
Katz-Wachtel phenomenon
Kaufman
    K. Assessment Battery for Children
      (KABC)
    K. Factor Score
    K. oculocerebrofacial syndrome
    K. pneumonia
    K. Survey of Early Academic and
      Language Skills (K-SEALS)
    K. Test of Educational
      Achievement (K-TEA)
Kaufman-McKusick syndrome
kava kava
Kaveggia syndrome
Kawasaki
    K. disease (KD)
    K. syndrome (KS)
Kay Ciel
Kayexalate
Kayser-Fleischer ring
Kaznelson syndrome
kb
    kilobase
    kb pair
KBG syndrome
kc
    kilocycle

kcal
    kilocalorie
K+ Care ET
K-cell
KCl
    potassium chloride
KD
    Kawasaki disease
    Krabbe disease
KDC-Healthdyne nonfluorescent spotlight 91kD cytochrome b peptide
KDF-2.3
    K. intrauterine catheter
    K. intrauterine insemination cannula
kDNA
    kinetoplast deoxyribonucleic acid
K-Dur
Kearns-Sayre syndrome (KSS)
KEDS
    Kids Eating Disorder Survey
keel chest
keeled breast
Keeler
    K. fiberoptic headlight
    K. loupe
keep vein open (KVO)
Keflex
Keftab
Kefurox Injection
Kefzol
Kegel exercises
Kehr
    K. incision
    K. sign for splenic injury
Keipert syndrome
Keith-Wagener retinopathy
Kell
    K. alloimmunization
    K. antibodies
    K. antigen
    K. autoantibody
    K. hydrops
    K. isoimmunization
    K. sensitization
    K. series
    K. test
Keller syndrome
Kelley-Seegmiller syndrome
Kelly
    K. clamp
    K. operation
    K. plication
    K. plication procedure
    K. retractor
    K. suture
    K. syndrome
    K. tissue forceps
    K. vulsellum forceps
Kelly-Gray curette

Kelly-Kennedy
  K.-K. plication
  K.-K. procedure
keloid
Kemadrin
Kempsey
  hemoglobin K.
Kenalog
  K. Injection
  K. in Orabase
  K. Topical
Kendall
  K. double-lumen catheter
  K. McGaw Intelligent pump
Kennedy-Pacey operation
Kennedy procedure
Kenny-Caffey syndrome
Kenny-Linarelli-Caffey syndrome
Kenny-Linarelli syndrome
Kenny syndrome
Kent Infant Development Scale (KIDS)
Keofeed tube
Keplerian parabola
keratan
  k. sulfate
  k. sulfaturia
keratin cyst
keratinization
keratinized
  k. cyst
  k. papule
keratinizing nasopharyngeal carcinoma
keratinocyte
  k. growth factor (KGF)
  k. growth factor receptor (KGFR)
keratinous
  k. cyst
  k. debris
  k. plug
keratitis
  Acanthamoeba k.
  bacterial k.
  dendritic k.
  disciform k.
  epithelial k.
  k. fugax hereditaria
  herpes k.
  herpetic k.
  k., ichthyosis, deafness (KID)
  interstitial k.
  neurotrophic k.

  palmar and plantar keratosis
    and k.
  punctate epithelial k.
  k. sicca
  syphilitic k.
  transient k.
keratoacanthoma
keratoconjunctivitis
  epidemic k. (EKC)
  microsporidial k.
  k. sicca
  tuberculous k.
keratoconus
keratocyst
  odontogenic k.
keratocyte
keratoderma
  k. blennorrhagicum
  mutilating k.
  palmoplantar k.
  k. palmoplantaris transgrediens
keratolysis
  k. neonatorum
  pitted k.
keratolytic gel
keratoma hereditarium mutilans
keratomalacia
keratopathy
  band k.
  herpetic k.
keratosis
  crusting telangiectasia k.
  k. follicularis
  k. follicularis spinulosa decalvans
  k. palmaris
  k. palmaris et plantaris
  k. palmaris et plantaris-corneal
    dystrophy syndrome
  k. palmoplantaris
  k. palmoplantaris-corneal dystrophy
    syndrome
  k. pilaris
  seborrheic k.
keratotic
  k. debris
  k. papule
  k. scaling
Kergaradec sign
kerion formation
Kerley B lines
Kerlix gauze bandage
kernicterus

K

NOTES

511

Kernig sign
Kernohan sign
Kerr cesarean
Keshan disease
Kessner Index
Kestrone
Ketalar
ketamine sedation
ketanserin
ketoacid
    k. accumulation
    branched-chain k.
    serum k.
    urine k.
ketoacidosis
    diabetic k. (DKA)
    severe k.
    starvation k.
ketoaciduria
    ADR syndrome with k.
    ataxia-deafness-retardation syndrome
      with k.
    branched-chain k.
ketoaciduria-mental deficiency syndrome
ketoconazole
3-ketodesogestrel
11-ketoetiocholanolone
ketogenic diet
17-ketogenic steroid
ketone
    k. body
    k. production
ketonemia
ketonuria
    branched-chain k.
ketoprofen
ketorolac tromethamine
ketosis
    starvation k.
ketosis-prone diabetes
ketosis-resistant diabetes
17-ketosteroid reductase deficiency
17-ketosteroids (17-KS)
ketotic
    k. hyperglycemia
    k. hyperglycinemia
    k. hypoglycemia
ketotifen
Kety-Schmidt cerebral blood flow
  measurement technique
Keutel syndrome (1, 2)
keV
    kilo-electronvolt
Kevorkian
    K. curette
    K. punch biopsy
Kevorkian-Younge
    K.-Y. biopsy forceps

    K.-Y. cervical biopsy instrument
    K.-Y. curette
Keyes
    K. biopsy instrument
    K. dermatologic punch
    K. punch biopsy
    K. vulvar punch
keyhole pupil
key-in-lock
    k.-i.-l. incontinence
    k.-i.-l. maneuver
Key-Pred Injection
Key-Pred-SP Injection
kg
    kilogram
KGF
    keratinocyte growth factor
KGFR
    keratinocyte growth factor receptor
KHD
    kinky-hair disease
KHQ
    King's Health Questionnaire
kHz
    kilohertz
Ki67 antibody
Kibrick
    K. method
    K. test
Kibrick-Isojima infertility test
kick count
Kicker Pavlik harness
KID
    keratitis, ichthyosis, deafness
    KID syndrome
Kidd blood group
Kidde
    K. cannula technique
    K. tubal insufflator
KidKart
kidney
    Ask-Upmark k.
    k. biopsy
    cystic k.
    k. dialysis
    k. disease
    duplex k.
    dysplastic k.
    k. failure
    k. function
    horseshoe k.
    hydronephrotic k.
    hypoplastic k.
    k. internal splint/stent (KISS)
    medullary sponge k.
    k. morphology
    multicystic k.
    multicystic dysplastic k. (MDK)
    palpable k.

palpably enlarged k.
pelvic k.
k. pole
polycystic k.
single k.
solitary k.
k. stone
supernumerary k.
k. transplantation
k.'s, ureters, bladder (KUB)
kidney-derived growth factor
KIDS
 Kent Infant Development Scale
Kids Eating Disorder Survey (KEDS)
Kienböck disease
Kiesselbach
 K. area
 K. plexus
 K. triangle
kifafa seizure disorder
Kikuchi disease
Kilian pelvis
kill
 cell k.
killed virus vaccine
killer
 k. cell
 natural k. cell (NK)
Killian syndrome
kilobase (kb)
kilocalorie (kcal)
kilocycle (kc)
kilo-electronvolt (keV)
kilogram (kg)
kilohertz (kHz)
kilohm
kilovolt (kV)
kilowatt (kW)
Kimmelstiel-Wilson
 K.-W. disease (KW)
 K.-W. syndrome
Kimura procedure
kinase
 creatine k. (CK)
 glycerol k. (GK)
 histone H1 k.
 myosin light-chain k.
 phosphoglycerate k. (PGK)
 protein k. C (PKC)
 pyruvate k. (PK)
 serine-threonine k.

tyrosine k.
viral thymidine k.
Kindercal formula
kindergarten
kindling
kindred
 degree of k.
Kinesed
kinesigenic paroxysmal dyskinesia
kinesiologic
kinesthesia
kinesthetic learner
kinetics
 cell k.
kinetochore
kinetoplast
 k. deoxyribonucleic acid (kDNA)
 k. DNA
King
 K. classification
 K.'s Health Questionnaire (KHQ)
 K. operation
kingae
 Haemophilus aphrophilus,
 Actinobacillus
 actinomycetemcomitans,
 Cardiobacterium hominis,
 Eikenella corrodens, Kingella
 kingae (HACEK)
kinin
kininogen
 high molecular weight k. (HMWK)
kinked
 k. cord
 k. midbrain
kinky-hair
 k.-h. disease (KHD)
 k.-h. syndrome
Kinsbourne syndrome
Kinyoun
 K. acid-fast stain
 K. acid-fast staining test
 K. carbol fuchsin stain
Kionex
KIO syndrome
Kirby-Bauer method
Kirghizian dermatoosteolysis
Kirner disease
Kirschner wire (K-wire)
Kish urethral illuminating catheter
KISS
 kidney internal splint/stent

NOTES

kiss
    angel's k.
kissing
    k. disease
    k. lesions
    k. patellae
    k. ulcer
kit
    ABI PRISM Dye Terminator Cycle Sequencing Ready Reaction K.
    Amplicor HIV-1 test k.
    Amplicor PCR k.
    Amplicor typing k.
    ApopTag Plus k.
    AutoDELFIA PRL molecule k.
    AutoDELFIA unconjugated E3 k.
    Centocor CA 125 radioimmunoassay k.
    cervical block k.
    Coat-A-Count neonatal 17 hydroxyprogesterone k.
    Confide HIV test k.
    FACE k.
    Ferritin IRMA k.
    Follistim/Antagon k.
    Hy-Gene seminal fluid collection k.
    InPouch TV subculture k.
    Male FactorPak seminal fluid collection k.
    Metra PS procedure k.
    newborn screening k.
    Ortho diaphragm k.
    Otovent autoinflation k.
    OvuDate fertility test k.
    OvuGen test k.
    OvuKIT Self-Test k.
    ovulation detection k.
    OvuQuick One-Step ovulation k.
    OvuQuick Self-Test k.
    Perkin Elmer rhodamine dye terminator k.
    PICC k.
    Pneumotest k.
    Preven emergency contraception k.
    Progesterone Radioimmunoassay K.
    QIAamp Tissue k.
    qualitative detection k.
    rape evidence k.
    SAFE k.
    SureCell Chlamydia Test k.
    Tago diagnostic k.
    TCI OcuLook saliva ovulation tester k.
    urinary ovulation detection k.
    urinary ovulation predictor k.
    Uri-Three urine culture k.
    Vesica sling k.
    Vidas Estradiol II assay k.
Kitano knot

Kitchen postpartum gauze packer
Kittner dissector
Kitzinger method of childbirth
Kiuchi histocytic necrotizing lymphadenitis
Kjelland
    K. forceps
    K. rotation
Kjelland-Barton forceps
Kjelland-Luikart forceps
Kjer-type dominant optic atrophy
KL-6 mucinous glycoprotein
Klavikordal
Klebsiella
    K. *oxytoca*
    K. *ozaenae*
    K. *pneumoniae*
***Klebsiella-Enterobacter* species**
kleeblattschädel
    k. deformity
    k. syndrome
Kleihauer
    K. fetomaternal hemorrhage estimation technique
    K. stain
    K. test
Kleihauer-Betke
    K.-B. stain
    K.-B. test
Kleine-Levin syndrome
Klein-Waardenburg syndrome
Kleppinger
    K. bipolar forceps
    K. envelope sign
kleptomania
Klinefelter
    K. syndrome
    K. variant
Klinefelter-Reifenstein-Albright syndrome
Klinefelter-Reifenstein syndrome
Kling bandage
Klippel-Feil syndrome
Klippel-Trenaunay-Parkes-Weber syndrome
Klippel-Trenaunay syndrome
Klippel-Trenaunay-Weber syndrome
Kloepfer syndrome
Klonopin
K-Lor
Klor-Con
Klor-Con/25
Klorvess
Klotrix
Klotz syndrome
Kluge method
Klumpke
    K. brachial palsy
    K. paralysis
Klumpke-Dejerine paralysis

Klüver-Bucy syndrome
KM-1 breast pump
K-Medic
KMS
 Kabuki makeup syndrome
knee
 k. angle
 anterior translation of k.
 breaststroker's k.
 k. height measuring device
 k. hinge
 housemaid's k.
 k. jerk reflex
 k. joint hyperextensibility
 jumper's k.
 knock k.'s
 k. presentation
knee-ankle-foot
knee-ankle-foot orthosis (KAFO)
knee-chest position
knee-elbow position
kneel-stand position
knemometry
Kniest
 K. dwarfism
 K. dysplasia
 K. syndrome
Kniest-like dysplasia
knife
 X-acto k.
knob
 aortic k.
 chromosome k.
knock
 k. knees
 pericardial k.
knock-knee
knot
 Aberdeen k.
 clinch k.
 Duncan k.
 false k.
 false k. of umbilical cord
 fisherman's k.
 granny k.
 Kitano k.
 laparoscopic slip k.
 modified Roeder k.
 primitive k.
 k. pusher
 Roeder k.

 4S k.
 square k.
 surgeon's k.
 syncytial k.
 Weston k.
knuckle of tube
Knudson two-hit tumorigenesis
 hypothesis
Koala intrauterine pressure catheter
Koate-DVI
Kobayashi vacuum extractor
Kobberling-Dunnigan syndrome
Köbner phenomenon
Koby syndrome
Koch
 K. postulates
 K. pouch diversion
Kocher clamp
Kocher-Debré-Sémélaigne syndrome
kocherize
Kock pouch
Kodak
 K. hCG serum test
 K. SureCell Chlamydia Test
 K. SureCell hCG-Urine Test
 K. SureCell Herpes (HSV) Test
 K. SureCell LCH in-office
 pregnancy test
 K. SureCell Strep A test
Koebner
 K. epidermolysis bullosa simplex
 K. reaction
 K. response
Koenen tumor
Koeppe iris nodule
Koerber-Salus-Elschnig syndrome
Koffex DM
Kogan endocervical speculum
Kogenate
KOH
 potassium hydroxide
 KOH colpotomizer system
 KOH prep
 KOH preparation
 KOH stain
 KOH test
Köhler bone disease
Kohn canal
koilocyte
koilocytic atypia
koilocytosis

K

NOTES

koilocytotic
- k. atypia
- k. cell

koilonychia
Kok disease
Kolmer test
Kolobow membrane lung
Kondremul
Kono procedure
Konsyl
Konsyl-D
Kontron electrode
Konyne 80
konzo
Kopan needle
Koplik spot
Korean hemorrhagic fever
Korenman estrogen window hypothesis
Koromex
Korotkoff
- K. phase
- K. sound
- K. test

Kosenow-Sinios syndrome
koseri
- *Citrobacter k.*

Kostmann
- K. disease
- K. infantile agranulocytosis
- K. neutropenia
- K. syndrome

Kovalevsky canal
Kowarski syndrome
Koyanagi procedure
Kozlowski
- K. disease
- K. spondylometaphysial dysplasia

K-Phos
- K-P. M.F.
- K-P. Neutral
- K-P. Original

Krabbe
- K. disease (KD)
- K. leukodystrophy
- K. syndrome

Kramer
- K. disease
- K. syndrome

Kraske position
K-*ras* oncogene
kraurosis vulvae
Krause
- K. disease
- K. lacrimal accessory gland
- K. syndrome

Krause-Kivlin syndrome
Krause-van Schooneveld-Kivlin syndrome
Krebs cycle
Kreiselman infant warmer

Kremer penetration test
Kristalose
Kristeller
- K. maneuver
- K. method

Kroner tubal ligation
Kronner
- K. Manipujector
- K. Manipujector uterine manipulator-injector
- K. manipulator

Kruger index
Krukenberg tumor
krusei
- *Candida k.*

KS
- Kabuki syndrome
- Kaposi sarcoma
- Kawasaki syndrome

17-KS
- 17-ketosteroids

K-SADS
- Schedule for Affective Disorders and Schizophrenia for School-Age Children

K-SADS-E
- Schedule for Affective Disorders and Schizophrenia for School-Age Children-Epidemiologic Version

K-SADS-P
- Schedule for Affective Disorders and Schizophrenia for School-Age Children-Present Episode

K-SEALS
- Kaufman Survey of Early Academic and Language Skills

KSS
- Kearns-Sayre syndrome

KT
- Orudis KT

K-Tab
K-TEA
- Kaufman Test of Educational Achievement

KTP
- potassium titanyl phosphate
- KTP laser

KUB
- kidneys, ureters, bladder

Kufs disease
Kugelberg-Welander (KW)
- K.-W. disease

Küntscher rod
Kupffer
- K. cell
- K. cell hyperplasia

Kupperman
- K. index
- K. menopausal distress test

kuru disease

Kurzrok-Miller test
Kurzrok-Ratner test
Kussmaul
    K. respiration
    K. sign
Küstner sign
Ku-Zyme HP
kV
    kilovolt
Kveim
    K. antibody
    K. test
KVO
    keep vein open
KW
    Kimmelstiel-Wilson disease
    Kugelberg-Welander
      KW disease
      KW test
kW
    kilowatt
kwashiorkor
    dermatosis of k.
    k. disease
Kwell
Kwellada

K-wire
    Kirschner wire
Kyasanur Forest disease
K-Y lubricating jelly
kynocephalus
kynurenine hydroxylation
Kyotest
kyphomelic dysplasia
kyphoscoliosis
    cataract, microcephaly, failure to
      thrive, k. (CAMFAK)
    k. dorsalis juvenilis
kyphoscoliotic heart disease
kyphosis
    cataract, microcephaly,
      arthrogryposis, k. (CAMAK)
    congenital k.
    dorsal k.
    k. dorsalis juvenilis
    flexible k.
    juvenile k.
    Scheuermann juvenile k.
    thoracic k.
    thoracolumbar k.
kyphotic pelvis
Kytril Injection

NOTES

L
>liter

L1
>neural cell adhesion molecule L1 (LICAM)

LA
>latex agglutination
>long-acting
>>Comhist LA
>>Dexone LA
>>Entex LA
>>Inderal LA
>>Zephrex LA

L-A
>Bicillin L-A

L.A.
>Humibid L.A.

La
>La Crosse (LAC)
>La Crosse encephalitis
>La Leche League
>La (SS-B) autoantigen

LAAH
>laparoscopic-assisted abdominal hysterectomy

lab
>Breathmobile mobile asthma testing l.

Laband syndrome
Labcath catheter
labeling
>primed in situ l. (PRINS)
>terminal deoxyribonucleotidyl transferase-mediated biotin-16-dUTP nick-end l. (TUNEL)

labetalol
labia (*pl. of* labium)
labial
>l. adhesion
>l. agglutination
>l. commissure
>l. edema
>l. fusion
>l. hernia
>l. hypertrophy
>l. reflex
>l. traction technique

labialis
>herpes simplex l.
>micropapillomatosis l.

labile
>l. asthma
>l. factor

lability
>emotional l.
>mood l.

labiodental speech sound
labioperineal pouch
labioscrotal
>l. fusion
>l. swelling
>l. Y-V plasty

labium, pl. **labia**
>caruncle of labia
>hypertrophy of labia
>hypoplastic labia
>labia majora
>l. majus
>l. majus pudendi
>labia minora
>l. minus
>l. minus pudendi

labor
>abnormal l.
>accelerated painless l. (APL)
>active phase of l.
>l. analgesia
>arrest of l.
>l. augmentation
>l. augmentation induction
>l. and delivery (L&D)
>l., delivery, and recovery (LDR)
>desultory l.
>dry l.
>false l.
>fetal distress in l.
>first stage of l.
>fourth stage of l.
>induced l.
>l. inhibition
>l. initiation
>latent phase of l.
>mimetic l.
>missed l.
>obstructed l.
>oxytocin stimulation of l.
>l. pains
>placental stage of l.
>postmature l.
>postponed l.
>precipitate l.
>precipitous l.
>premature l.
>preterm l. (PTL)
>primary dysfunctional l.
>prodromal l.
>prolonged l.
>second stage of l.

L

labor *(continued)*
    spontaneous l.
    stages of l.
    third stage of l.
    l. trial
    true l.
    vaginal birth after cesarean trial
      of l. (VBAC-TOL)
laboratory
    l. finding
    gait l.
    l. test
    Venereal Disease Research L.
      (VDRL)
Labotect catheter
labrum
    acetabular l.
labyrinth
labyrinthine
    l. afferent input
    l. concussion
    l. placenta
    l. reflex
    l. stimulation
labyrinthitis
    acute l.
    bacterial l.
    progressive l.
    suppurative l.
    traumatic l.
LAC
    La Crosse
    lupus anticoagulant
    LAC virus
laceration
    anal sphincter l.
    aortic l.
    birth canal l.
    bladder l.
    cerebral l.
    cervical l.
    falx l.
    first-degree l.
    fourth-degree l.
    perineal l.
    posterior pharyngeal l.
    scalp l.
    second-degree l.
    stellate l.
    suture penile l.
    tentorial l.
    third-degree l.
    vaginal l.
Lachman test
Lac-Hydrin
lack of natural killer cells
Lacks
    Henrietta L. (HeLa)
lacmoid staining solution

Lacri-Lube SOP lubricant eye ointment
lacrimal
    l. bone
    l. duct
    l. duct obstruction
    l. duct stenosis
    l. gland
    l. sac distention
    l. sac massage
lacrimation
    gustatory l.
lacrimoauriculodentodigital syndrome
lactacidemia
lactacidosis
Lactaid
    L. fat free milk
    L. reduced fat milk
    L. Ultra lactase enzyme supplement
Lact-Aid nursing trainer system
lactalbumin
    alpha l. (ALA)
lactamase
    beta l.
lactase
    congenital absence of l.
    l. deficiency
lactate
    ammonium l.
    amrinone l.
    arterial l.
    blood l.
    cyclizine l.
    l. dehydrogenase (LDH)
    plasma l.
    Ringer l.
lactated
    l. Ringer
    l. Ringer solution
lactating
    l. adenoma
    l. breast
    l. woman
lactation
    l. amenorrhea
    l. disorder
    inappropriate l.
    l. initiation
    l. letdown response
lactational
    l. amenorrhea method (LAM)
    l. amenorrhea method of
      contraception
    l. mastitis
lactea
    crusta l.
lacteal
    l. calculus
    l. cyst
    l. fistula

lactic
>l. acid
>l. acid dehydrogenase (LDH)
>l. acidemia
>l. acidosis

lacticacidemia
LactiCare
LactiCare-HC Topical
lactiferous duct
lactifugal
lactifuge
lactigenous
Lactina Select breast pump
Lactinex
Lactobacillus
>*L. acidophilus*
>*L. bifidus*
>*L. bulgaricus*
>*L. fermentum*
>*L. gasseri*
>*L. plantarum*
>*L. rhamnosus*
>*L. rhamnosus* strain GG (L-GG)

lactobacillus, pl. **lactobacilli**
>hydrogen peroxide-producing l.

lactobezoar
lactobionate
>erythromycin l.

lactocele
lactoferrin
>plasma l.

lactoflavin
LactoFree LIPIL formula
lactogen
>human placental l. (hPL, HPL)
>placental l.

lactogenesis
lactogenic
lactoovovegetarian
lactorrhea
lactose
>l. breath hydrogen test
>l. deficiency
>l. intolerance
>l. malabsorption
>l. monohydrate
>l. tolerance test

lactose-containing formula
lactose-free
>l.-f. diet
>l.-f. formula

Lactosorb

lactosuria
lactotropin
lactovegetarian
lactulose enema
lacuna, pl. **lacunae**
lacunar
>l. sinusoid
>l. skull

LAD
>left anterior descending
>leukocyte adhesion deficiency

LAD-1
>leukocyte adhesion deficiency-1

LAD-2
>leukocyte adhesion deficiency-2

Ladd
>L. band
>L. monitor
>L. operation
>L. procedure
>L. syndrome

Ladin sign
Laerdal
>L. mask
>L. resuscitator

laetrile
Lafora
>L. body
>L. body disease

Laforin
lag
>anaphase l.
>head l.
>homeostatic l.
>lid l.

lagophthalmia, lagophthalmos
Lahey
>L. clamp
>L. forceps

LA-HFOV
>liquid-assisted high-frequency oscillatory ventilation

LAI
LAIT
>latex agglutination inhibition test

lait
>café au l. (CAL)

LAK
>lymphokine-activated killer cell

lake
>subchorial l.
>venous l.

NOTES

lallation
Lalonde delicate hook forceps
LALT
    larynx-associated lymphoid tissue
LAM
    lactational amenorrhea method
    laser-assisted myringotomy
        LAM contraceptive method
Lamarck theory
Lamaze
    L. childbirth education
    L. method
LAMB
    lentigines, atrial myxomas, cutaneous
    papular myxomas, blue nevi
        LAMB syndrome
lambda
    l. sign
    l. suture line
lambdoid synostosis
Lambert-Eaton syndrome
Lambert syndrome
lamblia
    Giardia l.
Lambotte syndrome
lamellar
    l. body (LB)
    l. body count (LBC)
    l. body number density
    l. bone
    l. desquamation of newborn
    l. exfoliation
    l. ichthyosis
    l. inclusion body
lamellated appearance
Lamictal
lamina, pl. **laminae**
    basal l.
    l. cribrosa
    duplicated elastic l.
    elastic l.
    l. lucida
    l. propria
    l. terminalis
laminar airflow
laminaria
    l. cervical dilator
    L. digitata
    l. infusion
    L. japonica
    l. tent
    l. tent insertion
lamination
laminin
L-amino acid
Lamisil Cream
lamivudine
lamotrigine

lamp
    halogen l.
    Nightingale examining l.
    Sunnex Tri-Star l.
    Wood ultraviolet l.
lampbrush chromosome
Lamprene
Lanacaps
    Ferralyn L.
Lanacort Topical
lance
    heel l. (HL)
Lancefield streptococcal typing system
lancet
    Quikheel l.
Landau
    L. reflex
    L. response
    L. test
Landau-Kleffner
    L.-K. syndrome (LKS)
    L.-K. syndrome variant
Landing syndrome
Landmark catheter
Landouzy-Dejerine
    facioscapulohumeral syndrome
      of L.-D.
    L.-D. muscular dystrophy
Landouzy dystrophy
Landry
    L. palsy
    L. type of paralysis
Landry-Guillain-Barré syndrome
landscape
    adaptive l.
Langdon Down disease
Lange
    Brachmann-Cornelia de L. (BCDL)
    Cornelia de L. (CDL)
    L. test
Lange-Nielsen syndrome
Langer
    L. line
    L. mesomelic dwarfism
    L. mesomelic dysplasia
    L. syndrome
Langer-Giedion syndrome
Langerhans
    L. cell
    L. cell histiocytosis (LCH)
    L. granule
    L. islands
    islets of L.
Langer-Petersen-Spranger syndrome
Langer-Saldino syndrome
Langhans
    L. giant cell
    L. giant cell granuloma

L. layer
L. stria
language
American Sign L. (ASL)
body l.
l. delay
l. development
l. disorder
l. domain
expressive l.
l. milestone
receptive l.
sign l.
l. skill
language-based learning disability
lanolin
Lanophyllin
Lanoxicaps
Lanoxin
lansoprazole
Lanterman cleft
lanuginosa
hypertrichosis l.
lanuginous
lanugo
Lanvis
Lanz incision
LAO
left anterior oblique
lap
laparotomy
lap count
ex lap
Lap Sac
lap tape
laparoelytrotomy
laparohysterectomy
laparohystero-oophorectomy
laparohysteropexy
laparohysterosalpingo-oophorectomy
laparohysterotomy
Laparolift system
laparomyomectomy
LaparoSAC single-use obturator and cannula
laparosalpingectomy
laparosalpingo-oophorectomy
laparosalpingotomy
laparoscope
Lent l.
MiniSite l.

Storz l.
Surgiview l.
Weerda l.
Wolf l.
laparoscopic
l. cautery
l. cholecystectomy (LC)
l. cornual excision
l. Döderlein hysterectomy
l. electrocautery
l. evidence
l. fenestration
l. full-thickness intestinal biopsy
l. fundoplication (LF)
l. incision
l. insufflator
l. laser-assisted autoaugmentation
l. leash
l. lymphadenectomy
l. management
l. microsurgery
l. multiple-punch resection
l. myomectomy
l. oophorectomy
l. oophoropexy
l. ovarian diathermy
l. plasma forceps
l. retropubic colposuspension
l. sacrocolpopexy
l. slip knot
l. sonography
l. supracervical hysterectomy (LSH)
l. treatment
l. trocar
l. tubal ligation (LTL)
l. unipolar coagulation procedure
l. ureterosacral ligament resection (LUSLR)
laparoscopically
l. assisted anorectoplasty
l. assisted radical vaginal hysterectomy
laparoscopic-assisted
l.-a. abdominal hysterectomy (LAAH)
l.-a. vaginal hysterectomy (LAVH)
l.-a. vaginal hysteroscopy (LAVH)
laparoscopy
gasless l.
laser l.
pelvic l.

L

NOTES

laparoscopy *(continued)*
    l. port
    second-look l.
LaparoSonic coagulating shears (LCS)
laparotomy (lap)
    exploratory l.
    l. incision
    l. pad
    salvage l.
    second-look l.
laparotrachelotomy
laparouterotomy
lap-belt
    l.-b. compex
    l.-b. trauma
Lapides vesicourethropexy technique
Lapwall sponge
LAR
    laryngeal adductor reflex
    late asthmatic response
Largactil
large
    l. B-cell lymphoma
    l. bowel injury
    l. bowel stasis
    l. cell anaplastic Ki-1 lymphoma
    l. cell immunoblastic lymphoma
    l. cisterna magna
    l. endometrioma
    l. foreskin
    l. for gestational age (LGA)
    l. intestine
    l. intestine neoplasm
    l. loop excision
    l. loop excision of transformation zone (LLETZ)
    l. lysosome-like granule
    l. single copy
    l. tongue
large-bore catheter
large-for-dates
    l.-f.-d. infant
    l.-f.-d. uterus
large-volume
    l.-v. blood study
    l.-v. nonobstruction
L-arginine
lari
    Campylobacter l.
Laron
    L. dwarfism
    L. syndrome
Larsen syndrome
larva
    l. currens
    l. migrans
larval granulomatosis
larvicide

laryngeal
    l. abductor paralysis
    l. adductor paralysis
    l. adductor reflex (LAR)
    l. atresia
    l. atresia syndrome
    l. chemoreflex
    l. cleft
    l. closure
    l. diphtheria
    l. edema
    l. fracture
    l. hypoplasia
    l. mask airway (LMA)
    l. nerve
    l. nerve paralysis
    l. papilloma
    l. papillomatosis
    l. paresis
    l. spasm
    l. stenosis
    l. stridor
    l. vagal reflex
    l. wart
    l. web
larynges (*pl. of* larynx)
laryngitis
    acute spasmodic l.
    viral l.
laryngocele
laryngologist
laryngomalacia
laryngopharyngeal
    l. sensory stimulation (LPSS)
    l. sensory stimulation testing
laryngopharynx
laryngoscope
    Andrews infant l.
    l. blade
    l. handle
    Holinger infant l.
    pencil-handled l.
    Pentax l.
    Siker l.
laryngoscopy
    direct l.
    indirect l.
    mirror l.
laryngospasm
laryngotracheal
    l. reconstruction
    l. stenosis (LTS)
laryngotracheitis
laryngotracheobronchitis
    bacterial l.
    membranous l.
    viral l.
laryngotracheoesophageal
    l. cleft

laryngotracheomalacia
larynx, pl. **larynges**
    atresia of l.
    floppy l.
larynx-associated lymphoid tissue (LALT)
Larzel anemia
laser
    l. ablation
    alexandrite l.
    ArF excimer l.
    argon l.
    l. blanching
    Candela l.
    carbon dioxide l.
    l. cervical conization
    CO_2 l.
    l. ejecta
    Er:YAG l.
    l. excision
    l. excisional conization
    flashlamp-pulsed dye l.
    Ho:YAG l.
    Illumina Pro Series laparoscopic l.
    KTP l.
    l. laparoscopy
    Merrimack 1040 CO_2 l.
    l. method
    l. myringotomy
    Nd:YAG l.
    l. office ventilation of ears (LOVE)
    l. office ventilation of ears with insertion of tubes (LOVE IT)
    Opmilas CO_2 l.
    l. photocoagulation
    l. photocoagulation of the communicating vessels (LPCV)
    l. photovaporization
    l. plume
    l. reaction
    SPTL vascular lesion l.
    l. surgery
    Surgicenter 40 CO_2 l.
    Surgilase 55W l.
    l. therapy
    l. treatment
    l. uterosacral nerve ablation (LUNA)
    l. vaporization
    Xanar 20 Ambulase CO_2 l.

    YAG l.
    yttrium-aluminum-garnet l.
laser-assisted myringotomy (LAM)
laser-Doppler flowmeter
lasered
Lash
    L. operation
    L. procedure
Lasix
    L. Injection
    L. Oral
L-asparaginase
Lassa
    L. fever
    L. virus
La/SSB antigen
last
    l. menstrual period (LMP)
    l. normal menstrual period (LNMP)
LAT
    lateral atrial tunnel
    lidocaine, adrenaline, tetracaine
    LAT cavopulmonary anastomosis
latae
    tensor fasciae l. (TFL)
LATCH
    Lower Anchorages and Tethers for children
    LATCH system
latching-on process
late
    l. adolescence
    l. apnea
    l. arrhythmia
    l. asthmatic reaction
    l. asthmatic response (LAR)
    l. complication
    l. complication of transfusion
    l. congenital syphilis
    l. deceleration
    l. embryonic testicular regression syndrome
    l. hemorrhagic disease
    l. hypocalcemia
    l. infantile amaurotic idiocy
    l. infantile MLD
    l. infantile NCL
    l. infantile neural ceroid lipofuscinosis (LINCL)
    l. infantile systemic lipidosis
    l. luteal phase dysphoric disorder (LLPDD)

NOTES

late (*continued*)
    l. luteal phase syndrome
    l. mature
    l. neonatal hypocalcemia
    l. phase
    l. pregnancy
    l. radiation encephalopathy
    l. replicating chromosome
    l. uterine wedge resection
latency
    interpeak l.
    pudendal nerve terminal motor l.
    REM l.
    response l.
    sleep l.
    terminal motor l.
latent
    l. carrier
    l. celiac disease
    l. class analysis (LCA)
    l. diabetes
    l. herpes simplex virus infection
    l. nystagmus
    l. phase
    l. phase of labor
    l. syphilis
latent-stage syphilis
late-onset
    l.-o. congenital large ectopic gland
    l.-o. hyperplasia
    l.-o. hypogammaglobulinemia
    l.-o. local junctional epidermolysis bullosa-mental retardation syndrome
    l.-o. SED
    l.-o. sepsis
latera (*pl. of* latus)
lateral
    l. atrial tunnel (LAT)
    l. collateral ligament complex
    l. compartment
    l. condylar fracture
    l. condyle
    l. curvature
    l. curvature of spine
    l. displacement of inner canthus
    l. epicondylitis
    l. facial dysplasia (LFD)
    l. femoral torsion (LFT)
    l. geniculate
    l. geniculate body
    l. head displacement (LHD)
    l. head-righting
    l. head tilt
    l. hip rotation
    l. incisor
    l. lemniscus
    l. luxation
    l. malleolus

    l. nasal proboscis
    l. oblique view
    l. ovarian transposition
    l. pelvic wall
    l. plate mesoderm
    l. radiograph
    l. rectus muscle
    l. rectus palsy
    l. recumbent position
    l. resolution
    l. rotation (LR)
    l. shoulder sway
    l. sinus thrombosis
    l. sperm head displacement
    l. tibial bowing
    l. tibial torsion (LTT)
    l. transverse thigh flap
    l. umbilical fold
    l. wall retractor
lateralis
    proboscis l.
    vastus l.
laterality
    l. defect
    l. disorder
    l. sequence
lateralization process
lateralizing sign
laterally extended endopelvic resection
lateris (*gen. of* latus)
lateromedial oblique view
laterothoracic exanthem
lateroversion
latex
    l. agglutination (LA)
    l. agglutination assay
    l. agglutination inhibition test (LAIT)
    l. fixation test
    l. glove
    l. particle agglutination
    l. particle agglutination test
    l. sensitization
    l. test for *Pneumococcus*
lathyrism
latissimus dorsi flap
lato
    Borrelia burgdorferi sensu l.
latrodectism
LATS
    long-acting thyroid stimulator
    LATS hormone
    LATS protector
latum
    condyloma l.
    Diphyllobothrium l.
latus, gen. **lateris**, pl. **latera**
    fascia lata
    nevus unius lateris

Latzko
  L. cesarean
  L. colpocleisis
  L. operation
laudanum
Lauenstein
  L. lateral radiograph
  L. pelvic x-ray
Laufe-Piper forceps
Laufe polyp forceps
Lauge-Hansen mechanism of injury
Laugier-Hunziker syndrome
Launois-Cléret syndrome
Launois syndrome
Laurell (rocket) immune electrophoresis
Laurence-Moon-Biedl (LMB)
  L.-M.-B. syndrome
Laurence-Moon-Biedl-Bardet (LMBB)
  L.-M.-B.-B. syndrome (LMBBS)
Laurence-Moon syndrome
Laurer forceps
Laurus ND-260 needle driver
LAV
  lymphadenopathy-associated virus
lavage
  alveolar l.
  antral l.
  bronchoalveolar l. (BAL)
  bronchopulmonary l.
  diagnostic peritoneal l. (DPL)
  gastric l.
  nasal l.
  nonbronchoscopic bronchoalveolar l.
  oral colonic l. (OCL)
  peritoneal l.
  pulmonary l.
  saline l.
  surfactant l.
  therapeutic pulmonary l.
  tracheal l.
LAVH
  laparoscopic-assisted vaginal
    hysterectomy
  laparoscopic-assisted vaginal
    hysteroscopy
law
  Collins l.
  Hardy-Weinberg l.
  Hellin l.
  Hellin-Zeleny l.
  Leopold l.
  l. of mass action

  Mendel first l.
  Mendel second l.
  Pflüger l.
Lawford syndrome
Lawrence-Seip syndrome
Lawrence syndrome
lax
  l. joint
  l. ligament
laxa
  acquired cutis l.
  cutis l.
laxative
  bulk-forming l.
  osmotic l.
laxity
  anteroposterior l.
  joint l.
  ligamentous l.
  mental retardation, overgrowth,
    craniosynostosis, distal
    arthrogryposis, sacral dimple,
    joint l.
  pelvic floor l.
  suspensory ligament l.
layer
  Bowman l.
  l. of Brun
  buffy coat l.
  feeder l.
  germ l.
  glycosaminoglycan l.
  half-value l. (HVL)
  Langhans l.
  musculoaponeurotic l.
  myofascial l.
  Nitabuch l.
  Rauber l.
  skeletal muscle l.
  Waldeyer l.
lazaroid
Lazarus-Nelson closed peritoneal lavage technique
LazerSporin-C Otic
lazy
  l. bladder syndrome
  l. eye
  l. leukocyte syndrome
lazy-S incision
LB
  lamellar body

NOTES

527

LBC
    lamellar body count
LBM
    lean body mass
LBW
    low birth weight
      LBW infant
LBWC
    limb-body wall complex
LBWI
    low birth weight infant
LBW-MES
    low birth weight-maternal employment
      study
LC
    laparoscopic cholecystectomy
    living children
LCA
    latent class analysis
    Leber congenital amaurosis
LCAD
    long-chain acyl-CoA dehydrogenase
      LCAD deficiency
LCAD/MCAD
    long- and medium-chain acyl-CoA
      dehydrogenase
      LCAD/MCAD deficiency
LCAD/VLCAD
    long- and very-long-chain acyl-CoA
      dehydrogenase
      LCAD/VLCAD deficiency
L-Caine
L-carnitine
L-Cath peripherally inserted neonatal catheter
LCD
    L. cream
    L. ointment
LCH
    Langerhans cell histiocytosis
LCHAD
    long-chain 3-hydroxyacyl-CoA
      dehydrogenase
    long-chain hydroxyacyl-coenzyme A
      dehydrogenase
      LCHAD deficiency
lck protooncogene
LCL
    localized cutaneous leishmaniasis
LCMV
    lymphocytic choriomeningitis virus
      LCMV syndrome
LCP
    Legg-Calvé-Perthes
LCPD
    Legg-Calvé-Perthes disease
LCPUFA
    long-chain polyunsaturated fatty acid

LCR
    ligase chain reaction
      LCR assay
LCS
    LaparoSonic coagulating shears
LCx Probe System test
LD
    learning disability
L&D
    labor and delivery
LDH
    lactate dehydrogenase
    lactic acid dehydrogenase
      LDH deficiency
LDL
    low-density lipoprotein
      LDL apheresis
      LDL cholesterol
L-DOPA
LDR
    labor, delivery, and recovery
      LDR room
LDS
    ligate-divide-staple
      LDS clip applier
      LDS instrument
LE
    lower extremity
    lupus erythematosus
      LE cell preparation
Le
    Le Fort fracture
    Le Fort fracture pattern
    Le Fort operation
    Le Fort partial colpocleisis
LEA
    local education agency
lead
    l. agency
    l. block
    blood l.
    l. bra
    l. encephalopathy
    l. exposure
    l. ingestion
    l. intoxication
    limb l.
    l. line
    organic l.
    l. pipe stiffness
    l. pipe urethra
    l. point
    l. poisoning
    tetraethyl l.
    l. tracing
    l. triphosphate
    l. wire

Leadbetter-Politano
L.-P. procedure
L.-P. ureterovesicoplasty
LeadCare handheld blood lead analyzer
leading ancestor
leaf, pl. **leaves**
l. of broad ligament
cabbage leaves
leaflet
flail mitral l. (FML)
League
La Leche L.
leak
air l.
capillary l.
cerebrospinal fluid l.
staple line l.
leakage
placental l.
silicone implant l.
urine l.
leak-point
l.-p. pressure
l.-p. pressure test
leaky gene
lean
l. body mass (LBM)
l. spastic dwarfism
l. tissue mass (LTM)
Lear complex
learner
active l.
auditory l.
kinesthetic l.
visual l.
learning
l. disability (LD)
discrete-trial l.
l. disorder
L. to Eat manual
Mullen Scales of Early L. (MSEL)
situated l.
slow rate of l.
l. style
wide range assessment of memory
and l. (WRAML)
leash
laparoscopic l.
**Lea's shield female barrier
contraceptive**
least restrictive environment (LRE)
leather-bottle stomach

leaves (*pl. of* leaf)
Leber
L. abiotrophy
L. congenital amaurosis (LCA)
L. congenital retinal amaurosis
L. congenital tapetoretinal
degeneration
L. disease
L. disease 2
L. hereditary atrophy
L. hereditary optic neuropathy
(LHON)
L. optic neuropathy
Leboyer
L. episiotomy technique
L. method
LEC
life events checklist
lecanopagus
Lecat gulf
lecithin
disaturated l.
l.-sphingomyelin ratio (L/S)
Lecompte maneuver
lectin
Lectrolyte
Kao L.
Leder stain
LEDS
life events and difficulties schedule
LEDS interview
LEEP
loop electrosurgical excision procedure
LEEP Redi-kit
Lee-White clotting time
Leff forceps
left
l. anterior descending (LAD)
l. anterior hemiblock
l. anterior oblique (LAO)
l. arterial pressure
l. atrial hypertrophy
l. atrium
l. axis deviation
l. bundle branch block
l. common carotid
l. ear
l. frontoanterior position (LFA)
l. frontoposterior position (LFP)
l. frontotransverse position (LFT)
l. hemisyndrome
l. hepatectomy

NOTES

529

left *(continued)*
    l. lateral decubitus position (LLDP)
    l. lateral position
    l. lower quadrant (LLQ)
    l. main coronary artery
    l. mentoanterior position (LMA)
    l. mentoposterior position (LMP)
    l. mentotransverse position (LMT)
    l. occipitoanterior position (LOA)
    l. occipitoposterior position (LOP)
    l. occipitotransverse position (LOT)
    l. renal vein
    l. to right (L-R)
    l. sacroanterior
    l. sacroanterior position (LSA)
    l. sacroposterior position (LSP)
    l. sacrotransverse position (LST)
    l. scapuloanterior position (LScA)
    l. scapuloposterior position (LScP)
    l. upper quadrant (LUQ)
    l. ventricle (LV)
    l. ventricular (LV)
    l. ventricular apical aneurysm
    l. ventricular assist device (LVAD)
    l. ventricular dysfunction (LVD)
    l. ventricular ejection fraction
    (LVEF)
    l. ventricular end-diastolic
    dimension
    l. ventricular end-systolic dimension
    l. ventricular failure
    l. ventricular hypertrophy (LVH)
    l. ventricular outflow tract (LVOT)
    l. ventricular outflow tract
    obstruction (LVOTO)
    l. ventricular outlet obstruction
    l. ventricular paced beat
    l. ventricular stroke work index
    (LVSWI)
    l. vertical vein
left/right
    l. asymmetry
    l. dynein
left-sided lesion
left-sidedness
    bilateral l.-s.
left-to-right
    l.-t.-r. shunt
    l.-t.-r. shunting
    l.-t.-r. shunt lesion
Lefty-1, -2
leg
    l. atrophy
    baker's l.
    bayonet l.
    l. cramp
    l. edema
    l. length discrepancy (LLD)
    milk l.

    white l.
    W position of l.'s
legal
    l. intervention
    l. issue
legally blind
Legat point
Legatrin
leg-compression stocking
Legg-Calvé-Perthes (LCP)
    L.-C.-P. disease (LCPD)
leggings
Legg-Perthes disease
Legionella
    L. micdadei
    L. pneumophila
legionellosis
Legionnaires, Legionnaire
    L. disease
Leiden
    factor V L.
    L. mutation
Leigh
    L. disease
    encephalomyopathy of L.
    L. necrotizing encephalomyelopathy
    L. subacute necrotizing
    encephalopathy
    L. syndrome
Leiner
    L. disease
    L. syndrome
leiomyoblastoma
leiomyoma, pl. **leiomyomata**
    cervical l.
    endometrial metastasizing l.
    ovarian l.
    parasitic l.
    pedunculated l.
    submucous l.
    l. uteri
    uterine leiomyomata
    vascular l.
leiomyomatosis
    intravenous l.
    l. peritonealis disseminata (LPD)
leiomyosarcoma (LMS)
    epithelioid l.
Leisegang colposcope
Leishmania
    L. braziliensis
    L. infantum
    L. major
    L. mexicana
    L. panamensis
    L. tropica
leishmaniasis
    cutaneous l.
    diffuse cutaneous l. (DCL)

localized cutaneous l. (LCL)
mucocutaneous l.
mucosal l.
post-kala azar dermal l. (PKDL)
visceral l.

Leiter International Performance Scale
Lejeune syndrome
Lejour-type modified breast reduction
Lem-Blay circumcision clamp
Lemierre syndrome
Lemli-Opitz syndrome
lemniscus, pl. **lemnisci**
lateral l.
lemon
l. balm
l. sign
lemon-squeezer obstetrical elevator
length
birth l.
cervical l.
clitoral l.
crown-heel l. (CHL)
crown-rump l. (CRL)
cycle l.
femoral l.
femur l. (FL)
fetal foot l. (FFL)
functional urethral l. (FUL)
funnel l.
humerus l. (HL)
long bone l.
penile l.
sinus cycle l.
stretched penile l.
stretched phallic l.
subischial leg l. (SILL)
supine l.
lengthening
Achilles tendon l.
Evans calcaneal l.
hamstring l.
l. of hamstring
heel cord l.
muscle l.
l. osteotomy
tendo Achillis l. (TAL)
tendon l.
Lennox-Gastaut syndrome
Lennox syndrome
lens
Barkan infant l.
crystalline l.

L. culinaris agglutinin
30-degree l.
70-degree l.
l. dislocation
Morgan therapeutic l.
l. opacity
posterior chamber intraocular l.
(PC-IOL)
Sauflon PW contact l.
Silsoft extended wear contact l.
Lente Iletin II
lenticonus
anterior l.
posterior l.
lenticular
l. cataract
l. opacity
lentiform nucleus
lentigines (*pl. of* lentigo)
lentiginosis profusa
lentiginous nevus
lentigo, pl. **lentigines**
agminated l.
lentigines, atrial myxomas,
cutaneous papular myxomas, blue
nevi (LAMB)
lentigines (multiple),
electrocardiographic abnormalities,
ocular hypertelorism, pulmonary
stenosis, abnormalities of
genitalia, retardation of growth,
and deafness (sensorineural)
(LEOPARD)
l. simplex
lentis
ectopia l.
simple ectopia l.
lentivirus
Lent laparoscope
Lenz
L. dysmorphogenic syndrome
L. dysplasia
L. microphthalmia syndrome
Lenz-Majewski
L.-M. hyperostotic dwarfism
L.-M. syndrome
Leonard catheter
LEOPARD
lentigines (multiple), electrocardiographic
abnormalities, ocular hypertelorism,
pulmonary stenosis, abnormalities of

L

NOTES

LEOPARD *(continued)*
  genitalia, retardation of growth, and
  deafness (sensorineural)
  LEOPARD syndrome
Leopold
  L. law
  L. maneuver
Lepiota cristata
Lepore
  hemoglobin L.
  L. thalassemia
lepori
  Brugia l.
leprae
  Mycobacterium l.
leprechaunism
lepromatous leprosy
leprosum
  erythema nodosum l.
leprosy
  borderline lepromatous l.
  borderline tuberculoid l.
  dimorphous l.
  full lepromatous l.
  full tuberculoid l.
  indeterminate l.
  lepromatous l.
  tuberculoid l.
leprous salpingitis
leptin
  cord plasma l.
  maternal plasma l.
  l. receptor
  serum l.
  umbilical cord l.
leptomeningeal
  l. angioma
  l. angiomatosis
  l. cyst
  l. heterotopia
leptomeningitis
  acute syphilitic l.
  mumps l.
leptometacarpy
Leptospira
  L. canicola
  L. grippotyphosa
  L. icterohaemorrhagiae
  L. interrogans
  L. interrogans serovar *L.*
  L. pomona
leptospiral
  l. illness
  l. meningitis
leptospire
leptospirosis
  anicteric l.
  icteric l.

leptotene
  l. phase of meiosis
  l. stage
leptotrichosis
Leri
  L. pleonosteosis
  L. syndrome
Leri-Weill syndrome
Leroy syndrome
LeRoy ventricular catheter
LES
  lower esophageal sphincter
  LES pressure
lesbian relationship
lesbianism
Leschke syndrome
Lesch-Nyhan
  L.-N. disease
  L.-N. syndrome (LNS)
lesion
  acetowhite l.
  acquired hypothalamic l.
  acral skin l.
  acyanotic l.
  anal squamous intraepithelial l.
    (ASIL)
  anesthetic skin l.
  anular l.
  arciform l.
  axillary skin l.
  Bankart l.
  barrel-shaped l.
  benign l.
  blanching wheal and flare l.
  blueberry muffin skin l.
  brain l.
  brainstem l.
  brown skin l.
  cannonball l.
  cardiac l.
  cavitary white-matter l.
  central cord l.
  cervical l.
  cicatricial l.
  clastic l.
  coin l.
  collapse-consolidation l.
  confetti l.
  congenital l.
  coronary artery l. (CAL)
  correctable l.
  crescentic l.
  crusted l.
  cutaneous l.
  cyanotic congenital heart l.
  cystic l.
  dermatophyte l.
  Dieulafoy gastric l.
  discoid l.

discontinuous l.
ductal-dependent l.
ectocervical l.
eczematoid l.
eczematous skin l.
endometriotic l.
epileptogenic l.
erythematous satellite l.
exogastric l.
exophytic l.
extrapyramidal l.
flaccid l.
genital l.
gingival l.
glandular atypia l.
guttate l.
heart l.
high-grade squamous
  intraepithelial l. (HGSIL, HSIL)
HPV-associated l.
hyperpigmented l.
hypoesthesic skin l.
hypopigmented l.
hypothalamic l.
intestinal l.
intracavitary l.
intraepithelial l.
iris l.
isodense l.
Janeway l.
juxtapleural inflammatory l.
kissing l.'s
left-sided l.
left-to-right shunt l.
linear l.
local l.
low-grade squamous
  intraepithelial l. (LGSIL, LSIL)
lumbosacral plexus l.
lumbosacral root l.
Lynch and Crues type 2 l.
lytic l.
macular-papular-vesicular l.
maculopapular l.
mass l.
metaphysial l.
metastatic l.
microvascular l.
mixing l.
morphogenetic l.
mucosal l.

multifocal white matter
  inflammatory l.
multiple ring-enhancing mass l.
nipplelike l.
nodulocystic l.
Noonan-like giant cell l.
oculocutaneous l.
organic brain l.
osseous BA l.
osteochondrotic l.
palmar l.
papular l.
papulonodular l.
papulovesicular l.
parenchymal brain l.
pebbly skin l.
pedunculated l.
perineal l.
photodistributed l.
pigmented l.
plexus l.
plucked chicken skin l.
powder-burn endometrial l.
precancerous l.
precursor l.
preinvasive l.
premalignant l.
proliferative l.
pseudoencapsulated l.
psoriasiform l.
punched-out lytic l.
pyramidal l.
radial sclerosing l.
raised l.
right-sided l.
satellite l.
sclerosing l.
seborrheic-looking skin l.
SIL/ASCUS l.
Sinding-Larsen l.
single ring-enhancing mass l.
skin l.
skip l.
solitary bone l.
space-occupying l.
spiculated l.
squamous intraepithelial l. (SIL)
target l.
targetoid l.
total mixing l.
tubulointerstitial l.
umbilication of l.

NOTES

lesion *(continued)*
>   upper GI l.
>   urticarial raised l.
>   vascular proliferative l.
>   vasculitic skin l.
>   vermiform l.
>   vesicobullous skin l.
>   vesicopustular l.
>   vesicular palmar l.
>   vesicular skin l.
>   vesiculoulcerative l.
>   violaceous l.
>   vulvar pigmented l.
>   vulvovaginal l.
>   watershed l.
>   weeping l.
>   zosteriform l.

lesson
>   speech l.

LET
>   lidocaine, epinephrine, tetracaine

letalis
>   epidermolysis bullosa l.
>   Herlitz epidermolysis bullosa l.

letdown
>   milk l.
>   l. reflex

lethal
>   l. bone dysplasia
>   l. equivalent
>   l. gene
>   l. multiple pterygium syndrome
>   l. neonatal dwarfism

lethargic
lethargica
>   encephalitis l.

lethargy
>   postictal l.

letrozole
letter chart
Letterer-Siwe disease
LETZ
>   loop excision of the transformation zone
>   LETZ procedure

leucine
>   l. aminopeptidase
>   l. tolerance test

leucocoria
leucocyte detection strip
Leuconostoc
leucovorin
>   calcium l.

leukapheresis
leukemia
>   acute lymphatic l.
>   acute lymphoblastic l. (ALL)
>   acute lymphocytic l. (ALL)
>   acute megakaryoblastic l.
>   acute myeloblastic l.

>   acute myelogenous l.
>   acute myeloid l. (AML)
>   acute nonlymphoblastic l. (ANLL)
>   acute nonlymphocytic l.
>   amyeloid l.
>   aplastic l.
>   basophilic l.
>   chronic lymphocytic l. (CLL)
>   chronic myelocytic l.
>   chronic myelogenous l. (CML)
>   CNS l.
>   congenital l.
>   eosinophilic l.
>   granulocytic l.
>   hemoblastic l.
>   l. infiltrate
>   l. inhibitory factor (LIG)
>   juvenile myelomonocytic l. (JMML)
>   leukopenic l.
>   lymphatic l.
>   lymphoblastic l.
>   lymphocytic l.
>   lymphosarcoma cell l.
>   mast cell l.
>   megakaryoblastic l.
>   megakaryocytic l.
>   micromyeloblastic l.
>   myeloblastic l.
>   myelocytic l.
>   myelogenous l.
>   myeloid l.
>   myelomonocytic l.
>   nonlymphoblastic l.
>   nonlymphocytic l.
>   promyelocytic l.
>   testicular l.

leukemia/lymphoma
>   adult T-cell l./l. (ATLL)

leukemic
>   l. blast
>   l. cell

leukemicus
>   hiatus l.

leukemogenesis
leukemoid reaction
Leukeran
Leukine
leukoclastic angiitis
leukocoria, leukokoria
leukocyte
>   l. adhesion deficiency (LAD)
>   l. adhesion deficiency-1 (LAD-1)
>   l. adhesion deficiency-2 (LAD-2)
>   l. count
>   diapedetic l.
>   l. esterase dipstick
>   l. function
>   l. hexosaminidase A
>   l. histamine release test

l. infiltration
l. integrin lymphocyte function-associated antigen 1
l. interferon
polymorphonuclear l.
l. transfusion
leukocyte-depletion filter
leukocyte-removal filter
leukocytoclastic
l. angiitis
l. vasculitis
leukocytosis
extreme l.
granulocytic l.
mild l.
neutrophilic l.
leukocytospermia
leukocyturia
leukodepletion filter
leukoderma
l. acquisitum centrifugum
l. of vulva
leukodystrophy
adrenal l.
cerebral l.
demyelinogenic l.
fibrinoid l.
globoid cell l.
Krabbe l.
melanodermic l.
metachromatic l. (MLD)
sudanophilic l.
leukoencephalopathy
focal pontine l.
multifocal l.
perinatal telencephalic l.
progressive multifocal l. (PML)
l. syndrome
leukoerythroblastic syndrome
leukokoria (*var. of* leukocoria)
leukokraurosis
leukoma
corneal l.
leukomalacia
cerebral l.
cystic l.
cystic periventricular l. (cPVL)
periventricular l. (PVL)
leukopenia
leukopenic leukemia
leukophlegmasia dolens

leukoplakia
hairy l.
oral hairy l.
l. vulvae
leukoplakic vulvitis
leukorrhagia
leukorrhea
menstrual l.
physiologic l.
leukorrheal
l. discharge
l. disorder
leukospermia
leukostasis
pulmonary l.
Leukotrap red cell collector
leukotriene
l. C_4 (LTC_4)
l. D_4 (LTD_4)
l. E_4 (LTE_4)
l. inhibitor
l. receptor antagonist (LTRA)
leuprolide acetate
leuprorelin acetate
Leustatin
levalbuterol hydrochloride
levallorphan tartrate
levamisole
Levaquin
levarterenol
Levate
levator
l. ani
l. ani muscle
l. ani spasm
l. ani syndrome
l. palpebrae muscle
l. plate
l. sling

Levbid
LeVeen shunt
level
ACD l.
air-fluid l.
alpha antitrypsin l.
amniotic fluid l.
arachidonic acid l.
arousal l.
bile chenodeoxycholic acid l.
biparietal diameter l.
blood alcohol l. (BAL)
blood ammonia l.

L

NOTES

lexical-syntactic
   l.-s. deficit
   l.-s. syndrome (LSS)
lexicon
Leyden-Möbius muscular dystrophy
Leydig
   L. cell aplasia
   L. cell atrophy
   L. cell embryology
   L. cell hyperplasia
   L. cell hypoplasia
   L. cells
   L. cell tumor
Leyton Obsessional Inventory
LF
   laparoscopic fundoplication
   low frequency
LFA
   left frontoanterior position
LFD
   lateral facial dysplasia
LFP
   left frontoposterior position
LFT
   lateral femoral torsion
   left frontotransverse position
LG
   limb girdle
LGA
   large for gestational age
   LGA infant
   postterm LGA
   term LGA
LGD
   low-grade dysplasia
L-GG
   Lactobacillus rhamnosus strain GG
LGS
   limb girdle syndrome
LGSIL
   low-grade squamous intraepithelial lesion
LGV
   lymphogranuloma venereum
LH
   luteinizing hormone
   LH color test
   LH surge
LHD
   lateral head displacement
Lhermitte-Duclos
   L.-D. disease
   L.-D. syndrome

Lhermitte sign
LHON
   Leber hereditary optic neuropathy
   LHON syndrome
LHR
   right lung-head circumference ratio
LH-RH
   luteinizing hormone-releasing hormone
   LH-RH agonist therapy
   LH-RH analog
L-5 hydroxytryptophan
liability to pressure palsy
liberty
   reproductive l.
libidinal change
libido
   decreased l.
Libman-Sacks
   L.-S. disease
   L.-S. endocarditis
library
   arrayed l.
   cDNA l.
   DNA l.
   gene l.
   genomic l.
   l. ligation
Librax
Librium
LICAM
   neural cell adhesion molecule L1
   LICAM gene for X-linked hydrocephalus
lice (*pl. of* louse)
Licentiate in Midwifery (LM)
lichen
   l. infantum
   l. nitidus
   l. planus
   l. ruber planus (LRP)
   l. sclerosis of vulva
   l. sclerosus
   l. sclerosus et atrophicus (LS)
   l. scrofulosorum
   l. simplex
   l. simplex chronicus (LSC)
   l. spinulosus
   l. striatus
lichenification
lichenified plaque
lichenoides
   pityriasis l.

NOTES

537

lichenoid papule
Lich-Gregoire technique
Lich vesicoureteral reflux repair technique
Liddle
    L. syndrome
    L. test
Lidemol
Lidex-E
lid lag
lidocaine
    l., adrenaline, tetracaine (LAT)
    buffered l.
    l. and epinephrine
    l., epinephrine, tetracaine (LET)
    l. infiltration
    l. and prilocaine
    l. toxicity
lidocaine-prilocaine cream
Lidodex NS
lidofilcon B
lie
    abnormal l.
    anterior l.
    fetal l.
    longitudinal l.
    oblique l.
    posterior l.
    transverse fetal l.
    unstable l.
    vertical l.
Lieberkühn
    crypts of L.
lienorenal ligament
Liesegang LM-Flex 7 flexible hysteroscope
LIFE
    longitudinal interval followup evaluation
life
    day of l. (DOL)
    l. event
    l. events checklist (LEC)
    l. events and difficulties schedule (LEDS)
    l. expectancy
    extrauterine l.
    health-related quality of l. (HRQOL)
    Incontinence quality of l. (I-QOL)
    quality of l. (QOL)
    l. stress
    l. table method
    l. table survival
    wrongful birth and l.
Lifepak
    L. AEDS
    L. defibrillator
LifePak nutritional supplement
LifeScan blood glucose meter

lifestyle factor
life-support machine
life-threatening injury
Li-Fraumeni cancer syndrome
lift
    chin l.
    parasternal l.
LIG
    leukemia inhibitory factor
Ligaclip
ligament
    acromioclavicular l.
    Adams advancement of round l.'s
    anterior cruciate l. (ACL)
    anterior talofibular l. (ATFL)
    broad l.
    calcaneocuboid l.
    calcaneofibular l. (CFL)
    Carcassonne l.
    cardinal l.
    cardinal-uterosacral l.
    congenital laxity of l.
    coracoclavicular l.
    gastrophrenic l.
    Gilliam round l.
    Gimbernat reflex l.
    infundibulopelvic l.
    inguinal l.
    IP l.
    lax l.
    leaf of broad l.
    lienorenal l.
    Mackenrodt l.
    l. of Marshall
    medial collateral l. (MCL)
    median umbilical l.
    ovarian l.
    patellar l.
    Petit l.
    phrenoesophageal l.
    posterior talofibular l. (PTFL)
    posterior uterosacral l.
    Poupart l.
    pubovesical l.
    reflex l.
    round l.
    sacrospinous l.
    subcutaneous suspensory l.
    transverse cervical l.
    l. of Treitz
    triangular l.
    ulnar collateral l.
    umbilical l.
    uteroovarian l.
    uterosacral l.
    Waldeyer preurethral l.
ligamentopexis, ligamentopexy
ligamentous
    l. ectopic pregnancy

l. injury (grade I–III)
l. laxity

ligamentum
l. pubovesicam
l. teres
l. venosum

ligand
l. binding
l. receptor

ligase
l. chain reaction (LCR)
l. chain reaction assay
l. chain reaction testing
DNA l.

ligate-divide-staple (LDS)

ligation
l. of appendix
arterial l.
bilateral tubal l. (BTL)
bleeding site l.
Doppler-guided l.
endoscopic elastic band l.
endoscopic variceal l. (EVL)
hypogastric artery l.
Irving tubal l.
Kroner tubal l.
laparoscopic tubal l. (LTL)
library l.
liver lobe l.
modified Irving-type tubal l.
Parkland tubal l.
Pomeroy tubal l.
thoracic duct l.
tubal l. (TL)
Uchida tubal l.
uterine artery l.
in utero percutaneous umbilical
  cord l.
uterosacral nerve l.

ligature
chromic gut pelviscopic loop l.
Deschamps l.

light
ambient l.
bili l.
bilirubin l.'s
broad-spectrum white l.
l. chain
double-bank bili l.'s
green l.
l. microscopy
MultArray l.

narrow-spectrum blue l.
l. perception (LP)
Questran L.
Right Light examination l.
Sabre FreeHand high-intensity
  medical pocket l.
Solar Beam medical examination l.
Speculite chemiluminescent l.
super blue l.
l. therapy
ultraviolet l.
Wood l.

light-emitting diode
lightening
LightMat surgical illuminator
lightning
l. attack
l. pain
l. seizure

LighTouch Neonate thermometer
Lightwood-Albright syndrome
Lignac syndrome
lignocaine
Likert scale
Liley
L. curve
L. three-zone chart

Lilliput neonatal oxygenator
limb
l. abnormality syndrome
l. actigraphy
l. bud
circumferential ringed creases
  of l.'s
circumferential skin crease of l.'s
l. disproportion
efferent l.
fetal l.
l. girdle (LG)
l. girdle muscular dystrophy
l. girdle muscular weakness and
  atrophy
l. girdle syndrome (LGS)
ileal l.
l. infarction
l. lead
l. length inequality
l. motion
multiple benign circumferential skin
  creases on l.'s
l. pain of childhood
phantom l.

NOTES

limb *(continued)*
    l. reduction
    l. reduction deformity (LRD)
    l. salvage
    short l.
    tripus l.
limb-body wall complex (LBWC)
Limberg flap technique
limbi (*pl. of* limbus)
limbic
    l. bands
    l. GABAergic system
    l. status epilepticus
    l. structure
Lim broth
limbus, pl. **limbi**
liminal
limit
    l. dextrans
    l. dextrinosis
    fetal dose l.
    radiation dose l.
limited
    l. neck motion
    l. support
    l. systemic scleroderma
    l. venography
limited-exposure intravenous pyelogram
limp
    antalgic l.
    gluteus medius l.
    l. infant syndrome
    psychogenic l.
    Trendelenburg l.
limulus
    l. amebocyte lysate assay
    l. lysate test
LINCL
    late infantile neural ceroid lipofuscinosis
Lincocin
lincomycin
lindane shampoo
line
    arcuate l.
    art l.
    arterial l. (A-line, art line)
    Beau l.
    black l.
    Blaschko l.
    breeding l.
    Burton gum lead l.
    canthomeatal l.
    central venous l. (CVL)
    Chamberlain l.
    CVP l.
    cytogenetic l.
    Dennie l.
    Dennie-Morgan l.
    dentate l.

    l. drawing
    Farre white l.
    genetic l.
    germ l.
    Harris growth arrest l.
    Hart l.
    hemostatic staple l.
    Hilgenreiner l.
    iliopectineal l.
    indwelling venous l. (IVL)
    intravenous l.
    Kerley B l.'s
    lambda suture l.
    Langer l.
    lead l.
    long l.
    midaxillary l.
    midclavicular l.
    milk l.'s
    multiple resistant cell l.'s
    murine myeloid leukemia cell l.
    neonatal l.
    Pastia l.
    pectinate l.
    percutaneous l.
    peripheral arterial l.
    Perkin l.
    PICC l.
    l. placement
    radial arterial l.
    radiolucent l.
    railroad track l.
    recombinant substitution l.
    sagittal suture l.
    Shenton l.
    simian l.'s
    Sydney l.
    tympanomastoid suture l.
    tympanosquamous suture l.
    umbilical l.
    umbilical artery l. (UAL)
    umbilical venous l. (UVL)
    V l.
    venous l.
linea, pl. **lineae**
    l. alba
    l. alba hernia
    lineae albicantes
    lineae atrophicae
    l. nigra
    l. semicircularis
    l. terminalis
lineage
    B-cell l.
    neural crest-derived cell l.
linear
    l. accelerator
    l. atelectasis
    l. atrophy

l. branching pattern
l. energy transfer
l. gingival erythema
l. growth
l. growth retardation
l. growth velocity
l. hyperkeratotic plaque
l. hypocalcification
l. hypoplasia
l. IgA dermatosis
l. IgA disease
l. IgM disease of pregnancy
l. in-line ligature carrier
l. Koebner reaction
l. lesion
l. nevus sebaceus syndrome
l. probe
l. salpingostomy
l. scleroderma
l. sebaceous nevus syndrome
l. skull fracture
l. verrucous epidermal nevus
l. visual analog scale

linearis
nevus sebaceus l.

linezolid
Lin-Gettig syndrome
lingua, pl. **linguae**
apex linguae
dorsum linguae
folia linguae
frenulum linguae
l. nigra
l. plicata
short frenulum linguae

lingual
l. appliance
l. frenulum
l. surface

linguistic
lingula, pl. **lingulae**
lingular effusion
linguofacialis
dysplasia l.

linitis plastica
linkage
l. analysis
complete l.
l. disequilibrium
l. equilibrium
genetic l.
l. group

l. map
partial l.
Y l.

link antibody
linogram
linoleic acid
linolenic acid
Linton tube
Lion's Claw grasper
Lioresal
liothyronine
liotrix
LIP
lipoid interstitial pneumonitis
lymphocytic interstitial pneumonitis
lymphoid interstitial pneumonitis

lip
cleft l. (CL)
l. closure
Cupid's bow upper l.
double l.
fissured l.'s
frozen smile puckered l.'s
nodular blueberry l.'s
l. phenomenon
l. pit
l. pseudocleft-hemangiomatous
branchial cyst syndrome
l. reflex
l. scar revision
vermilion border of l.

lipase
bile salt-stimulated l. (BSSL)
lipoprotein l. (LPL)
l. unit

lipemia
lipid
l. accumulation
l. cell
l. cell neoplasm
l. cell ovarian tumor
l. envelope
l. inclusion
l. metabolism
l. metabolism disorder
myelin l.
l. myopathy
l. peroxidation
l. peroxide
l. storage disease
l. storage disorder

lipid-associated sialic acid

NOTES

L

541

lipid-laden macrophage
lipidosis, pl. **lipidoses**
    cerebroside l.
    familial neurovisceral l.
    galactosylsphinogosine l.
    juvenile dystonic l.
    late infantile systemic l.
    neurovisceral l.
    psychosine l.
Lipidox
lipiduria
Lipiodol
Lipisorb
lipoatrophic diabetes
lipoatrophy
    human insulin-induced l.
    insulin l.
    localized l.
lipoblastoma
    primitive l.
lipochondrodystrophy
lipodystrophy
    congenital generalized l.
    familial l.
    generalized l.
    partial l.
    protease inhibitor-induced l.
**lipodystrophy-acromegaloid gigantism
  syndrome**
lipofuscin material
lipofuscinosis
    ceroid l.
    Haltia-Santavuori neural ceroid l.
    hypoadrenalism neural ceroid l.
    Jansky-Bielschowsky neural
      ceroid l.
    late infantile neural ceroid l.
      (LINCL)
    neural ceroid l.
    neuronal ceroid l. (CLN, NCL)
    Spielmeyer-Vogt neural ceroid l.
lipogenic dyshepatia
lipoglycan antigen
lipogranulomatosis
    Farber l.
    l. subcutanea
lipohypertrophy
lipoic acid
lipoid
    l. adrenal gland hypoplasia
    l. adrenal hyperplasia
    l. interstitial pneumonitis (LIP)
    l. ovarian neoplasm
    l. ovarian tumor
    l. pneumonia
    l. proteinosis
lipoidica
    necrobiosis l.

lipolysis
lipoma, pl. **lipomata**
    cord l.
    lumbosacral l.
    vulvar l.
lipomatosis
    encephalocraniocutaneous l. (ECCL)
    familial multiple l.
lipomeningocele
Lipomul
lipomyelomeningocele
    skin-covered l.
liponecrosis microcystica calcificans
lipooligosaccharide (LOS)
lipophilic fungus
lipoplasty
    suction-assisted l. (SAL)
lipopolysaccharide (LPS)
    l. coat
    l. endotoxin
    Shiga l.
lipoprotein
    l. concentration
    high-density l. (HDL)
    l. lipase (LPL)
    low-density l. (LDL)
    l. receptor-related protein (LRP)
    very low density l. (VLDL)
lipoprotein(a) (Lp(a))
lipoprotein-cholesterol metabolism
liposarcoma
    myxoid l.
liposomal amphotericin B
Liposyn
    L. formula
    L. II
lipotropin
    beta-l.
    mu-l.
5-lipoxygenase
lip-palate syndrome
Lippes loop
Lippes-type intrauterine device
lipreading
Lipschütz ulcer
liquefaction
    semen l.
liquefactive necrosis
Liquibid
Liqui-Char
liquid
    chylous l.
    End Lice L.
    l. feeding
    fetal lung l.
    Gordofilm L.
    Lotrimin AF Spray L.
    l. nitrogen
    Occlusal-HP L.

perfluorochemical l.
l. petrolatum
Pyrinyl II L.
Rid l.
Ryna L.
Sklar Kleen l.
Tisit L.
Titralac Plus L.
Triple X L.
l. ventilation (LV)
X-Prep L.
liquid-assisted high-frequency oscillatory ventilation (LA-HFOV)
liquified powder cocaine
Liquifilm
HMS L.
Poly-Pred L.
Liqui-Gel
Liquiprin
LiquiVent
liquor
l. amnii
l. carbonis detergens
l. carbonis detergens ointment
l. cerebrospinalis
l. cotunii
l. entericus
l. folliculi
meconium staining of l.
LIS1 gene for lissencephaly
Lisch nodule
lisinopril
Lison syndrome
lisp
lispro
insulin l.
Lissauer tract
lissencephaly
classical l.
hydrocephalic l.
ILS17 gene for isolated l.
ILSX gene for X-linked l.
LIS1 gene for l.
l. (type I, II)
list
Amsterdam Depression L. (ADL)
Interpersonal Support Evaluation L.
national recipient waiting l.
listening
dichotic l.
Listeria
L. meningitis

L. monocytogenes
L. monocytogenes sepsis
listeriosis
congenital l.
neonatal l.
Lister scissors
listless
listlessness
litem
guardian ad l.
liter (L)
milliequivalent per l. (mEq/L)
l.'s per minute (L/min)
lithiasis
biliary l.
uric acid l.
lithium
l. carbonate
l. citrate
l. resistance
Lithobid
lithokelyphopedion, lithokelyphopedium
lithopedion, lithopedium
lithotomy
marian l.
l. position
vaginal l.
Little
L. area
L. disease
L. League elbow
L. League shoulder
Littmann ECG electrode
Littre gland
Litzmann obliquity
Livaditis circular myotomy
live
l. attenuated
l. poliovirus vaccine
live-attenuated
l.-a. virus
l.-a. virus vaccine
livebirth, live birth, live birth
liveborn infant
livedo reticularis
liver
acute fatty l.
l. biopsy
l. bud
l. cirrhosis
cirrhosis of l.
cut-down l.

L

NOTES

liver *(continued)*
    l. disease
    enlarged l.
    fatty l.
    fetal l.
    l. flap
    l. function tests
    l. infiltrate
    l. lobe ligation
    l. lobe resection
    l. metastasis
    l. parenchyma
    l. phosphorylase deficiency
    shock l.
    l. span
    l. steatosis
    l. transplant
    l. transplantation
    l. tumor
Livernois-McDonald forceps
live-virus vaccine
lividity
    postmortem l.
living
    activities of daily l. (ADL)
    l. children (LC)
Livostin
LJP
    localized juvenile periodontitis
LKS
    Landau-Kleffner syndrome
LLD
    leg length discrepancy
LLDP
    left lateral decubitus position
LLETZ
    large loop excision of transformation zone
LLETZ-LEEP active loop electrode
l-loop
Llorente dissecting forceps
Lloyd-Davies stirrups
Lloyd-Still index
LLPDD
    late luteal phase dysphoric disorder
LLQ
    left lower quadrant
LM
    Licentiate in Midwifery
LMA
    laryngeal mask airway
    left mentoanterior position
LMB
    Laurence-Moon-Biedl
    LMB syndrome
LMBB
    Laurence-Moon-Biedl-Bardet
LMBBS
    Laurence-Moon-Biedl-Bardet syndrome

L/min
    liters per minute
LMP
    last menstrual period
    left mentoposterior position
    low malignant potential
LMS
    leiomyosarcoma
LMT
    left mentotransverse position
LMW
    low molecular weight
    LMW dextran
    LMW proteinuria
LMWD
    low molecular weight dextran
LMWH
    low molecular weight heparin
LNMP
    last normal menstrual period
LNS
    Lesch-Nyhan syndrome
LOA
    left occipitoanterior position
load
    axial l.
    plasma viral l.
    potential renal solute l. (PRSL)
    pressure l.
    renal solute l. (RSL)
    task l.
    viral l.
    volume l.
loading
    familial l.
lobar
    l. consolidation
    l. emphysema
    l. holoprosencephaly
    l. panniculitis
    l. pneumonia
    l. sclerosis
lobe
    hepatic l.
    mesial temporal l.
    quadrate hepatic l.
    Riedel l.
    sequestered l.
    temporal l.
lobectomy
    fetal l.
Lobstein
    L. disease
    L. syndrome
lobster-claw
    l.-c. deformity
    l.-c. hand
    l.-c. with ectodermal defects syndrome

lobular
- l. architecture
- l. capillary hemangioma
- l. carcinoma
- l. carcinoma in situ
- l. distortion
- l. neoplasia

lobulation defect
lobulation-polydactyly syndrome
lobule
- placental l.
- sebaceous gland l.
- tense l.

LOC
- level of consciousness

local
- l. anesthesia
- l. anesthetic
- l. education agency (LEA)
- l. excision
- l. inflammatory response
- l. irradiation
- l. lesion
- l. methotrexate injection
- l. ovarian condition
- l. seizure
- l. treatment

localization
- epithelial autoantibody l.
- estrogen receptor l.
- needle l.
- placental l.

localization-related epilepsy seizure
localize
localized
- l. albinism
- l. cutaneous leishmaniasis (LCL)
- l. juvenile periodontitis (LJP)
- l. lipoatrophy
- l. pachygyria
- l. peritonitis
- l. scleroderma
- l. vulvar pemphigoid of childhood (LVPC)

localizing sign
location
- breech l.
- extraembryonic l.
- gene l.
- noncornual placental l.
- placental l.

lochia
- l. alba
- l. cruenta
- l. purulenta
- l. rubra
- l. sanguinolenta
- l. serosa

lochial
lochiometra
lochiometritis
lochioperitonitis
lochiorrhagia
lochiorrhea
loci (*pl. of* locus)
lock
- English l.
- French l.
- German l.
- heparin l. (hep lock)
- pivot l.
- sliding l.

locked
- l. facet
- l. twins

Locke solution
Locke-Wallace Marital Adjustment test
locking twins
lockjaw
Locoid Topical
locomotion
locomotor
locoregional node
loculate
locus, pl. **loci**
- l. caeruleus
- L. of Control Scale
- gene l.
- genetic l.
- GUSB l.
- l. heterogeneity
- operator l.
- quantitative trait l. (QTL)

locus-specific probe
locutionary stage
LOD
- logarithm of odds
- LOD score

lodoxamide tromethamine
Loeb deciduoma
Loehlein diameter
Loestrin
- L. 1.5/30

NOTES

Loestrin *(continued)*
    L. 21 1/20
    L. Fe
Löffler syndrome
Löfgren syndrome
Lofstrand crutches
Log-a-Rhythm Signal Acquisition unit
logarithm of odds (LOD)
logroll maneuver
LOH
    loss of heterogeneity
**Lohman-Brozek body fat percentage
    formula**
lollipop
    fentanyl l.
    Oralet l.
lomefloxacin
Lomotil
lomustine
Lonalac formula
Lone
    L. Star retractor system
    L. Star tick
loneliness
long
    l. arm of chromosome (q)
    l. arm of Y chromosome
    l. atraumatic retractor
    l. axis
    l. bone
    l. bone length
    l. course
    l. leg cast
    l. leg sitting
    l. line
    l.- and medium-chain acyl-CoA
      dehydrogenase (LCAD/MCAD)
    l. Q-T syndrome (LQTS)
    l. thin extremity
    l.- and very-long-chain acyl-CoA
      dehydrogenase (LCAD/VLCAD)
    l. weighted speculum
long-acting (LA)
    l.-a. contraception
    l.-a. contraceptive
    l.-a. contraceptive steroid
    Sinex L.-a.
    l.-a. thyroid stimulator (LATS)
long-axis view
long-chain
    l.-c. acyl-CoA dehydrogenase
      (LCAD)
    l.-c. fatty acid
    l.-c. 3-hydroxyacyl-CoA
      dehydrogenase (LCHAD)
    l.-c. hydroxyacyl-coenzyme A
      dehydrogenase (LCHAD)
    l.-c. polyunsaturated fatty acid
      (LCPUFA)

longitudinal
    l. deficiency
    l. dense striation
    l. growth
    l. interval followup evaluation
      (LIFE)
    l. lie
    l. oval pelvis
    l. presentation
    l. proton MR spectroscopy
    l. scan
    l. study
long-segment
    l.-s. aganglionosis
    l.-s. congenital tracheal stenosis
      (LSCTS)
long-term
    l.-t. followup
    l.-t. sequelae
    l.-t. survival
long-tract sign
longum
    Bifidobacterium l.
Loniten Oral
Lonox
look
    anxious l.
loop
    bipolar cutting l.
    bipolar urological l.
    capillary end l.
    cine l.
    cutting l.
    l. diathermy cervical conization
    dilated intestinal l.
    l. diuretic
    l. diversion
    dropout of capillary end l.
    l. electrode
    l. electrosurgical excision procedure
      (LEEP)
    l. excision of the transformation
      zone (LETZ)
    flow-volume l.
    free-floating l.
    l. of Henle
    ileal l.
    Lippes l.
    low-voltage diathermy l.
    Medevice surgical l.
    obstructed bowel l.
    physiologic endometrial
      ablation/resection l. (PEARL)
    polysomnogram with flow-volume l.
    Schroeder tenaculum l.
    sentinel l.
    somatic nervous system feedback l.
    tenaculum hook l.
    vaginal speculum l.

looping
    cardiac l.
loose body
Loosett maneuver
Lo/Ovral contraceptive pill
LOP
    left occipitoposterior position
lop ear
loperamide hydrochloride
lophosphamide
Lopressor
Loprox
Lorabid
loracarbef
Lorain-Lévi
    L.-L. dwarfism
    L.-L. infantilism
    L.-L. syndrome
loratadine
lorazepam
Lorber criteria
Lorcet
    L. 10/650
    L. Plus
Lorcet-HD
lordosis
    lumbar l.
lordotic
    l. deformity
    l. gait
Lorenz night splint
Lorenzo's
    L. oil
    L. oil diet
Loroxide
Lortab
    L. 2.5/500
    L. 5/500
    L. 10/500
    L. Elixir
LOS
    lipooligosaccharide
Los Angeles variant galactosemia
Losec
losoxantrone
loss
    acute interpersonal l.
    autosomal dominant nonsyndromic
      hearing l. (DFNA3)
    autosomal recessive nonsyndromic
      hearing l. (DFNB1)
    average blood l.

    blood l.
    bone l.
    conductive hearing l.
    congenital hearing l.
    l. of consciousness
    consecutive l.
    l. of correction
    covert l.
    dialysate protein l.
    early embryonic l.
    early pregnancy l.
    electrolyte l.
    embryonic l.
    estrogen l.
    excessive blood l.
    fecal water l.
    fetal l.
    gastrointestinal l.
    hair l.
    hearing l.
    heat l.
    l. of heterogeneity (LOH)
    high-frequency hearing l.
    high-tone hearing l.
    hysterical visual l.
    insensible fluid l.
    insensible water l. (IWL)
    menstrual blood l.
    mixed hearing l.
    nephron l.
    normal blood l.
    overt l.
    perioral tissue l.
    permanent hearing l. (PHL)
    postmenopausal bone l.
    pregnancy l.
    protein l.
    range l.
    rapid bone l.
    recurrent pregnancy l.
    renal l.
    repeated pregnancy l. (RPL)
    repetitive pregnancy l.
    RP with progressive sensorineural
      hearing l.
    sensorineural hearing l. (SNHL)
    sensory l.
    spinal bone l.
    status l.
    stocking-glove sensory l.
    stool l.
    surgical weight l.

L

NOTES

loss *(continued)*
    third space l.
    tissue l.
    tooth l.
    transepidermal water l. (TEWL)
    vertebral bone l.
    visual l.
    water l.
    weight l.
Lossen rule
loss-of-resistance technique
Lostorfer body
lost surgical specimen
LOT
    left occipitotransverse position
lotion
    calamine l.
    Ovide l.
    Polysonic ultrasound l.
    Sarna l.
    thiosulfate l.
    Total Eclipse moisturizing skin l.
Lotrimin
    L. AF Spray Liquid
    L. AF Spray Powder
    L. Topical
Lotronex
LOU
    lower obstructive uropathy
    fetal LOU
loudness
Lou Gehrig disease
Louis-Bar syndrome
loupe
    Keeler l.
    l. magnification
louse, pl. **lice**
    body l.
    crab l.
    head l.
    l. infestation
    pubic lice
louse-borne
    l.-b. fever
    l.-b. typhus
Lovaas
    L. method
    L. program
    L. training
LOVE
    laser office ventilation of ears
LOVE IT
    laser office ventilation of ears with
    insertion of tubes
Lovenox
Lovset maneuver
low
    l. birth weight (LBW)
    l. birth weight infant (LBWI)

    l. birth weight-maternal employment
    study (LBW-MES)
    l. blood sugar
    l. cardiac output syndrome
    l. cervical cesarean
    l. forceps
    l. forceps delivery
    l. frequency (LF)
    l. imperforate anus
    l. malignant potential (LMP)
    l. molecular weight (LMW)
    l. molecular weight dextran
    (LMWD)
    l. molecular weight heparin
    (LMWH)
    l. muscle tone
    l. nasal bridge
    l. occipital hairline
    l. output
    l. power field (lpf)
    l. pressure bladder
    l. rectal resection
    l. sensory threshold
    l. steroid content combined oral
    contraceptive
    l. transverse cesarean (LTC)
    l. transverse hysterotomy
    l. transverse uterine incision
    l. T3 syndrome
    l. vertical uterine incision
    l. vision
low-back pain
low-branched-chain amino acid diet
low-cholesterol diet
low-density lipoprotein (LDL)
low-dose
    l.-d. danazol
    l.-d. heparin
    l.-d. involved-field irradiation
    l.-d. oral contraceptive
    l.-d. splenic irradiation
    l.-d. steroids
Lowe
    fetal oculocerebrorenal syndrome
    of L.
    oculocerebrorenal disease of L.
    oculocerebrorenal syndrome of L.
    L. oculocerebrorenal syndrome
    L. syndrome (LS)
Löwenstein-Jensen medium
lower
    l. abdominal pain
    l. abdominal tenderness
    l. airway disease
    L. Anchorages and Tethers for
    children (LATCH)
    l. collecting system
    l. esophageal sphincter (LES)
    l. esophageal transection

l. extremity (LE)
l. genital tract
l. genital tract infection
l. limb ossification center
l. lip paralysis
l. motor neuron palsy
l. obstructive uropathy (LOU)
l. respiratory illness (LRI)
l. respiratory infection (LRI)
l. respiratory tract
l. respiratory tract disorder
l. respiratory tract infection (LRTI)
l. segment cesarean (LSCS)
l. segment scar
l. segment transverse cesarean section (LSTCS)
l. segment vertical cesarean section (LSVCS)
l. triceps skinfold Z score
l. urinary tract infection
l. uterine segment
l. uterine segment fibroid
l. uterine segment transverse (LUST)
Lowe-Terry-MacLachlan syndrome
low-fat diet
low-flow
l.-f. cardiopulmonary bypass
l.-f. sidestream capnography
low-grade
l.-g. B-cell lymphoma
l.-g. diffuse astrocytoma
l.-g. dysplasia (LGD)
l.-g. fibrillary astrocytoma
l.-g. mosaicism
l.-g. positive smear
l.-g. squamous intraepithelial lesion (LGSIL, LSIL)
Lowila soap
low-lying previa
Lown-Ganong-Levine syndrome
Low-Ogestrel-21, -28
low-phenylalanine diet
low-pressure
l.-p. breast pump
l.-p. urethra
low-protein diet
Low-Quel
low-residue diet
low-resolution banding
Lowry-Maclean syndrome

Lowry syndrome
Lowry-Wood syndrome (LWS)
low-salt diet
low-segment transverse incision
low-set ears
low-sodium
l.-s. diet
l.-s. syndrome
low-vision aid
low-voltage
l.-v. diathermy loop
l.-v. electrocortical activity (LV ECoG, LVECoG)
loxapine
Loxitane
lozenge
benzocaine l.
Cough-X l.
Suppress l.'s
Lozol
LP
light perception
lumbar puncture
Lp(a)
lipoprotein(a)
L-PAM
L-phenylalanine mustard
LPCV
laser photocoagulation of the communicating vessels
LPD
leiomyomatosis peritonealis disseminata
luteal phase defect
lpf
low power field
LPL
lipoprotein lipase
LPL deficiency
LPS
lipopolysaccharide
LPSS
laryngopharyngeal sensory stimulation
LPSS testing
LQTS
long Q-T syndrome
LR
lateral rotation
L-R
left to right
LRD
limb reduction deformity

NOTES

L

549

LRE
least restrictive environment
LRI
lower respiratory illness
lower respiratory infection
LRP
lichen ruber planus
lipoprotein receptor-related protein
LRTI
lower respiratory tract infection
LS
lichen sclerosus et atrophicus
Lowe syndrome
L/S
lecithin-sphingomyelin ratio
LSA
left sacroanterior position
LSC
lichen simplex chronicus
LScA
left scapuloanterior position
LScP
left scapuloposterior position
LSCS
lower segment cesarean
LSCTS
long-segment congenital tracheal stenosis
LSD
lysergic acid diethylamide
LSH
laparoscopic supracervical hysterectomy
lutein-stimulating hormone
L-shaped cautery
LSIL
low-grade squamous intraepithelial lesion
LSIL Pap smear
LSO
lumbosacral orthosis
LSP
left sacroposterior position
L/S ratio
LSS
lexical-syntactic syndrome
LST
left sacrotransverse position
LSTCS
lower segment transverse cesarean
section
LSVCS
lower segment vertical cesarean section
LTC
low transverse cesarean
LTC$_4$
leukotriene C$_4$
LTD$_4$
leukotriene D$_4$
LTE$_4$
leukotriene E$_4$

L-TGA
L-transposition of great arteries
L-thyroxine
L-t. therapy
LTL
laparoscopic tubal ligation
LTM
lean tissue mass
LTRA
leukotriene receptor antagonist
L-transposition
levotransposition
L-transposition of great arteries (L-TGA)
LTS
laryngotracheal stenosis
LTT
lateral tibial torsion
Lubchenco nomogram
lube
Sklar l.
Lübke uterine vacuum cannula
lubricant
Astroglide personal l.
Maxilube personal l.
ocular l.
Replens l.
vaginal l.
lubrication
vaginal l.
Lubri-Flex stent
Lub syndrome
Lucarelli bone marrow transplant risk group
lucency
white matter l.
lucent band
Lucey-Driscoll syndrome
lucida
lamina l.
luciferase assay
lucinactant
Lucite
L. dilator
L. form
Lückenschadel
Ludiomil
Ludorum
Ludwig angina
Luekens trap
Luer
L. lock site
L. Lok syringe
L. retractor
lues ascites
luetic
LUFS
luteinized unruptured follicle syndrome
Luft disease

Lugol
  L. iodine solution
  L. iodine stain
Luikart forceps
Luikart-Simpson forceps
Lujan-Fryns syndrome
luliberin
Lumadex-FSI test
lumbar
  l. artery
  l. curve
  l. epidural anesthesia
  l. extensor muscle
  l. gibbus
  l. lordosis
  l. meningocele
  l. puncture (LP)
  l. puncture manometry
  l. theca
lumboperitoneal shunt
lumbosacral
  l. agenesis
  l. dimple
  l. junction
  l. lipoma
  l. meningomyelocele
  l. neurofibroma
  l. orthosis (LSO)
  l. plexus injury
  l. plexus lesion
  l. root lesion
  l. sinus
  l. skin pigment change
  l. tuft of hair
lumbricoides
  Ascaris l.
lumen, pl. **lumina, lumens**
  appendiceal l.
  decidual l.
  l. dilation
  urethral l.
Lumex PT fiberoptic cystometry system
luminal epithelium
Lumopaque
lump
lumpectomy
lumpy jaw
LUNA
  laser uterosacral nerve ablation
Luna-Parker acid fuscin stain
Lunar DPX dual-energy absorptiometer

lunata
  Curvularia l.
Lund and Browder chart for burn assessment
Lundh test
Lunelle
lung
  l. abscess
  l. aeration
  agenesis of l.
  azygos lobe of l.
  bubbly l.'s
  l. cancer
  l. capacity (CL)
  l. carcinoma
  l. compliance (CL)
  l. consolidation
  cystic adenomatoid malformation of l.
  l. edema
  farmer's l.
  l. fluke
  granular l.
  l. growth and development
  hazy l.
  l. hernia
  honeycomb l.
  hyperlucent l.
  hypoplasia of l.
  hypoplastic l.
  idiopathic diffuse interstitial fibrosis of l.
  l. infiltrate
  junky l.
  Kolobow membrane l.
  lymphangiomyomatosis of l.
  malt worker's l.
  l. morphogenesis
  l. overdistention
  paraquat l.
  premature l.
  l. profile
  l. recruitment
  SciMed-Kolobow membrane l.
  sequestered l.
  shock l.
  SP-A of l.'s
  SP-B of l.'s
  SP-C of l.'s
  l. strip
  surfactant-deficient l.
  l. surgery

L

NOTES

lung *(continued)*
    l. tap
    l. transplantation
    unilateral hyperlucent l.
    l. volume
Lupron
    L. add-back therapy
    L. Depot
    L. Depot-3 Month
    L. Depot-4 Month
    L. Depot-Ped
lupus
    ANA-negative l.
    l. angiitis
    l. anticoagulant (LAC)
    l. anticoagulant activity
    l. anticoagulant antibody
    l. anticoagulant syndrome
    l. cerebritis
    l. crisis
    discoid l.
    l. erythematosus (LE)
    l. erythematosus disseminatus
    l. erythematosus profundus
    gestational l.
    l. inhibitor
    l. miliaris disseminatum faciei
    neonatal l.
    l. nephritis
    l. obstetric syndrome
    l. pernio
    l. vulgaris
lupus-like syndrome
LUQ
    left upper quadrant
lurch
    abductor l.
Luride
Lurline PMS
Luschka
    foramen of L.
Lusk instrument
LUSLR
    laparoscopic ureterosacral ligament
    resection
LUST
    lower uterine segment transverse
        LUST cesarean section
        LUST C-section
lutea
    corpora l.
    macula l.
luteal
    l. cell
    l. function
    l. ovarian cyst
    l. phase
    l. phase defect (LPD)
    l. phase deficiency

    l. phase inadequacy
    l. phase support
luteectomy
luteinalis
    hyperreactio l.
lutein cell
luteinization
    l. inhibition
    l. inhibitor
    l. stimulator
luteinized
    l. thecoma
    l. unruptured follicle
    l. unruptured follicle syndrome
      (LUFS)
luteinizing
    l. hormone (LH)
    l. hormone receptor-binding
      inhibitor
    l. hormone-releasing hormone (LH-
      RH)
    l. hormone secretion
luteinoma
lutein-stimulating hormone (LSH)
Lutembacher syndrome
luteolysis
luteolytic action
luteoma
    pregnancy l.
    l. of pregnancy
    stromal l.
luteoplacental shift
luteotropic hormone
luteum
    corpus l.
    ruptured corpus l.
Lutheran blood group
Lutrepulse
Lutz-Jeanselme nodule
Lutz-Splendore-Almeida blastomycosis
luxation
    dental extrusion/lateral l.
    extrusion/lateral l.
    extrusive l.
    intrusive l.
    lateral l.
    rotary atlantoaxial l.
luxury perfusion
LV
    left ventricle
    left ventricular
    liquid ventilation
      LV afterload
      LV contractility
      LV dysfunction
      LV preload
LVAD
    left ventricular assist device
L-valine ester

LVD
left ventricular dysfunction
LV ECoG
low-voltage electrocortical activity
LVECoG
low-voltage electrocortical activity
LVEF
left ventricular ejection fraction
LVFA
LVH
left ventricular hypertrophy
LVN
LVOT
left ventricular outflow tract
LVOTO
left ventricular outflow tract obstruction
LVPC
localized vulvar pemphigoid of childhood
LVSI
lymphovascular space invasion
LVSWI
left ventricular stroke work index
lwoffi
Achromobacter l.
Acinetobacter l.
LWS
Lowry-Wood syndrome
lyase
Lyderm
Lyell
L. disease
L. syndrome
Lyer
side L.
Lyme
L. arthritis
L. disease
L. disease vaccine
L. ELISA
L. meningitis
L. neuroborreliosis
L. radiculoneuritis
Lyme-associated peripheral facial nerve palsy
lymph
l. node
l. node biopsy
l. node drainage
l. node endometriotic adenoacanthoma
l. node enlargement
l. node involvement

l. node metastasis
l. node positivity
lymphadenectomy
inguinal l.
laparoscopic l.
Meigs pelvic l.
paraaortic l.
pelvic l.
retroperitoneal l.
lymphadenitis
cervical l.
chronic pyogenic l.
granulomatous l.
histocytic necrotizing l.
inguinal l.
Kiuchi histocytic necrotizing l.
mediastinal l.
mesenteric l.
necrotizing granulomatous l.
periauricular l.
pyogenic l.
recurrent pyogenic l.
regional l.
submental l.
suppurative l.
tuberculous cervical l.
lymphadenopathy
acute suppurative cervical l.
l.-associated virus (LAV)
axillary l.
cervical l.
diffuse nonmalignant l.
hilar l.
mediastinal l.
shotty cervical l.
submental l.
Toxoplasma l.
lymphangiectasia, lymphangiectasis
congenital pulmonary l.
pulmonary l.
lymphangiography
bipedal l.
lymphangioma
alveolar l.
cavernous l.
l. circumscriptum
cystic l.
l. cysticum
lymphangiomatosis
lymphangiomyomatosis of lung
lymphangiosarcoma
lymphangitis

L

NOTES

lymphatic
- l. drainage
- l. drainage of genitalia
- l. dysplasia
- l. leukemia
- l. obstruction
- paracervical l.'s
- l. spread
- l. system

lymphedema
- congenital extremity l.
- extremity l.
- hereditary l.
- intrauterine l.
- l. praecox
- primary l.
- secondary l.
- l. tarda

lymphoblastic
- l. leukemia
- l. lymphoma

lymphoblastoid
- l. cell
- l. interferon

lymphocyst
- l. omentum
- pelvic l.

lymphocytapheresis
lymphocyte
- l. activator
- B l.
- cytotoxic T l. (CTL)
- l. depleted
- l. dysfunction
- l. function-associated antigen 1
- l. immune globulin
- natural killer l.
- peripheral blood l. (PBL)
- polymorphonuclear l.
- l. predominant
- T l.
- T1–T10 l.

lymphocyte-activating factor
lymphocyte-depleted Hodgkin disease
lymphocyte-predominant Hodgkin disease
lymphocytic
- l. adenohypophysitis
- l. choriomeningitis
- l. choriomeningitis virus (LCMV)
- l. gastritis
- l. hypophysitis
- l. interstitial pneumonitis (LIP)
- l. leukemia
- l. meningitis
- l. meningoradiculoneuritis
- l. myocarditis
- l. pleocytosis
- l. thyroiditis
- l. vasculitis

lymphocytosis
- infectious l.

lymphogranuloma
- l. inguinale
- venereal l.
- l. venereum (LGV)

lymphography
lymphohematogenous disease
lymphohistiocytic infiltration
lymphohistiocytosis
- erythrophagocytic l.
- familial erythrophagocytic l. (FEL)
- familial hemophagocytic l. (FHLH)
- hemophagocytic l.

lymphoid
- l. cell
- l. hyperplasia
- l. interstitial pneumonitis (LIP)
- l. tissue

lymphokine
lymphokine-activated killer cell (LAK)
lymphoma
- African Burkitt l.
- AIDS-related l.
- American Burkitt l.
- anaplastic large cell l.
- B-cell l.
- Burkitt l. (BL)
- central nervous system l.
- colonic B-cell l.
- diffuse small cell cleaved l.
- EBV-related B-cell l.
- endemic Burkitt l.
- extranodal marginal zone B-cell l.
- histiocytic l.
- Hodgkin l.
- immunoblastic l.
- intraocular l.
- large B-cell l.
- large cell anaplastic Ki-1 l.
- large cell immunoblastic l.
- low-grade B-cell l.
- lymphoblastic l.
- malignant l.
- Mediterranean l.
- metastatic l.
- non-Hodgkin l. (NHL)
- ovarian l.
- primary central nervous system l. (PCNSL)
- recurrent l.
- retroorbital l.
- small cell cleaved l.
- small noncleaved cell l. (SNCCL)
- sporadic Burkitt l.
- T-cell l.
- true histiocytic l. (THL)

lymphomatous infiltration

lymphonodular
- l. hyperplasia
- l. pharyngitis

lymphopenia

lymphoplasmacytic
- l. colitis
- l. infiltration
- l. inflammation

lymphopoietic differentiation

lymphoproliferative
- l. disease
- l. disorder
- l. process
- l. syndrome

lymphoproliferative/myeloproliferative disease

lymphoreticular
- l. malignancy
- l. neoplasia
- l. system

lymphoreticulosis

lymphorrhage

lymphosarcoma cell leukemia

lymphotoxin antitumor activity

lymphovascular
- l. space
- l. space invasion (LVSI)
- l. space involvement

Lynch
- L. and Crues type 2 lesion
- L. syndrome

lynestrenol

lyn protooncogene

Lyodura sling procedure

Lyon hypothesis

lyonization

lyophilize

lyosomal

Lyphocin

lypressin

lysate
- cell l.
- endothelial cell l.

lysergic
- l. acid
- l. acid diethylamide (LSD)

lysine
- l. malabsorption syndrome
- l. 6-oxidase

lysinuric protein intolerance

lysis
- l. of adhesion
- l. test

Lysodren

lysome
- hepatocellular l.

lysoPC diagnostic ovarian cancer test

lysosomal
- l. enzyme disorder
- l. hydrolase enzyme assay
- l. metabolite
- l. storage disease
- l. storage disorder

lysosome

lysozyme

lyssa body

lysyl bradykinin

lytic
- l. cocktail
- l. infection
- l. lesion

Lytren formula

L

NOTES

M
　　M antigen
　　M protein factor
M2 inhibitor
MA
　　metatarsus adductus
mA
　　milliampere
MAA
　　microphthalmia or anophthalmos with
　　　associated anomalies
Maalox
　　M. Anti-Gas
MAAP
　　multiple arbitrary amplicon profiling
MAb
　　monoclonal antibody
　　　enhanced-potency MAb
　　　OvaRex MAb
MABP
　　mean arterial blood pressure
MAC
　　midarm circumference
　　Mycobacterium avium complex
　　Mycobacterium avium-intracellulare
　　　complex
MacArthur
　　M. Longitudinal Twin Study
　　M. Story Stem Battery (MSSB)
MacCallum patch
MacConkey II agar
MacDermot-Winter syndrome
MACDP
　　Metropolitan Atlanta Congenital Defects
　　Program
Macer abdominal cystocele repair
macerate
macerated fetus
maceration
　　fetal m.
Macewen sign
Machado-Joseph
　　M.-J. ataxia
　　M.-J. disease
Mach band effect
Macherey-Nagel strep test
machine
　　Acuson Model 128XP m.
　　Berkeley suction m.
　　BiPAP m.
　　cobalt megavoltage m.
　　CPAP m.
　　life-support m.
　　Mayo-Gibbon heart-lung m.
　　megavoltage m.

machinery
　　m. murmur
　　m. murmur in patent ductus
　　　arteriosus
Machupo virus
MacIntosh
　　English M. (E-Mac)
Mackenrodt ligament
MacLean
Macleod syndrome
macrencephaly, macrencephalia
macroadenoma
　　prolactin-secreting m.
macrobead
　　methyltestosterone m.
Macrobid
macroblepharon
macrocalcification
　　breast m.
macrocardius
macrocarpon
　　Vaccinium m.
macrocephaly
　　benign familial m. (BFM)
　　m., cutis marmorata, telangiectatica
　　　congenita syndrome
　　m., facial abnormalities,
　　　disproportionate tall stature,
　　　mental retardation syndrome
　　familial m.
　　m., hypertelorism, short limbs,
　　　hearing loss, developmental delay
　　　syndrome
　　m., multiple lipomas, hemangiomata
　　　syndrome
　　m., pseudoepithelioma, multiple
　　　hemangiomas syndrome
　　m. with feeblemindedness and
　　　encephalopathy with peculiar
　　　deposits
macrocephaly-hamartomas syndrome
macrocirculatory
macrocrania
macrocrystal
　　monohydrate m.
　　nitrofurantoin monohydrate m.
macrocytic
　　m. anemia of pregnancy
　　m. megaloblastic anemia
macrocytosis
macrodactyly
　　primary m.
　　secondary m.
Macrodantin
Macrodex

M

macrodontia
macroevolution
macrogamete
macrogenitosomia praecox
macroglobinemia
    Waldenström m.
macroglobulin
    alpha-2 m.
macroglossia
    relative m.
    true m.
macroglossia-omphalocele syndrome
macroglossia-omphalocele-visceromegaly
  syndrome
macrognathia
macrogyria
macrolecithal
macrolide therapy
macromastia, macromazia
macromelus
macromineral
macromolecular damage
macronodular cirrhosis
macronutrient balance
macroorchidism-marker X (MOMX)
macrophage
    m. activation syndrome (MAS)
    m. colony-stimulating factor
    hemosiderin laden m.
    m. inflammatory protein (MIP)
    m. inflammatory protein-1 alpha
      (MIP-1 alpha)
    lipid-laden m.
    peritoneal m.
    m. tropic
macrophage-activating factor (MAF)
macrophage-inhibition factor
macrophage-targeted glucocerebrosidase
macrophage-tropic strain
macrophallus
Macroplastique implantable device
macroprolactinoma
macrorestriction map
macroscopic hematuria
macrosomia
    m. adiposa congenita
    fetal m.
    neonatal m.
    m., obesity, macrocephaly, ocular
      abnormality (MOMO)
macrosomia-mental retardation syndrome
macrosomic infant
macrostomia
macrothrombocytopenia
macrovascular
MACS
    magnetically activated cell sorter
    Multicenter AIDS Cohort Study
macula, pl. maculae

    m. cerulea
    m. communis
    m. corneae
    m. cribosa
    m. flava
    m. gonorrhoica
    m. lutea
    m. pellucida
    m. of retina
    m. retinae
macular
    m. atrophy
    m. cherry-red spot
    m. dystrophy
    m. hemangioma
    m. light reflex
    m. pseudocoloboma
    m. rash
    m. stain
    m. star formation
macular-papular-vesicular lesion
macule
    ash-leaf m.
    blanching m.
    bluish-black m.
    cherry-red m.
    crop of m.'s
    erythematous m.
    hypopigmented m.
maculopapular
    m. eruption
    m. exanthem
    m. lesion
    m. nodosa
    m. rash
maculosus
    dystrophia bullosa hereditaria,
      typus m.
MadaJet XL needle-free injector
madarosis
mad cow disease
MADD
    Mothers Against Drunk Driving
    multiple acyl-coenzyme A dehydrogenase
      deficiency
Maddacrawler walker
Madelung deformity
Madlener operation
Madonna finger
madurae
    Actinomadura m.
Madura foot
Maestre de San Juan-Kallmann-de
  Morsier syndrome
MAF
    macrophage-activating factor
mafenide
Mafucci syndrome
Mag-200

mag
magnesium
MAG-3 diuretic renogram
magaldrate
Magan
Mag-Carb
Magendie
atresia of the foramina of Luschka and M.
foramen of M.
Maggi disposable biopsy needle guide for ultrasound
magic mouthwash
magma reticulare
magna
chorea m.
cisterna m.
coxa m.
dilated cisterna m.
large cisterna m.
mega cisterna m.
Magnacal formula
magnesia
Milk of M. (MOM)
Phillips' Milk of M.
magnesium (mag)
m. chloride
m. citrate
m. deficiency
m. hydroxide
intratracheal m. (ITMg)
ionized m.
m. level
m. oxide
m. pemoline
m. salicylate
m. sulfate (MgSO$_4$)
m. supplement
total m.
magnesium-containing cathartic
magnetic
m. resonance angiography (MRA)
m. resonance cholangiography (MRC)
m. resonance cholangiopancreatography (MRCP)
m. resonance elastography (MRE)
m. resonance imaging (MRI)
m. resonance mammography (MRM)
m. resonance spectroscopy (MRS)
m. resonance urography (MRU)
m. source imaging (MSI)
magnetically
m. activated cell sorter (MACS)
m. responsive microsphere
magnetite (Fe$_3$O$_4$)
magnetoencephalography (MEG)
magnification
area of interest m. (AIM)
loupe m.
m. mammography
spot m.
magnum
asymmetric small foramen m.
foramen m.
Magnus and de Kleijn tonic neck reflex
Magonate
Mag-Ox 400
MAGPI
meatal advancement and glansplasty incorporation
meatal advancement and glanuloplasty incorporation
MAGPI operation
MAGPI procedure
Magsal
Mag-Tab SR
Magtrate
MAH
minimal acceptable height
Maher disease
ma huang
MAI
Mycobacterium avium-intracellulare
MAI infection
MAID
mesna, Adriamycin, Ifosfamide, Dacarbazine
maidenhead
Maigret-50
main
m. bronchus
m. duct of Wirsung
m. renal vein
Maine
coast of M. café au lait spots
Mainstay urologic soft tissue anchor
mainstreaming
maintenance
m. fluid

NOTES

maintenance *(continued)*
  m. medication
  m. therapy
Mainz
  M. pouch
  M. pouch diversion
  M. pouch urinary reservoir
Maisonneuve fracture
Majewski
  M. short rib polydactyly
  M. syndrome
Majocchi granuloma
major
  m. aortopulmonary collateral artery
    (MAPCA)
  m. basic protein (MBP)
  m. capsid protein gene
  m. depressive disorder (MDD)
  m. detoxificating enzyme
  m. dysmorphism
  m. histocompatibility antigen
  m. histocompatibility complex
    (MHC)
  Leishmania m.
  m. motor seizure
  pelvis m.
  thalassemia m.
majus, pl. **majora**
  labia majora
Makler
  M. insemination
  M. insemination device
  M. reusable semen analysis
    chamber
mal
  m. de Meleda
  grand m.
  myoclonic petit m.
  petit m.
malabsorption
  bile acid m.
  carbohydrate m.
  congenital carbohydrate m.
  congenital folate m.
  fat m.
  glucose-galactose m.
  isolated congenital folate m.
    (ICFM)
  lactose m.
  methionine m.
  primary bile acid m.
  starch m.
  m. syndrome
  tryptophan m.
  m. workup
malacia
malacoplakia
maladaptation
  immunologic m.

maladaptive coping strategy
maladie
  m. de Roger
  m. des tics
malaise
malalignment
  patellofemoral m.
  rotational m.
  m. syndrome
malar
  m. distribution
  m. eminence
  m. fat pad
  m. flush
  m. hypoplasia
  m. rash
malaria
  cerebral m.
  chloroquine-resistant m.
  m. endemic
  falciparum m.
malariae
  Plasmodium m.
Malassezia
  M. furfur
  M. furfur pustulosis
  M. pachydermatitis
malate
malathion
maldescensus testis
male
  m. condom
  m. factor
  m. factor infertility
  M. FactorPak seminal fluid
    collection kit
  m. genital duct
  m. genital duct development
  m. karyotype
  m. pseudohermaphroditism (MPH)
  m. pseudohermaphroditism,
    persistent müllerian structures,
    mental retardation syndrome
  m. reproductive system
  m. sex differentiation
  m. Turner syndrome
  46,XX m.
  XXY m.
  XYY m.
  ZZ m.
maleate
  ergonovine m.
  fluvoxamine m.
  methylergonovine m.
  methysergide m.
  timolol m.
Malecot
  M. catheter
  M. tube

male-pattern hirsutism
male pseudohermaphroditism (MPH)
malformation
    adenomatoid m.
    airway m.
    aortic arch m.
    Arnold-Chiari m.
    arteriovenous m. (AVM)
    arteriovenous fistula m. (AVFM)
    AV m.
    body stalk m.
    bronchopulmonary m.
    cardiac m.
    cardiovascular m. (CVM)
    cerebral arteriovenous m. (CAVM)
    Chiari m. (type I–IV)
    cloacal m.
    clomiphene fetal m.
    congenital bronchopulmonary m.
    congenital cardiovascular m.
      (CCVM)
    congenital cystic adenomatoid m.
      (CCAM)
    congenital lung m.
    congenital obstructive müllerian m.
    congenital upper airway m.
    conotruncal cardiac m.
    craniooculofrontonasal m.
    cystic adenomatoid m. (CAM)
    cystic adenomatous m. (CAM)
    cystic congenital adenomatoid m.
      (CCAM)
    Dandy-Walker m.
    diabetes-related congenital m.
    ductal plate m.
    dural arteriovenous m.
    Ebstein m.
    embryologic m.
    extracardiac m.
    faciotelencephalic m.
    fetal m.
    fetal structural m.
    foregut m.
    GI tract venous m.
    gyral m.
    hamartomatous m.
    intracranial m.
    obstructive m.
    ocular m.
    pelvic arteriovenous m.
    pictures of syndromes and
      undiagnosed m.'s (POSSUM)

    pulmonary arteriovenous m.
      (PAVM)
    Rieger m.
    m. sequence
    split cord m. (SCM)
    split spinal cord m. (SSCM)
    submucosal arterial m.
    m. syndrome
    teratogen-induced m.
    thyroid gland m.
    urinary tract m.
    uterine arteriovenous m.
    vascular m.
    vein of Galen m.
    venous m. (VM)
    Walker-Warburg m.
malformed
    m. ear
    m. pinna
    m. radial head
malfunction
    congenital cystic adenomatoid m.
    shunt m.
Malgaigne fracture
malignancy
    borderline m. (BLM)
    breast m.
    CNS m.
    extrapelvic m.
    gastrointestinal m.
    genital tract m.
    gynecologic m.
    inflammatory bowel m.
    intraocular m.
    lymphoreticular m.
    metastatic m.
    ovarian m.
    vulvar m.
malignant
    m. arrhythmia
    m. brain edema
    m. brain tumor
    m. calcification
    m. cytotrophoblast
    m. degeneration
    m. epithelial tumor
    m. extrarenal rhabdoid tumor
    m. fibrous histiocytoma (MFH)
    m. germ cell tumor
    m. histiocytosis
    m. hyperphenylalaninemia
    m. hyperpyrexia

NOTES

M

malignant *(continued)*
 m. hypertension
 m. hyperthermia (MH)
 m. hyperthermic rhabdomyolysis
 m. lymphoma
 m. melanoma
 m. mesenchymal stroma
 m. mesodermal tumor
 m. mesothelioma (MM)
 m. mixed müllerian tumor
 (MMMT)
 m. nephrosclerosis
 m. nerve sheath tumor
 m. neurilemoma
 m. osteoid
 m. otitis externa
 m. ovarian germ cell tumor
 m. ovarian neoplasm
 m. ovarian teratoma
 m. phenylalaninemia
 m. pilocytic astrocytoma
 m. pleural effusion
 m. schwannoma
 m. syncytiotrophoblast
 m. transformation
 m. tumor of cervix
malignum
 adenoma m.
malingering
Malis CMC-II bipolar coagulator
Mallamint
Mallazine Eye drop
malleable
 m. retractor
 m. splint
mallei
 Burkholderia m.
malleolar ossification center
malleolus, pl. **malleoli**
 lateral m.
 medial m.
Mallergan-VC With Codeine
mallet
 m. finger
 m. toe
malleus
 short process of m.
Mall formula
Mallory-Weiss
 M.-W. syndrome
 M.-W. tear (MWT)
malmoense
 Mycobacterium m.
Malmstrom
 M. cup
 M. vacuum extractor
malnourished
malnutrition
 fetal m.

 protein-calorie m.
 protein-energy m.
malocclusion
malodorous
 m. breath
 m. urine
malondialdehyde (MDA)
Malouf syndrome
malplacement
malposition
 cardiac m.
 uterine m.
malpositioned catheter
malpresentation
 fetal m.
Malpuech facial clefting syndrome
malrotation
 m. of bowel
 intestinal m. (IM)
 renal m.
 volvulus m.
 m. with midgut volvulus
MALT
 mucosa-associated lymphoid tissue
 MALT type
malt
 barley m.
 m. soup extract
 m. worker's lung
maltase
 acid m.
maltophilia
 Stenotrophomonas m.
 Xanthomonas m.
maltreatment
Maltsupex
malunion
 pancreaticobiliary m.
MAMC
 mean arm muscle circumference
 midarm muscle circumference
mamma, pl. **mammae**
 m. accessoria
 m. erratica
 supernumerary m.
mammaglobin
mammal
mammalgia
mammalian transgenesis
mammaplasty
 augmentation m.
 postreduction m.
 reconstructive m.
 reduction m.
mammary
 m. calculus
 m. duct ectasia
 m. dysplasia
 m. fistula

m. galactogram
m. gland
m. neuralgia
m. sclerosing adenosis
m. souffle
mammectomy
Mammex TR computer-aided mammography diagnosis system
mammillaplasty
mammillitis
mammitis
mammogram
cephalocaudal film-screen m.
x-ray m.
mammographic
m. abnormality
m. detection
m. screening
mammography
computed tomography laser m. (CTLM)
contoured tilting compression m.
Corometrics Model 900SC in-office m.
CT laser m.
diagnostic m.
digital m.
Egan m.
heavy-ion m.
magnetic resonance m. (MRM)
magnification m.
preaspiration m.
screening m.
x-ray m.
Mammomat C3 mammography system
mammoplasty
MammoReader computer-aided detection system
MammoScan digital imaging system
mammose
Mammotest breast biopsy system
Mammotome breast biopsy system
mammotomy
mammotropic, mammotrophic
man
azoospermic m.
elephant m.
Mendelian Inheritance in M. (MIM)
managed care organization (MCO)
management
active third-stage m.

airway m.
antenatal m.
antepartum m.
anxiety m.
behavioral m.
brace m.
burn m.
conservative m.
epilepsy m.
expectant m.
Family Inventory of Resources for M. (FIRM)
home m.
home conservative m.
infertility m.
inpatient m.
intensive diabetes m. (IDM)
intrapartum m.
invasive m.
laparoscopic m.
metabolic m.
noninvasive m.
operative m.
pharmacologic m.
physiologic third-stage m.
postevacuation m.
pregnancy m.
m. protocol
risk m.
routine wound m.
surgical m.
total quality m. (TQM)
manager
case m.
Manchester
M. operation
M. ovoid
Manchester-Fothergill operation
Mancini plate
mandated reporter (of child abuse)
Mandelamine
mandelate
methenamine m.
mandelic acid
mandible
acroosteolysis with osteoporosis and changes in skull and m.
dislocated m.
hypoplastic m.
prominent m.
underdeveloped m.

M

NOTES

mandibular
    m. advancement
    m. dislocation
    m. hypoplasia
    m. prognathism
mandibular-acral dysplasia
mandibuloacral dysplasia
mandibulofacial
    m. dysostosis (MFD)
    m. dysostosis with epibulbar
      dermoids syndrome
    m. dysostosis with limb
      malformations syndrome
mandibulofacialis
    dysostosis m.
mandibulo-oculofacial
    m.-o. dyscephaly
    m.-o. dysmorphism
mandibulo-oculofacialis
    dyscephalia m.
Mandol
mandrel, mandril
    intrauterine insemination cannula
      with m.
mandrillaris
    Balamuthia m.
maneuver
    all-fours m.
    Barlow m.
    Bill m.
    Bracht m.
    Brandt-Andrews m.
    corkscrew m.
    Credé m.
    DeLee m.
    diagnostic m.
    Dix-Hallpike m.
    doll's eye m.
    doll's head m.
    forceps m.
    Frenzel m.
    Gaskin m.
    Gowers m.
    Hallpike m.
    heel-to-ear m.
    Heimlich m.
    Hillis-Müller m.
    Hodge m.
    jaw thrust-spine stabilization m.
    key-in-lock m.
    Kristeller m.
    Lecompte m.
    Leopold m.
    Levret m.
    logroll m.
    Loosett m.
    Lovset m.
    Massini m.
    Mauriceau m.

    Mauriceau-Levret m.
    Mauriceau-Smellie-Veit m.
    McDonald m.
    McRoberts m.
    midforceps m.
    modified Ritgen m.
    modified Zavanelli m.
    Müller-Hillis m.
    Munro-Kerr m.
    Nylen m.
    Ortolani m.
    ostrich m.
    Pajot m.
    physical m.
    Pinard m.
    Prague m.
    reverse form McRoberts m.
    Ritgen m.
    Rubin m.
    Saxtorph m.
    Scanzoni m.
    Scanzoni-Smellie m.
    scarf m.
    Schatz m.
    Sellick m.
    vagal m.
    vagotonic m.
    Valsalva m.
    Wigand m.
    Woods corkscrew m.
    Zavanelli m.
manganese intoxication
mange
    sarcoptic m.
mania
    prepuberal m.
manic
manic-depressive
    m.-d. disorder
    m.-d. illness
manifestation
    cardiovascular m.
    congenital m.
    endocrine m.
    extraintestinal m. (EIM)
    extrapyramidal m.
    gastrointestinal m.
    hypervigilance m.
    metabolic m.
    ocular m.
    renal m.
    systemic m.
manifold
Manipujector
    Kronner M.
manipulation
    gamete m.
    hormonal m.
    preorthognathic surgery m.

manipulative examination
manipulator
>ClearView uterine m.
>Kronner m.
>uterine m.
>Valtchev uterine m.

manipulator-injector
>Harris-Kronner uterine m.-i. (HUMI)
>Kronner Manipujector uterine m.-i.
>Rowden uterine m.-i. (RUMI)
>Zinnanti uterine m.-i. (ZUMI)

Manning score of fetal activity
Mann isthmic cerclage
mannitol
mannose-type sugar
mannosidase
mannosidosis
manometer
manometric
manometry
>anal m.
>anorectal perfusion m.
>esophageal m.
>lumbar puncture m.
>rectal balloon m.

mansoni
>*Schistosoma m.*

Mantel-Haenszel
>M.-H. procedure

mantle
>acid m.
>cortical m.
>m. sclerosis
>visible cortical m.

Mantoux
>M. method
>M. tuberculin skin test

manual
>m. alphabet
>m. breast pump
>m. cleavage
>m. detorsion
>m. differential
>m. English
>m. healing method
>*Learning to Eat* m.
>m. muscle testing
>m. pelvimetry
>m. reduction
>m. rotation
>m. splinting of thoracic cage

>m. thrust
>m. vacuum aspirator
>m. ventilation bag (MVB)

manubrium, pl. **manubria**
manuum
>tinea m.

MAO
>monoamine

MAOA
>monoamine oxidase type A

MAOI
>monoamine oxidase inhibitor

MAP
>mean airway pressure
>mean arterial pressure

map
>brain electrical activity m. (BEAM)
>chromosome m.
>contig m.
>cytogenetic m.
>cytological m.
>gene m.
>genetic m.
>linkage m.
>macrorestriction m.
>physical m.
>recombination m.
>restriction m.

Mapap
MAPCA
>major aortopulmonary collateral artery

maple
>m. leaf flap
>m. syrup urine
>m. syrup urine disease (MSUD)

maplike skull
MapMarkers fluorescent DNA sizing standard
mapping
>brain m.
>brain electrical activity m. (BEAM)
>chromosome m.
>comparative m.
>fate m.
>gene m.
>intraoperative lymphatic m.
>pressure m.

maprotiline
MAR
>mixed agglutination reaction
>MAR test

M

NOTES

mar22
    marker 22
Marañón syndrome
Maranox
marantic endocarditis
marasmic
marasmus
Marbaxin
marble
    m. bone disease
    m. bones
marbled hypopigmented streak
Marburg
    M. disease
    M. variant multiple sclerosis
    M. virus
Marcaine with epinephrine
marcescens
    Serratia m.
march
    m. hemoglobinuria
    jacksonian m.
Marchand
    M. adrenals
    M. rest
Marchetti test
Marcillin
Marckwald operation
Marcus
    M. Gunn jaw-winking ptosis
    M. Gunn phenomenon
    M. Gunn pupil
    M. Gunn sign
Marden-Walker syndrome
Marezine
Marfan
    M. sign
    M. syndrome
marfanoid
    m. craniosynostosis syndrome
    m. habitus
    m. habitus, mental retardation
      syndrome
    m. habitus, microcephaly,
      glomerulonephritis syndrome
**Margarita Island type ectodermal
  dysplasia**
Margesic
    M. A-C
    M. H
margin
    anal m.
    blurring of left psoas m.
    costal m.
    placental m.
    psoas m.
    tentorial m.
marginal
    m. alopecia

m. cord insertion
obtuse m.
m. previa
m. sinus
m. sinus rupture
m. zone
marginatum
    eczema m.
    erythema m.
Margulies coil
marian lithotomy
Marie-Sainton syndrome
Marie-Strümpell encephalitis
Marie syndrome
Marie-Unna hypotrichosis
marijuana effect
Marinesco-Garland syndrome
Marinesco-Sjögren-Garland syndrome
Marinesco-Sjögren-like syndrome
Marinesco-Sjögren syndrome
Marinol
marinum
    Mycobacterium m.
Marion disease
Marion-Moschcowitz culdoplasty
marital
    M. Dyadic Inventory
    m. introitus
mark
    belt m.
    Caitlin m.
    choke m.
    port-wine m.
    strawberry m.
    stretch m.
    Unna m.
marked asynchrony
markedly decreased reflex
marker
    m. 22 (mar22)
    adrenal hyperandrogenism m.
    Anderson m.
    assay m.
    biallelic m.
    CA 15-3 breast cancer m.
    CA 125 endometrial cancer m.
    CA 549 tumor m.
    chromosomal m.
    chromosome 22 supernumerary m.
      (SMG22)
    DNA m.
    fecal m.
    Freeman cookie cutter areola m.
    m. gene
    genetic m.
    infection m.
    maternal serum m.
    neonatal m.
    pericentromeric m.

peripheral androgen activity m.
protein m.
radiopaque m.
serologic m.
sigma tumor m.
tumor m.
m. X (marX)
m. X chromosome
m. X syndrome

marking
pulmonary vascular m.
m. time pattern

Marlex
Marlow
M. disposable cannula
M. disposable trocar

Marmine Oral
Marmo method
marmorata
cutis m.

marmoratus
status m.

marneffei
Penicillium m.

Maroteaux-Lamy
M.-L. disease
M.-L. syndrome

Maroteaux-Malamut syndrome
Marplan
marrow
adult bone m. (ABM)
bone m.
, fetal bone m. (FBM)
m. transplantation

marrow-ablative chemotherapy
MARS
mixed antiinflammatory syndrome
molecular adsorbent recirculating system
motion artifact rejection system

Marshall
ligament of M.
M. syndrome
M. test

Marshall-Marchetti-Krantz (MMK)
M.-M.-K. operation
M.-M.-K. procedure

Marshall-Marchetti procedure
Marshall-Smith syndrome (MSS)
Marshall-Tanner
M.-T. pubertal stage (1–5)
M.-T. pubertal staging (1–5)

Marshall-Taylor vacuum extraction

Mars pulse oximetry
Marsupial
M. belt
M. pouch

marsupialization
Spence and Duckett m.
m. technique
transurethral m.

Marthritic
Martin-Bell-Renpenning syndrome
Martin-Bell syndrome (MBS)
Martin modification
Martius
M. bulbocavernosus fat flap
M. flap and fascial sling
M. graft
M. procedure

Martsolf syndrome
marX
marker X
marX syndrome

Mary Jane breast pump
Maryland dissector
MAS
macrophage activation syndrome
Maternal Attitude Scale
meconium aspiration syndrome

MASA
mental retardation, aphasia, shuffling
gait, adducted thumb
MASA syndrome

masculine pelvis
masculinization
masculinovoblastoma
MAS-ECMO
meconium aspiration syndrome
extracorporeal membrane oxygenation
MAS-ECMO infant

Masimo
M. SET home monitor
M. SET signal extraction pulse
oximetry

mask
m. of atopic dermatitis
bag and m.
bag, valve, m. (BVM)
m. and bag ventilation
face m.
m. inhalation anesthesia
Laerdal m.
Neutrogena Acne M.
nonrebreather face m.

M

NOTES

mask *(continued)*
    N95 particulate respirator
      surgical m.
    m. of pregnancy
    ventilation by m.
    Venturi m.
Maslach Burnout Inventory
masquerade syndrome
MASS
    mitral valve, aorta, skeleton, skin
    MASS phenotype
mass
    abdominal m.
    m. accretion
    adnexal m.
    benign m.
    bilateral flank m.'s
    bone m.
    bone mineral m. (BMM)
    calcified m.
    cervical m.
    circumscribed m.
    complex m.
    cortical m.
    cystic adnexal m.
    cystic ovarian m.
    doughnut-shaped m.
    doughy m.
    m. effect
    exophytic m.
    extravesical m.
    extrinsic extravesical m.
    fallopian tube m.
    fat m. (FM)
    fat-free m. (FFM)
    flank m.
    fungating m.
    hamartomatous m.
    hyperechoic m.
    hypoxia, intussusception, brain m.
      (HIB)
    ill-defined m.
    inner cell m.
    intramyometrial m.
    lean body m. (LBM)
    lean tissue m. (LTM)
    m. lesion
    maternal pelvic m.
    mediastinal m.
    mixed-density m.
    neonatal abdominal m.
    noncalcified nodular m.
    ovarian m.
    paraspinal m.
    pelvic m.
    persistent ovarian m.
    poorly marginated m.
    postmenopausal body m.
    potato-like m.
    pyloric m.
    scrotal m.
    m. spectrometer
    m. spectrometry (MS)
    spongy m.
    stellate m.
    submucosal m.
    suprapubic m.
    total fat m. (TFM)
    tubal m.
    tumor m.
    umbilical cord m.
    unilateral flank m.
    unilocular cystic ovarian m.
    uterine m.
    vertebral bone m. (VBM)
    virilizing ovarian m.
    well-defined m.
massage
    bimanual m.
    cardiac m.
    closed chest m.
    heart m.
    lacrimal sac m.
    perineal m.
    Shiatsu therapeutic m.
    m. therapy
    uterine m.
Masse Breast Cream
Massengill douche
masseter muscle
Massini maneuver
massive
    m. ascites
    m. atelectasis
    m. breast hypertrophy
    m. genital prolapse
    m. intravascular hemolysis
    m. ovarian cyst
    m. pulmonary embolus
    m. transfusion
Masson-Fontana stain
MAST
    military antishock trousers
    MAST suit
mast
    m. cell
    m. cell disease
    m. cell leukemia
    m. cell stabilizer
mastadenitis
mastadenoma
mastalgia
    cyclic m.
mastatrophy, mastatrophia
mastectomy
    Auchincloss modified radical m.
    extended radical m.
    Halsted m.

McWhirter m.
modified radical m.
prophylactic m.
radical m.
simple m.
skin-sparing m.
subcutaneous m.
total m.
Willy Meyer m.
MasterFlex fetal perfusion pump
Masters-Allen syndrome
mastitis
chronic cystic m.
gargantuan m.
glandular m.
granulomatous m.
interstitial m.
lactational m.
m. neonatorum
nonpuerperal m.
parenchymatous m.
phlegmonous m.
plasma cell m.
puerperal m.
retromammary m.
stagnation m.
submammary m.
suppurative m.
mastocytoma
mastocytosis
bullous m.
cutaneous m.
diffuse cutaneous m.
nasal m.
primary nasal m.
systemic m.
mastodynia, mazodynia
mastoid
m. air cell
m. bone fracture
cloudy m.
m. cortex
m. drainage
m. fontanelle
m. osteitis
m. process
mastoidectomy
mastoiditis
acute coalescent m.
acute surgical m.
chronic m.
coalescent m.

pneumococcal m.
surgical m.
mastology
mastoncus
mastopathy
mastopexy, mazopexy
Benelli m.
mastoplasia, mazoplasia
mastoplasty
mastoptosis
mastorrhagia
mastoscirrhus
mastotomy
masturbation
MAT
microscopic agglutination test
mat
mycelial m.
matching
M. Familiar Figures (MFF)
feature m.
V/Q m.
Mateer-Streeter ovum
mater
dura m.
pia m.
material
absorbent gelling m. (AGM)
Avitene hemostatic m.
coffee-grounds m.
dextran-70 barrier m.
didactic m.
elective abortion m.
Endo-Avitene hemostatic m.
FlowGel barrier m.
genetic m.
hyperechogenic m.
Interceed barrier m.
lipofuscin m.
metal suture m.
mobile hyperechogenic m.
nonionic contrast m.
nylon suture m.
other potentially infectious m. (OPIM)
Poloxamer 407 barrier m.
polyester suture m.
polyethylene suture m.
polypropylene suture m.
radiocontrast m.
spontaneous abortion m.
suture m.

NOTES

material *(continued)*
    synthetic suture m.
    white pseudomembranous m.

Materna
    M. prenatal vitamin
    M. Tablet

maternal
    m. abdominal pressure
    m. activity restriction
    m. age
    m. age-related risk
    m. age screening
    m. alcohol consumption
    m. alcoholism
    m. anesthesia
    m. antiplatelet antibody
    m. antithyroid antibody
    m. assessment
    m. asthma
    M. Attitude Scale (MAS)
    m. Bernard-Soulier syndrome
    m. birthing position
    m. blood clot patch therapy
    m. breast milk
    m. care
    m. central hemodynamics
    m. cholestasis
    m. coagulopathy
    m. cocaine use
    m. cortical vein
    m. cortical vein thrombosis
    m. cotyledon
    m. cyanotic heart disease
    m. cytokinemia
    m. death
    m. death rate
    m. deprivation syndrome
    m. diabetes
    m. douche
    m. drug abuse
    m. dystocia
    m. effect
    m. estriol level
    m. estrogen withdrawal
    m. exercise
    m. exhaustion
    m. factor
    m. febrile morbidity
    m. fever
    m. floor infarction
    m. fracture
    m. gonads
    m. hemopathy
    m. hepatitis
    m. HLA haplotype
    m. hydration
    m. hydrops
    m. hydrops fetalis
    m. hydrops syndrome

    m. hypercalcemia
    m. hyperparathyroidism
    m. hypertension
    m. hypotension
    m. hypoxia
    m. IgG antibody
    m. illness
    m. immune response
    m. immunocompetence
    m. immunology
    m. indications
    m. infection
    m. inflammatory response
    m. inheritance
    m. insulin
    M. Interview of Substance Use (MISU)
    m. intravascular inflammation
    m. karyotype
    m. meiosis I (MMI)
    m. meiosis II (MMII)
    m. mercury exposure
    m. mortality
    m. mortality rate
    m. nutrition
    m. ocular adaptation
    m. outcome
    m. parvovirus fetalis
    m. pelvic mass
    m. peripheral blood
    m. phenylketonuria
    m. physiology
    m. plasma leptin
    m. plasma volume
    m. position
    m. pulse
    m. pyrexia
    m. serum
    m. serum alpha fetoprotein (MSAFP)
    m. serum marker
    m. serum marker level
    m. serum screening
    m. serum triple screen
    m. size
    m. smoking
    m. sperm antibody
    m. stature
    m. steroid concentration
    m. stress
    m. substance abuse
    m. surveillance
    m. systemic condition
    m. tachycardia
    m. thrombocytopenia
    m. thyrotropin receptor blocking antibody-induced congenital hypothyroidism
    m. tissue

m. titer
m. trauma
m. undernourishment
m. uniparental heterodisomy
m. vascular response
m. weight
m. weight gain
m. well-being

maternal-fetal

m.-f. hemorrhage
m.-f. histocompatibility
m.-f. histoincompatibility
m.-f. HLA compatibility
m.-f. interface
m.-f. medicine
m.-f. medicine unit (MFMU)
m.-f. microtransfusion
m.-f. transmission
m.-f. transmission of antibody

maternal-infant

m.-i. attachment
m.-i. bonding

maternally inherited myopathy and cardiomyopathy (MIMyCA)
maternal-placental-fetal unit
maternal-placental unit
maternity

m. blues
disputed m.

maternofetal transfusion
mating

assortative m.
backcross m.
consanguineous m.
nonrandom m.
random m.
m. type

matrices (*pl. of* matrix)
matrilineal
matrilysin
Matritech NMP22 bladder cancer test
matrix, pl. **matrices**

bone m.
calcified m.
extracellular m.
germinal m.
identity m.
m. metalloproteinase (MMP)
myxoid m.
nail m.
Raven Progressive Matrices (RPM)
square m.

telencephalic subependymal
  germinal m.
uncalcified bone m.

matroclinous inheritance
matted

m. omentum
m. peritoneum

matter

gray m.
heterotopic gray m.
particulate m.
spongy degeneration of white m.
supratentorial white m.
white m.

mattress

apnea alarm m.
Dräger thermal gel m.

Matulane
maturation

adrenal m.
m. of cell
delayed sexual m.
excessive villous m.
fetal lung m.
follicular m.
ovum m.
premature accelerated lung m.
  (PALM)
pulmonary m.
sexual m.
skeletal m.
terminal m.
vaginal cellular m.
m. value
in vitro m.

maturation-promoting factor (MPF)
mature

m. burst-forming unit erythroid (M-BFU-E)
m. cystic ovarian teratoma
m. cystic teratoma
early m.
m. infant
late m.
m. neutrophil
m. teratoma

maturity

chronic lung disease of m.
Dubowitz Scale for Infant M.
fetal lung m. (FLM)
fetal pulmonary m.
neuromuscular m.

M

NOTES

maturity *(continued)*
  m. onset deafness
  physical m.
  social m.
maturity-onset
  m.-o. diabetes
  m.-o. diabetes of the young
    (MODY)
  m.-o. diabetes of youth (MODY)
Maturna bra system
Maunoir hydrocele
Mauriac syndrome
Mauriceau-Levret maneuver
Mauriceau maneuver
Mauriceau-Smellie-Veit maneuver
Maxafil
Maxalt
Maxaquin
Maxeran
Maxidex Ophthalmic
Maxiflor
maxilla, pl. **maxillae**
  short m.
maxillary
  m. advancement
  m. bone
  m. hypoplasia
  m. sinus
  m. sinus aspiration
  m. sinus mucosal specimen
maxillofacial dysostosis
maxillonasal dysplasia
Maxilube personal lubricant
maximal
  m. cardiac width
  m. chest width
  m. electroshock (MES)
  m. oxygen intake (MOI)
  m. permissible dose
maximum
  m. breathing capacity
  m. likelihood estimator
  m. oxygen uptake (VO_2max)
  m. temperature (T-max)
  m. urethral closure pressure
    (MUCP)
maximum-intensive phototherapy
Maxipime
Maxitrol Ophthalmic
Maxivate Topical
Maxon delayed-absorbable suture
Mayaro virus
Mayer
  M. pessary
  M. sign
  M. wave
Mayer-Rokitansky-Küster-Hauser
  syndrome
May-Hegglin anomaly

Maylard incision
Mayo
  M. culdoplasty
  M. hook
  M. hysterectomy
  M. scissors
Mayo-Fueth inversion procedure
Mayo-Gibbon heart-lung machine
Mayo-Hegar needle holder
mazindol
mazodynia *(var. of* mastodynia)
mazolysis
mazopexy *(var. of* mastopexy)
mazoplasia *(var. of* mastoplasia)
Mazzariello-Caprini forceps
Mazzini test
MB
  myocardial band
    creatine kinase MB
    MB isoenzyme
m-BACOD
  methotrexate, bleomycin, doxorubicin,
    cyclophosphamide, Oncovin,
    dexamethasone
MBC
  minimal bacterial concentration
MBD
  minimal brain dysfunction
M-BFU-E
  mature burst-forming unit erythroid
MBM
  mother's breast milk
MBP
  major basic protein
  modified Bagshawe protocol
MBPP
  modified biophysical profile
MBS
  Martin-Bell syndrome
  modified barium swallow
MCA
  middle cerebral artery
MCAD
  medium-chain acyl-CoA dehydrogenase
    MCAD deficiency
McAllister grading system
MCAO
  middle cerebral artery occlusion
McArdle disease
McBurney
  M. incision
  M. point
McCall
  M. culdoplasty
  M. stitch
McCall-Schumann procedure
McCaman-Robins test
McCarthy
  M. Memory Scale

M. reflex
M. Scales of Children's Abilities
McCraw gracilis myocutaneous flap
McCune-Albright syndrome
MCD
metastatic Crohn disease
molybdenum cofactor deficiency
MCDD
multiple complex developmental disorder
McDonald
M. cervical cerclage
M. maneuver
M. measurement
M. operation
M. procedure
M. rule
McDonough syndrome
MCDU
mercaptolactate-cysteine disulfiduria
MCF-7 breast cancer cell
MCFA
medium-chain fatty acid
mcg
microgram
McGee forceps
McGill forceps
mcg/kg min, mcg/kg/min
microgram per kilogram per minute
McGoon index
McGovern nipple
McGrath scale
MCH
mean cell hemoglobin
mean corpuscular hemoglobin
MCHC
mean cell hemoglobin concentration
mean corpuscular hemoglobin
concentration
MCi
megacurie
McIndoe
M. operation
M. procedure
McIndoe-Hayes procedure
McKernan-Adson forceps
McKernan-Potts forceps
McKusick-Kaufman syndrome
MCL
medial collateral ligament
McLane forceps
McLeod syndrome

MCLS
mucocutaneous lymph node syndrome
McMaster Family Assessment Device
McMurray
M. sign
M. test
McNemar test
MCNS
minimal change nephrotic syndrome
MCO
managed care organization
MCP
medical control physician
metacarpophalangeal
McPherson forceps
MCR
metabolic clearance rate
m-cresyl acetate
McRoberts maneuver
MCS
Miles-Carpenter syndrome
MCT
medium-chain triglyceride
MCT oil
MCT oil formula
MCTD
mixed connective tissue disease
M-cup
M-c. vacuum extraction device
MCV
mean corpuscular volume
methotrexate, cisplatin, vinblastine
molluscum contagiosum virus
McWhirter mastectomy
MD
medical doctor
muscular dystrophy
myotonic dystrophy
MDA
malondialdehyde
Multichannel discrete analyzer
MDAC
multidose activated charcoal
MDD
major depressive disorder
MDI
mental development index
MDK
multicystic dysplastic kidney
MDLS
Miller-Dieker lissencephaly syndrome

M

NOTES

MDMA
methylenedioxymethamphetamine
MDR
minimum daily requirement
multidrug resistance
MDR-TB
multidrug-resistant tuberculosis
MDS
myelodysplastic syndrome
MDT
multidrug therapy
M:E
myeloid to erythroid ratio
MEA
mercaptoethylamine
microwave endometrial ablation
multiple endocrine abnormalities
multiple endocrine adenomatosis
Mead Johnson
M. J. bottle
M. J. formula
Meadows syndrome
meal-time skill
mean
m. age
m. airway pressure (MAP)
m. aortic pressure
m. arm muscle circumference (MAMC)
m. arterial blood pressure (MABP)
m. arterial pressure (MAP)
m. birth weight
m. cell hemoglobin (MCH)
m. cell hemoglobin concentration (MCHC)
m. corpuscular hemoglobin (MCH)
m. corpuscular hemoglobin concentration (MCHC)
m. corpuscular volume (MCV)
m. developmental quotient
m. hemoglobin concentration
m. intercriterion correlation (MIC)
m. left atrial pressure
m. length of utterance (MLU)
m. length of utterance in morphemes (MLUm)
m. menstrual cycle hematocrit
m. plasma iron concentration
m. platelet volume (MPV)
m. pulmonary artery pressure
regression of the m.
m. right atrial pressure
means-end problem solving (MEPS)
measles
atypical m.
black m.
m. exanthem
German m.

m. inclusion body encephalitis (MIBE)
modified m.
m., mumps, rubella (MMR)
m. pneumonia
three-day m.
typical m.
uncomplicated m.
m. vaccine
m. virus
m. virus enzyme-linked immunosorbent assay (MV(c)ELISA)
measure
anthropometric m.
first-line m.
gross motor function m.
Prematurity Risk Evaluation M. (PREM)
process-oriented m.
second-line m.
third-line m.
measurement
acid-base m.
anthropometric m.
anthropomorphic m.
blood pressure m.
body proportion m.
bone density m.
bone mineral m.
bone strength m.
fetal fibronectin m.
fetal growth m.
fundal height m.
intrauterine pressure m.
McDonald m.
midluteal progesterone m.
noninvasive blood pressure m. (NIBPM)
nuchal translucency m.
optical density m.
peak flow m.
POWSBP m.
sequential peak flow m.
somatic growth m.
third trimester m.
transcutaneous m.
measuring hat
meatal
m. advancement and glansplasty incorporation (MAGPI)
m. advancement and glanuloplasty
meatal advancement and glanuloplasty incorporation (MAGPI)
m. stenosis
meatus
auditory m.

bilateral atresia of external
    auditory m.
external auditory m.
external urethral m.
fishmouth m.
glanular urethral m.
penile urethral m.
penopubic urethral m.
urethral m.

MEB
muscle-eye-brain
MEB disease

mebanazine
Mebaral
mebendazole
MEBS
muscle-eye-brain syndrome

MECA
Methods for Epidemiology of Child and
    Adolescent Mental Disorders
MECA study
MECA T score

mecamylamine
mechanical
m. birth injury
m. buttress
m. cervical dilator
m. compression
m. dead space
m. dysmenorrhea
m. hemolysis
m. obstruction
m. respirator
m. suffocation
m. ventilation

mechanic's hand
mechanism
alloimmune m.
autoimmune m.
bypass continence m.
cellular cytotoxic m.
cerebroprotective m.
Douglas m.
Duncan m.
excitotoxic m.
Frank-Starling m.
heat transfer m.
host defense m.
host response m.
neural m.
normal flap-valve m.
ovum pickup m.

pathophysiologic m.
peptide growth factor signaling m.
Schultze m.
Starling m.
two-cell m.

mechanobullous
mechlorethamine
m. hydrochloride
m., Oncovin, procarbazine,
    prednisone
m., Oncovin (vincristine),
    procarbazine, prednisone (MOPP)

Meckel
M. cave
M. diverticulum
M. scan
M. syndrome

Meckel-Gruber syndrome
meclizine
meclofenamate
mecometer
meconial colic
meconiorrhea
meconium
m. aspiration
m. aspiration syndrome (MAS)
m. aspiration syndrome
    extracorporeal membrane
    oxygenation (MAS-ECMO)
m. blockage syndrome
m. corpuscle
m. ileus (MI)
m. ileus appearance
m. ileus equivalent
m. obstruction
passage of m.
m. passage
m. peritonitis
m. plug
m. plug syndrome
m. stain
m. stained
m. staining
m. staining of liquor

meconium-stained
m.-s. amniotic fluid (MSAF)
m.-s. skin

MeCP2
methyl-CpG-binding protein 2

MED
minimal effective dose

Meda-Cap

M

NOTES

MedaSonics first beat ultrasound stethoscope
Meda Tab
Medela
    M. Dominant vacuum delivery pump
    M. manual breast pump
    M. membrane regulator
Medevice
    M. surgical loop
    M. surgical paws
Medex
Medfusion 1001 syringe infusion pump
media (*gen. of* medius) (*pl. of* medium)
medial
    m. collateral ligament (MCL)
    m. collateral ligament syndrome
    m. compartment
    m. condyle
    m. epicondylar fracture
    m. femoral torsion (MFT)
    m. hip rotation
    m. hip rotation in extension
    m. longitudinal arch
    m. longitudinal arch support
    m. malleolus
    m. metaphyseal beak
    m. necrosis
    m. oblique view
    m. rotation (MR)
    m. rotation clubfoot
    m. snapping hip syndrome
    m. talocalcaneal facet
    m. tibial torsion (MTT)
medialis
    vastus m.
median
    m. alveolar notch
    m. cleft upper lip, mental retardation, pugilistic facies syndrome
    m. eminence
    m. episiotomy
    m. facial cleft syndrome
    m. fecal calprotectin
    multiples of the appropriate gestational m. (MoM)
    m. plane
    m. raphe
    m. umbilical fold
    m. umbilical ligament
mediana
    diameter m.
mediastinal
    m. air drainage
    m. collagenosis
    m. crunch
    m. granuloma

    m. imaging
    m. lymphadenitis
    m. lymphadenopathy
    m. mass
    m. teratoma
    m. tumor
    m. widening
mediastinitis
    fibrosing m.
    pyogenic m.
    suppurative m.
mediastinum
    narrow m.
mediating action
mediator
    herpes virus entry m. (HVEM)
    intracellular m.
Medibottle
Medicaid
medical
    m. control physician (MCP)
    m. doctor (MD)
    m. geneticist
    m. genetics
    M. Manager software
    m. noncompliance
    m. oophorectomy
    m. optical spectroscopy (MOS)
    m. optimal imaging (MOI)
    m. termination
    m. worry beads
MedicAlert
    M. bracelet
    M. Foundation
medicalization
medically fragile
medicamentosa
    rhinitis m.
Medicare
medicated
    Zilactin-B M.
medication
    aerosolized m.
    anticholinesterase m.
    antiemetic m.
    antipruritic m.
    antiretroviral m.
    antispastic m.
    antitussive m.
    anxiolytic m.
    base m.
    exogenous m.
    intrathecal m.
    intravenous m.
    iodide-containing m.
    maintenance m.
    neuroleptic m.
    opioid m.
    organ-specific m.

over-the-counter m.
parenteral m.
postcoital contraceptive m.
pressor m.
prophylactic m.
psychostimulant m.
rescue m.
teratogenic m.
medication-induced stuttering
medicine
adolescent m.
Alka-Seltzer Plus Children's
Cold M.
American Institute of Ultrasound
in M. (AIUM)
Chinese m.
community m.
complementary and alternative m.
(CAM)
digital imaging and communication
in m. (DICOM)
doctor of m.
emergency m.
fetal-maternal m.
folk m.
herbal m.
maternal-fetal m.
neonatal m.
osteopathic m.
pediatric emergency m. (PEM)
pediatric pulmonary m.
perinatal m.
pulmonary m.
Reese's Pinworm M.
medicolegal
Medicone
Rectal M.
MED-IDDM
multiple epiphyseal dysplasia-early onset
diabetes mellitus syndrome
Medilium
Medilog 9000 polysomnography device
medinensis
Dracunculus m.
mediolateral
m. episiotomy
m. view
Mediplast Plaster
Medipore H soft cloth surgical tape
MediPort catheter
Medi-Quick Topical Ointment
meditation

Mediterranean
M. anemia
M. fever
M. lymphoma
M. myoclonus
Medi-Trace electrode
MediTran
medium, pl. **media**
Biggers m.
Bordet-Gengoi m.
charcoal-blood m.
CPS ID chromogenic m.
dermatophyte test m. (DTM)
Dulbecco m.
Earle culture m.
gallium-67 citrate contrast m.
Gibco BRL sperm preparation m.
Ham F10 m.
HEPES-buffered Ham F10 m.
ionic contrast m.
Löwenstein-Jensen m.
Nickerson m.
nonionic contrast m.
OncoScint CR/OV contrast m.
Regan-Lowe m.
Sabouraud m.
selective broth m. (SBM)
sperm capacitation m.
Thayer-Martin m.
thioglycollate broth m.
transfer m.
transmission m.
transport m.
Whitten m.
Whittingham m.
medium-chain
m.-c. acyl-CoA dehydrogenase
(MCAD)
m.-c. fatty acid (MCFA)
m.-c. triglyceride (MCT)
medius, gen. **media**
acute otitis media (AOM)
acute suppurative otitis media
chronic otitis media (COM)
chronic suppurative otitis media
(CSOM)
clostridial otitis media
draining otitis media
mucoid otitis media (MOM)
mucoid otitis media (MOM)
otitis media (OM)
recurrent otitis media

M

NOTES

medius *(continued)*
    saccus m.
    secretory otitis media
    serous otitis media
    suppurative otitis media
Med-Neb respirator
medorrhea
Medrol Oral
medroxyprogesterone
    m. acetate (MPA)
    depot m.
    m. injection
medrysone
MEDS
    microsurgical extraction of ductal sperm
Medscan
medulla
    adrenal m.
    m. oblongata
    rostral ventromedial m.
medullaris
    tethered conus m.
medullary
    m. canal
    m. cord
    m. cystic disease
    m. dysplasia
    m. necrosis
    m. parenchyma
    m. recycling
    m. sponge kidney
    m. thyroid carcinoma
medulloblastoma
    classic m.
    desmoplastic m.
    melanotic m.
    primitive neuroectodermal tumor m.
        (PNET/MB)
medullomyoblastoma
medusae
    caput m.
MedWatch form
MEE
    middle ear effusion
Meesmann corneal dystrophy
MEF
    middle ear fluid
mefenamic acid
mefloquine hydrochloride
Mefoxin
MEG
    magnetoencephalography
megabase
megabladder
megacalicosis
megacalycosis
megacardia
Megace
megacephaly

Megacillin Susp
mega cisterna magna
megacolon
    aganglionic m.
    congenital aganglionic m.
    toxic m.
megacurie (MCi)
megacystis
    m., microcolon, intestinal
        hypoperistalsis (MMIH)
megacystis-megaureter syndrome
megadosing
megaelectron volt (MeV)
megaesophagus
megahertz (MHz)
megakaryoblastic leukemia
megakaryocyte
megakaryocytic
    m. leukemia
    m. thrombocytopenia
megakaryocytopoiesis
megakaryopoiesis
megalencephaly
    benign familial m.
    m., cranial sclerosis, osteopathia
        striata syndrome
    idiopathic m.
    primary m.
    unilateral m.
    m. with hyaline panneuropathy
megaloblastic
    m. anemia
    m. crisis
    m. erythropoiesis
megaloblastoid
megaloblastosis
megalocardia
megalocephalia
megalocephaly
megaloclitoris
megalocornea
    m., developmental retardation,
        dysmorphic syndrome
    m., macrocephaly, mental and
        motor retardation syndrome
        (MMMM)
    m.-mental retardation syndrome
        (MMR)
megalodactyly
megaloencephaly
megalomelia
Megalone
megalopenis
megalophthalmos
megalosyndactyly
megaloureter, megaureter
    obstructive m.
megalourethra
meganeurite

megarectum
megaterium
    Bacillus m.
megaureter (*var. of* megaloureter)
megaureter
megavitamin therapy
megavolt (MV)
megavoltage machine
megestrol acetate
meglumine
    m. diatrizoate
    Hypaque M.
meibomian gland
meibomianitis, meibomitis
Meier-Gorlin syndrome
Meigs
    M. pelvic lymphadenectomy
    M. syndrome
Meigs-Kass syndrome
Meigs-Okabayashi procedure
Meigs-Werthein hysterectomy
Meinecke-Peper syndrome
meiosis
    diakinesis stage of oocyte m.
    dictyate stage of oocyte m.
    diplotene phase of m.
    m. I (MI)
    m. II (MII)
    leptotene phase of m.
    maternal m. I (MMI)
    maternal m. II (MMII)
    oocyte m.
    pachytene phase of m.
    paternal m. I (PMI)
    paternal m. II (PMII)
    zygotene phase of m.
meiotic division
Meissner plexus
mekongi
    Schistosoma m.
melancholia
    involutional m.
melancholic depression
Melanex topical solution
melanin-like pigment
melaninogenicus
    Bacteroides m.
melanization
melanoblastoma
    Bloch-Sulzberger m.
melanoblastosis cutis linearis sive systematisata

melanocyte
    epidermal m.
    pigmented m.
melanocyte-stimulating hormone
melanocytic nevus
melanocytosis
    congenital dermal m.
    dermal m.
    meningeal m.
melanoderma
melanodermic leukodystrophy
melanoma
    benign juvenile m.
    Clark classification of vulvar m.
    cutaneous m.
    juvenile m.
    malignant m.
    metastatic m.
    nodular m.
    m. specific antigen
    superficial spreading m.
    vulvar m.
melanosarcoma
melanosis
    Becker m.
    m. corii degenerativa
    cutaneous m.
    neonatal pustular m.
    m. oculi
    pustular m.
    transient neonatal pustular m.
    m. vaginae
    m. vulvae
melanotic medulloblastoma
melanura
    Culiseta m.
MELAS
    mitochondrial encephalomyopathy, lactic
      acidosis, strokelike episodes
    MELAS syndrome
melasma gravidarum
melatonin
    m. secretion
    urinary excreted m.
Meleda
    mal de M.
melena
    m. neonatorum
    m. spuria
Meleney synergistic gangrene
Melfiat
melioidosis

M

NOTES

melitensis
  Brucella m.
Melkersson-Rosenthal syndrome
Melkersson syndrome
Mellaril
mellituria
mellitus
  adult-onset diabetes m. (AODM)
  diabetes m. (type 1, 2) (DM)
  gestational diabetes m. (GDM)
  insulin-dependent diabetes m.
    (IDDM)
  juvenile diabetes m. (JDM)
  juvenile-onset diabetes m. (JDM,
    JODM)
  new-onset diabetes m.
  non-insulin-dependent diabetes m.
    (NIDDM)
  overt insulin-dependent diabetes m.
  pregestational diabetes m. (PDM)
  transient neonatal diabetes m.
    (TNDM)
  type 1, 2 diabetes m.
Melnick-Fraser syndrome
Melnick-Needles
  M.-N. disease
  M.-N. syndrome
melorheostosis
melphalan
membrana granulosa
membrane
  allograft m.
  amniotic m.
  artificial rupture of m.'s (ARM,
    AROM)
  m. attack complex
  basal m. (BM)
  basement m.
  m. bridge
  chorioallantoic m. (CAM)
  cloacal m.
  cracked mucous m.
  cricothyroid m.
  cuprophane hemodialyzer m.
  cytoplasmic m.
  Descemet m.
  diphtheritic m.
  dry mucous m.
  Duralon-UV nylon m.
  dysmenorrheal m.
  egg m.
  erythrocyte m.
  exocelomic m.
  extraembryonic fetal m.
  extraplacental m.
  fetal m.
  floating m.
  germinal m.
  glomerular basement m. (GBM)

m. glycoprotein IB/IX
Gore-Tex surgical m.
m. granulosa
Heuser m.
hyaline m.
hymenal m.
intact m.
interfetal m.
Jackson m.
milk fat globule m. (MFGM)
mucous m.
otitis media with perforated
  tympanic m.
parched mucous m.
perforated tympanic m.
perineal m.
persistent pupillary m.
placental m.
plasma m.
platelet m.
Preclude peritoneal m.
prelabor rupture of m.'s (PROM)
premature rupture of m.'s (PROM)
preterm premature rupture of m.'s
  (PPROM)
preterm rupture of m.'s (PROM)
preterm spontaneous rupture
  of m.'s (PSROM)
prolonged premature rupture
  of m.'s (PPROM)
prolonged rupture of m.'s (PROM)
m. protein
pupillary m.
red blood cell m.
Reissner m.
retained m.
m. rupture
Seprafilm bioresorbable m.
Slavianski m.
spontaneous rupture of m.'s
  (SROM)
m. stripping
subaortic m.
tympanic m.
ultrafiltration m.
vernix m.
Viresolve ultrafiltration m.
vitelline m.
Wachendorf m.
yolk m.
membranoproliferative glomerulonephritis
  (MPGN)
membranous
  m. conjunctivitis
  m. croup
  m. dysmenorrhea
  m. glomerulonephritis
  m. laryngotracheobronchitis
  m. lupus nephritis

m. nephropathy
m. septum
m. twins
memory
autobiographical m.
m. cell
episodic m.
m. phenomenon
recovered m.
rote m.
semantic m.
sequential m.
spatial m.
visual sequential m.
visual spatial m.
MEMR
multiple exostosis-mental retardation
MEMR syndrome
MEMS 6 TrackCap Monitor medication monitoring system
MEN
multiple endocrine neoplasia, (type I, II, III)
menacme
menadiol sodium diphosphate
menadione
Menadol
menarche
delayed m.
m. factor
isolated premature m.
premature m.
menarcheal, menarchial
MenCon vaccine
Mendel
M. first law
M. second law
mendelian
m. genetic disorder
m. inheritance
M. Inheritance in Man (MIM)
m. syndrome
m. trait
mendelizing
Mendelson syndrome
Mendenhall syndrome
Menest
Menetrier disease
Menge pessary
Mengert
M. index
M. shock syndrome

Meni-D
Ménière
M. disease
M. syndrome
M. vertigo
meningeal
m. capillary angiomatosis
m. carcinomatosis
m. fibrosis
m. irritation
m. melanocytosis
m. sign
meninges (*pl. of* meninx)
meningioma
acoustic m.
optic nerve sheath m.
perioptic m.
suprasellar m.
meningis
meningism
meningismus
meningitidis
Neisseria m.
meningitis, pl. **meningitides**
aseptic m.
bacillary m.
bacterial m.
basilar m.
Candida m.
chronic lymphocytic m.
chronic syphilitic m.
coccidioidomycosis m.
cryptococcal m.
echoviral m.
echovirus 9 m.
enteroviral m.
eosinophilic m.
experimental pneumococcal m.
exudative m.
fulminating m.
fungal m.
GBS m.
Haemophilus influenzae m.
herpes aseptic m.
herpes zoster m.
influenzal m.
leptospiral m.
Listeria m.
Lyme m.
lymphocytic m.
meningococcal m.
Mollaret m.

M

NOTES

581

meningitis *(continued)*
    neonatal m.
    nosocomial bacterial m.
    pneumococcal m.
    postnatal bacterial m.
    purulent m.
    pyogenic m.
    recurrent bacterial m.
    recurrent fungal m.
    recurrent purulent m.
    Salmonella m.
    septic m.
    serous form of tuberculous m.
    streptococcal m.
    syphilitic m.
    tuberculous m.
    viral m.
meningocele
    cranial m.
    lumbar m.
    spinal m.
meningococcal
    m. conjugate
    m. conjugate vaccine
    m. endotoxin
    m. meningitis
    m. multifocal osteomyelitis
    m. polysaccharide
    m. polysaccharide vaccine (MENps)
    m. septicemia
meningococcemia
    chronic m.
meningococcus, pl. **meningococci**
    serogroup B m.
meningoencephalitic stage
meningoencephalitis
    amebic m.
    aseptic m.
    bacterial m.
    Balamuthia m.
    enteroviral m.
    eosinophilic m.
    granulomatous amebic m.
    mumps m.
    primary amebic m.
    m. syndrome
    viral m.
meningoencephalocele
meningoencephalomyelitis
meningomyelocele
    lumbosacral m.
    sacral m.
meningooculofacial angiomatosis
meningoradiculomyelitis
    chronic m.
meningoradiculoneuritis
    lymphocytic m.
meningoulofacialis
    angiomatosis m.

meningovascular syndrome
meningoventriculitis
meninx, pl. **meninges**
meniscal injury
meniscoplasty
meniscus, pl. **menisci**
    discoid lateral m.
    m. tear
Menkes
    M. kinky hair
    M. kinky hair syndrome (MKHS)
    M. syndrome
Menkes-Kaplan syndrome
menocelis
menometrorrhagia
menopausal
    m. estrogen replacement therapy
    m. syndrome
menopause
    iatrogenic m.
    premature m.
menophania
menorrhagia
menorrhalgia
menoschesis
menostasis, menostasia, menostaxis
menotropin
menotropins
menouria
menoxenia
MENps
    meningococcal polysaccharide vaccine
    MENps vaccine
menses
    absent m.
    irregular m.
    m. phase
menstrual
    m. age
    m. aspiration
    m. blood loss
    m. colic
    m. cramps
    m. cycle hemodynamic response
    m. cycle induction
    m. cycle regulation
    m. cycle resumption
    m. disturbance
    m. edema
    m. endometrium
    m. extraction
    m. extraction abortion
    m. flow
    m. formula
    m. history
    m. irregularity
    m. leukorrhea
    m. migraine
    m. molimina

m. ovarian cycle
m. pain
m. pattern
m. period (MP)
m. phase
m. prodrome
m. reflux
m. sclerosis
m. state

menstrual-associated periodic hypersomnia
menstrual-like cramp
menstruant
menstruate
menstruation

abnormal m.
anovular m.
delayed m.
retained m.
retrograde m.
supplementary m.
suppressed m.
vicarious m.

mentagrophytes

Trichophyton m.

mental

m. age
m. arithmetic test
m. clouding
m. deficiency
m. deficiency, spasticity, congenital ichthyosis syndrome
m. development
m. development index (MDI)
m. disturbance
m. and growth retardation-amblyopia syndrome
m. handicap
m. health
m. illness
m. and physical retardation, speech disorders, peculiar facies syndrome
m. retardation
m. retardation-absent nails of hallux and pollex syndrome
m. retardation-adducted thumbs syndrome
m. retardation, aphasia, shuffling gait, adducted thumb (MASA)

m. retardation, ataxia, hypotonia, hypogonadism, retinal dystrophy syndrome
m. retardation, blepharonasofacial abnormalities, hand malformations syndrome
m. retardation-clasped thumb syndrome
m. retardation, coarse face, microcephaly, epilepsy, skeletal abnormalities syndrome
m. retardation, coarse facies, epilepsy, joint contracture syndrome
m. retardation, congenital contracture, low fingertip arches syndrome
m. retardation, congenital heart disease, blepharophimosis, blepharoptosis, hypoplastic teeth
m. retardation-distal arthrogryposis syndrome
m. retardation, dysmorphism, cerebral atrophy syndrome
m. retardation, dystonic movements, ataxia, seizures syndrome
m. retardation, epilepsy, short stature, skeletal dysplasia syndrome
m. retardation, facial anomalies, hypopituitarism, distal arthrogryposis syndrome
m. retardation, gynecomastia, obesity syndrome
m. retardation, hearing impairment, distinctive facies, skeletal anomalies syndrome
m. retardation, hip luxation, G6PD variant syndrome
m. retardation, macroorchidism syndrome
m. retardation, microcephaly, blepharochalasis syndrome
m. retardation, mitral valve prolapse, characteristic face syndrome
m. retardation, optic atrophy, deafness, seizures syndrome
m. retardation, overgrowth, craniosynostosis, distal arthrogryposis, sacral dimple, joint laxity

NOTES

M

mental *(continued)*
m. retardation-overgrowth sequence
m. retardation-overgrowth syndrome
m. retardation, polydactyly, phalangeal hypoplasia, syndactyly, unusual face, uncombable hair
m. retardation, pre- and postnatal overgrowth, remarkable face, acanthosis nigricans syndrome
m. retardation-psoriasis syndrome
m. retardation, retinopathy, microcephaly syndrome
m. retardation, scapuloperoneal muscular dystrophy, lethal cardiomyopathy syndrome
m. retardation, short stature, hypertelorism syndrome
m. retardation, short stature, obesity, hypogonadism syndrome
m. retardation, skeletal dysplasia, abducens palsy syndrome (MRSD)
m. retardation-sparse hair syndrome
m. retardation, spasticity, distal transverse limb defects syndrome
m. retardation, spastic paraplegia, palmoplantar hyperkeratosis syndrome
m. retardation, typical facies, aortic stenosis syndrome
m. scale
m. status evaluation
m. subnormality
mentalis habit
mentoanterior
left m. position (LMA)
m. position
m. presentation
right m. position (RMA)
mentoposterior
left m. position (LMP)
m. position
m. presentation
right m. position (RMP)
Mentor
M. catheter
M. female self-catheter
mentotransverse
left m. position (LMT)
m. position
right m. position (RMT)
mentum
m. anterior position
m. posterior position
m. transverse position
Mentzer index
MEP
motor evoked potential
mepenzolate bromide

meperidine hydrochloride
mephentermine
mephenytoin
mephobarbital
Mephyton Oral
mepivacaine
m. hydrochloride
m. intoxication
meprobamate
conjugated estrogen and m.
Mepron
MEPS
means-end problem solving
mepyramine
mEq
milliequivalent
mEq/L
milliequivalent per liter
MER
methanol extraction residue
meralgia paresthetica
mercaptoacetyl triglycine
2-mercaptoethane sulfonate (mesna)
mercaptoethylamine (MEA)
mercaptolactate-cysteine disulfiduria (MCDU)
mercaptopurine
6-mercaptopurine
mercaptotriglycine
Merchant view
Mercier bar
Merck respirator
mercurial diuretic
mercuric chloride
mercury-free vaccine
mercury vapor poisoning
Meritene formula
Merkel
M. cell
M. cell carcinoma
M. tactile disc
meroacrania
meroanencephaly
merocyte
merogastrula
merogenesis
merogony
diploid m.
meromelia
meromicrosomia
meropenem
merorachischisis
merosin deficiency
merozygote
Merrem I.V.
MERRF
myoclonic epilepsy with ragged red fibers

myoclonus epilepsy with ragged red
    fibers
    MERRF syndrome
Merrill program
Merrimack 1040 CO$_2$ laser
Mersilene
    M. fascial strip
    M. gauze hammock
    M. mesh
    M. mesh sling
    M. suture
Merthiolate spray
Meruvax II
merycism
Méry gland
Merzbacher-Pelizaeus disease
MES
    maximal electroshock
MESA
    microsurgical epididymal sperm
    aspiration
mesalamine
mesangial
    m. cell proliferation
    m. hypercellularity
    m. lupus nephritis
    m. proliferative glomerulonephritis
    m. sclerosis
**mesangiocapillary glomerulonephritis
    (type I, II) (MPGN)**
mesangium
mesaraic (*var. of* mesenteric)
mesaraica (*var. of* mesenterica)
mesareic (*var. of* mesenteric)
mesatipellic pelvis
mesectodermal dysplasia
mesencephalic-diencephalic junction
mesencephalic tectum
mesencephalon
mesenchymal
    m. cell
    m. hamartoma
    m. neoplasm
mesenchyme
    nonspecific m.
    portal m.
mesenchymoma
mesenteric, mesaraic, mesareic
    m. adenitis
    m. artery
    m. lymphadenitis
    m. root

m. stalk
    m. vein
mesenterica, mesaraica
    tabes m.
mesenteroaxial volvulus
mesentery
    intestinal m.
    ventral m.
mesh
    Brennen biosynthetic surgical m.
    Dexon m.
    m. erosion
    Mersilene m.
mesial
    m. temporal lobe
    m. temporal sclerosis (MTS)
mesiodens-cataracts syndrome
mesna
    2-mercaptoethane sulfonate
    mesna, Adriamycin, Ifosfamide,
        Dacarbazine (MAID)
Mesnex
mesoappendix
**mesoaxial hexadactyly-cardiac
    malformation syndrome**
mesoblast
mesoblastic nephroma
mesoblastoma
    m. ovarii
    m. vitellinum
mesocardia
mesocaval shunt
mesocephalic
mesoderm
    extraembryonic m.
    head m.
    lateral plate m.
    paraxial m.
mesodermal
    m. dysgenesis of anterior segment
    m. heterotopia
    m. sarcoma
    m. tumor
mesogaster
mesogastrium
mesolimbic dopamine tract
mesomelic
    m. dwarfism-small genitalia
        syndrome
    m. dysplasia
    m. shortening
mesometanephric carcinoma

M

NOTES

mesometric pregnancy
mesometritis
mesonephric
    m. adenocarcinoma
    m. carcinoma
    m. cyst
    m. duct
    m. rest
    m. ridge
    m. tubule
mesonephroi (*pl. of* mesonephros)
mesonephroid
    m. clear-cell carcinoma
    m. tumor
mesonephroma
mesonephros, pl. **mesonephroi**
mesoporphyrin
    tin m. (SnMP)
mesorchium
mesoridazine besylate
mesosalpingeal
mesosalpinx, pl. **mesosalpinges**
mesothelioma
    benign m. of genital tract
    malignant m. (MM)
mesothelium
    peritoneal m.
mesovarium, pl. **mesovaria**
messenger
    m. ribonucleic acid (mRNA)
    m. RNA
    second m.
Mestatin
Mestinon Oral
mestranol
    m. and norethindrone
    m. and norethynodrel
mesylate
    benztropine m.
    2-Br-alpha-ergocryptine m.
    bromocriptine m.
    deferoxamine m.
    Desferal M.
    desferrioxamine m.
    dihydroergotamine m.
    dimethothiazine m.
meta-analysis, metaanalysis
metabolic
    m. abnormality
    m. acidemia
    m. acidosis
    m. acidosis syndrome
    m. alkalosis
    m. bone disease
    m. clearance rate (MCR)
    m. disease in newborn
    m. disorder
    m. disorder with hepatic
      dysfunction

    m. disorder with neurologic
      dysfunction
    m. encephalopathy
    m. error
    m. management
    m. manifestation
    m. myopathy
    m. response
    m. syndrome X
    m. test
metabolism
    aberrant vitamin D m.
    aerobic m.
    amino acid m.
    ammonia m.
    androgen m.
    bone mineral m.
    brain m.
    carbohydrate m.
    cerebral glucose m.
    copper m.
    defective purine m.
    energy m.
    estrogen m.
    fat m.
    fetal m.
    glycolipid m.
    inborn error of m. (IEM)
    m. in intraperitoneal chemotherapy
    lipid m.
    lipoprotein-cholesterol m.
    methionine m.
    mineral m.
    neonatal m.
    organic acid m.
    partition of energy m.
    progesterone m.
    prostaglandin m.
    purine m.
    steroid m.
    vitamin m.
    water m.
metabolite
    arachidonic acid m.
    lysosomal m.
    steroid m.
metacarpal
    m. fracture
    m. shortening
metacarpophalangeal (MCP)
    m. dislocation
    m. joint
metacentric
    m. chromosome
    m. metaphase
metacercaria excyst
metachromatic
    m. cytoplasmic granule
    m. leukodystrophy (MLD)

metachromosome
metacognition
metacognitive
metacyesis
Metadate ER tablets
metaepiphysaria
    dysostosis enchondralis m.
metafemale
metagaster
metaiodobenzylguanidine (MIBG, MIGB)
metal
    m. coil
    m. intoxication
    m. metabolism disorder
    m. poisoning
    m. suture material
    trace m.
metallic
    m. bead-chain cystourethrography
    m. skin staple
metalloenzyme
metalloproteinase
    matrix m. (MMP)
    tissue inhibitors of m.
metalloprotein dimer
metamorphopsia
Metamucil Instant Mix
metamyelocyte
    m. cell
    giant m.
Metandren
metanephric
    m. blastema
    m. bud
    m. duct
metanephros, pl. metanephroi
metaphase
    m. chromosome
    metacentric m.
metaphoric dysplasia
metaphyses (pl. of metaphysis)
metaphysial
    m. anadysplasia
    m. aspiration
    m. cortex
    m. dysostosis
    m. dysplasia
    m. fibrous defect
    m. flaring
    m. fracture
    m. lesion

    m. lesion of distal femur
    m. sclerosis
metaphysial-diaphyieal angle
metaphysis, pl. metaphyses
    m. angulation
    cupped m.
    popcorn m.
    rachitic m.
    tibial m.
    widened m.
metaplasia
    agnogenic myeloid m. (AMM)
    apocrine m.
    celomic m.
    ciliated m.
    intestinal m.
    squamous m.
    squamous m. of amnion
    tubal m.
    vaginal squamous m.
metaplastic carcinoma
metaproterenol sulfate
metaraminol bitartrate
metastasis, pl. metastases
    adnexal m.
    aortic node m.
    bony m.
    fallopian tube m.
    floxuridine in hepatic m.
    hematogenous m.
    hepatic m.
    inguinal lymph node m.
    liver m.
    lymph node m.
    ovarian cancer m.
    placental m.
    pulmonary m.
    stomach cancer m.
    trocar implantation m.
    tumor, node, metastases (TNM)
    uterine sarcoma m.
    vascular m.
metastatic
    m. adenocarcinoma
    m. axillary involvement
    m. carcinoma
    m. Crohn disease (MCD)
    m. gynecologic tumor
    m. implant
    m. lesion
    m. lymphoma
    m. malignancy

M

NOTES

metastatic *(continued)*
    m. melanoma
    m. neuroblastoma
    m. tuberculous abscess
Metastron
metatarsal
    m. head osteochondritis
    m. shortening
metatarsophalangeal joint
metatarsus
    m. adductus (MA)
    m. primus varus
    rigid m.
    m. varus
metatropic
    m. dwarfism
    m. dysplasia
metencephalon
Metenier sign
metenkephalin
meter
    Airshields jaundice m.
    Astech Peak Flow M.
    glucose m.
    Health Scan Assess Plus peak
        flow m.
    LifeScan blood glucose m.
    Mini-Wright Peak Flow M.
    Parkinson-Cowan dry gas m.
    peak flow m. (PFM)
    Pocketpeak peak flow m.
    transcutaneous jaundice m.
    US 1005 uroflow m.
    Wright peak flow m.
metergoline
metformin
methacholine
    m. challenge
    m. provocation testing
methacycline hydrochloride
methadone hydrochloride
methamphetamine exposure
methandrostenolone
methanol extraction residue (MER)
methantheline bromide
methapyrilene
methaqualone
metharbital
methazolamide
methdilazine hydrochloride
methemoglobin
    m. level
    m. reduction test
methemoglobinemia
    hereditary m.
methemoglobinuria
methenamine
    m. hippurate

    m. mandelate
    m. silver stain
Methergine
methergoline
methicillin-resistant *Staphylococcus*
    aureus **(MRSA)**
methicillin sodium
methimazole
methionine
    m. malabsorption
    m. malabsorption syndrome
    m. metabolism
    m. synthase
    m. synthase deficiency
methioninemia
Methitest tablet
methixene hydrochloride
methocarbamol
method
    amniotomy plus oxytocin m.
    arithmetic m.
    Astrand 30-beat stopwatch m.
    Attwood staining m.
    barrier m.
    Bayley and Pinneau height-
        predicting m.
    Billings m.
    bone-age determination m.
    Bonnaire m.
    Bradley m.
    brine flotation m.
    bromelin m.
    Buist m.
    caloric m.
    cluster-stratified sampling m.
    Cobb m.
    cold knife m.
    contraceptive m.
    Corning m.
    CorrTest m.
    cotton swab m.
    cutdown m.
    Döderlein m.
    Douglas m.
    encu m.
    end-point dilution m.
    ensu m.
    M.'s for Epidemiology of Child
        and Adolescent Mental Disorders
        (MECA)
    Ferber m.
    Fick m.
    flush m.
    forward roll m.
    Gamper m.
    Gibson-Coke m.
    Grantley Dick-Read m.
    growth-remaining m.
    Hamilton m.

Harrison m.
hemoglobin subtype m.
Irving m.
Ito m.
Johnson m.
Kaplan-Meier m.
Kibrick m.
Kirby-Bauer m.
Kluge m.
Kristeller m.
lactational amenorrhea m. (LAM)
Lamaze m.
LAM contraceptive m.
laser m.
Leboyer m.
life table m.
Lovaas m.
Mantoux m.
manual healing m.
Marmo m.
Narula m.
oscillometric m.
per square meter m.
pilocarpine iontophoresis m.
Plastibell circumcision m.
m. of Politzer
Pomeroy m.
Prochownik m.
Puzo m.
reverse dot blot sequence-specific
  oligonucleotide m.
rhythm m.
Rodeck m.
shotgun m.
simplistic m.
Smellie m.
Smellie-Veit m.
sperm washing insemination m.
  (SWIM)
Spiegel m.
Strauss m.
Stroganoff m.
symptothermal m.
symptothermic contraceptive m.
Tanner-Whitehouse II bone/age
  determination m.
Tarkowski m.
terminal heating m.
thermodilution m.
Towako m.
twin m.
Uchida m.

Vecchietti m.
Victor Gomel m.
Video Overlay M.
Volpe m.
Wardill four-flap m.
Wardill-Kilner advancement flap m.
Watson m.
Yuzpe contraceptive m.
methodology study
**Methods for the Epidemiology of Child
  and Adolescent Disorders score**
methohexital
methotrexate (MTX)
Adriamycin, fluorouracil, m. (AFM)
m., bleomycin, doxorubicin,
  cyclophosphamide, Oncovin,
  dexamethasone (m-BACOD)
m., cisplatin, vinblastine (MCV)
cytosine arabinoside, etoposide, m.
  (CEM)
Cytoxan, Oncovin, fluorouracil plus
  Cytoxan, Oncovin, m.
  (COF/COM)
intrathecal m.
methotrimeprazine
methoxamine hydrochloride
methoxyflurane
methscopolamine
methsuximide
methyclothiazide
methyl
methylation
methylbenzethonium chloride
methylbromide
hyoscine m.
scopolamine m.
methylbutyrate
hydroxy beta m. (HMB)
methyl-CCNU
methylcellulose drops
methylcobalamin
methyl-CpG-binding protein 2 (MeCP2)
methyldopa
methylene
m. blue
m. blue dye
m. tetrahydrofolate reductase
  (MTHFR)
**methylenedioxymethamphetamine
  (MDMA)**
5,10-methylenetetrahydrofolate
methylergometrine maleate

M

NOTES

methylergonovine maleate
3-methylglutaconic aciduria
Methylin C, ER
methylmalonic
    m. acid
    m. acidemia
    m. aciduria (MMA)
methylmercury
    m. intoxication
    m. neurotoxicity
    m. toxicity
methylphenidate (MPH)
    extended-release m.
    m. hydrochloride
methylprednisolone
    m. acetate
    m. base
    pulse m.
15-methyl prostaglandin
15-methylprostaglandin $F_{2\alpha}$
α-methyl-*p*-tyrosine
methylsuccinic acid
methyltestosterone
    estrogens with m.
    m. macrobead
    Premarin with M.
    Premarin with M. Oral
methyltransferase
    thiopurine m. (TPMT)
methylxanthine
methysergide maleate
Meticorten
metoclopramide hydrochloride
metolazone
metopagus
metopic
    m. craniosynostosis
    m. ridging
Metopirone test
metopopagus
metoprolol tartrate
Metra PS procedure kit
MetraGrasp ligament grasper
MetraPass suture passer
MetraTie knot pusher
metratonia
metratrophy, metratrophia
metrectomy
Metreton Ophthalmic
metria
metritis
    postpartum m.
metrizamide
metrizoate sodium
Metrodin
metrodynamometer
metrodynia
MetroGel Topical
MetroGel-Vaginal gel

metrography
Metro I.V.
metrolymphangitis
metromalacia
metromalacoma, metromalacosis
metromenorrhagia
metronidazole vaginal gel
metroparalysis
metropathia hemorrhagica
metropathic
metropathy
metroperitoneal fistula
metroperitonitis
metrophlebitis
metroplasty
    abdominal m.
    hysteroscopic m.
    Jones wedge m.
    Strassman m.
    Tompkins m.
Metropolitan Atlanta Congenital Defects Program (MACDP)
metrorrhagia
    m. myopathica
metrorrhea
metrorrhexis
metrosalpingitis
metrosalpingography
metroscope
metrostaxis
metrostenosis
metrotomy
metyrapone test
metyrosine
Metzenbaum scissors
MeV
    megaelectron volt
MEVA
    multiplane endovaginal
    MEVA probe
    MEVA Probe for endovaginal scanning
mevalonic
    m. acidemia
    m. aciduria
mexicana
    Leishmania m.
Mexican cardiomelic dysplasia
mexiletine
Mexitil
meyeri
    Actinomyces m.
Meyer-Schwickerath and Weyers syndrome
Meyerson nevus
Mezlin
mezlocillin sodium
M.F.
    K-Phos M.F.

MFD
mandibulofacial dysostosis
MFF
Matching Familiar Figures
MFG
milk fat globule
MFGM
milk fat globule membrane
MFH
malignant fibrous histiocytoma
M-FISH
multispectral fluorescent in situ
hybridization
M-FISH cytogenetic technique
MFMU
maternal-fetal medicine unit
MFNS
mometasone furoate aqueous nasal spray
MFPR
multifetal pregnancy reduction
MFT
medial femoral torsion
mg
milligram
mg%
milligram percent
MGD
mixed gonadal dysgenesis
MgSO₄
magnesium sulfate
MH
malignant hyperthermia
MHA
microhemagglutination assay
MHA-TP
microhemagglutination assay for
antibodies to *Treponema pallidum*
MHC
major histocompatibility complex
MHC antigen
MHC class I antigen deficiency
MHP
hyperphenylalaninemia
MHz
megahertz
MI
meconium ileus
meiosis I
migration index
myocardial infarction
Miacalcin Nasal Spray
Miami Moss instrumentation

MIBE
measles inclusion body encephalitis
Mibelli
angiokeratoma of M.
M. angiokeratoma
porokeratosis of M.
MIBG
metaiodobenzylguanidine
MIBG scan
MIC
mean intercriterion correlation
minimal inhibitory concentration
minimum inhibitory concentration
MICA
microinvasive carcinoma
Micardis
Micatin
M. Topical
micdadei
Legionella m.
micelle
Michaelis-Menten dissociation constant
Michel
M. anomaly
M. aplasia
M. deformity
Michelin-tire baby syndrome
Michels syndrome
**Michigan four-wall sacrospinous
suspension**
Miconazole
M. 7 vaginal insert
miconazole
m. gel
m. nitrate
m. nitrate vaginal cream
Micral
M. Chemstrip
M. urine dipstick test
micrencephaly
MICRhoGAM
microabscess
Munro m.
microadenoma
microaerophilic
microalbuminuria
microangiopathic
m. hemolysis
m. hemolytic anemia
m. hemolytic uremic syndrome
m. process

M

NOTES

microangiopathy
>HIV m.
>mineralizing m.
>thrombotic m. (TMA)

microarousal

microaspiration

microassisted fertilization

microatelectasis

microbe

microbial
>m. factor
>m. flora
>m. sensitivity

microbiology

microbrachia

microbrachycephaly

microbubble
>gelatin-encapsulated m.

microcalcification

microcephalia (*var. of* microcephaly)

microcephalic
>m. idiocy
>m. primordial dwarfism 1
>m. primordial dwarfism-cataracts
>syndrome

microcephalus

microcephaly, microcephalia
>m., hiatus hernia, nephrotic
>syndrome
>m., hypergonadotropic
>hypogonadism, short stature
>syndrome
>m., infantile spasm, psychomotor
>retardation, nephrotic syndrome
>m., mental retardation, cataract,
>hypogonadism syndrome
>m., mental retardation, retinopathy
>syndrome
>m. mesobrachyphalangy,
>tracheoesophageal fistula
>m. microphthalmia, ectrodactyly,
>prognathism syndrome (MMEP)
>m., mild developmental delay,
>short stature, distinctive face
>syndrome
>m., mild mental retardation, short
>stature, skeletal anomalies
>syndrome
>m., muscular build, rhizomelia-
>cataracts syndrome
>primary m.
>secondary m.
>m., sparse hair, mental retardation,
>seizures syndrome

**microcephaly-calcification of cerebral
white matter syndrome**

microcephaly-cardiomyopathy syndrome

**microcephaly-cervical spine fusion
anomalies**

microcephaly-chorioretinopathy syndrome

microcephaly-deafness syndrome

microcephaly-digital anomalies syndrome

**microcephaly, oculo-digito-esophageal,
duodenal syndrome (MODED)**

microcephaly-spastic diplegia syndrome

microcirculation

microcirculatory
>m. compromise
>m. dysfunction

microcolon

microcolpohysteroscope
>Hamou m.

microcolpohysteroscopy

microcomedone

microcoria

microcornea

microcrania

microcrystalline
>griseofulvin m.

microcurettage
>Accurette m.

microcurette
>HemoCue m.

microcyst
>milk of calcium m.

microcystica

microcytic anemia

microcytosis

microdactyly

microdeletion
>chromosome m.
>m. of chromosome 22q11
>m. syndrome

microdialysis

**microdontia, microcephaly, short stature
syndrome**

microdysgenesis

microembolization

microencephaly

microendoscopic optical catheter

microendoscopy

microenvironment

microfibrillar collagen

microfilament

microflora
>fecal m.
>neonate gut m.
>vaginal m.

microfracture
>vertebral m.

microgastria

microgenitalism

Microgestin
>M. Fe 1.5/30
>M. Fe 1/29

microglandular
>m. adenosis

m. cervical hyperplasia
m. dysplasia
microglia
microglobulin
beta-2 m.
microglossia
micrognathia
severe m.
micrognathia-glossoptosis syndrome
microgram (mcg)
**microgram per kilogram per minute
(mcg/kg min, mcg/kg/min)**
microgyria
microhamartoma
biliary m.
microhemagglutination
m. assay (MHA)
m. assay for antibodies to
Treponema pallidum (MHA-TP)
m. test
microhematometra
microhyphema
Microhysteroflator
Hamou M.
microhysteroscope
Hamou contact m.
microimmunofluorescence (MIF)
m. test
microimplant
silicone m.
microinfarct
microinjection
microinvasion
stromal m.
microinvasive
m. adenocarcinoma
m. carcinoma (MICA)
m. carcinoma classification
m. cervical cancer
MicroIron II carbonyl iron
Micro-K 10 Extencaps
MicroLap
M. endoscope
M. Gold system
microlaparoscopic sterilization
microlaparoscopy
**Microline Re-New II 5-mm modular
laparoscopic scissors**
Microlipid formula
microlithiasis
biliary m.
pulmonary alveolar m.

micromanipulation
gamete m.
micromanipulator
micromazia
micromelia
micromelic dwarfism
Micro-Mist disposable nebulizer
micromyeloblastic leukemia
Micronase
microneedle
micronized
m. 17beta estradiol
m. progesterone
micronodular
m. gastritis
m. liver cirrhosis
Micronor
micronutrient deficiency
microorchidism
microorganism
micropapillomatosis labialis
microparticle enzyme immunoassay
micropenis
microperforate hymen
microphallus
m., imperforate anus,
hamartoblastoma, abnormal lung
lobulation, polydcactyly syndrome
m., imperforate anus, syndactyly,
hamartoblastoma, abnormal lung
lobulation, polydactyly (MISHAP)
**microphthalmia, microphthalmos,
microphthalmus**
m. or anophthalmos with associated
anomalies (MAA)
anterior m.
m.-arhinia
m., dermal aplasia, sclerocornea
(MIDAS)
m. with linear skin defects (MLS)
**microphthalmia-mental deficiency
syndrome**
micropinocytosis
micropodia
micropolygyria
m. with muscular dystrophy
micropreemie
microprosopus
microretrognathia
microsatellite
sequence tagged m.

M

NOTES

microscope
> H-7000 electron m.
> Optiphot-2UD m.

microscopic
> m. agglutination test (MAT)
> m. confirmation
> m. fat
> m. polyarteritis

microscopy
> dark-field m.
> direct m.
> electron m.
> light m.
> phase-contrast m.
> scanning electron m. (SEM)
> transmission electron m. (TEM)

microsomia
> hemifacial m. (HM)
> unilateral facial m.

MicroSpan
> M. microhysterescopy system
> M. sheath

microspectroscopy
> Fourier transform infrared m.

microsphere
> degradable starch m. (DSM)
> Embosphere m.
> magnetically responsive m.
> perflutren m.
> radioactive m.

microspherocyte
microspherophakia
microsporidial keratoconjunctivitis
Microsporum
> *M. audouinii*
> *M. canis*

microstomia
Microstream capnograph
Microsulfon
microsurgery
> distal tubal m.
> endoscopic m.
> laparoscopic m.
> transanal endoscopic m. (TEM)
> tubal m.
> tubocornual m.

microsurgical
> m. epididymal sperm aspiration (MESA)
> m. extraction of ductal sperm (MEDS)
> m. tubal reanastomosis (MTR)
> m. tubocornual anastomosis

microthelia
microthrombocytopenia
microthromboembolism
microti
> *Babesia m.*

microtia
> m., absent patellae, micrognathia syndrome
> aural atresia and m.
> unilateral m.

Microtip catheter
Micro-Touch Platex medical glove
MicroTrak test
Micro-Transducer catheter
microtransfusion
> maternal-fetal m.

microtrauma
microvascular
> m. complication
> m. lesion

microvasculopathy
microvesicular steatosis
microvessel
microvillus, pl. **microvilli**
> m. atrophy (MVA)
> m. inclusion disease (MID)

microviscometry
microwave endometrial ablation (MEA)
Microzide
micturition
> diurnal m.
> nocturnal m.
> m. syncope

MID
> microvillus inclusion disease

mid
> midposition

Midamor
midarm
> m. circumference (MAC)
> m. muscle circumference (MAMC)

MIDAS
> microphthalmia, dermal aplasia, sclerocornea
> MIDAS syndrome

midaxillary line
midazolam
> m. nasal spray
> transmucosal m.

midbrain
> m. abnormality
> m. herniation
> kinked m.

midclavicular line
midcycle
> m. cervical mucus
> m. spotting
> m. surge

middiastolic
> m. murmur
> m. rumble

middle
> m. adolescence
> m. cerebellar peduncle

m. cerebral artery (MCA)
m. cerebral artery occlusion (MCAO)
m. ear
m. ear effusion (MEE)
m. ear fluid (MEF)
m. ear infection
m. finger
m. hypospadias
m. meatus nasal antral window
m. sacral artery
m. third of clavicle fracture
m. third of face underdevelopment
midface hypoplasia
midfacial hypoplasia
midfetal testicular regression syndrome
midfoot breech
midforceps
m. delivery
m. maneuver
midgestational
midgut volvulus
midline
m. cleft palate
m. cleft syndrome
m. craniofacial tumor
m. episiotomy
m. facial defect
m. heart
m. incision
m. shift
m. vertical uterine extension
midluteal
m. phase progesterone level
m. progesterone measurement
Midmark 413 power female procedure chair
midmenstrual
midodrine
Midol IB
midpain
midparental height
midpelvis
midplane
midposition (mid)
m. uterus
midsecretory
midshaft hypospadias
midstream
m. catch
m. urine sample
m. urine specimen

midsystolic click
midtemporal epilepsy
midtrimester ultrasonographic evaluation
midureteral stricture
midurethra
midvaginal transverse septum
midwife, pl. **midwives**
American College of Nurse Midwives
midwifery
Licentiate in M. (LM)
Miege disease
Miescher syndrome
Mietens syndrome
Mietens-Weber syndrome
MIF
microimmunofluorescence
migration inhibitory factor
müllerian inhibiting factor
müllerian inhibitory factor
MIF test
Mifeprex
mifepristone
MIGB
metaiodobenzylguanidine
MIGB imaging
miglitol
migraine
abdominal m.
acute confusional m.
basilar artery m.
classic m.
classical m.
common m.
complicated m.
confusional m.
m. diet
familial hemiplegic m. (FHM)
footballer's m.
m. generator
m. headache
hemiplegic m.
menstrual m.
ophthalmoplegic m.
m. sine hemicrania
m. syndrome
m. variant
m. with aphasia
m. with aura
m. without aura
migraine-type headache

M

NOTES

595

migrainous
    m. attack
    m. headache
migrans
    cutaneous larva m.
    erythema m.
    erythema chronicum m. (ECM)
    larva m.
    ocular larva m.
    visceral larva m.
migration
    cellular m.
    m. index (MI)
    m. inhibitory factor (MIF)
    placental m.
migrational disorder
migratory
    m. path
    m. peripheral arthritis
    m. polyarthritis
MIH
    müllerian inhibiting hormone
MII
    meiosis II
Mikity-Wilson syndrome
Mikulicz
    M. disease
    M. procedure
    M. syndrome
mild
    m. acetabular dysplasia
    m. anemia
    m. anorexia nervosa
    m. dehydration
    m. downslant to palpebral fissure
    m. leukocytosis
    m. mental retardation
    m. pulmonic stenosis
    m. scoliosis
    m. spastic diplegic cerebral palsy
    m. ulcerative colitis
    m. X-linked recessive muscular
    dystrophy
mild-to-moderate obesity
Miles
    M. Nervine caplets
    M. syndrome
Miles-Carpenter syndrome (MCS)
milestone
    anticipated behavioral m.
    anticipated developmental m.
    behavioral m.
    cognitive developmental m.
    developmental m.
    Early Language M. (ELM)
    emotional m.
    fine motor m.
    gross motor m.
    language m.

    motor m.
    puberal m.
    social m.
    social-adaptive m.
Milex
    M. cervical cup
    M. spatula
milia (*pl. of* milium)
miliaria
    apocrine m.
    m. crystalloid
    m. profunda
    m. pustulosa
    m. rubra
    sebaceous m.
    sudoral m.
miliary
    m. calcified necrosis
    m. infiltrate
    m. sudamina
    m. tuberculosis
milieu
    endometrial m.
    m. therapy
military
    m. antishock trousers (MAST)
    m. presentation
milium, pl. **milia**
    milia neonatorum
milk
    m. abscess
    m. allergy
    atomic m.
    banked breast m.
    m. bolus obstruction
    breast m.
    m. of calcium bile
    m. of calcium microcyst
    m. cyst
    m. ejection
    m. ejection reflex
    evaporated m.
    m. fat globule (MFG)
    m. fat globule membrane (MFGM)
    m. fever
    fluorescein-labeled m.
    human m.
    hydrolyzed cow's m.
    icterogenic breast m.
    Lactaid fat free m.
    Lactaid reduced fat m.
    m. leg
    m. letdown
    m. lines
    m. lines of abdomen
    m. lines of thorax
    M. of Magnesia (MOM)
    maternal breast m.
    mother's breast m. (MBM)

nonfat m.
nuclear m.
m. precipitin disease
m. protein hydrolysate (MPH)
m. protein intolerance
m. scan
soy m.
m. stool
m. supply
m. teeth
m. triglyceride
uterine m.
volume percent of cream in m. (CRCT)
witch's m.
milk-alkali syndrome
milk-based formula
milk-fed
human m.-f.
milking of umbilical cord
milkmaid's
m. grip
m. hand
m. sign
milk-plasma ratio
milk-protein allergy
milk/soy-protein allergy
milky fluid
Millar microtransducer urethral catheter
Millen-Read modification
Miller
M. Assessment for Preschoolers
M. blade (#0, #1)
M. ovum
M. syndrome
Miller-Abbott tube
Miller-Dieker
M.-D. lissencephaly syndrome (MDLS)
M.-D. syndrome
Miller-Fisher variant of Guillain-Barré syndrome
milleri
Streptococcus m.
milliampere (mA)
milliequivalent (mEq)
m. per liter (mEq/L)
milligram (mg)
milligram percent (mg%)
millijoule (mJ)
milliliter (mL)

million
parts per m. (ppm)
Millipore filter
millirad (mrad)
milliroentgen (mR)
millivolt (mV)
mill wheel murmur
milrinone
Milroy disease
MILTA
mucosal intact laser tonsillar ablation
Miltex disposable biopsy punch
Miltown
Milwaukee brace
MIM
Mendelian Inheritance in Man
Mima polymorpha
Mi-Mark
Mi-M. disposable endocervical curette
Mi-M. endocervical curette set
Mi-M. endometrial curette set
mimetic labor
mimicry
antigenic m.
molecular m.
Mims
nevus sebaceus of Feuerstein and M.
MIMyCA
maternally inherited myopathy and cardiomyopathy
MIMyCA syndrome
Minamata disease
mind
theory of m.
mind-body intervention
mineral
m. balance study
bone m.
m. metabolism
m. oil
m. requirement
mineralization
bone tissue m.
skeletal m.
mineralizing microangiopathy
mineralocorticoid
mineralocorticoid-deficiency RTA
mineralocorticosteroid
Minesse
minicore myopathy

M

NOTES

minidose heparin
Mini-Flex
>M.-F. flexible Harris uterine
>injector
>HUI M.-F.

mini fluoroscopy
miniform
MiniGuard CO₂ sensor
minilap
>minilaparotomy

minilaparoscope
>Aslan 2 mm m.
>Pixie m.

minilaparotomy (minilap)
minima
minimal
>m. acceptable height (MAH)
>m. bacterial concentration (MBC)
>m. brain damage
>m. brain dysfunction (MBD)
>m. cerebral dysfunction
>m. change disease
>m. change nephrotic syndrome
>(MCNS)
>m. deviation adenocarcinoma
>m. effective dose (MED)
>m. inhibitory concentration (MIC)
>m. lesion nephrotic syndrome
>(MLNS)

minimal-incision pubovaginal suspension
minimally invasive surgical technique
>(MIST)

minimal-stimulation in vitro fertilization
MiniMed continuous glucose monitoring
>system
Mini-Med tubing
Minims
minimum
>m. daily requirement (MDR)
>m. inhibitory concentration (MIC)
>m. lethal dose (MLD)

MiniOX I, II, III, 100-IV oxygen
>monitor
mini-Pena procedure
minipill
Minipress
minisatellite
MiniSite laparoscope
Minitran Patch
mini Vidas automated immunoassay
>system
Mini-Wright Peak Flow Meter
Minizide
Minkowski-Chauffard syndrome
Minnesota
>M. Multiphasic Personality
>Inventory (MMPI)
>M. Multiphasic Personality
>Inventory-Adolescent (MMPI-A)

Minocin IV Injection
minocycline
minor
>m. cerebral dysfunction
>chorea m.
>m. dysmorphism
>emancipated m.
>m. group antigen incompatibility
>m. motor seizure
>pelvis m.
>thalassemia m.
>m. vestibular gland duct

minora (*pl. of* minus)
Minot disease
Minot-von Willebrand syndrome
minoxidil
Mintezol
minus, pl. **minora**
>labium m., pl. labia minora
>*Spirillum m.*

minute
>beats per m. (bpm)
>breaths per m. (bpm)
>liters per m. (L/min)
>microgram per kilogram per m.
>(mcg/kg min, mcg/kg/min)
>m. oxygen uptake
>m. ventilatory volume

minutissimum
>*Corynebacterium m.*

Miocarpine
Miochol-E
miodidymus
miopus
miosis
>congenital m.
>ipsilateral m.

Miostat
miotic division
MIP
>macrophage inflammatory protein
MIP-1 alpha
>macrophage inflammatory protein-1 alpha
>recombinant human MIP-1 alpha
mirabilis
>*Proteus m.*

Miradon
MiraLax
Miraluma test
Mircette tablet
Mirena
Mirhosseini-Holmes-Walton syndrome
mirror
>m. duplication
>m. image breast biopsy
>m. image interpretation
>m. laryngoscopy
>pharyngeal m.
>m. syndrome

mirror-image dextrocardia
MIS
    müllerian inhibiting substance
misarticulation
misbehavior
miscarriage
    missed m.
    recurrent m.
    spontaneous m.
    threatened m.
    unexplained recurrent m.
miscarry
MISHAP
    microphallus, imperforate anus,
    syndactyly, hamartoblastoma, abnormal
    lung lobulation, polydactyly
    MISHAP syndrome
mismatch
    ventilation/perfusion m.
    V̇/Q̇ m.
misonidazole
misoprostol
    oral m.
    vaginal m.
mispairing
MISS
    Modified Injury Severity Score
missed
    m. abortion
    m. labor
    m. miscarriage
    m. period
missense mutation
missing teeth
Mission
    M. Prenatal F.A.
    M. Prenatal H.P.
    M. Prenatal Rx
missionary position
MIST
    minimally invasive surgical technique
mist
    Ayr saline nasal m.
    child-adult m. (CAM)
    hood m.
    Ocean Nasal M.
    Primatene M.
    m. tent
    m. therapy
MISU
    Maternal Interview of Substance Use

mite
    dust m.
    house dust m.
    scabies m.
Mitex GII/mini anchor
Mithracin
mithramycin
mitis
    Streptococcus m.
    m. type Ehlers-Danlos syndrome
mitochondrial
    m. chromosome
    m. cytopathy
    m. deoxyribonucleic acid (mtDNA)
    m. disease
    m. DNA (mtDNA)
    m. encephalomyelopathy
    m. encephalomyelopathy, lactic
    acidosis, strokelike episodes
    m. encephalomyopathy
    m. encephalomyopathy, lactic
    acidosis, strokelike episodes
    (MELAS)
    m. encephalopathy
    m. encephalopathy, lactic acidosis,
    stroke
    m. function
    m. glycine cleavage system
    m. inheritance
    m. injury
    m. myopathy
    m. myopathy, encephalopathy, lactic
    acidosis, strokelike episodes
    m. myopathy and sideroblastic
    anemia (MLASA)
    m. oxidative phosphorylation
    m. respiratory chain defect
mitochondrion, pl. **mitochondria**
    abnormal m.
mitogen
    pokeweed m. (PWM)
mitogenic
    m. activity
    m. effect
    m. peptide
mitomycin C
mitoplasm
mitosis
    crypt cell m.
    m. phase
mitosis-promoting factor (MPF)
mitotane

M

NOTES

mitotic
- m. chromosome
- m. figure

mitoxantrone hydrochloride
mitral
- m. arcade
- m. commissurotomy
- m. regurgitation
- m. stenosis
- m. valve
- m. valve, aorta, skeleton, skin (MASS)
- m. valve atresia
- m. valve disease
- m. valve insufficiency
- m. valve prolapse (MVP)

Mitrofanoff
- M. appendicovesicotomy
- M. continent urinary diversion technique
- M. neourethral procedure
- M. principle

Mitsuda reaction
mittelschmerz
mitten
- m. hand
- m. hand deformity

Mittendorf dot
Mittendorf-Williams rule
Mityvac
- M. obstetric vacuum extractor cup
- M. reusable vacuum pump
- M. Super M cup
- M. vacuum delivery system
- M. vacuum extractor

Mivacron
mivacurium
mix
- CeraLyte drink m.
- Metamucil Instant M.
- preMA prenatal drink m.

mixed
- m. agglutination reaction (MAR)
- m. antiinflammatory syndrome (MARS)
- m. cellularity Hodgkin disease
- m. cerebral palsy
- m. connective tissue disease (MCTD)
- m. cystic/solid architecture
- m. flexor/extensor fit
- m. germ cell tumor
- m. gonadal dysgenesis (MGD)
- m. hearing impairment
- m. hearing loss
- m. hyperlipidemia
- m. hypothyroidism
- m. incontinence
- m. infantile spasm
- m. iron and folate deficiency anemia
- m. lymphocyte reaction blocking factor
- m. mesodermal sarcoma (MMS)
- m. mesodermal tumor
- m. müllerian sarcoma
- m. müllerian tumor (MMT)
- m. obstructive apnea/hypopnea index (MOAHI)
- m. ovarian mesodermal sarcoma
- m. pattern
- m. porphyria
- m. receptive-expressive language disorder (MRELD)
- m. sclerosing bone dysplasia, small stature, seizures, mental retardation syndrome
- m. sensory polyneuritis
- m. sleep apnea
- m. umbilical arterial acidemia
- m. uterine tumor
- m. venous oxygen content

mixed-density mass
mixed-type cerebral palsy
mixing lesion
mixoploid
mixoploidy
- diploid/tetraploid m.
- diploid/triploid m.

Mixtard
Miya hook ligature carrier
Miyazaki-Bonney test for stress incontinence
Miyazaki technique
mizoribine
mJ
- millijoule

MKHS
- Menkes kinky hair syndrome

ML
- mucolipidosis

mL
- milliliter

ML-II
- mucolipidosis II

ML-III
- mucolipidosis III

MLASA
- mitochondrial myopathy and sideroblastic anemia
  - MLASA syndrome

MLD
- metachromatic leukodystrophy
- minimum lethal dose
  - juvenile MLD
  - late infantile MLD

MLNS
  minimal lesion nephrotic syndrome
  mucocutaneous lymph node syndrome
MLS
  microphthalmia with linear skin defects
MLU
  mean length of utterance
MLUm
  mean length of utterance in morphemes
MM
  malignant mesothelioma
    MM band
10-mm umbilical port
MMI
  maternal meiosis I
MMII
  maternal meiosis II
MMA
  methylmalonic aciduria
MMEP
  microcephaly, microphthalmia,
    ectrodactyly, prognathism syndrome
    MMEP syndrome
MMIH
  megacystis, microcolon, intestinal
    hypoperistalsis
    MMIH syndrome
MMK
  Marshall-Marchetti-Krantz
    MMK procedure
MMMM
  megalocornea, macrocephaly, mental and
    motor retardation syndrome
MMMT
  malignant mixed müllerian tumor
M-mode
    M.-m. display
    M.-m. echocardiogram
    M.-m. echocardiography
    M.-m. echogram
    M.-m. imaging
    M.-m. ultrasound
MMP
  matrix metalloproteinase
MMPI
  Minnesota Multiphasic Personality
    Inventory
MMPI-A
  Minnesota Multiphasic Personality
    Inventory-Adolescent
MMR
  measles, mumps, rubella

  megalocornea-mental retardation
    syndrome
    MMR II vaccine
    MMR immunization
MMS
  mixed mesodermal sarcoma
5-mm suprapubic trocar
MMT
  mixed müllerian tumor
  MMT syndrome
    MMT syndrome (MMT)
MNBCC
  multiple nevoid-basal cell carcinoma
    MNBCC syndrome
M-O
  Haley's M-O
MOAHI
  mixed obstructive apnea/hypopnea index
Moban
Mobenol
Mobidin
mobile hyperechogenic material
mobility
    m. aid
    bladder neck m.
    m. disability
    Q-tip test for determining
      urethral m.
    m. specialist
mobilization
    gastric m.
    tarsometatarsal m.
Mobiluncus
    M. mulieris
    M. vaginitis
Mobitz I, II block
Möbius, Moebius
    M. anomaly
    M. sequence
    M. syndrome
modafinil acetamide
modality
Modane Bulk
mode
    delivery m.
    multiplanar display m.
    polygenic m.
    pressure support m.
    transparency m.
Modecate

NOTES

MODED
microcephaly, oculo-digito-esophageal, duodenal syndrome
model
APLS m.
cognitive-diathesis m.
Cox proportional hazard m.
Gail breast cancer m.
genetic m.
Gesell Developmental M.
pathological m.
random regression m.
Rossavik growth m.
M. 5315 sequential compression device
statistical m.
modeling
generalized linear interactive m. (GLIM)
moderate
m. dehydration
m. hirsutism
m. mental retardation
m. ulcerative colitis
modern genetics
Modicon
modification
behavior m.
Burch m.
Gesell test with Knobloch m.
Martin m.
Millen-Read m.
posttranslational m.
modified
m. Bagshawe protocol (MBP)
m. barium swallow (MBS)
m. barium swallow with videofluoroscopy
m. Beighton criteria
m. biophysical profile (MBPP)
m. Blalock-Taussig shunt
m. bovine surfactant extract
m. BPP
m. Burch colpourethropexy
m. Dieterle stain
m. Fontan operation
m. Fontan procedure
m. Gomori trichrome reaction
m. Ham F-10 solution
M. Injury Severity Score (MISS)
m. Irving-type tubal ligation
m. Kinyoun acid-fast stain
m. measles
m. Pomeroy tubal ligation technique
m. radical hysterectomy
m. radical mastectomy
m. Ritgen maneuver
m. Roeder

m. Roeder knot
m. sling
m. trichrome stain
m. Zavanelli maneuver
modifier
biologic response m. (BRM)
Moditen
MODS
multiorgan dysfunction syndrome
multiple organ dysfunction syndrome
Moducal formula
modulation
antigenic m.
cardiac autonomic m.
sex steroid m.
modulator
benzothiophene-derived selective estrogen receptor m.
cytokine m.
selective estrogen receptor m. (SERM)
triphenylethylene selective estrogen receptor m.
MODY
maturity-onset diabetes of the young
maturity-onset diabetes of youth
Moebius (*var. of* Möbius)
Moeller-Barlow disease
mofetil
mycophenolate m.
Mogen
M. circumcision
M. clamp
Mohr-Claussen syndrome
Mohr syndrome
Mohr-Tranebjaerg syndrome (MTS)
MOI
maximal oxygen intake
medical optimal imaging
multiplicity of infection
moiety, pl. **moieties**
moist
Nasal M.
moisture
vaginal m.
moisturizer
Vagisil intimate m.
molar
m. degeneration
m. destruens
m. evacuation
first permanent m.
first primary m.
hutchinsonian m.
Moon m.'s
mulberry m.
permanent m.
m. pregnancy
primary m.

second permanent m.
second primary m.
third permanent m.

mold
Counsellor vaginal m.
m. spore

molding of head

mole
amniography in hydatidiform m.
blood m.
Breus m.
carneous m.
complete hydatidiform m.
cystic m.
false m.
fleshy m.
grape m.
hydatid m.
hydatidiform m.
invasive hydatidiform m.
partial hydatidiform m.
prior complete m.
prior partial m.
repeated complete m.
tuberous m.
vesicular m.

molecular
m. adsorbent recirculating system (MARS)
m. clone
m. genetic analysis
m. genetic study
m. genetic technique
m. mimicry
m. regulation

molecule
adhesion m.
cell adhesion m. (CAM)
inflammatory m.
intercellular adhesion m. 1 (ICAM1)
vascular cell adhesion m. (VCAM)

molestation
sexual m.

molimina
menstrual m.

molindone

Mol-Iron

Moll
apocrine gland of M.
M. gland

Mollaret meningitis
Mollica-Pavone-Anterer syndrome
Mollica syndrome
Mollifene Ear Wax Removing Formula
Mollison formula

molluscum
m. contagiosum
m. contagiosum virus (MCV)
m. contagiosum of the vulva
m. fibrosum
m. fibrosum gravidarum
m. fibrosum pendulum
Staphylococcus aureus m.

molybdenum
m. cofactor
m. cofactor deficiency (MCD)
m. rotating anode x-ray tube

Molypen

MOM
Milk of Magnesia
mucoid otitis media

MoM
multiples of the appropriate gestational median

mometasone
m. furoate
m. furoate aqueous nasal spray (MFNS)

MOMO
macrosomia, obesity, macrocephaly, ocular abnormality
MOMO syndrome

MOMP gene

MOMX
macroorchidism-marker X
MOMX syndrome

Monafed
Monaghan respirator
monarticular arthritis
Monday morning colic
Mondini
M. anomaly
M. aplasia

Mondor disease

mongolian
m. idiot
m. spot

mongolism

mongoloid
m. features
m. slant

NOTES

603

monilethrix
> sex-linked neurodegenerative disease with m.

Monilia
monilia
monilial
> m. diaper dermatitis
> m. diaper rash
> m. esophagitis
> m. vaginitis

moniliasis
> oral m.

moniliform hair
moniliformis
> *Streptobacillus m.*

Monistat
> M. 1 Combination Pack vaginal insert
> M. 1 1-day vaginal ointment
> M. Dual-Pak
> M. I.V.
> M. Vaginal
> M. 3 vaginal cream
> M. 3 vaginal cream combination pack
> M. 3 vaginal suppository

Monistat-Derm Topical
monitor
> Accu-Chek Easy glucose m.
> Accu-Chek II Freedom blood glucose m.
> Aequitron 9200 apnea m.
> antepartum m.
> apnea m.
> Arvee model 2400 infant apnea m.
> Baby Dopplex 3000 antepartum fetal m.
> Baby Sense m.
> BASC m.
> Bear NUM-1 tidal volume m.
> Behavior Assessment System for Children m.
> blood pressure m.
> CA m.
> Camino m.
> cardiac-apnea m.
> cardiac event m.
> cardiorespiratory m.
> cerebral function m. (CFM)
> ClearPlan Easy fertility m.
> Corometrics fetal m.
> Corometrics 118 maternal/fetal m.
> Cue Fertility M.
> Dinamap blood pressure m.
> EdenTec 2000W in-home cardiorespiratory m.
> Endotek OM-3 Urodata m.
> Endotek UDS-1000 m.
> event m.

> Fetal Dopplex m.
> fetal heart rate m.
> FetalPulse Plus m.
> Fetasonde fetal m.
> Finapres blood pressure m.
> Healthdyne apnea m.
> Holter m.
> home cardiorespiratory m. (HCRM)
> home uterine activity m. (HUAM)
> Imex antepartum m.
> intrapartum m.
> Ladd m.
> Masimo SET home m.
> MiniOX I, II, III, 100-IV oxygen m.
> Nellcor N-499 fetal oxygen saturation m.
> Nellcor N-200 home m.
> Nellcor N-3000 home m.
> Nellcor Puritan Bennett home m.
> Nellcor Puritan Bennett oxygen saturation m.
> neonatal m.
> Neo-trak 515A neonatal m.
> Neotrend premature infant blood gas/temperature m.
> Omron m.
> Oxisensor fetal oxygen saturation m.
> peak flow meter m.
> Pocket-Dop 3 m.
> Press-Mate model 8800T blood pressure m.
> ProDynamic m.
> Profilomat m.
> Propaq Encore vital signs m.
> QuietTrak m.
> Quik Connect fetal m.
> Toitu MT-810 cardiographic m.
> Tokos m.
> transcutaneous blood gas m.
> uterine activity m.
> VersaLab APM2 portable antepartum m.
> virtual labor m. (VLM)
> VitaGuard m.

monitored anesthesia care
monitoring
> ambulatory m.
> ambulatory blood pressure m. (ABPM)
> ambulatory urodynamic m. (AUM)
> beat-to-beat continuous blood pressure m.
> blood sugar m.
> cardiac m.
> continuous blood gas m.
> continuous fetal heart m.
> continuous long-term m. (CLTM)

critical care m.
distal esophageal pH m.
domiciliary m.
EEG/polygraphic/video m.
electronic fetal m. (EFM)
electronic fetal heart rate m.
end-tidal CO_2 m.
external fetal m. (EFM)
fetal heart rate m.
fetal oximetry m.
fetal scalp m.
glucose m.
heart rate m.
hemodynamic m.
home blood glucose m.
home uterine m. (HUM)
home uterine activity m. (HUAM)
ICP m.
inpatient m.
internal m.
intracranial pressure m.
intrapartum fetal m.
intrauterine fetal m.
invasive hemodynamic m.
jugular bulb m.
prolonged EEG m.
pulmonary artery pressure m.
Series 50 XMO fetal/maternal
  monitor with integrated fetal
  oxygen saturation m.
tactile sensory m.
telefetal m.
tissue pH m.
transcutaneous blood gas m.
transcutaneous oxygen tension m.
transtelephonic m. (TTM)
video m.
monitrice
monkeybars
monkey polyoma virus
mono
  mononucleosis
monoamine (MAO)
  m. oxidase
  m. oxidase A deficiency
  m. oxidase inhibitor (MAOI)
  m. oxidase type A (MAOA)
monoaminergic
monoamnionicity
monoamniotic
  m. sac
  m. twins

monoarticular synovitis
monobactam
monobrachius
monocaprin
monocephalus
monochorial twins
monochorionic
  m. gestation
  m. monoamniotic placenta
  m. placentation
  m. twin pregnancy
  m. twins
monochorionic-diamniotic
  m.-d. gestation
  m.-d. placenta
  m.-d. twins
monochromatism
  blue cone m.
  pi cone m.
Monoclate-P
monoclonal
  m. antibody (MAb)
  m. antibody coagglutination test
  m. antibody therapy
  m. antiendotoxin antibody
  m. anti-IgE antibody
monoclonic seizure
monocranius
Monocryl suture
monocular
  m. diplopia
  m. nystagmus
monocyte
monocytogenes
  Listeria m.
monocytopenia
monocytosis
monodactyly
monodermal tumor
Monodox
monoecious
monofactorial inheritance
monofluorophosphate
monogamous
monogamy
monogenic disorder
Mono-Gesic
monoglutamate
monohybrid cross
monohydrate
  cefadroxil m.
  doxycycline m.

M

NOTES

monohydrate *(continued)*
    lactose m.
    m. macrocrystal
    nitrofurantoin m.
monokine
monolaurin
monomelic
monomorphous papular eruption
mononeuritis, pl. **mononeuritides**
    m. multiplex
    m. with paralysis
mononeuropathy
    multiple m.'s
    peripheral m.
Mononine
mononuclear
    m. phagocyte
    m. pleocytosis
mononucleosis (mono)
    infectious m. (IM)
mononucleosis-type syndrome
4-monooxygenase
    phenylalanine 4-m.
monophasic
    m. oral contraceptive
    m. regimen
monophonic wheeze
monophosphate
    adenosine m. (AMP)
    cyclic adenosine m. (cAMP)
    cyclic guanosine m. (cGMP)
    cytidine m.
monoplegia
    spastic m.
monoploid
monopodia
monopolar cautery
monops
monopus
monorchidic
monosialoganglioside
monosodium glutamate poisoning
monosome
monosomy
    m. 1–22
    autosomal m.
    chromosome 1p–22p m.
    chromosome 1q–22q m.
    chromosome Xp21 m.
    chromosome Xq m.
    m. G
    m. G syndrome
    partial m. 1p–22p
    partial m. Xp21, Xp22
    partial m. Xq
    m. 1p–22p
    m. 1p36 syndrome
    m. 11q23
    m. 22q13,3 deletion syndrome

    m. 7 syndrome
    m. X
    m. Xp21
    m. Xp22
    m. Xq
Monospot
    M. screen
    M. test
Monosticon
    M. Dri-Dot
    M. Dri-Dot test
monostotic
Mono-Sure
monosymptomatic delusional
  pseudocyesis
Mono-Test
monotherapy
    digoxin m.
    zidovudine m.
monotonically
monotropins for injection
Mono-Vacc Test (O.T.)
monovular twins
monoxide
    carbon m. (CO)
    end-tidal breath carbon m.
monozygosity
monozygotic twins
monozygous
Monro
    foramen of M.
Monro-Kellie doctrine of intracranial
  pressure
mons
    m. pubis
    m. veneris
Monsel
    M. gel
    M. paste
    M. solution
monsplasty
monster
    m. cell
    hair m.
monstrosity
Montefiore syndrome
Monteggia
    M. fracture
    M. fracture dislocation
montelukast
Montenegro skin test
Montgomery
    M. County virus
    M. gland
    M. strap
    M. tubercle
month
    Lupron Depot-3 M.
    Lupron Depot-4 M.

Monurol
mood
 m. disorder
 dysphoric m.
 m. fluctuation
 m. lability
 m. state
mood-congruent psychotic feature
moodiness
Moon
moon
 m. facies
 M. molars
 M. teeth
moon-shaped facies
Moore-Federman syndrome
MOPP
 mechlorethamine, Oncovin (vincristine),
  procarbazine, prednisone
 MOPP chemotherapy protocol
Morand foot
Moraxella catarrhalis
morbidity
 antenatal m.
 asthma m.
 childbirth-related m.
 febrile m.
 fetal m.
 infant m.
 maternal febrile m.
 neonatal m.
 perinatal m.
 postpartum febrile m.
 m. predictor
 puerperal febrile m.
morbilliform
 m. eruption
 m. skin rash
Morbillivirus
morbillorum
 Gemella m.
morbus Down
morcellation
 electromechanical m.
 m. operation
 uterine m.
 vaginal m.
morcellator
 Diva laparoscopic m.
 motorized m.
 OPERA Star m.
 Steiner electromechanical m.

morcellize, morselize
Morch respirator
More-Dophilus acidophilus powder
Morel ear
Morgagni
 anterior retrosternal hernia of M.
 foramen of M.
 M. hernia
 hydatid cyst of M.
 M. tubercle
Morgagni-Adams-Stokes syndrome
morgagnian
Morgagni-Turner-Albright syndrome
Morgagni-Turner syndrome
Morganella morganii
morganii
 Morganella m.
 Proteus m.
Morgan therapeutic lens
moribund
moricizine
Morison pouch
morning
 m. glory disc anomaly
 m. glory syndrome
 m. osmolality
 m. sickness
morning-after
 m.-a. contraception
 m.-a. pill
Moro
 M. reflex
 M. response
Moro-Heisler diet
morphea
morpheme
 mean length of utterance in m.'s
  (MLUm)
morphine
 epidural m.
 m. sulfate
morphogen
morphogenesis
 branching m.
 lung m.
 parenchymal lung m.
morphogenetic lesion
morphologic
 m. assessment
 m. data

M

NOTES

morphological
    m. characteristic
    m. sex
morphology
    adrenal gland m.
    endometrial m.
    kidney m.
morphometric
morphometrics
    body m.
Morquio
    M. disease
    M. syndrome
Morquio-Brailsford
    M.-B. disease
    M.-B. syndrome
Morquio-Ullrich
    M.-U. disease
    M.-U. syndrome
Morrow
    M. myotomy-myectomy
    M. procedure
morselize (*var. of* morcellize)
mortality
    anesthesia-related maternal m.
    m. data
    fetal m.
    high altitude perinatal m.
    infant m.
    maternal m.
    neonatal m.
    Pediatric Risk of M. (PRISM)
    perinatal m.
    postneonatal m.
    m. predictor
    prenatal m.
    m. rate
    reproductive m.
    m. risk factor
mortiferum
    Fusobacterium m.
mortise view
morula
MOS
    medical optical spectroscopy
mosaic
    m. aneuploidy
    gene m.
    m. pattern
    m. perfusion
    m. tetrasomy 8p syndrome
    m. translocation
    m. trisomy 14
    Turner m.
    m. Turner syndrome
    m. verruca
mosaicism
    chromosomal m.
    erythrocyte m.

    germ cell m.
    germ line m.
    gonadal m.
    low-grade m.
    placental m.
    somatic m.
    trisomy 8 m.
    Turner m.
    m. for XXX
    45,X/46,XY m.
Moschcowitz
    M. fashion
    M. procedure
Moschowitz
MOSF
    multiple organ system failure
***mos* protooncogene**
Moss
    M. classification
    M. tube
mossy fiber sprouting
mothball
    naphthalene m.
mother
    M.'s Against Drunk Driving
      (MADD)
    m. and baby endoscope
    m. burnout
    diabetic m.
    Du-positive m.
    gestational m.
    high-risk m.
    hysterical m.
    infant of diabetic m. (IDM)
    infant of substance-abusing m.
      (ISAM)
    Rh-negative m.
    rubella-immune m.
    rubella-negative m.
    serology-negative m.
    surrogate m.
    m. wort
Mother2Be
    M. breast nourishing cream
    M. nipple restoration cream
mother-child interaction
motherese speech
motherhood
    surrogate gestational m.
mother-infant
    m.-i. bonding
    m.-i. transmission
mother's
    m. breast milk (MBM)
**Mothers Against Drunk Driving
(MADD)**
moth patch
motif
motile sperm

motilin receptor agonist
motility
>altered gastric m.
decreased gastrointestinal m.
m. disorder
gut m.
intestinal m.
ocular m.
receptor for hyaluronan-mediated m.
(RHAMM)
sperm m.

motility-related dysphagia
motion
>active range of m. (AROM)
m. artifact rejection system
(MARS)
chest wall m.
early cardiac m.
embryonic heart m. (EHM)
fetal cardiac m.
limb m.
limited neck m.
paradoxical chest wall m.
passive range of m.
range of m. (ROM)
scapulothoracic m.
m. sickness

motion-resistant pulse oximetry
motoneuron
motor
>m. automatism
m. control
m. cortex
m. disability
m. evoked potential (MEP)
fine m.
gross m.
m. hyperactivity
m. milestone
m. nerve
m. neuron
m. neuron disease
m. neuron palsy
m. neuron sign
oral m.
m. pattern
m. perception
m. perception dysfunction
m. planning
m. restlessness
m. scale
m. seizure

>m. sensory neuropathy (MSN)
m. skill
m. tic

motor-axonal neuropathy
motorized morcellator
motor-sensory
>m.-s. axonal neuropathy (MSN)
m.-s. neuropathy, X-linked type II,
with deafness and mental
retardation

Motrin
>Children's M.
Ibu-Tab Junior Strength M.
Junior Strength M.

MOTT
>mycobacteria other than tuberculosis

mottled
>m. enamel
m. retina

mottling of skin
mount
>chest m.
direct wet m.
wet m.

mountain sickness
mouse
>peritoneal m.

mousse
>Rid M.

mouth
>m. breathing
carp m.
carp-like m.
downturned m.
fish-shaped m.
m. guard
inverted-V m.
open m.
purse-string m.
tapir m.
trench m.

Mouth-Aid
>Orajel M.-A.

mouth-and-hand synkinesia
mouthing
mouthpiece
mouth-to-mask breathing
mouth-to-mouth resuscitation
mouth-to-nose/mouth resuscitation
mouthwash
>magic m.

Movat stain

NOTES

M

609

movement
    adventitious choreiform m.
    angular m.
    athetoid m.
    bicycling m.
    cardinal m.
    chaotic eye m.
    choreic m.
    choreiform m.
    choreoathetoid m.
    choreoathetotic m.
    circumduction m.
    clonic m.
    compensatory m.
    dancing eye m.
    deviant volitional m.
    dissociated m.
    equal ocular m. (EOM)
    extraocular m. (EOM)
    extrapyramidal m.
    eye m.
    fetal body m.
    fetal breathing m. (FBM)
    gliding m.
    hand-to-mouth m.
    hand-wringing m.
    involuntary m.
    irregular stereotyped m.
    multifocal clonic m.
    nonrapid eye m. (NREM)
    opposition m.
    pedaling m.
    rapid alternating m.
    rapid eye m. (REM)
    rapid succession m.
    reciprocal m.
    respiratory m.
    rotation m.
    sleep with rapid eye m.
    sound-stimulated fetal m.
    stereotypical m.
    swimming m.
    symmetrical m.
    tonic-clonic m.'s
    unifocal clonic m.
    vibroacoustic-induced fetal m.
    volitional m.
moxa herb
moxalactam disodium
moxibustion
moyamoya
    m. disease
    m. syndrome
Moynahan alopecia syndrome
Moynihan
    M. respirator
    M. syndrome
Mozart ear

MP
    menstrual period
MPA
    medroxyprogesterone acetate
MPF
    maturation-promoting factor
    mitosis-promoting factor
MPGN
    membranoproliferative
      glomerulonephritis
    mesangiocapillary glomerulonephritis
      (type I, II)
MPH
    male pseudohermaphroditism
    methylphenidate
    milk protein hydrolysate
M-phase-promoting factor
MPHD
    multiple pituitary hormone deficiency
MPIAS
    multiparameter intraarterial sensor
MPO
    myeloperoxidase
      MPO deficiency
MPQ
    Multidimensional Personality
      Questionnaire
MPR
    multifetal pregnancy reduction
    multiple pregnancy reduction
MPS
    mucopolysaccharide
    mucopolysaccharidosis
    myofascial pain syndrome
      MPS I
      MPS II
        mucopolysaccharide
        mucopolysaccharidosis
        myofascial pain syndrome
      MPS III
      MPS IV
      MPS VI
      MPS VII
        mucopolysaccharide
        mucopolysaccharidosis
        myofascial pain syndrome
MPT
    multipuncture test
MPV
    mean platelet volume
MR
    medial rotation
mR
    milliroentgen
MRA
    magnetic resonance angiography
mrad
    millirad

MRC
  magnetic resonance cholangiography
MRCP
  magnetic resonance
    cholangiopancreatography
    MRCP using HASTE with a
      phased array coil
MRE
  magnetic resonance elastography
MRELD
  mixed receptive-expressive language
    disorder
MRI
  magnetic resonance imaging
    diffuse tensor brain MRI
    functional MRI (fMRI)
    GRASS MRI
    ^{31}P MRI
    Siemens Vision MRI
    ultrafast MRI
MRM
  magnetic resonance mammography
mRNA
  messenger ribonucleic acid
    posttranslational modification of
      mRNA
MRS
  magnetic resonance spectroscopy
    phosphorus MRS
    proton MRS
MRSA
  methicillin-resistant *Staphylococcus*
    aureus
MRSD
  mental retardation, skeletal dysplasia,
    abducens palsy syndrome
MRU
  magnetic resonance urography
MRX
  X-linked mental retardation (1-47)
MRXA
  X-linked mental retardation-aphasia
    syndrome
MRXS1–6
  X-linked mental retardation syndrome
    1–6
MS
  mass spectrometry
  multiple sclerosis
    acute MS
    MS Contin
    MS Contin Oral

MSAF
  meconium-stained amniotic fluid
MSAFP
  maternal serum alpha fetoprotein
MSBP
  Münchausen syndrome by proxy
MSD
  multiple sulfatase deficiency
    MSD Enteric Coated ASA
MSEL
  Mullen Scales of Early Learning
MSI
  magnetic source imaging
MSIR Oral
MSK
  musculoskeletal
MSLSS
  Multidimensional Student Life
    Satisfaction Scale
MSLT
  Multiple Sleep Latency Test
MSN
  motor-sensory axonal neuropathy
  motor sensory neuropathy
    MSN syndrome
MSP
  Münchausen syndrome by proxy
MSPS
  musculoskeletal pain syndrome
MSPSS
  Multidimensional Scale of Perceived
    Social Support
MSS
  Marshall-Smith syndrome
MSSB
  MacArthur Story Stem Battery
MST
  multiple subpial transection
  multisystemic therapy
MSUD
  maple syrup urine disease
3M syndrome
MT
    Pancrease MT
MTC
  multilocular thymic cyst
mtDNA
  mitochondrial deoxyribonucleic acid
  mitochondrial DNA
M.T.E.-4, -5, -6
MTHFR
  methylene tetrahydrofolate reductase

NOTES

M

MTHFR *(continued)*
  MTHFR gene
  MTHFR thermolability
MTMX
  X-linked myotubular myopathy
MTR
  microsurgical tubal reanastomosis
M-tropic strain
MTS
  mesial temporal sclerosis
  Mohr-Tranebjaerg syndrome
MTT
  medial tibial torsion
MTX
  methotrexate
M-type extractor
Mucat
  M. cervical sampling
  M. cervical sampling device
Mucha-Habermann disease
mucin clot test
mucinous
  m. cancer
  m. carcinoma
  m. cystadenocarcinoma
  m. cystadenoma
  m. ovarian neoplasm
  m. tumor
mucociliary
  m. clearance
  m. function
mucocolpos
mucocutaneous
  m. bleeding
  m. candidiasis
  m. candidosis
  m. junction
  m. leishmaniasis
  m. lymph node
  m. lymph node syndrome (MCLS, MLNS)
  m. pigmentation
  m. ulcer
mucoepidermoid carcinoma
Muco-Fen-LA
mucoid
  m. myoma degeneration
  m. otitis media (MOM)
  m. sputum
mucolipidosis (ML)
  m. II (ML-II)
  m. III (ML-III)
mucolytic
Mucomyst
Mucomyst solution
mucopeptide
mucoperichondrium
mucopolysaccharide (MPS II, MPS, MPS VII)

  aggregated m.
  m. pattern
  m. protein
  m. storage disease (I–VIII)
  urine m.
mucopolysaccharidosis,
  pl. mucopolysaccharidoses (MPS II, MPS, MPS VII)
  beta-glucuronidase deficiency m.
  m. F
  focal m.
  m. II
  m. I, IH, IH/s, IS
  m. IIIA, B, C, D
  m. IVA, B
  m. unclassified types
  m. V-VIII
mucoprotein
  Tamm-Horsfall m.
mucopurulent cervicitis
mucopus
Mucor
mucormycosis
  cutaneous m.
  pulmonary m.
  rhinocerebral m.
mucorrhea
  cervical m.
mucosa
  atrophic vaginal m.
  buccal m.
  cervical m.
  ectopic gastric m.
  endocervical m.
  estrogenized m.
  gastric m.
  genital m.
  intestinal m.
  necrotic m.
  palatal m.
  rugated vaginal m.
  thin vaginal m.
  unestrogenized vaginal m.
  vaginal m.
mucosa-associated lymphoid tissue (MALT)
mucosae
  hyalinosis cutis et m.
mucosal
  m. biopsy
  m. bleeding
  m. ganglioneuromatosis
  m. intact laser tonsillar ablation (MILTA)
  m. leishmaniasis
  m. lesion
  m. neuroma syndrome
  m. rosette

m. sloughing
m. transudate
mucosalis
   Campylobacter m.
Mucosil
mucositis
mucosotropic
mucosulfatidosis
mucous
m. discharge
m. inspissation
m. membrane
m. membrane provocation
m. membrane wart
m. patch
m. plug
m. plugging
m. retention cyst
mucoviscidosis
MUCP
maximum urethral closure pressure
mucus
m. aspirator
cervical m.
m. extractor
inspissated m.
midcycle cervical m.
ovulatory m.
m. plug
mu dimeric protein
Mueller (*var. of* Müller)
muffled heart sound
MUGA
multiple gated acquisition
MUGA scan
mulberry
m. molar
m. ovary
m. tumor
mulibrey
muscle, liver, brain, eye
mulibrey nanism
mulibrey nanism or dwarfism
mulieris
Mullen Scales of Early Learning (MSEL)
Müller, Mueller
M. syndrome
M. tubercle
Müller-Hillis maneuver
müllerian
m. abnormality

m. adenosarcoma
m. agenesis
m. cyst
m. duct
m. duct anomaly
m. duct aplasia, renal agenesis/ectopia, cervical somite dysplasia (MURCS)
m. duct aplasia, unilateral renalagenesis, and cervicothoracic somite abnormalities
m. duct fusion
m. duct inhibitory factor
m. dysgenesis
m. fusion defect
m. hypoplasia
m. inhibiting factor (MIF)
m. inhibiting hormone (MIH)
m. inhibiting substance (MIS)
m. inhibitory factor (MIF)
m. tumor
Mullins long transseptal sheath
MultArray light
multicelled embryo
Multicenter AIDS Cohort Study (MACS)
multicentric
m. carcinoma
m. Castleman disease
m. lower genital tract neoplasia
multichannel
m. cystometrogram
M. discrete analyzer (MDA)
m. recorder
multicolor FISH cytogenetic technique
multicore myopathy
multicystic
m. dysplastic kidney (MDK)
m. encephalomalacia
m. kidney
m. kidney disease
m. renal dysplasia
Multidex gel
multidimensional
M. Personality Questionnaire (MPQ)
M. Scale of Perceived Social Support (MSPSS)
M. Student Life Satisfaction Scale (MSLSS)
multidisciplinary team
multidose activated charcoal (MDAC)

NOTES

multidrug
    m. chemotherapy
    m. resistance (MDR)
    m. therapy (MDT)
multidrug-resistant tuberculosis (MDR-TB)
multielectrode
    ESA Coulochem m.
multifactorial
    m. disorder
    m. inheritance
    m. trait
multifetal
    m. gestation
    m. pregnancy
    m. pregnancy reduction (MFPR, MPR)
multifetation
multifocal
    m. atrial tachycardia
    m. clonic convulsion
    m. clonic movement
    m. clonic seizure
    m. leukoencephalopathy
    m. osteomyelitis
    m. spike
    m. white matter inflammatory lesion
multifollicular ovary
multiforme
    bullous erythema m.
    erythema m. (EM)
    glioblastoma m.
multigenerational
multigenic disorder
multigravida
multihandicapped
Multiload Cu-375 intrauterine device
multiloba
    placenta m.
multilocal genetics
multilocular
    m. cyst
    m. thymic cyst (MTC)
multilocularis
    Echinococcus m.
multilocular thymic cyst (MTC)
multiloculated cyst
multimammae
multimodal treatment plan
multinuclearity
    hereditary erythroblastic m.
multinucleate
multinucleated
    m. cell encephalitis
    m. giant cell
multinucleation parakeratosis
multiorgan
    m. dysfunction syndrome (MODS)

    m. system failure
    m. thrombosis
Multi-Pak-4
multipara
    grand m.
    great-grand m.
multiparameter intraarterial sensor (MPIAS)
multiparity
    grand m.
multiparous
multiplanar display mode
multiplane
    m. endovaginal (MEVA)
    m. intracavitary probe
multiple
    m. acyl-coenzyme A dehydrogenase deficiency (MADD)
    m. alleles
    m.'s of the appropriate gestational median (MoM)
    m. arbitrary amplicon profiling (MAAP)
    m. articular contracture
    m. articular rigidity
    m. basal cell carcinoma syndrome
    multiple basal cell nevus syndrome
    m. basal cell nevoid syndrome
    m. benign circumferential skin creases on limbs
    m. births
    m. bone enchondromata
    m. carboxylase deficiency
    m. cartilaginous exostoses
    m. cervix
    m. complex developmental disorder (MCDD)
    m. congenital anomalies
    m. cyst
    m. dislocations
    m. endocrine abnormalities (MEA)
    m. endocrine adenomatosis (MEA)
    m. endocrine neoplasia, (type I, II, III) (MEN)
    m. epiphyseal dysplasia
    m. epiphyseal dysplasia-early onset diabetes mellitus syndrome (MED-IDDM)
    m. epiphyseal dysplasia tarda syndrome
    m. exostosis-mental retardation (MEMR)
    m. gastrointestinal polyps
    m. gated acquisition (MUGA)
    m. gated acquisition scan
    m. gestation
    m. hamartoma syndrome

m. hereditary cutaneomandibular polyoncosis
m. lentigines syndrome
m. marker screening
m. mononeuropathies
m. myeloma
m. myofibromatosis
m. neuroma syndrome
m. nevoid-basal cell carcinoma (MNBCC)
m. nevoid-basal cell carcinoma syndrome
m. nevoid, basal cell epithelioma, jaw cysts, bifid rib syndrome
m. opportunistic pathogen infection
m. oral frenula
m. organ dysfunction syndrome (MODS)
m. organ failure
m. organ system failure (MOSF)
m. osteomas
m. pituitary hormone deficiency (MPHD)
m. pregnancy
m. pregnancy reduction (MPR)
m. pterygium syndrome
m. resistant cell lines
m. ring-enhancing mass lesion
m. sclerosis (MS)
M. Sleep Latency Test (MSLT)
m. subpial transection (MST)
m. sulfatase deficiency (MSD)
m. synostoses
m. synostoses syndrome
m. tics
m. villous infarction
m. X syndrome
multiple-punch resection
multiplex
arthrogryposis m.
dysostosis m.
mononeuritis m.
myodysplasia fibrosa m.
paramyoclonus m.
steatocystoma m.
synostosis m.
multiplexing
multiplicity of infection (MOI)
multipuncture
m. technique
m. test (MPT)

multisite
m. BRACA
m. lower genital tract involvement
Multispatula cervical sampling device
multispectral fluorescent in situ hybridization (M-FISH)
multisymptomatic
multisystemic therapy (MST)
multivalent
multivitamin
multivorans
Burkholderia m.
MultiVysion PB assay test
multocida
Pasteurella m.
Prevotella m.
Mulvihill-Smith syndrome
mummified fetus
mummy wrap
mumps
m. arthritis
m. encephalitis
m. leptomeningitis
m. meningoencephalitis
m. orchitis
m. vaccine
m. virus
Mumpsvax
Münchausen
M. disease
M. syndrome
M. syndrome by proxy (MSBP, MSP)
munching pattern
munity
Munro
M. microabscess
M. and Parker classification for laparoscopic hysterectomy
M. point
Munro-Kerr maneuver
Munson sign
mupirocin
mural
m. endocardium
m. pregnancy
m. thrombosis
MURCS
müllerian duct aplasia, renal agenesis/ectopia, cervical somite dysplasia
MURCS syndrome

M

NOTES

Murine
  M. Ear Drops
  M. Plus Ophthalmic
Murless
  M. head extractor
  M. head retractor
  M. vacuum extractor
murmur
  aortic ejection m.
  apical presystolic m.
  Austin Flint m.
  blowing decrescendo diastolic m.
  cardiac m.
  continuous shunt m.
  crescendo m.
  decrescendo diastolic m.
  diamond-shaped m.
  diastolic m.
  ejection m.
  flow m.
  functional m.
  Gibson m.
  Graham Steell m.
  harsh pansystolic m.
  heart m.
  holosystolic m.
  innocent m.
  machinery m.
  middiastolic m.
  mill wheel m.
  musical m.
  pansystolic m.
  presystolic m.
  pulmonary ejection m.
  pulmonic m.
  regurgitant m.
  rumbling m.
  Still m.
  systolic continuous m.
  systolic ejection m. (SEM)
  to-and-fro m.
  m. of valvulitis
  vibratory m.
muromonab-CD3
Muro 128 Ophthalmic
Muroptic-5
Murphy
  M. hole
  M. sign
muscarinic
  m. action
  m. effect
muscle
  abdominis m.
  absence of rectal m.'s
  accessory m.
  m. actin
  m. adenosine monophosphate
    deaminase deficiency

airway smooth m.
antagonistic m.
m. atrophy
m. atrophy-contracture-oculomuscle
  apraxia syndrome
biceps femoris m.
m. biopsy
bulbocavernosus m.
bulbospongiosus m.
m. bulk
m. carnitine palmityltransferase
  deficiency
ciliary m.
coccygeal m.
coccygeus m.
conal m.
concave temporalis m.
m. cylinder
deltoid m.
depressor anguli oris m.
detrusor m.
diarthrodial m.
divergent rectus m.
m. enlargement
m. enzyme test
external oblique m.
external sphincter m.
extraocular m.
eyelid m.
m. fasciculation
gastrocnemius m.
genioglossus m.
gluteal m.
gluteus maximus m.
gluteus medius m.
gluteus minimus m.
m. glycogen storage disorder
gracilis m.
Guthrie m.
m. herniation
hypertrophic bundle of smooth m.
hypoplasia of anguli oris
  depressor m. (HAODM)
m. hypotonia
iliococcygeal m.
iliococcygeus m.
internal oblique m.
ipsilateral lateral rectus m.
ischiocavernosus m.
lateral rectus m.
m. lengthening
levator ani m.
levator palpebrae m.
m., liver, brain, eye (mulibrey)
lumbar extensor m.
masseter m.
m. necrosis
oblique flank m.
obturator internus m.

papillary m.
m. paralysis
pectoralis major m.
peroneus brevis m.
peroneus longus m.
pharyngeal m.
m. phosphofructokinase deficiency
m. proprioceptor
pubococcygeal m.
pubococcygeus m.
puborectal m.
puborectalis m.
pubovisceral m.
pyramidalis m.
quadratus labiae superioris m.
rectus abdominis m.
rectus femoris m.
m. relaxant
m. rigidity
scalene m.
scalloped temporalis m.
SCM m.
semimembranosus m.
semitendinosus m.
smooth m.
sphincter m.
m. splitting
sternocleidomastoid m.
m. strength grading scale
striated circular m.
superficial transverse perineal m.
superior oblique m.
m. surgery
temporalis m.
m. testing
thyroarytenoid m.
m. tone
m. transposition
transversus abdominis m.
unilateral hypoplastic pectoral m.
urethrovaginal sphincter m.
vastus lateralis m.
vertical m.
zygomatic head of quadratus labii
    superioris m.
muscle-brain
muscle-eye-brain (MEB)
m.-e.-b. disease of Santavuori
m.-e.-b. syndrome (MEBS)
muscular
m. atrophy
m. cuff

m. dystrophy (MD)
m. hypertrophy syndrome
m. hypotonia
m. infantilism
m. injury
m. torticollis
m. ventricular septum
muscularis
musculature
perineal m.
musculoaponeurotic layer
musculocutaneous nerve
musculofascial supply
musculoperitoneal
transverse rectus abdominis m.
    (TRAMP)
musculoskeletal (MSK)
m. disorder
m. injury
m. pain syndrome (MSPS)
m. system
Muse pellet
mushroom
Amanita m.
m. gyrus
m. poisoning
mushrooming of fimbria
musical murmur
mustard
M. atrial switch procedure
nitrogen m.
M. operation
L-phenylalanine m. (L-PAM)
M. TGA technique
Mustardé
M. cheek flap
M. cheek flap procedure
M. hypospadias procedure
(M. ratio) inner canthal
    distance/interpupillary distance
    (ICD/IPD)
Mustargen Hydrochloride
musty odor
mutagen
mutagenesis
insertional m.
mutagenic treatment
Mutamycin
mutans
Streptococcus m.
mutant
m. allele

M

NOTES

617

mutant *(continued)*
    m. cell
    m. gene
    m. homoplasmy
mutation
    autosomal recessive m.
    BRCA1 gene m.
    BRCA2 gene m.
    chromosome 17 m.
    Drosophila m.
    dynamic m.
    factor V Leiden m.
    frameshift m.
    full m.
    function-enhancing m.
    gene m.
    genetic m.
    germ-line m.
    G-to-T transversion m.
    HBS m.
    heparin-binding site m.
    hew m.
    121ins2 m.
    Leiden m.
    missense m.
    mutator m.
    new m.
    nonsense m.
    point m.
    prothrombin gene m.
    reactive site m.
    RS m.
    m. testing
    trinucleotide repeat expansion m.
mutational dysostosis
mutator mutation
Mutchinick syndrome
mute
mutilans
    keratoma hereditarium m.
mutilating keratoderma
mutilation
    female genital m. (FMG)
    female genital tract m. (FGTM)
mutism
    akinetic m.
    cerebellar m.
    selective m.
    transient m.
muzzled sperm
MV
    megavolt
mV
    millivolt
MVA
    microvillus atrophy
MVB
    manual ventilation bag

MV(c)ELISA
    measles virus enzyme-linked
      immunosorbent assay
MVP
    mitral valve prolapse
MWT
    Mallory-Weiss tear
MX2-300 xenon quality light source
myalgia
    m. cruris epidemica
    febrile m.
    tension m.
Myambutol
Myapap
myasthenia
    congenital m.
    m. gravis
    juvenile m.
    transient neonatal m.
myasthenia-like syndrome
myasthenic syndrome
Mycelex
mycelial mat
mycelium, pl. **mycelia**
mycetoma
    renal m.
Myciguent
Mycinettes
Mycitracin Topical
Myclo-Derm
Myclo-Gyne
mycobacteria (*pl. of* mycobacterium)
mycobacterial
    m. disease
    m. organism
Mycobacterium
    M. abscessus
    M. africanum
    M. avium
    M. avium complex (MAC)
    M. avium-intracellulare (MAI)
    M. avium-intracellulare complex
      (MAC)
    M. bovis
    M. chelonae
    M. fortuitum
    M. fortuitum complex
    M. kansasii
    M. leprae
    M. malmoense
    M. marinum
    M. scrofulaceum
    M. tuberculosis
    M. ulcerans
    M. xenopi
mycobacterium, pl. **mycobacteria**
    atypical mycobacteria
    nontuberculous m. (NTM)

mycobacteria other than tuberculosis (MOTT)
Mycobutin
Mycogen II Topical
Mycolog-II Topical
mycophenolate mofetil
mycophenolic acid
Mycoplasma
    M. fermentans
    M. genitalium
    M. hominis
    M. penetrans
    M. pneumonia
    M. pneumoniae
mycoplasma
    genital m.
    T strain m.
mycoplasmal
    m. antibody
mycosis
    m. fungoides
    hypopigmented m.
Mycostatin
mycotic
    m. aneurysm
    m. infection
    m. vaginosis
Myco-Triacet II
Mydfrin
    M. Ophthalmic
    M. Ophthalmic Solution
Mydriacyl
mydriasis
    congenital m.
    unilateral m.
mydriatic
myelencephalon
myelin
    m. lipid
    m. sheath
myelination
myelinization
myelinoclastic diffuse cerebral sclerosis
myelinolysis
    central pontine m.
myelitis
    acute transverse m.
    transverse m.
    viral m.
    zoster m.
myeloblast cell
myeloblastic leukemia

myelocele
myelocyte cell
myelocytic leukemia
myelodysplasia
    pediatric m.
myelodysplastic syndrome (MDS)
myelodystrophy
myelofibrosis
myelogenous leukemia
myelogram
myelograph
myelography
myeloid
    m. to erythroid ratio (M:E)
    m. leukemia
myelokathexis
myeloma
    multiple m.
    m. protein
myelomalacia
myelomeningocele
myelomonocytic leukemia
myeloneuropathy
    human T-cell lymphotropic virus 1 tropic m.
myelo-opticneuropathy
    subacute m.-o.
myelopathy
    compression m.
    craniocervical m.
    delayed m.
    human T-cell lymphotrophic virus type I associated m. (HAM)
    postirradiation m.
    schistosomal m.
    tropical spastic paraparesis/HTLV-I associated m. (TSP/HAM)
    vacuolar m.
    vascular m.
myeloperoxidase (MPO)
    m. deficiency
myelophthisis
myelopoiesis
    ineffective m.
myeloproliferative
    m. disorder
    m. syndrome
myeloradiculitis
    acute m.
myeloschisis
    dorsal m.
myelosuppression

M

NOTES

myelosuppressive agent
myelotoxicity
myenteric
> m. plexus
> m. plexus neuropathy

Myhre syndrome
myiasis
Mykrox
Mylanta Gas
Mylar glove
Myleran
Mylicon drops
Mylocel tablet
myoblastoma
> granular cell m.

myoblast transfer therapy
myocardial
> m. abscess
> m. band (MB)
> m. blood flow
> m. contusion
> m. fiber degeneration
> m. function
> m. hypertrophy
> m. infarction (MI)
> m. ischemia
> m. muscle creatine kinase
>   isoenzyme (CK-MB)
> m. siderosis
> m. steal syndrome
> m. stunning

myocarditis
> acute interstitial m.
> diphtheritic toxic m.
> enteroviral m.
> eosinophilic m.
> Fiedler m.
> giant cell m.
> granulomatous m.
> infectious m.
> interstitial m.
> lymphocytic m.
> silent m.
> toxic m.
> viral m.

myocardium
> stunned m.

Myochrysine
myoclonia
myoclonic
> m. absence
> m. ataxia
> m. convulsion
> m. dystonia
> m. encephalopathy
> m. epilepsy
> m. epilepsy with ragged red fibers
>   (MERRF)
> m. jerk
> m. petit mal
> m. seizure
> m. spasm

myoclonic-astatic seizure
myoclonus
> Baltic m.
> cortical reflex m.
> m. epilepsy
> m. epilepsy with ragged red fibers
>   (MERRF)
> epileptic m.
> essential m.
> intention m.
> jaw m.
> Mediterranean m.
> nocturnal m.
> nonepileptic m.
> ocular m.
> reflex m.
> reticular reflex m.
> sleep m.
> m. syndrome

myocolpitis
myocutaneous
> m. flap
> transverse rectus abdominis m.
>   (TRAM)

myocytic hypertrophy
myocytolysis
> coagulative m.

myodysplasia
> m. fetalis deformans
> m. fibrosa multiplex

myodystrophia fetalis deformans
myodystrophy
> Duchenne m.

myoepithelial cell
myofascial
> m. layer
> m. pain
> m. pain syndrome (MPS II, MPS,
>   MPS VII)
> m. release
> m. release technique

myofiber disarray
myofibril
myofibromatosis
> congenital multiple m.
> infantile m.
> multiple m.
> periorbital infantile m.
> renal m.
> solitary renal m.

myofilament
myogenic
myoglobin
myoglobinuria
> recurrent m.
> sporadic m.

myognathus
myography
myoinositol
myokymia
  interictal m.
myoma, pl. **myomata**
  asymptomatic m.
  calcified m.
  cervical m.
  degenerating m.
  m. fixation instrument
  intracavitary m.
  intraligamentous m.
  intramural m.
  myoma m.
  parasitic m.
  retained m.
  m. screw
  subendometrial m.
  submucosal m.
  submucous m.
  subserosal pedunculated m.
  subserous m.
  m. uteri
  uterine m.
myomectomy
  abdominal m.
  hysteroscopic m.
  laparoscopic m.
  vaginal m.
  vaginal birth after m.
myometrial
  m. contraction
  m. coring
  m. fiber
  m. invasion
  m. neurofibroma
myometritis
myometrium
  hypotonic m.
  m. of pregnancy
  uterine m.
myomotomy
myonecrosis
  clostridial m.
myoneural junction disorder
myopathic limb-girdle syndrome
myopathy
  Batten-Turner congenital m.
  Bethlem m.
  cardioskeletal m.
  centronuclear m. (CNM)

congenital m.
dysmaturative m.
dystrophic m.
familial visceral m.
fatal infantile m.
genetic m.
hypothyroid m.
infantile myofibrillar m.
inflammatory m.
m., lactic acidosis, sideroblastic
  anemia
lipid m.
metabolic m.
minicore m.
mitochondrial m.
multicore m.
myotonic m.
myotubular m.
nemaline m.
nemaline rod m.
nonfamilial visceral m.
ocular m.
Proteus syndrome m.
ragged red m.
rod m.
Sengers mitochondrial m.
steroid-induced m.
visceral m.
X-linked cardioskeletal m.
X-linked centronuclear m.
X-linked myotubular m. (MTMX,
  XLMTM)
X-linked recessive centronuclear m.
X-linked recessive myotubular m.
myopathy-myxedema syndrome
myopericarditis
myophosphorylase deficiency
myopia
  high m.
  severe m.
myosalpingitis
myosalpinx
myosin
  m. filament
  m. light-chain kinase
  m. light-chain phosphorylation
myosis
myositis
  eosinophilic m.
  inflammatory m.
  intrauterine viral m.
  m. ossificans

M

NOTES

myositis *(continued)*
    m. ossificans circumscripta
    m. ossificans progressiva
myotomy
    Heller m.
    Livaditis circular m.
myotomy-myectomy
    Morrow m.-m.
Myotonachol
myotonia
    chondrodystrophic m.
    m. chondrodystrophica
    cold-induced m.
    m. congenita
    grip m.
    m. neonatorum
    percussion m.
    spondyloepimetaphyseal dysphasia
     with m.
myotonic
    m. chondrodystrophy
    m. dystrophy (MD)
    m. muscular dystrophy
    m. myopathy
myotonica
    chondrodystrophia m.
MyoTrac EMG
myotubular myopathy
Myphetapp
myringitis
    bullous m.

myringotomy
    laser m.
    laser-assisted m. (LAM)
    Otoscan laser-assisted m. (OtoLAM)
    m. tube
    wide-field m.
myrtiform caruncle
Mysoline
mystery syndrome
Mytelase
Mytrex F Topical
Mytussin DM
myxedema
    m. coma
    infantile m.
myxedema-myotonic dystrophy syndrome
myxedematous infantilism
myxoid
    m. dysplasia
    m. histopathologic subtype
    m. liposarcoma
    m. matrix
myxoma
    familial cardiac m.
myxorrhea
M-Zole
    M-Z. 3 combination pack
    M-Z. 7 combination pack

N
    nitrogen
N95 particulate respirator surgical mask
NA
    nosocomially acquired
Na
    sodium
NAA
    nucleic acid amplification
        NAA technique
        NAA test
Nabi-HB
    N.-H. hepatitis B immune globulin human
Naboth
        N. cyst
        N. follicle
        N. gland
nabothian
        n. cyst
        n. follicle
        n. gland
        n. vesicle
N-acetylaspartate
N-acetylaspartic acid
N-acetylcysteine
N-acetyl-galactosamine
N-acetylgalactosamine-4-sulfatase deficiency
N-acetyl-glucosamine
N-acetylglutamate
        N.-a. synthetase
        N.-a. synthetase deficiency
N-acetylneuraminic
        N-a. acid (NANA)
        N-a. acid storage disease (NSD)
NaCl
    sodium chloride
NACS
    Neurologic and Adaptive Capacity Score
nadir
Nadler forceps
nadolol
Nadopen-V
Nadostine
NADPH
    nicotinamide adenine dinucleotide phosphate
        NADPH oxidase
Naegeli
        chromatophore nevus of N.
        N. syndrome

thrombasthenia of Glanzmann and N.
Naegeli-Franceschetti-Jadasshon (NJF)
Naegleria fowleri
naeslundii
        Actinomyces n.
nafarelin acetate
nafcillin sodium
naftifine hydrochloride
Naftin
Nägele
        N. forceps
        N. obliquity
        N. pelvis
        N. rule
Nager
        N. anomaly
        N. sign
        N. syndrome
        N. type acrofacial dysostosis
Nager-de Reynier syndrome
NaHCO$_3$
        sodium bicarbonate
nail
        n. bed cyanosis
        n. bed telangiectasia
        brittle n.
        clubbing of n.'s
        n. defect
        dystrophic n.
        n. dystrophy
        n. fold telangiectasia
        hippocratic n.
        hypertrophic n.
        hypoplastic n.'s
        n. matrix
        n. pitting
        n. ringworm
        shedding of n.'s
        spoon-shaped n.
        titanium elastic n.
        n. trephination
        yellow n.'s
nail-fold
        n.-f. capillary
        n.-f. infection
nailing
        titanium elastic n. (TEN)
nail-patella syndrome
naive
Najjar syndrome
nalbuphine
Nalcrom
Nalfon
Nalgest

N

Nal-Glu
nalidixic
n. acid
n. acid agar
nalorphine
naloxone hydrochloride
NALS
neonatal adjuvant life support
NALT
nasopharyngeal-associated lymphoid
tissue
naltrexone
NAMCS
National Ambulatory Medical Care
Survey
NAME
nevi, atrial myxoma, myxoid
neurofibromas, ephilides
NAME syndrome
naming speed deficit
NANA
N-acetylneuraminic acid
NANBH
non-A, non-B hepatitis
Nance-Horan syndrome (NHS)
nandrolone
nanism
mulibrey n.
Russell n.
Seckel n.
nanism-constrictive pericarditis syndrome
nanocephalic dwarfism
nanocephaly
nanogram
nanoid
nanomelia
nanosomia
nape nevus
naphazoline
naphthalene mothball
naphthoquinone
NAPI
Neurodevelopmental Assessment of
Preterm Infants
NAPNAP
National Association of Pediatric Nurse
Associates and Practitioners
nappy test
Naprosyn
naproxen sodium
Na⁺ pump
Naqua
narasin
naratriptan
Narcan
narcissus
narcolepsy

narcoleptic
n. attack
n. sleep
narcosis
narcotic
n. analgesia
n. analgesic
n. antagonist
n. depression
n. drug
intrathecal n.
n. withdrawal syndrome
Nardil
naris, pl. **nares**
anteverted n.
Naropin
NARP
neuropathy, ataxia, retinitis pigmentosa
NARP syndrome
narrow
n. band spectrophotometer
n. bifrontal diameter
n. complex supraventricular
tachycardia
n. foot
n. hand
n. mediastinal waist
n. mediastinum
n. mesenteric stalk
n. palate
n. pubic arch
n. pulmonary outflow tract (NPOT)
narrowing
vaginal n.
narrowness
intermaxillary n.
narrow-spectrum blue light
Narula method
NAS
neonatal abstinence syndrome
NAS score
Nasacort AQ
NaSal
nasal
n. air emission
n. ala
n. alar cartilage cleft
n. antral window
n. antrum
Ayr N.
n. bone
n. bridge
n. cannula
n. cauterization
n. consonant
n. continuous positive airway
pressure (nCPAP)
n. CPAP
n. decongestant

n. diphtheria
n. encephalocele
n. flaring
n. hypoplasia, peripheral dysostosis, mental retardation syndrome
n. lavage
n. mastocytosis
N. Moist
n. obstruction
n. packing
n. polyp
n. polyposis
Privine N.
n. prong continuous positive airway pressure (NP-CPAP)
n. pyriform aperture stenosis
n. regurgitation
n. retractor
n. root
n. septum
n. smear
n. speculum
n. swab
n. swab culture
n. tampon
n. tip thermistor
n. tube intubation
n. turbinate
Tyzine N.
n. ulceration
n. voice
n. wash
NasalCrom
Nasalide
N. Nasal Aerosol
N. Nasal Inhaler
Nasarel Nasal Spray
NASBA
nucleic acid sequence-based amplification
nascentium
trismus n.
NASH
nonalcoholic steatohepatitis
nasi
ala n.
flaring of ala n.
nasion
nasoduodenal feeding
nasoendoscopy
nasofrontal suture
nasogastric (NG)
n. aspirate

n. decompression
n. drainage
n. drip feeding
n. tube (NGT)
n. tube feeding
nasojejunal tube
nasolabial
n. fold asymmetry
n. reflex
nasolacrimal
n. duct
n. duct obstruction
n. sac
Nasonex
nasoorbitoethmoid (NOE)
nasopharyngeal
n. airway obstruction
n. aspirate (NPA)
n. carcinoma
n. fibroma
n. reflux (NPR)
n. suction
n. suctioning
n. swab
n. wash
nasopharyngeal-associated lymphoid tissue (NALT)
nasopharyngitis
nasopharyngolaryngoscopy (NPL)
nasopharynx
nasotracheal intubation
NASPGN
North American Society for Pediatric Gastroenterology and Nutrition
NASS
Neonatal Abstinence Scoring System
natal
n. cleft
n. teeth
NatalCare Plus film-coated tablet
natality
NataTab
N. CFe film-coated tablet
N. FA film-coated tablet
N. Rx film-coated tablet
natiform skull
natimortality
national
N. Acute Spinal Cord Injury Study
N. Ambulatory Medical Care Survey (NAMCS)

NOTES

national *(continued)*
>>N. Association of Pediatric Nurse Associates and Practitioners (NAPNAP)
>>N. Cancer Institute (NCI)
>>N. Center for Child Abuse and Neglect (NCCAN)
>>N. Clearing House on Child Abuse and Neglect (NCCANH)
>>N. Collaborative Diethylstilbestrol Adenosis Project (DESAD)
>>N. Collaborative Perinatal project
>>N. Committee for Quality Assurance (NCQA)
>>N. Educational Longitudinal Survey (NELS)
>>N. Fertility Clinic
>>N. Health Interview Survey (NHIS)
>>N. Health and Nutrition Examination Survey (NHANES)
>>N. Hospital Discharge Survey (NIDS)
>>N. Institute of Child Health and Human Development (NICHD)
>>N. Institute of Mental Health (NIMH)
>>N. Institutes of Health (NIH)
>>N. Joint Committee on Learning Disabilities (NJCLD)
>>N. Maternal and Infant Health Survey
>>N. Organization for Rare Disorders (NORD)
>>N. Osteoporosis Foundation
>>N. Pediatric Trauma Registry (NPTR)
>>n. recipient waiting list
>>N. Surgical Adjuvant Breast Project (NSABP)
>>N. Vaccine Advisory Committee (NVAC)
>>N. Wilms Tumor Study Group (NWTS)

native
>>n. ileum
>>n. squamous epithelium

NATP
>neonatal alloimmune thrombocytopenic purpura

natriuresis
natriuretic peptide
natural
>>n. antibody
>>n. childbirth
>>n. conception
>>n. delivery
>>n. environment
>>n. family planning
>>n. fecundity

>>n. hormone replacement therapy
>>n. killer cell (NK)
>>n. killer lymphocyte
>>n. killer T cell
>>n. penicillin
>>n. resistance
>>n. selection

nature of specimen
Naturetin
naturopath (NP)
nausea
>>n. gravidarum
>>n. and vomiting (N/V)

Navajo brainstem syndrome
Navane
navel
>>blue n.

Navelbine
navicular
>>accessory n.
>>n. bone
>>carpal n.

navicularis
>>fossa n.

naviculocuneiform joint
Naxen
NB
>>neuroblastoma

NBAS
>>Neonatal Behavioral Assessment Scale
>>Newborn Behavior Assessment Scale

NBCC
>>nevoid basal cell carcinoma

NBCCS
>>nevoid basal cell carcinoma syndrome

NBI
>>nosocomial bacterial infection

NBIC
>>newborn intensive care

NBICU
>>newborn intensive care unit

NBRS
>>Neurobiologic Risk Scale
>>>nursery NBRS

NBS
>>neonatal Bartter syndrome
>>nevoid basal cell carcinoma syndrome
>>new Ballard score
>>Nijmegen breakage syndrome

NBSCU
>>newborn special care unit

NBT
>>nitroblue tetrazolium
>>>NBT dye test

NBTV
>>nonbacterial thrombotic vegetation

NC
>>Histussin NC

NCAH
  nonclassic adrenal hyperplasia
NC-CAH
  nonclassic congenital adrenal hyperplasia
NCCAN
  National Center for Child Abuse and
  Neglect
NCCANH
  National Clearing House on Child Abuse
  and Neglect
NCCDS
  North American Collaborative Crohn
  Disease Study
NCCPC-R
  Noncommunicating Children's Pain
  Checklist-Revised
NCI
  National Cancer Institute
NCL
  neuronal ceroid lipofuscinosis
    adult NCL
    infantile NCL
    juvenile NCL
    late infantile NCL
nCPAP
  nasal continuous positive airway pressure
NCQA
  National Committee for Quality
  Assurance
NCSE
  nonconvulsive status epilepticus
NCV
  nerve conduction velocity
NDH
  neurogenic dysplasia of hip
ND-Stat
NDT
  neurodevelopment therapy
NDW
  number of different words
Nd:YAG
    Nd:YAG laser
    Nd:YAG laser ablation
NE
  neonatal encephalopathy
NE-8000 analyzer
near
    n. drowning
    n. gaze reflex
    n. infrared photoplethysmography
    (NIRP)

    n. infrared spectrophotometry
    (NIRS, NIS)
    n. infrared spectroscopy (NIRS,
    NIS)
    n. vision
near-anhydramnios
near-drowning
near-miss
    n.-m. SIDS
    n.-m. sudden infant death
    syndrome
near-myeloablative chemotherapy
nearsightedness
near-term
    n.-t. delivery
    n.-t. pregnancy
near-viable fetus
neat pincer grasp
Nebcin Injection
Nebules
    Ventolin N.
nebulization
    ipratropium n.
    n. ventilator
nebulized prostacyclin
nebulizer
    compressed air-driven n.
    DuraNeb portable n.
    Hudson T Up-Draft II
    disposable n.
    jet n.
    Micro-Mist disposable n.
    Pari LC Plusjet n.
    PulmoMate n.
    Respirgard II n.
    Schuco n.
NebuPent Inhalation
NEC
    necrotizing enterocolitis
    Neurological Examination for Children
Necator americanus
necessitatis
    empyema n.
neck
    bladder n.
    femoral n.
    n. reflex
    n. response
    short n.
    stiff n.
    thick n.
    twisted n.

NOTES

neck *(continued)*
    vesical n.
    webbed n.
necklace
    Casal n.
neck-righting reflex
neck-shaft angle (NSA)
necrobiosis
    n. lipoidica
    n. lipoidica diabeticorum (NLD)
necrolysis
    erythema multiforme/toxic
      epidermal n. (EM/TEN)
    toxic epidermal n. (TEN)
necrophorum
    Fusobacterium n.
necropsy
necrosis
    acute tubular n. (ATN)
    aseptic n.
    avascular n. (AVN)
    basal ganglia n.
    bone avascular n.
    caseating n.
    centrilobular n.
    cerebral cortical n.
    cortical n.
    cystic medial n.
    decidual fibrinoid n.
    excitotoxic n.
    fascial n.
    fat n.
    fibrinoid n.
    full-thickness n.
    hepatic n.
    idiopathic juvenile avascular n.
    intrauterine facial n.
    ischemic decidual n.
    juvenile avascular n.
    liquefactive n.
    medial n.
    medullary n.
    miliary calcified n.
    muscle n.
    neuronal n.
    papillary n.
    periportal hemorrhagic n.
    pituitary n.
    pontosubicular neuron n. (PSN)
    postpartum pituitary n.
    postsurgical fat n.
    posttraumatic fat n.
    progressive outer retinal n. (PORN)
    pulp n.
    radiation n.
    renal cortical n.
    renal tubular n.
    selective neuronal n.
    spotty n.

    subcutaneous fat n.
    superficial n.
    tissue n.
    tubular n.
    tumor n.
    unilateral intrauterine facial n.
    uterine n.
    white matter n.
necrospermia
necrotic
    n. arachnidism
    n. coagulum
    n. facial dysplasia
    n. mucosa
necrotizing
    n. adrenalitis
    n. arteriolitis
    n. arteritis
    n. colitis
    n. encephalopathy
    n. enterocolitis (NEC)
    n. erysipelas
    n. factor
    n. funisitis
    n. gingivitis
    n. glomerulonephritis
    n. granulomatous lymphadenitis
    n. granulomatous vasculitis
    n. jejunitis
    n. myositis/fasciitis
    n. pneumonia
    n. ulcerating gingivitis (NUG)
necrozoospermia
nedocromil
    n. sodium
    n. sodium ophthalmic solution
N.E.E. 1/35
need
needle
    Adair-Veress n.
    n. aspiration
    Bard Biopty cut n.
    Biopty cut n.
    butterfly scalp vein n.
    Chiba n.
    coaxial sheath cut-biopsy n.
    Cobb-Ragde n.
    n. cricothyroidotomy
    n. cricothyrotomy
    CUSALap accessory n.
    n. cystourethropexy
    Dieckmann intraosseous n.
    disposable 23-gauge butterfly n.
    D-Tach removal n.
    Echotip Norfolk aspiration n.
    Echotip percutaneous entry n.
    Endopath Ultra Veress n.
    Ethiguard n.
    Euro-Med FNA-21 aspiration n.

eXcel-DR Glasser laparoscopic n.
n. excision
n. excision of the transformation zone
FNA-21 n.
21-gauge hypodermic n.
GraNee n.
Hawkins breast localization n.
n. holder
Howell biopsy aspiration n.
insufflation n.
intraosseous n.
J n.
Kopan n.
n. localization
n. localization breast biopsy
Osgood bone marrow n.
Pereyra n.
Potocky n.
scalp vein n.
screw-tipped intraosseous n.
short-bevel 21-gauge n.
SonoVu US aspiration n.
spinal n.
splittable n.
Stamey n.
stereotactic breast biopsy n.
Sur-Fast n.
n. suspension
n. thoracentesis
n. tip
Tuohy spinal n.
Ultra-Vue amniocentesis n.
Veress n.
Vim-Silverman n.
Virginia n.
Wolf-Veress n.

needle holder
Crile-Wood n. h.
Endo-Assist endoscopic n. h.
Heaney n. h.
Mayo-Hegar n. h.
Wangensteen n. h.
Wolf-Castroviejo n. h.

needlestick exposure

needs
Carolina Curriculum for Infants and Toddlers with Special N.'s
Children with Special Health Care N. (CWSN)
special n.

NEEP
negative end-expiratory pressure

Neer view

nefazodone

negative
n. affectivity
n. balance
n. balance of body fluid
n. end-expiratory pressure (NEEP)
false n.
n. inspiratory pressure
n. interference
polyarthritis, RF n.
n. punch biopsy
n. reinforcement

negative-pressure
n.-p. box
n.-p. respirator

negativism

negevensis
Simkania n.

NegGram

neglect
child abuse and n.
National Center for Child Abuse and N. (NCCAN)
National Clearing House on Child Abuse and N. (NCCANH)
suspected child abuse or n. (SCAN)

negligence

Negri body

Neill-Dingwall syndrome

Neisseria
N. gonorrhea
N. meningitidis

neisserial infection

nelfinavir

Nellcor
N. FS-10 oximeter sensor
N. FS-14 oximeter sensor
N. N-499 fetal oxygen saturation monitor
N. N-400/FS system
N. N-200 home monitor
N. N-3000 home monitor
N. N20, N200 pulse oximeter
N. Puritan Bennett home monitor
N. Puritan Bennett oxygen saturation monitor

N

NOTES

NELS
    National Educational Longitudinal
    Survey
Nelson
    N. sign
    N. syndrome
nemaline
    n. myopathy
    n. rod
    n. rod disease
    n. rod myopathy
Nemasole
nematode endophthalmitis
nem (breast milk nutritional unit)
Nembutal
NEMD
    nonspecific esophageal motility disorder
neoadjuvant
    n. chemotherapy
    n. hormonal therapy (NHT)
neoaneurysm
neoantigen
neoaorta formation
neoaortic valve
neobladder diversion procedure
Neocate One+ formula
Neo-Codema
NeoCure cryoablation system
neocystostomy
neodarwinism
neodymium:yttrium-aluminum-garnet
Neo-Estrone
neofetus
neoformans
    Cryptococcus neoformans var. *n.*
Neo-fradin
neogala
Neo-Gen screening
neologism
Neoloid
Neolon surgical glove
neomucosa
neomycin
    n. (bacitracin), polymyxin B,
      hydrocortisone
    n. and polymyxin B
    n., polymyxin B, bacitracin
    n., polymyxin B, prednisolone
    n. sulfate
neomycin-polymycin combination otic solution
neonatal
    n. abdominal mass
    N. Abstinence Scoring System (NASS)
    n. abstinence sign
    n. abstinence syndrome (NAS)
    n. acne
    n. adjuvant life support (NALS)

n. adrenoleukodystrophy
n. alloimmune thrombocytopenia
n. alloimmune thrombocytopenic purpura (NATP)
n. amblyogenic stimulus
n. apnea
n. asphyxia
n. assessment
n. autoimmune neutropenia
n. autoimmune thrombocytopenia
n. Bartter syndrome (NBS)
N. Behavioral Assessment Scale (NBAS)
n. blood volume
n. brain injury
n. breast hyperplasia
n. bullous dermatitis
n. candidiasis
n. cardiomyopathy
n. chest disease
n. cholestasis
n. cholestatic hepatitis
n. cholestatic jaundice
n. chronic idiopathic neutropenia
n. cold injury
n. condition
n. conjunctivitis
n. convulsion
n. cuff
n. cyanotic congenital heart disease
n. death
n. dermatology
n. diagnosis
n. distress
n. elastin deposition
n. encephalopathy (NE)
Exosurf N.
n. facial coding system (NFCS)
n. gonococcal disease
n. Guillain-Barré syndrome
n. Guthrie card
n. gynecomastia
n. hemochromatosis (NH)
n. hepatitis syndrome
n. herpes
n. herpes simplex
n. herpes simplex virus infection
n. HMD
n. HSV-1, -2 encephalitis
n. hyperbilirubinemia
n. hyperparathyroidism
n. hyperthermia
n. hypocalcemia
n. hypoglycemia
n. hypomagnesemia
n. hypoxic-ischemic encephalopathy
N. Infant Pain Scale (NIPS)
n. intensive care unit (NICU)
n. intubation

n. iron-storage disease (NISD)
n. isoimmune hemolytic anemia
n. isoimmune thrombocytopenia
n. leukemoid reaction
n. line
n. listeriosis
n. lupus
n. lupus erythematosus (NLE)
n. lupus syndrome
n. macrosomia
n. Marfan syndrome
n. marker
n. maturity classification of Dubowitz
n. medicine
n. meningitis
n. metabolism
n. midgut volvulus
n. monitor
n. morbidity
n. mortality
n. mortality rate
n. mortality risk (NMR)
n. myasthenia gravis
n. myasthenic syndrome
n. narcotic pack
n. neuroblastoma
n. nongoitrous hypothyroidism
n. ocular prophylaxis
n. OPCA
n. ophthalmia
n. osseous dysplasia
n. outcome
n. pemphigus vulgaris
N. Perception Inventory (NPI)
n. period
n. pneumonia
n. polycythemia
n. progeroid syndrome
n. pseudohydrocephalic progeroid syndrome
n. purpura fulminans
n. pustular melanosis
n. pustule
n. RDS
n. respiratory depression
n. resuscitation
N. Resuscitation Program (NRP)
n. ring
n. scabies
n. scalp abscess
n. screening

n. seizure
n. sepsis
n. septic arthritis
N. Skin Assessment Score
n. small left colon syndrome
n. stadiometer
n. stress
n. teeth
n. tetanus
n. tetany
n. thymectomy
n. thyrotoxicosis
n. thyrotropin
n. torticollis
n. transport
n. varicella
n. vascular accident
N. Withdrawal Inventory (NWI)

neonate
athyrotic n.
cola-colored n.
dysmature n.
early n.
n. examination
n. gut microflora
N. One Plus
postmature n.
preterm n.
seronegative n.
stress n.
surgical n.

neonatologist
neonatology
neonatorum
acne n.
adiponecrosis subcutanea n.
anemia n.
apnea n.
asphyxia n.
diabetes n.
eczema n.
edema n.
erythema toxicum n.
erythroblastosis n.
gonococcal ophthalmia n.
herpes n.
icterus gravis n.
impetigo n.
keratolysis n.
mastitis n.
melena n.
milia n.

NOTES

N

neonatorum *(continued)*
    myotonia n.
    noma n.
    ophthalmia n. (type 1, 2)
    pemphigus n.
    sclerema n.
    sepsis n.
    tetania n.
    tetanus n.
    trismus n.
    volvulus n.
Neopap
NeoPath
neoplasia
    anal intraepithelial n. (AIN)
    cervical epithelial n.
    cervical intraepithelial n. (CIN)
    endometrial n.
    endometrial intraepithelial n. (EIN)
    estrogen-dependent n.
    gestational trophoblastic n. (GTN)
    glandular n.
    hematologic n.
    intraepithelial n.
    invasive n.
    lobular n.
    lymphoreticular n.
    multicentric lower genital tract n.
    multiple endocrine n., (type I, II, III) (MEN)
    syndrome of multiple endocrine n.
    thyroid n.
    trophoblastic n.
    vaginal intraepithelial n. (VAIN)
    vulvar intraepithelial n. (VIN)
neoplasm
    adrenal n.
    benign ovarian n.
    benign vascular n.
    bilateral ovarian n.
    borderline epithelial ovarian n.
    borderline malignant epithelial n.
    cerebellar n.
    cervix n.
    cystic cerebellar n.
    endometrial n.
    epithelial stromal ovarian n.
    germ cell ovarian n.
    gonadal germ cell n.
    hepatic n.
    hormone-producing n.
    indigenous n.
    isologous n.
    large intestine n.
    lipid cell n.
    lipoid ovarian n.
    malignant ovarian n.
    mesenchymal n.
    mucinous ovarian n.

    neural n.
    ovarian lipid cell n.
    ovarian malignant epithelial n.
    ovarian sex-cord stromal n.
    papillary n.
    posterior fossa n.
    primary intrapulmonary n.
    serous ovarian n.
    sex cord stromal n.
    soft tissue ovarian n.
    testicular n.
    uterine n.
    vascular n.
    vulvar n.
neoplastic
    n. cyst
    n. fibrosis
    n. sequela
    n. trophoblastic disease
neopterin
Neoral
neosalpingostomy
    terminal n.
Neosar
Neo-Sert
    N.-S. umbilical vessel catheter
    N.-S. umbilical vessel catheter insertion set
Neosporin
    N. Cream
    N. G.U. Irrigant
    N. Ophthalmic Ointment
    N. Topical Ointment
neostigmine
NeoSure nutritional supplement
Neo-Synephrine
    N.-S. 12 Hour Nasal Solution
    N.-S. Ophthalmic Solution
Neo-Therm neonatal skin temperature probe
Neotrace-4
Neo-trak 515A neonatal monitor
Neotrend
    N. premature infant blood gas/temperature monitor
    N. sensor
    N. system
neoumbilicus
neourethra
neovagina
    gracilis flap n.
    reconfiguration for n.
neovascularization of disc (NVD)
neovascular tissue
Nephramine
nephrectomy
nephrin (NPHN)
nephritic factor
nephritis, pl. **nephritides**

acute interstitial n.
acute postinfectious n.
Alport syndrome-like n.
autoimmune interstitial n.
diffuse proliferative lupus n.
focal lupus n.
n. gravidarum
hemorrhagic familial n.
hemorrhagic hereditary n.
hereditary familial congenital n.
interstitial n.
lupus n.
membranous lupus n.
mesangial lupus n.
postinfectious n.
proliferative lupus n.
pyoderma-associated n.
shunt n.
tubulointerstitial n. (TINU)
nephritogenic
nephroblastoma
nephroblastomatosis
Nephro-Calci
nephrocalcinosis
Nephrocaps
Nephro-Fer
nephrogenesis
nephrogenic
n. cord
n. diabetes insipidus
n. fibrosing dermopathy
n. rest
nephrolithiasis
uric acid n.
X-linked hypercalciuric n. (XLHN)
X-linked recessive n.
nephrologist
nephroma
congenital mesoblastic n.
cystic n.
mesoblastic n.
nephron
cortical n.
n. loss
Nephronex
nephronophthisis (NPH)
n. type 1 (NPH1)
nephropathy
diabetic n.
familial juvenile hyperuricemic n.
HIV-associated n.
immunoglobulin A n.

membranous n.
pediatric lupus n.
reflux n.
renal cortical n.
sickle cell n.
thin basement membrane n.
urate n.
nephrophthisis
familial juvenile n. (FJN)
nephrosclerosis
malignant n.
nephrosis
congenital n.
n., microcephaly, hiatus hernia
syndrome
nephrosis-microcephaly syndrome
nephrosis-neural dysmigration syndrome
nephrosis-neuronal dysmigration syndrome
nephrostomy
percutaneous n.
nephrotic syndrome
nephrotoxicity
aminoglycoside n.
nephrotoxin
nephroureterectomy
nepiology
Neptazane
NERICP
New England Regional Infant Cardiac
Program
neridronate
nerve
abducens n.
accessory n.
acoustic n.
anterior labial n.'s
auditory n.
n. block
ciliary n.
clitoral n.
n. conduction study
n. conduction velocity (NCV)
cranial n. (II–XII)
n. dysplasia
facial n.
femoral cutaneous n.
genitofemoral n.
glioma of optic n.
glossopharyngeal n.
n. growth factor (NGF)
hemorrhoidal n.

NOTES

nerve *(continued)*
    hypoglossal n.
    inferior hemorrhoidal n.
    inferior rectal n.
    infraorbital n.
    n. injury
    laryngeal n.
    motor n.
    musculocutaneous n.
    nociceptive sensory n.
    obturator n.
    oculomotor n.
    optic n.
    n. palsy
    n. paralysis
    paralysis of superior laryngeal n.
    parasympathetic n.
    pelvic floor n.
    perineal n.
    phrenic n.
    postauricular n.
    preauricular n.
    presacral n.
    pudendal n.
    sacral n.
    saphenous n.
    sciatic n.
    sensory n.
    n. sheath tumor
    n. sprouting
    superior laryngeal n.
    n. thickening
    thoracolumbar sympathetic n.
    n. tract
    trigeminal n.
    trochlear n.
    vagus n.
    vestibular n.
    vestibulocochlear n.
nerve-muscle pedicle
nervi (*pl. of* nervus)
Nervine
Nervocaine
nervorum
    vasa n.
nervosa
    anorexia n. (AN)
    bulimia n. (BN)
    mild anorexia n.
nervous
    n. colon
    n. system
    n. system sarcoidosis
    n. tissue nevus
nervus, pl. **nervi**
    nervi erigentes
nesidioblastosis
nest
    cancer n.
    crow's n.
    Walthard n.
Nestabs FA
net
    Chiari n.
    n. ultrafiltration pressure
NET-EN
    norethindrone enanthate
Netherton syndrome
netilmicin sulfate
netting
    Baby Air mesh n.
Nettleship-Falls ocular albinism
Nettleship syndrome
network
    American College of Obstetrics & Gynecology n.
    Cooperative Human Tissue N. (CHTN)
    Human Genome Epidemiology N. (HuGENET)
    SEER n.
    support n.
    trans-Golgi n.
Neubauer
    N. chamber
    N. hemocytometer
Neugebauer-LeFort procedure
Neuhauser syndrome
neu/HER2 oncogene
neuii
    Actinomyces n.
Neu-Laxova syndrome (NLS)
Neupogen
neural
    n. arch
    n. arch joint
    n. axis
    n. cell adhesion molecule L1 (LICAM)
    n. ceroid lipofuscinosis
    n. crest
    n. crest cell
    n. crest-derived cell lineage
    n. crest tissue
    n. crest tumor
    n. discharge
    n. groove
    n. index
    n. mechanism
    n. neoplasm
    n. plate
    n. reflex pathway
    n. retina
    n. tissue accretion
    n. tube
    n. tube closure
    n. tube defect (NTD)

n. tube disorder
n. tube rupture
neuralgia
mammary n.
postherpetic n.
neurally
n. mediated hypotension
n. mediated syncope (NMS)
neural plate
neuraminic acid
neuraminidase
n. deficiency
n. inhibitor
neuraxial anesthesia
neuraxis tumor imaging
neurectomy
presacral n.
neurenteric
n. canal
n. cyst
neurilemoma, neurilemmoma
malignant n.
neurinoma
neurinomatosis
n. centralis
n. universalis
neuritic cytoplasmic process
neuritis
acute n.
bilateral optic n.
cranial n.
intraocular optic n.
optic n.
peripheral n.
retrobulbar n.
subacute n.
unilateral optic n.
neuritogenesis
neuroacanthocytosis
neuroanatomical
neuroangiomatosis
encephalocraniofacial n.
n. encephalofacialis
neuroarthromyodysplasia
neuroaxonal dystrophy
neurobehavioral abnormality
neurobiological
neurobiologic influence
Neurobiologic Risk Scale (NBRS)
neuroblastoma (NB)
n. cell
central n.

familial n.
metastatic n.
neonatal n.
occult n.
peripheral n.
neuroborreliosis
Lyme n.
neurocardiogenic syncope
neurochemical
neurocognitive
n. impairment
n. potential
neurocristopathy
neurocutaneous
n. disorder
n. melanosis syndrome
NeuroCybernetic prosthesis
neurocysticercosis
intraventricular n.
neurodermatitis
circumscribed n.
neurodevelopmental
n. assessment
N. Assessment of Preterm Infants (NAPI)
n. complication
n. deficit
n. delay
n. disability
n. disease
n. handicap
n. problem
n. sequela
n. treatment
neurodevelopment therapy (NDT)
neuroectoderm
neuroectodermal
n. hamartoma
n. tumor
neuroendocrine
n. response
n. system
neuroendocrinology
neuroepithelioma
peripheral n.
neuroepithelium
telencephalic n.
neurofaciodigitorenal (NFDR)
n. syndrome
neurofibroma
abdominal n.
clitoral n.

N

NOTES

neurofibroma *(continued)*
> lumbosacral n.
> myometrial n.
> ovarian n.
> plexiform n.
> subcutaneous n.
> vaginal n.
> vulvar n.

neurofibromatosis (NF)
> bilateral acoustic n.
> central type n.
> familial spinal n.
> peripheral n.
> plexiform n.
> segmental n.
> spinal n.
> n. type 1 (NF1)
> n. type 2 (NF2)
> vaginal n.
> von Recklinghausen n.
> n. with Noonan phenotype

neurofibromatosis-Noonan syndrome (NF-NS, NFNS)
neurofibrosarcoma
neurofilament antibody
neurofunctional
neurogenic
> n. atrophy
> n. bladder
> n. bladder dysfunction
> n. bowel
> n. clubfoot
> n. dysplasia of hip (NDH)
> n. equinus deformity
> n. hip disease
> n. hip dysplasia
> n. polydipsia
> n. pulmonary edema
> n. respiratory failure
> n. sarcoma
> n. shock
> n. stuttering
> n. talipes equinovarus
> n. tumor

neuroglial heterotopia
neurogram
> pudendal n.

neurohormonal
neurohypophysis
neuroichthyosis-hypogonadism syndrome
neuroid
> n. cell
> n. nevus

neuroimaging study
neuroleptic
> n. drug
> n. malignant syndrome (NMS)
> n. medication

neurologic
> n. abnormality
> N. and Adaptive Capacity Score (NACS)
> n. adverse effect
> n. complication
> n. demyelinating disease
> n. development
> n. disability
> n. disorder
> n. examination
> n. impairment
> n. involvement
> n. shellfish poisoning

neurological
> n. disease syndrome
> n. disorder
> N. Examination for Children (NEC)
> n. injury

neurologist
> pediatric n.

neurology
> American Board of Psychiatry and N. (ABPN)

neurolysis
> transcutaneous n.

neuroma
> acoustic n.
> bilateral acoustic n.'s
> incisional n.

neuromelanin
neuromelanogenesis
neuromodulator
neuromotor dysfunction
neuromuscular
> n. blockade
> n. blockage
> n. blocking agent
> n. disease
> n. disorder
> n. imbalance
> n. injury
> n. junction (NMJ)
> n. maturity
> n. maturity assessment
> n. scoliosis
> n. scoliosis syndrome

neuromyelitis optica
neuron
> Cajal-Retzius n.
> hippocampal n.
> motor n.
> oxytocin-secreting n.
> n. palsy
> parasympathetic n.

neuronal
> n. ceroid lipofuscinosis (CLN, NCL)

n. damage
n. dysplasia
n. GM1 gangliosidosis
n. heterotopia
n. migration disorder
n. necrosis

neuronitis
vestibular n.

neuronophagia

neuronophagy

neuronotmesis (*var. of* neurotmesis)

neuron-specific enolase (NSE)

Neurontin

neurooculocutaneous angiomatosis

neuropathic
n. anhidrosis
n. bladder
n. cystinosis

neuropathy
acute motor-axonal n. (AMAN)
acute motor-sensory axonal n. (AMSAN)
n., ataxia, retinitis pigmentosa (NARP)
autonomic n.
bulbar hereditary motor n. (type I, II)
chronic peripheral n.
congenital hypomyelinating n. (CHN)
congenital sensory n.
distal symmetric sensorimotor n.
familial visceral n.
femoral n.
giant axonal n.
glue-sniffing n.
hereditary autonomic n.
hereditary motor-sensory n. (type IA, II–VII) (HMSN)
hereditary sensory autonomic n.
hereditary sensory radicular n.
Leber hereditary optic n. (LHON)
Leber optic n.
motor-axonal n.
motor sensory n. (MSN)
motor-sensory axonal n. (MSN)
myenteric plexus n.
nutritional n.
obstetric n.
optic n.
peripheral entrapment n.
porphyric n.

postdiphtheritic n.
pudendal n.
radicular n.
reflux n. (RN)
retractor n.
sensory n.
tomaculous n.
toxic n.
tropical ataxic n.
ulnar n.

neuropeptide
enteric n.

neuropharmacology

neurophysin I, II

neurophysiologic

neurophysiology

neuropore
caudal n.
rostral n.

neuroprotection

neuropsychiatric
n. behavior
n. disorder
n. syncope

neuropsychiatry

neuropsychologic

neuropsychological profile

neuropsychology
clinical assessment in n.

neuropsychopharmacology

neuroradiographic study

neuroretinitis
optic n.

neuroretinoangiomatosis

neurosarcoidosis

neuroschisis

neurosecretion

neurosecretory

neurosensory
n. deafness
n. impairment (NSI)

neurosis, pl. **neuroses**
battle n.

neurosonographic

neurospongioblastosis diffusa

neurosteroid

neurosurgeon

neurosurgical
n. closure
n. shunt

neurosyphilis
congenital paretic n.

N

NOTES

neurosyphilis *(continued)*
    congenital tertiary n.
    tabetic n.
neurotensin
neurotic
neurotmesis, neuronotmesis
neurotoxicity
    methylmercury n.
neurotoxic shellfish poisoning
neurotoxin
    botulinus n.
    tetanus n.
neurotransmission
neurotransmitter
    n. precursor
    n. release
    substance P pain n.
neurotrauma
neurotrichocutaneous syndrome
neurotrophic keratitis
neurovascular
    n. compromise
    n. dystrophy
neurovegetative functioning or symptom
neurovirulence
neurovisceral lipidosis
neurula, pl. **neurulae**
neurulation
Neut Injection
neutral
    K-Phos N.
    n. lipid storage disease
    n. pH
    n. pH of vagina
    n. position
    n. protamine Hagedorn (NPH)
    n. protamine Hagedorn insulin
    n. rotation
neutralization
neutralize
Neutra-Phos
Neutra-Phos-K
Neutrogena
    N. Acne Mask
    N. T/Derm
neutron
    fast n.
    n. therapy
neutropenia
    alloimmune neonatal n. (ANN)
    autoimmune n. (AIN)
    benign n.
    cardioskeletal n.
    chemotherapy-related n.
    chronic benign n.
    chronic idiopathic n.
    congenital n.
    cyclic n.
    drug-induced n.

    idiopathic n.
    immune n.
    immune-mediated n.
    Kostmann n.
    neonatal autoimmune n.
    neonatal chronic idiopathic n.
    peripheral n.
    persistent n.
    severe chronic n. (SCN)
    severe congenital n.
    transient n.
    X-linked cardioskeletal myopathy
      and n.
neutropenic
neutrophil
    n. actin deficiency
    n. actin dysfunction
    n. apoptosis
    band form n.
    n. chemotactic deficiency
    circulating n.'s
    n. egress
    n. G6PD deficiency
    n. granulopoiesis
    hypersegmented n.
    mature n.
    n. protease-3
    segmented n.
    n. transfusion
neutrophilia
    acute acquired n.
neutrophilic
    n. leukocytosis
    n. pleocytosis
    n. rhinitis
NEV
    noninvasive extrathoracic ventilator
nevi (*pl. of* nevus)
Neville-Barnes forceps
nevirapine
nevocellular nevus
nevoid
    n. amentia
    n. basal cell carcinoma (NBCC)
    n. basal cell carcinoma syndrome
      (NBCCS, NBS)
    n. basal cell epithelioma, jaw
      cysts, bifid rib syndrome
    n. hyperkeratosis of the nipple and
      areola
nevomelanocyte
Nevo syndrome
nevoxanthoendothelioma
nevus, pl. **nevi**
    achromic n.
    acquired melanocytic n. (AMN)
    n. anemicus
    angiomatous involuting n.
    n. araneus

nevi, atrial myxoma, myxoid
  neurofibromas, ephilides (NAME)
atypical melanocytic n.
bathing trunk n.
Becker n.
benign n.
blue rubber bleb n.
cellular blue n.
combined n.
n. comedonicus
common blue n.
compound n.
congenital n.
congenital hairy n.
congenital melanocytic n.
congenital nevomelanocytic n.
congenital pigmental n.
conjunctival n.
connective tissue n.
cutaneous n.
depigmented n.
n. depigmentosus
dermal n.
dysplastic n.
eczematous halo n.
n. elasticus of Lewandowsky
epidermal n.
epithelioid cell n.
eruptive n.
faun tail n.
n. flammeus
giant congenital pigmented n.
hairy n.
halo n.
intradermal n.
involuting n.
n. of Ito
Ito n.
n. of Jadassohn
Jadassohn-Tieche n.
junctional n.
lentigines, atrial myxomas,
  cutaneous papular myxomas, blue
  nevi (LAMB)
lentiginous n.
linear verrucous epidermal n.
melanocytic n.
Meyerson n.
nape n.
nervous tissue n.
neuroid n.
nevocellular n.

organoid n.
n. of Ota
Ota n.
pigmented n.
n. pigmentosus systematicus
port-wine n.
rubber bleb n.
satellite melanocytic n.
sebaceous n.
n. sebaceus
n. sebaceus of Feuerstein and
  Mims
n. sebaceus of Jadassohn (SNJ)
n. sebaceus linearis
n. simplex
speckled lentiginous n.
spider n.
n. spilus
spindle cell epithelioid n.
Spitz n.
strawberry n.
telangiectatic n.
n. unius lateris
Unna n.
n. varicosus osteohypertrophicus
vascular n.
n. vasculosus osteohypertrophicus
verrucous streaky epidermal n.
vulvar nevomelanocytic n.
white sponge n.
woolly hair n.
zosteriform lentiginous n.

new
n. Ballard score (NBS)
N. England Regional Infant
  Cardiac Program (NERICP)
n. MacArthur emotion story-stems
N. Moves obesity-prevention
  program
n. mutation
n. variant CJD
n. variant Creutzfeldt-Jakob disease
  (nvCJD)
N. York Heart Association
  (NYHA)
newborn
N. Behavior Assessment Scale
  (NBAS)
congenital anemia of n.
congenital epulis of the n.
cyanotic n.
epulis of n.

NOTES

newborn *(continued)*
  n. euglycemia
  n. examination
  full-term n.
  n. genetic screening test
  genital crisis of n.
  gingival cyst of n.
  gonococcal arthritis of n.
  hemolytic disease of n. (HDN)
  hemorrhagic disease of n. (HDN)
  horizontal suspension in n.
  hyperthermia in n.
  n. intensive care (NBIC)
  n. intensive care unit (NBICU)
  jaundice of n.
  lamellar desquamation of n.
  metabolic disease in n.
  n. narcotic withdrawal syndrome
  nonfollicular pustulosis of n.
  n. nursery
  Parrot atrophy of n.
  n. period
  persistent pulmonary hypertension
    of n. (PPHN)
  physiologic jaundice of the n.
  n. platelet antigen typing
  pulmonary hypertension of n.
  n. rehospitalization after early
    discharge
  respiratory distress syndrome of
    the n.
  n. respiratory distress syndrome
  n. resuscitation
  retinopathy of n.
  Rh disease of n.
  n. screening kit
  n. special care unit (NBSCU)
  transient bullous dermolysis of
    the n.
  transient tachypnea of n. (TTN)
  transient tyrosinemia of n.
  transitory fever of n.
new-onset
  n.-o. diabetes mellitus
  n.-o. hydrocephalus
  n.-o. JDM
newport
  N. medical instrument
  Salmonella n.
  N. Wave ventilator
newtonian aberration
Newtrition
  N. Isofiber formula
  N. Isotonic formula
**NexPill SmartCap medication
  monitoring system**
Nezelof syndrome

Nezhat-Dorsey
  N.-D. aspirator
  N.-D. suction-irrigator
NF
  neurofibromatosis
NF1
  neurofibromatosis type 1
  NF1 gene
NF2
  neurofibromatosis type 2
NFAT
  nuclear factor of activated T cell
NFCS
  neonatal facial coding system
NFDR
  neurofaciodigitorenal
  NFDR syndrome
NF-NS, NFNS
  neurofibromatosis-Noonan syndrome
NG
  nasogastric
  NG tube
NGF
  nerve growth factor
NGHD-SS
  non-growth hormone-deficient short
    stature
NGT
  nasogastric tube
N.G.T. Topical
NH
  neonatal hemochromatosis
NHANES
  National Health and Nutrition
    Examination Survey
NHIS
  National Health Interview Survey
NHL
  non-Hodgkin lymphoma
NHS
  Nance-Horan syndrome
NHT
  neoadjuvant hormonal therapy
**N-[2-hydroxyethyl]piperazine N′-[2-
  ethanesulfonic acid] (HEPES)**
niacin poisoning
niacinamide
nialamide
Niaspan
NIBPM
  noninvasive blood pressure measurement
nicardipine
NICHD
  National Institute of Child Health and
    Human Development
niche
  ontogenetic n.

Nichols
> N. procedure
> N. sacrospinous fixation

nicked human chorionic gonadotropin
nickel dermatitis
Nickerson
> N. BiGGY vials
> N. medium

nick translation
niclosamide
Nico-400
Nicobid
Nicoderm
Nicolas-Favre disease
nicotinamide adenine dinucleotide phosphate (NADPH)
nicotine patch therapy
Nicotinex
nicotinic acid
nicotinyl alcohol
nicoumalone
NICU
> neonatal intensive care unit

nidation
NIDDM
> non-insulin-dependent diabetes mellitus

nidi (*pl. of* nidus)
NIDS
> National Hospital Discharge Survey

nidulans
> *Aspergillus n.*

nidus, pl. **nidi**
Niemann-Pick
> N.-P. cell
> N.-P. disease type A (NPA)
> N.-P. disease type B (NPB)
> N.-P. disease type C (NPC)
> N.-P. disease type D (NPD)
> N.-P. disease (type I, II)

nifedipine
nifurtimox
niger
> *Aspergillus n.*
> *Peptococcus n.*

night
> n. blindness
> n. pain
> n. splint
> n. splinting
> n. sweat
> n. terror

Nightingale examining lamp

nightmare
nigra
> lingua n.
> substantia n.

nigricans
> acanthosis n.
> hirsutism, androgen excess, insulin resistance, acanthosis n. (HAIR-AN, HAIRAN)
> hyperandrogenism, insulin resistance, acanthosis n. (HAIR-AN, HAIRAN)
> pseudoacanthosis n.
> n. syndrome

nigricans-hyperinsulinemia syndrome
nigripalpus
> *Culex n.*

nigrostriatal tract
NIH
> National Institutes of Health

NIHF
> nonimmune hydrops fetalis

Niikawa-Kuroki syndrome
Nijmegen breakage syndrome (NBS)
Nikolsky sign
Nilandron
nilutamide
Nimbex
NIMH
> National Institute of Mental Health
> NIMH global scale

nimodipine
NIMV
> noninvasive motion ventilation

nine
> rule of n.'s

Niplette device
nipple
> accessory n.
> n. discharge
> n. eczema
> extranumerary n.
> n. fed
> n. feeding
> n. flow rate
> inverted n.
> McGovern n.
> O₂ flowmeter n.
> out-of-profile n.
> Paget disease of n.
> preemie n.
> n. retraction

NOTES

nipple *(continued)*
    n. shield
    n. soreness
    n. stimulation
    n. stimulation test
    supernumerary n.
nipple-areola complex
nipple-fed baby
nipplelike lesion
nippling
Nipride
NIPS
    Neonatal Infant Pain Scale
NIRP
    near infrared photoplethysmography
NIRS, NIS
    near infrared spectrophotometry
    near infrared spectroscopy
NIS-2
    Second National Incidence Study
NISD
    neonatal iron-storage disease
Nisentil
Nissen fundoplication
Nissl
    N. bodies
    N. granule
nit
Nitabuch layer
Nite Train'r Alarm
nitidus
    lichen n.
nitrate
    butoconazole n.
    miconazole n.
    silver n.
Nitrazine
    fern-positive N.
    N. paper
    N. test
nitric
    n. oxide (NO)
    n. oxide oxidation
nitrite
    plasma n.
    n. urine test
Nitro-Bid Ointment
nitroblue
    n. tetrazolium (NBT)
    n. tetrazolium dye reduction test
Nitrocap
nitrocellulose
Nitro-Dur Patch
nitrofurantoin
    n. monohydrate
    n. monohydrate macrocrystal
Nitrogard Buccal
nitrogen (N)
    blood urea n. (BUN)

    n. dioxide inhalation
    liquid n.
    n. mustard
    n. partial pressure (PN_2)
    serum urea n. (SUN)
    urea n.
    n. washout
    n. washout test
nitrogenous base
nitroglycerin (NTG)
    n. paste
    topical n.
Nitroglyn Oral
nitroimidazole compound
Nitrolingual Translingual Spray
Nitrol Ointment
Nitronet
Nitrong
Nitropress
nitroprusside
    sodium n. (SNP)
    n. sodium
nitrosourea
Nitrospan
Nitrostat Sublingual
nitrotyrosine
nitrous oxide (N_2O)
nitrovasodilator
Nivea cream
Nix Creme Rinse
nizatidine
Nizoral
NJCLD
    National Joint Committee on Learning
    Disabilities
NJF
    Naegeli-Franceschetti-Jadasshon
    NJF syndrome
NJ tube
NK
    natural killer cell
NKC
NKH
    nonketotic hyperglycinemia
NLD
    necrobiosis lipoidica diabeticorum
NLE
    neonatal lupus erythematosus
NLGCLS
    Noonan-like giant cell lesion syndrome
N2-L-lysylbradkinin
NLP
    no light perception
NLS
    Neu-Laxova syndrome
NMGTD
    nonmetastatic gestational trophoblastic
    disease

NMJ
neuromuscular junction
NMN
Novy-McNeal-Nicolle
NMR
neonatal mortality risk
nuclear magnetic resonance
NMR spectroscopy
NMS
neurally mediated syncope
neuroleptic malignant syndrome
N-Multistix
n,n-diethyl-m-toluamide (DEET)
NNRTI
nonnucleoside reverse transcriptase
inhibitor
NO
nitric oxide
N₂O
nitrous oxide
No. 1
Valertest No. 1
no
no light perception (NLP)
no tears
Noack syndrome
Noble-Mengert perineal repair
Nocardia
  N. asteroides
  N. brasiliensis
  N. caviae
  N. farcinica
  N. nova
  N. otitidiscaviarum
  N. transvalensis
nocardiosis
nociception
nociceptive
  n. pathway
  n. sensory nerve
  n. stimulus
nociferous cortex
nocturia
nocturnal
  n. angina
  n. asthma
  n. enuresis
  n. epilepsy
  n. leg cramp
  n. micturition
  n. myoclonus
  n. pulse oximetry

  n. retrosternal chest pain
  n. sweating
nocturnus
pavor n.
nodal
  n. involvement
  n. tachycardia
nodding spasm
node
  aortic n.
  atrioventricular n.
  axillary lymph n.
  caseous n.
  Cloquet n.
  femoral lymph n.
  gluteal lymph n.
  Hensen n.
  hypogastric lymph n.
  iliac n.
  inguinal lymph n.
  intramammary lymph n.
  locoregional n.
  lymph n.
  mucocutaneous lymph n.
  Osler n.
  paraaortic n.
  parapharyngeal lymph n.
  parauterine lymph n.
  pelvic lymph n.
  peracervical n.
  periaortic lymph n.
  rectal n.
  retroperitoneal n.
  retropharyngeal lymph n.
  sacral lymph n.
  Schmorl n.
  sentinel lymph n.
  shotty n.
  signal n.
  sinoatrial n. (SA)
  subaortic lymph n.
  ureteral n.
  vulvar lymph n.
nodosa
  distal trichorrhexis n.
  infantile periarteritis n. (IPN)
  infantile polyarteritis n. (IPAN)
  maculopapular n.
  periarteritis n.
  polyarteritis n. (PAN)
  salpingitis isthmica n. (SIN)
  trichorrhexis n.

NOTES

N

nodosum
  amnion n.
  erythema n.
nodular
  n. adrenal hyperplasia
  n. blueberry lips
  n. cortical sclerosis
  n. embryo
  n. fasciitis
  n. gastritis
  n. infiltration
  n. lymphoid hyperplasia
  n. melanoma
  n. nerve thickening
  n. nonsuppurative panniculitis
  n. renal blastoma
  n. sclerosing Hodgkin disease
  n. thyroid disease
nodularity
  uterosacral n.
nodule
  Albini n.
  Aschoff n.
  blueberry muffin n.
  Bohn n.
  Brown n.
  Busacca iris n.
  cold n.
  cutaneous n.
  Hoboken n.
  hot n.
  iris Lisch n.
  Koeppe iris n.
  Lisch n.
  Lutz-Jeanselme n.
  palpable n.
  parenchymal n.
  pearly-white n.
  placental site n.
  rheumatoid n.
  Sister Mary Joseph n.
  subcutaneous n.
  subserosal n.
  thyroid n.
  vocal n.
nodulocystic lesion
NOE
  nasoorbitoethmoid
  NOE fracture
NOFT, NOFTT
  nonorganic failure to thrive
Noguchi test
noir
  tache n.
noise
  expiratory n.
  upper airway n.
Nolahist
Nolvadex

noma
  n. neonatorum
  n. pudendi
  n. vulvae
nomenclature
  FIGO n.
  Fisher-Race Rh system n.
  TNM n.
nomogram
  body mass index n.
  Done n.
  gestation-specific n.
  Lubchenco n.
  Rumack-Matthew n.
  Siggaard-Andersen n.
non-A
  n.-A hepatitis
  n.-A, non-B hepatitis (NANBH)
  n.-A, non-B hepatotropic virus
non-ABCDE hepatitis
nonaccidental spiral tibial fracture
nonalcoholic steatohepatitis (NASH)
nonalkylating agent
nonallele
nonallergenic
  n. perrenial rhinitis
  n. rhinitis with eosinophilia
nonallergic rhinitis
nonalpha cell tumor
nonambulatory
nonangiitic vasculopathic condition
nonanion gap metabolic acidosis
nonappendiceal carcinoid
nonatopic wheezer
nonautoimmune myasthenic syndrome
nonautologous reconstruction
nonautonomous attachment
nonbacterial
  n. thrombotic endocarditis
  n. thrombotic vegetation (NBTV)
non-B hepatitis
nonbilious vomiting
nonbranching pseudohypha
non-breathhold MR cholangiography
nonbronchoscopic bronchoalveolar lavage
nonbullous
  n. congenital ichthyosiform
    erythroderma
  n. impetigo
noncalcific vasculopathy
noncalcified nodular mass
noncalculous
noncarbonic acid
noncardiac pulmonary edema
noncarrier
noncaseating sarcoidlike granuloma
non-casein-based diet
noncategorical placement
noncirrhotic ascitic disease

nonclassic, nonclassical
- n. adrenal hyperplasia (NCAH)
- n. congenital adrenal hyperplasia (NC-CAH)
- n. 21-hydroxylase deficiency

noncleft median face syndrome

noncoiled cord

noncoital
- n. sexual pain
- n. sexual stimulation

noncommunicating
- N. Children's Pain Checklist-Revised (NCCPC-R)
- n. cyst
- n. hydrocephalus
- n. uterine horn

noncompliance
- medical n.

noncontact ultrasound

nonconvulsive
- n. seizure
- n. status epilepticus (NCSE)

noncornual placental location

noncosmetic panniculectomy

noncovalent

noncyanotic congenital heart disease

nondeciduous placenta

nondeletion

nondepolarizing paralyzing agent

nondiagnostic culdocentesis

nondirective
- n. counseling
- n. supportive psychotherapy

nondisjunction
- chromosomal n.
- n. trisomy 21

nondisplaced lateral condylar fracture

nondysgerminomatous germ cell tumor

nonencephalitogenic cell

nonepileptic
- n. myoclonus
- n. seizure

nonessential amino acid

nonestrogen drug

nonestrogen-regulated growth

nonexercise activity thermogenesis

nonexudative conjunctival injection

nonfamilial
- n. aniridia
- n. hyperinsulinemic hypoglycemia
- n. hyperinsulinism of infancy
- n. visceral myopathy

nonfat milk

nonfenestrated forceps

nonfixing eye

nonfollicular
- n. pustulosis
- n. pustulosis of newborn

nonfrank breech

nonfrosted tip

nonfunctional
- n. pituitary tumor
- n. streak

nongamma Coombs test

nongenetic syndrome

nongenital pelvic organ

nongenotoxic

nongestational choriocarcinoma

nongonococcal
- n. cervicitis
- n. urethritis

nongranulomatous salpingitis

non-growth hormone-deficient short stature (NGHD-SS)

nonhematogenous tumor

nonheme iron

nonhemolytic
- n. aerobic organism
- n. reaction

nonhistone

non-Hodgkin lymphoma (NHL)

nonhomologous chromosome

nonhydropic fetus

nonhyperinsulinemic hypoglycemia

non-IgE-mediated food allergy

nonimmune
- n. fetal hydrops
- n. hemolysis
- n. hydrops fetalis (NIHF)

non-insulin-dependent
- n.-i.-d. diabetes
- n.-i.-d. diabetes mellitus (NIDDM)
- n.-i.-d. diabetic

noninvasive
- n. blood pressure measurement (NIBPM)
- n. detection of trisomy 18
- n. extrathoracic ventilator (NEV)
- n. management
- n. motion ventilation (NIMV)
- n. respiratory support
- n. test

NOTES

N

645

nonionic
- n. contrast material
- n. contrast medium

nonionizing nonthermal application
nonirritating
nonisomorphic presentation
nonketotic
- n. hyperglycemia
- n. hyperglycinemia (NKH)
- n. hyperosmolar coma
- n. hypoglycemia

nonkinesigenic
nonlactating breast
nonleukocytospermic
nonlinkage
nonlocking closure
nonlymphoblastic leukemia
nonlymphocytic leukemia
nonmaleficence
nonmaternal death
nonmendelian disorder
nonmetastatic gestational trophoblastic disease (NMGTD)
nonmigrainous headache
nonmonogamous partner
nonmotile sperm
nonmusical wheeze
nonmutogenic
nonnarcotic abstinence syndrome
Nonne-Milroy-Meige syndrome
nonneoplastic epithelial disorder
nonneural congenital defect
nonneurogenic
- n. dysphagia
- n. neurogenic bladder

nonnucleoside reverse transcriptase inhibitor (NNRTI)
nonnutritional rickets
nonnutritive
- n. sucking
- n. sucking opportunity (NSO)

nonobstruction
- large-volume n.

nonobstructive
- n. pattern
- n. pyelonephritis

nonoliguric ARF
nonorganic failure to thrive (NOFT, NOFTT)
nonossifying fibroma
nonoxynol-9/octoxynol-9
nonpalpable
- n. abnormality
- n. testis

nonparalytic
- n. hypotonia
- n. poliomyelitis
- n. strabismus

nonparous

nonpathologic fracture
nonphotogenic seizure
nonpigmented endometriosis
nonpitting induration
non-PKU phenylalaninemia
nonpolio enterovirus
nonpregnant endometrium
nonprimary
- n. first episode
- n. infection

nonprogressive
- n. cerebellar disorder with mental retardation
- n. hypoplastic syndrome
- n. motor impairment syndrome
- n. ventriculomegaly

nonproliferative
- n. diabetic retinopathy
- n. fibrocystic change

nonproteinuric hypertension
nonpsychotic
nonpuerperal
- n. endometritis
- n. mastitis

nonpurging
- bulimia nervosa n. (BN-NP)

non-Q-wave AMI
nonradioactive immunoassay
nonrandom mating
nonrapid eye movement (NREM)
nonreactive
- n. immunoassay
- n. NST

nonreassuring
- n. fetal heart beat pattern
- n. fetal heart rate pattern
- n. fetal status
- n. fetal testing
- n. FHR

nonrebreather
- n. face mask
- high-flow n.

nonreciprocal gait
non-REM sleep
nonresting energy expenditure (NREE)
nonrhabdomyogenic soft tissue sarcoma
nonrhabdomyomatous sarcoma
nonrhabdomyosarcoma soft tissue sarcoma (NRSTS)
non-Rh D/non-ABO hemolytic disease
nonsalt-losing adrenogenital syndrome
nonsecreting pituitary tumor
nonsense mutation
nonseptated
non-sex hormone-binding globulin bound testosterone
nonspastic paraparesis
nonspecific
- n. arrhythmia (NSA)

n. encephalopathy
n. esophageal motility disorder (NEMD)
n. ileitis
n. immunotherapy
n. mental retardation
n. mesenchyme
n. urethritis (NSU)
n. vaginitis
n. vulvovaginitis

nonspherical congruent hips
nonspherocytic anemia
nonsteroidal antiinflammatory drug (NSAID)
nonstreptococcal pharyngitis
nonstressed fetus
nonstress test (NST)
nonstructural gene
nonsuppurative panniculitis
nonsusceptible
nonsustained ventricular tachycardia
non-syncytium-inducing (NSI)

n.-s.-i. strain
n.-s.-i. variant of AIDS virus

nonsyndromic bile duct paucity
nontension pneumothorax
nonthyroidal illness (NTI)
nontoxic
nontreponemal

n. serology
n. test

non-*Treponema* titer
nontubal ectopic pregnancy
nontuberculous

n. mycobacterial infection
n. mycobacterium (NTM)

nontumoral hyperprolactinemia
nontypeable organism
non-typhi *Salmonella* (NTS)
nontyphoidal *Salmonella*
nontyphoid *Salmonella*
nonulcer dyspepsia
nonunion
nonvalent pneumococcal conjugate vaccine (PnCV)
nonvascular
nonverbal

n. communication
n. developmental index
n. learning disability (NVLD)
n. perceptual-organization-output disorder

nonvertex fetus
nonvertex-nonvertex
nonvertex-vertex
nonvertiginous condition
nonvesicular rash
nonviable fetus
nonvolatile acid
non-Wessel colic
Noonan-Ehmke syndrome
Noonan-like

N.-l. giant cell lesion
N.-l. giant cell lesion syndrome (NLGCLS)

Noonan syndrome
noradrenaline

plasma n.

noradrenergic

n. locus ceruleus
n. system

Norcept-E 1/35
Norcuron
NORD

National Organization for Rare Disorders

Nordette contraceptive pill
Norditropin Injection
norelgestromin
norepinephrine
Norethin

N. 1/35M
N. 1/50M

norethindrone

n. acetate
n. acetate and ethinyl estradiol
n. enanthate (NET-EN)
ethinyl estradiol and n.
mestranol and n.

norethisterone
norethynodrel

mestranol and n.

Norflex
norfloxacin
norgestimate

ethinyl estradiol and n.
n. and ethinyl estradiol
n. progestin

norgestrel

ethinyl estradiol and n.

***d*-norgestrel**
norgestrel/ethinyl estradiol combination
norimbergensis

Burkholderia n.

NOTES

Norinyl
- N. 1+35
- N. 1+50

Norisodrine

Norlestrin
- N. 1/50
- N. 2.5/50
- N. Fe

normal
- n. blood loss
- n. blood pressure
- n. female sex chromosome type (XX)
- n. fetal development
- n. flap-valve mechanism
- n. gastroesophageal reflux of infancy
- n. intelligence
- n. male sex chromosome type (XY)
- n. ovariotomy
- n. placentation
- n. pressure hydrocephalus (NPH)
- n. saline
- n. saline solution (NSS)
- n. spontaneous vaginal delivery (NSVD)
- n. temperature
- n. transformation zone
- n. vaginal delivery

normally progressing pregnancy (NPP)
Norman-Landing syndrome
Norman Miller vaginopexy
Norman-Roberts lissencephaly syndrome
Norman-Wood syndrome
Normegon
Nor-Mil
normoactive bowel sounds
normobaric oxygen
normoblast cell
normoblastemia
normocalcemic
normocapnia
normocephalic
normochromic anemia
normocytic anemia
Normodyne
normoglycemia
normophosphatemic
normoprolactinemia
normospermic
normotensive intrauterine growth restriction
Normotest
normothermia
norm-referenced test
Noroxin
Norpace CR

Norplant
- N. implant
- N. system

Norpramin
Nor-QD
Norrbottnian Gaucher disease
Norrie
- N. disease
- N. syndrome

Norrie-Warburg syndrome
Norris-Carroll criteria
19-nortestosterone derivative
Nor-tet Oral
North
- N. American Collaborative Crohn Disease Study (NCCDS)
- N. American Society for Pediatric Gastroenterology and Nutrition (NASPGN)
- N. Asian tick typhus

Northern
- N. blot
- N. blot test

Northway staging
Norton operation
Nortrel 7/7/7
nortriptyline hydrochloride
Nortussin
Norvir
- N. capsule
- N. oral solution

Norwalk
- N. agent
- N. virus

Norwalk-like virus
Norwegian scabies
Norwood
- N. operation
- N. palliation
- N. procedure
- N. stage

nose
- beaked n.
- bifid n.
- broad flat n.
- flat n.
- prominent n.
- rabbit n.
- saddle n.
- short beaked n.

nosebleed
nose-breather
- obligate n.-b.

nosocomial
- n. bacterial infection (NBI)
- n. bacterial meningitis
- n. diarrhea
- n. infection

n. pneumonia
n. sepsis
nosocomially acquired (NA)
nosology
nostril
anteverted n.
N. Nasal Solution
reverse n.'s
Nostrilla
notch
alveolar n.
interarytenoid n.
intercondylar n.
median alveolar n.
N. receptor
sacrosciatic n.
suprasternal n.
notching
rib n.
note
hyperresonant calvarial
percussion n.
notochord
notogenesis
notomelus
Nottingham breast cancer grading
system
nova
Nocardia n.
Novafed
Novafil
Novahistine
Novak curette
Novamoxin
Novantrone
Novapren
Nova Rectal
Novasome
NovaSure
N. endometrial ablation procedure
N. impedance-controlled endometrial
ablation system
novo
N.-AZT
N.-Cimetidine
N.-Clobetasol
N.-Cloxin
N.-Cromolyn
de n.
N.-Difenac
N.-Difenac-SR
N.-Diflunisal

N.-Dipam
N.-Doxylin
N.-Famotidine
N.-Fibrate
N.-Flurazine
N.-Flurprofen
N.-Hydrazide
N.-Keto-EC
N.-Lexin
N.-Naprox
N.-Nidazol
N.-Pen-VK
N.-Piroxicam
N.-Pramine
N.-Profen
N.-Ranidine
N.-Reserpine
N.-Ridazine
N.-Rythro Encap
N.-Seven
N.-Soxazole
stress incontinence de n.
N.-Tamoxifen
N.-Terfenadine
N.-Tetra
N.-Trimel
novobiocin
Novolin
N. 70/30
N. insulin
N. L, N, R
N. N, R PenFil
N. 70/30 PenFil
Novopropamide
Novy-McNeal-Nicolle (NMN)
N.-M.-N. biphasic blood agar
noxa, pl. **noxae**
embryonic noxae
Nozinan
NP
naturopath
NPA
nasopharyngeal aspirate
Niemann-Pick disease type A
NPB
Niemann-Pick disease type B
NPC
Niemann-Pick disease type C
NP-CPAP
nasal prong continuous positive airway
pressure

N

NOTES

NPD
Niemann-Pick disease type D
NPH
nephronophthisis
neutral protamine Hagedorn
normal pressure hydrocephalus
NPH Iletin I, II
NPH insulin
NPH-N
pork NPH
NPH1
nephronophthisis type 1
NPHN
nephrin
NPI
Neonatal Perception Inventory
NPL
nasopharyngolaryngoscopy
NPOT
narrow pulmonary outflow tract
NPP
normally progressing pregnancy
NPR
nasopharyngeal reflux
NPTR
National Pediatric Trauma Registry
NR
Organidin NR
Tussi-Organidin DM NR
NREE
nonresting energy expenditure
NREM
nonrapid eye movement
NREM arousal parasomnia
NRP
Neonatal Resuscitation Program
NRSTS
nonrhabdomyosarcoma soft tissue
sarcoma
NRTI
nucleoside reverse transcriptase inhibitor
thymidine analog NRTI
NS
Lidodex NS
NSA
neck-shaft angle
nonspecific arrhythmia
NSA of femur
NSABP
National Surgical Adjuvant Breast
Project
NSAID
nonsteroidal antiinflammatory drug
NSD
N-acetylneuraminic acid storage disease
NSE
neuron-specific enolase
NSI
neurosensory impairment

non-syncytium-inducing
NSI strain
NSO
nonnutritive sucking opportunity
NSS
normal saline solution
NST
nonstress test
antepartum fetal NST
fetal NST
nonreactive NST
NST tracing
NSU
nonspecific urethritis
NSVD
normal spontaneous vaginal delivery
NT
N-telopeptide
NTD
neural tube defect
N-telopeptide (NT)
N-t. cross-links (NTx)
N-t. test
NTG
nitroglycerin
NTI
nonthyroidal illness
NTM
nontuberculous mycobacterium
NTS
non-typhi *Salmonella*
NTT
nuchal translucency thickness
NTx
N-telopeptide cross-links
NTx test
Nu
Nu-Amoxi
Nu-Ampi
Nu-Cephalex
Nu-Cimet
Nu-Cloxi
Nu-Cotrimox
Nu-Diclo
Nu-Diflunisal
Nu-Doxycycline
Nu-Famotidine
Nu-Flurprofen
Nu Gauze dressing
Nu-Ibuprofen
Nu-Ketoprofen
Nu-Ketoprofen-E
Nu-Naprox
Nu-Pen-VK
Nu-Pirox
Nu-Ranit
Nu-Tetra
Nubain

nuchal
n. arm
n. cord
n. cystic hygroma
n. fold
n. pad thickening
n. rigidity
n. translucency
n. translucency in a fetus
n. translucency measurement
n. translucency screening
n. translucency thickness (NTT)
nuchal-spinal sign
Nuck
canal of N.
N. canal
N. diverticulum
N. hydrocele
nuclear
n. agenesis
n. antigen
n. aplasia
n. atypia
n. debris
n. degeneration
n. dust
n. factor of activated T cell
(NFAT)
n. jaundice
n. magnetic resonance (NMR)
n. milk
n. radiation
n. scintigraphy
n. sex
nuclease
nucleated red blood cell
nucleatum
Fusobacterium n.
nuclei (*pl. of* nucleus)
nucleic
n. acid
n. acid amplification (NAA)
n. acid hybridization
n. acid probe
n. acid sequence-based amplification
(NASBA)
nucleoid
nucleolar chromosome
nucleolus, pl. **nucleoli**
nucleoside
n. analog
n. pair

n. phosphorylase
n. reverse transcriptase inhibitor
(NRTI)
nucleosome
nucleotide
adenine n.
antisense n.
cytosine n.
guanine n.
thymine n.
nucleotide-fortified formula
nucleotidylexotransferase
DNA n.
nucleotidyltransferase
DNA n.
RNA n.
nucleus, pl. **nuclei**
n. accumbens
arcuate n.
Béclard n.
caudate n.
cerebellar n.
cranial nerve n.
dentate n.
disorganized brainstem nuclei
Edinger-Westphal n.
inferior olivary n.
lentiform n.
olivary nuclei
owl's eye n.
red n.
n. reticularis gigantocellularis
n. retroambiguus
steroid n.
superior olivary n.
n. tractus solitarius
X-linked congenital recessive
muscle hypotrophy with central
nuclei
NucliSens assay
NUG
necrotizing ulcerating gingivitis
Nu-Gel dressing
Nugent criteria
Nu-Knit
Surgical N.-K.
null
n. cell tumor
n. zone
nulligravida
nullipara
nulliparity

NOTES

nulliparous woman
NuLYTELY
number
>n. of different words (NDW)
>fetal n.
>n. of needle passes
>ovulation n.
>Reynolds n.

numbing
Numby Stuff
nummular
>n. dermatitis
>n. eczema

Numorphan
Nunn engorged corpuscles
Nupercainal cream
Nuprin
Nuromax Injection
nurse
>wet n.

nursemaid's elbow
nursery
>intensive care n. (ICN)
>intensive special care n. (ISCN)
>level 1–3 n.
>n. NBRS
>newborn n.
>well-baby n. (WBN)

Nursette prefilled disposable bottle
nursing
>Association of Women's Health, Obstetrics, and Neonatal N. (AWHONN)

nurturant
nurture
Nuss concave chest correction technique
nutans
>eclampsia n.
>spasmus n.

nutcracker esophagus
Nutracort Topical
Nutraderm cream
Nutramigen formula
Nutren
>N. 1.0, 1,5, 2.0 formula
>N. 1.0 with Fiber formula

nutrient
>intraluminal n.
>n. requirement

Nutrilipid
nutrition
>central venous n. (CVN)
>diet and n.
>fetal n.
>fluids, electrolytes, n. (FEN)
>home parenteral n. (HPN)
>inadequate maternal n.
>maternal n.

>North American Society for Pediatric Gastroenterology and N. (NASPGN)
>parenteral n. (PN)
>PediaSure liquid n.
>pediatric n.
>ProBalance liquid n.
>total parenteral n. (TPN)
>total peripheral parenteral n. (TPPN)

nutritional
>n. assessment
>n. deprivation syndrome
>n. hepatotoxicity
>n. immunology
>n. neuropathy
>n. problem
>n. requirement
>n. rickets
>n. supplement
>n. support
>n. surveillance

nutrition-associated
>parenteral n.-a. (PNAC)

nutritionist
Nutropin AQ Injection
NuvaRing vaginal contraceptive ring
N/V
>nausea and vomiting

NVAC
>National Vaccine Advisory Committee

nvCJD
>new variant Creutzfeldt-Jakob disease

NVD
>neovascularization of disc

NVLD
>nonverbal learning disability

NWI
>Neonatal Withdrawal Inventory

NWTS
>National Wilms Tumor Study Group

NX
>Talwin NX

Nyaderm
nyctalopia
Nydrazid Injection
NYHA
>New York Heart Association
>>NYHA classification of heart disease

Nylen maneuver
nylidrin hydrochloride
nylon suture material
nympha, pl. **nymphae**
nymphectomy
nymphitis
nymphomania
nymphoncus
nymphotomy

NyQuil
Vicks Children's N.
Nyquist frequency
nystagmus
acquired n.
asymmetric n.
congenital jerky n.
congenital pendular n.
convergent n.
downbeat n.
fixation n.
gaze-evoked n.
gaze-paretic n.
horizontal n.
jerk n.
latent n.
monocular n.
optokinetic n.
pendular n.

positional n.
railroad n.
retractive n.
n. retractorius
seesaw n.
spontaneous n.
unilateral optokinetic n.
upbeat n.
vertical n.
vestibular n.
nystatin
n. and triamcinolone cream
n. and triamcinolone ointment
Nystat-Rx
Nystop topical powder
Nytilax
Nytol
Nytone enuretic control unit

NOTES

N

O₂
>oxygen
>>O₂ flowmeter nipple
>>hood O₂
>>O₂ saturation

OA
>occipitoanterior
>occiput anterior
>ocular albinism
>osteoarthritis

OAAS
>Observer Assessment of Alertness and Sedation

OAB
>overactive bladder

OAC
>optical aspirating curette

OAD
>overanxious disorder

OADP-CDS
>Oregon Adolescent Depression Project-Conduct Disorder Screener

OAE
>otoacoustic emission
>>OAE test
>>OAE testing

O antigen

OAR
>Ottawa Ankle Rules

oasthouse urine disease

oat cell carcinoma

OATS
>oligoasthenoteratozoospermia syndrome

OAV
>oculoauriculovertebral
>>OAV syndrome

OAVS
>oculoauriculovertebral spectrum

OB
>obstetrician
>obstetrics
>osteoblast
>osteoblastoma
>>Chemstrip 4 The OB
>>OB Gees maternity orthotic
>>Sil-K OB

obese

obesity
>adolescent o.
>age-adjusted o.
>android o.
>o. in endometrial sarcoma
>exogenous o.
>experimental o.
>gynecoid o.

hypotonia, hypopigmentia, hypogonadism, o. (HHHO)
>mild-to-moderate o.
>o., short stature, mental deficiency, hypogonadism, micropenis, finger contracture, cleft lip-palate syndrome
>progressive o.
>truncal o.

obesity-hypotonia syndrome

obesity-hypoventilation syndrome

obesity-related hyposomatotropism

Obetrol

Obeval

Obezine

OBG
>OBG Clinical Records Manager software
>OBG LabTrack software

OB/GYN
>obstetrician-gynecologist
>obstetrics and gynecology

obidoxime chloride

object
>o. assembly test
>o. constancy
>o. permanence
>unidentified bright o.

objective probability

obligate
>o. carrier
>o. heterozygote
>o. nose-breather

obligatory
>o. heel valgus
>o. primitive reflex
>o. tonic neck reflex

oblique
>o. diameter
>o. flank muscle
>o. fracture
>left anterior o. (LAO)
>o. lie
>o. presentation
>o. radiograph
>right anterior o. (RAO)
>o. view

obliquity
>antimongoloid o.
>Litzmann o.
>Nägele o.

obliterans
>bronchiolitis o.

obliterated
>o. processus vaginalis

O

obliterated *(continued)*
 o. umbilical artery
 o. urachus
 o. vein
obliteration
 o. of apophyseal space
 cul-de-sac o.
 vessel o.
obliterative
 o. arachnoiditis
 o. bronchitis
 o. coronary artery disease
 o. endarteritis
 o. fibroproliferative bronchiolitis
oblongata
 medulla o.
Obrinsky syndrome
observation
 o. hip
 prelinguistic autism diagnostic o.
  (PL-ADOS)
Observer Assessment of Alertness and Sedation (OAAS)
obsession
obsessionality
obsessive-compulsive
 o.-c. behavior (OCB)
 o.-c. disorder (OCD)
 o.-c. personality disorder (OCPD)
obstetric
 o. accident
 o. analgesia
 o. anesthesia
 o. auscultation
 o. binder
 o. brachial plexus palsy
 o. canal
 o. care
 o. complication
 o. conjugate
 o. conjugate diameter
 o. conjugate of outlet
 o. damage
 o. emergency room
 o. forceps
 o. history
 o. hysterectomy
 o. neuropathy
 o. operation
 o. outcome
 o. paralysis
 o. position
 o. risk factor
 o. traction injury
 o. ultrasonography
 o. ultrasound
 o. ultrasound examination

obstetrical
 o. palsy
 o. paralysis
obstetric-gynecologic care
obstetrician (OB)
 high-risk o.
obstetrician-gynecologist (OB/GYN)
obstetricopediatric
obstetrics (OB)
 ambulatory o.
 defensive o.
 family-centered o.
 general o.
 o. and gynecology (OB/GYN)
 International Federation of
  Gynecology and O. (FIGO)
obstipation
obstructed
 o. bowel loop
 o. calyx
 o. labor
obstructing periureteral fibrosis
obstruction
 airway o.
 o. of appendix
 arterial o.
 bilateral ureteral o. (BUO)
 bladder neck o.
 bowel o.
 cervical stenosis o.
 check valve o.
 closed-loop o.
 colonic o.
 congenital lacrimal duct o.
 congenital nasolacrimal duct o.
  (CNLDO)
 congenital urinary tract o.
 distal intestinal o.
 distal tubal o.
 ductal o.
 duodenal o.
 extrahepatic portal vein o.
 extrahepatic presinusoidal o.
 extramural upper airway o.
 extrathoracic o.
 fimbrial o.
 functional outlet o.
 gastrointestinal o.
 glottal o.
 hypopharyngeal-glottal o.
 iatrogenic urethral o.
 incomplete bowel o.
 infravesical o.
 intestinal o.
 intrabronchial o.
 intrabronchiolar o.
 intraluminal upper airway o.
 intramural upper airway o.
 intrathoracic airway o.

intrauterine ureteral o.
lacrimal duct o.
left ventricular outflow tract o.
 (LVOTO)
left ventricular outlet o.
lymphatic o.
mechanical o.
meconium o.
milk bolus o.
nasal o.
nasolacrimal duct o.
nasopharyngeal airway o.
outflow o.
pelviureteric junction o.
portal vein o. (PVO)
positional airways o.
presinusoidal o.
proximal tubal o.
pseudointestinal o.
pulmonary venous o.
renal o.
right ventricular outflow tract o.
 (RVOTO)
strangulating o.
o. syndrome
systemic outflow o.
tracheobronchial o.
tubal o.
unilateral ureteral o. (UUO)
UPJ o.
ureteral o.
ureterovesical o.
urinary outlet o.
urinary tract o.
uterine outflow o.
UVJ o.
valve o.
variable o.
vein o.
venous o.
ventricular outflow o.

obstructive
o. apnea
o. atelectasis
o. azoospermia
o. dysmenorrhea
o. hydrocephalus
o. jaundice
o. lung disease
o. malformation
o. megaloureter

o. overinflation
o. respiratory disease
o. shock
o. sleep apnea (OSA)
o. sleep apnea/hypoventilation
 (OSA/H)
o. sleep apnea syndrome (OSAS)
o. symptom
o. uropathy

obtundation
obtunded
obturator
o. artery
Endopath Optiview optical
 surgical o.
o. fascia
o. internus
o. internus muscle
o. nerve
o. nerve damage
Optiview optical surgical o.
plastic o.
o. sign
obtuse marginal
OB-View imaging
OC
oral contraceptive
OC-125
OCA
oculocutaneous albinism
 yellow OCA
OCB
obsessive-compulsive behavior
OCC
oculocerebrocutaneous
 OCC syndrome
occasional bacteria
occipital
o. bossing
o. horn syndrome
o. osteodiastasis
o. plagiocephaly
occipitoanterior (OA)
left o. position (LOA)
o. position
right o. position (ROA)
occipitoatlantal instability
occipitofrontal
o. circumference (OFC)
o. diameter

O

NOTES

occipitomental
    o. diameter
    o. view
occipitoposterior (OP)
    left o. position (LOP)
    o. position
    right o. position (ROP)
occipitotransverse (OT)
    left o. position (LOT)
    o. position
    right o. position (ROT)
occiput
    o. anterior (OA)
    flattened o.
    o. posterior (OP)
    o. posterior position
    o. presentation
    o. transverse (OT)
Occlucort
occludens
    zonula o.
occluder
    Amplatzer septal o.
occluding spring embolus
occlusal
    o. problem
    o. radiograph
Occlusal-HP Liquid
occlusion
    airway o.
    o. amblyopia
    Angle classification of o.
    arteriolar o.
    basal arterial o.
    cerebral artery o.
    coil o.
    constant flow end-inspiratory airway o.
    o. dermatitis
    distal o.
    end-inspiratory airway o.
    fetal endoscopic tracheal o. (fentendo)
    fetal tracheal o.
    isthmic o.
    middle cerebral artery o. (MCAO)
    proximal o.
    roller o.
    salpingitis after previous tubal o. (SPOT)
    surgical tape o.
    tracheal o.
    tubal o.
    tuboovarian abscess after previous tubal o. (TOAPOT)
occlusive
    o. dressing
    o. vascular disease
    o. vasculitis

occult
    o. bacteremia
    o. blood
    o. cancer
    o. cord prolapse
    o. focus
    o. neuroblastoma
    o. neurogenic bladder
    o. spinal dysraphism
occulta
    spina bifida o.
occultum
    cranium bifidum o.
occupational
    o. acne
    o. history
    o. therapy (OT)
occurrence
    inconsequential o.
OCD
    obsessive-compulsive disorder
    osteochondritis dissecans
Ocean Nasal Mist
Ochoa syndrome
Ochrobactrum anthropi
ochronosis
Ochsner forceps
Ockelbo virus
OCL
    oral colonic lavage
O'Connor-O'Sullivan retractor
OCP
    oral contraceptive pill
OCPD
    obsessive-compulsive personality disorder
OCR
    oculocerebrorenal
    OCR syndrome
OCRL syndrome
OCT
    oral contraceptive therapy
    ornithine carbamoyltransferase
    oxytocin challenge test
    OCT deficiency
octaploidy
Octocaine Injection
Octostim
octoxynol 9
octreotide
    o. acetate
    o. therapy
OcuClear Ophthalmic
Ocufen Ophthalmic
Ocuflox ophthalmic solution
Ocugram
ocular
    o. adnexa
    o. albinism (OA)

o. alignment
o. aspergillosis
o. bobbing
o. coloboma
o. coloboma-imperforate anus
   syndrome
o. erythema
o. flutter
o. hypertelorism
o. hypotelorism
o. hypotony
o. involvement
o. larva migrans
o. lubricant
o. malformation
o. manifestation
o. motility
o. motor dysmetria
o. muscular dystrophy
o. myoclonus
o. myopathy
o. nonnephropathic cystinosis
o. oscillation
o. pain
o. paresis
o. prophylaxis
o. prosthesis
o. sarcoidosis
o. toxoplasmosis
oculi (*pl. of* oculus)
oculoauricular dysplasia
oculoauriculofrontonasal syndrome
oculoauriculovertebral (OAV)
o. dysplasia
o. spectrum (OAVS)
oculocephalic reflex
oculocephalogyric reflex
oculocerebral
o. dystrophy
o. hypopigmentation syndrome
oculocerebrocutaneous (OCC)
oculocerebrofacial syndrome
oculocerebrorenal (OCR)
o. disease of Lowe
o. dystrophy
o. syndrome of Lowe
oculocutaneous
o. albinism (OCA)
o. lesion
o. telangiectasia
o. tyrosinemia
o. tyrosinosis

oculodental syndrome
oculodentodigital (ODD)
o. dysplasia
o. syndrome
oculodentodigitalis
dysplasia o.
oculodentoosseous dysplasia (ODOD)
oculo-digito-esophagoduodenal (ODED)
oculofacial paralysis
oculogenitolaryngeal syndrome
oculoglandular tularemia
oculogyration
oculogyria
oculogyric crisis
oculomandibular dyscephaly
oculomandibulodyscephaly (OMD)
oculomandibulodyscephaly-hypotrichosis
   syndrome
oculomandibulofacial (OMF)
oculomelic amyoplasia
oculomotor
o. apraxia
o. dysfunction
o. nerve
oculomuscular
oculopalatoskeletal syndrome
oculopharyngeal muscular dystrophy
oculoplethysmography
oculosympathetic paresis
oculovestibular response
oculus, pl. **oculi**
adnexa oculi
melanosis oculi
Ocu-Sol
OD$_{450}$
delta OD$_{450}$
ODD
oculodentodigital
oppositional defiant disorder
osteodental dysplasia
ODD syndrome
odd
o. chromosome
o.'s ratio
ODED
oculo-digito-esophagoduodenal
ODED syndrome
od gene
ODOD
oculodentoosseous dysplasia
O'Donnell operation
odontogenesis

NOTES

odontogenic
> o. keratocyst
> o. keratocytosis-skeletal anomalies
>   syndrome

odontoid
> o. process
> o. process hypoplasia

odontoideum
> os o.

odontolyticus
> *Actinomyces o.*

odontoonychodermal dysplasia
odor
> acrid o.
> amine o.
> fishy o.
> fruity breath o.
> musty o.

odorant
odorous
ODT
> Zofran ODT

odynophagia
OE
> otitis externa

OEC
> ovarian epithelial cancer

Oedipus complex
Oestrilin
OFC
> occipitofrontal circumference

OFD
> orofaciodigital
> OFD syndrome, type I–IV, VI–IX
> OFD with tibial dysplasia

offender
> extrafamily o.
> intrafamily o.

office
> o. cystometrics
> o. laparoscopy under local
>   anesthesia (OLULA)
> O. of Special Education Programs
>   (OSEP)

officer
> guidance o.

offspring psychopathology
ofloxacin
OG
> orogastric
> OG tube

OGCT
> oral glucose challenge test

Ogen
> O. Oral
> O. Vaginal

Ogino-Knaus rule
Ogita test

OGTT
> oral glucose tolerance test
> oral glucose tolerance testing

Oguchi disease
OH
> hydroxyl radical

Ohdo blepharophimosis syndrome
Ohio
> O. bed
> O. humidifier
> O. warmer

Ohmeda
> O. Care-Plus incubator
> O. Minx pulse oximeter
> O. 3800 pulse oximeter
> O. SoftProbe probe

21-OH nonclassical adrenal hyperplasia
17-OHP
> 17-hydroxyprogesterone

OHSS
> ovarian hyperstimulation syndrome

Ohtahara syndrome
OI
> osteogenesis imperfecta (type I–IV)
> oxygenation index

OIA
> optical immunoassay
> BioStar Flu OIA

oil
> algal o.
> BAL in O.
> camphorated o.
> castor o.
> cod liver o.
> o. cyst
> o. enema
> ethiodized o.
> evening primrose o. (EPO)
> fish o.
> fungal o.
> glycerin, lanolin and peanut o.
> immersion o.
> Lorenzo's o.
> MCT o.
> mineral o.
> peanut o.
> Progesterone O.

Oilatum soap
ointment
> A and D O.
> Calmoseptine o.
> Centany o.
> Cormax O.
> hydrophilic o.
> Lacri-Lube SOP lubricant eye o.
> LCD o.
> liquor carbonis detergens o.
> Medi-Quick Topical O.
> Monistat 1 1-day vaginal o.

Neosporin Ophthalmic O.
Neosporin Topical O.
Nitro-Bid O.
Nitrol O.
nystatin and triamcinolone o.
oxytetracycline/polymyxin o.
Pazo hemorrhoid o.
Polysporin o.
Protopic o.
salicylic acid o.
Sutilains O.
tioconazole 6.5% o.
Topicort o.
triamcinolone acetonide o.
Triple Paste o.
undecylenic acid o.
Whitfield o.
Xylocaine Topical O.
zinc oxide o.

OIS
Organ Injury Scaling
Oka
O. strain
O. strain varicella vaccine
Okazaki fragment
Oklahoma ankle joint
OKT3
Orthoclone OKT3
OKT8
olanzapine
OLB
open lung biopsy
Olean
oleandomycin phosphate
oleate-condensate
triethanolamine polypeptide o.-c.
olecranon
o. apophysitis
o. fossa
o. fracture
olestra
olfaction
olfacto-ethmoidohypothalamic
o.-e. dysplasia
o.-e. dysraphia
olfactogenital
o. dysplasia
o. syndrome
olfactory
o. hallucination
o. placode
oligamnios (*var. of* oligoamnios)

oligemia
oligo
allele specific o.
oligoamnios, oligamnios
oligoanuria
oligoarthritis
oligoarticular
o. arthritis
o. disease
oligoasthenospermia
oligoasthenoteratozoospermia syndrome (OATS)
oligoclonal bands
oligoclonality
oligodactyly
postaxial o.
oligodendrocyte
oligodendroglia
oligodendroglial degeneration
oligodendroglioma
anaplastic o.
oligodeoxynucleotide
antisense o.
oligogalactia
oligogenic inheritance
oligohydramnios
oligomeganephronia
oligomenorrhea
oligonucleotide
antisense o.
o. probe analysis
oligoovulation
oligophrenia
growth retardation, ocular
abnormalities, microcephaly,
brachydactyly, o. (GOMBO)
oligophrenia-ichthyosis syndrome
oligosaccharide
oligospermia
eugonadotropic o.
reversible o.
oligoteratoasthenozoospermia syndrome
oligozoospermia
oligozoospermic
oliguria
transient o.
oliguric ARF
olivary nuclei
olive
pyloric o.
superior o.
Oliver-McFarlane syndrome

NOTES

O

Oliver syndrome
olivopontocerebellar
    o. atrophy (OPCA)
    o. degeneration
Ollier
    O. disease
    O. syndrome
Ollier-Klippel-Trenaunay-Weber
  syndrome
olopatadine hydrochloride
olpadronate
olsalazine sodium
Olshausen
    O. procedure
    O. sign
    O. suspension
OLTx
   orthotopic liver transplantation
OLULA
   office laparoscopy under local anesthesia
olympian brow
Olympic Neostraint immobilizer
Olympus
    O. disposable cannula
    O. disposable trocar
    O. flexible hysterofiberscope
    O. GIF-XP10 video endoscope
    O. hysteroscope
OM
   otitis media
OMD
   oculomandibulodyscephaly
OME
   otitis media with effusion
omega-3 fatty acid
omega fatty acid
omega-shaped epiglottis
Omenn syndrome
omenta (*pl. of* omentum)
omental
    o. adhesion
    o. biopsy
    o. cake
    o. cyst
omentectomy
    partial o.
omentum, pl. omenta
    lymphocyst o.
    matted o.
omeprazole
OMF
   oculomandibulofacial
    OMF syndrome
OMI
   oocyte maturation inhibitor
OMM
   ophthalmomandibulomelic
Ommaya reservoir

Omnicef oral suspension
Omnipaque
Omniprobe test
Omni-Tract vaginal retractor
omovertebral bone
omphalitis
omphaloangiopagous twins
omphaloangiopagus
omphalocele
omphalocele-cleft palate syndrome
omphalomesenteric
    o. artery
    o. canal
    o. cord
    o. cyst
    o. duct
    o. duct remnant
omphalopagus
omphalorrhagia
omphalorrhea
omphalorrhexis
omphalotomy
omphalotripsy
Omron monitor
Omsk
    O. hemorrhagic fever
    O. virus
OMS Oral
onanism
Onat syndrome
Oncaspar
Onchocerca volvulus
onchocerciasis
oncofetal
    o. antigen
    o. fibronectin
oncogene
    Bcl-2 o.
    c-*erb* B-2 o.
    c-*myc* o.
    o. expression
    H-*ras* o.
    human epidermal growth factor-
      2 o.
    K-*ras* o.
    neu/HER2 o.
oncogenous rickets
oncologist
   Society of Gynecologic O.'s (SGO)
oncology
   gynecologic o.
On-Command catheter
oncoprotein
    c-*erb* B-2 o.
OncoScint
    O. CR103 monoclonal antibody
    O. CR/OV contrast medium
    O. test

oncotic
>   o. force
>   o. pressure

Oncovin

ondansetron HCl

Ondine curse

Ondine-Hirschsprung syndrome

Ondogyne

one-child sterility

one-egg twins

one-horned uterus

one-hour
>   o.-h. glucose tolerance test
>   o.-h. PG
>   o.-h. prostaglandin

O'Neil
>   O. cup
>   O. vacuum extractor

One Step Button gastrostomy device

one-way valve

ONH
>   optic nerve hypoplasia

onion bulb formation

onion-skin appearance

onion skinning

onlay
>   o. island flap
>   o. patch anastomosis

onset
>   infantile o.
>   juvenile o.
>   optic atrophy 2 (OPA 2) with
>   early o.

ontogenesis

ontogenetic
>   o. niche
>   o. shift

ontogeny

ontology

OnTrak

onychatrophia

onychia

onychodystrophy-congenital deafness
  syndrome

onycholysis
>   distal o.

onychomycosis
>   candidal o.
>   proximal white subungual o.
>   sublingual o.
>   superficial o.
>   white superficial o.

onychoosteodysplasia

onychophagia

Ony-Clear Spray

o'nyong-nyong virus

ooblast

oocyesis

oocyte
>   aspiration of mature o.
>   o. atresia
>   o. collection
>   o. cryopreservation
>   o. culture
>   o. donation
>   donor o.
>   o. donor
>   o. extrusion
>   o. fertilization
>   fertilized o.
>   GV o.'s
>   o. maturation inhibitor (OMI)
>   o. meiosis
>   primary o.
>   o. production
>   o. recovery
>   o. retrieval
>   sibling o.

oogenesis

oogonia, sing. oogonium

oolemma

oophoralgia

oophorectomy
>   laparoscopic o.
>   medical o.
>   prophylactic o.
>   surgical o.

oophoritic cyst

oophoritis
>   autoimmune o.

oophorocystectomy

oophorocystosis

oophorohysterectomy

oophoroma

oophoropathy

oophoropeliopexy

oophoropexy
>   laparoscopic o.

oophoroplasty

oophororrhaphy

oophorosalpingectomy

oophorosalpingitis

oophorostomy

oophorotomy

NOTES

O

oophorrhagia
ooplasm
oozing
    venous o.
OP
    occipitoposterior
    occiput posterior
O&P
    ova and parasites
    stool culture for O&P
Op
    osmotic pressure
opacification
    corneal o.
opacity
    abnormal o.
    corneal o.
    fine lens o.
    lens o.
    lenticular o.
    punctate lenticular o.
Opalski cell
opaque white exudate
OPC
    oropharyngeal candidiasis
OPCA
    olivopontocerebellar atrophy
    neonatal OPCA
    X-linked OPCA
OPD
    otopalatodigital
    OPD syndrome
open
    o. biopsy
    o. bite
    o. comedo
    o. crib
    o. dermal sinus
    o. endotracheal suction
    o. endotracheal suctioning
    o. flap drainage
    o. fracture
    o. gastrostomy tube placement
    o. heart surgery
    keep vein o. (KVO)
    o. lung biopsy (OLB)
    o. mouth
    o. neural tube defect
    o. pericardial drainage
    o. pneumothorax
    o. reading frame
OpenGene automated DNA sequencing system
opening
    gland duct o.
    glottic o.
    high hymenal o.
    hymenal o.
    Skene duct o.

    tentorial o.
    urethral o.
    vaginal o.
    o. wedge osteotomy
open-mouth view
open-tube bronchoscopy
OPERA
    outpatient endometrial resection/ablation
    OPERA procedure
    OPERA Star morcellator
    OPERA Star SL hysteroscope
operant
    o. conditioning theory
    o. level
operation (*See also* procedure, technique)
    Alexander o.
    arterial switch o.
    atrial switch o.
    Bacon-Babcock o.
    Baldy o.
    Ball o.
    Band-Aid o.
    Baudelocque o.
    Blalock-Hanlon o.
    Blalock-Taussig o.
    Bozeman o.
    cesarean o.
    Cotte o.
    Counsellor-Davis artificial vagina o.
    Damus-Kaye-Stansel o.
    Döderlein roll-flap o.
    Donald-Fothergill o.
    Doyle o.
    Emmet o.
    Estes o.
    Falk-Shukuris o.
    Fontan o.
    Fothergill o.
    Fothergill-Donald o.
    Fothergill-Hunter o.
    Fredet-Ramstedt o.
    Freund o.
    Gigli o.
    Gilliam o.
    Gilliam-Doleris o.
    Giordano o.
    Gittes o.
    Glenn o.
    Grant-Ward o.
    Halsted o.
    Haultain o.
    Heaney o.
    Heller-Belsey o.
    Heller-Nissen o.
    Jatene o.
    Kasai o.
    Kelly o.
    Kennedy-Pacey o.
    King o.

Ladd o.
Lash o.
Latzko o.
Le Fort o.
Madlener o.
MAGPI o.
Manchester o.
Manchester-Fothergill o.
Marckwald o.
Marshall-Marchetti-Krantz o.
McDonald o.
McIndoe o.
modified Fontan o.
morcellation o.
Mustard o.
Norton o.
Norwood o.
obstetric o.
O'Donnell o.
partial exenteration o.
Pomeroy o.
Porro o.
Ramstedt o.
Rastelli o.
Récamier o.
Ross o.
Ross-Konno o.
Ross-Konno-Switch o.
Saenger o.
Schauta vaginal o.
Schroeder o.
Schuchardt o.
second-look o.
Senning o.
sex change o.
Shirodkar o.
Sistrunk o.
Spinelli o.
Stamey o.
Strassman o.
Sturmdorf o.
suprapubic urethrovesical
   suspension o.
suspensory sling o.
switch o.
TeLinde o.
Tessier craniofacial o.
Thiersch o.
transsphenoidal o.
two-stage arterial switch o.
Urban o.
vaginal switch o.

Vecchietti o.
Waters o.
Way o.
Webster o.
Wertheim o.
Wertheim-Schauta o.
window o.
operative
   o. management
   o. site complication
   o. vaginal delivery
operator
   o. gene
   o. locus
opercular syndrome
operculum, pl. **opercula**
operon
OPG
   osteoprotegerin
ophiasis
Ophthacet
Ophthalgan
ophthalmia
   gonococcal o.
   gonorrheal o.
   neonatal o.
   o. neonatorum (type 1, 2)
ophthalmic
   Achromycin O.
   Acular O.
   Akarpine O.
   AK-Con O.
   AK-Dex O.
   AK-Poly-Bac O.
   AK-Pred O.
   AKTob O.
   AK-Tracin O.
   AK-Trol O.
   Albalon Liquifilm O.
   Atropine-Care O.
   Atropisol O.
   Collyrium Fresh O.
   Dexacidin O.
   Dexasporin O.
   Econopred Plus O.
   Eyesine O.
   Geneye O.
   o. herpes
   Infectrol O.
   Inflamase Forte O.
   Inflamase Mild O.
   Isopto Atropine O.

O

NOTES

ophthalmic *(continued)*
    Isopto Carpine O.
    Maxidex O.
    Maxitrol O.
    Metreton O.
    Murine Plus O.
    Muro 128 O.
    Mydfrin O.
    OcuClear O.
    Ocufen O.
    Optigene O.
    Osmoglyn O.
    Pilocar O.
    Pilopine HS O.
    Piloptic O.
    Polysporin O.
    Pred Forte O.
    Pred Mild O.
    Timoptic O.
    Timoptic-XE O.
    Tobrex O.
    VasoClear O.
    Vira-A O.
    Viroptic O.
    Visine Extra O.
    Visine L.R. O.
    Voltaren O.
ophthalmicus
    herpes zoster o. (HZO)
ophthalmitis
ophthalmoacromelic syndrome
ophthalmologic
ophthalmologist
ophthalmomandibulomelic (OMM)
    o. dysplasia
ophthalmopathy
    thyroid o.
    thyroid-related o. (TRO)
ophthalmoplegia
    chronic progressive external o. (CPEO)
    external o.
    fibrotic o.
    internal o.
    internuclear o.
    o. plus
    progressive external o. (PEO)
ophthalmoplegic migraine
ophthalmoscope
    direct o.
    indirect o.
    indirect laser o.
ophthalmoscopy
    indirect o.
Ophthetic
opiate
    endogenous o.
    o. poisoning
    o. receptor

OPIM
    other potentially infectious material
opioid
    o. activity
    o. addiction
    endogenous o.
    epidural o.
    o. medication
    o. peptide
    o. receptor antagonist
opioidergic control impairment
opipramol hydrochloride
opisthorchiasis
Opisthorchis
opisthotonic posturing
opisthotonos, opisthotonus
    o. fetalis
Opitz
    O. BBBG syndrome
    O. G/BBB syndrome
    O. trigonocephaly syndrome
Opitz-Christian syndrome
Opitz-Frias syndrome
Opitz-Kaveggia syndrome
opium
    alcoholic tincture of o.
    o. tincture
Opmilas CO$_2$ laser
opocephalus
opodidymus
Oppenheim
    O. congenital hypotonia
    O. disease
    O. reflex
    O. syndrome
opponens splint
opportunistic infection
opportunity
    nonnutritive sucking o. (NSO)
opposing wall
opposition
    finger o.
    o. movement
    precise finger o.
oppositional
    o. defiant disorder (ODD)
    o. disorder
oppositionalism
OPS
    orthogonal polarization spectral
    osteoporosis-pseudoglioma syndrome
    OPS imaging
opsoclonus
    o. disorder
    transient o.
opsoclonus-myoclonus
    o.-m. etiology
    syndrome of o.-m.
opsomyoclonus

opsonin defect
opsonization
>poor o.
>o. system

opsonophagocytosis
optic
>o. atrophy-ataxia syndrome
>o. atrophy 2 (OPA 2) with early onset
>o. chiasma
>o. disc
>o. disc hyperemia
>o. fundus
>o. nerve
>o. nerve aplasia
>o. nerve atrophy
>o. nerve cupping
>o. nerve disease
>o. nerve dysplasia
>o. nerve edema
>o. nerve glioma
>o. nerve hypoplasia (ONH)
>o. nerve sheath
>o. nerve sheath meningioma
>o. nerve tumor
>o. neuritis
>o. neuropathy
>o. neuroretinitis
>o. pathway glioma
>o. pathway tumor

optica
>neuromyelitis o.

optical
>o. aspirating curette (OAC)
>o. density
>o. density measurement
>o. immunoassay (OIA)
>o. prism
>o. spectroscopy
>o. tomography

optician
Opticrom
Opti-Flow catheter
Optigene Ophthalmic
optimal debulking
optimality score
Optimal Observation Score
Optimine
Optimox
>O. C-500
>O. Mag 200

Optimyd

option
>therapeutic o.

Optiphot-2UD microscope
Optiview optical surgical obturator
Optivite PMT
Optochin-resistant *Streptococcus pneumoniae* **(ORSP)**
Optochin test
optode
>indwelling o.

optokinetic nystagmus
optometrist
OPUS immunoassay system
OPV
>oral polio vaccine
>oral poliovirus vaccine
>>Sabin OPV
>>OPV vaccine

ora (*pl. of* os (mouth, opening))
Orabase
>O. gel
>O. HCA Topical
>Kenalog in O.

Orabase-B, -O
Oracit
Oragrafin
Orajel
>O. Maximum Strength
>O. Mouth-Aid
>O. Perioseptic

oral
>o. administration
>o. allergy syndrome
>AllerMax O.
>Ansaid O.
>o. aphthous ulcer
>Apresoline O.
>Aquasol E O.
>Aristocort O.
>Asacol O.
>o. attenuated *Salmonella typhi* vaccine
>Benadryl O.
>Bentyl Hydrochloride O.
>o. bronchodilator
>Calm-X O.
>o. candidiasis
>o. candidosis
>Catapres O.
>o. cavity
>Ceftin O.
>Celestone O.

NOTES

O

oral *(continued)*

Chlor-Trimeton O.
Cipro O.
Cleocin HCl O.
Cleocin Pediatric O.
o. colonic lavage (OCL)
o. conjugated estrogen
o. contraception
o. contraceptive (OC)
o. contraceptive efficacy
o. contraceptive pill (OCP)
o. contraceptive therapy (OCT)
o. contraceptive use
Cortef O.
o. Crohn disease
Curretab O.
Cytomel O.
Decadron O.
Delta-Cortef O.
Demadex O.
Dexameth O.
Dilaudid O.
Dormin O.
Doxy O.
Dynacin O.
Edecrin O.
o. enanthem
o. epithelium
Estrace O.
Estratest O.
o. estrone
o. exploration
Flagyl O.
Flumadine O.
o. gastric tube
Genahist O.
o. glucose challenge test (OGCT)
o. glucose tolerance test (OGTT)
o. glucose tolerance testing (OGTT)
Gly-Oxide O.
o. hairy leukoplakia
o. hormone replacement therapy
Hydrocortone O.
o. hypoglycemic
Indocin SR O.
o. intake
Lasix O.
o. leukokeratosis
Levothroid O.
Loniten O.
Marmine O.
Medrol O.
Mephyton O.
Mestinon O.
o. misoprostol
o. moniliasis
o. motor
MS Contin O.

MSIR O.
o. mucosa cyanosis
o. mucous membrane graft
Nitroglyn O.
Nor-tet O.
Ogen O.
OMS O.
Oramorph SR O.
Ortho-Est O.
o. osmotic (OROS)
Panmycin O.
PediaCare O.
Pediapred O.
Pentasa O.
Phenergan O.
o. play
o. polio vaccine (OPV)
o. poliovirus vaccine (OPV)
Prelone O.
Proglycem O.
Provera O.
Proxigel O.
o. reflex
o. rehydration solution (ORS)
o. rehydration therapy (ORT)
Rheumatrex O.
Salagen O.
o. sex
Siladryl O.
Sinequan O.
Sominex O.
o. steroid contraceptive
o. stimulation
Sumycin O.
Synthroid O.
o. tactile defensiveness
o. temperature
o. thrush
Toradol O.
o. transmucosal fentanyl citrate (OTFC)
o. tube intubation
Twilite O.
Ucephan O.
o. ulceration
Urolene Blue O.
Valium O.
Vancocin O.
Vasotec O.
Videx O.
Vistaril O.
Voltaren O.
Voltaren-XR O.
Xylocaine O.

Oralet lollipop
oral-facial-digital syndrome with retinal abnormalities
orally administered estrogen
oral-motor dysfunction

Oramide
Oraminic II
Oramorph
    O. SR
    O. SR Oral
orange
    Agent O.
oranienburg
    Salmonella o.
Orap
Orapred solution
Orasept
Orasol
OraSure
    O. device
    O. oral HIV-1 antibody testing
    system
    O. oral HIV test
Orazinc
Orbeli syndrome
Orbenin
orbiculare
    Pityrosporum o.
orbit
    shallow o.'s
orbital
    o. blowout
    o. blowout fracture
    o. bone hypoplasia
    o. cellulitis
    o. floor
    o. hemorrhage
    o. hypotelorism
    o. inflammation
    o. septum
    o. subperiosteal abscess
    o. tumor
    o. wall fracture
Orbit blade
orbitofrontal gyri
orbitopagus
orchidectomy
orchiditis
orchidoblastoma
orchidoepididymitis
orchidometer, orchiometer
    Prader o.
orchiopexy, orchidopexy
    Fowler-Stephens o.
    scrotal o.
orchiorrhaphy, orchidorrhaphy

orchitis
    mumps o.
orciprenaline oral suspension
orciprenaline sulfate
order
    high fetal o.
Ordinal Scales of Intellectual Development
Oregon Adolescent Depression Project-Conduct Disorder Screener (OADP-CDS)
Oregon-type tyrosinemia
Oretic
organ
    O. Injury Scaling (OIS)
    internal generative o.
    nongenital pelvic o.
    pelvic o.
    reproductive o.
    o. of Rosenmüller
    sensory o.
    o. situs
    o. transplant
    o. transplantation
    Zuckerkandl o.
organelle
organic
    o. acidemia
    o. acid metabolism
    o. acidosis
    o. acid screen
    o. aciduria
    o. arsenical
    o. brain disease
    o. brain lesion
    o. heart disease
    o. hyperkinetic syndrome
    o. lead
    o. mental syndrome
    o. mercury poisoning
    o. tricuspid incompetence
Organidin NR
organism
    antibiotic-resistant gram-negative o. (ARGNO)
    coliform o.
    comma-shaped o.
    gram-negative o.
    gram-positive o.
    mycobacterial o.
    nonhemolytic aerobic o.
    nontypeable o.

NOTES

O

organism *(continued)*
  parasitic o.
  transgenic o.
organization
  health maintenance o. (HMO)
  managed care o. (MCO)
  preferred provider o. (PPO)
  World Health O. (WHO)
organoaxial volvulus
organochlorine pesticide
organogenesis
  fetal o.
organoid
  o. nevus
  o. nevus syndrome
organoleptic characteristic
organomegaly
Organon percutaneous E2 implant
organophosphate
  o. ingestion
  o. insecticide
  o. poisoning
organ-specific medication
orgasm
orgasmic
  o. disorder
  o. flush
  o. motor response
  o. plateau
O'Riain wrinkle test
Oriental
  O. spotted fever
orientation
  child-centered literary o. (CCLO)
  sexual o.
  spatial o.
Orientia tsutsugamushi
orienting
orifice
  eccentric o.
orificial tuberculosis
origin
  O. balloon
  congenital amaurosis of retinal o.
  fever of undetermined o. (FUO)
  fever of unknown o. (FUO)
  histoimmunological o.
  parental o.
  Somatropin of rDNA o.
  O. Tacker
  O. trocar
original
  O. Doan's
  K-Phos O.
Orimune poliovirus vaccine
oris (*gen. of* os (mouth, opening))

ORLAU
  Orthotic Research and Locomotor
  Assessment Unit
    ORLAU swivel walker
Ornade
ornidazole
ornipressin
ornithine
  o. to citrulline ratio
  o. decarboxylase
  difluoromethyl o. (DFMO)
  o. transcarbamylase (OTC)
  o. transcarbamylase deficiency
   (OTCD)
ornithine carbamoyltransferase (OCT)
**ornithine-ketoacid aminotransferase
  deficiency**
ornithosis
orocecal transit time
orocraniodigital syndrome
orodigitofacial
  o. dysostosis
  o. syndrome
orofacial
  o. cleft
  o. dyskinesia
orofaciodigital (OFD)
orogastric (OG)
orogenital
  o. sexual practices
  o. syndrome
orolabial herpes
orol leukokeratosis
oromandibular
  o. dystonia
  o. limb hypoplasia
oromandibuloauricular syndrome
oromandibulootic syndrome
oromotor
  o. function
  o. sign
oronasal
oroorbital cleft
oropharyngeal
  o. candidiasis (OPC)
  o. colonization
  o. tularemia
oropharynx
OROS
  oral osmotic
    OROS methylphenidate
     hydrochloride
orotic
  o. acid
  o. acidemia
  o. aciduria
orotracheal intubation
Oroya fever

orphan
- o. drug
- enteric cytopathogenic human o. (ECHO)
- enterocytopathogenic human o. (ECHO)
- respiratory enteric o.

orphanage
orphenadrine
Orr rectal prolapse repair
ORS
- oral rehydration solution

ORSP
- Optochin-resistant *Streptococcus pneumoniae*

ORT
- oral rehydration therapy

Ortho
- O. All-Flex diaphragm
- O. diaphragm kit
- O. Evra
- O. Evra transdermal patch
- O. Personal Pak
- O. Tri-Cyclen

Ortho-Cept
Orthoclone OKT3
Ortho-Creme
Ortho-Cyclen
orthodeoxia
orthodiagram
Ortho-Dienestrol Vaginal
orthodontic appliance
orthodontist
orthodromic conduction
Ortho-Est Oral
Orthoglass splint
orthognathic surgery
orthogonal
- o. lead system
- o. plane
- o. polarization spectral (OPS)

orthographic
Ortho-Gynol
orthology
orthomolecular therapy
orthomyxovirus
Ortho-Novum
- O.-N. 1/35
- O.-N. 1/50
- O.-N. 7/7/7
- O.-N. 10/11

orthopedic, orthopaedic
- o. anomaly
- o. appliance
- o. condition

orthopedically disabled
orthopedics
orthopedist
orthophoria
Orthoplast jacket
orthoplasty
orthopnea
orthopoxvirus
Ortho-Prefest
orthoroentgenogram
orthosis, pl. **orthoses**
- ankle-foot o. (AFO)
- Atlanta Scottish Rite Hospital o.
- Boston o.
- cranial o.
- CranioCap cranial o.
- foot o. (FO)
- hip-knee-ankle-foot o. (HKAFO)
- knee-ankle-foot o. (KAFO)
- lumbosacral o. (LSO)
- reciprocating gait o. (RGO)
- soft Boston o.
- supramalleolar o. (SMO)
- thoracolumbosacral o. (TLSO)

orthostasis
orthostatic
- o. dizziness
- o. hypotension
- o. intolerance
- o. proteinuria
- o. syncope
- o. tachycardia syndrome
- o. test

orthosympathetic
orthotic
- OB Gees maternity o.

Orthotic Research and Locomotor Assessment Unit (ORLAU)
orthotonos, orthotonus
orthotopic
- o. heart transplantation
- o. liver transplantation (OLTx)

orthovoltage radiation
Orthoxine
Ortolani
- O. click
- O. congenital hip dislocation technique

O

NOTES

Ortolani *(continued)*
    O. maneuver
    O. sign
    O. test
Orudis KT
Oruvail
OSA
    obstructive sleep apnea
OSA/H
    obstructive sleep apnea/hypoventilation
OSAS
    obstructive sleep apnea syndrome
os (bone), gen. **ossis**, pl. **ossa**
    o. odontoideum
    o. pubis
    o. subfibulare
    o. trigonum
Osborne wave
Os-Cal 500
oscillation
    o. amplitude
    anal sphincter o.
    flutter-like o.
    high-frequency o. (HFO)
    ocular o.
oscillator
    Babylog 8000 o.
    high-frequency o.
    Infant Star 8000 o.
    Sensormedic 3100A 8000 o.
    Stephanie 8000 o.
oscillatory
    high-frequency o. (HFO)
    o. ventilation
oscillometric
    o. method
    o. technique
oscilloscope
    cathode ray o. (CRO)
OSD
    Osgood-Schlatter disease
Osebold-Remondini syndrome
oseltamivir
OSEP
    Office of Special Education Programs
Osgood bone marrow needle
Osgood-Schlatter
    O.-S. disease (OSD)
    O.-S. syndrome
Osler node
Osler-Weber-Rendu
    O.-W.-R. disease (OWRD)
    O.-W.-R. syndrome (OWRS)
Osler-Weber syndrome
osmiophilic body
Osmitrol Injection
OsmoCyte pillow
Osmoglyn Ophthalmic

osmolality
    morning o.
    plasma o.
    serum o.
osmolarity
Osmolite HN formula
osmoregulation
osmotic
    o. diarrhea
    o. dilator
    o. diuresis
    o. fragility test
    o. gap
    o. laxative
    oral o. (OROS)
    o. pressure (Op)
    o. UF
os (mouth, opening), gen. **oris**, pl. **ora**
    cervical o.
    depressor anguli oris
    external o.
    fetor oris
    internal o.
    parous o.
    Scanzoni second o.
    ora serrata retinae
Osp
    outer surface protein
OspA
    outer surface protein A
    recombinant OspA
ossa (*pl. of* os (bone))
osseous
    o. BA lesion
    o. coalition
osseous-oculodental dysplasia
ossicle
    Andernach o.
    anlagen of the auditory o.
    auditory o.'s
ossicular
    o. discontinuity
    o. disruption
ossiculum terminale
ossificans
    myositis o.
ossification
    appositional o.
    enchondral o.
    endochondral o.
    extra o.
ossified ear cartilages, mental deficiency, muscle wasting, bony changes syndrome
ossifying fibroma
ossis (*gen. of* os (bone))
ossium
    fragilitas o.

OSSUM
>   O. database
>   O. database of skeletal dysplasias

ostectomy

osteitis
>   acute mastoid o.
>   alveolar o.
>   o. condensans generalisata
>   o. fibrosa
>   o. fibrosis cystica
>   mastoid o.
>   o. pubis
>   rarefying o.

OsteoAnalyzer densitometer

osteoangiohypertrophy

osteoarthritis (OA)
>   degenerative o.

osteoarthroophthalmopathy
>   hereditary o.

osteoblast (OB)

osteoblastic osteosarcoma

osteoblast-like cell

osteoblastoma (OB)

osteocalcin
>   serum o.

osteochondral fracture

osteochondritis
>   capitellar o.
>   o. of capitellum
>   o. deformans juvenilis
>   o. dissecans (OCD)
>   o. ischiopubica
>   metatarsal head o.
>   radial head o.
>   tarsal navicular o.

osteochondrodysplasia
>   hereditary o.
>   hypertrichotic o.

osteochondrodystrophia deformans

osteochondrodystrophy
>   familial o.

osteochondroma

osteochondromuscular dystrophy

osteochondrosis, pl. **osteochondroses**
>   o. deformans tibiae

osteochondrotic lesion

osteoclast

osteoclastic

osteoclast-mediated bone resorption

osteoclastogenesis

osteocranium

osteocystoma

osteodental dysplasia (ODD)

osteodiastasis
>   occipital o.

osteodysplasia

osteodysplastic primordial dwarfism

osteodystrophia juvenilis

osteodystrophy
>   Albright hereditary o. (AHO)
>   azotemic o.
>   renal o.

osteofibrous dysplasia

osteogenesis
>   o. imperfecta congenita syndrome
>   o. imperfecta cystica
>   o. imperfecta, optic atrophy,
>   retinopathy, developmental delay
>   syndrome
>   o. imperfecta (type I–IV) (OI)

osteogenic sarcoma

osteoglophonic
>   o. dwarfism
>   o. dysplasia

OsteoGram bone density test

osteohypertrophicus
>   nevus varicosus o.
>   nevus vasculosus o.

osteohypertrophic varicose syndrome

osteoid
>   malignant o.
>   o. osteoma
>   o. seam

osteoma
>   multiple o.'s
>   osteoid o.

osteomalacia
>   juvenile o.

Osteomark NTx serum test

Osteomeasure computer-assisted image analyzer

osteomyelitis
>   acute hematogenous o.
>   calvarial o.
>   chronic o.
>   chronic recurrent multifocal o.
>   (CRMO)
>   diaphysial o.
>   hematogenous o.
>   meningococcal multifocal o.
>   multifocal o.
>   *Pasteurella multocida* o.
>   o. pubis

O

NOTES

osteomyelitis *(continued)*
> pyogenic o.
> *Salmonella* o.
> sclerosing o.
> spinal o.
> subacute o.
> tuberculous o.
> vertebral o.

osteonecrosis
osteooarthropathy
> hypertrophic o. (HOA)

osteo-onchodysostosis
Osteopatch
osteopathia
> o. dysplastica familiaris
> o. striata
> o. striata, deafness, cranial osteopetrosis syndrome
> o. striata, macrocephaly, cranial sclerosis syndrome
> o. striata with cranial sclerosis

osteopathic medicine
osteopedion
osteopenia
> ground-glass o.
> juxtaarticular o.
> relative o.
> o., sparse hair, mental retardation syndrome

osteopenic halo
osteopetrosis
> congenital o.
> infantile o.
> o. tarda

osteopoikilosis
osteopontin
osteoporosis
> corticosteroid-induced o.
> juvenile o.
> postmenopausal o.

osteoporosis-pseudoglioma syndrome (OPS)
osteoporotic fracture
osteoprotegerin (OPG)
osteopsathyrosis
osteoradionecrosis
osteorhabdotosis
Osteosal test
osteosarcoma
> chondroblastic o.
> femoral o.
> fibroblastic o.
> osteoblastic o.
> secondary o.
> small cell o.
> telangiectatic o.

osteotabes
osteotomy
> derotation femoral o.

> diaphysial fibular o.
> femoral o.
> fibular o.
> innominate o.
> lengthening o.
> opening wedge o.
> pelvic lengthening o.
> plantarflexion o.
> proximal humeral derotation o.
> rotational o.
> Salter o.
> shortening dorsal wedge radial o.
> tibial valgus o.
> transiliac lengthening o.
> valgus o.
> varus o.
> wedge o.

OsteoView
> O. device
> O. 2000 system

ostiomeatal complex
ostium, pl. **ostia**
> abdominal o.
> follicular o.
> o. primum
> o. primum ASD
> o. secundum
> o. secundum ASD
> tubal o.
> o. venosus ASD
> vessel o.

ostomy
> intestinal o.

ostrich maneuver
Ostrum-Furst syndrome
O'Sullivan-O'Connor retractor
OT
> occipitotransverse
> occiput transverse
> occupational therapy

O.T.
> Mono-Vacc Test (O.T.)

Ota
> nevus of O.
> O. nevus

otalgia
OTC
> ornithine transcarbamylase
> over-the-counter

OTCD
> ornithine transcarbamylase deficiency

OTFC
> oral transmucosal fentanyl citrate

other
> o. cerebral palsy
> o. potentially infectious material (OPIM)

otic
> Acetasol HC o.

AntibiOtic O.
Cerumenex O.
Cipro HC O.
Cortisporin O.
Cortisporin-TC o.
Debrox O.
O. Domeboro
Drotic O.
Floxin O.
LazerSporin-C O.
Otic-Care o.
Otocort O.
Otomycin-HPN O.
VoSol o.
VoSol HC o.
Otic-Care otic
oticus
herpes zoster o.
Otis-Lennon Intelligence Test
otitic hydrocephalus
otitidiscaviarum
Nocardia o.
otitis
adhesive o.
Alloiococcus o.
o. externa (OE)
external o.
o. media (OM)
o. media with effusion (OME)
o. media without effusion
o. media with perforated tympanic membrane
otitis-conjunctivitis syndrome
otoacoustic emission (OAE)
Otobiotic
Otocalm Ear
Otocort Otic
otocyst
otofacial dysostosis
otofaciocervical syndrome
otogenic brain abscess
OtoLAM
Otoscan laser-assisted myringotomy
otolaryngologist
otolaryngology
pediatric o.
otologist
otomandibular
o. dysostosis
o. facial dysmorphogenesis
o. syndrome
Otomycin-HPN Otic

otomycosis
otopalatodigital (OPD)
o. syndrome
otorhinolaryngologist
otorrhea
CSF o.
Otoscan laser-assisted myringotomy (OtoLAM)
otosclerosis syndrome
otoscope
Siegel o.
otoscopy
pneumatic o.
otospondylomegaepliphyseal dysplasia
otospongiosis syndrome
Ototemp 3000 thermometer
ototoxic drug
ototoxicity
Otovent
O. autoinflation kit
O. negative pressure treatment
Oto-Wick
Pope O.-W.
Ottawa Ankle Rules (OAR)
Otto
O. pelvis
O. syndrome
ouabain
Oucher scale
ounce (oz)
calorie per o. (cal/oz)
out
toeing o.
outbreak
recurrent herpetic o.
outbreeding
outcome
adverse o.
Bayley cognitive o.
fetal o.
maternal o.
neonatal o.
obstetric o.
perinatal o.
poor pregnancy o.
pregnancy o.
teratogenic o.
outer
o. canthus
o. chorion
o. ear

NOTES

outer *(continued)*
    o. surface protein (Osp)
    o. surface protein A (OspA)
outercourse
outflow
    o. obstruction
    o. tract
outlet
    conjugate of pelvic o.
    o. foramina
    o. forceps
    o. forceps delivery
    parous o.
    pelvic o.
    o. septum
    vaginal o.
    vulvovaginal o.
outline
    fetal o.
out-of-phase endometrial biopsy
out-of-profile nipple
outpatient
    o. anticoagulation
    o. endometrial resection/ablation
    (OPERA)
    o. fetal nonstress testing
    o. postpartum care
output
    cardiac o.
    decreased urine o.
    elevated cardiac o.
    high o.
    hyperdynamic ventricle with
     high o.
    intake and o. (I&O, I/O)
    low o.
    urine o.
    urine acid o. (UAO)
outtoe gait
outtoeing, out-toeing
outward menstrual flow
ova (*pl. of* ovum)
oval
    o. scaling
    o. window
ovale
    foramen o.
    patent foramen o. (PFO)
    Pityrosporum o.
    Plasmodium o.
ovalis
    fossa o.
ovalocytary anemia
ovalocytosis
    Southeast Asian o. (SAO)
OvaRex
    O. MAb
    O. vaccine
ovaria (*pl. of* ovarium)

ovarialgia
ovarian
    o. ablation
    o. abnormality
    o. abscess
    o. activity
    o. agenesis
    o. amenorrhea
    o. androgen secretion
    o. antibody
    o. aplasia
    o. artery
    o. axis dysfunction
    o. cancer
    o. cancer metastasis
    o. carcinoma antigen
    o. carcinoma debulking
    o. cautery
    o. clear cell adenocarcinoma
    o. colic
    o. cortex
    o. cycle
    o. cycle change
    o. cyst
    o. cystadenocarcinoma
    o. cystectomy
    o. cystic teratoma
    o. disorder
    o. dwarfism
    o. dysgenesis
    o. dysgenesis-sensorineural deafness
    syndrome
    o. dysgerminoma
    o. dysmenorrhea
    o. embryonal teratoma
    o. endometrioma
    o. endometriosis
    o. epithelial cancer (OEC)
    o. estrogen synthesis
    o. excrescence
    o. factor
    o. failure
    o. fibroma
    o. fibromatosis
    o. follicle exhaustion
    o. function
    o. gametogenesis
    o. germinal epithelium
    o. gonadoblastoma
    o. hormone
    o. hyperandrogenism
    o. hyperstimulation
    o. hyperstimulation syndrome
    (OHSS)
    o. hypertrophy
    o. leiomyoma
    o. ligament
    o. lipid cell neoplasm
    o. lymphoma

o. malignancy
o. malignant epithelial neoplasm
o. malignant germ cell tumor
o. mass
o. neurofibroma
o. plexus
o. pregnancy
o. preservation
o. proliferative cystadenoma
o. remnant syndrome
o. retention
o. retrieval
o. rupture
o. seminoma
o. sex-cord stromal neoplasm
o. short stature syndrome
o. small-cell carcinoma
o. sonography
o. steroid
o. steroidogenesis
o. stimulation
o. stroma
o. stromal hyperthecosis
o. thecoma
o. torsion
o. tubular adenoma
o. varicocele
o. vasculitis
o. vein
o. vein syndrome
o. vein thrombosis (OVT)
o. vessel
o. wedge resection
ovarian-sparing irradiation
ovariectomy
ovarii (*gen. of* ovarium)
ovarioabdominal pregnancy
ovariocele
ovariocentesis
ovariocyesis
ovariodysneuria
ovariogenic
ovariohysterectomy
ovariolytic
ovarioncus
ovariopathy
ovariorrhexis
ovariosalpingectomy
ovariosalpingitis
ovarioscopy
ovariosteresis
ovariostomy

ovariotomy
Beatson o.
normal o.
ovaritis
ovarium, gen. **ovarii**, pl. **ovaria**
o. bipartitum
o. disjunctum
o. gyratum
hyperthecosis ovarii
o. lobatum
mesoblastoma ovarii
struma ovarii
ovary
accessory o.
autoamputation of o.
contralateral o.'s
cystic teratoma of o.
o. in inguinal hernia
JGCT of o.
mulberry o.
multifollicular o.
oyster o.
palpable postmenopausal o. (PPO)
polycystic o. (PCO)
resistant o.
Stein-Leventhal type of
polycystic o.
strumal carcinoid of o.
supernumerary o.
suspensory ligament of o.
torsion of o.
transposition of o.
tubes and o.'s (T&O)
wandering o.
Ovation falloposcopy system
ovatus
Bacteroides o.
O-Vax vaccine
Ovcon 35, 50
over
crossing o.
overactive bladder (OAB)
overactivity
detrusor o.
overaeration
overanxious
o. disorder (OAD)
o. disorder of childhood
overcirculation
pulmonary o.
overcorrection
overcrowding

O

NOTES

overdistention, overdistension
    lung o.
    o. syndrome
overdose syndrome
overfeeding
overflow
    o. incontinence
    o. proteinuria
    tear o.
overgrowth
    cyclosporine-induced gingival o.
    gingival o.
    phenytoin-induced gingival o.
    small bowel o.
    o. syndrome
overhead warmer
overheating
overhydration
overinflation
    congenital lobar o. (CLO)
    generalized obstructive o.
    obstructive o.
overlap
    criterion o.
overlapping
    o. clones
    o. closure of peritoneum
    o. toe
overload
    diastolic o.
    fluid o.
    iron o.
    o. pattern
    sensory o.
    systolic o.
    volume o.
overloading
    carbohydrate o.
overmature gamete
overpressuring
overprotection
overriding
    o. aorta
    o. finger
    o. of sutures
    o. toe
oversewing placental bed
overshadowing
    diagnostic o.
overstimulated
overt
    o. bilirubin encephalopathy
    o. insulin-dependent diabetes
      mellitus
    o. loss
over-the-counter (OTC)
    o.-t.-c. drug
    o.-t.-c. medication
over-the-needle catheter

overtraining syndrome
overuse
    o. injury
    o. syndrome
overwhelming infection
Oves Cervical Cap
ovicidal
Ovide
    O. lotion
    O. Topical
Ovidrel powder
oviduct
    ampulla of o.
    angiomyoma of o.
ovigenesis
ovoid
    Delclos o.
    Fleming o.
    Manchester o.
ovotestis, pl. **ovotestes**
    dysgenetic o.
Ovral contraceptive pill
Ovrette contraceptive pill
O-V Staticin
OVT
    ovarian vein thrombosis
OvuDate
    O. fertility test kit
    O. hCG
OvuGen test kit
OvuKIT
    O. Self-Test kit
    O. test
ovular transmigration
ovulation
    contralateral o.
    o. detection kit
    incessant o.
    o. induction
    o. number
    paracyclic o.
    o. rate
    spontaneous o.
    o. stimulation
ovulational sclerosis
ovulation-associated hemoperitoneum
ovulation-inducing drug
ovulatory
    o. age
    o. defect
    o. disturbance
    o. menstrual cycle
    o. mucus
Ovules
    Cleocin Vaginal O.
ovulocyclic porphyria
ovum, pl. **ova**
    blighted o.
    Bryce-Teacher o.

o. capture
o. donation
fertilized o.
o. forceps
frozen o.
Hertig-Rock o.
holoblastic o.
Mateer-Streeter o.
o. maturation
Miller o.
ova and parasites (O&P)
Peters o.
o. pickup mechanism
primitive o.
primordial o.
o. transport
trapped o.
ovum-capture inhibitor
ovumeter
OvuQuick
O. One-Step ovulation kit
O. Self-Test
O. Self-Test kit
O. Self-Test ovulation predictor
OvuStick
owl's
o. eye cell
o. eye inclusion body
o. eye nucleus
o. eyes view of hydrocele
OWRD
Osler-Weber-Rendu disease
Owren disease
OWRS
Osler-Weber-Rendu syndrome
oxacillin sodium
oxalate
oxalosis
primary o.
Oxandrin
oxandrolone
oxazepam
Oxepa formula
Oxford
O. diagnostic criteria
O. Family Planning Association
Contraceptive Study
oxiconazole
oxidase
catechol o.
cholesterol o.

monoamine o.
monoamine o. type A (MAOA)
NADPH o.
6-oxidase
lysine 6-o.
oxidation
o. disorder
fatty acid o. (FAO)
nitric oxide o.
oxidative
o. brain injury
o. phosphorylation (OXPHOS)
o. stress
oxidative-reductase activity
oxide
inhalation of nitrous o.
inhaled nitric o. (iNO, I-NO)
magnesium o.
nitric o. (NO)
nitrous o. (N_2O)
zinc o.
oxime
hexamethyl propylene amine o.
(HMPAO)
technetium
hexamethylpropyleneamine o. (Tc
HMPAO)
oximeter
Healthdyne o.
Invos 3100 cerebral o.
Nellcor N20, N200 pulse o.
Ohmeda Minx pulse o.
Ohmeda 3800 pulse o.
OxyShuttle pulse o.
Oxytrak pulse o.
pulse o.
RPO o.
oximetric data
oximetry
cerebral o.
fetal pulse o.
Mars pulse o.
Masimo SET signal extraction
pulse o.
motion-resistant pulse o.
nocturnal pulse o.
pulse o.
reflectance pulse o. (RPO)
signal extraction pulse o.
stress o.
transcutaneous o.

O

NOTES

Oxisensor
> O. fetal oxygen saturation monitor
> O. transducer

Oxistat Topical
5-oxoprolinase deficiency
Ox-Pam
OXPHOS
> oxidative phosphorylation
> OXPHOS disease

oxprenolol
ox's eye
oxtriphylline
Oxy-10 Advanced Formula for Sensitive Skin
oxybutynin chloride
oxycardiorespirogram
Oxycel
> O. cautery
> O. gauze

oxycephaly
oxychlorosene sodium
oxycodone
> o. and acetaminophen
> o. and aspirin

oxy-CR gram
Oxydess II
oxygen (O$_2$)
> blow-by o.
> o. consumption
> o. consumption per minute (Vo$_2$)
> o. delivery
> o. deprivation
> o. dissociation curve
> fraction of inspired o. (FIO$_2$, FiO$_2$)
> free-flow o.
> helium and o. (heliox)
> home o.
> hood o.
> o. hood
> hyperbaric o.
> inspired o.
> normobaric o.
> partial pressure o. (PO$_2$)
> partial pressure alveolar o. (PaO$_2$)
> partial pressure arterial o. (PaO$_2$)
> o. saturation (SaO$_2$)
> supplemental o.
> o. tent
> o. therapy
> o. toxicity
> o. toxicity lung disease
> transcutaneous partial pressure of o. (tCpO$_2$)

oxygenase
> heme o.

oxygenated fetal blood
oxygenation
> congenital diaphragmatic hernia-extracorporeal membrane o. (CDH-ECMO)
> extracorporeal membrane o. (ECMO)
> fetal cerebral o.
> fetal scalp o.
> o. index (OI)
> meconium aspiration syndrome extracorporeal membrane o. (MAS-ECMO)

oxygenator
> Lilliput neonatal o.

oxygen-diffusing capacity
oxygen-free radical
Oxygent temporary blood substitute
oxyhemoglobin
> o. saturation
> total o.

Oxy-Hood oxygen hood
oxymetazoline
oxymetholone
oxymorphone
oxyphenbutazone
oxyphencyclimine
oxyphenonium bromide
OxyShuttle pulse oximeter
oxytetracycline HCl
oxytetracycline/polymyxin ointment
oxytoca
> *Klebsiella o.*

oxytocia
oxytocic stimulation
oxytocin
> o. administration
> o. analog
> o. augmentation
> o. challenge test (OCT)
> o. secretion
> o. stimulation of labor
> o. stress test

oxytocinase
oxytocin-secreting neuron
Oxytrak pulse oximeter
Oxy 10 Wash
Oyst-Cal 500
Oystercal 500
oyster ovary
oz
> ounce

ozaenae
> *Klebsiella o.*

P
>partial pressure
>phosphorus
>>P protein

³²P
>phosphorus-32

P_ao
>airway opening pressure

p
>short arm of chromosome

p53
>>p53 gene
>>p53 tumor suppressor gene

P32 intraperitoneal treatment
P450 cytochrome
p55 soluble tumor necrosis factor receptor
p75 soluble tumor necrosis factor receptor
PA
>alveolar partial pressure
>pernicious anemia
>plasminogen activator
>posteroanterior
>pulmonary artery
>>PA pressure

P&A
>protection and advocacy

Pa
>arterial partial pressure
>pascal

PAAS
>pediatric acute admission severity
>>PAAS classification

Paas disease
PAB
>passenger air bag

Pabanol
PAB-equipped vehicle
PAC
>papular acrodermatitis of childhood

pacchionian granulation
PACE-2C DNA probe test
paced auditory serial addition test
pacemaker
>artificial p.
>wandering atrial p.

pachydermatitis
>*Malassezia* p.

pachygyria
>localized p.

pachyonychia
>p. congenita
>p. congenita syndrome

pachysalpingitis

pachysalpingoovaritis
pachytene
>p. phase of meiosis
>p. stage

pachyvaginitis cystica
Pacific
>P. Islander
>P. yew

pacificus
>*Ixodes p.*

pacifier
>sucrose p.
>sugar-dipped p.
>sweetened p.
>water p.

pacing
>epicardial p.
>phrenic nerve p.
>transvenous p.

Pacis
>P. BCG bladder cancer treatment
>P. BCG immunotherapy

pack
>barrier p.
>E-Z Heat hot p.
>Flents breast comfort p.
>Monistat 3 vaginal cream combination p.
>M-Zole 3 combination p.
>M-Zole 7 combination p.
>neonatal narcotic p.
>Peri-Cold P.
>Peri-Gel P.
>perineal cold p.
>perineal warm p.
>Peri-Warm P.
>respiratory therapy p.
>vaginal p.

packaging RNA
packed
>p. erythrocyte
>p. RBC transfusion
>p. red blood cells (PRBC)
>p. red blood cell transfusion

packer
>Bernay uterine p.
>Kitchen postpartum gauze p.

packing
>anterior nasal p.
>impregnated vaginal p.
>iodoform gauze p.
>Kaltostat p.
>nasal p.
>posterior nasal p.

P

packing *(continued)*
    uterine p.
    vaginal p.
paclitaxel
PACNS
    primary angiitis of CNS
PaCO₂
    partial pressure of arterial carbon dioxide
PAD
    pelvic adhesive disease
pad
    Aquaflex ultrasound gel p.
    arch insole p.
    p. and bell technique for enuresis
    Breathe Easy foam p.
    buccal fat p.
    Bumpa Bed crib bumper p.
    InSync miniform p.
    laparotomy p.
    malar fat p.
    Padette interlabial p.
    pronator fat p.
    scaphoid p.
    Sleep Guardian foam p.
    Soothies glycerin gel breast p.
    sucking p.
    suctorial p.
    suprapubic fat p.
    p. test
    Triaz benzoyl peroxide p.
paddle forceps
Padette interlabial pad
PadKit sample collection system
Paecilomyces
paediatric *(var. of pediatric)*
paediatrics *(var. of pediatrics)*
PAG
    pictorial anticipatory guidance
Paget
    P. disease
    P. disease of anus
    P. disease of breast
    P. disease of nipple
    P. disease of vulva
pagetic
pagetoid
Pagon syndrome
pagophagia
PAH
    phenylalanine hydroxylase
PAI
    partial (incomplete) androgen
     insensitivity
    plasminogen activator inhibitor
     PAI deficiency
PAI-1
    plasminogen-activator inhibitor-1
PAI-2
    plasminogen-activator inhibitor-2

pain
    abdominal p.
    abdominopelvic p.
    acyclic pelvic p.
    after-p.'s
    afterbirth p.
    asymbolia for p.
    bearing-down p.
    bone p.
    chest p.
    chronic pelvic p. (CPP)
    colicky abdominal p.
    congenital insensitivity to p.
    p. crisis
    p. disorder
    epigastric p.
    expulsive p.'s
    facial p.
    false p.'s
    flank p.
    functional abdominal p.
    heel p.
    hypogastric p.
    incapacitating p.
    intermenstrual p.
    intractable p.
    labor p.'s
    lightning p.
    low-back p.
    lower abdominal p.
    menstrual p.
    myofascial p.
    night p.
    nocturnal retrosternal chest p.
    noncoital sexual p.
    ocular p.
    patellofemoral malalignment p.
    pelvic p.
    periumbilical p.
    pleuritic p.
    postoperative p.
    psychogenic pelvic p.
    recurrent abdominal p. (RAP)
    referred pelvic p.
    retrosternal chest p.
    Rome criteria for functional
     abdominal p.
    round ligament p.
    somatic p.
    splanchnic pelvic p.
    suprapubic p.
    p. threshold
    visceral p.
Paine syndrome
painful joint
painless hematuria
paint, painting
    chromosome p.
    whole chromosome p. (wcp)

whole chromosome 1-22 p.
whole chromosome X, Y p.

PAIR
percutaneous aspiration, instillation of
hypertonic saline, respiration

pair
base p.
chromosome p.
kb p.
nucleoside p.
vertex-nonvertex p.
vertex-vertex p.

paired
p. allosome
P. Associate Learning Task
(PALT)
p. box
p. crura

pairing
chromosome p.

Pai syndrome

PAIVS
pulmonary atresia with intact ventricular
septum

Pajot maneuver

Pak
Ortho Personal P.
Pedi-Boro Soak P.'s
Trovan/Zithromax Compliance P.

Palant cleft palate syndrome

palatal
p. expansion
p. fistula
p. fistula closure
p. mucosa
p. paresis
p. petechia

palatal-digital-oral syndrome

palate
abnormal p.
cleft p. (CP)
cleft lip and p. (CLP)
conotruncal cardiac defect,
abnormal face, thymic hypoplasia,
cleft p. (CATCH 22)
high-arched p.
isolated cleft p.
midline cleft p.
narrow p.
p. repair
soft p.
submucous cleft p.

palatine tonsil
palatognathous
palatopharyngeal incompetence
palatorespiratory dysfunction
palatoschisis
paleartica
pale stool
palilalia
palisading granuloma
palivizumab
palliation
p. of great vessels
Norwood p.

palliative
p. procedure
p. shunt
p. surgery

pallid
p. breathholding spells
p. complexion

pallidal degeneration
pallidin
pallidotomy
pallidum
microhemagglutination assay for
antibodies to *Treponema p.*
(MHA-TP)
Treponema p.

pallidus
globus p.

Pallister
P. mosaic aneuploidy
P. mosaic syndrome
P. W syndrome

Pallister-Hall syndrome
Pallister-Killian syndrome
pallor
blanching p.
circumoral p.
placental p.
p. of skin
white matter p.
yellow-green p.

PALM
premature accelerated lung maturation

palm
p. leaf pattern
tripe p.

palmar
p. crease
p. erythema
p. grasp

NOTES

palmar *(continued)*
    p. grasping reflex
    p. grasp reflex
    p. hyperlinearity
    p. lesion
    p. and plantar keratosis and
      keratitis
    p. and plantar punctate
      hyperkeratosis
    p. pustulosis
    p. xanthoma
palmaris
    keratosis p.
    pustulosis p.
    tinea nigra p.
    xanthoma striata p.
palmar-plantar sign
palmatae
    plicae p.
Palmaz stent
palm-chin reflex
Palmer ovarian biopsy forceps
palmitate
    colfosceril p.
Palmitate-A 5000
palmitic acid
palmitoyltransferase
    carnitine p. (CPT)
    carnitine p. I (CPT I)
    carnitine p. II (CPT II)
palmomental reflex
palmoplantar
    p. keratoderma
    p. pustulosis
palmoplantaris
    keratosis p.
PalmVue system
palpable
    p. bony abnormality
    p. cord
    p. gonad
    p. kidney
    p. nodule
    p. postmenopausal ovary (PPO)
    p. purpura
    p. spongy mass sign
palpably enlarged kidney
palpate
palpation
    spoke-wheel p.
    vaginal p.
palpebral
    p. conjunctiva
    p. conjunctivitis
    p. fissure
    p. reflex
    p. slant
palpebrum
    pediculosis p.

palpitation
PALS
    pediatric advanced life support
palsy
    abducens p.
    abducent p.
    acquired abducens p.
    acquired 6th nerve p.
    ataxic cerebral p.
    athetoid cerebral p.
    atonic cerebral p.
    Bell p.
    brachial birth p.
    brachial plexus p.
    bulbar p.
    cerebellar cerebral p.
    cerebral p. (CP)
    choreoathetoid cerebral p.
    congenital 6th nerve p.
    cranial nerve p.
    diaphragm p.
    double elevator p.
    Duchenne p.
    dyskinetic cerebral p.
    dystonic cerebral p.
    Erb p.
    Erb-Duchenne p.
    Erb-Klumpke p.
    extrapyramidal cerebral p.
    facial nerve p.
    familial congenital fourth cranial
      nerve p.
    familial congenital superior oblique
      oculomotor p.
    familial congenital trochlear
      nerve p.
    fourth nerve p.
    gaze p.
    hemiparetic cerebral p.
    hemiplegic cerebral p.
    hereditary neuropathy with liability
      to pressure p. (HNPP)
    horizontal supranuclear gaze p.
    hypotonic cerebral p.
    Klumpke brachial p.
    Landry p.
    lateral rectus p.
    liability to pressure p.
    lower motor neuron p.
    Lyme-associated peripheral facial
      nerve p.
    mild spastic diplegic cerebral p.
    mixed cerebral p.
    mixed-type cerebral p.
    motor neuron p.
    nerve p.
    neuron p.
    obstetrical p.
    obstetric brachial plexus p.

other cerebral p.
peripheral facial nerve p. (PFNP)
phrenic nerve p.
postinfectious abducens p.
pressure p.
progressive bulbar p.
pseudobulbar p.
pyramidal cerebral p.
rectus p.
rigid cerebral p.
spastic cerebral p.
supranuclear p.
trochlear nerve p.
vertical gaze p.

PALT
Paired Associate Learning Task

Pam
E Pam

pamabrom

PAMBA
paraaminomethylbenzoic acid

Pamelor

pamidronate

Pamine

pamoate
pyrantel p.

pampiniform plexus

PAN
polyarteritis nodosa

panagglutinin

panamensis
Leishmania p.

pANCA
perinuclear antineutrophil cytoplasmic
antibody

pancarditis
acute p.

pancreas
anular p.
direct stimulation of p.
p. divisum
p. sufficient (PS)

Pancrease MT

pancreatic
p. agenesis
p. duct stent
p. dysfunction
p. enzyme replacement
p. enzyme replacement therapy
(PERT)
p. exocrine deficiency
p. exocrine insufficiency

p. head resection
p. hypoplasia
p. insufficiency syndrome
p. islet cell
p. oncofetal antigen (POA)
p. panniculitis
p. pseudocyst
p. ring
p. sequestrum
p. tumor
p. ultrasound

pancreaticobiliary
p. anomaly
p. malunion

pancreaticojejunostomy

pancreatin

pancreatitis
acute hemorrhagic p.
choledochal cyst-induced p.
chronic p.
cyst-induced p.
drug-induced p.
gallstone p.
hereditary p.
idiopathic p.
infectious p.

pancreatoblastoma

Pancrecarb

pancrelipase

panculture

pancuronium bromide

pancytopenia
aplastic p.
Fanconi p.
p. syndrome

PANDAS
pediatric autoimmune neuropsychiatric
disorders associated with streptococcus

pandemic

Pander islands

Pandoraea
P. apista
P. pnomenusa
P. pulmonicola
P. sputorum

Panectyl

panel
streptococcal antigen p.
von Willebrand p.

panencephalitis
progressive rubella p.
rubella p.

NOTES

panencephalitis *(continued)*
    sclerosing p.
    subacute sclerosing p. (SSPE)
Paneth cell inclusion
Panex
Panhematin
panhypogammaglobulinemia
panhypopituitarism
    familial p.
panhysterectomy
panic
    p. attack
    p. disorder
panlobar disarray
Panmycin Oral
Panner disease
panneuropathy
    megalencephaly with hyaline p.
panniculectomy
    noncosmetic p.
panniculitis
    cold p.
    factitial p.
    lobar p.
    nodular nonsuppurative p.
    nonsuppurative p.
    pancreatic p.
    popsicle p.
    poststeroid p.
    relapsing nodular nonsuppurative p.
    septal p.
panniculus
    hanging p.
pannus
Panogauze
panopacification
panophthalmitis
PanoPlex dressing
panoramic radiograph
Panorex view
PanOxyl-AQ
PanOxyl Bar
Panretin topical gel
pansystolic murmur
pantothenate
    calcium p.
pantothenic acid
pants-over-vest technique
panty spica
panuveitis
PaO$_2$
    partial pressure alveolar oxygen
    partial pressure arterial oxygen
PAOP
    pulmonary artery occluded pressure
PAP
    pulmonary alveolar proteinosis
      acquired PAP

    primary PAP
    secondary PAP
Pap
    Papanicolaou
    Pap Plus HPV screen
    Pap plus speculoscopy (PPS)
    Pap smear
PAPA
    preschool-age psychiatric assessment
Papanicolaou (Pap)
    P. smear
PAPase
    phosphatidic acid phosphohydrolase
papaverine
paper
    filter p. (FP)
    Nitrazine p.
paper-doll fetus
Papette
    P. cervical collector
    P. device
papG allele
Papile grading
papilla, pl. **papillae**
    Bergmeister p.
    columnar epithelium p.
    p. of columnar epithelium
    edematous p.
    fungiform p.
    p. of Vater
papillary
    p. adenocarcinoma
    p. dermis
    p. endometrial carcinoma
    p. hidradenoma
    p. muscle
    p. muscle dysfunction
    p. necrosis
    p. neoplasm
    p. serous cervical carcinoma
    p. serous cystadenocarcinoma
    p. variant
papilledema
    chronic p.
papilliferum
    syringocystadenoma p.
papillitis
papillocarcinoma
    choroid plexus p.
papilloma
    choroid plexus p. (CPP)
    ductal p.
    intraductal p.
    laryngeal p.
    pathognomonic p.
    raised raspberry-like p.
    raspberry-like p.
    respiratory p.
    tan p.

papillomacular bundle
papillomatosis
>benign p.
>juvenile p.
>laryngeal p.
>recurrent respiratory p. (RRP)
>respiratory p.
>subareolar duct p.
>vulvar p.

Papillomavirus
papillomavirus
>human p. (HPV)
>p. hybridization
>p. infection
>p., polyoma virus, simian virus 40 vacuolating virus (PAPOVA)
>transcriptionally active human p.
>type 16 p.

Papillon-Léage-Psaume syndrome
Papillon-Lefèvre syndrome
Pap-Kaps
PapNet
>P. automated cervical cystology system
>P. reader
>P. test
>P. testing
>P. testing system

papoose board
PAPOVA
>papillomavirus, polyoma virus, simian virus 40 vacuolating virus

PAPP-A
>pregnancy-associated plasma protein A

PAPP-C
>pregnancy-associated plasma protein C

PAPP-D
>pregnancy-associated plasma protein D

Pap-Perfect
>P.-P. plastic spatula
>P.-P. supply system

PapSure
papular
>p. acrodermatitis
>p. acrodermatitis of childhood (PAC)
>p. dermatitis of pregnancy (PDP)
>p. eruption
>p. exanthem
>p. lesion
>p. rash
>p. urticaria

papule
>acral keratotic p.
>acuminate p.
>blue p.
>crop of p.'s
>erythematous p.
>filiform p.
>flesh-colored p.
>genital p.
>Gottron p.
>keratinized p.
>keratotic p.
>lichenoid p.
>polygonal p.
>pruritic urticarial p.
>satellite p.
>urticarial p.
>verrucous p.
>violaceous polygonal p.
>white p.

papulonecrotica
>tuberculosis p.

papulonecrotic tuberculid
papulonodular lesion
papulosa
>deciduas tuberosa p.

papulosis
>bowenoid p.
>introital p.

papulosquamous
>p. eruption
>p. rash
>p. skin change

papulovesicle
papulovesicular
>p. acrodermatitis
>p. lesion

PAPVR
>partial anomalous pulmonary venous return

papyraceous fetus
papyraceus
>fetus p.

PAQLQ
>Pediatric Asthma Quality of Life Questionnaire

PAR
>population-attributable risk calculation

para 1, 2
paraaminomethylbenzoic acid (PAMBA)
paraaminosalicylate
paraaminosalicylic acid (PAS)

NOTES

P

paraaortic
  p. lymphadenectomy
  p. node
  p. node irradiation
  p. positivity
parabasal cell
paraben
parabiosis
  dialytic p.
  vascular p.
parabola
  Keplerian p.
parabolic twins
paracentesis
paracentric inversion
paracervical
  p. anesthesia
  p. area
  p. block
  p. blockade
  p. extension
  p. injection
  p. lymphatics
paracetamol suppository
parachute
  p. mitral valve
  p. reflex
  p. response
Paracoccidioides brasiliensis
paracoccidioidin skin testing
paracoccidioidomycosis
paracolic gutter
paracolpitis
paracolpium
paracrine-acting growth factor
paracrine communication
paracrystalline inclusion
paracyclic ovulation
paracyesis
paradoxical, paradoxic
  p. aciduria
  p. breathing
  p. chest wall motion
  p. incontinence
  p. pulse
  p. pupil reaction
  p. respiration
paradoxus
  pulsus p.
paraductal acanthosis
paraduodenal hernia
paraesophageal hiatal hernia
Parafon Forte DSC
paraganglioma
  gastrointestinal p.
ParaGard
  P. T380A intrauterine copper
    contraceptive
  P. T380 copper IUD

paragonimiasis
  cerebral p.
Paragonimus westermani
parahaemolyticus
  Vibrio p.
parahemophilia
parainfluenza
  p. virus (PIV)
  p. virus (type 1–4)
parakeratosis
  multinucleation p.
Paral
paraldehyde
parallel
  p. circulation
  p. play
  p. speech
  p. study arm
paralogy
paralysis, pl. paralyses
  abducens facial p.
  acute flaccid p.
  anal sphincter p.
  antigenic p.
  birth p.
  bladder sphincter p.
  bulbar p.
  ciliary p.
  congenital abducens facial p.
  congenital oculofacial p.
  congenital unilateral lower lip p.
  p. of conjugate upward gaze
  deltoid p.
  diaphragm p.
  Duchenne p.
  Erb-Duchenne p.
  facial nerve p.
  familial hypokalemic periodic p.
  flaccid p.
  fleeting p.
  hereditary abductor vocal cord p.
  hyperkalemic periodic p.
  hypokalemic periodic p.
  hysterical p.
  idiopathic facial p.
  immunologic p.
  infantile p.
  Klumpke p.
  Klumpke-Dejerine p.
  Landry type of p.
  laryngeal abductor p.
  laryngeal adductor p.
  laryngeal nerve p.
  lower lip p.
  mononeuritis with p.
  muscle p.
  nerve p.
  obstetric p.
  obstetrical p.

oculofacial p.
parturient p.
phrenic nerve p.
poliomyelitis-like p.
postictal p.
pseudohypertrophic muscular p.
recurrent laryngeal nerve p.
respiratory ciliary p.
sleep p.
spastic spinal p.
sphincter p.
p. spinalis spastica
p. of superior laryngeal nerve
tick p.
Todd p.
total muscle p.
unilateral lower lip p.
unilateral partial facial p.
vocal cord p.
Werdnig-Hoffmann p.

paralytic
p. hypotonia
p. idiocy
p. ileus
p. poliomyelitis
p. rabies
p. shellfish poisoning
p. strabismus

paramagnetic particle
paramedian incision
paramenia
parameningeal infection
paramesonephric duct
parameter
fetal growth p.'s
growth p.'s
paramethadione syndrome
parametrectomy
radical p.
parametrial
p. extension
p. phlegmon
parametritic abscess
parametritis
parametrium
paramyoclonus multiplex
paramyotonia congenita
paramyxovirus
paranasal sinus
paraneoplastic
p. amyloidosis

p. symptom
p. syndrome
paraneoplastica
acrokeratosis p.
paranoid
p. ideation
p. personality disorder
paraovarian
p. adhesion
p. cyst
paraparesis
acute spastic p.
areflexic p.
familial spastic p.
flaccid p.
HTLV-I associated
myelopathy/tropical spastic p.
(HAM/TSP)
nonspastic p.
spastic p.
tropical spastic p. (TSP)
parapertussis
Bordetella p.
parapharyngeal
p. abscess
p. lymph node
paraphasia
paraphimosis
Paraplatin
paraplegia
congenital spastic p.
familial spastic p. (FSP)
flaccid p.
hereditary spastic p.
infantile spastic p.
spastic p. (SP)
p. spastica
paraplegic
paraplegin
parapneumonic pleural effusion
parapodium
Toronto p.
paraprofessional
parapsilosis
Candida p.
parapsoriasis guttata
paraquat
p. ingestion
p. lung
pararectal space

NOTES

P

parasagittal
    p. cerebral injury
    p. cortical infarction
parasalpingitis
parasite
    intestinal p.
    ova and p.'s (O&P)
parasitemia
parasitic
    p. fetus
    p. gastroenteritides
    p. infection
    p. leiomyoma
    p. myoma
    p. organism
    p. pregnancy
parasiticus
    dipygus p.
    janiceps p.
parasitized cecal pouch
parasomnia
    NREM arousal p.
    REM p.
paraspadias
paraspinal mass
parasternal
    p. lift
    p. short-axis view
parastremmatic dwarfism
parasuicide
parasympathetic
    p. fiber
    p. nerve
    p. nervous system
    p. neuron
    p. tone
parasympatholytic drug
parasympathomimetic drop
paratesticular tumor
parathyroid
    p. adenoma
    p. disease
    p. disorder
    p. gland
    p. gland immaturity
    p. hormone (PTH)
    p. hormone-related peptide (PTHrP)
parathyroidectomy
parathyromatosis
Paratrol shampoo
paratropicalis
    Candida p.
paratubal cyst
paratyphi
    Salmonella p.
paratyphoid fever
paraumbilical defect
paraurethral
    p. cyst

    p. duct
    p. gland
parauterine
    p. abscess
    p. lymph node
paravaginal
    p. cystocele
    p. cystocele repair
    p. defect
    p. hysterectomy
    p. soft tissue
    p. suspension
paravaginitis
paraventricular tachycardia
paravertebral abscess
paravesical space
paraxial
    p. fibular hemimelia
    p. mesoderm
    p. tibial hemimelia
parched mucous membrane
parchment skin
paregoric
parencephalia
parencephalous
parenchyma
    liver p.
    medullary p.
    patchy infiltration of medullary p.
    placental p.
    renal p.
parenchymal
    p. abscess
    p. brain lesion
    p. cyst
    p. damage
    p. lung disease
    p. lung morphogenesis
    p. nodule
parenchymatous
    p. cerebral cysticercosis
    p. congenital syphilis
    p. form
    p. mastitis
parent
    p. child
    consanguineous p.'s
    Coping Health Inventory for P.'s (CHIP)
    p. effectiveness training (PET)
    p. guidance work
    rearing p.'s
    social p.'s
    P. and Teacher Conners Scale
parentage
    coefficient of p.
    p. determination
parental
    p. chromosomal abnormality

p. chromosome abnormality
p. consanguinity
p. karyotype
p. origin
P. Stress Index (PSI)
parent-child
p.-c. interaction
p.-c. interaction problem
parenteral
p. administration
p. alimentation
p. aqueous penicillin G
p. fluid therapy
p. hyperalimentation
p. medication
p. nutrition (PN)
p. nutrition-associated (PNAC)
p. progesterone
Parenti-Fraccaro syndrome
parenting
attachment p.
parent-professional partnership
Parent's Choice formula
paresis
apparent p.
asymmetric palatal p.
cochleovestibular p.
congenital suprabulbar p.
flaccid p.
horizontal saccadic gaze p.
laryngeal p.
ocular p.
oculosympathetic p.
palatal p.
spastic p.
suprabulbar p.
Todd p.
paresthesia
Berger p.
pargyline
Pari
P. LC Plusjet nebulizer
P. Proneb Turbo compressor
paricalcitol
parietal
p. bone
p. bulge
p. cell antibody
p. cell hyperplasia
p. encephalocele
p. foramina

p. foramina, brachymicrocephaly,
mental retardation syndrome
p. pericardiectomy
p. peritoneum
p. shunt
parietooccipital region
Parinaud
P. oculoglandular syndrome
P. sign
parity
vaginal p.
park
hemoglobin M Hyde P.
Parkes Weber-Dimitri syndrome
Parkinson-Cowan dry gas meter
Parkinson disease
parkinsonian
p. movement disorder
p. rigidity
parkinsonian-like
parkinsonism
rapid-onset dystonia, parkinsonism
Parkland
P. formula
P. Hospital technique
P. tubal ligation
Parlodel
Parnate
parodynia perversa
paromomycin sulfate
paronychia
candidal p.
paronychial infection
paroophoritis
paroöphoron
parotid
p. enlargement
p. gland
parotitis
acute p.
bacterial p.
epidemic p.
suppurative p.
parous
p. introitus
p. os
p. outlet
vaginally p.
p. woman
parovarian tumor
parovariotomy
parovaritis

NOTES

P

parovarium
paroxetine hydrochloride
paroxysm
    febrile p.
paroxysmal
    p. atrial tachycardia (PAT)
    p. blinking
    p. coughing
    p. depolarization shift (PDS)
    p. dystonia
    p. emotional state
    p. hypercyanotic attack
    p. hypoxic spell
    p. kinesigenic choreoathetosis
    p. nocturnal dyspnea (PND)
    p. nocturnal hemoglobinuria (PNH)
    p. tachycardia
    p. torticollis
    p. vertigo
parrot
    P. artery
    P. atrophy
    P. fever
    P. jaw
    P. pseudoparalysis
    P. sign
    P. syndrome
Parry-Jones vulvectomy
Parry-Romberg syndrome
PARS
    Personal Adjustment and Role Skills
    PARS III questionnaire
    PARS scale
pars
    p. interarticularis
    p. tuberalis
part
    fetal small p.'s
    p.'s per million (ppm)
    presenting p.
parthenogenesis
partial
    p. agenesis
    p. agenesis of vermis
    p. anomalous pulmonary venous
      return (PAPVR)
    p. auxiliary orthotopic liver
      transplantation
    p. breech extraction
    p. colpectomy
    p. complex epilepsy
    p. complex seizure
    p. DiGeorge anomaly
    p. DiGeorge syndrome
    p. epileptogenic discharge
    p. exchange transfusion
    p. exenteration operation
    p. external biliary diversion
      (PEBD)

    p. gonadal dysgenesis
    p. hepatectomy
    p. hydatidiform mole
    p. (incomplete) androgen
      insensitivity (PAI)
    p. linkage
    p. lipodystrophy
    p. liquid ventilation (PLV)
    p. monosomy 1p–22p
    p. monosomy Xp21, Xp22
    p. monosomy Xq
    p. oculocutaneous albinism
    p. omentectomy
    p. pressure (P)
    p. pressure alveolar oxygen (PaO$_2$)
    p. pressure of arterial carbon
      dioxide (PaCO$_2$)
    p. pressure arterial oxygen (PaO$_2$)
    p. pressure carbon dioxide (PCO$_2$)
    p. pressure oxygen (PO$_2$)
    p. previa
    p. rollerball endometrial ablation
    p. salpingectomy
    p. sitting position
    p. squatting position
    p. status epilepticus
    p. tetrasomy 10p
    p. thromboplastin time (PTT)
    p. trisomy 1p–22p
    p. trisomy 10q syndrome
    p. trisomy Xq
    p. villus atrophy
    p. vulvectomy
    p. zona dissection (PZD)
partialis
    rachischisis p.
partially
    p. duplicated ureter
    p. sighted
partial-syndrome eating disorder
partial-thickness burn
particle
    alpha p.
    Dane p.
    paramagnetic p.
particulate
    p. matter
    p. radiation
Partington-Anderson syndrome
Partington X-linked mental retardation
    syndrome (PRTS)
partition of energy metabolism
partner
    p. gene
    intimate p.
    nonmonogamous p.
partnership
    parent-professional p.
partograph

parturient
- p. apoplexy
- p. canal
- p. fever
- p. paralysis

parturifacient

parturiometer

parturition

Parvolex

parvoviral infection

parvovirus
- p. B19
- p. B19-induced red blood cell aplasia
- p. B19 red blood cell aplasia
- human p. (HPV)

parvula
- *Veillonella p.*

parvum
- *Cryptosporidium p.*

PAS
- paraaminosalicylic acid
- periodic acid-Schiff
- PAS stain

pascal (Pa)

Pashayan-Pruzansky syndrome

Pashayan syndrome

Pasini variant

passage
- meconium p.
- p. of meconium
- transplacental p.

passenger air bag (PAB)

passer
- MetraPass suture p.

passes
- number of needle p.

passive
- p. head-up tilt test
- p. immunity
- p. immunization
- p. incontinence
- p. range of motion
- p. supination
- p. venous congestion

passivity

Passos-Bueno syndrome

paste
- Bipp p.
- Boudreaux's Butt p.
- Butt p.
- Monsel p.

- nitroglycerin p.
- Triple P.
- zinc oxide p.

Pasteurella
- *P. canis*
- *P. multocida*
- *P. multocida* osteomyelitis

Pasteur pipette

Pastia
- P. line
- P. sign

PAT
- paroxysmal atrial tachycardia
- preventive allergy treatment

Patanol

Patau syndrome

patch
- Alora Transdermal p.
- atrophic p.
- blood p.
- bovine pericardium p.
- Climara estradiol transdermal system p.
- corporal cavernosal p.
- Dacron p.
- EMLA p.
- Esclim p.
- fentanyl p.
- Gore-Tex Soft Tissue P.
- hair p.
- hairy p.
- herald p.
- MacCallum p.
- Minitran P.
- moth p.
- mucous p.
- Nitro-Dur P.
- Ortho Evra transdermal p.
- pericardium p.
- Peyer p.
- salmon p.
- shagreen p.
- spontaneous atrophic p.
- strawberry p.
- transdermal fentanyl p.
- transdermal glyceryl trinitrate p.
- transdermal medication p.
- Transderm-Nitro P.
- Trans-Ver-Sal Transdermal P.
- p. unroofing
- p. unroofing of outflow tract

patching

NOTES

P

patchy
>p. infiltrate
>p. infiltration
>p. infiltration of medullary
>parenchyma

patella, pl. **patellae**
>absent p.
>aplastic p.
>bipartite p.
>chondromalacia p.
>congenital dislocation of p.
>dislocated p.
>dislocating p.
>hypoplastic p.
>kissing patellae
>sleeve fracture of p.
>subluxating p.

patellar
>p. fracture
>p. ligament
>p. reflex
>p. tendinitis

patellofemoral
>p. malalignment
>p. malalignment pain
>p. pain syndrome (PFPS)
>p. stress syndrome

patency
>probe p.
>tubal p.
>ureteral p.

patent
>p. anus
>p. ductus arteriosis coil
>embolization
>p. ductus arteriosus (PDA)
>p. ductus venosus
>p. foramen ovale (PFO)
>p. omphalomesenteric duct
>p. processus vaginalis peritonei
>p. urachus

paternal
>p. age
>p. factor
>p. karyotype
>p. meiosis I (PMI)
>p. meiosis II (PMII)
>p. postnatal depression
>p. status
>p. uniparenteral isodisomy

paternity

path
>migratory p.

pathergy sign
Pathfinder DFA test
pathogen
>blood-borne p.

pathogenesis
pathogenic bacteria

pathogenicity
pathognomonic
>p. Koplik spot
>p. papilloma
>p. symptom

pathologic
>p. amenorrhea
>p. apnea
>p. discharge
>p. finding
>p. fracture
>p. reflex
>p. retraction ring
>p. retraction ring of Bandl

pathological
>p. apnea
>p. cavus
>p. gynecomastia
>p. model

pathologist
>Cancer Committee of College of
>American P.'s
>International Society of
>Gynecologic p.'s (ISGYP)
>perinatal/placental p.
>speech-language p.

pathology
>anaplastic p.
>hilar cell p.
>International Society for
>Gynecologic P.
>intracranial p.
>perinatal p.
>speech p.
>speech-language p.
>uterine p.

pathophysiologic mechanism
pathophysiology
pathotropic
pathway
>COX p.
>Embden-Meyerhof p.
>neural reflex p.
>nociceptive p.
>pericardial p.
>postchiasmal visual p.
>reflex p.
>visual p.

PATI
>Penetrating Abdominal Trauma Index

patient
>adolescent-onset p.
>amenorrheic p.
>analbuminemic p.
>anovulatory p.
>antenatal p.
>CMV-seronegative transplant p.
>gynecologic cancer p.
>high-risk p.

infertile p.
P. Outcomes Research Team
(PORT)
pregnant cardiac p.
thalassemic p.
transplant p.
Zoladex in premenopausal p.'s
(ZIPP)
patient-controlled analgesia (PCA)
patient-triggered ventilation
patter
cocktail party p.
pattern
abnormal respiratory p.
abnormal vasculature flow p.
age-to-dose p.
android p.
apple p.
atypical vessel colposcopic p.
banding p.
behavior p.
bimodal p.
biphasic temperature p.
branching p.
breathing p.
burst-suppression p.
capillary p.
central fat distribution p.
characteristic
electroencephalogram p.
chessboard p.
Christmas tree p.
chromosomal p.
complete suppression p.
dermatoglyphic p.
developmental p.
diastolic overload p.
distribution p.
dysfunctional labor p.
eggbeater running p.
extensor thrust p.
fat distribution p.
ferning p.
fern leaf p.
fetal heart rate p.
fleur-de-lis breast reconstruction p.
flow p.
four-leaf clover p.
fracture p.
genetic inheritance p.
ground-glass p.
gynecoid fat distribution p.

gyral p.
heliotrope p.
herringbone p.
hyperkinetic behavior p.
hypsarrhythmic p.
inactivation p.
interweaving p.
Le Fort fracture p.
linear branching p.
marking time p.
menstrual p.
mixed p.
mosaic p.
motor p.
mucopolysaccharide p.
munching p.
nonobstructive p.
nonreassuring fetal heart beat p.
nonreassuring fetal heart rate p.
overload p.
palm leaf p.
pear p.
persistent primitive reflex p.
primitive reflex p.
prominent ductal p.
prosodic p.
reflex p.
respiratory p.
restrictive breathing p.
reticulogranular p.
reticulonodular p.
silent fetal heart rate p.
silent oscillatory p.
sinusoidal heart rate p.
skin ridge p.
sleep p.
snowflake p.
startle p.
subpleural reticulonodular p.
sun-seeking p.
systolic overload p.
temperature p.
temporospatial p.
tonic neck p.
urinary mucopolysaccharide p.
vasculature flow p.
voiding p.
patterned breathing
patterning therapy
Patterson pseudoleprechaunism syndrome
Patterson-Stevenson-Fontaine syndrome

NOTES

P

695

patty
   Cellolite p.
patulous rectal sphincter
pauciarticular
   p. JRA
   p. juvenile chronic arthritis
pauciarticular-onset
   p.-o. JRA
   p.-o. juvenile arthritis
paucicellular
pauciimmune glomerulonephritis
paucity
   bile duct p.
   p. of gas
   p. of interlobular bile duct
      (PILBD)
   intrahepatic bile duct p.
   nonsyndromic bile duct p.
   syndromic p.
Paul-Bunnell
   P.-B. antibody test
   P.-B. reaction
Paul-Bunnell-Davidsohn test
Pavacap
Pavacen
Pavatest
Pavlik harness
PAVM
   pulmonary arteriovenous malformation
pavor
   p. diurnus
   p. nocturnus
PAW
   pulmonary artery wedge
Pawlik fold
PAWP
   pulmonary artery wedge pressure
paws
   Medevice surgical p.
PAX3 gene
Paxil
Pazo
   P. Hemorrhoid
   P. hemorrhoid ointment
PBC
   periodic breathing cycle
   plasma bilirubin concentration
   primary biliary cirrhosis
PBF
   percent body fat
   pulmonary blood flow
PBL
   peripheral blood lymphocyte
PBMC
   peripheral blood mononuclear cell
PBS
   phosphate buffered saline
      isotonic PBS

PBSC
   peripheral blood stem cell
PCA
   patient-controlled analgesia
   postconceptional age
PCC
   Poison Control Center
   postcoital contraception
PCC-R
   Percentage of Consonants Correct-
      Revised
PCD
   primary ciliary dyskinesia
PCDAI
   Pediatric Crohn Disease Activity Index
PCE
   physical capacity evaluation
PCEC
   purified chick embryo cell culture
      PCEC vaccine
4p+ chromosome
PC-IOL
   posterior chamber intraocular lens
PCNSL
   primary central nervous system
      lymphoma
PCO
   polycystic ovary
PCO$_2$
   partial pressure carbon dioxide
PCOD
   polycystic ovarian disease
   polycystic ovary disease
PCOS
   polycystic ovarian syndrome
   polycystic ovary syndrome
PCP
   phencyclidine
   Pneumocystis carinii pneumonia
PCR
   polymerase chain reaction
      allele-specific PCR
      PCR assay
      PCR test
PCr
   phosphocreatine
PCT
   postcoital test
   procalcitonin
      serum PCT
PCV7
   pneumococcal 7-valent conjugate vaccine
PCVC
   percutaneous central venous catheter
PCWP
   pulmonary capillary wedge pressure
PD
   peritoneal dialysis
   personality disorder

postural drainage
Bromfenex PD
Iofed PD
PDA
patent ductus arteriosus
bidirectional PDA
P.D. Access with Peel-Away needle introducer
PDD
pervasive developmental disorder
PDD-NOS
pervasive developmental disorder not otherwise specified
PDE
personality disorder examination
PDE5
phosphodiesterase 5
PdE
pediatric endocrinology
PDHC
PDHC deficiency
PDI
phosphodiesterase inhibitor
psychiatric diagnostic interview
psychomotor development index
PDM
pregestational diabetes mellitus
PDMS
Peabody Developmental Motor Scale
PDP
papular dermatitis of pregnancy
positive distending pressure
PDS
paroxysmal depolarization shift
PE
preeclampsia
pressure equalization
pulmonary embolism
AT3 type II PE, RS
PE tube
Peabody
P. Developmental Motor Activity Cards
P. Developmental Motor Scale (PDMS)
P. Picture Vocabulary Test (PPVT)
P. Picture Vocabulary Test-Revised (PPVT-R)
Peacock bromide
peak
adaptive p.
p. admittance

Bragg p.
p. end-expiratory pressure
p. expiratory flow rate (PEFR)
p. flow measurement
p. flow meter (PFM)
p. flow meter monitor
p. flow rate
p. growth velocity
p. inspiratory pressure (PIP)
p. instantaneous gradient
p. and trough
p. and trough levels
Webb-McCall p.
Péan
P. clamp
P. forceps
peanut oil
PEARL
physiologic endometrial ablation/resection loop
pearl
Bohn epithelial p.'s
collar of p.'s
epithelial p.
Epstein p.'s
perineal p.'s
Pearl index
pearly-white nodule
pear pattern
pear-shaped uterus
Pearson marrow-pancreas syndrome
pea soup stool
peau
p. d'orange
p. d'orange appearance
p. d'orange appearance of the breast
pebbly skin lesion
PEBD
partial external biliary diversion
PEC
protein-induced eosinophilic colitis
pecorum
Chlamydia p.
pectin
kaolin and p.
pectinate line
pectoralis major muscle
pectoriloquy
whispered p.
pectus
p. bar

NOTES

697

pectus *(continued)*
    p. carinatum
    p. excavatum
    p. gallinatum
    p. recurvatum
peculiar facies
PED
    pediatric emergency department
    prenatally exposed to drugs
pedaling movement
pedal pulse
Pedameth
Pedersen speculum
Pederson vaginal speculum
PEDI
    Pediatric Evaluation of Disability
    Inventory
PediaCare
    P. Cough-Cold
    P. Fever
    P. Night Rest
    P. Oral
Pediacof
Pediaflor
Pedialyte
    P. formula
    P. oral electrolyte maintenance
    solution
Pediamist
Pediapred Oral
PediaSure
    P. liquid nutrition
    P. with Fiber formula
pediatric, paediatric
    p. acquired immunodeficiency
    syndrome
    p. acute admission severity (PAAS)
    p. advanced life support (PALS)
    p. anesthesiologist
    p. aphakia
    P. Asthma Quality of Life
    Questionnaire (PAQLQ)
    p. autoimmune neuropsychiatric
    disorders associated with
    streptococcus (PANDAS)
    p. balloon
    Benylin p.
    p. bone rongeur
    p. bronchoscopy
    p. bulldog clamp
    p. cocktail
    P. Crohn Disease Activity Index
    (PCDAI)
    p. dermatology
    p. dosing information
    P. Early Elemental Examination
    (PEEX)
    p. EKG
    p. emergency department (PED)

    p. emergency medicine (PEM)
    p. endocrinology (PdE)
    P. Evaluation of Disability
    Inventory (PEDI)
    P. Examination at Three (PEET)
    P. Examination of Educational
    Readiness (PEER)
    p. exanthem
    p. gonococcal conjunctivitis
    p. gonococcal infection
    p. gynecology
    p. hypertension
    p. infectious disease (PID)
    p. intensive care unit (PICU)
    p. labial agglutination
    P. Liver Transplant-Specific Scale
    (PLTSS)
    p. lung surgery
    p. lupus nephropathy
    p. myelodysplasia
    p. neurocritical care
    p. neurologist
    p. nutrition
    P. Oncology Group
    p. otolaryngology
    p. ovarian teratoma
    Prostin VR P.
    p. public health
    p. pulmonary medicine
    p. radiologist
    P. Risk of Mortality (PRISM)
    Robitussin p.
    Rynatan p.
    p. sedation
    p. sedation unit (PSU)
    p. self-retaining retractor
    p. spectrum of disease (PSD)
    p. surgeon
    P. Symptom Checklist (PSC)
    p. thyroid carcinogenesis
    P. Trauma Score (PTS)
    p. tuberculosis
    p. vaginoscopy
    p. vascular clamp
    Vicks P. 44E, 44M
    Vicks Formula 44 P.
    p. viral diarrhea
    Vivonex p.
Pediatrician infant dietary supplement
pediatrics, paediatrics
    American Academy of p. (AAP)
    behavioral p.
Pediatrix vaccine
Pediazole
Pedi-Bath Salts
Pedi-Boro Soak Paks
Pedi-cap detector
pedicle
    p. clamp

nerve-muscle p.
renal p.
uterosacral ligament p.
Pedicran with Iron
pedicterus
pediculosis
    p. capitis
    p. corporis
    p. corpus
    p. palpebrum
    p. pubis
Pediculus
    P. humanus
    P. humanus corporis
    P. humanus var capitis
Pedi-Dri Topical
pedigree
    CEPH p.
    p. chart
Pediotic
Pedi PEG tube
Pedi-Pro Topical
pedis
    dorsalis p.
    tinea p.
Pedituss Cough
pedodontist
pedologist
pedometer
Pedric
Pedte-Pak-4
Pedtrace-4 hyperalimentation
peduncle
    cerebral p.
    inferior p.
    middle cerebellar p.
pedunculated
    p. leiomyoma
    p. lesion
    p. molluscum fibrosum
    p. polyp
PedvaxHIB vaccine
PEEP
    positive end-expiratory pressure
        PEEP ventilator
PEER
    Pediatric Examination of Educational
        Readiness
peer
    p. conformity inventory
    p. relation

PEET
    Pediatric Examination at Three
PEEX
    Pediatric Early Elemental Examination
pefloxacin
PEFR
    peak expiratory flow rate
PEG
    percutaneous endoscopic gastrostomy
        PEG tube
peg
    rete p.
PEG-ADA
    polyethylene glycol-modified adenosine
        deaminase
pegademase bovine
Peganone
pegaspargase
pegboard
    grooved p.
peglike teeth
peg-shaped upper central incisor
PEHO
    progressive encephalopathy, edema,
        hypsarrhythmia, optic atrophy
        PEHO syndrome
Peiper reflex
Pel-Ebstein fever
Pelger-Huet anomaly
peliosis
    bacillary p.
    p. hepatis
Pelizaeus-Merzbacher disease (PMD)
pellagra
pellagralike skin rash
pellet
    Muse p.
    YAG p.
Pelletier-Leisti syndrome
Pellizzi syndrome
pellucida
    agenesis of septa p.
    macula p.
    zona p. (ZP)
pellucidum
    cavum septum p.
    enlarged cavum septum p.
    septum p.
Pelosi
    P. hysterotomy
    P. vaginal hysterectomy
pelves (*pl. of* pelvis)

NOTES

P

pelvic
- p. abscess
- p. actinomycosis
- p. adhesive disease (PAD)
- p. appendicitis
- p. architecture
- p. arterial embolization
- p. arteriogram
- p. arteriovenous malformation
- p. artery
- p. axis
- p. band
- p. bleeding
- p. boost radiotherapy
- p. brim
- p. Castleman disease
- p. cavity
- p. cellulitis
- p. congestion syndrome
- p. connective tissue
- p. contraction
- p. diaphragm
- p. direction
- p. endometriosis
- p. examination
- p. exenteration
- p. exostosis
- p. fibromatosis
- p. floor
- p. floor damage
- p. floor electrical stimulation (PFS)
- p. floor laxity
- p. floor nerve
- p. forceps
- p. fracture
- p. girdle relaxation (PGR)
- p. gutter
- p. hematocele
- p. inclination
- p. index
- p. infection
- p. inflammation
- p. inflammatory disease (PID)
- p. inlet
- p. involvement
- p. irradiation
- p. joint
- p. kidney
- p. laparoscopy
- p. lengthening osteotomy
- p. lymphadenectomy
- p. lymph node
- p. lymphocyst
- p. malignancy in pregnancy
- p. mass
- p. muscle exercise
- p. muscle-strengthening exercise
- p. nerve injury
- p. node dissection
- p. organ
- p. organ prolapse
- P. Organ Prolapse-Quantified (POPQ)
- p. organ prolapse quantitation
- p. outlet
- p. ovarian vein thrombosis (POVT)
- p. pain
- p. peritonitis
- p. plane of greatest dimensions
- p. plane of inlet
- p. plane of least dimensions
- p. plane of outlet
- p. plexus
- p. pole
- p. presentation
- p. reconstruction surgeon
- p. reconstructive surgery
- p. recurrence
- p. relaxation
- p. rest
- p. score
- p. side wall
- p. support defect
- p. support index (PSI)
- p. tenderness
- p. tilt
- p. tuberculosis
- p. tumor
- p. ultrasound
- p. vein congestion
- p. vein incompetence
- p. vein thrombophlebitis
- p. venous congestion syndrome
- p. version

pelvicephalography
pelvicephalometry
pelvic-floor surgery
pelvicocleidocranial dysostosis
pelviectasis
pelvifixation
pelvigraph
pelvimeter
pelvimetry
- clinical p.
- CT p.
- manual p.
- planographic p.
- radiographic p.
- stereoscopic p.
- x-ray p.

pelvioperitonitis
pelvioplasty
pelvioscopy, pelviscopy, pelvoscopy
pelviotomy
pelviperitonitis
pelvis, pl. **pelves**
- android p.
- anthropoid p.

arcus tendineus fasciae p.
assimilation p.
axis of p.
beaked p.
bifid p.
bowl of p.
breech location out of p.
calcified phleboliths in p.
p. capsular dysplasia
concrete p.
conjugata anatomic p.
conjugata diagonalis p.
conjugata externa p.
conjugata vera p.
contracted p.
cordate p.
cordiform p.
Deventer p.
dilated renal p.
dwarf p.
elephant p.
p. enlargement
false p.
flat p.
flying-T p.
frozen p.
funnel-shaped p.
gynecoid p.
heart-shaped p.
inverted p.
p. justo major
p. justo minor
juvenile p.
Kilian p.
kyphotic p.
longitudinal oval p.
p. major
masculine p.
mesatipellic p.
p. minor
Nägele p.
p. nana
Otto p.
p. plana
platypellic p.
Prague p.
renal p.
reniform p.
Robert p.
Rokitansky p.
round p.
sweep the p.

transverse oval p.
trefoil p.
true p.
well engaged in p.
pelviscope
pelviscopic intrafascial hysterectomy
pelviscopy (*var. of* pelvioscopy)
pelvis-shoulder dysplasia
pelvitherm
pelviureteric junction obstruction
pelvocephalography
pelvoscopy (*var. of* pelvioscopy)
PEM
    pediatric emergency medicine
Pemberton
    P. acetabuloplasty
    P. procedure
pemirolast potassium
pemoline
    magnesium p.
Pemoline C-IV
pemphigoid
    bullous p.
    childhood cicatricial p.
    p. gestationis
pemphigus
    benign familial chronic p.
    p. foliaceus
    p. neonatorum
    syphilitic p.
    p. vulgaris
pen
    P. A/N
    Epi E-Z P.
    Humalog P.
    Humulin P.
    insulin p.
Pena
    P. midsagittal anorectoplasty
    P. procedure
Pena-Shokeir
    P.-S. phenotype
    P.-S. syndrome (I, II)
Penbritin
penciclovir cream
pencil
    Conmed electrosurgical p.
    Valleylab p.
pencil-handled laryngoscope
pendelluft
Pendred syndrome
pendular nystagmus

NOTES

P

pendulous
> p. abdomen
> p. breast

pendulum
> molluscum fibrosum p.

Penecort Topical
Penetrak test
penetrance
penetrans
> *Mycoplasma p.*

penetrant
> p. gene
> p. trait

penetrating
> P. Abdominal Trauma Index (PATI)
> p. brain injury
> p. trauma

penetration
> accidental p.
> anal p.
> cercarial skin p.
> skin p.

Penetrex
PenFill
> Novolin 70/30 P.
> Novolin N, R P.

penicillamine
penicillin
> antistaphylococcal p.
> aqueous crystalline p.
> aqueous crystalline p. G
> benzathine p.
> benzathine p. G (BPG)
> extended-spectrum p.
> p. G
> p. G benzathine
> p. G procaine
> natural p.
> parenteral aqueous p. G
> penicillinase-resistant p.
> phenoxymethyl p.
> procaine p.
> procaine p. G
> semisynthetic p.
> p. V potassium
> p. V, VK

penicillinase-producing gonococcus
penicillinase-resistant penicillin
penicillin-nonsusceptible *Streptococcus pneumoniae* (PNSP)
penicillin-resistant
> p.-r. *Staphylococcus* pneumonia (PRSP)
> p.-r. *Streptococcus pneumoniae* (PRSP)

penicilliosis
Penicillium marneffei

penile
> p. agenesis
> p. chordee
> p. curvature
> p. duplication
> p. dysgenesis
> p. erection
> p. flaccidity
> p. ischemia
> p. Kaposi sarcoma
> p. length
> p. torsion
> p. ulceration
> p. urethra
> p. urethral meatus
> p. zipper entrapment

penis
> bulbus p.
> buried p.
> concealed p.
> corona of p.
> fracture of p.
> glans p.
> hidden p.
> hypoplastic p.
> inconspicuous p.
> webbed p.

penischisis
Pen-Jr
> Epi E-Z P.-Jr

Pen Kera moisturizing cream
Penlon infant resuscitator
Pennington
> P. clamp
> P. forceps

Penn pouch procedure
penopubic urethral meatus
penoscrotal
> p. hypospadias
> p. Kaposi sarcoma
> p. transposition

Penrose drain
Pentacef
pentaerythritol tetranitrate
pentagastrin
pentalogy
> p. of Cantrell
> Fallot p.
> p. of Fallot

Pentam-300 Injection
pentamidine isethionate
Pentamycetin
pentane
> exhaled p.

Pentasa Oral
pentasomy
> chromosome X p.
> p. X syndrome

pentastarch

pentavalent vaccine
Pentax
    P. EG-2430 video endoscope
    P. FG 24-x video endoscope
    P. laryngoscope
penta-X
    p.-X. chromosomal aberration
    p.-X. syndrome
Pentazine
pentazocine
Pentids-P AS
pentobarbital
    p. coma
    sodium p.
pentobarbitone
pentosifylline
Pentostam
pentosuria
    essential benign p.
Pentothal Sodium
pentoxifylline
Pentrax
Pentritol
penumbra
Pen-Vee
Pen-Vee K
PEO
    progressive external ophthalmoplegia
    PEO syndrome
PEP
    postexposure prophylaxis
    progestogen-dependent endometrial
      protein
Pepcid
    P. AC
    P. AC Acid Controller
    P. Complete
    P. RPD
PEPCK
    phosphoenolpyruvate carboxykinase
    PEPCK deficiency
PEPI
    postmenopausal estrogen and progestin
      intervention
    PEPI study
Pepper syndrome
Peptamen
    P. Jr.
    P. Jr. formula
peptic
    p. esophagitis

    p. gastritis
    p. ulcer
    p. ulcer disease (PUD)
peptide
    amino-terminal p.
    atrial natriuretic p. (ANP)
    brain p.
    carboxyl terminal p. (CTP)
    corticotropin-like intermediate
      lobe p.
    endogenous opioid p.
    glucose-dependent insulinotropic p.
    gonadotropin-releasing hormone-
      associated p. (GAP)
    p. growth factor receptor signal
    p. growth factor signaling
      mechanism
    helix termination p.
    p. hormone
    insulinotropic p.
    91kD cytochrome b p.
    mitogenic p.
    natriuretic p.
    opioid p.
    parathyroid hormone-related p.
      (PTHrP)
    PTH-derived p.
    synthetic gliadin p.
    thrombin receptor-activating p.
      (TRAP)
    trypsin activation p. (TAP)
    vasoactive intestinal p. (VIP)
Pepto-Bismol
Peptococcus
    P. anaerobius
    P. asaccharolyticus
    P. niger
Peptostreptococcus
per
    per os (by mouth) (p.o.)
    per rectum (p.r.)
    per square meter method
    per vaginam
    per vias naturales
peracervical node
Perative formula
Perceived Stress Scale
percent
    p. body fat (PBF)
    p. fractional shortening
    p. of ideal body weight (%IBW)

NOTES

P

percentage
P. of Consonants Correct-Revised (PCC-R)
high oxygen p. (HOPE)
percentile
perception
deficits in attention, motor control, p. (DAMP)
depth p.
light p. (LP)
motor p.
no light p. (NLP)
perceptual
p. domain
p. skill
perchlorate
perchloroethylene
Percocet
Percodan
Percoll sperm preparation technique
percreta
placenta p.
Percuflex Plus stent
percussion
abdominal p.
chest p.
costovertebral angle tenderness to p.
dullness to p.
flatness to p.
hyperresonance to p.
p. myotonia
p. therapy
percutaneous
p. adductor tenotomy
p. aspiration, instillation of hypertonic saline, respiration (PAIR)
p. blood sampling
p. catheter drainage
p. central venous catheter (PCVC)
p. central venous catheterization
p. cholangiography
p. cyst aspiration
p. endoscopic gastrostomy (PEG)
p. endoscopic gastrostomy tube
p. epididymal sperm aspiration (PESA)
p. femoral venous catheter
p. fetal transfusion
p. line
p. lung tap
p. multipuncture technique
p. nephrostomy
p. nephrostomy catheter
p. patent ductus arteriosus closure
p. pin fixation
p. renal biopsy
p. retrograde scleroembolization

p. Seldinger technique
p. Stoller afferent nerve stimulation (PerQ SANS)
p. suprapubic telescopy
p. therapy
p. tracheostomy
p. transluminal angioplasty (PTA)
p. transluminal coronary rotational ablation (PTCRA)
p. umbilical blood sampling (PUBS)
percutaneously inserted central line catheter (PICC)
Perdiem
P. Fiber
P. Plain
perennial
allergic rhinitis p.
p. allergic rhinitis
p. asthma
p. rye grass
Pereyra
P. needle
P. needle suspension
P. procedure
Pereyra-Lebhertz modification of Frangenheim-Stoeckel procedure
Perez-Castro forceps
Perez reflex
perfectionism
rigid p.
Perfectoderm Gel
perflubron emulsion temporary blood substitute
perfluorocarbon (PFC)
perfluorocarbon-assisted gas exchange
perfluorochemical (PFC)
p. liquid
perfluorodecaline (PFD)
perflutren microsphere
perforated
p. appendicitis
p. bowel
p. eardrum
p. tympanic membrane
p. viscus
perforating
p. collagenosis
p. granuloma annulare
p. wound
perforation
appendiceal p. (AP)
biliary p.
eardrum p.
esophageal p.
gastric p.
ileal p.
small bowel p.
spontaneous biliary p. (SBP)

tympanic membrane p.
uterine p.
perforator
Baylor amniotic p.
Performa
P. Acoustic Imaging system
P. diagnostic ultrasound imaging system
P. ultrasound
performance
reproductive p.
perfringens
Clostridium p.
perfused twins
perfusion
fallopian tube sperm p. (FTSP)
luxury p.
mosaic p.
peripheral p.
placental p.
pulmonary p.
renal p.
twin reversed arterial p. (TRAP)
uteroplacental p.
pergolide
Pergonal
Perheentupa syndrome
periadenitis mucosa necrotica recurrens
perianal
p. abscess
p. aphthosis
p. candidosis
p. dermatitis
p. fistula
p. hypopigmentation
p. pruritus
p. skin tag
p. suture
perianastomotic ulceration
periaortic lymph node
periappendiceal abscess
periappendicitis decidualis
periaqueductal tumor
periarteritis nodosa
periarticular
periauricular lymphadenitis
periaxial encephalitis
peribronchial
p. fibrosis
p. infiltration
peribronchiolar infiltration
pericanalicular fibroadenoma

pericapillary inflammatory cuffing
pericardial
p. constriction-growth failure syndrome
p. cyst
p. effusion
p. friction rub
p. knock
p. pathway
p. puncture
p. tamponade
pericardiectomy
parietal p.
visceral p.
pericardiocentesis
pericardiotomy
pericarditis
acute fibrinous p.
bacterial p.
constrictive p.
dry p.
fibrinous p.
immune complex-mediated p.
infectious p.
purulent p.
pericardium patch
pericentric inversion
pericentromeric marker
perichondritis
perichondrium
Peri-Colace
Peri-Cold Pack
pericolpitis
periconceptional rubella
periconceptual intake
pericoronitis
acute p.
pericranium
pericyte
periderm
Peridex
Peridin-C
Peridol
peridural
p. analgesia
p. anesthesia
perifascicular atrophy
perifollicular accentuation
perifolliculitis
Peri-Gel Pack
perihepatitis
gonococcal p.

NOTES

705

perihilar
    p. infiltrate
    p. shadow
    p. streaking
periimplantation
perikaryon, pl. **perikarya**
perilobular connective tissue
perilymph
perilymphatic fistula (PLF)
perimembranous
    p. septum
    p. VSD
perimenopausal woman
perimenopause
perimenstrual tenesmus
perimesencephalic region
perimetritic
perimetritis
perimolysis
perimortem
    p. delivery
    p. sampling
perinatal
    p. acidosis
    p. asphyxia
    p. assessment
    p. cerebral hemorrhage
    p. death
    p. distress prediction
    p. effect
    p. grief
    p. herpes
    p. hydronephrosis
    p. hypoxemia
    p. hypoxia
    p. insult
    p. lethal osteogenesis imperfecta
    p. medicine
    p. morbidity
    p. mortality
    p. mortality rate (PMR, PNMR)
    p. outcome
    p. pathology
    p. period
    p. risk factor
    p. stroke
    p. telencephalic leukoencephalopathy
    p. transmission
    p. trauma
perinatally acquired HIV infection
perinatal/placental pathologist
perinate
perinatologist
perinatology
perineal
    p. analgesia
    p. anesthesia
    p. body
    p. body integrity

    p. cold pack
    p. defect
    p. desquamation
    p. fistula
    p. hygiene
    p. hypospadias
    p. infiltration
    p. irritation
    p. itching
    p. laceration
    p. lesion
    p. massage
    p. membrane
    p. musculature
    p. nerve
    p. pearls
    p. repair
    p. resection
    p. scar
    p. sphincter disruption
    p. surgical apron
    p. testis
    p. trauma
    p. warm pack
perineometer
perineoplasty
perineorrhaphy
    vaginal p.
perineoscrotal hypospadias
perineotomy
perineovaginal fistula
perinephric
    p. abscess
    p. phlegmon
perinephritis
perineum
    central tendon of p.
    dashboard p.
perineurium, pl. **perineuria**
perinuclear antineutrophil cytoplasmic
    antibody (pANCA)
PerioChip
period
    rest/sleep p.'s
period
    antepartum p.
    blastogenic p.
    canalicular p.
    effective refractory p.
    embryonic p.
    fertile p.
    incubation p.
    intrapartum p.
    last menstrual p. (LMP)
    last normal menstrual p. (LNMP)
    menstrual p. (MP)
    missed p.
    neonatal p.
    newborn p.

perinatal p.
postictal p.
postpartum p.
postseizure p.
previous menstrual p. (PMP)
pseudoglandular p.
puerperal p.
saccular p.
terminal saccular p.
window p.

periodic
p. acid-Schiff (PAS)
p. auscultation
p. breathing
p. breathing cycle (PBC)
p. breathing in infants
p. fever
p. fever, aphthous stomatitis, pharyngitis, cervical adenitis (PFAPA)
p. movement disorder
p. patient assessment

periodicity
periodontal disease
periodontitis
juvenile p.
localized juvenile p. (LJP)
prepuberal p.

PerioGard
perioophoritis
perioophorosalpingitis
perioperative
perioptic meningioma
perioral
p. cyanosis
p. rash
p. tissue loss

periorbital
p. ecchymosis
p. edema
p. fullness
p. hyperpigmentation
p. infantile myofibromatosis
p. puffiness
p. skin cellulitis
p. violaceous erythema

periorificial
p. dermatitis
p. rhagades

Perioseptic
Orajel P.

periosteal
p. cloaking
p. elevation
p. reaction
p. stripping

periosteum
periostitis
pubic symphysis p.

periovaritis
peripancreatic fluid
peripartal heparin anticoagulation
peripartum
p. cardiomyopathy
p. symphysis separation

peripheral
p. ablative surgery
p. acrocyanosis
p. airway structure
p. androgen activity
p. androgen activity marker
p. arterial cannulation
p. arterial catheter
p. arterial disease
p. arterial line
p. arteriovenous fistula
p. arthritis
p. auditory disorder
p. blood
p. blood lymphocyte (PBL)
p. blood mononuclear cell (PBMC)
p. blood smear
p. blood stem cell (PBSC)
p. cyanosis
p. dysostosis, nail hypoplasia, mental retardation (PNM)
p. entrapment neuropathy
p. eosinophilia
p. facial nerve palsy (PFNP)
p. fractional oxygen extraction (PFOE)
p. hormone level
p. hyperalimentation
p. instantaneous X-ray imager (PIXI)
p. insulin resistance
p. intravenous (PIV)
p. intravenous catheter
p. jaundice
p. mononeuropathy
p. myelin protein (PMP)
p. nerve block
p. nerve injury

NOTES

peripheral *(continued)*
    p. neuritis
    p. neuroblastoma
    p. neuroectodermal tumor
    p. neuroepithelioma
    p. neurofibromatosis
    p. neutropenia
    p. perfusion
    p. placental separation
    p. precocious puberty
    p. primitive neuroectodermal tumor
     (PPNET)
    p. pulmonary stenosis
    p. pulmonic stenosis
    p. stem cell transplantation
    p. thrombophlebitis
    p. vascular shock
    p. venous catheterization
    p. vertigo
    p. vision
peripherally
    p. inserted catheter (PIC)
    p. inserted central catheter (PICC)
periphery
periportal hemorrhagic necrosis
peripubertal examination
perirectal
    p. abscess
    p. fascia
perirenal abscess
perisalpingitis
perisphincteric factor
perissodactylous
peristalsis
    intestinal p.
    ureteral p.
    visible p.
peristaltic wave
perisulcal topography
perisylvian
    p. abnormality
    p. syndrome
peritomy
peritoneal
    p. biopsy
    p. button
    p. catheter
    p. cavity
    p. cytology
    p. dialysis (PD)
    p. dissemination
    p. drain
    p. envelope
    p. exudate
    p. fibrosis
    p. fluid
    p. hernia
    p. implant
    p. insufflation

    p. lavage
    p. macrophage
    p. mesothelium
    p. mouse
    p. oocyte sperm transfer (POST)
    p. reflection
    p. serosa
    p. serous papillary carcinoma
    p. sign
    p. studding
    p. tap
    p. venous shunt
    ventricular p. (VP)
    p. washing
peritonei
    gliomatosis p.
    patent processus vaginalis p.
    persistent processus vaginalis p.
    processus vaginalis p.
peritoneoscopy
peritoneum
    abdominal p.
    Blake closure of p.
    matted p.
    overlapping closure of p.
    parietal p.
    visceral p.
peritonitis
    acute secondary localized p.
    bacterial p.
    bile p.
    chemical p.
    infectious p.
    localized p.
    meconium p.
    pelvic p.
    primary p.
    secondary localized p.
    spontaneous bacterial p. (SBP)
    tuberculous p.
peritonsillar
    p. abscess
    p. cellulitis
    p. edema
peritubal adhesion
peritubular fibrosis
periumbilical
    p. incision
    p. pain
periungual
    p. avascularity
    p. desquamation
    p. erythema
    p. fibroma
    p. flaking
    p. wart
periurethral
    p. collagen injection
    p. gland

perivaginitis
perivascular
  p. calcification
  p. emphysema
  p. eosinophilic infiltrate
  p. inflammatory infiltrate
  p. polymorphonuclear infiltrate
  p. pseudorosette formation
perivasculitis
  granulomatous p.
periventricular
  p. echolucency (PVEL)
  p. encephalomalacia
  p. hemorrhage (grade 1–4) (PVH)
  p. infarction
  p. leukomalacia (PVL)
  p. nodular gray matter heterotopia
periventricular-intraventricular
  hemorrhage (PIVH)
perivitelline space
Peri-Warm Pack
Perkin
  P. Elmer rhodamine dye terminator
  kit
  P. line
perlèche
Perlman nephroblastomatosis syndrome
perlocutionary stage
Perls iron stain
permanence
  object p.
permanent
  p. dentition
  p. hearing loss (PHL)
  p. molar
  p. posthemorrhagic hydrocephalus
  p. sterilization
  p. suture
  p. teeth
permanganate
  potassium p.
Permanone
Permapen Isoject
PermCath catheter
permeability
  intestinal p. (IP)
  vascular p.
permethrin
  p. 5% cream
  p. creme rinse

permission, limited information, specific
  suggestions and intensive therapy
  (PLISSIT)
permissive hypercapnia
permutation
pernicious
  p. anemia (PA)
  p. anemia of pregnancy
  p. vomiting
pernio
  lupus p.
Pernox
perocormus
perodactyly
peromelia
peroneal
  p. atrophy, X-linked recessive
  p. dislocation
  p. muscle atrophy
  p. muscular atrophy
  p. muscular atrophy, axonal type
  p. muscular dystrophy
  p. nerve function
  p. retinaculum
  p. rupture
  p. sign
  p. spastic flatfoot
peroneus
  p. brevis muscle
  p. brevis tendon
  p. longus muscle
  p. longus tendon
peropus
perosomum
perosplanchnia
peroxidase
  p. defect
  eosinophil p.
  glutathione p.
  streptavidin p.
peroxidation
  lipid p.
  plasma lipid p.
peroxidative enzyme
peroxide
  benzoyl p.
  carbamide p.
  hydrogen p.
  lipid p.
  zinc p.
peroxisomal
  p. congenital disorder

NOTES

peroxisomal *(continued)*
    p. deficiency
    p. disease
    p. ghost
peroxisome import disorder
Peroxyl
peroxynitrite
peroxyoxalate
perphenazine
Per-Q-Cath catheter
PerQ SANS
    percutaneous Stoller afferent nerve
      stimulation
    PerQ SANS system
Perrault syndrome
Persantine
perseveration
persistence
    p. of fetal circulation
    foramen ovale p.
persistens
    ductus arteriosus p.
persistent
    p. alkaline urine
    p. anovulation
    p. ectopic pregnancy
    p. estrogen secretion
    p. fetal circulation (PFC)
    p. gastrocutaneous fistula
    p. hyperinsulinemic hypoglycemia
      of infancy (PHHI)
    p. hyperplastic primary vitreous
      (PHPV)
    p. müllerian duct syndrome
    p. neutropenia
    p. occiput posterior position
    p. occiput posterior presentation
    p. ovarian mass
    p. postmolar gestational
      trophoblastic tumor
    p. primitive reflex pattern
    p. processus vaginalis peritonei
    p. proteinuria
    p. pulmonary hypertension (PPH)
    p. pulmonary hypertension of
      newborn (PPHN)
    p. pupillary membrane
    p. right umbilical vein
    p. tachycardia
    p. trismus
    p. trophoblastic tissue
    p. urachus
    p. vegetative state (PVS)
    p. ventricular dilation
personal
    P. Adjustment and Role Skills
      (PARS)
    p. hygiene history
    p. probability

personality
    p. change
    p. disorder (PD)
    p. disorder examination (PDE)
    P. Inventory for Children (PIC)
personal-social skill
perstans
    telangiectasia macularis eruptiva p.
persulcatus
    Ixodes p.
Persutte and Lenke study
PERT
    pancreatic enzyme replacement therapy
pertactin
pertechnetate
    technetium-99m p.
pertenue
    Treponema p.
Perthes disease
pertubation
    cardiovascular p.
Pertussin ES
pertussis
    acellular p.
    Bordetella p.
    diphtheria, tetanus, p.
    diphtheria, tetanus toxoid, p. (DTP)
    diphtheria, tetanus toxoid,
      acellular p.
    diphtheria, tetanus toxoid, whole-
      cell p. (DTPw)
    p. toxin (PT)
    p. toxoid (PT)
peruana
    verruca p.
pervasive
    p. developmental disorder (PDD)
    p. developmental disorder not
      otherwise specified (PDD-NOS)
    p. support
perversa
    parodynia p.
perversus
    situs p.
pes
    p. anserina bursitis
    p. anserinus
    p. cavus
    p. cavus deformity
    p. equinovarus
    p. planus
PESA
    percutaneous epididymal sperm aspiration
pessary
    Albert-Smith p.
    Biswas Silastic vaginal p.
    blue ring p.
    cube p.
    diaphragm p.

doughnut p.
Dumontpallier p.
Dutch p.
Emmett-Gellhorn p.
Findley folding p.
Gariel p.
Gehrung p.
Gelhorn p.
Hodge p.
inflatable ball p.
p. injection
Mayer p.
Menge p.
PGE$_2$ p.
Prentif p.
Prochownik p.
prostaglandin p.
ring p.
Smith p.
Smith-Hodge p.
vaginal p.
Zwanck p.

pesticide
organochlorine p.

pestis
Yersinia p.

PET
parent effectiveness training
positron emission tomography
postexposure treatment
preeclamptic toxemia
pressure equalization tube

Petasites hybridus
petechia, pl. **petechiae**
palatal p.
petechial
p. hemorrhage
p. rash
Peters
P. anomaly
P. anomaly, corneal clouding,
growth and mental retardation
syndrome
P. anomaly-short limb dwarfism
syndrome
P. ovum
Peters-plus syndrome
pethidine
petit
P. canals
P. hernia

P. herniotomy
P. ligament
P. lumbar triangle
p. mal
p. mal attack
p. mal epilepsy
p. mal-like seizure disorder
p. mal seizure
p. mal status
p. mal variant
P. sinus
Petri cast
petrolatum
liquid p.
petroleum
p. distillate poisoning
p. jelly
petrositis
Pettigrew syndrome (PGS)
Peutz-Jeghers
P.-J. polyp
P.-J. syndrome
Peyer patch
Peyronie disease
Pezzer
P. catheter
P. tube
PF
Astramorph PF
Pfannenstiel incision
PFAPA
periodic fever, aphthous stomatitis,
pharyngitis, cervical adenitis
Pfaundler-Hurler syndrome
PFC
perfluorocarbon
perfluorochemical
persistent fetal circulation
PFD
perfluorodecaline
Pfeiffer syndrome
PFGE
pulsed field gel electrophoresis
PFIC
progressive familial intrahepatic
cholestasis
P-fimbriae
PFK
phosphofructokinase
PFK deficiency
Pflüger law

NOTES

P

711

PFM
  peak flow meter
    TruZone PFM
PFNP
  peripheral facial nerve palsy
PFO
  patent foramen ovale
PFOE
  peripheral fractional oxygen extraction
PFP
  purified fusion protein
    PFP vaccine
PFPS
  patellofemoral pain syndrome
PFS
  pelvic floor electrical stimulation
    Adriamycin PFS
    Idamycin PFS
    Vincasar PFS
PFT
  placentofetal transfusion
  pulmonary function test
pfu
  plaque-forming unit
PG
  phosphatidylglycerol
  prostaglandin
    one-hour PG
P/G
    Fulvicin P/G
P&G
  Procter and Gamble
pg
  picogram
PGD
  preimplantation genetic diagnosis
PGE
  prostaglandin E
PGE$_2$
  prostaglandin E$_2$
    PGE$_2$ pessary
PGE$_1$
  prostaglandin E$_1$
PGF
  placental growth factor
PGF2 alpha
  prostaglandin F$_{2\ alpha}$
PGG
  prostaglandin G
PGH
  placental growth hormone
  prostaglandin H
PGI$_2$
  prostacyclin 2
PGK
  phosphoglycerate kinase
    PGK deficiency
    PGK hereditary nonspherocytic
      anemia

P-glycoprotein
PGR
  pelvic girdle relaxation
    symptom-giving PGR
PgR
  progesterone receptor
PGS
  Pettigrew syndrome
  prolapse-gastropathy syndrome
PGSI
  prostaglandin synthetase inhibitor
PGWB
  Psychological General Well-Being Index
PH-1
  primary hyperoxaluria type 1
Ph1
  Philadelphia chromosome
pH
  hydrogen in concentration
    endoesophageal pH
    fetal scalp blood pH
    intracellular pH (pHi)
    intragastric pH
    neutral pH
    pH probe
    scalp pH
    umbilical arterial pH
    venous pH
PHA
  phytohemagglutinin
PHACE
  posterior fossa malformation,
    hemangiomas, arterial anomalies,
    coarctation of aorta and cardiac defects,
    eye abnormalities
    PHACE syndrome
phacomatosis
    fifth p.
    fourth p.
Phaedra complex
phage phenotype
phagocyte
    mononuclear p.
    polymorphonuclear p.
phagocytic
phagocytophilia
    Ehrlichia p.
phagocytosis
    poor p.
phakoma, pl. **phakomata**
phakomatosis, pl. **phakomatoses**
    Jadassohn nevus p. (JNP)
phalangectomy
phalanx, pl. **phalanges**
    delta p.
phalli (*pl. of* phallus)
phalloides
    Amanita p.
phalloidin

phallometric assessment
phalloplasty
phallus, pl. **phalli**
Phaneuf-Graves repair
Phaneuf uterine artery forceps
phantom
    p. limb
    p. pregnancy
    Schultze p.
pharaonic circumcision
pharmacodynamic response
pharmacokinetic
pharmacokinetics
pharmacologic
    p. immunosuppression
    p. intervention
    p. management
    p. treatment
pharmacologically induced hypomania
pharmacotherapy
    stand-alone p.
Pharmaflur
Pharmaseal
    P. disposable cervical dilator
    P. disposable uterine sound
Pharsight
    P. Trial Designer
    P. Trial Designer simulation
      program
pharyngeal
    p. diphtheria
    p. diverticulum
    p. gonococcal infection
    p. gonorrhea
    p. incompetence
    p. mirror
    p. muscle
    p. pouch syndrome
    p. space
pharynges (*pl. of* pharynx)
pharyngitis
    acute lymphonodular p.
    bacterial p.
    exudative p.
    GABHS p.
    group C p.
    lymphonodular p.
    nonstreptococcal p.
    purulent p.
    streptococcal p.
    viral p.
pharyngoconjunctival fever

pharyngoplasty
pharyngotonsillitis
pharynx, pl. **pharynges**
phase
    acceleration p.
    active p.
    p. advance treatment
    aqueous p.
    beta p.
    deceleration p.
    deep tendon reflex delayed
      relaxation p.
    p. delay chronotherapy
    delayed relaxation p.
    p. delay treatment
    early proliferative p.
    end-expiratory p. (EEP)
    equilibrium p.
    fertile p.
    follicular p.
    hair growth p.
    hyperprolactinemia-associated
      luteal p.
    icteric p.
    immune p.
    implantation p.
    inadequate luteal p.
    Korotkoff p.
    late p.
    latent p.
    luteal p.
    menses p.
    menstrual p.
    mitosis p.
    polyuric p.
    postictal p.
    pre-pulseless p.
    proliferative p.
    prolonged expiratory p.
    pulseless p.
    S p.
    secretory p.
    stance p.
    telogen p.
    viremic p.
phase-contrast microscopy
phased array probe
Phazyme infant drops
PHC
    primary hepatocellular carcinoma
PHCO$_3$
    plasma bicarbonate

NOTES

P

PHE
    phenylalanine
        blood PHE
        serum PHE
phenacetin
phenanthrene
phenazocine
phenazone
phenazopyridine
    p. HCl
    p. hydrochloride
phencyclidine (PCP)
phendimetrazine
phenelzine
Phenergan
    P. Injection
    P. Oral
    P. Rectal
    P. VC
phenindamine
phenindione
pheniramine
phenobarbital
    hyoscyamine, atropine,
      scopolamine, p.
phenobarbitone
phenocopy
phenogenetics
phenolphthalein
phenolsulfonphthalein test
phenomenology
phenomenon, pl. **phenomena**
    all-or-none p.
    Arias-Stella p.
    clasp-knife p.
    crankshaft p.
    dawn p.
    dissociative p.
    doll's eye p.
    Hata p.
    intrapsychic p.
    Kasabach-Merritt p.
    Katz-Wachtel p.
    Köbner p.
    lip p.
    Marcus Gunn p.
    memory p.
    pseudo-Köbner p.
    Raynaud p. (RP)
    rebound p.
    recall p.
    ritualistic p.
    Rumpel-Leede p.
    Schwartzman p.
    Somogyi p.
    squatting p.
    steal p.
    stuck twin p.
    tension-discharging p.

    trigger p.
    Wenckebach phenomena
    X-linked p.
phenothiazine
    p. intoxication
    p. poisoning
phenotype
    body p.
    Bombay erythrocyte p.
    cardiac abnormality, T-cell deficit,
      clefting, hypocalcemia p.
    CATCH 22 p.
    fibroblast growth factor-10 null p.
    hemoglobin SC, SS p.
    hemoglobin S-Thal p.
    Hunter-Hurler p.
    MASS p.
    neurofibromatosis with Noonan p.
    Pena-Shokeir p.
    phage p.
    Potter p.
    Turner p.
    XX and XY Turner p.
phenotypic
    p. female
    p. sex
    p. threshold
    p. variance
phenoxybenzamine
phenoxymethyl penicillin
phenprocoumon
phensuximide
phentermine
phentolamine
phenylacetate
    sodium p.
phenylacetic acid
phenylacetylglutamine
phenylalanine (PHE)
    p. dehydroxylase
    p. hydroxylase (PAH)
    p. 4-monooxygenase
phenylalaninemia
    malignant p.
    non-PKU p.
L-phenylalanine mustard (L-PAM)
phenylbutazone
phenylbutyrate
    sodium p.
phenylephrine
    guaifenesin, phenylpropanolamine, p.
    promethazine and p.
phenylethylamine
phenylhydantoin
phenylketonuria (PKU)
    maternal p.
    preconceptionally treated p.
    p. test
phenylpiperazine

phenylpropanolamine
>bromopheniramine and p.

phenylpyruvate
phenylpyruvic acid
phenyl salicylate
phenyltoloxamine
phenytoin
>p. encephalopathy
>p. therapy

phenytoin-associated adenopathy
phenytoin-induced gingival overgrowth
pheochromocytoma
>extrarenal p.

PHH
>posthemorrhagic hydrocephalus

PHHI
>persistent hyperinsulinemic hypoglycemia
>of infancy

pH (hydrogen ion concentration)
>fetal blood pH
>vaginal pH

PHI
>Prehospital Index

pHi
>intracellular hydrogen ion concentration
>intracellular pH

Phialophora
Philadelphia
>P. chromosome (Ph1)
>P. collar

Philip gland
Philips SensorTouch temple
thermometer
Phillips' Milk of Magnesia
philtrum
>hypoplastic p.
>short p.
>smooth p.

phimosis, pl. **phimoses**
>p. clitoridis
>secondary p.
>p. vaginalis

phimotic ring
pHisoHex
>p. bath
>p. soap

PHL
>permanent hearing loss

phlebarteriectasis
phlebectasia
>congenital generalized p.
>generalized p.

phlebitis
>infective p.
>puerperal p.
>string p.
>suppurative p.
>syphilitic p.

phlebography
phlebometritis
phlebothrombosis
phlebotomum
>*Bunostomum p.*

phlebotomus fever
phlebotomy
phlegmasia
>p. alba dolens
>cellulitic p.
>p. dolens
>thrombotic p.

phlegmon
>parametrial p.
>perinephric p.
>postcesarean p.

phlegmonous mastitis
phlyctenule
PHMB
>polyhexamethyl biguanide

PHN
>public health nurse

phobia
>fever p.
>school p.
>simple p. (SPh)
>social p.
>specific p.

phobic
>p. avoidance
>p. hallucination

Phocas
>P. disease
>P. syndrome

phocomelia syndrome
pholcodine
phonation
>abnormal p.

phoneme segmentation task
phonemic
>p. awareness
>p. awareness task

phonetics
phonocardiography
phonological
>p. coding

NOTES

P

phonological *(continued)*
    p. development
    p. disorder
phonologic-syntactic syndrome
phonology
phonophobia
phorbol ester
phoria
Phos-Flur
phosphatase
    acid p.
    alkaline p. (ALP)
    bone alkaline p. (BAP)
    bone-specific alkaline p.
    placental alkaline p. (PLAP)
    tyrosine p.
phosphate
    p. buffered saline (PBS)
    calcium p.
    chloroquine p.
    chromic p.
    Cleocin P.
    clindamycin p.
    p. enema
    etoposide p.
    nicotinamide adenine dinucleotide p. (NADPH)
    plasma p.
    polyestradiol p.
    polyribosylribitol p. (PRP)
    potassium titanyl p. (KTP)
    primaquine p.
    pyridoxal p.
    sodium hydrogen p.
    p. supplement
    p. toxicity
    p. wasting
phosphate-buffered
    p.-b. saline
    p.-b. saline solution
phosphatidic acid phosphohydrolase (PAPase)
phosphatidylcholine
    dipalmitoyl p. (DPPC)
    disaturated p.
    unsaturated p.
phosphatidylethanolamine
phosphatidylglycerol (PG)
    p. level
phosphatidylinositol (PI)
phosphaturia
phosphene
5-phospho-alpha-d-ribosyl pyrophosphate (PRPP)
phosphocreatine (PCr)
phosphodiesterase
    p. 5 (PDE5)
    cGMP-specific p.

    cGMP-specific p. 5
    p. inhibitor (PDI)
phosphoenolpyruvate
    p. carboxykinase (PEPCK)
phosphofructokinase (PFK)
    congenital defect of p.
    p. deficiency
phosphoglycerate
    p. kinase (PGK)
phosphohydrolase
    phosphatidic acid p. (PAPase)
phosphokinase
    creatine p. (CPK)
    creatinine p.
phospholipase
    p. A_2
    p. activity
    p. C
phospholipid
    p. antibody
    egg p.
phospholipidosis
phosphoribosylpyrophosphate synthetase superactivity
phosphoribosyltransferase
    adenine p.
phosphorus (P)
    p.-31 magnetic resonance imaging (^{31}P MRI)
    p.-32 (^{32}P)
    p. MRS
phosphoryl
phosphorylase
    p. kinase deficiency
    nucleoside p.
    purine nucleoside p. (PNP)
phosphorylated drug form
phosphorylation
    mitochondrial oxidative p.
    myosin light-chain p.
    oxidative p. (OXPHOS)
    protein p.
    sperm tail protein p.
Phospho-Soda
    Fleet P.-S.
photic stimulation
photoallergic reaction
photobilirubin
photochemotherapy
photocoagulation
    infrared p. (IRC)
    laser p.
PhotoDerm PL handpiece
photodistributed lesion
photodynamic therapy
Photofrin
photogenic seizure
photometabolism

photometer
    HemoCue hemoglobin p.
    reflectance p.
photometric analysis
photometry
    scanning p.
photomicrograph
photon
photophobia
    ichthyosis, follicularis, atrichia (or alopecia), p. (IFAP)
photophobic iritis
photophoresis
photoplethysmography (PPG)
    near infrared p. (NIRP)
    red p.
Photoplex
photoretinopathy
photoscreening
photosensitive
    p. dermatitis
    p. epilepsy
    p. porphyria
    p. seizure
photosensitivity
photostethoscope
phototesting
phototherapy
    p. bulb
    double-bank p.
    double-blanket p.
    fiberoptic p. (FO-PT)
    halogen spotlight p.
    intensive p.
    maximum-intensive p.
    PUVA p.
photothermal sclerosis
photothermolysis
    selective p. (SPTL)
phototoxic reaction
photovaporization
    laser p.
PHPV
    persistent hyperplastic primary vitreous
phrenic
    p. nerve
    p. nerve pacing
    p. nerve palsy
    p. nerve paralysis
phrenoesophageal ligament

PHS
    pseudoprogeria/Hallermann-Streiff PHS syndrome
phthalate
    dimethyl p.
phthalylsulfacetamide
phthalylsulfathiazole
Phthirus pubis
PHVD
    posthemorrhagic ventricular dilation
PHVM
    posthemorrhagic ventriculomegaly
phycomycosis
pHydrion strip
phygogalactic
Phyllocontin
phyllodes
    cystosarcoma p.
    p. tumor
phylloides
    Demodex p.
phylloquinone
phylogenesis
physial, physeal
    p. arrest
    p. bridge
    p. closure
    p. destruction
    p. fracture
    p. injury
    p. separation
physiatrist
physical
    p. abuse
    p. capacity evaluation (PCE)
    p. maneuver
    p. map
    p. maturity
    p. sexual abuse (PSA)
    p. therapy (PT)
    p. victimization
physician
    medical control p. (MCP)
    p. payment review commission (PPRC)
physician-applied force
physiognomy
physiologic, physiological
    p. addiction/abstinence syndrome
    p. amenorrhea
    p. anemia
    p. anemia of infancy

NOTES

physiologic *(continued)*
    p. anemia of pregnancy
    p. bowleg
    p. cavus
    p. childbirth
    p. delay
    p. delay of puberty
    p. derangement
    p. discharge
    p. endometrial ablation/resection
     loop (PEARL)
    p. flatfoot
    p. follicular regulation
    p. genu valgum
    p. genu varum
    p. gynecomastia
    p. hypogammaglobulinemia
    p. icterus
    p. jaundice
    p. jaundice of the newborn
    p. leukorrhea
    p. neonatal withdrawal bleed
    p. reflex
    p. reflux
    p. regurgitation
    p. replacement dose
    p. retraction ring
    p. saline
    p. salt solution (PSS)
    p. sclerosis
    P. Stability Index (PSI)
    p. third-stage management
    p. transient hypoparathyroidism
    p. tumescence
physiologically corrected transposition
physiologist
    fetal p.
physiology
    Eisenmenger p.
    maternal p.
    pregnancy p.
    Score for Neonatal Acute P.
     (SNAP)
physiopathologic
physiotherapist
physiotherapy (PT)
    chest p. (CPT)
physis
    bridging p.
    broad p.
    radial p.
    serpiginous cephalad curved p.
physometra
physopyosalpinx
physostigmine
phytanic
    p. acid
    p. acid oxidation disorder
    p. acid storage disease

phytoagglutinin
phytobezoar
phytoestrogen
phytohemagglutinin (PHA)
phytomenadione
phytonadione
phytophotodermatitis
phytosterol (PS)
PI
    phosphatidylinositol
    ponderal index
    premature infant
    present illness
    protease inhibitor
    pulsatility index
     alpha-1 PI
Pi
    P. type
    P. type gene
    P. type 2 gene
    P. type 22 gene
    P. type ZZ gene defect
pi
    p. cone monochromatism
    p. dimeric protein
pial thickening
pia mater
piano-wire adhesion
PIC
    peripherally inserted catheter
    Personality Inventory for Children
PICA
    Pictorial Instrument for Children and
     Adolescents
    posterior inferior cerebellar artery
pica craving
PICC
    percutaneously inserted central line
     catheter
    peripherally inserted central catheter
     PICC kit
     PICC line
pickettii
    Burkholderia p.
    Ralstonia p.
pickups
    Adson p.'s
    rat tooth p.'s
pickwickian syndrome
picky eater
picogram (pg)
picornavirus
PICP
    carboxyterminal propeptide of type 1
     procollagen
picrotoxin
pictorial
    p. anticipatory guidance (PAG)

P. Instrument for Children and
Adolescents (PICA)
picture
p. chart
p. completion test
postencephalitic parkinsonian p.
p.'s of syndromes and undiagnosed
malformations (POSSUM)
PICU
pediatric intensive care unit
PID
pediatric infectious disease
pelvic inflammatory disease
primary immune deficiency
primary immunodeficiency
PID consultant
PIE
postinfectious encephalomyelitis
preimplantation embryo
pulmonary infiltrate with eosinophilia
pulmonary interstitial emphysema
PIE syndrome
piebald
piebaldism
Pie Medical ultrasound
piercing
cartilage p.
Pierre
P. Robin malformation sequence
P. Robin sequence
P. Robin syndrome
**Piers-Harris Children's Self-Concept
Scale**
Piersol point
PIF
prolactin inhibiting factor
pigeon
p. breast
p. toe
pigeon-toed, pigeontoed
Pigg-O-Stat
pigment
bile p.
melanin-like p.
p. stone
pigmentary
p. retinopathy, hypogonadism,
mental retardation, nerve deafness,
glucose intolerance syndrome
p. stage
pigmentation
black p.

contiguous p.
p. disorder of vulva
mucocutaneous p.
reticulated p.
pigmented
p. lesion
p. melanocyte
p. nevus
p. nodular adrenal hyperplasia
pigmenti
Block-Sulzberger incontinentia p.
incontinentia p. (type I, II)
pigmentosa
autosomal dominant retinitis p.
(adRP)
congenital bullous urticaria p.
congenital retinitis p.
neuropathy, ataxia, retinitis p.
(NARP)
retinitis p.
urticaria p.
pigmentosum
xeroderma p.
pigtail catheter
PIH
pregnancy-induced hypertension
PIH symptom
pilar cyst
pilaris
keratosis p.
pityriasis rubra p. (PRP)
PILBD
paucity of interlobular bile duct
pileus
pili (*pl. of* pilus)
pill
birth control p. (BCP)
combined birth control p.
emergency contraception p. (ECP)
emergency contraceptive p. (ECP)
Levlen contraceptive p.
Lo/Ovral contraceptive p.
morning-after p.
Nordette contraceptive p.
oral contraceptive p. (OCP)
Ovral contraceptive p.
Ovrette contraceptive p.
progestin-only p. (POP)
Seasonale birth control p.
Tri-Levlen contraceptive p.
Triphasil contraceptive p.

NOTES

P

pillar
    bladder p.
    rectal p.
pill-free week
pillow
    Crescent p.
    OsmoCyte p.
Pilocar
    P. Ophthalmic
pilocarpine
    p. iontophoresis
    p. iontophoresis method
pilocytic fibrillary astrocytoma
piloid tumor
pilomatricoma
pilonidal
    p. cyst
    p. dimple
    p. sinus
Pilopine HS Ophthalmic
Piloptic Ophthalmic
pilosebaceous
    p. duct
    p. gland
    p. gland of Zeis
    p. unit
Pilot
    P. audiometer
    P. suturing guide
pilus, pl. **pili**
    pili anulati
    bulbus pili
    pili torti
    pili trianguli et canaliculi
pimagedine
pimozide
pin
    Beath p.
    Surgin hemorrhage occluder p.
    p. tract
Pinard
    P. maneuver
    P. sign
pincer grasp
pindolol
pineal
    p. body
    p. cyst
    p. germinoma
    p. gland
    p. tumor
pinealoblastoma
pinealoma
    ectopic p.
pineoblastoma
ping-pong
    p.-p. ball deformity
    p.-p. ball depression

    p.-p. fracture
    p.-p. spread of disease
pinguecula, pinguicula
pinhole
    p. collimated scan
    p. collimation
    p. test
pink
    p. diaper syndrome
    p. disease
    p. tetralogy of Fallot
pinked up
pinkeye
pinna, pl. **pinnae**
    anteverted p.
    displaced p.
    malformed p.
pinning
    in situ p.
pinopode
pinpoint hemorrhage
pinworm
    p. infestation
    p. vaginitis
Pin-X
PIP
    peak inspiratory pressure
pipecolic acidemia
Pipelle
    P. biopsy
    P. endometrial suction curette
    Unimar P.
Piper
    P. fatigue scale
    P. forceps
piperacetazine
piperacillin
    p. sodium/tazobactam sodium
    p. and tazobactam
piperazine
    p. dione
    p. estrone sulfate
piperidolate hydrochloride
piperonyl butoxide
pipestem urethra
Pipet Curette
pipette
    Pasteur p.
pipiens
    Culex p.
PIPP
    Premature Infant Pain Profile
piracetam
pirbuterol
Pirie syndrome
piriform aperture stenosis
piriformis syndrome
piroxicam
Piskacek sign

Pistofidis cervical biopsy forceps
pit
>commissural lip p.
>congenital lip p.
>lip p.
>preauricular p.

pitch
pitcher's elbow
Pitocin
>P. augmentation
>P. induction

Pitressin
Pitrex
pitted
>p. keratolysis
>p. teeth

pitting
>digital p.
>p. edema
>nail p.

Pitt-Rogers-Danks syndrome (PRDS)
Pitt syndrome
Pitt-Williams brachydactyly
pituitary
>p. adenoma
>p. axis
>p. cell
>p. desensitization
>p. disorder
>p. dwarfism
>p. forceps
>p. gigantism
>p. gland
>p. gland function
>p. gland gumma
>p. gland transplantation
>p. gland tumor
>p. gonadotropin
>p. gonadotropin effect
>p. gonadotropin inhibition
>p. gonadotropin regulation
>p. gonadotropin secretion
>p. gonadotropin suppression
>p. hormone
>p. hormone release
>p. necrosis

pituitary-adrenal function
pituitary-hypothalamic circulation
pituitary-ovarian function
pityriasis
>p. alba
>p. lichenoides

>p. lichenoides chronica (PLC)
>p. lichenoides et varioliformis acuta (PLEVA)
>p. rosea
>p. rotunda
>p. rotunda treatment
>p. rubra pilaris (PRP)
>p. versicolor

Pityrosporum
>P. disease
>P. *orbiculare*
>P. *ovale*
>P. yeast

PIV
>parainfluenza virus
>peripheral intravenous
>PIV catheter

pivampicillin
Piver type II procedure
PIVH
>periventricular-intraventricular hemorrhage

PIVKA
>protein-induced vitamin K absence

PIVKA-II assay
pivoting
>prone p.

pivot lock
pixel
PIXI
>peripheral instantaneous X-ray imager
>PIXI bone densitometer

Pixie minilaparoscope
PK
>pyruvate kinase
>PK activity
>PK deficiency
>PK factor

Pk
>Synsorb Pk

PKC
>protein kinase C

PKD
>polycystic kidney disease
>infantile PKD

PKDL
>post-kala azar dermal leishmaniasis

PKU
>phenylketonuria
>PKU test

placebo
placebo-controlled study

NOTES

P

721

placement
　　categorical p.
　　catheter tip p.
　　central venous catheter p.
　　cerclage p.
　　external jugular vein catheter p.
　　extraovular p.
　　gastrostomy tube p.
　　internal jugular vein catheter p.
　　intraosseous line p.
　　intravenous line p.
　　irregular tooth p.
　　J-wire p.
　　line p.
　　noncategorical p.
　　open gastrostomy tube p.
　　stent p.
　　tooth p.
　　tube p.

placenta, gen. and pl. **placentae**
　　ablatio placentae
　　abruptio placentae (AP)
　　accessory p.
　　accessory lobe of p.
　　p. accreta
　　p. accreta vera
　　adherent p.
　　amotio placentae
　　anular p.
　　battledore p.
　　bidiscoidal p.
　　p. biloba
　　bilobate p.
　　bilobed p.
　　p. bipartita
　　central p. previa
　　chorioallantoic p.
　　chorioamnionic p.
　　choriovitelline p.
　　circummarginate p.
　　p. circumvallata
　　circumvallate p.
　　cotyledonary p.
　　p. creta
　　deciduate p.
　　diamniotic dichorionic p.
　　dichorionic p.
　　dichorionic-diamniotic p.
　　p. diffusa
　　p. dimidiata
　　disperse p.
　　Duncan p.
　　p. duplex
　　endotheliochorial p.
　　endothelio-endothelial p.
　　epitheliochorial p.
　　p. extrachorales
　　p. fenestrata
　　hemochorial p.

　　horseshoe p.
　　immature p.
　　incarcerated p.
　　p. increta
　　labyrinthine p.
　　p. marginata
　　p. membranacea
　　monochorionic-diamniotic p.
　　monochorionic monoamniotic p.
　　p. multiloba
　　nondeciduous p.
　　p., ovary, uterus (POU)
　　p. panduraformis
　　p. percreta
　　p. previa (PP)
　　p. previa centralis
　　p. previa creta
　　p. previa marginalis
　　p. previa partialis
　　p. reflexa
　　p. reniformis
　　retained p.
　　Schultze p.
　　p. in situ
　　p. spuria
　　Stallworth p.
　　succenturiate p.
　　supernumerary p.
　　total p. previa
　　p. triloba
　　p. tripartita
　　p. triplex
　　twin p.
　　p. velamentosa
　　velamentous p.
　　villous p.
　　zonary p.

placentaire
　　bruit p.

placental
　　p. abnormality
　　p. abruption
　　p. adaptive angiogenesis
　　p. alkaline phosphatase (PLAP)
　　p. barrier
　　p. bed
　　p. bleeding
　　p. bleeding site
　　p. blood flow
　　p. bruit
　　p. cotyledon
　　p. damage
　　p. disc
　　p. dysfunction
　　p. dysfunction syndrome
　　p. dystocia
　　p. edema
　　p. extrusion
　　p. fragment

p. function
p. giant cell
p. grade
p. grading
p. growth
p. growth factor (PGF)
p. growth hormone (PGH)
p. hemangioma syndrome
p. hemorrhage
p. hormone
p. hydrops
p. immunology
p. implantation
p. infarction
p. insufficiency
p. interface
p. lactogen
p. leakage
p. lobule
p. localization
p. location
p. margin
p. maturity index
p. membrane
p. metastasis
p. migration
p. mosaicism
p. mosaicism for triploidy
p. oxygen transfer
p. pallor
p. parenchyma
p. perfusion
p. polyp
p. presentation
p. profusion
p. progesterone deficiency
p. protein
p. respiration
p. secretion
p. separation
p. septa
p. sign
p. site gestational trophoblastic disease
p. site nodule
p. site trophoblastic tumor (PSTT)
p. site tumor
p. souffle
p. stage
p. stage of labor
p. steroid
p. sulfatase deficiency

p. thickness
p. thrombosis
p. tissue transplant
p. transfer
p. transfusion
p. transfusion syndrome
p. trophoblastic tissue
p. vascular anastomosis
p. vasopressin
p. villus
p. weight
placentascan
placentation
abnormal p.
p. abnormality
dichorionic p.
fundal p.
monochorionic p.
normal p.
placentitis
coccidioidal p.
placentofetal transfusion (PFT)
placentography
indirect p.
placentology
placentoma
placentotherapy
Placidyl
placing
p. reflex
p. response
placode
olfactory p.
PL-ADOS
prelinguistic autism diagnostic observation
plagiocephalic
plagiocephaly
deformational occipital p.
frontal p.
p. headband
p. helmet
occipital p.
unilateral occipital p.
plague vaccine
plain
p. abdominal radiograph
Perdiem P.
plan
Asthma Action P.
cleavage p.
exit p.

NOTES

plan *(continued)*
    Individualized Family Service P.
      (IFSP)
    multimodal treatment p.
    transition p.

plana
    coxa p.
    verruca p.
    vertebra p.

planar bone scan

plane
    equatorial p.
    fat p.
    first parallel pelvic p.
    fourth parallel pelvic p.
    p. of greatest diameter
    p. of least diameter
    median p.
    p. of midpelvis
    orthogonal p.
    p. of pelvic canal
    pelvic p. of greatest dimensions
    pelvic p. of inlet
    pelvic p. of least dimensions
    pelvic p. of outlet
    sagittal p.
    second parallel pelvic p.
    soft-tissue fat p.
    third parallel pelvic p.
    wide p.

planning
    family p.
    motor p.
    natural family p.
    poor motor p.

planographic pelvimetry

planovalgus
    flexible pes p.
    talipes p.

plant
    p. alkaloid
    anticholinergic p.
    p. thorn synovitis

plantar
    p. crease
    p. dermatosis
    p. eccrine bromhidrosis
    p. fascia
    p. fasciitis
    p. grasp
    p. grasp reflex
    p. imaging
    p. response
    p. wart

plantarflexion osteotomy

plantaris
    keratosis palmaris et p.
    pustulosis palmaris et p.
    verruca p.

plantarum
    Lactobacillus p.

plantigrade

planum temporale

planus
    acute eruptive lichen p.
    eruptive lichen p.
    hypermobile pes p.
    lichen p.
    lichen ruber p. (LRP)
    pes p.
    talipes p.

PLAP
    placental alkaline phosphatase

plaque
    acuminate p.
    bacterial p.
    calcified bacterial p.
    confluent p.
    erythematous confluent p.
    erythematous cutaneous p.
    filiform p.
    honey-crusted p.
    hyperpigmented lichenified p.
    lichenified p.
    linear hyperkeratotic p.
    p. of nummular eczema
    pruritic urticarial p.
    pruritic urticarial papules and p.'s
      (PUPP)
    pulmonary p.
    p. radiotherapy
    sclerose en p.
    p. of thrush
    uncalcified bacterial p.
    verrucous p.
    white p.
    white-yellow p.

plaque-forming unit (pfu)

plaquelike rash

Plaquenil Sulfate

plaque-type psoriasis

Plasbumin

plasma
    p. albumin
    p. amino acid concentration
    p. aminogram
    p. ammonia
    p. anion gap
    p. arginine
    p. bicarbonate ($PHCO_3$)
    p. bilirubin concentration (PBC)
    p. cell
    p. cell balanitis
    p. cell infiltrate
    p. cell mastitis
    p. cell pneumonia
    p. cell vulvitis
    p. cholesterol

p. citrulline
p. coagulation factor VIII, IX
p. cortisol
p. dissector
p. estrogen level
p. exchange
p. fibrinogen
p. fraction
fresh frozen p. (FFP)
frozen p.
p. glucose
p. histamine concentration
p. inorganic pyrophosphate
p. iron-binding capacity
p. iron concentration
p. lactate
p. lactoferrin
p. linoleic acid
p. lipid peroxidation
p. membrane
p. nitrite
p. noradrenaline
p. oncotic pressure
p. ornithine level
p. osmolality
p. phosphate
p. phosphate concentration
platelet-poor p. (PPP)
platelet-rich p. (PRP)
postingestion p.
p. prolactin
p. prorenin
p. prorenin increase
p. protein
p. renin activity
p. retinol concentration
seminal p.
p. testosterone
p. theophylline concentration
p. thromboplastin
p. thromboplastin antecedent (PTA)
p. thromboplastin antecedent factor
p. TPO
p. transfusion
p. very-long-chain fatty acid
p. viral load
p. viremia
p. vitamin A concentration
p. volume
p. volume expansion
p. volume regulation

plasmacellularis
    balanitis circumscripta p.
plasmacrit test
plasma-free iron
PlasmaKinetic instrument
Plasmanate
plasma neuropeptide Y
plasmapheresis
plasmatic
    progesterone p.
plasmid
    p. DNA
    p. fingerprinting
plasmin
plasminogen
    p. activator (PA)
    p. activator inhibitor (PAI)
    p. activator inhibitor deficiency
    p. level
plasminogen-activator
    p.-a. inhibitor-1 (PAI-1)
    p.-a. inhibitor-2 (PAI-2)
Plasmodium
    chloroquine-resistant *P. falciparum*
    chloroquine-sensitive *P. falciparum*
    P. falciparum
    P. malariae
    P. ovale
    P. vivax
plaster
    Mediplast P.
    Sal-Acid P.
    urea p.
Plastibell circumcision method
plastic
    p. blanket
    p. bronchitis
    p. cup vacuum extractor
    p. deformation
    p. deformation fracture
    p. heat shield
    p. obturator
    p. pleurisy
plastica
    linitis p.
    rectal linitis p. (RLP)
plasticity
plastid
plasty
    labioscrotal Y-V p.
plate
    agar p.

NOTES

P

plate *(continued)*
    basal p.
    breast p.
    Brucella agar p.
    chocolate agar p.
    chorionic p.
    cribriform p.
    epiphyseal growth p.
    p. fracture
    growth p.
    hemineural p.
    levator p.
    Mancini p.
    neural p.
    tarsal p.
    trigonal p.
    tubularized incised p. (TIP)
    urethral p.
    vaginal p.
    widened growth p.
plateau
    p. encephalopathy
    orgasmic p.
platelet (PLT)
    p. abnormality
    p. adhesion
    p. aggregation
    p. antigen
    p. calmodulin level
    p. cofactor I
    p. concentrate
    p. concentration
    p. count
    p. cyclooxygenase
    p. disorder
    p. function test
    p. membrane
    p. neutralization procedure
    p. neutralizing procedure
    p. plugging
    single donor apheresis p. (SDAP)
    p. transfusion
    TRAP-activated neonatal p.
    p. trapping
platelet-activating factor
platelet-antigen incompatibility
platelet-associated antibody
platelet-derived growth factor
platelet-poor plasma (PPP)
platelet-rich plasma (PRP)
platelet-type von Willebrand disease
plate-like atelectasis
Platelin Plus Activator
platform
    Aspen ultrasound p.
    wedge-shaped p.
Platinol
    bleomycin, Eldisine, mitomycin, P. (BEMP)

    bleomycin, etoposide, P. (BEP)
    bleomycin, ifosfamide, P. (BIP)
platinum
platinum-based regimen
platybasia
platypellic, platypelloid
    p. pelvis
platypnea
platyspondyly
play
    p. activity
    imitative p.
    oral p.
    parallel p.
    p. therapy
    vocal p.
PLC
    pityriasis lichenoides chronica
pleasure
    sexual p.
Pleatman
    P. pouch
    P. sac
pleconaril
pledget
    cotton p.
pleiotropia
pleiotropic
    p. cytokine
    p. functional defect
    p. gene
pleiotropy
pleocytosis
    CSF lymphocytic p.
    eosinophilic p.
    lymphocytic p.
    mononuclear p.
    neutrophilic p.
pleomastia, pleomazia
pleomorphic
    p. cellular infiltrate
    p. gram-negative rod
    p. spindle cell tumor
pleomorphism of hepatocyte
pleonosteosis
    Leri p.
Plesiomonas shigelloides
plethora
plethoric
plethysmograph
    face-out, whole-body p.
plethysmography
    finger p.
    impedance p.
    jugular occlusion p.
    respiratory inductive p. (RIP)

Respitrace inductance p.
venous occlusion p.
pleura, pl. **pleurae**
stripping of p.
pleural
p. abrasion
p. biopsy
p. decortication
p. effusion
p. fluid analysis
p. friction rub
pleurectomy
Pleur-evac chest catheter
pleurisy
dry p.
plastic p.
serofibrinous p.
pleuritic pain
pleuritis
pleuroamniotic shunt
pleurocentesis
pleurodesis
chemical p.
surgical p.
tetracycline p.
pleurodynia
epidemic p.
pleuromelus
pleuropericardial
pleuroperitoneal
p. fold
p. foramen
p. hernia
pleuropulmonary
p. blastoma (PPB)
p. involvement
pleuropulmonic
pleuroscopy
pleurosomus
PLEVA
pityriasis lichenoides et varioliformis acuta
plexectomy
plexiform
p. neurofibroma
p. neurofibromatosis
plexopathy
brachial p.
plexus, pl. **plexus, plexuses**
Auerbach p.
brachial p.
branchial p.

cavernous p.
choroid p.
Frankenhäuser p.
hypogastric p.
Kiesselbach p.
p. lesion
Meissner p.
myenteric p.
ovarian p.
pampiniform p.
pelvic p.
submucosal p.
superior mesenteric p.
vaginal venous p.
PLF
perilymphatic fistula
PLH
pulmonary lymphoid hyperplasia
plica, pl. **plicae**
plicae palmatae
plicamycin
plicata
lingua p.
plicate
plication
p. of diaphragm
diaphragmatic p.
fundal p.
Kelly p.
Kelly-Kennedy p.
transverse p.
PLISSIT
permission, limited information, specific suggestions and intensive therapy
ploidy
DNA p.
plosive
Plott syndrome
PLP
proteolipid protein
PLT
platelet
PLTSS
Pediatric Liver Transplant-Specific Scale
plucked chicken skin lesion
PLUG
plug the lung until it grows
plug
anorectal p.
Avina female urethral p.
colonic p.
copulation p.

NOTES

727

plug *(continued)*
    epithelial p.
    fentendo p.
    intraluminal p.
    keratinous p.
    p. the lung until it grows (PLUG)
    meconium p.
    mucous p.
    mucus p.
    silicone p.
plugging
    follicular p.
    mucous p.
    platelet p.
plumbism
plume
    electrosurgical p.
    laser p.
    smoke p.
plural pregnancy
pluripotentiality
plus
    Answer P.
    Betadine PrepStick P.
    Cenafed P.
    Duramist P.
    Fact P.
    GentleLASE P.
    P. Jet
    Lorcet P.
    Neonate One P.
    ophthalmoplegia p.
    Riopan P.
1-plus
    ALGO 1-p.
PLV
    partial liquid ventilation
PM
    polymyositis
PM-60/40
    Similac P.
PMB
    postmenopausal bleeding
    PMB 200. 400
PMD
    Pelizaeus-Merzbacher disease
PMDD
    premenstrual dysphoric disorder
PM/DM
    polymyositis/dermatomyositis
PMF
    protein modified fast
PMI
    point of maximal impulse
    point of maximum impulse
PMI
    paternal meiosis I
PMII
    paternal meiosis II

PML
    progressive multifocal leukoencephalopathy
PMN
    polymorphonuclear
PMP
    peripheral myelin protein
    previous menstrual period
PMR
    perinatal mortality rate
^{31}P MRI
    phosphorus-31 magnetic resonance imaging
PMS
    premenstrual syndrome
    PMS-Cyproheptadine
    PMS-Diazepam
    PMS-Erythromycin
    PMS-Imipramine
    PMS-Ketoprofen
    PMS-Lindane
    Lurline PMS
    PMS-Methylphenidate
    PMS-Nystatin
    PMS-Progesterone
    PMS-Pseudoephedrine
    PMS-Sodium Cromoglycate
PMS-Amantadine
Pm-Scl antigen
PMT
    point of maximum tenderness
    postmenstrual tension
    Optivite PMT
PMVP
    pulmonary microvascular permeability to protein
PN
    parenteral nutrition
    pronucleus
PN$_2$
    nitrogen partial pressure
PNAC
    parenteral nutrition-associated
    PNAC liver disease
PncD
    pneumococcal conjugate diphtheria toxoid
    PncD vaccine
PNCRM7 vaccine
PncT
    pneumococcal conjugate tetanus protein
    PncT vaccine
PnCV
    nonvalent pneumococcal conjugate vaccine
PND
    paroxysmal nocturnal dyspnea
    postnatal depression
pneogaster

PNET
primitive neuroectodermal tumor
PNET/MB
primitive neuroectodermal tumor
medulloblastoma
pneumatic
p. cell
p. compression
p. compression stocking
p. dilation
p. otoscopy
pneumatic-otoscope
pneumatocele formation
pneumatosis
p. cystoides intestinalis
p. intestinalis
pneumocapillary infusion pump
pneumocardiogram
pneumocele
pneumocephalus
tension p.
pneumococcal
p. conjugate diphtheria toxoid (PncD)
p. conjugate tetanus protein (PncT)
p. conjugate vaccine
p. facial cellulitis
p. mastoiditis
p. meningitis
p. pneumonia
p. polysaccharide vaccine
p. protein conjugate vaccine
p. sepsis
p. 7-valent conjugate vaccine (PCV7)
pneumococcus, pl. **pneumococci**
cephalosporin-resistant p.
latex test for *P.*
resistant p.
pneumocystiasis
Pneumocystis
P. carinii
P. carinii pneumonia (PCP)
pneumocystography
pneumocystosis
pneumocyte
type II p.
pneumoencephalogram
pneumoencephalography
pneumogram
2-channel p.

pneumography
impedance p.
pneumohydrometra
pneumomediastinum
pneumonia
acquired p.
acute interstitial p.
adenoviral p.
p. alba
p. alba of Virchow
aspiration p.
bacteremia-associated pneumococcal p. (BAPP)
bacterial p.
bronchiolitis obliterans organizing p. (BOOP)
chemical p.
chickenpox p.
chlamydial p.
Chlamydia trachomatis p.
congenital p.
desquamative interstitial p. (DIP)
Enterobacter p.
eosinophilic p.
exogenous lipoid p. (ELP)
fulminant early-onset neonatal p.
giant cell p.
gram-negative p.
group B streptococcal p.
Hecht p.
herpes simplex p.
hydrocarbon p.
hypostatic p.
interstitial plasma cell p.
intrauterine p.
Kaufman p.
lipoid p.
lobar p.
measles p.
Mycoplasma p.
necrotizing p.
neonatal p.
nosocomial p.
penicillin-resistant *Staphylococcus* p. (PRSP)
plasma cell p.
pneumococcal p.
Pneumocystis carinii p. (PCP)
postinfluenza p.
postviral p.
recurrent aspiration p.
respiratory syncytial virus p.

NOTES

P

pneumonia *(continued)*
    rheumatic p.
    staphylococcal p.
    streptococcal p.
    Streptococcus p.
    suppurative p.
    thrush p.
    tuberculous p.
    vaccine-associated p.
    varicella p.
    ventilator-associated p. (VAP)
    viral p.
pneumoniae
    Chlamydia p.
    Diplococcus p.
    drug-resistant *Streptococcus* p.
      (DRSP)
    Klebsiella p.
    Mycoplasma p.
    Optochin-resistant *Streptococcus* p.
      (ORSP)
    penicillin-nonsusceptible
      Streptococcus p. (PNSP)
    penicillin-resistant *Streptococcus* p.
      (PRSP)
    Streptococcus p.
pneumonic
    p. consolidation
    p. tularemia
pneumonitis
    acute p.
    aspiration p.
    chemical p.
    desquamative interstitial p. (DIP)
    hypersensitivity p.
    interstitial p.
    lipoid interstitial p. (LIP)
    lymphocytic interstitial p. (LIP)
    lymphoid interstitial p. (LIP)
    radiation p.
    RSV p.
    secondary p.
    varicella p.
    viral p.
pneumonocyte
    type II p.
pneumootoscope
pneumoparotiditis
pneumopericardium
pneumoperitoneum
pneumophila
    Legionella p.
pneumotachography
pneumotachygraph
pneumotaxic center
Pneumotest kit
pneumothorax, pl. **pneumothoraces (PTX)**
    catamenial p.
    iatrogenic p.

    nontension p.
    open p.
    simple p.
    spontaneous p.
    tension p.
    traumatic p.
Pneumovax 23
Pneumo-Wrap
PNH
    paroxysmal nocturnal hemoglobinuria
PNM
    peripheral dysostosis, nail hypoplasia,
      mental retardation
PNMR
    perinatal mortality rate
pnomenusa
    Pandoraea p.
PNP
    purine nucleoside phosphorylase
      PNP deficiency
PNSP
    penicillin-nonsusceptible *Streptococcus*
      pneumoniae
PO$_2$
    partial pressure oxygen
      simultaneous preductal-postductal
        PO$_2$
p.o.
    per os (by mouth)
    p.o. feeding
POA
    pancreatic oncofetal antigen
POADS
    postaxial acrofacial dysostosis syndrome
POAH
    posterior occipitoatlantal hypermobility
POC
    products of conception
pocket
    amniotic fluid p.
Pocket-Dop 3 monitor
Pocketpeak peak flow meter
POD
    polycystic ovary disease
podalic
    p. extraction
    p. version
podencephalus
Podocon-25
podocyte
podofilox
podophyllin
    topical p.
podophyllotoxin
    purified p.
podophyllum resin
POE
    prone on elbows
      POE position

POEMS
: polyneuropathy, organomegaly, endocrinopathy, M protein, skin changes
: POEMS syndrome

POF
: premature ovarian failure

Pogosta virus

poikilocyte
: fragmented p.

poikilocytosis

poikiloderma
: p. congenitale
: infantile p.

poikiloploidy

point
: p. A, subspinale
: p. B, supramentale
: cardinal p.'s
: Halle p.
: hypothalamic set p.
: infection p.
: lead p.
: Legat p.
: p. of maximal impulse (PMI)
: p. of maximum impulse (PMI)
: p. of maximum tenderness (PMT)
: McBurney p.
: Munro p.
: p. mutation
: Piersol p.
: pressure p.
: set p.
: p. tenderness
: trigger p.

pointer
: hip p.
: p. syndrome

pointes
: torsade de p.

point-spread artifact

Poiseville-Hagen relationship

Poison Control Center (PCC)

poisoning
: accidental p.
: acute iron p.
: aflatoxin p.
: amnesic shellfish p.
: anticholinergic p.
: antidepressant p.
: antimalarial p.
: antinauseant p.
: antipsychotic p.
: antispasmodic p.
: arsenic p.
: barbiturate p.
: carbon monoxide p.
: castor bean p.
: ciguatera fish p.
: cobalt p.
: cyclic antidepressant p.
: diarrheal shellfish p.
: ethanol p.
: fish p.
: food p.
: heavy metal p.
: histamine fish p.
: intentional p.
: iron p.
: lead p.
: mercury vapor p.
: metal p.
: monosodium glutamate p.
: mushroom p.
: neurologic shellfish p.
: neurotoxic shellfish p.
: niacin p.
: opiate p.
: organic mercury p.
: organophosphate p.
: paralytic shellfish p.
: petroleum distillate p.
: phenothiazine p.
: rodenticide p.
: salicylate p.
: salt p.
: scombroid p.
: scopolamine p.
: sedative p.
: shellfish p.
: strychnine p.
: tetrodotoxin p.
: thallium p.
: vapor p.
: zinc p.

pokeweed mitogen (PWM)

Poland
: P. anomalad
: P. anomaly
: P. malformation sequence
: P. syndrome

polar
: p. body

NOTES

polar *(continued)*
 p. body in-situ hybridization
 p. presentation
Polaris
 P. reusable cutters
 P. reusable dissector
 P. reusable forceps
 P. reusable grasper
 P. reusable instrument
polarity
polarization
 amniotic fluid fluorescence p.
 fluorescent p.
pole
 caudal p.
 cephalic p.
 fetal p.
 germinal p.
 head p.
 kidney p.
 pelvic p.
police
 food p.
polio
 poliomyelitis
 polio immunization
 vaccine-associated paralytic polio
 (VAPP)
poliodystrophia cerebri progressiva infantilis
poliodystrophy
polioencephalitis
 bulbar p.
poliomyelitis (polio)
 abortive p.
 bulbar p.
 bulbospinal p.
 inapparent p.
 nonparalytic p.
 paralytic p.
 pure bulbar p.
 spinal paralytic p.
 vaccine-associated paralytic p.
 (VAPP)
poliomyelitis-like
 p.-l. paralysis
 p.-l. syndrome
poliosis
Poliovirus hominis
poliovirus
 inactivated p.
 p. vaccine
 vaccine-acquired p.
polish
 Sklar instrument p.
Politano-Leadbetter
 P.-L. ureteroneocystostomy
 P.-L. ureteroneocystostomy
 technique

Politzer
 method of P.
pollakiuria
pollen
 p. allergy
 birch tree p.
 grass p.
 ragweed p.
 tree p.
pollen-induced rhinitis
pollical ray
pollicization of index finger
pollination
pollinosis
 seasonal p.
Pollitt syndrome
Pollock forceps
pollution
 air p.
Poloxamer 407 barrier material
poly
 p. A RNA
 P. CS device
polyacrylamide gel electrophoresis
polyamine
polyarteritis
 microscopic p.
 p. nodosa (PAN)
polyarthritis
 juvenile p.
 migratory p.
 p., RF negative
 RF-negative juvenile p.
 p., RF positive
polyarticular
 p. JRA
 p. juvenile chronic arthritis
polybutester
polycarbophil
 calcium p.
polycheiria
polychlorinated biphenyl
polychondritis
polychotomous
polychromasia
polychromatophilia
Polycitra K
Polycitra-LC
polyclonal
 p. antiendotoxin anticore antibody
 p. B cell activation
 p. cryoglobulin
 p. hypergammaglobulinemia
polyclonal-monoclonal antibody
Polycose
 P. liquid formula
 P. powder
 P. powder formula
polycyesis

polycystic
    p. encephalomalacia
    p. fibrous dysplasia
    p. kidney
    p. kidney disease (PKD)
    p. ovarian disease (PCOD)
    p. ovarian syndrome (PCOS)
    p. ovary (PCO)
    p. ovary disease (PCOD, POD)
    p. ovary syndrome (PCOS, POS)
    p. renal disease
polycythemia
    neonatal p.
    primary p.
    relative p.
    p. rubra vera
    secondary p.
polycythemia-hyperviscosity syndrome
polydactylism
polydactyly
    Majewski short rib p.
    microphallus, imperforate anus,
      hamartoblastoma, abnormal lung,
      lobulation, polydactyly p.
    microphallus, imperforate anus,
      syndactyly, hamartoblastoma,
      abnormal lung lobulation, p.
      (MISHAP)
    postaxial p.
    preaxial p.
    Saldino-Noonan short rib-p.
    short rib-p. (type I, II)
polydactyly-chondrodystrophy syndrome
polydactyly-craniofacial
    p.-c. anomalies syndrome
    p.-c. dysmorphism syndrome
polydactyly-imperforate anus syndrome
polydimethylsiloxane
polydioxanone
polydipsia
    neurogenic p.
    primary p.
    psychogenic p.
polydysplasia
    hereditary ectodermal p.
polydysspondylism
polydystrophic dwarfism
polydystrophy
    pseudo-Hurler p.
polyembryoma
polyembryony
polyester suture material

polyestradiol phosphate
polyethylene
    p. catheter
    p. feeding tube
    p. glycol
    p. glycol-ADA
    p. glycol-electrolyte solution
    p. glycol-modified adenosine
      deaminase (PEG-ADA)
    p. glycol solution
    p. suture material
polygalactia
Polygam S/D
Polygeline colloid solution
polygene
polygenic
    p. disorder
    p. inheritance
    p. mode
polygenic/multifactorial disorder
polyglactic acid suture
polyglactin 910 suture
polyglandular
    p. autoimmune disease (type I, II)
    p. autoimmune syndrome
polyglutamate
polyglutamation
polyglutamine-expanded Huntington
polyglycolic acid
polyglycol suture
polyglyconate suture
polygnathus
polygonal papule
polygraphy
PolyHeme blood substitute
polyhexamethyl biguanide (PHMB)
Poly-Histine DM
polyhydramnios
polyhypermenorrhea
polyhypomenorrhea
polymastia, polymazia
PolyMem dressing
polymenorrhea
polymer
    sodium polyacrylate p.
polymerase
    p. chain reaction (PCR)
    DNA p.
    DNA-directed RNA p.
    RNA p.
    RNA-directed DNA p.
    viral DNA p.

NOTES

P

polymeric diet
polymetacarpalia
polymetatarsalia
polymicrobial
    p. bacteremia
    p. coverage
    p. pelvic infection
polymicrogyria
    syndrome of symmetric parasagittal
      parietooccipital p.
polymicrogyric
polymorpha
    Mima p.
polymorphic light eruption of
  pregnancy
polymorphism
    amplified fragment length p.
    genetic p.
    restriction fragment length p.
     (RFLP)
    single nucleotide p.
    single stranded conformational p.
    TGFA p.
polymorphonuclear (PMN)
    p. infiltrate
    p. leukocyte
    p. lymphocyte
    p. phagocyte
polymorphonucleocyte
polymorphous
    p. exanthem
    p. light eruption
    p. rash
polymyalgia rheumatica
polymyositis (PM)
    juvenile p.
    primary idiopathic p.
polymyositis/dermatomyositis (PM/DM)
polymyxin
    p. B, E
    p. B sulfate
    neomycin and p. B
polyneuritiformis
    heredopathia atactica p.
polyneuritis
    acute infectious p.
    infantile p.
    infectious p.
    mixed sensory p.
    purely sensory p.
    relapsing infectious p.
    sensory p.
polyneuropathy
    acute inflammatory demyelinating p.
     (AIDP)
    p., cataract, deafness syndrome
    chronic inflammatory
     demyelinating p. (CIDP)
    erythredema p.

    p., organomegaly, endocrinopathy,
     M protein, skin changes
     (POEMS)
    spinal p.
polynomial
polyomavirus JC
polyoncosis
    hereditary cutaneomandibular p.
    multiple hereditary
     cutaneomandibular p.
polyostotic, polystotic
    p. fibrous dysplasia
polyotia
polyp
    adenomatous p.
    allergic p.
    antral choanal p.
    aural p.
    cervical p.
    charcoal p.
    cobblestone sessile p.
    colonic p.
    diffuse intestinal p.
    endocervical p.
    endometrial p.
    fibrinous p.
    fibroepithelial p.
    fundic gland p.
    gastrointestinal p.
    hydatid p.
    hyperplastic p.
    inflammatory p.
    intestinal p.
    juvenile colonic p.
    multiple gastrointestinal p.'s
    nasal p.
    pedunculated p.
    Peutz-Jeghers p.
    placental p.
    prolapsing p.
    retention p.
    sessile p.
    umbilical p.
polypectomy
polypeptide
    factor V p.
    gastric inhibitory p. (GIP)
    small nuclear ribonucleoprotein-
     associated p. (SNRPN)
    S-methionine-labeled p.
    vasoactive intestinal p. (VIP)
polyphagia
    Acanthamoeba p.
polypharmacy
Polyphenon E
polyphonic wheeze
polyphosphatidylinositide
polyphosphol inositide
polyploid

polyploidy
polypoid
> p. epithelial tumor
> p. hyperplasia

polyposis
> adenomatous colonic p.
> colonic p.
> familial adenomatous p.
> intestinal p.
> nasal p.
> small bowel intestinal p.
> p. syndrome

Poly-Pred Liquifilm
polypropylene
> p. fascial strip
> p. suture material

polyradiculoneuritis
> epidemic motor p.

polyradiculoneuropathy
> chronic inflammatory
>   demyelinating p. (CIDP)
> chronic relapsing p.
> chronic unremitting p.

polyribosylribitol phosphate (PRP)
polysaccharide (PS)
> anti-O-specific p.
> p. group-specific antigen
> meningococcal p.
> purified p.

polyscelia
polyserositis
> idiopathic p.

polysiloxane cast
polysomia
polysomnogram (PSG)
> p. with flow-volume loop

polysomnographic
polysomnography (PSG)
> ambulatory p.
> 8-hour p.

polysomy
> sex chromosomal p.

Polysonic ultrasound lotion
Polysorb suture
polyspermy, polyspermia
polyspike discharge
polysplenia syndrome
Polysporin
> P. ointment
> P. Ophthalmic
> P. Topical

polystotic (*var. of* polyostotic)
polysymbrachydactyly
polysyndactyly
> crossed p.

polysyndactyly-dyscrania syndrome
polysyndactyly-peculiar skull syndrome
polysynostoses syndrome
Polytar shampoo
polytef
> polytetrafluoroethylene

polytene chromosome
polytetrafluoroethylene (polytef)
> p. graft

polythelia
polytherapy
polythiazide
polytrauma
Polytrim eye drops
polyunsaturate
polyunsaturated fatty acid (PUFA)
polyurethane
> p. catheter
> p. dressing

polyuria
polyuric phase
polyvalent
> antivenin (Crotalidae) p.
> p. immunoglobulin therapy
> p. pneumococcal vaccine

Poly-Vi-Flor vitamins
polyvinyl chloride
polyvinylidene fluoride (PVDF)
polyvinylpyrrolidone (PVP)
Poly-Vi-Sol vitamins
PolyWic
POMC
> proopiomelanocortin

Pomeroy
> P. method
> P. operation
> P. tubal ligation
> P. tubal ligation technique

pommel
pomona
> *Leptospira p.*

Pompe
> P. glycogen storage disease (type I, II)
> P. syndrome

pompholyx

NOTES

735

POMS
Profile of Mood States
POMS score
ponderal index (PI)
pond fracture
Pondocillin
pons
Ponstan
Ponstel
Ponten fasciocutaneous flap
Pontiac fever
pontile hypertrophy
pontine
p. glioma
p. tumor
pontis
basis p.
pontobulbar palsy with neurosensory deafness
Pontocaine
pontocerebellar hypoplasia
pontomedullary junction
pontosubicular neuron necrosis (PSN)
PONV
postoperative nausea and vomiting
pool
gene p.
pooling
dependent p.
venous p.
poor
p. adaptability
p. attention span
p. caloric intake
p. capillary refill
p. convergence
p. coordination
p. dental hygiene
p. feeding
p. feeding interaction
p. head control
p. linear growth
p. man's clot test
p. motor planning
p. muscle tone
p. opsonization
p. oral intake
p. phagocytosis
p. pregnancy outcome
p. suck
p. weight gain
poorly marginated mass
POP
progestin-only pill
popcorn
p. formation
p. metaphysis
popcorn-like calcification

Pope
P. night splint
P. Oto-wick
popliteal
p. angle
p. cyst
p. pterygium syndrome
p. space
p. web syndrome
pop-off valve
popping
eye p.
skin p.
POPQ
Pelvic Organ Prolapse-Quantified
popsicle
p. injury
p. panniculitis
population-attributable risk calculation (PAR)
poractant alfa
Porak-Durante syndrome
porcine
p. surfactant
p. valve
porcupine skin
porencephalic
p. cyst
p. diverticulum
porencephaly
central p.
p., cerebellar hypoplasia, internal malformations syndrome
p. cortical dysplasia
porfimer sodium
Porges-Meier test
pork
p. insulin
p. NPH
p. Regular Iletin II
p. tapeworm
PORN
progressive outer retinal necrosis
porokeratosis of Mibelli
porphyria
acute intermittent p. (AIP)
congenital erythropoietic p. (CEP)
congenital photosensitive p.
p. cutanea tarda
p. cutanea tarda hereditaria
p. cutanea tarda symptomatica
cutaneous hepatic p.
erythrohepatic p.
erythropoietic p.
hepatic p.
hepatoerythropoietic p. (HEP)
intermittent p.
mixed p.
ovulocyclic p.

photosensitive p.
South African genetic p.
Swedish p.
symptomatic p.
p. variegata
variegate p. (VP)
porphyric neuropathy
porphyrin
p. metabolism disorder
stool p.
Porphyromanus gingivalis
Porro
P. cesarean section
P. hysterectomy
P. operation
PORT
Patient Outcomes Research Team
port
laparoscopy p.
10-mm umbilical p.
p. site hernia
portable respirator
Port-A-Cath catheter
Portagen formula
Portage project
porta hepatis
portal
p. fibrosis
p. hypertension
p. inflammation
p. mesenchyme
p. pyelophlebitis
p. system
p. vein obstruction (PVO)
p. vein sepsis
p. venous pressure
Porta-Lung noninvasive extrathoracic
ventilator
Porteous syndrome
Porter-Silber reaction
portio, pl. **portiones**
p. supravaginalis
p. vaginalis
Portland
hemoglobin P.
portoaortal shunt
portocaval shunt
portoenterostomy
Kasai p.
portosystemic shunt
Portuguese disease

port-wine
p.-w. hemangioma
p.-w. mark
p.-w. nevus
p.-w. stain
p.-w. stained angioma
POS
polycystic ovary syndrome
Posiero effect
POSIT
Problem-Oriented Screening Instrument
for Teenagers
position (*See also* presentation)
Adam p.
alternative birthing p.
antigravity p.
arm p.
asynclitic p.
back-up p.
batrachian p.
birthing p.
Bozeman p.
breech p.
brow p.
brow-anterior p.
brow-down p.
brow-posterior p.
brow-up p.
cervical p.
chin p.
coaxial p.
cock-robin p.
coital p.
decubitus p.
dorsal birthing p.
dorsal lithotomy p.
dorsal supine p.
Duncan p.
en face p.
English p.
equinus p.
face-to-pubes p.
fencing p.
fetal head p.
fetal spine p.
four-point p.
Fowler p.
frogleg p.
frontanterior p.
frontoposterior p.
frontotransverse p.
genucubital p.

NOTES

P

position *(continued)*
- genupectoral p.
- half-kneeling p.
- hands-feet p.
- intrauterine p.
- jackknife p.
- knee-chest p.
- knee-elbow p.
- kneel-stand p.
- Kraske p.
- lateral recumbent p.
- left frontoanterior p. (LFA)
- left frontoposterior p. (LFP)
- left frontotransverse p. (LFT)
- left lateral p.
- left lateral decubitus p. (LLDP)
- left mentoanterior p. (LMA)
- left mentoposterior p. (LMP)
- left mentotransverse p. (LMT)
- left occipitoanterior p. (LOA)
- left occipitoposterior p. (LOP)
- left occipitotransverse p. (LOT)
- left sacroanterior p. (LSA)
- left sacroposterior p. (LSP)
- left sacrotransverse p. (LST)
- left scapuloanterior p. (LScA)
- left scapuloposterior p. (LScP)
- lithotomy p.
- maternal p.
- maternal birthing p.
- mentoanterior p.
- mentoposterior p.
- mentotransverse p.
- mentum anterior p.
- mentum posterior p.
- mentum transverse p.
- missionary p.
- neutral p.
- obstetric p.
- occipitoanterior p.
- occipitoposterior p.
- occipitotransverse p.
- occiput posterior p.
- partial sitting p.
- partial squatting p.
- persistent occiput posterior p.
- POE p.
- prone sleep p.
- puppy p.
- right acromiodorsoposterior p.
- right frontoanterior p. (RFA)
- right frontoposterior p. (RFP)
- right frontotransverse p. (RFT)
- right lateral p.
- right mentoanterior p. (RMA)
- right mentoposterior p. (RMP)
- right mentotransverse p. (RMT)
- right occipitoanterior p. (ROA)
- right occipitoposterior p. (ROP)
- right occipitotransverse p. (ROT)
- right sacroanterior p. (RSA)
- right sacroposterior p. (RSP)
- right sacrotransverse p. (RST)
- right scapuloanterior p. (RScA)
- right scapuloposterior p. (RScP)
- sacroanterior p.
- sacroposterior p.
- sacrotransverse p.
- scissored p.
- scrotal p.
- semi-Fowler p.
- semilithotomy p.
- semiprone p.
- Simon p.
- Sims p.
- sitting p.
- sleep p.
- sleeping p.
- sniffing p.
- squatting p.
- standing p.
- supine sleep p.
- supranormal scrotal p.
- swimming p.
- three-point p.
- Trendelenburg p.
- tripod p.
- tripod-supporting p.
- tube p.
- uterine p.
- Valentine p.
- vertex p.
- Walcher p.
- wearing p.
- withdrawal p.
- W sitting p.

positional
- p. airways obstruction
- p. cloning
- p. clubfoot
- p. nystagmus

positioner
- head p.

positioning
- intrauterine p.

positive
- p. airway pressure
- Coombs p.
- p. distending pressure (PDP)
- p. end-expiratory pressure (PEEP)
- false p.
- Hematest p.
- p. interference
- polyarthritis, RF p.
- p. pressure urethrography
- p. reinforcement

P. Reinforcement in the
Menopausal Experience (PRIME)
p. support reflex
positive-pressure
high-frequency p.-p. (HFPP)
positive-pressure ventilation (PPV)
positivity
lymph node p.
paraaortic p.
positron emission tomography (PET)
possible migrational abnormality
POSSUM
pictures of syndromes and undiagnosed
malformations
POSSUM database
POSSUM database of genetic
syndromes
POST
peritoneal oocyte sperm transfer
post
p. cordocentesis bradycardia
p. dates
postabortal
p. pelvic inflammatory disease
p. syndrome
postadolescence
postalveolar cleft
postanesthetic apnea
postanginal sepsis
postanoxic dystonic syndrome
postasphyxial
p. apoptosis
p. cerebral edema
p. change
p. encephalopathy
p. seizure
postaugmentation
postauricular
p. ecchymosis
p. nerve
postaxial
p. acrofacial dysostosis syndrome
(POADS)
p. hexadactyly
p. oligodactyly
p. polydactyly
postcesarean
p. hemorrhage
p. phlegmon
postchiasmal visual pathway
postcoartectomy syndrome

postcoital
p. bleeding
p. contraception (PCC)
p. contraceptive medication
p. douching
p. estrogen
p. spotting
p. test (PCT)
p. testing
postconceptional age (PCA)
postconcussion syndrome
postconvulsive hemiparesis
postdate pregnancy
postdatism
postdiphtheritic neuropathy
postdose serum
postdouching
p. bleeding
p. spotting
postductal
p. coarctation
p. oxygen saturation
postdural puncture headache
postdysenteric arthritis
postembolization syndrome
postencephalitic parkinsonian picture
postenteritis arthritis
posterior
anterior and p. (A&P)
p. asynclitism
p. chamber intraocular lens (PC-
IOL)
p. colpoperineorrhaphy
p. colporrhaphy
p. column sensory deficit
p. commissure
p. cranial fossa
p. cul-de-sac
p. cul-de-sac gutter
dysplasia marginalis p.
p. embryotoxon
p. exenteration
p. fontanelle
p. fornix
p. fossa anaplastic ependymoma
p. fossa arachnoid cyst
p. fossa arachnoiditis
p. fossa hemorrhage
p. fossa malformation,
hemangiomas, arterial anomalies,
coarctation of aorta and cardiac

NOTES

739

posterior *(continued)*
    defects, eye abnormalities (PHACE)
    p. fossa neoplasm
    p. fossa tumor
    p. fourchette
    p. hypospadias
    p. iliac crest
    p. inferior cerebellar artery (PICA)
    p. knee capsulotomy
    p. lenticonus
    p. leukoencephalopathy syndrome
    p. lie
    p. nasal packing
    p. neural tube closure
    p. occipitoatlantal hypermobility (POAH)
    occiput p. (OP)
    p. pelvic exenteration
    p. pharyngeal laceration
    p. pharyngeal pseudodiverticulum
    p. pharyngeal wall elevation
    p. pituitary disorder
    p. probability
    rachischisis p.
    p. rectal wall resection
    p. rectus sheath
    p. repair
    p. rhizotomy
    p. sagittal anorectoplasty
    p. sagittal diameter
    p. segmental fixation instrumentation
    p. splenium
    p. superior iliac spine
    p. synechia
    p. talofibular ligament (PTFL)
    p. tibial artery cannulation
    p. tibial pulse
    p. triangle
    p. urethra
    p. urethral valve (PUV)
    p. urethral valves, unilateral reflux, renal dysplasia (VURD)
    p. urethritis
    p. uterosacral ligament
    p. uveitis
    p. vagina
    p. vaginal cuff
    p. vaginal fornix
    p. vaginismus
posteroanterior (PA)
posterolateral fontanelle
posteromedial
    p. articular depression
    p. bow
    p. bow of tibia
    p. tibial bowing
postevacuation management

postexchange transfusion syndrome
postexposure
    p. prophylaxis (PEP)
    p. treatment (PET)
postextubation stridor
postganglionic acetylcholine release
postgastroenteritis malabsorption syndrome
posthemorrhagic
    p. hydrocephalus (PHH)
    p. ventricular dilation (PHVD)
    p. ventriculomegaly (PHVM)
posthepatic aplastic anemia
postherpetic neuralgia
posthetomy
posthitis
posthysterectomy
    p. infection
    p. prolapse
postictal
    p. confusion
    p. depression
    p. lethargy
    p. paralysis
    p. period
    p. phase
    p. weakness
posticus
    saccus p.
postinfectious
    p. abducens palsy
    p. arthritis
    p. cerebellitis
    p. encephalitis
    p. encephalomyelitis (PIE)
    p. glomerulonephritis
    p. ileus
    p. immune response
    p. nephritis
    p. secondary lactase deficiency
postinflammatory
    p. adenopathy
    p. depigmentation
postinfluenza
    p. pneumonia
    p. vaccination encephalitis
postingestion plasma
postirradiation
    p. destruction
    p. myelopathy
    p. syndrome
postischemic stenosis
post-kala azar dermal leishmaniasis (PKDL)
postlumbar puncture headache
postlumpectomy
postmature
    p. fetus
    p. infant

p. labor
p. neonate

postmaturity syndrome
postmeasles encephalitis
postmeiotic segregation
postmembrane

p. pressure
p. rupture

postmenarchal

p. bleeding
p. cyclicity

postmenopausal

p. amenorrhea
p. atrophy
p. bleeding (PMB)
p. body mass
p. bone loss
p. estrogen and progestin
  intervention (PEPI)
p. estrogen replacement therapy
p. hirsutism
p. level
p. osteoporosis
p. palpable ovary syndrome
p. urogenital symptom
p. woman

postmenopause
postmenstrual

p. stress
p. tension (PMT)

postmigrainous stroke hemiplegia
postmolar persistent gestational
  trophoblastic tumor
postmortal pregnancy
postmortem

p. cesarean section
p. delivery
p. lividity
p. sampling
p. study

postnasal drip
postnatal

p. age
p. bacterial meningitis
p. depression (PND)
p. factor
p. gonadotropin surge
p. penicillin prophylaxis (PPP)
p. septicemia
p. year

postnatally
postnecrotic cirrhosis

postneonatal mortality
postoperative

p. apnea
p. bladder dysfunction
p. care
p. chemotherapy
p. complication
p. congestive epididymitis
p. cuff cellulitis
p. cystitis
p. nausea and vomiting (PONV)
p. pain
p. pelvic radiation
p. radiotherapy
p. sepsis
p. seroma
p. shock
p. sudden death
p. symptom analysis
p. voiding dysfunction

postovulatory age
postpartum

p. amenorrhea
p. attitude
p. blues
p. cardiomyopathy
p. care
p. confinement
p. depression
p. endometritis
p. endomyometritis
p. evaluation
p. febrile morbidity
p. hemodynamic change
p. hemolytic uremic syndrome
p. hemorrhage (PPH)
p. hypertension
p. incontinence
p. infection
p. metritis
p. partial salpingectomy
p. period
p. pituitary necrosis
p. pituitary necrosis syndrome
p. pleuropulmonary and cardiac
  disease
p. psychosis
p. sterilization
p. tetanus
p. thyroiditis
p. visit

NOTES

P

postperfusion syndrome
postpericardiotomy syndrome (PPS)
postphlebitic syndrome (PPS)
postpill amenorrhea
postpolio syndrome
postponed labor
postponing sexual involvement (PSI)
postprandial
    p. glucose
    p. hyperemia
    p. plasma cholecystokinin
postpuberal, postpubertal
postpuberty
postpubescent
postrabies vaccine encephalomyelitis
postradiation
    p. cystitis
    p. fistula
    p. periureteral fibrosis
postreduction mammaplasty
postrenal ARF
postrheumatic valve disease
postrubella syndrome
postscabetic syndrome
postseizure period
postsplenectomy
poststeroid panniculitis
poststreptococcal
    p. glomerulonephritis
    p. reactive arthritis
postsurgical fat necrosis
postsynaptic fiber
postterm
    p. AGA
    p. infant
    p. LGA
    p. pregnancy
    p. SGA
postthoracotomy pulmonary edema
posttransfusion hematocrit
posttranslational
    p. modification
    p. modification of mRNA
posttransplant
    p. lymphoproliferative disease
    (PTLD)
    p. lymphoproliferative disorder
    (PTLD)
posttraumatic
    p. amnesia
    p. epilepsy
    p. fat necrosis
    p. hyperemia
    p. signs or symptoms (PTSS)
    p. stress disorder (PTSD)
    p. stress syndrome
posttreatment
    p. evaluation
    p. surveillance

posttubal ligation syndrome
posttussive
    p. apnea
    p. emesis
postulate
    Koch p.'s
postural
    p. deformity
    p. drainage (PD)
    p. orthostatic tachycardia syndrome
    (POTS)
    p. proteinuria
    p. reaction
    p. reflex
    p. round-back
    p. scoliosis
    p. tachycardia
    p. version
posture
    bipedal p.
    extensor leg p.
    fetal p.
    frogleg p.
    hemiparetic p.
    scissoring p.
    surrender p.
    waiter tip p.
posturing
    athetotic p.
    decerebrate p.
    decorticate p.
    dystonic p.
    opisthotonic p.
    transient dystonic p.
posturography
    dynamic p.
postvaccinal encephalopathy
postvaginal fusion
postvagotomy dumping syndrome
postviral
    p. encephalitis
    p. pneumonia
    p. subacute thyroiditis
postvoid
    p. residual
    p. residual urine test
potable
potassium (K)
    p. bromide
    p. chloride (KCl)
    p. chloride stain
    p. citrate
    clavulanate p.
    diclofenac p.
    extracellular plasma p.
    p. gluconate
    p. hydroxide (KOH)
    p. hydroxide preparation
    p. iodide

p. iodide Enseals
pemirolast p.
penicillin V p.
p. permanganate
p. supplement
ticarcillin and clavulanate p.
p. titanyl phosphate (KTP)
total body p. (TBK)
potassium-sparing diuretic
potato-like mass
potbelly
potent
potential
auditory evoked p. (AEP)
brainstem auditory evoked p.
  (BAEP)
brief, small, abundant motor-unit
  action p. (BSAP)
event-related p. (ERP)
evoked p.
fetal brain stem auditory evoked p.
fibrillation p.
insertion p.
low malignant p. (LMP)
motor evoked p. (MEP)
neurocognitive p.
p. renal solute load (PRSL)
resting membrane p.
somatosensory evoked p. (SSEP)
stage IIIc papillary tumor of low
  malignant p.
vertex p.
visual evoked p. (VEP)
Potocky needle
POTS
postural orthostatic tachycardia syndrome
Pott
P. disease
P. puffy tumor
Potter
P. disease
P. facies
P. oligohydramnios sequence
P. phenotype
P. syndrome
P. version
Potts shunt
potty-train
potty-trained
potty-training

POU
placenta, ovary, uterus
POU theory of Ishihara
pouce flottant
pouch
blind vaginal p.
branchial p.
Broca p.
cecal p.
colon p.
continent urinary p.
Denis Browne p.
Douglas p.
Florida p.
Indiana p.
intravaginal p.
kangaroo p.
Kock p.
labioperineal p.
Mainz p.
Marsupial p.
Morison p.
parasitized cecal p.
Pleatman p.
Rathke p.
Reality vaginal p.
rectal p.
rectouterine p.
right colon p.
Rowland p.
Seessel p.
sigmoid p.
utriculovaginal p.
vaginal p.
vulvovaginal p.
wallaby p.
pouchitis
pouchogram
Poupart ligament
Pourcelot index
poverty of content
povidone-iodine
p.-i. douche
p.-i. gel
p.-i. solution
p.-i. wipe
POVT
pelvic ovarian vein thrombosis
Powassan encephalitis
powder
p. burn spot
Casec p.

NOTES

P

powder *(continued)*
    cocaine hydrochloride p.
    Fiberall P.
    fluticasone propionate inhalation p.
    Lotrimin AF Spray P.
    Nystop topical p.
    Ovidrel p.
    Polycose p.
    p. pseudocalcification
    Questran p.
    salicylic sugar p.
    salmeterol p.
    Secretin-Ferring P.
    Sklar Kleen p.
    talcum p.
    Zeasorb p.
    Zeasorb-AF P.
    zinc stearate p.
powder-burn
    p.-b. endometrial lesion
    p.-b. visual appearance
powdered
    p. casein
    p. milk formula
powder-free glove
POWER
    PTH for osteoporotic women on estrogen replacement
power
    p. Doppler sonography
    p. spectral analysis (PSA)
POWSBP
    pulse oximetry waveform systolic blood pressure
        POWSBP measurement
pox
***Poxviridae* family**
Pozzi procedure
PP
    placenta previa
    precocious pubarche
PPB
    pleuropulmonary blastoma
PPC
    primary peritoneal carcinoma
PPD
    primary peritoneal drainage
    purified protein derivative
PPG
    photoplethysmography
PPH
    persistent pulmonary hypertension
    postpartum hemorrhage
PPHN
    persistent pulmonary hypertension of newborn
PPHP
    pseudopseudohypoparathyroidism

PPI
    proton pump inhibitor
ppm
    parts per million
PPNET
    peripheral primitive neuroectodermal tumor
PPO
    palpable postmenopausal ovary
    preferred provider organization
        PPO syndrome
PPP
    platelet-poor plasma
    postnatal penicillin prophylaxis
PPRC
    physician payment review commission
PPROM
    preterm premature rupture of membranes
    prolonged premature rupture of membranes
        PPROM UCI
PPS
    Pap plus speculoscopy
    postpericardiotomy syndrome
    postphlebitic syndrome
PPSH
    pseudovaginal perineoscrotal hypospadias
PPTT
    prepuberal testicular tumor
PPV
    positive-pressure ventilation
PPVT
    Peabody Picture Vocabulary Test
PPVT-R
    Peabody Picture Vocabulary Test-Revised
PR
    progesterone receptor
        PR interval
p.r.
    per rectum
    by way of rectum
practice
    Advisory Committee on Immunization P.'s (ACIP)
    orogenital sexual p.'s
    P. Parameters for the Assessment and Treatment of Anxiety Disorders
    sexual p.
practitioner
    general p.
    National Association of Pediatric Nurse Associates and P.'s (NAPNAP)
Prader
    P. balls
    P. orchidometer
Prader-Labhart-Willi-Fanconi syndrome

Prader-Labhart-Willi syndrome
Prader-Willi
  P.-W. habitus, osteopenia,
    camptodactyly syndrome
  P.-W. habitus, osteoporosis, hand
    contracture syndrome
  P.-W. syndrome (PWS)
  P.-W. syndrome critical region
    (PWSCR)
praecox
  dentia p.
  familial lymphedema p.
  icterus p.
  lymphedema p.
  macrogenitosomia p.
  pubertas p.
pragmatics
**pragmatic and semantic-pragmatic
  deficits**
Prague
  P. maneuver
  P. pelvis
pralidoxime chloride
PrameGel
Pramosone
pramoxine
PRAMS
  Pregnancy Risk Assessment Monitoring
    System
Pratt
  P. dilator
  sigmoid pouch of P.
Prax
praxis
prazepam
praziquantel
prazosin
PRBC
  packed red blood cells
pRb tumor suppressor gene
PRDS
  Pitt-Rogers-Danks syndrome
preadolescent vaginal bleeding
prealbumin
preantral follicle
preaspiration mammography
preauricular
  p. adenopathy
  p. nerve
  p. pit
  p. sinus
  p. tag

preaxial
  p. acrofacial dysostosis
  p. hexadactyly
  p. mandibulofacial dysostosis
  p. polydactyly
precancerous lesion
precapillary
PreCare Conceive
precautions
  airway and cervical spine p.
Precef
Prechtl test
precipitable
precipitant
precipitate
  p. labor
  p. labor and delivery
precipitating factor
precipitation
  aragonite p.
precipitin
precipitous
  p. delivery
  p. labor
precise
  P. disposable skin stapler
  p. finger opposition
  P. pregnancy test
precision
preclinical carcinoma
Preclude peritoneal membrane
precocious
  p. adrenarche
  p. pseudopuberty
  p. pubarche (PP)
  p. puberty
  p. teeth
precocity
  complete isosexual p.
  contrasexual p.
  GnRH-independent sexual p.
  isosexual p.
  sexual p.
  true p.
preconception
  p. care
  p. counseling
  p. immunization
  p. risk assessment
  p. visit
**preconceptionally treated
  phenylketonuria**

NOTES

preconceptual workup
precordial
    p. bulge
    p. catch syndrome
    p. thump
precordium
    hyperdynamic p.
    quiet p.
    silent p.
Precose
precursor
    cell p.
    p. lesion
    neurotransmitter p.
Pred
    P. Forte Ophthalmic
    P. Mild Ophthalmic
predecidual
predeciduous teeth
Pred-G
prediction
    perinatal distress p.
    prenatal risk p.
    scar p.
predictive value of test
predictor
    ClearPlan Easy ovulation p.
    Conceive Ovulation P.
    First Response ovulation p.
    morbidity p.
    mortality p.
    OvuQuick Self-Test ovulation p.
    Q-test ovulation p.
predigested formula
predisposing factor
predisposition
    genetic p.
prednicarbate
prednisolone
    p. and gentamicin
    neomycin, polymyxin B, p.
    p. sodium
Prednisol TBA Injection
prednisone
    cyclophosphamide, doxorubicin (Adriamycin), Oncovin (vincristine), p.
    cyclophosphamide, hydroxydaunorubicin, methotrexate, p. (CHOP)
    cyclophosphamide, methotrexate, 5-fluorouracil, and p. (CMFP)
    cyclophosphamide, Oncovin, methotrexate, p. (COMP)
    Cytoxan, methotrexate, fluorouracil, p. (CMFP)
    Cytoxan, methotrexate, fluorouracil, vincristine, p. (CMFVP)

    mechlorethamine, Oncovin, procarbazine, p.
    mechlorethamine, Oncovin (vincristine), procarbazine, p. (MOPP)
    vincristine, actinomycin D, methotrexate, p. (VAMP)
    vincristine, cyclophosphamide, and p. (VCP)
predominance
predominant
    lymphocyte p.
preductal coarctation
preeclampsia (PE)
    early-onset p.
    p. headache
    superimposed p.
preeclamptic
    p. state
    p. toxemia (PET)
preeclamptic toxemia (PET)
pre-embryo
    triploid p.
preemie, premie
    premature
    preemie nipple
    preemie Simpson forceps
preexcitation syndrome
preexisting maternal medical condition
preference
    hand p.
preferred provider organization (PPO)
prefilled disposable bottle
preformation
Prefrin Ophthalmic Solution
prefrontal
pregenesis
pregestational
    p. diabetes
    p. diabetes mellitus (PDM)
Pregestimil formula
pregnancy
    abdominal p.
    aborted ectopic p.
    accidental p.
    acute fatty liver of p. (AFLP)
    adolescent p.
    ampullar p.
    anaphylactoid syndrome of p.
    anembryonic p.
    at-risk p.
    Besnier prurigo of p.
    bichorial p.
    bigeminal p.
    bilateral ectopic p.
    bilateral simultaneous tubal p.'s
    biochemical p.
    broad ligament p.
    p. category A, B, C, D, X

p. cell
cervical ectopic p.
chemical p.
cholestatic hepatosis of p.
clinical p.
coincident p.
combined p.
p. complication
compound p.
cornual p.
p. dating
diabetogenic effect of p.
direct agglutination p. (DAP)
dyspnea of p.
ectopic p. (EP)
epulis of p.
euploid p.
extraamniotic p.
extrachorial p.
extramembranous p.
extrauterine p.
failed intrauterine p.
fallopian p.
false p.
fatty liver of p.
p. fear
fimbrial ectopic p.
first-cycle clinical p.
full-term p.
gemellary p.
grand p.
hemolytic uremia syndrome
  associated with p.
hepatic p.
heterotopic p.
heterotropic p.'s
high-risk p.
p. hormone
hydatid p.
iatrogenic multiple p. (IMP)
idiopathic cholestasis of p.
idiopathic recurrent jaundice of p.
inherited thrombophilia in p.
interstitial p.
intrahepatic cholestasis of p.
intraligamentary ectopic p.
intramural p.
intraperitoneal p.
intrauterine p. (IUP)
isoimmunization in p.
IVF-induced abdominal p.
late p.

ligamentous ectopic p.
linear IgM disease of p.
p. loss
p. luteoma
luteoma of p.
p. management
mask of p.
mesometric p.
molar p.
monochorionic twin p.
multifetal p.
multiple p.
mural p.
myometrium of p.
near-term p.
nontubal ectopic p.
normally progressing p. (NPP)
p. outcome
ovarian p.
ovarioabdominal p.
papular dermatitis of p. (PDP)
parasitic p.
pelvic malignancy in p.
pernicious anemia of p.
persistent ectopic p.
phantom p.
physiologic anemia of p.
p. physiology
plural p.
polymorphic light eruption of p.
postdate p.
postmortal p.
postterm p.
previous p.
primary abdominal p.
prolonged p.
prurigo of p.
pruritic folliculitis of p.
pruritic urticarial papules and
  plaques of p. (PUPPP)
recurrent jaundice of p.
recurrent molar p.
p. reduction
refractory anemia of p.
rhinitis of p.
P. Risk Assessment Monitoring
  System (PRAMS)
p. risk factor (PRF)
sarcofetal p.
secondary abdominal p.
singleton p.
Spangler papular dermatitis of p.

NOTES

pregnancy *(continued)*
    splenic p.
    spurious p.
    successful p.
    SureCell rapid test kit for p.
    term p.
    p. termination
    p. test
    toxemia of p.
    toxemic rash of p.
    transient hypertension of p.
    treatment-associated p.
    treatment-independent p.
    triplet p.
    tubal p.
    tuboabdominal p.
    tuboovarian p.
    tubouterine p.
    p. tumor
    twin p.
    unplanned p.
    unrecognized p.
    uterine p.
    p., uterine, not delivered (PUND)
    uteroabdominal p.
    voluntary interruption of p. (VIP)
    p. wastage
    Working Group on Asthma and P.
    p. workup
    p. zone protein
pregnancy-associated
    p.-a. gingivitis
    p.-a. globulin
    p.-a. hypertension
    p.-a. hypoplastic anemia
    p.-a. plasma protein
    p.-a. plasma protein A (PAPP-A)
    p.-a. plasma protein C (PAPP-C)
    p.-a. plasma protein D (PAPP-D)
    p.-a. thrombosis
    p.-a. urinary stasis
pregnancy-induced
    p.-i. hypertension (PIH)
    p.-i. hypertension symptom
pregnancy-specific protein
pregnane
pregnanediol
pregnanetriol
pregnant
    p. cardiac patient
    p. diabetic
pregnenolone
Pregnosis
Pregnyl
pregranulosa cell
pre-hCG estradiol
prehension
Prehn sign
Prehospital Index (PHI)

preicteric stage
preimplantation
    p. diagnosis
    p. embryo (PIE)
    p. genetic diagnosis (PGD)
preinvasive
    p. cervical disease
    p. lesion
prekallikrein deficiency
prelabor
    p. membrane rupture
    p. rupture of membranes (PROM)
preleukemic syndrome
Prelief
prelingual deafness
**prelinguistic autism diagnostic
  observation (PL-ADOS)**
preload
    LV p.
    ventricular p.
Prelone Oral
Prelu-2
PREM
    Prematurity Risk Evaluation Measure
    PREM score
premalignant
    p. disease
    p. lesion
premammary abscess
preMA prenatal drink mix
Premarin
    P. with Methyltestosterone
    P. with Methyltestosterone Oral
premature (preemie, premie)
    p. accelerated lung maturation
      (PALM)
    p. adrenarche
    p. aging
    p. airway closure
    p. amnion rupture
    p. atrial contraction
    p. birth
    p. centromere division
    p. cervical dilation
    p. closure of coronal suture
    p. delivery
    p. ductus arteriosus closure
    p. ejaculation
    p. infant (PI)
    P. Infant Pain Profile (PIPP)
    p. labor
    p. lung
    p. luteal regression
    p. membrane rupture
    p. menarche
    p. menopause
    p. ovarian failure (POF)
    p. placental separation
    p. pubarche

pulmonary insufficiency of p.
p. rupture of membranes (PROM)
p. senility
p. suture synostosis
p. thelarche
p. uterine contraction inhibition
p. ventricular contraction (PVC)

prematurity
anemia of p.
anetoderma of p.
apnea of p. (AOP)
fetal p.
high oxygen percentage in
   retinopathy of p. (HOPE-ROP)
hypothyroxinemia of p. (HOP)
idiopathic apnea of p.
p. prevention program
pulmonary insufficiency of p.
retinopapillitis of p.
retinopathy of p. (ROP)
P. Risk Evaluation Measure
   (PREM)
sequelae of extreme p.
spontaneous atrophic patch of p.
Supplemental Therapeutic Oxygen
   for Prethreshold Retinopathy
   of P. (STOP-ROP)

premembrane
p. pressure
p. rupture

premenarchal
p. age
p. girl
p. vulvovaginitis

premenstrual
p. dysphoria
p. dysphoric disorder (PMDD)
p. edema
p. salivary syndrome
p. symptoms
p. syndrome (PMS)
p. tension
p. tension syndrome

premenstruum
PremesisRx
premie (*var. of* preemie)
**Premier Platinum HpSA enzyme
   immunoassay, The**
Premphase
Prempro
premutation allele

prenatal
p. appointment
p. asphyxia
p. care
p. cytogenetic analysis
p. cytomegalovirus
p. detection
p. diethylstilbestrol exposure
p. fibroelastosis
p. genetic counseling
p. genetic diagnosis
p. genetics
p. growth retardation
p. history
p. hydronephrosis
p. infection
p. interphase fluorescence in situ
   hybridization
p. interview
p. magnetic resonance imaging
p. mortality
p. placement of thoracoamniotic
   shunt
p. risk
p. risk factor
p. risk prediction
p. screen
p. screening
p. selection
p. sex determination
p. smoking
p. smoking intervention
p. stroke
p. surgery
p. tocolysis
p. treatment
p. ultrasound

prenatally exposed to drugs (PED)
Prenate
P. 90
P. GT delayed-release gel-coated
   tablet
P. Ultra

Prentif
P. cavity-rim cervical sap
P. pessary

prenylamine
preoperational stage
preorthognathic surgery manipulation
preovulatory
p. follicle
p. LH surge

NOTES

P

prep
    preparation
        KOH prep
        Tzanck prep
        wet prep
Pre-Par
preparation (prep)
    aseptic p.
    bowel p.
    P. H
    hemorrhoidal p.
    improper formula p.
    International Reference P. (IRP)
    KOH p.
    LE cell p.
    potassium hydroxide p.
    recombinant FSH p.
    sickle cell p.
    site p.
    wet p.
Preparation-H hydrocortisone cream
PREPARE
    prevent postmenopausal Alzheimer with
        replacement estrogens
prepared semen
preparticipation sports examination
    (PSE)
prepartum
prepatellar bursitis
Pre-Pen
prepenile testis
preperitoneal fat
Prepidil
    P. Gel cervical ripener
    P. Vaginal Gel
prepregnancy
    p. body mass index
    p. care
    p. level
prepuberal, prepubertal
    p. depression
    p. examination
    p. mania
    p. periodontitis
    p. testicular tumor (PPTT)
    p. vaginal flora
prepuberal-onset bipolarity
prepuberty
prepubescent vagina
prepuce
pre-pulseless phase
preputial
    p. flap
    p. sac
    p. washings
prereading stage
prerenal
    p. ARF

p. azotemia
p. insufficiency
prereproductive
presacral
    p. fascia
    p. nerve
    p. neurectomy
    p. space
    p. sympathectomy
preschool
preschool-age psychiatric assessment
    (PAPA)
preschooler
    Miller Assessment for P.'s
prescription (Rx)
    p. drug
    P. Strength Desenex
preseizure state
presence
    family member p. (FMP)
present
    p. episode
    p. illness (PI)
presentation (See also position)
    acromion p.
    arm p.
    breech p.
    brow p.
    brow-down p.
    cephalic p.
    complete breech p.
    compound p.
    p. of cord
    double breech p.
    double footling p.
    Duncan p.
    face p.
    face/chin p.
    fetal p.
    p. of fetus
    foot p.
    footling breech p.
    frank breech p.
    full breech p.
    funic p.
    hand and head p.
    head p.
    incomplete breech p.
    incomplete foot p.
    incomplete knee p.
    isomorphic p.
    knee p.
    longitudinal p.
    mentoanterior p.
    mentoposterior p.
    military p.
    nonisomorphic p.
    oblique p.
    occiput p.

pelvic p.
persistent occiput posterior p.
placental p.
polar p.
right occipitoposterior p.
shoulder p.
sincipital p.
single breech p.
single footling p.
singleton breech p.
torso p.
transverse lie p.
trunk p.
umbilical p.
unstable fetal p.
vertex p.
vertex-breech twin p.
vertex-transverse twin p.
presenting part
preseptal cellulitis
preservation
 ovarian p.
PreservCyt
presinusoidal
 p. hypertension
 p. obstruction
Preslip SCFE
presomite embryo
press-in
 p.-i. bone anchor
 p.-i. bone anchor system
Press-Mate model 8800T blood pressure monitor
pressor
 p. agent
 p. medication
 p. response
pressure
 abdominal leak point p. (ALPP)
 airway opening p. (P_{ao})
 airway transmural p.
 ambulatory blood p. (ABP)
 aortic blood p.
 arterial p.
 arterial blood p. (ABP)
 auto-positive end-expiratory p.
  (auto-PEEP)
 bilevel positive airway p. (BiPAP, B-PAP)
 bladder p.
 blood p. (BP)
 p. of carbon dioxide

carotid sinus p.
central venous p. (CVP)
cerebral perfusion p. (CPP)
colloid oncotic p.
colloid osmotic p. (COP)
constant positive airway p.
continuous distending p. (CDP)
continuous distending airway p.
 (CDAP)
continuous negative airway p.
 (CNAP)
continuous negative extrathoracic p.
 (CNEP)
continuous positive airway p.
 (CPAP)
cricoid p.
detrusor p.
diastolic arterial p. (DAP)
diastolic blood p.
distending p.
elevated intracranial p.
end-expiratory p. (EEP)
p. equalization (PE)
p. equalization tube (PET)
erratic blood p.
esophageal p.
p., facial expression, sleeplessness
fetal hydrostatic p.
finger arterial blood p. (FABP)
fundal p.
p. gradient
high bladder p.
hydrostatic p.
increased intracranial p.
inspiratory p.
intraabdominal p.
intracranial p. (ICP)
intraluminal p.
intraocular p. (IOP)
intravascular oncotic p.
intravesical p.
jugular venous p. (JVP)
leak-point p.
left arterial p.
LES p.
p. load
p. mapping
maternal abdominal p.
maximum urethral closure p.
 (MUCP)
mean airway p. (MAP)
mean aortic p.

NOTES

P

pressure *(continued)*
 mean arterial p. (MAP)
 mean arterial blood p. (MABP)
 mean left atrial p.
 mean pulmonary artery p.
 mean right atrial p.
 Monro-Kellie doctrine of
  intracranial p.
 nasal continuous positive airway p.
  (nCPAP)
 nasal prong continuous positive
  airway p. (NP-CPAP)
 negative end-expiratory p. (NEEP)
 negative inspiratory p.
 net ultrafiltration p.
 nitrogen partial p. (PN_2)
 normal blood p.
 p. of CO_2
 oncotic p.
 osmotic p. (Op)
 PA p.
 p. palsy
 partial p. (P)
 peak end-expiratory p.
 peak inspiratory p. (PIP)
 plasma oncotic p.
 p. point
 portal venous p.
 positive airway p.
 positive distending p. (PDP)
 positive end-expiratory p. (PEEP)
 postmembrane p.
 premembrane p.
 pulmonary artery occluded p.
  (PAOP)
 pulmonary artery wedge p.
  (PAWP)
 pulmonary capillary wedge p.
  (PCWP)
 pulse p.
 pulse oximetry waveform systolic
  blood p. (POWSBP)
 rectal p.
 resting anal sphincter p.
 right atrial p.
 p. support mode
 p. support ventilation
 suprapubic p.
 systolic arterial p. (SAP)
 systolic blood p.
 p. transducer
 p. transmission
 transpulmonary p.
 tubal perfusion p. (TPP)
 urethral closure p.
 p. urticaria
 vacuum p.
 venous p.

 wide pulse p.
 zero end-expiratory p.
pressure-cycled ventilator
pressured speech
pressure-preset ventilator
pressure-separator tubing
Pressyn
presternal edema
PreSun
presyncope
presystolic
 p. murmur
 p. thrill
preterm
 p. birth
 p. delivery
 p. formula
 p. infant
 p. labor (PTL)
 p. labor arrest
 p. neonate
 P. Prediction Study
 p. premature rupture of membranes
  (PPROM)
 p. rupture of membranes (PROM)
 p. spontaneous rupture of
  membranes (PSROM)
prethickened formula
pretibial skin dimple
Pretz
Pretz-D
prevaccination
Prevacid
prevalence rate
Prevalite
Preven emergency contraception kit
prevention
 Centers for Disease Control and P.
  (CDC)
 injury p.
 primary p.
 secondary prematurity p.
 tertiary p.
preventive
 p. allergy treatment (PAT)
 p. antibiotic
 p. antioxidant
prevent postmenopausal Alzheimer with
 replacement estrogens (PREPARE)
Preveon
prevesical space
Prevex
 P. Baby Diaper Rash
 P. HC
previa
 central placenta p.
 complete placenta p.
 low-lying p.
 marginal p.

partial p.
placenta p. (PP)
total p.
vasa p. (VP)
previable fetus
Prevident
previllous embryo
previous
p. maternal immunity
p. menstrual period (PMP)
p. pregnancy
p. transfundal uterine surgery
Prevnar pneumococcal vaccine
Prevotella
P. bivia
P. disiens
P. multocida
prezygotic
PRF
pregnancy risk factor
prolactin releasing factor
Pribnow box
prickly heat
prick test
Prieto syndrome (PRS)
prilocaine
lidocaine and p.
Prilosec
Primacor
primaquine phosphate
primary
p. abdominal pregnancy
p. acquired urticaria
p. adrenal insufficiency
p. amebic meningoencephalitis
p. amenorrhea
p. anastomosis
p. angiitis of CNS (PACNS)
p. antiphospholipid antibody
syndrome
p. aqueductal stenosis
p. atelectasis
p. bile acid malabsorption
p. biliary cirrhosis (PBC)
p. bubo
p. bullous disorder
p. cardiac arrhythmia
P. Care Evaluation of Mental
Disorders (PRIME-MD)
p. caregiver
p. caretaker
p. carnitine deficiency

p. central nervous system
lymphoma (PCNSL)
p. cesarean section
p. chondrodystrophy
p. ciliary dyskinesia (PCD)
p. circular reaction
p. cleft palate repair
p. closure
p. congenital glaucoma
p. craniosynostosis
p. cytoreductive surgery
p. dentition
p. dysfunctional labor
p. dysmenorrhea
p. dystonia
p. EFE
p. embryonic cell
p. empty sella syndrome
p. follicle
p. generalized epilepsy
p. generalized seizure
p. headache
p. hepatocellular carcinoma (PHC)
p. herpetic gingivostomatitis
p. hyperoxaluria
p. hyperoxaluria type 1 (PH-1)
p. hypersomnia
p. hyperuricemia syndrome
p. hypoalphalipoproteinemia
p. hypochondriasis
p. hypogonadism
p. hypomagnesemia
p. hypophosphatemic rickets
p. hypothyroidism
p. idiopathic dermatomyositis
p. idiopathic polymyositis
p. immune deficiency (PID)
p. immunodeficiency (PID)
p. immunodeficiency disorder
p. infection
p. infertility
p. insomnia
p. intraocular tumor
p. intrapulmonary neoplasm
p. lactic acidosis
p. lactose intolerance
p. lung bud formation
p. lymphedema
p. macrodactyly
p. macular atrophy
p. megalencephaly
p. microcephaly

NOTES

P

primary *(continued)*
    p. molar
    p. nasal mastocytosis
    p. nephrotic syndrome
    p. neuraminidase deficiency
    p. nocturnal enuresis
    p. oocyte
    p. ovarian insufficiency
    p. oxalosis
    p. PAP
    p. peritoneal carcinoma (PPC)
    p. peritoneal drainage (PPD)
    p. peritonitis
    p. polycythemia
    p. polydipsia
    p. prevention
    p. prophylaxis
    p. pulmonary hemosiderosis
    p. pulmonary hypertension
    p. pulmonary tuberculosis
    p. repair of esophageal atresia
    p. sclerosing cholangitis
    p. snoring
    p. syphilis
    p. teeth
    p. testicular failure
    p. testis-determining factor
    p. thrombocythemia (PT)
    p. tracheal tumor
    p. tracheomalacia
    p. uterine inertia
    p. vesicoureteral reflux
    p. writing tremor
    p. xanthomatosis
Prima Series LEEP speculum
Primatene Mist
Primaxin
PRIME
    Positive Reinforcement in the
      Menopausal Experience
    PRIME patient support program
primed in situ labeling (PRINS)
PRIME-MD
    Primary Care Evaluation of Mental
      Disorders
primer
    allele specific associated p.
    arbitrarily p.
    degenerate consensus p.
    degenerate oligonucleotide p. (DOP)
    p. pair system
primidone
primigravida
    elderly p.
priming
    cervical p.
    p. dose
    gastrointestinal p.
primipara

primiparity
primiparous
primitive
    p. blastoma
    p. fetal hemoglobin (HbP)
    p. groove
    p. knot
    p. lipoblastoma
    p. neuroectodermal tumor (PNET)
    p. neuroectodermal tumor
      medulloblastoma (PNET/MB)
    p. ovum
    p. reflex
    p. reflex pattern
    p. streak
primordial
    p. cephalization
    p. dwarfism
    p. follicle
    p. germ cell
    p. ovum
    p. pluripotent stem cell
    vesicourethral p.
primordium, pl. **primordia**
    choroid plexus primordia
    esophagotracheal p.
    thymus p.
    uterovaginal p.
Primrose syndrome
Primsol solution
primum
    foramen p.
    ostium p.
    septum p.
Principen
principle
    ALARA p.
    Doppler p.
    Fick p.
    Fontan p.
    Frank-Starling p.
    Mitrofanoff p.
Pringle disease
Prinivil
PRINS
    primed in situ labeling
prion disease
prior
    p. complete mole
    p. low transverse uterine incision
    p. low vertical uterine incision
    p. partial mole
    p. probability
**Priscilla White classification of diabetes
in pregnancy system (class A, A1,
A2, B, C, D, F, R, H, T)**
PRISM
    Pediatric Risk of Mortality
    PRISM score

prism
  optical p.
Pritchard intramuscular regimen
private blood group
Privine Nasal
PRL
  prolactin
p.r.n.
  pro re nata (as the occasion arises)
PRO
  P. 2000 Gel
  P. infusion catheter
proaccelerin
Pro-Amox
Pro-Ampi
proanthocyanidin
probability
  conditional p.
  joint p.
  objective p.
  personal p.
  posterior p.
  prior p.
  subjective p.
Probalan
ProBalance liquid nutrition
proband
probe
  bacterial artificial chromosome p.
  BICAP p.
  BiLAP bipolar laparoscopic p.
  biopsy p.
  biplane intracavitary p.
  Bipolar Circumactive P.
  blunt p.
  convex p.
  dedicated Doppler p.
  DNA dual color p.
  Doppler p.
  Endopath needle tip
    electrosurgery p.
  endovaginal p.
  Envision endocavity p.
  gene p.
  in-line p.
  IntraDop p.
  linear p.
  locus-specific p.
  MEVA p.
  multiplane intracavitary p.
  Neo-Therm neonatal skin
    temperature p.

  nucleic acid p.
  Ohmeda SoftProbe p.
  p. patency
  pH p.
  phased array p.
  ribonucleic acid p.
  p. sheath
  Spencer p.
  p. system
  transrectal p.
  transvaginal transducer p.
  Universal vaginal p.
  ViraType p.
  V33W Endocavity p.
  YSI neonatal temperature p.
probenecid
probiotic
PROBIT
  promotion of breastfeeding intervention
  trial
problem
  acid-base p.
  attention-distractibility p.
  chronic behavior p.
  dietary p.
  feeding p.
  growth p.
  internalizing p.
  intersex p.
  neurodevelopmental p.
  nutritional p.
  occlusal p.
  parent-child interaction p.
  psychosexual p.
  sensory p.
  sexual p.
  p. solving
  speech p.
  toileting p.
  urologic p.
  V code rational p.'s
**Problem-Oriented Screening Instrument
  for Teenagers (POSIT)**
proboscis, pl. **proboscides, proboscises**
  disruptive p.
  holoprosencephalic p.
  p. lateralis
  lateral nasal p.
  supernumerary p.
Probst
  bundle of P.
procainamide

NOTES

P

procaine
    p. penicillin
    penicillin G p.
    p. penicillin G
procalcitonin (PCT)
    cerebrospinal fluid p.
    serum p.
procarbazine
Procardia XL
procaterol
procedural sedation and analgesia
  (PSA)
procedure (*See also* operation, technique)
    Abbe-McIndoe p.
    Abbe-McIndoe-Williams p.
    Abbe-Wharton-McIndoe p.
    abdominopelvic p.
    ACE p.
    ACS p.
    Aldridge sling p.
    Altemeier p.
    American Cancer Society p.
    antegrade continence enema p.
    anterior cricoid split p.
    Aries-Pitanguy p.
    arterial switch p.
    atrial inversion p.
    atrial septoplasty p.
    atrial septostomy p.
    atrial switch p.
    Baden p.
    Baldy-Webster p.
    Ball-Burch p.
    Barbero-Marcial p.
    Bastiaanse-Chiricuta p.
    bidirectional Glenn p.
    Bishop-Koop p.
    Blair-Brown p.
    Blalock-Hanlon atrial septostomy p.
    Blalock-Taussig shunt p.
    Boix-Ochoa p.
    bowel lengthening p.
    Bricker p.
    Burch p.
    buried vaginal island p.
    Castaneda p.
    Chassar Moir-Sims p.
    Chassar Moir sling p.
    Chiari p.
    Coblation-Channeling surgical p.
    Cohen p.
    Cole intubation p.
    cricoid split p.
    cyclodestructive p.
    Cyclops p.
    Dall-Miles cable grip p.
    Damus-Kaye-Stansel p.
    Danus-Fontan p.
    Davydov p.

    Delorme p.
    diagnostic p.
    diverting colostomy with pull-
      through p.
    Donald p.
    dot-blot p.
    double-switch p.
    drainage p.
    Duckett p.
    Duhamel p.
    enema p.
    Estes p.
    Evans-Steptoe p.
    Everard Williams p.
    EXIT p.
    fascial sling p.
    female sterilization p.
    fetal surgical p.
    Fontan p.
    Frank p.
    Fredet-Ramstedt p.
    Gittes p.
    GITUP p.
    glans-cavernosal p.
    Goebell p.
    Goebell-Stoeckel-Frangenheim p.
    Halban p.
    heel-stick p.
    hemi-Fontan p.
    Heyman-Herndon clubfoot p.
    Hoffer p.
    Hood p.
    Ilizarov limb-lengthening p.
    Ingelman-Sundberg gracilis
      muscle p.
    interventional p.
    intestinal bypass p.
    Jatene arterial switch p.
    Jones p.
    Kaliscinski ureteral p.
    Kasai p.
    Kelly-Kennedy p.
    Kelly plication p.
    Kennedy p.
    Kimura p.
    Kono p.
    Koyanagi p.
    Ladd p.
    laparoscopic unipolar coagulation p.
    Lash p.
    Leadbetter-Politano p.
    LETZ p.
    loop electrosurgical excision p.
      (LEEP)
    Lyodura sling p.
    MAGPI p.
    Mantel-Haenszel p.
    Marshall-Marchetti p.
    Marshall-Marchetti-Krantz p.

Martius p.
Mayo-Fueth inversion p.
McCall-Schumann p.
McDonald p.
McIndoe p.
McIndoe-Hayes p.
Meigs-Okabayashi p.
Mikulicz p.
mini-Pena p.
Mitrofanoff neourethral p.
MMK p.
modified Fontan p.
Morrow p.
Moschcowitz p.
Mustard atrial switch p.
Mustardé cheek flap p.
Mustardé hypospadias p.
neobladder diversion p.
Neugebauer-LeFort p.
Nichols p.
Norwood p.
NovaSure endometrial ablation p.
Olshausen p.
OPERA p.
palliative p.
Pemberton p.
Pena p.
Penn pouch p.
Pereyra p.
Pereyra-Lebhertz modification of
  Frangenheim-Stoeckel p.
Piver type II p.
platelet neutralization p.
platelet neutralizing p.
Pozzi p.
psoas hitch p.
pubovaginal sling p.
pull-through p.
Ramstedt p.
Rashkind atrial septostomy p.
Rastelli p.
Ravitch p.
Raz-Leach p.
Raz sling p.
Récamier p.
retroperitoneal laparoscopic p.
retropubic suspension p.
retropubic urethropexy p.
Richter and Albrich p.
Ross p.
Rotazyme diagnostic p.
Salter p.

Schauffler p.
selective embolization p.
selective tubal occlusion p. (STOP)
semidefinitive p.
Senning atrial switch p.
Seton p.
Shauta-Aumreich p.
Shirodkar p.
sling p.
Soave abdominal pull-through p.
SPARC urological sling p.
Spence p.
split p.
Stamey modification of Pereyra p.
Stamm p.
Stanley Way p.
Steele p.
Sting p.
Sugiura p.
surgical sterilization p.
Sutherland p.
Swenson pull-through p.
tension-free vaginal tape p.
three-stage Norwood-Fontan p.
Tompkins p.
Tonnis hip dysplasia p.
Torkildsen p.
triangular vaginal patch sling p.
Uchida p.
UPLIFT p.
urinary unidiversion p.
vaginal tubal p.
vaginal wall sling p.
valvulotomy p.
van Ness p.
ventricular shunt p.
WAMBA p.
Waterston-Cooley p.
Waterston shunt p.
Whipple p.
Winter glans-cavernosal p.
W-stapled urinary reservoir p.
procedure-related pyrexia
process
  acromion p.
  antenatal disease p.
  attaching p.
  binary p.
  cleft premaxillary p.
  CytoRich p.
  freezing p.
  grieving p.

NOTES

process *(continued)*
    immune p.
    inflammatory p.
    latching-on p.
    lateralization p.
    lymphoproliferative p.
    mastoid p.
    microangiopathic p.
    neuritic cytoplasmic p.
    odontoid p.
    quality assurance p.
    short p.
    tapering cytoplasmic p.
processed blood product
processing
    slow cognitive p.
    visuoperceptual/simultaneous
      information p.
processor
    ThinPrep p.
process-oriented measure
processus
    p. vaginalis
    p. vaginalis peritonei
prochlorperazine
Prochownik
    P. method
    P. pessary
procidentia uteri
procoagulant protein
procollagen
    carboxyterminal propeptide of type
      1 p. (PICP)
    serum type III p.
procollagenase
proconvertin
PRO/Covers ultrasound probe sheath
procreation
    assisted medical p. (AMP)
Procrit
Procter and Gamble (P&G)
proctitis
    HSV2 p.
proctocolpoplasty
Proctocort Rectal
ProctoCream-HC
proctoelytroplasty
proctoepisiotomy
ProctoFoam-HC
ProctoFoam NS
proctogram
    defecating p.
proctography
    evacuation p.
proctoscopy
proctosigmoiditis
proctosigmoidoscopy
proctotomy
procyclidine

procyonis
    Baylisascaris p.
Procytox
prodromal
    p. illness
    p. labor
    p. symptom
prodrome, prodroma, pl. **prodromata**
    menstrual p.
    viral p.
Prodrox
prodrug
product
    P. 80056
    advanced oxidation protein p.
    alpha-1 thymosin p.
    blood p.
    clearance of fetal p.
    p.'s of conception (POC)
    fibrin degradation p.
    fibrinogen degradation p. (FDP)
    fibrinogen-fibrin degradation p.
    fibrinogen split p.
    fibrin split p. (FSP)
    gene p.
    processed blood p.
    red blood cell p.
    Repliform alternative p.
    unpasteurized milk p.
production
    cyclic hormone p.
    endogenous hormonal p.
    extraglandular testosterone p.
    ketone p.
    oocyte p.
    sebum p.
    speech p.
    in vitro antibody p. (IVAP)
productivity
ProDynamic monitor
prodynorphin
proemial breast
proencephalus
proenkephalin A, B
proenzyme
Profasi HP
profenamine
Profiber formula
proficiency
    Bruininks-Oseretsky Test of
      Motor P.
profilaggrin
Profilate OSD
profile
    acylcarnitine p.
    Alpern-Boll Developmental P.
    anatomic p. (AP)
    biometric p.
    biophysical p. (BPP)

coagulation p.
fatty acid p.
fetal biophysical p.
fetal movement p.
Hawaii Early Learning P. (HELP)
lung p.
modified biophysical p. (MBPP)
P. of Mood States (POMS)
neuropsychological p.
Premature Infant Pain P. (PIPP)
protein p.
rectilinear p.
Sickness Impact P. (SIP)
torsional p.
urethral pressure p.
urethral pressure cough p.
P. viral probe test

Profile-II
Developmental P.-II (DP-II)
profiling
multiple arbitrary amplicon p.
(MAAP)
Profilnine
P. Heat-Treated
P. SD
Profilomat monitor
profilometry
urethral pressure p.
profound mental retardation
profunda
miliaria p.
tinea p.
profundus
lupus erythematosus p.
profusa
lentiginosis p.
profusion
placental p.
PRO/Gel ultrasound transmission gel
progenitor
erythroid p.
fetal erythroid p.
progeny
progeria
adult p.
p. syndrome
progeria-like syndrome
progeroid
p. facies
p. short stature-pigmented nevi
syndrome
Progestasert intrauterine device

progestational
p. activity
p. agent
p. challenge
p. compound
p. effect
p. protection
p. state
p. therapy
progesterone
p. antagonist
p. breakthrough bleeding
p. challenge test
p. dermatitis
first-generation p.
p. metabolism
micronized p.
p. myometrial level
P. Oil
parenteral p.
p. plasmatic
P. Radioimmunoassay Kit
p. receptor (PgR, PR)
second-generation p.
p. secretion
serum p.
p. synthesis
third-generation p.
urinary free p.
p. withdrawal bleeding
progesterone-releasing T-shaped device
progestin
C_{21} p.
norgestimate p.
p. oral contraceptive
progestin-impregnated vaginal ring
progestin-only
p.-o. implant
p.-o. injectable contraceptive
p.-o. oral contraceptive
p.-o. pill (POP)
progestogen
C_{21} p.
p. support therapy
progestogen-dependent endometrial protein (PEP)
Proglycem Oral
prognathism
mandibular p.
prognosis
clinical p.

NOTES

P

prognostic
>p. factor
>p. indicator
>p. scoring system

prognostication

prognosticator

Prognosticon Dri-Dot

Prograf

program
>antepartum surveillance p.
>bed rest support p.
>Bridge Reading P.
>Childhood Asthma Management P.
>(CAMP)
>Children's Health Insurance P.
>(CHIP)
>chronic hypertransfusion p.
>Early Childhood Special
>Education P.
>early-discharge p.
>early intervention p. (EIP)
>Epidemiologic Catchment P.
>EPSDT p.
>expanded food nutrition
>education p. (EFNEP)
>Free to Be Me body image p.
>Fria muscle training device & p.
>Individualized Education P. (IEP)
>infant development p.
>infant stimulation p.
>Lovaas p.
>Merrill p.
>Metropolitan Atlanta Congenital
>Defects P. (MACDP)
>Neonatal Resuscitation P. (NRP)
>New England Regional Infant
>Cardiac P. (NERICP)
>New Moves obesity-prevention p.
>Office of Special Education P.'s
>(OSEP)
>Pharsight Trial Designer
>simulation p.
>prematurity prevention p.
>PRIME patient support p.
>PSI p.
>residential p.
>Restore p.
>Special Supplemental Nutrition P.
>SRA Basic Reading P.
>State Children's Health
>Insurance P. (SCHIP)
>STEPS p.
>The Injury Prevention P. (TIPP)
>universal newborn hearing
>screening p. (UNHSP)

progress
>cessation of p.
>failure to p.

progression
>intraepithelial disease p.
>tumor p.

progressiva
>fibrodysplasia ossificans p. (FOP)
>myositis ossificans p.

progressive
>p. biliary cirrhosis
>p. bulbar palsy
>p. bulbar palsy with epilepsy
>p. bulbar palsy with perceptive
>deafness
>p. bulbar paralysis of childhood
>p. central nervous system failure
>p. deforming osteogenesis
>imperfecta
>p. dystonia
>p. encephalitis
>p. encephalopathy
>p. encephalopathy, edema,
>hypsarrhythmia, optic atrophy
>(PEHO)
>p. external ophthalmoplegia (PEO)
>p. facial hemiatrophy
>p. familial intrahepatic cholestasis
>(PFIC)
>p. familial scleroderma
>p. granuloma
>p. hydronephrosis
>p. labyrinthitis
>p. multifocal leukoencephalopathy
>(PML)
>p. muscular dystrophy of childhood
>p. myoclonic epilepsy
>p. obesity
>p. obliterative cholangiopathy
>p. outer retinal necrosis (PORN)
>p. primary pulmonary tuberculosis
>p. renal failure
>p. rubella panencephalitis
>p. systemic sclerosis

proguanil hydrochloride

prohormone

proinflammatory cytokine

project
>Breast Cancer Detection p.
>Breast Cancer Detection
>Demonstration P. (BCDDP)
>Diana P.
>Fort Bragg evaluation p. (FBEP)
>genome p.
>Human Genome P.
>National Collaborative
>Diethylstilbestrol Adenosis P.
>(DESAD)
>National Collaborative Perinatal p.
>National Surgical Adjuvant
>Breast P. (NSABP)
>Portage p.

social interaction and perinatal
  addiction p. (SIPAP)
P. TEACCH
projectile vomiting
projection
  bony p.
  red blood cell spiny p.
projective assessment
prokaryote
prokaryotic reaction
prokinetic agent
prolactin (PRL)
  p. deficiency
  p. inhibiting factor (PIF)
  p. level
  plasma p.
  p. regulation
  p. releasing factor (PRF)
  p. secretion
  serum p.
  p. stimulation
  p. suppression
prolactinoma
  bromocriptine p.
  bromocriptine-resistant p.
  estrogen-induced p.
prolactin-producing adenoma
prolactin-secreting
  p.-s. adenoma
  p.-s. macroadenoma
prolan
prolapse
  aortic cusp p.
  cervical p.
  complete rectal p.
  concealed rectal p.
  cord p.
  p. of corpus luteum
  fallopian tube p.
  fimbrial p.
  first degree p.
  p.-gastropathy syndrome (PGS)
  genital p.
  incomplete rectal p.
  intrapartum cord p.
  massive genital p.
  mitral valve p. (MVP)
  occult cord p.
  pelvic organ p.
  posthysterectomy p.
  rectal p.
  second-degree p.

p. stage I–IV
third-degree p.
total vaginal vault p.
umbilical cord p.
p. of umbilical cord
urethral p.
uterine p.
uterovaginal p.
p. of uterus
vaginal stump p.
vaginal vault p.
valve p.
vault p.
prolapsed
  p. cord
  p. ectopic ureterocele
  p. uterus
Prolapse-Quantified
  Pelvic Organ P.-Q. (POPQ)
prolapsing
  p. apex
  p. apex of intussusception
  p. polyp
Prolastin
Prolene suture
prolidase deficiency
proliferating hemangioma
proliferation
  beta FGF-stimulated cell p.
  endometrial p.
  epithelial cell p.
  mesangial cell p.
proliferative
  p. change
  p. endometrium
  p. glomerulonephritis
  p. histology
  p. lesion
  p. lupus nephritis
  p. phase
  p. retinitis
  p. vasculopathy
  p. zone (PZ)
proline
  p. aminopeptidase activity
  p. hydroxyproline
prolinemia
  encephalopathy with p.
Prolixin
prolongation
  excessive QT p.
  QTc p.

NOTES

P

prolonged
    p. bradycardia
    p. capillary refill
    p. delivery hospitalization
    p. EEG monitoring
    p. expiratory apnea
    p. expiratory phase
    p. gestation
    p. indirect hyperbilirubinemia
    p. jaundice
    p. labor
    p. partial asphyxia
    p. pregnancy
    p. premature rupture of membranes (PPROM)
    p. QT interval
    p. QT syndrome
    p. regard
    p. rupture
    p. rupture of membranes (PROM)
    p. unconjugated hyperbilirubinemia
Proloprim
PROM
    prelabor rupture of membranes
    premature rupture of membranes
    preterm rupture of membranes
    prolonged rupture of membranes
Promensil
prometaphase
promethazine
    p. hydrochloride
    p. and phenylephrine
    p., phenylephrine, codeine
    unP. VC Plain Syrup
Prometrium
prominence
    calcaneal p.
    cephalic p.
    Rokitansky p.
prominent
    p. ductal pattern
    p. ear
    p. heart sound
    p. incisors-obesity-hypotonia syndrome
    p. mandible
    p. maxillary incisor
    p. nose
    p. quadrigeminal plate cistern
    p. skin discoloration
ProMod formula
promontory
    sacral p.
promoter
    AIRE p.
Promote with Fiber formula
promotion of breastfeeding intervention trial (PROBIT)
promyelocyte cell

promyelocytic leukemia
pronate
pronated foot
pronation
pronator
    p. fat pad
    p. sign
prone
    p. board
    p. extension test
    p. on elbows (POE)
    p. pivoting
    p. sleep position
    p. stander
pronephros
Pronestyl-SR
prong
    binasal p.'s
    Hudson p.'s
pronormoblast cell
Pronto Shampoo
pronuclear embryo
pronucleate
    p. stage embryo transfer (PROST)
    p. stage tubal transfer (PROST)
pronucleus, pl. **pronuclei (PN)**
proopiomelanocortin (POMC)
prooxyphysin
PROP
    propranolol
Propac Plus formula
Propaderm
Propadrine
propagation
propamidine
propantheline
propantheline bromide
Propaq Encore vital signs monitor
proparacaine
propeptide
    carboxyterminal p.
properdin
    p. deficiency
    p. factor B
property
    teratogenic p.'s
prophase
prophylactic
    p. antibiotic
    p. antibiotic therapy
    p. aspirin use
    p. bed rest
    p. cerclage
    p. chemotherapy
    p. culdoplasty
    p. episiotomy
    p. heparin
    p. immunization
    p. isoniazid

p. mastectomy
p. medication
p. oophorectomy
p. red-cell transfusion
p. tetracycline
p. treatment
prophylaxis
antibiotic p.
antimicrobial p.
aspiration p.
Credé p.
drug p.
intrapartum antibiotic p. (IAP)
neonatal ocular p.
ocular p.
postexposure p. (PEP)
postnatal penicillin p. (PPP)
primary p.
rabies p.
SBE p.
secondary p.
silver nitrate eye p.
tetanus p.
trimethoprim-sulfamethoxazole p.
vitamin K p.
propidium iodide
Propine
propionate
beclomethasone p.
clobetasol p.
fluticasone p.
Propionibacterium
P. acnes
P. propionicus
propionic acidemia
propionicus
Propionibacterium p.
propionyl CoA carboxylase deficiency
Pro-Piroxicam
Proplex SX-T
Proplex T
propofol
propositus
propoxyphene and acetaminophen
propping
bottle p.
p. reflex
2-propranol
propranolol (PROP)
p. hydrochloride
propressophysin

propria
lamina p.
substantia p.
proprioception
proprioceptive
p. input
p. sensation
proprioceptor
muscle p.
proptosis
spinal p.
Propulsid
propulsion
decreased p.
propylene
p. glycol
p. glycol diacetate
propylthiouracil
Propyl-Thyracil
pro re nata (as the occasion arises) (p.r.n.)
prorenin
plasma p.
prorenin-renin-angiotensin system
Prorex Injection
Prosed/DS
prosencephalon
ProSobee formula
prosocial behavior scale
prosodic pattern
prosody
prosogaster
prosopoanoschisis
prosopopagus
prosoposchisis
prosoposternodymus
prosopothoracopagus
ProSound SSD-5500 ultrasound
PROST
pronucleate stage embryo transfer
pronucleate stage tubal transfer
prostacyclin
p. 2 (PGI$_2$)
p. assay
p. deficiency
nebulized p.
prostacyclin-stimulating factor (PSF)
prostaglandin (PG)
p. biosynthesis
p. D$_2$
p. E (PGE)
p. E$_2$ (PGE$_2$)

NOTES

P

prostaglandin *(continued)*
  p. E$_1$ (PGE$_1$)
  p. E analog
  p. E$_2$ gel
  p. endoperoxide synthase
  p. F
  p. F$_{2\ alpha}$ (PGF2 alpha)
  p. F$_2$
  p. G (PGG)
  p. H (PGH)
  p. I$_2$
  intravaginal p.
  p. metabolism
  15-methyl p.
  one-hour p.
  p. pessary
  serum p.
  p. suppository
  p. synthesis inhibition
  p. synthetase inhibitor (PGSI)
  vaginal p.
  vasoactive p.
prostanoid
  cyclooxygenase-2-derived p.
prostate
  absent p.
  high-riding p.
  hypoplastic p.
prostatic utricle
Pro-Step hCG
prosthesis, pl. **prostheses**
  Becker breast p.
  breast p.
  Introl bladder neck support p.
  NeuroCybernetic p.
  ocular p.
  vaginal prolapse p.
  valvular p.
prosthetic
  p. attachment
  p. graft implantation
  p. patch aortoplasty
prosthodontist
Prostigmin
Prostin
  P. E2 Vaginal Suppository
  P. VR Pediatric
Prostin/15M
protamine
  p. insulin zinc suspension
  p. sulfate
protease
  p. inhibitor (PI)
  p. inhibitor-induced lipodystrophy
  p. inhibitor type
  vitamin K-dependent serine p.
protease-3
  neutrophil p.-3
ProtectaCap cap

Protectaid
  P. contraceptive sponge
  P. contraceptive sponge with F-5
    gel
protection
  p. and advocacy (P&A)
  airway p.
  progestational p.
protective
  p. colostomy
  p. extension
  p. protein
  p. service agency
protector
  LATS p.
proteiform syndrome
protein
  accessory p.
  agouti p.
  alpha dimeric p.
  bactericidal/permeability-increasing p.
    (BPI)
  Bcl-2 p.
  Bence Jones p.
  p. binding
  binding p.
  p. C
  carrier p.
  cartilage oligomeric matrix p.
    (COMP)
  p. C concentrate
  chimeric p.
  Clara cell 16 p.
  congenital absence of iron-
    binding p.
  cow's milk p. (CMP)
  C-reactive p. (CRP)
  p. C, S coagulation inhibitor
  p. C, S deficiency
  deficiency of C4-binding p.
  dimeric p.
  E-cadherin p.
  endometrial p.
  eosinophilic cationic p. (ECP)
  fetoneonatal estrogen-binding p.
  FK binding p.
  follicle regulatory p. (FRP)
  fragile X mental retardation p.
    (FMRP)
  G p.
  glial fibrillary acidic p. (GFAP)
  gonadotropin-releasing
    hormonelike p.
  gp120 viral p.
  growth hormone-binding p. (GHBP)
  H p.
  heat shock p.
  H-*ras* p21 p.
  p. hydrolysate

p. hydrolysate formula
hydrolyzed p.
I IFG-binding p.
implantation p.
insulinlike growth factor-binding p. (IGFBP)
p. intolerance
iron-binding p.
KAL p.
p. kinase C (PKC)
lipoprotein receptor-related p. (LRP)
p. loss
macrophage inflammatory p. (MIP)
major basic p. (MBP)
p. marker
membrane p.
methyl-CpG-binding p. 2 (MeCP2)
p. modified fast (PMF)
mucopolysaccharide p.
mu dimeric p.
myeloma p.
outer surface p. (Osp)
outer surface p. A (OspA)
P p.
peripheral myelin p. (PMP)
p. phosphorylation
pi dimeric p.
placental p.
plasma p.
pneumococcal conjugate tetanus p. (PncT)
pregnancy-associated plasma p.
pregnancy-associated plasma p. A (PAPP-A)
pregnancy-associated plasma p. C (PAPP-C)
pregnancy-associated plasma p. D (PAPP-D)
pregnancy-specific p.
pregnancy zone p.
procoagulant p.
p. profile
progestogen-dependent endometrial p. (PEP)
protective p.
proteolipid p. (PLP)
pulmonary microvascular permeability to p. (PMVP)
pulmonary surfactant p.
purified fusion p. (PFP)
receptor-associated p. (RAP)

recombinant outer surface p. A (rOspA)
retinol-binding p.
p. S
p. S antithrombin
Schwangerschafts p. 1
p. solder
p. standard
steroidogenic acute regulatory p. (StAR)
surfactant-associated p. (SAP)
T p.
Tamm-Horsfall p.
theta dimeric p.
thrombus precursor p. (TpP)
thyroid-specific enhancer binding p. (T4/ebp-1)
thyroxine-binding p. (TBP)
transmembrane conductance regulatory p.
transport-associated p. (TAP)
urinary excretion of p. (UEP)
vitamin D-binding p.
zona p.

protein-1
sphingolipid activator p.-1 (SAP1)
protein-3
insulinlike growth factor-binding p.-3 (IGFBP-3)
protein-A
surfactant p.-A (SP-A)
proteinaceous subretinal fluid
proteinase
p. factor
p. K
serine p.
protein-B
surfactant p.-B (SP-B)
protein-C
surfactant p.-C (SP-C)
protein-calorie malnutrition
protein-conjugated vaccine
protein-energy malnutrition
protein-induced
p.-i. eosinophilic colitis (PEC)
p.-i. vitamin K absence (PIVKA)
protein-losing enteropathy
proteinosis
alveolar p.
congenital alveolar p.

NOTES

P

765

proteinosis *(continued)*
    lipoid p.
    pulmonary alveolar p. (PAP)
protein-sparing modified fast (PSMF)
protein-to-urine creatinine ratio
proteinuria
    gestational p.
    glomerular p.
    idiopathic low molecular weight p.
    LMW p.
    orthostatic p.
    overflow p.
    persistent p.
    postural p.
    renal p.
    selective p.
    transient p.
    treatment-resistant p.
    tubular p.
proteinuric
Proteobacteria
    alpha P.
proteoglycans
proteolipid protein (PLP)
proteolysis
    cellular p.
proteolytic enzyme
Proteus
    P. mirabilis
    P. morganii
    P. syndrome (PS)
    P. syndrome myopathy
prothrombic tendency
prothrombin
    p. gene mutation
    p. time (pro-time, PT)
    p. time coagulation test
prothrombin^{G20210A}
prothrombokinase
pro-time
    prothrombin time
ProTime microcoagulation system
protirelin
protoblast
protocol
    AIDS Clinical Trials Group p.
    Bagshawe p.
    chemotherapy p.
    management p.
    modified Bagshawe p. (MBP)
    MOPP chemotherapy p.
    rape p.
    Reese Clark p.
    wean and feed p.
protocoproporphyria
Protocult stool sampling device
protodiastolic gallop
protodyssomnia

protogaster
proton
    p. MRS
    p. MR spectroscopy
    p. pump antagonist
    p. pump inhibitor (PPI)
proto-oncogene
    c-*erb* B-2 p.-o.
    c-fms p.-o.
    fes p.-o.
    fgr p.-o.
    fyn p.-o.
    hck p.-o.
    HER-2/neu p.-o.
    lck p.-o.
    lyn p.-o.
    mos p.-o.
    raf p.-o.
    RET p.-o.
    Scr p.-o.
    yes p.-o.
Protopic ointment
protoporphyria
    erythrohepatic p.
    erythropoietic p. (EPP)
protoporphyrin
    free erythrocyte p. (FEP)
    tin p. (SnPP)
    zinc p. (ZnPP)
Protozoa
protracted
    p. depressive episode
    p. diarrhea
    p. diarrhea of infancy
protraction disorder
Pro-Trin
protriptyline
Protropin Injection
protruding tongue
protrusio acetabuli
protrusion
    reduction of p.
protuberance
    Rokitansky p.
protuberans
    dermatofibrosarcoma p.
protuberant step deformity
Proud syndrome
Proval
Proventil HFA
Provera Oral
Providencia rettgeri
provisional calcification
provocation
    bronchial p.
    epinephrine p.
    mucous membrane p.
    p. test

provocative
p. bronchial challenge testing
p. stress test
prowazekii
Rickettsia p.
proXeed
proxetil
cefpodoxime p.
Proxigel Oral
proximal
p. bowel
p. convoluted tubule
p. enterostomy
p. femoral epiphysis
p. femoral focal deficiency
p. humeral derotation osteotomy
p. humeral stress fracture
p. jejunum
p. occlusion
p. outflow tract
p. pattern weakness
p. pulmonary artery
p. pulmonary artery banding
p. row carpectomy
p. RTA
p. shaft hypospadias
p. splenorenal shunt
p. tibial epiphysis
p. transverse septum
p. tubal blockage
p. tubal obstruction
p. tubulopathy
p. urethra
p. white subungual onychomycosis
proxy
factitious disorder by p. (FDP)
Münchausen syndrome by p.
   (MSBP, MSP)
Prozac
Prozine-50
PRP
pityriasis rubra pilaris
platelet-rich plasma
polyribosylribitol phosphate
PRPP
5-phospho-alpha-d-ribosyl pyrophosphate
   PRPP synthetase superactivity
PRS
Prieto syndrome
PRSL
potential renal solute load

PRSP
penicillin-resistant *Staphylococcus*
   pneumonia
penicillin-resistant *Streptococcus*
   pneumoniae
PRTS
Partington X-linked mental retardation
   syndrome
prune
p. belly
p. belly syndrome
pruning
synaptic p.
prurigo
actinic p.
p. gestationis
p. of pregnancy
pruritic
p. folliculitis of pregnancy
p. rash
p. urticarial papule
p. urticarial papules and plaques
   (PUPP)
p. urticarial papules and plaques
   of pregnancy (PUPPP)
p. urticarial plaque
p. vesiculopapular eruption
pruritus
anal p.
p. ani
drug reaction p.
genital p.
p. gravidarum
perianal p.
p. vulvae
vulvar p.
PS
pancreas sufficient
phytosterol
polysaccharide
Proteus syndrome
pulmonic stenosis
PSA
physical sexual abuse
power spectral analysis
procedural sedation and analgesia
   PSA test
psammoma body
PSC
Pediatric Symptom Checklist
P450scc
cytochrome P.

NOTES

PSD
pediatric spectrum of disease
PSE
preparticipation sports examination
Pseudallescheria boydii
pseudarthrosis
clavicular p.
congenital p.
pseudautonomy
pseudencephalus
pseudoacanthosis nigricans
pseudoacephalus
pseudoachondroplasia syndrome
pseudoachondroplastic dysplasia
pseudoaddiction
pseudoallele
pseudoaminopterin syndrome
pseudoaneurysm
uterine artery p.
pseudoappendicitis
pseudoappendicular syndrome
pseudoarthrosis
congenital p.
p. of tibia
tibial p.
pseudoautosome
pseudobulbar palsy
pseudocalcification
powder p.
pseudocholinesterase deficiency
pseudochromosome
pseudochylous milky fluid
pseudocoagulopathy
pseudocoloboma
macular p.
pseudoconstipation
pseudo-Crouzon disease
pseudocyesis
monosymptomatic delusional p.
pseudocyst
pancreatic p.
pseudodeciduosis
pseudodiastrophic dysplasia
pseudodiverticulum
posterior pharyngeal p.
pseudoencapsulated lesion
pseudoephedrine
carbinoxamine and p.
p. hydrochloride
triprolidine and p.
pseudoepitheliomatous hyperplasia
pseudoesotropia
pseudoexstrophy
pseudofemale
hairless p.
pseudogene
pseudo-genu varum
pseudogestational sac

pseudoglandular
p. period
p. stage
p. stage of lung development
p. synovial sarcoma
pseudoglioma congenita
pseudogynecomastia
pseudohermaphrodite
pseudohermaphroditism
female p.
male p. (MPH)
pseudo-Hurler
p.-H. deformity
p.-H. polydystrophy
p.-H. syndrome
pseudohypertrophic
p. adult muscular dystrophy
p. muscular paralysis
p. progressive muscular dystrophy
pseudohypertrophy
pseudohypha, pl. **pseudohyphae**
nonbranching p.
pseudohypoaldosteronism
pseudohyponatremia
pseudohypoparathyroidism (type I, Ia, II)
pseudohypopyon
pseudoinfarction
pseudointestinal obstruction
pseudointraligamentous
pseudo-Köbner phenomenon
pseudoleukemia
pseudolithiasis
reversible biliary p.
pseudolobular cirrhosis
pseudolymphoma
pseudomallei
Burkholderia p.
Pseudomonas p.
pseudomembrane
adherent p.
pseudomembranous
p. colitis
p. conjunctivitis
p. enterocolitis
p. trigonitis
pseudomenopause
pseudomenstruation
Pseudomonas
P. aeruginosa
P. cepacia
P. exotoxin
P. fluorescens
P. pseudomallei
P. septic arthritis
pseudomonoamniotic cavity
pseudomosaicism
pseudomucinous tumor
pseudomyxoma peritonei

pseudonuchal infantilism
pseudoobstruction
  chronic idiopathic intestinal p. (CIIP)
  chronic intestinal p.
  intestinal p.
pseudoovulation
pseudopapilledema
pseudoparalysis
  Parrot p.
pseudoperoxidation
  iron-catalyzed p.
pseudopili anulati
pseudopolyp
pseudoporencephalic cyst
pseudoporphyria
pseudoprecocious puberty
pseudopregnancy
pseudoprogeria/Hallermann-Streiff (PHS)
pseudoprogeria syndrome
pseudopseudohypoparathyroidism (PPHP)
pseudopuberty
  precocious p.
pseudorabies
pseudoreaction
pseudo-Roth spots
pseudosarcoma
  botryoid p.
pseudoscleroderma
pseudosclerosis
pseudoscurvy
pseudoseizure
pseudostrabismus
pseudosubluxation
pseudothalidomide syndrome
pseudotoxemia
pseudotoxoplasmosis syndrome
pseudotrisomy 13 syndrome
pseudotropicalis
  Candida p.
pseudotruncus
pseudotuberculosis
  Yersinia p.
pseudotumor
  p. cerebri
  inflammatory p. (IPT)
  retinal p.
  trophoblastic p.
pseudo-Turner syndrome
pseudo-Ullrich-Turner syndrome

pseudovagina
pseudovaginal perineoscrotal hypospadias (PPSH)
pseudovertigo
pseudo-von Willebrand disease
pseudo-Wernicke syndrome
pseudoxanthoma elasticum
PSF
  prostacyclin-stimulating factor
PSG
  polysomnogram
  polysomnography
PSI
  Parental Stress Index
  pelvic support index
  Physiologic Stability Index
  postponing sexual involvement
    PSI program
psittaci
  Chlamydia p.
psittacosis
PSMF
  protein-sparing modified fast
    PSMF diet
PSN
  pontosubicular neuron necrosis
psoas
  p. abscess
  p. hitch procedure
  p. margin
  p. sign
psoralen and ultraviolet A (PUVA)
Psorcon
psoriasiform lesion
psoriasis
  classic plaque p.
  generalized pustular p.
  p. guttata
  guttate p.
  plaque-type p.
  p. vulgaris
  vulvar p.
psoriasis-associated arthritis
psoriatic
  p. arthritis
  p. dermatitis
  p. diaper rash
PsoriGel
PSROM
  preterm spontaneous rupture of membranes

NOTES

P

769

PSS
physiologic salt solution
P&S Shampoo
PSTT
placental site trophoblastic tumor
PSU
pediatric sedation unit
psychedelic drug
psychiatric
p. diagnostic interview (PDI)
p. drug
p. illness
psychiatrist
child and adolescent p.
psychiatry
American Academy of Child and
Adolescent P. (AACAP)
child and adolescent forensic p.
psychoactive drug
psychodynamic
p. psychotherapy
p. therapy
psychogenic
p. arthralgia
p. cough
p. cough tic
p. impotence
p. limp
p. pelvic pain
p. polydipsia
p. seizure
psychological
p. abuse
p. causes, excessive urine
production, restricted mobility,
stool impaction
p. comorbidity
p. distress
p. effect
P. General Well-Being Index
(PGWB)
p. sex
p. stress
p. trauma
psychologic nonneuropathic bladder
psychologist
psychometric
p. assessment
p. test
psychometrist
psychomotor
p. development index (PDI)
p. epilepsy
p. evaluation
p. retardation
p. seizure
p. status
psychopathology
offspring p.

psychopharmacogenetic
psychopharmacological intervention
psychopharmacology
psychoprophylaxis
psychoses (*pl. of* psychosis)
psychosexual
p. dysfunction
p. problem
psychosine lipidosis
psychosis, pl. **psychoses**
brief reactive p.
climacteric p.
psychoses cum encephalatides
gestational p.
involutional p.
postpartum p.
puerperal p.
reactive p.
symbiotic p.
psychosocial
p. adjustment
p. development
p. dwarfism
p. factor
p. support
psychosomatic
p. complaint
p. disease
psychostimulant medication
psychotherapy
cognitive-behavioral p.
nondirective supportive p.
psychodynamic p.
supportive p.
psychotic depression
psychotropic drug (PTD)
psyllium
4p syndrome
5p syndrome
9p syndrome
PT
pertussis toxin
pertussis toxoid
physical therapy
physiotherapy
primary thrombocythemia
prothrombin time
PT coagulation test
PTA
percutaneous transluminal angioplasty
plasma thromboplastin antecedent
pure-tone average
PTC
pulmonary tissue concentration
PTCRA
percutaneous transluminal coronary
rotational ablation
PTD
psychotropic drug

P.T.E.-4, -5
PTEN gene
pteridine ring compound
pterin
- synthetic p.
- urinary p.

pteroylglutamic acid
pterygium
- p. colli
- p. colli, mental retardation, digital anomalies syndrome
- congenital p.
- p. universale

pterygoarthromyodysplasia congenita
PTFL
- posterior talofibular ligament

PTH
- parathyroid hormone
  - PTH for osteoporotic women on estrogen replacement (POWER)

PTH-derived peptide
PTHrP
- parathyroid hormone-related peptide

PTK gene
PTL
- preterm labor

PTLD
- posttransplant lymphoproliferative disease
- posttransplant lymphoproliferative disorder

ptosis, pl. **ptoses**
- bilateral congenital p.
- congenital p.
- p., downslanting palpebral fissures, hypertelorism, seizures, mental retardation syndrome
- p. of eyelids, diastasis recti, hip dysplasia
- Marcus Gunn jaw-winking p.
- unilateral congenital p.
- upside-down p.

PTS
- Pediatric Trauma Score

PTSD
- posttraumatic stress disorder
  - Screening Tool for Early Predictors of PTSD (STEPP)

PTSS
- posttraumatic signs or symptoms

PTT
- partial thromboplastin time

PTX
- pneumothorax

ptyalism
pubarche
- precocious p. (PP)
- premature p.

puberal, pubertal
- p. aberrancy
- p. arrest
- p. delay
- p. growth
- p. gynecomastia
- p. milestone

pubertas praecox
puberty
- abnormal p.
- asynchronous p.
- central precocious p. (CPP)
- complete precocious p.
- constitutional delay of p.
- constitutional precocious p.
- delayed p.
- factitious precocious p.
- familial male precocious p.
- gonadotropin-dependent precocious p.
- gonadotropin-independent precocious p.
- heterosexual precocious p.
- iatrogenic precocious p.
- idiopathic isosexual precocious p.
- incomplete precocious p.
- p. initiation
- isosexual idiopathic precocious p.
- peripheral precocious p.
- physiologic delay of p.
- precocious p.
- pseudoprecocious p.
- true precocious p.

pubescence
pubescent
pubic
- p. arch
- p. hair
- p. hairline
- p. lice
- p. ramus
- p. ramus stress fracture
- p. symphysis
- p. symphysis periostitis
- p. triangle
- p. tubercle

NOTES

P

pubiotomy
pubis
> arcuate ligament of p.
> mons p.
> os p.
> osteitis p.
> osteomyelitis p.
> pediculosis p.
> *Phthirus p.*
> ruptured symphysis p.
> symphysis p.
> widened symphysis p.

public health nurse (PHN)
pubocervical fascia
pubococcygeal muscle
pubococcygeus muscle
puborectalis
> p. muscle
> p. sling

puborectal muscle
pubourethral
pubovaginal sling procedure
pubovesical ligament
pubovisceral muscle
PUBS
> percutaneous umbilical blood sampling

PUD
> peptic ulcer disease

puddle sign
pudendal
> p. anesthesia
> p. apron
> p. area
> p. artery
> p. block
> p. canal
> p. hematocele
> p. nerve
> p. nerve terminal motor latency
> p. neurogram
> p. neuropathy
> p. sac

pudendum, gen. pudendi, pl. pudenda
> frenulum labiorum pudendi
> labium majus pudendi
> labium minus pudendi
> noma pudendi

Pudenz
> P. reservoir
> P. shunt

puerorum
> hydroa p.

puerpera, pl. puerperae
puerperal
> p. convulsion
> p. eclampsia
> p. endometritis
> p. febrile morbidity
> p. fever

> p. hematoma
> p. infection
> p. inversion
> p. mastitis
> p. period
> p. phlebitis
> p. psychosis
> p. pyemia
> p. sepsis
> p. septicemia
> p. tetanus

puerperant
puerperium, pl. puerperia
PUFA
> polyunsaturated fatty acid

puffiness
> periorbital p.

puff-of-smoke disease
puffy skin
pug nose-peripheral dysostosis syndrome
Pulec and Freedman classification
pullback
> catheter p.

pull-down
> testicular p.-d.

pulled elbow
pulling
> hair p.

pull-through
> endorectal p.-t.
> ileoanal p.-t.
> p.-t. procedure
> retrorectal transanal p.-t.
> p.-t. surgery
> p.-t. technique

pull-to-sit reflex
pull-up
> gastric p.-u.

Pulmicort
> P. Respules
> P. Turbuhaler

Pulmo-Aid ventilator
Pulmocare
> P. diet
> P. formula

PulmoMate nebulizer
pulmonale
> cor p.

pulmonary
> p. acinar aplasia
> p. agenesis
> p. alveolar microlithiasis
> p. alveolar proteinosis (PAP)
> p. alveolus
> p. angiography
> p. anthrax
> p. arborization
> p. arterial banding
> p. arterial flow

p. arterial oxygen content
p. arterial trunk
p. arteriogram
p. arteriole
p. arteriovenous malformation (PAVM)
p. artery (PA)
p. artery angioplasty
p. artery atresia
p. artery banding
p. artery catheterization
p. artery/ductus view
p. artery occluded pressure (PAOP)
p. artery pressure monitoring
p. artery sling
p. artery thermodilution
p. artery wedge (PAW)
p. artery wedge pressure (PAWP)
p. ascariasis
p. aspergillosis
p. aspiration
p. atresia with intact ventricular septum (PAIVS)
p. bleb
p. blood flow (PBF)
p. bud
p. capillary wedge pressure (PCWP)
p. compliance
p. complication
p. contusion
p. cryptococcosis
p. cyanosis
p. diffusing capacity
p. disorder
p. dysmaturity syndrome
p. dysplasia
p. edema
p. ejection click
p. ejection murmur
p. ELF
p. embolism (PE)
p. embolus
p. endometriosis
p. eosinophilia
p. fat embolism
p. function
p. function test (PFT)
p. function testing
p. gangrene
p. hemangiomatosis
p. hemorrhage

p. hemosiderosis
p. histoplasmosis
p. hypertension
p. hypertension of newborn
p. hypoplasia
p. immaturity
p. infarction
p. infiltrate
p. infiltrate with eosinophilia (PIE)
p. infiltrate with eosinophilia syndrome
p. injury
p. insufficiency
p. insufficiency of premature
p. insufficiency of prematurity
p. interstitial emphysema (PIE)
p. interstitial fibrosis
p. lavage
p. leukostasis
p. lymphangiectasia
p. lymphoid hyperplasia (PLH)
p. maturation
p. medicine
p. metastasis
p. microvascular permeability to protein (PMVP)
p. mucormycosis
p. overcirculation
p. parenchymal disease
p. perfusion
p. plaque
p. porcine valve
p. recurrence
p. resection
p. sequestration
p. shunt
p. sound
p. suppuration
p. surfactant
p. surfactant protein
p. thermodilution catheter
p. thromboembolism
p. time constant
p. tissue concentration (PTC)
p. toilet
p. tuberculosis
p. tularemia
p. undervascularity
p. valve disease
p. valve stenosis
p. vascular bed
p. vascular congestion

NOTES

P

pulmonary *(continued)*
 p. vascular development
 p. vascular marking
 p. vascular resistance (PVR)
 p. vascular tone
 p. vasodilation
 p. vein
 p. venoocclusive disease
 p. venous drainage
 p. venous obstruction
 p. venous oxygen content
 p. ventilation
pulmonic
 p. murmur
 p. regurgitation
 p. stenosis (PS)
 p. stenosis-café-au-lait spots
   syndrome
 p. valve
pulmonicola
 Pandoraea p.
Pulmozyme
pulp
 digital p.
 p. necrosis
pulpal degeneration
pulpectomy
pulsatile
 p. air jet
 p. discharge
 p. fontanelle
 p. GnRH administration
 p. human menopausal gonadotropin
 p. release
pulsatility
 p. index (PI)
 intrinsic p.
pulsating exophthalmos
pulse
 apical p.
 bounding p.
 cutaneous pressure p.
 p. dexamethasone
 dorsalis pedis p.
 p. frequency
 p. interval
 jugular venous p.
 maternal p.
 p. methylprednisolone
 p. oximeter
 p. oximeter sensor N-25 and I-20
 p. oximetry
 p. oximetry waveform systolic
   blood pressure (POWSBP)
 paradoxical p.
 pedal p.
 posterior tibial p.
 p. pressure
 sharp p.

 p. steroid therapy
 thready p.
 p. width
pulsed
 p. Doppler ultrasound
 p. electromagnetic wave
 p. field gel electrophoresis (PFGE)
 p. intervention
 p. wave Doppler
pulsed-wave ultrasound
pulseless
 p. disease
 p. electrical activity
 p. phase
pulsion
 p. enterocele
 p. theory
pulsus
 p. alternans
 p. bisferiens
 p. paradoxus
pulvinar
Pulvule
 Seromycin P.'s
pump
 Advanced Collection breast p.
 Barron p.
 Basis breast p.
 battery-operated breast p.
 bilateral breast p.
 breast p.
 Chicco breast p.
 Chid breast p.
 Clarus model 5169 peristaltic p.
 Egnell breast p.
 electric breast p.
 Elmed peristaltic irrigation p.
 Grafco breast p.
 infusion p.
 insulin p.
 Kangaroo enteral feeding p.
 Kangaroo infusion p.
 Kendall McGaw Intelligent p.
 KM-1 breast p.
 Lactina Select breast p.
 low-pressure breast p.
 manual breast p.
 Mary Jane breast p.
 MasterFlex fetal perfusion p.
 Medela Dominant vacuum
   delivery p.
 Medela manual breast p.
 Medfusion 1001 syringe infusion p.
 Mityvac reusable vacuum p.
 Na$^+$ p.
 pneumocapillary infusion p.
 Pump In Style breast p.
 Salem p.
 servocontrolled ventilation p.

suction p.
p. twins
Unicare breast p.
Zyklomat infusion p.

punch
baby Tischler biopsy p.
Baker p.
p. biopsy forceps
Eppendorfer biopsy p.
Keyes dermatologic p.
Keyes vulvar p.
Miltex disposable biopsy p.
p. skin biopsy
Tischler-Morgan biopsy p.
Townsend biopsy p.
Wittner biopsy p.

punched-out lytic lesion
puncta (*pl. of* punctum)
punctata
chondrodysplasia p.
chondrodystrophia congenita p.
dysplasia epiphysealis p.
recessive X-linked
  chondrodysplasia p.
rhizomelic chondrodysplasia p.
  (RCDP)

punctate
p. epiphyseal dysplasia
p. epithelial keratitis
p. hyperkeratosis
p. lenticular opacity
p. wheal

punctation
punctum, pl. **puncta**
puncture
accidental dural p.
arterial p.
bone marrow p.
cisternal p.
lumbar p. (LP)
pericardial p.
p. punch site
subdural p.
transparenchymal needle p.
transvaginal amniotic p. (TAP)
ventricular p.

PUND
pregnancy, uterine, not delivered
punishment
corporal p.
Punnett square

pupil
Adie p.
Argyll Robertson p.
cat's eye p.
conjugate p.
keyhole p.
Marcus Gunn p.
p. reaction
white p.

pupillae
ectopia lentis et p.
pupillary
p. change
p. light response
p. membrane
p. red reflex
p. syndrome

PUPP
pruritic urticarial papules and plaques
puppet children
puppetlike
p. appearance
p. syndrome

PUPPP
pruritic urticarial papules and plaques of
  pregnancy
puppy position
pure
p. bulbar poliomyelitis
p. esophageal atresia
p. gonadal dysgenesis
p. random drift
p. red blood cell aplasia

pureed diet
Puregene DNA extraction system
Puregon
purely sensory polyneuritis
pure-tone average (PTA)
purging
anorexia nervosa with binging
  and p. (AN-BP)
p. rate

Puri-Clens
purified
p. chick embryo cell culture
  (PCEC)
p. fusion protein (PFP)
p. gamma globulin
p. hormone
p. human factor IX
p. podophyllotoxin
p. polysaccharide

NOTES

P

purified *(continued)*
    p. protein derivative (PPD)
    p. urinary FSH
    urofollitropin for injection, p.
purine
    p. metabolism
    p. metabolism disorder
    p. nucleoside phosphorylase (PNP)
Purinethol
Puritan swab
Purkinje
    P. cell
    P. cell tumor
    P. fibers
puromycin
purple
    p. hallux
    p. hue
    p. toes syndrome
Purpose cream
purpura
    alloimmune neonatal
      thrombocytopenic p.
    anaphylactic p.
    anaphylactoid p.
    autoimmune thrombocytopenic p.
      (AITP)
    childhood idiopathic
      thrombocytopenic p.
    drug-related p.
    p. fulminans
    p. hemorrhagica
    Henoch-Schönlein p. (HSP)
    idiopathic thrombocytopenic p.
      (ITP)
    immune thrombocytopenic p. (ITP)
    neonatal alloimmune
      thrombocytopenic p. (NATP)
    palpable p.
    Schönlein-Henoch p.
    thrombocytopenic p.
    thrombotic p.
    thrombotic thrombocytopenic p.
      (TTP)
    wet p.
purpuric
    p. light eruption
    p. rash
purse
    shepherd's p.
purse-string
    p.-s. mouth
    p.-s. suture
Purtilo syndrome
Purtscher retinopathy
purulent
    p. arthritis
    p. conjunctivitis
    p. meningitis
    p. nasal discharge
    p. pericarditis
    p. pharyngitis
    p. rhinitis
    p. sputum
    p. venous thrombosis
pus
    p. burrow
    sterile p.
    p. tube
pusher
    Endo-Assist endoscopic knot p.
    knot p.
    MetraTie knot p.
    Ranfac knot p.
pustular
    p. melanosis
    p. varicella
pustule
    neonatal p.
    satellite p.
pustulosa
    miliaria p.
    varicella p.
pustulosis
    infantile p.
    Juliusberg p.
    Malassezia furfur p.
    nonfollicular p.
    palmar p.
    p. palmaris
    p. palmaris et plantaris
    palmoplantar p.
    staphylococcal p.
    p. vacciniformis acuta
putamen
putrefaciens
    Alteromonas p.
putrescence
putrescine
PUV
    posterior urethral valve
PUVA
    psoralen and ultraviolet A
      PUVA phototherapy
Puzo method
PVC
    premature ventricular contraction
P.V. Carpine Liquifilm
PVDF
    polyvinylidene fluoride
PVEL
    periventricular echolucency
PVF K
PVH
    periventricular hemorrhage (grade 1–4)
PVL
    periventricular leukomalacia
      cystic PVL

PVO
portal vein obstruction
PVP
polyvinylpyrrolidone
PVP solution
PVR
pulmonary vascular resistance
PVS
persistent vegetative state
P-wave axis
PWM
pokeweed mitogen
PWS
Prader-Willi syndrome
PWSCR
Prader-Willi syndrome critical region
pycnodysostosis
Pycnogenol
pyelectasis
fetal p.
pyelitis
pyelocaliectasis
pyelogram
dragon p.
intravenous p. (IVP)
limited-exposure intravenous p.
retrograde p.
single-shot intravenous p.
washout p.
pyelography
intravenous p. (IVP)
retrograde p.
pyelonephritis
acute p.
antepartum p.
p. in exenteration
hereditary interstitial p.
nonobstructive p.
xanthogranulomatous p.
pyelophlebitis
portal p.
pyeloplasty
pyelostomy
cutaneous p.
pyemia
puerperal p.
pygoamorphus
pygodidymus
pygomelus
pygopagus
pyknocyte

pyknocytosis
infantile p.
pyknodysostosis syndrome
pyknoepilepsy
pyknotic cell
Pyle
bone age standard of Greulich and P.
P. disease
P. syndrome
pylephlebitis
pylori
Campylobacter p.
Helicobacter p.
PYtest for *Helicobacter p.*
pyloric
p. atresia
p. mass
p. nitric oxide synthase
p. olive
p. sphincter relaxation
p. stenosis
p. string sign
pyloromyotomy
Ramstedt p.
Ramstedt-Fredet p.
pyloroplasty
Heineke-Mikulicz p.
pylorospasm
pylorus
congenital double p.
double p.
pyocolpocele
pyocolpos
pyoderma
p. alopecia
blastomycosis-like p.
p. gangrenosum
streptococcal p.
p. vegetans
pyoderma-associated nephritis
pyogenes
Actinomyces p.
Staphylococcus p.
Streptococcus p.
pyogenic
p. abscess
p. arthritis
p. bacteria
p. granuloma
p. infection
p. lymphadenitis

NOTES

P

pyogenic *(continued)*
    p. mediastinitis
    p. meningitis
    p. osteomyelitis
    p. salpingitis
pyogranulomatous response
pyometra
pyometritis
pyomyoma
    uterine p.
pyomyositis
    tropical p.
pyoovarium
Pyopen
pyophysometra
pyopneumothorax
    iatrogenic p.
pyosalpingitis
pyosalpingo-oophoritis
pyosalpingo-oothecitis
pyosalpinx
Pyramid
    Food Guide P.
pyramidal
    p. cerebral palsy
    p. lesion
    p. tract
    p. tract disease
    p. tract sign
pyramidalis muscle
pyrantel pamoate
pyrazinamide
pyrethrins and piperonyl butoxide
pyrethroid
pyrethrum extract
pyrexia
    maternal p.
    procedure-related p.
Pyribenzamine
pyribenzamine
Pyridiate
pyridinoline
Pyridium
pyridostigmine bromide
pyridoxal
    p. phosphate
    p. 5-phosphate
pyridoxine
    p. deficiency
    p. dependency

pyridoxine-dependency syndrome
pyridoxine-dependent seizure
pyridoxine-refractory sideroblastic anemia
pyridoxine-responsive anemia
pyrilamine maleate
Pyrilinks-D assay
pyrimethamine
    sulfadoxine and p.
pyrimethamine-sulfadoxine
pyrimidine
Pyrinex Pediculicide Shampoo
Pyrinyl
    P. II Liquid
    P. Plus Shampoo
pyrogen
    endogenous p.
pyrogenicity
pyroglutamic acidemia
Pyronema domesticum
pyrophosphate
    5-phospho-alpha-d-ribosyl p. (PRPP)
    plasma inorganic p.
pyrophosphorylase
pyropoikilocytosis
    hereditary p. (HPP)
pyrosis
pyrroloporphyria
pyruvate
    p. decarboxylase
    p. dehydrogenase
    p. dehydrogenase complex
    p. dehydrogenation
    p. kinase (PK)
pyruvic acid
6-pyruvoyl tetrahydropteridine synthetase
pyrvinium pamoate
PYtest for *Helicobacter pylori*
pyuria
    amicrobic p.
    sterile p.
PZ
    proliferative zone
PZD
    partial zona dissection

Q

quotient
Q angle
Q band
Q fever

Q10

coenzyme Q10

Q̇

blood flow

q

long arm of chromosome

21q

tetrasomy 21q

22q11

microdeletion of chromosome 22q11

22q11.2 deletion syndrome

Qa (series of loci)

QCT

quantitative computed tomography

QDR

quantitative digital radiography

QDR-1500 bone densitometer

qEEG

quantitative electroencephalography

Qf

rate of fluid filtration

QIAamp Tissue kit

QNS

quantity not sufficient

QOL

quality of life

qr

quadriradial

QS complex

Qs/Qt

intrapulmonary shunt ratio
right-to-left shunt ratio

QTc

QTc prolongation

Q-test ovulation predictor

QTest Strep test

QT interval

Q-tip test for determining urethral mobility

QTL

quantitative trait locus

QT-Watch messaging wristwatch

quadrant

q. assessment
left lower q. (LLQ)
left upper q. (LUQ)
right lower q. (RLQ)
right upper q. (RUQ)

quadrantectomy, axillary dissection, radiation therapy (QUART)

quadrate hepatic lobe

quadratum

caput q.

quadratus labiae superioris muscle

quadriceps femoris muscle biopsy

quadrigemina

corpora q.

quadripara

quadriparesis

flaccid q.
spastic q.

quadriplegia

spastic q.
transient q.

quadriplegic

quadriradial (qr)

quadruped

quadruple-contrast study

quadruplet

quai

dong q.

qualitative

q. detection kit
q. developmental assessment
q. disorder
q. urine screen

quality

q. assurance process
q. of life (QOL)
Q. of Upper Extremities Test (QUEST)

Quan-Smith syndrome

quantification

Quantikine

Q. human IL-6 Immunoassay
Q. IVD

quantitation

amniotic fluid q.
pelvic organ prolapse q.

quantitative

q. analysis of fat content
q. beta hCG level
q. Bethesda assay
q. computed tomography (QCT)
q. digital radiography (QDR)
q. disorder
q. electroencephalography (qEEG)
q. immunoglobulin
q. inheritance
q. insulin sensitivity check index (QUICKI)
q. intradermal skin test
q. serum drug assay

quantitative *(continued)*
    q. sudomotor axon-reflex test
    q. trait locus (QTL)
    q. ultrasound (QUS)
quantity not sufficient (QNS)
quarantine
QUART
    quadrantectomy, axillary dissection,
    radiation therapy
quarter-strength formula
quartipara
Quarzan
quasicontinuous inheritance
quasidiploid
quasidominance
Queckenstedt test
Queensland
    Q. fever
    Q. tick typhus
Quelicin
query fever
QUEST
    Quality of Upper Extremities Test
questionnaire
    Achenbach q.
    Ages and Stages Q. (ASQ)
    attitude behavior q. (ABQ)
    autism spectrum screening q.
     (ASSQ)
    BFLUTS q.
    child health q. (CHQ)
    childhood trauma q. (CTQ)
    Conners Abbreviated Parent Q.
    Denver Home Screening Q.
    Dominic-R q.
    Harter self-esteem q.
    HRQOL q.
    human health and behavior q.
     (HBQ)
    Q. for Identifying Children with
     Chronic Conditions (QuICCC)
    Incontinence Impact Q. (IIQ)
    Incontinence Impact Q.-Revised
     (IIQ-R)
    Incontinence Stress q. (ISQ)
    Inflammatory Bowel Disease Q.
     (IBDQ)
    King's Health Q. (KHQ)
    Multidimensional Personality Q.
     (MPQ)
    PARS III q.
    Pediatric Asthma Quality of
     Life Q. (PAQLQ)
    Reynolds suicide ideation q.
    Seasonal Pattern Assessment Q.
     (SPAQ)
    SF-36 Health Status q.
    Terry q.
    Wolraich q.

Questran
    Q. Light
    Q. powder
Quetelet body mass index
quetiapine fumarate
Queyrat erythroplasia
Quibron-T
Quibron-T/SR
QuICCC
    Questionnaire for Identifying Children
    with Chronic Conditions
quickening
QUICKI
    quantitative insulin sensitivity check
    index
Quick test
QuickVue
    Q. *Chlamydia* test
    Q. In-Line One-Step Strep A test
    Q. one-step hCG-Combo pregnancy
     test
    Q. One-Step hCG-urine test
    Q. One-Step *H. pylori* test
    Q. UrinChek 10+ urine test strip
Quidel group B strep test
quiescence
    uterine q.
quiescent endometrium
quiet
    q. alertness
    q. and alert state
    q. precordium
    q. sleep
QuietTrak monitor
Quik Connect fetal monitor
Quikheel lancet
QuikPac-II OneStep hCG pregnancy
    test
quinacrine
    q. banding
    q. hydrochloride
Quinaglute Dura-Tabs
quinalbarbitone sodium
quinate
quinestrol
quinethazone
quingestanol acetate
Quinidex Extentabs
quinidine gluconate
quinine
    q. dihydrochloride
    q. sulfate
quinolinic acid
quinolone
Quinones uterine-grasping forceps
quinquefasciatus
    Culex q.
Quinsana Plus Tropical
quinsy

Q

quintana
> *Bartonella q.*
quintessence
quintipara
Quinton dual-lumen catheter
quintuplet
quintuple-X syndrome
quinupristin
Quips genetic imaging system
Quisling hammer
quivering
> chin q.

quotidian fever
quotient (Q)
> developmental q. (DQ)
> developmental motor q. (DMQ)
> Griffith General Q.
> intelligence q. (IQ)
> mean developmental q.
> respiratory q.
> ventilation/perfusion q.

QUS
> quantitative ultrasound

NOTES

R
radius
roentgen
R band
R & C Shampoo
R$_{AW}$
regional gas exchange
R$_{rs}$
respiratory system resistance
R$_{int}$
intrinsic flow resistance
RA
rheumatoid arthritis
^{226}Ra
radium-226
RA27/3 rubella strain
RAA
right aortic arch
Raaf catheter
RAB
remote afterloading brachytherapy
RABA
radioantigen-binding assay
rabbit nose
rabeprazole
rabies
r. immune globulin (RIG)
paralytic r.
r. prophylaxis
r. vaccine
r. vaccine, absorbed (RVA)
Rabson-Mendenhall syndrome
raccoon eyes
racemic
r. ephedrine
r. epinephrine
racemose form
Racephedrine
rachiopagus
rachischisis
craniospinal r.
r. partialis
r. posterior
thoracolumbar r.
r. totalis
rachitic
r. bone deformity
r. change
r. metaphysis
r. rosary
rachitis fetalis
racial difference
RAD
reactive airways disease

rad
radiation absorbed dose
radial
r. aplasia-thrombocytopenia syndrome
r. arterial catheter
r. arterial line
r. artery
r. artery catheter
r. artery catheterization
r. clubhand
r. curettage
r. digital grasp
r. dysplasia
r. epiphysis
r. head dislocation
r. head fracture
r. head osteochondritis
r. head subluxation (RHS)
r. jaw biopsy forceps
r. neck fracture
r. nerve block
r. palmar grasp
r. physis
r. ray aplasia
r. ray defect
r. ray defects, triangular face, telecanthus, sparse hair, dwarfism, mental retardation syndrome
r. scar
r. sclerosing lesion
radial-femoral delay
radial-renal syndrome
radiant warmer
radiata
corona r.
radiation
r. absorbed dose (rad)
adaptive r.
r. carcinogenesis
r. cystitis
r. danger
diagnostic r.
r. dose
r. dose limit
r. dysplasia
electromagnetic r.
r. encephalopathy
r. exposure
IF r.
intraoperative r.
involved-field r.
ionizing r.
r. necrosis
nuclear r.

R

radiation *(continued)*
  orthovoltage r.
  particulate r.
  r. pneumonitis
  postoperative pelvic r.
  state-of-the-art r.
  supervoltage r.
  r. syndrome
  r. therapy (RT)
  tissue tolerance to r.
  r. tolerance
  whole abdominal r.
radiation-induced
  r.-i. heart disease (RIHD)
  r.-i. physial injury
radical
  r. excision
  free hydroxyl r.
  hydroxyl r. (OH)
  r. hysterectomy
  intrarenal venous r.
  r. local excision
  r. mastectomy
  oxygen-free r.
  r. parametrectomy
  r. posteromedial and plantar release
    (RPMPR)
  superoxide r.
  r. surgery
  r. surgical therapy
  r. vaginal trachelectomy
  r. vulvectomy
radicular neuropathy
radiculitis
  dorsal r.
radiculomyelitis
  acute ascending r.
  ascending r.
radiculoneuritis
  Lyme r.
radii *(pl. of* radius)
radioactive
  r. applicator
  r. cobalt
  r. colloid
  r. gold
  r. immunoassay
  r. implant
  r. isotope
  r. microsphere
  r. ribbons
  r. seed
  r. seed implantation
  r. tracer
  r. uptake
radioallergosorbent test (RAST)
radioantigen-binding assay (RABA)
radiocisternography
radiocontrast material

radiocurable
radiodermatitis
radiofibrinogen uptake scan
radiofrequency
  r. catheter ablation
  r. interstitial tissue ablation system
    (RITA)
radiogram
  sinus r.
radiograph
  abdominal r.
  cephalometric r.
  chest r.
  flat abdominal r.
  frogleg lateral r.
  intercondylar r.
  lateral r.
  Lauenstein lateral r.
  oblique r.
  occlusal r.
  panoramic r.
  plain abdominal r.
  scout r.
  serial r.
  sinus r.
  skyline view r.
  stress view r.
  upright abdominal r.
radiographic
  r. absorptiometry
  r. bone strength index (RBSI)
  r. pelvimetry
radiography
  chest r.
  digital r.
  quantitative digital r. (QDR)
  stereotactic r.
  tunnel-view r.
radioimmunoassay (RIA)
  Raji cell r.
  solid phase r.
radioimmunodetection (RAID)
radioimmunoprecipitation assay (RIPA)
radioimmunosorbent test (RIST)
radioiodination
radioiodine ablative therapy
radioisotope
  r. angiography
  r. cisternography
  r. milk scan
radioisotopic reperfusion and excretion study
radiolabeled
  r. fibrinogen
  r. white blood cell scan
radiological examination
radiologic stigmata
radiologist
  pediatric r.

radiolucent
 r. circular shadow in bladder
 r. line
radiomutation
radionuclide
 r. bone scan
 r. cineangiography
 r. heart scan
 r. imaging
 r. scanning
 r. scintigraphy
 r. venography
 r. voiding cystography (RVC)
radiopaque marker
radioreceptor assay
radioreceptor-guided surgery
radio-reno-ocular syndrome
radioresistant yolk sac tumor
radiosensitivity
radiosensitization
radiosurgery
 stereotactic r.
radiotherapy
 abdominal strip r.
 adjuvant r.
 fractionated sterotactic r.
 hyperfractionated r.
 pelvic boost r.
 plaque r.
 postoperative r.
 split-course hyperfractionated r.
radiotracer
radioulnar
 r. synostosis
 r. synostosis, developmental
 retardation, hypotonia syndrome
 r. synostosis, short stature,
 microcephaly, scoliosis, mental
 retardation syndrome
radium
 r.-226 (^{226}Ra)
 r. implant
 intracavitary r.
RADIUS
 routine antenatal diagnostic imaging with
 ultrasound
 RADIUS trial
radius, pl. **radii (R)**
 absent r.
 hypoplastic r.

 thrombocytopenia absent radii
 thrombocytopenia absent r. (TAR)
radon-222 (^{222}Rn)
Radovici
 R. reflex
 R. sign
raf protooncogene
RAG
 recombinase activating gene
 RAG deficiency
rage
 violent r.
ragged
 r. red fiber (RRF)
 r. red myopathy
ragweed pollen
RAID
 radioimmunodetection
railroad
 r. nystagmus
 r. track line
Raimondi catheter
Raine syndrome
raised
 r. lesion
 r. raspberry-like papilloma
 r. red-black telangiectasia
Raji
 R. cell
 R. cell assay
 R. cell radioimmunoassay
rale
 coarse r.
 crackling r.
 crepitant r.
 wet r.
raloxifene
 Study of Tamoxifen and R.
 (STAR)
RALPH
 renal, anus, lung, polydactyly,
 hamartoblastoma
 RALPH syndrome
Ralstonia pickettii
Rambam-Hasharon syndrome
rami (*pl. of* ramus)
ramipril
Ramon syndrome
ramosum
 Clostridium r.
RAMP hCG assay
Ramsay Hunt syndrome (I–III)

NOTES

Ramses Condom
Ramstedt
    R. disease
    R. operation
    R. procedure
    R. pyloromyotomy
Ramstedt-Fredet pyloromyotomy
ramus, pl. **rami**
    infrapubic r.
    ischiopubic r.
    pubic r.
    superior r.
rancid butter syndrome
Randall
    R. stone forceps
    R. suction curette
random
    r. mating
    r. regression model
    r. sampling
    r. X inactivation
randomization
randomized
randomly amplified polymorphic DNA
Ranfac knot pusher
range
    cervical tissue impedance r.
    chromatofocusing pH r.
    r. loss
    r. of motion (ROM)
range-gated Doppler (RGD)
ranitidine hydrochloride
RANS
    retinal arterial narrowing and straightening
Ranson criteria
RANTES
    regulated upon activation, normal T-cell expressed and secreted
ranula
RAO
    right anterior oblique
RAP
    receptor-associated protein
    recurrent abdominal pain
rapamycin
rape
    r. crisis evaluation
    r. evidence
    r. evidence kit
    r. kit use
    r. protocol
    statutory r.
    r. trauma syndrome
    r. treatment
raphe
    anococcygeal r.
    fused r.

    median r.
    r. of scrotum
rapid
    r. acquisition with resolution enhancement (RARE)
    r. alternating movement
    r. antigen detection test
    r. blinking
    r. bone loss
    r. descent
    r. dissolution formula (RDF)
    r. eye movement (REM)
    r. eye movement sleep
    r. filter testing
    r. filter testing for bacteriuria
    r. plasma reagin (RPR)
    r. plasma reagin card test
    r. rehydration
    r. sequence induction
    r. sequence intubation (RSI)
    r. slide test
    R. Strep screen
    r. strep test
    r. succession movement
    r. UF
rapidly
    first abarelix depot study for treating endometriosis r. (FASTER)
    r. progressive glomerulonephritis
rapid-onset dystonia, parkinsonism
Rapp-Hodgkin
    R.-H. ectodermal dysplasia
    R.-H. ectodermal dysplasia syndrome
RARE
    rapid acquisition with resolution enhancement
rare-cutter enzyme
rarefaction
rarefying osteitis
RARS
    refractory anemia with ring sideroblasts
RAS
    renin-angiotensin system
rasa
    tabula r.
rash
    allergic diaper r.
    ampicillin r.
    angiectatic skin r.
    atopic diaper r.
    blueberry muffin r.
    butterfly r.
    candidal diaper r.
    collarette of r.
    r. crop
    diaper r.
    diffuse morbilliform r.

discoid r.
drug-induced r.
ECM r.
eczematoid skin r.
eczematous r.
erythematous r.
evanescent maculopapular r.
friction diaper r.
heliotrope r.
irritation diaper r.
macular r.
maculopapular r.
malar r.
monilial diaper r.
morbilliform skin r.
nonvesicular r.
papular r.
papulosquamous r.
pellagralike skin r.
perioral r.
petechial r.
plaquelike r.
polymorphous r.
Prevex Baby Diaper R.
pruritic r.
psoriatic diaper r.
purpuric r.
roseola r.
salmon-pink r.
sandpaper r.
scarlatiniform r.
seborrheic diaper r.
skin r.
slapped cheek r.
truncal r.

Rashkind
R. atrial septostomy procedure
R. balloon
R. balloon atrial septostomy

Rasmussen
R. encephalitis
R. syndrome

raspberry-like papilloma
raspberry tongue
RAST
radioallergosorbent test
Rastelli
R. operation
R. procedure
R. repair
rat-bite fever

rate
aldosterone excretion r. (AER)
basal metabolic r. (BMR)
baseline fetal heart r.
beat-to-beat variability of fetal heart r.
birth r.
cerebral metabolic r.
contraceptive failure r.
cumulative conception r. (CCR)
detection r.
erythrocyte sedimentation r. (ESR)
fertility r.
fetal death r.
fetal heart r. (FHR)
flow r.
r. of fluid filtration (Qf)
glomerular filtration r. (GFR)
glucose production r. (GPR)
growth r.
heart r. (HR)
infant mortality r.
maternal death r.
maternal mortality r.
metabolic clearance r. (MCR)
mortality r.
neonatal mortality r.
nipple flow r.
ovulation r.
peak expiratory flow r. (PEFR)
peak flow r.
perinatal mortality r. (PMR, PNMR)
prevalence r.
purging r.
recurrence r.
resting metabolic r. (RMR)
sedimentation r.
seroprevalence r.
sinusoidal fetal heart r.
sinusoidal heart r. (SHR)
stillbirth r.
survival r.
ventricular response r.

Rathke pouch
rating
Apgar r.
sexual maturity r. (SMR)
Tanner sex maturity r.
ratio
albumin-globulin r. (A/G)

NOTES

ratio *(continued)*
  arterial to alveolar oxygen tension r.
  calcium-creatinine r. (Ca:Cr)
  cardiothoracic r.
  CD4:CD8 r.
  cerebral-placental r.
  corpus-to-cervix r.
  cough-pressure transmission r.
  crude risk r.
  estrogen/progesterone r.
  expiratory to inspiratory r.
  HC/AC r.
  head circumference/abdominal circumference r. (HC/AC)
  inspiratory to expiratory r. (I/E, I:E)
  intensity/duration r. (I/T)
  intensity/time r. (I/T)
  international normalized r. (INR)
  intrapulmonary shunt r. (Qs/Qt)
  lecithin-sphingomyelin r. (L/S)
  L/S r.
  milk-plasma r.
  myeloid to erythroid r. (M:E)
  odds r.
  ornithine to citrulline r.
  protein-to-urine creatinine r.
  right lung-head circumference r. (LHR)
  right-to-left shunt r. (Qs/Qt)
  risk-benefit r.
  S/D r.
  sex r.
  standardized incidence r. (SIR)
  systolic/diastolic r. (S/D)
  testosterone/dihydrotestosterone r.
  triene-to-tetraene r.
  umbilical artery pulsatility index to middle cerebral artery pulsatility index r.
  umbilical velocity r.
  upper body segment to lower body segment r. (U/L)
  urinary lactate:creatinine r.
  variance r.
  ventilation/perfusion r. (V̇/Q̇)
  waist:hip r. (WHR)
  zinc protoporphyrin to heme r. (ZnPP/H)
rationalize
rat tooth pickups
Rauber layer
Raven
  R. IQ
  R. Progressive Matrices (RPM)
Ravitch procedure
raw score

ray
  beta r.
  gamma r.
  intercalary defect of pollical r.
  pollical r.
Rayleigh-Tyndall scattering
Raynaud
  R. disease
  R. phenomenon (RP)
  R. sign
  R. syndrome
Ray-Tec sponge
Raz
  R. bladder neck suspension
  R. double-prong ligature carrier
  R. sling procedure
Raz-Leach procedure
Razoxane
RBBB
  right bundle branch block
RBC
  red blood cell
    RBC adenosine deaminase level
    fresh-packed RBCs
    RBC P antigen
RBF
  renal blood flow
RBM **gene**
RBSI
  radiographic bone strength index
RCCA
  right common carotid artery
RCDP
  rhizomelic chondrodysplasia punctata
    RCDP syndrome
RCF
  Ross carbohydrate-free
    RCF formula
RCM
  restrictive cardiomyopathy
RCMAS, RCMASA
  Revised Children's Manifest Anxiety Scale
RD1000 resuscitator
RDA
  recommended daily allowance
  recommended dietary allowance
  right ductus arteriosus
RDEB
  recessive dystrophic epidermolysis bullosa
RDF
  rapid dissolution formula
    Adriamycin RDF
RDFC
  recurring digital fibroma of childhood
RDS
  respiratory distress syndrome
    neonatal RDS

REA
rollerball endometrial ablation
reabsorption
REACH
rehabilitation among women with
coronary artery disease
reactant
acute-phase r.
Reactine
reaction
acetowhite r.
acrosome r.
acute transfusion r.
adverse drug r. (ADR)
adverse food r.
anaphylactic r.
anaphylactoid r.
anorectic r.
arbitrarily primed polymerase
chain r.
Arias-Stella r.
Arthus r.
association r.
automatic movement r.
balance r.
biphasic anaphylactic r.
bullous r.
chain r.
Chlamydia trachomatis ligase
chain r.
circular r.
coccidioidin r.
conversion r.
cortical r.
decidual r.
delayed transfusion r.
dermatophytid r.
diazo r.
dysphoric r.
dystonic r.
early asthmatic r.
equilibrium r.
febrile nonhemolytic transfusion r.
Felix-Weil r.
ferric chloride r.
fetomaternal transfusion r.
fungal id r.
gliotic r.
Gomori trichrome r.
harlequin r.
hypersensitivity r.
id r.

immediate hypersensitivity r.
immunologic r.
insect sting r.
intrusive stress r.
inverse polymerase chain r.
Jarisch-Herxheimer r.
Koebner r.
laser r.
late asthmatic r.
leukemoid r.
ligase chain r. (LCR)
linear Koebner r.
Mitsuda r.
mixed agglutination r. (MAR)
modified Gomori trichrome r.
neonatal leukemoid r.
nonhemolytic r.
paradoxical pupil r.
Paul-Bunnell r.
periosteal r.
photoallergic r.
phototoxic r.
polymerase chain r. (PCR)
Porter-Silber r.
postural r.
primary circular r.
prokaryotic r.
pupil r.
reverse transcription polymerase
chain r. (RT-PCR)
righting r.
secondary circular r.
serum sickness-like r.
Shwartzman r.
single primer amplification r.
startle r.
Staudinger r.
stranger r.
stress r.
transfusion r.
twin-to-twin transfusion r.
urine ligase chain r.
vagal r.
van den Bergh r.
Weil-Felix r.
wheal and flare r.
zona r.
reactivation tuberculosis
reactive
r. adenopathy
r. airway
r. airways disease (RAD)

NOTES

reactive *(continued)*
    r. arthritis
    r. attachment disorder of infancy
      or early childhood
    r. epilepsy
    r. oxygen species (ROS)
    r. perforating collagenosis (RPC)
    r. psychosis
    r. site (RS)
    r. site mutation
reactivity
    fetal heart rate r.
    skin test r. (STR)
    substance P immune r.
    vascular r.
reactogenicity
reader
    AutoPap r.
    PapNet r.
readiness
    fetal lung r.
    Pediatric Examination of
      Educational R. (PEER)
reading
    r. disability
    r. frame
reagent
    antiimmunoglobulin r.
    r. strip
    TRIzol r.
reagin
    rapid plasma r. (RPR)
Reality
    R. condom
    R. vaginal pouch
real-time
    r.-t. B-scanner
    r.-t. echocardiography
    r.-t. imaging on ultrasound
    r.-t. sonography
    r.-t. ultrasonography
reanastomosis
    microsurgical tubal r. (MTR)
    tubocornual r.
REAR
    renal-ear-anal-radial
    REAR syndrome
rearfoot
    r. valgus
    r. varus
rearing parents
rearrangement
    balanced chromosome r.
    de novo balanced chromosome r.
rebelliousness
rebound
    behavioral r.
    r. dermatitis
    r. edema

    r. hyperglycemia
    r. hypertension
    r. phenomenon
    r. tenderness
recalcitrant condyloma
recall phenomenon
Récamier
    R. operation
    R. procedure
recanalization
    tubal r.
receiver operating characteristic (ROC)
receptive
    r. aphasia
    r. language
    r. language development
Receptive-Expressive
    R.-E. Emergent Language Scale
      (REEL)
    R.-E. Emergent Language Scale,
      2nd Edition (REEL-2)
receptivity
    vaginal r.
receptor
    activated estrogen r.
    adrenergic r.
    alpha-adrenergic r.
    alpha-chemokine r.
    androgen r.
    r. assay
    AT1, AT2 r.
    beta r.
    beta-adrenergic r.
    beta-chemokine r.
    calcitonin r.
    complement r.
    cough r.
    r. coupling
    r. cross talk
    endogenous opiate r.
    endometrial r.
    epidermal growth factor r. (EGFR)
    E-rosette r.
    estradiol r.
    estrogen r. (ER)
    fibroblast growth factor r. (FGFR,
      FGF-R)
    fibronectin r.
    G-protein-coupled r.
    granulocyte colony-stimulating
      factor r. (G-CSF-R)
    growth hormone r. (GHR)
    H1 r.
    hormone complex r.
    human EP1 r.
    r. for hyaluronan-mediated motility
      (RHAMM)
    iC3b r.
    r. internalization

irritant r.
J pulmonary r.
keratinocyte growth factor r.
(KGFR)
leptin r.
ligand r.
Notch r.
opiate r.
progesterone r. (PgR, PR)
p55 soluble tumor necrosis
factor r.
p75 soluble tumor necrosis
factor r.
soluble tumor necrosis factor r.
steroid hormone r.
transferrin r. (TfR)
type A IL-8 r.
type B IL-8 r.
tyrosine kinase r.
vitamin D r. (VDR)
receptor-associated protein (RAP)
receptor-mediated endocytosis
recess
epitympanic r.
suprapineal r.
recession
sternal r.
recessive
r. allele
autosomal r. (AR)
r. deafness-onychodystrophy
syndrome
r. disorder
r. disorder defect
r. dystrophic epidermolysis bullosa
(RDEB)
r. enhanced S-cone syndrome
r. gene
r. inheritance
r. Leber congenital amaurosis
peroneal atrophy, X-linked r.
r. trait
r. Usher syndrome
X-linked r. (XLR)
r. X-linked chondrodysplasia
punctata
rechallenge
recidivism
recipient twin
reciprocal
r. cross
r. gene

r. movement
r. translocation
reciprocating
r. gait
r. gait orthosis (RGO)
recirculation
enterohepatic r.
Recklinghausen
R. disease (type I, II)
R. tumor
Reclomide
Reclus disease
recognition
facial affect r.
recognizable viral syndrome (RVS)
recoil
arm r.
Recombigen assay
recombinant
r. antihemophilic factor
r. chromosome 8 syndrome
r. clone
r. DNA
r. DNA technique
r. DNA technology
r. enzyme
r. enzyme replacement therapy
r. factor VIIa
r. follicle stimulating hormone
(rFSH)
r. FSH preparation
r. hepatitis B immunization series
r. hepatitis B vaccine
r. human erythropoietin (r-EPO,
rHuEPO, rHuEpo)
r. human growth hormone (rhGH)
r. human insulin-like growth factor-
1 (rhIGF-1)
r. human MIP-1 alpha
r. human superoxide dismutase
(rhSOD)
r. immunosorbent assay (RIBA)
r. inbred strain
r. interleukin 2 (rIL-2)
r. OspA
r. outer surface protein A (rOspA)
r. substitution line
r. tissue type plasminogen activator
(rt-PA)
recombinase
r. activating gene (RAG)
Recombinate

NOTES

R

recombination
    r. fraction
    r. frequency
    homologous r.
    r. map
Recombivax
    R. HB
    R. HB immunization
recommendation
    diet r.
    exercise r.
    screening r.
    treatment r.
recommended
    r. daily allowance (RDA)
    r. dietary allowance (RDA)
reconfiguration for neovagina
reconstitute
reconstitution
reconstruction
    Abbe-McIndoe vaginal r.
    autologous r.
    cleft lip-nasal r.
    Dibbell cleft lip-nasal r.
    fascial r.
    laryngotracheal r.
    nonautologous r.
    right ventricular outflow tract r.
    transvaginal ultrasound-guided
      urethral r.
    umbilicus r.
    uterine r.
    ventricular outflow tract r.
    Young-Dees-Leadbetter bladder
      neck r.
reconstructive
    r. mammaplasty
    r. pelvic surgery
record
    bring-your-own medical r.
    daily fetal movement r.
    delivery r.
    Infant Behavior R. (IBR)
    women-held antenatal r.
recorder
    Digitrapper portable pH r.
    Dopcord r.
    multichannel r.
    VitaGuard 1000 event r.
recording
    closed-circuit video r.
    gastroesophageal reflux-reflex
      apnea r.
recovered memory
recovery
    bacterial r.
    fluid-attenuated inversion r.
      (FLAIR)
    labor, delivery, and r. (LDR)

    oocyte r.
    r. score
    r. time
    ultrasonic egg r.
recreational drug
recrudescence of fever
recrudescent typhus
recruitment
    alveolar r.
    lung r.
rec 8 syndrome
rectal
    r. administration
    r. balloon manometry
    r. canal
    r. cancer
    r. compliance testing
    r. examination
    r. fissure
    Fleet Babylax R.
    Hemet R.
    r. injury
    r. linitis plastica (RLP)
    R. Medicone
    r. node
    Phenergan R.
    r. pillar
    r. pouch
    r. pressure
    Proctocort R.
    r. prolapse
    RMS R.
    Rowasa R.
    r. sensation
    r. stump
    r. suppository
    r. swab
    r. temperature
    Tigan R.
    r. vault
    r. wall resection
rectal-fourchette fistula
recti
    diastasis r.
rectilinear profile
rectoabdominal examination
rectoanal inhibitory reflex
rectocele
    r. repair
rectocolonic saline enema
rectolabial fistula
rectopexy
    abdominal r.
    anterior resection r.
rectosacral space
rectoscopic endometrial ablation
rectoscopy
rectosigmoid
    r. carcinoma

r. colon
r. colon endometriosis
rectosigmoidectomy
Altemeier perineal r.
rectosphincteric
r. reflex
r. reflux
rectourethral fistula
rectouterine
r. cul-de-sac
r. fold
r. pouch
rectovaginal
r. examination
r. fascia defect repair
r. fistula
r. septum
r. space
rectovestibular fistula
rectovulvar fistula
rectum
aganglionic r.
by way of r. (p.r.)
rectus
r. abdominis
r. abdominis muscle
r. femoris
r. femoris muscle
r. palsy
r. sheath
recumbent infant board
recurrence
pelvic r.
pulmonary r.
r. rate
r. risk
recurrens
periadenitis mucosa necrotica r.
recurrent
r. abdominal pain (RAP)
r. ADEM
r. affective disorder
r. anaphylaxis
r. aneuploidy
r. angioedema
r. aphthous stomatitis
r. aspiration pneumonia
r. bacterial meningitis
r. blister
r. candida
r. carcinoma
r. cholangitis

r. coarctation
r. convulsive seizure
r. epistaxis
r. euploidic abortion
r. fungal meningitis
r. genital aphthous ulcer
r. gross hematuria (RGH)
r. headache
r. hemolytic uremia syndrome
r. hernia formation
r. herpetic outbreak
r. ITP
r. Japanese encephalitis virus
r. jaundice of pregnancy
r. laryngeal nerve paralysis
r. lymphoma
r. miscarriage
r. molar pregnancy
r. myoglobinuria
r. nonconvulsive seizure
r. otitis media
r. pregnancy loss
r. purulent meningitis
r. pyogenic lymphadenitis
r. respiratory papillomatosis (RRP)
r. sinusitis
r. spontaneous abortion (RSA)
r. staphylococcal infection
r. vaginitis
recurrentis
Borrelia r.
recurring digital fibroma of childhood (RDFC)
recurvatum
r. deformity
genu r.
pectus r.
recycling
medullary r.
red
r. blood cell (RBC)
r. blood cell antigen
r. blood cell cast
r. blood cell enzyme deficiency
r. blood cell membrane
r. blood cell membrane defect
r. blood cell phosphoglycerate kinase deficiency
r. blood cell product
r. blood cell sickling
r. blood cell spiny projection
r. blood cell tagged scan

NOTES

red *(continued)*
    r. blood cell transfusion
    r. blood cell volume
    r. degeneration
    r. desaturation
    r. fundus
    r. glass test
    r. nucleus
    r. photoplethysmography
    r. reflex
    r. reflex test
    r. rubber catheter
    r. strawberry tongue
red-black telangiectasia
Reddick-Saye forceps
Redi-kit
    LEEP R.-k.
redirection
    intraatrial r.
RediTab
    Claritin R.
Redi+Wash cleansing system
reduced
    r. bladder capacity
    r. hemoglobin
    r. liver transplant (RLT)
reduced-size liver transplant (RSLT)
reducer
    Axid AR Acid R.
reducible hernia
reducing substance
reductase
    5-alpha r.
    dihydrofolate r.
    dihydropteridine r.
    17-ketosteroid r. deficiency
    methylene tetrahydrofolate r.
      (MTHFR)
reduction
    air r.
    chromosome r.
    embryo r.
    failed r.
    fetal r.
    fracture r.
    funic r.
    hydrostatic r.
    Lejour-type modified breast r.
    limb r.
    r. mammaplasty
    manual r.
    multifetal pregnancy r. (MFPR,
      MPR)
    multiple pregnancy r. (MPR)
    pregnancy r.
    r. of protrusion
    selective transvaginal embryo r.
    in utero r.
    weight r.

redundant
    r. hymen
    r. skin
REE
    resting energy expenditure
Reed-Sternberg cell
Reed syndrome
REEL
    Receptive-Expressive Emergent
      Language Scale
REEL-2
    Receptive-Expressive Emergent
      Language Scale, 2nd Edition
reel foot
reentrant supraventricular tachycardia
Reese Clark protocol
Reese-Ellsworth classification
Reese's Pinworm Medicine
reexperiencing
refeeding
reference
    ambiguous r.
referential cohesion
referred pelvic pain
Refetoff syndrome
refill
    capillary r.
    poor capillary r.
    prolonged capillary r.
reflectance
    r. photometer
    r. pulse oximetry (RPO)
reflection
    bladder r.
    corneal light r.
    peritoneal r.
reflectometry
    acoustic r.
    spectral gradient acoustic r.
      (SGAR)
reflex
    acoustic blink r.
    anal wink r.
    anocutaneous r.
    r. anoxic seizure
    asymmetric tonic neck r. (ATNR)
    automatic r.
    autonomic walking r.
    axon r.
    Babinski r.
    Babkin r.
    Bezold-Jarisch r.
    biceps r.
    bite r.
    blink r.
    bowing r.
    brachioradialis r.
    bregmocardiac r.
    Breuer-Hering inflation r.

bulbocavernosus r.
bulbocavernous r.
cat's eye r.
cochleopalpebral r.
conditioned orientation r. (COR)
cremasteric r.
crossed adductor r.
crossed extension r.
darkened r.
darwinian r.
dazzle r.
deep tendon r. (DTR)
delayed deep tendon r.
diving r.
doll's eye r.
ear-cough r.
ejection r.
embrace r.
r. epilepsy
esophago-UES-contractile r.
extrusion r.
fencing r.
Ferguson r.
flexion r.
forced grasp r.
forced grasping r.
gag r.
Gallant r.
Gamper bowing r.
gastrocolic r.
Gordon r.
grasp r.
Grünfelder r.
Head r.
Hering-Breuer inflation r. (HBIR)
Hoffmann r.
r. HPV test
r. incontinence
r. irritability
knee jerk r.
labial r.
labyrinthine r.
Landau r.
laryngeal adductor r. (LAR)
laryngeal vagal r.
letdown r.
r. ligament
lip r.
macular light r.
Magnus and de Kleijn tonic
 neck r.
markedly decreased r.

McCarthy r.
milk ejection r.
Moro r.
r. myoclonus
nasolabial r.
near gaze r.
neck r.
neck-righting r.
obligatory primitive r.
obligatory tonic neck r.
oculocephalic r.
oculocephalogyric r.
Oppenheim r.
oral r.
palmar grasp r.
palmar grasping r.
palm-chin r.
palmomental r.
palpebral r.
parachute r.
patellar r.
pathologic r.
r. pathway
r. pattern
Peiper r.
Perez r.
physiologic r.
placing r.
plantar grasp r.
positive support r.
postural r.
primitive r.
propping r.
pull-to-sit r.
pupillary red r.
Radovici r.
rectoanal inhibitory r.
rectosphincteric r.
red r.
rhinobronchial r.
righting r.
rooting r.
Rossolimo r.
sacral r.
snout r.
startle r.
stepping r.
r. stepping
sucking r.
suckling r.
support r.
swallow r.

NOTES

reflex *(continued)*
    swallowing r.
    swimming r.
    symmetrical tonic neck r. (STNR)
    r. sympathetic dystrophy (RSD)
    r. syncope
    tendon stretch r.
    tongue protrusion r.
    tonic labyrinthine r.
    tonic neck r. (TNR)
    triceps r.
    truncal incurvation r.
    walking r.
    white pupillary r.

reflexology

reflex-placing response

reflux
    acid r.
    r. of air
    alkaline r.
    complicated gastroesophageal r.
    contralateral r.
    dilating r.
    esophageal r.
    r. esophagitis
    extraesophageal r. (EER)
    gastroesophageal r. (GER)
    gastrointestinal r.
    intrarenal r.
    menstrual r.
    nasopharyngeal r. (NPR)
    r. nephropathy
    r. neuropathy (RN)
    physiologic r.
    primary vesicoureteral r.
    rectosphincteric r.
    secondary vesicoureteral r.
    silent gastroesophageal r.
    ureterovesical r.
    urinary r.
    vesicoureteral r. (grade 1–4) (VUR)
    vesicoureteric r. (grade 1–4) (VUR)

refractile body

refraction

refractive error

refractory
    r. anemia of pregnancy
    r. anemia with ring sideroblasts (RARS)
    r. ascites
    r. Crohn disease
    r. depressive symptom
    r. dyserythropoietic anemia
    r. epistaxis
    r. hypoglycemia
    r. sprue
    r. status epilepticus (RSE)

Refsum
    R. disease
    R. syndrome

refusal to bear weight

Regan-Lowe medium

regard
    prolonged r.
    visual r.

Regenbogen-Donnai syndrome

regeneration
    aberrant r.
    tissue r.

regimen
    add-back r.
    COMP drug r.
    conditioning r.
    downregulation r.
    feeding r.
    hypertransfusion r.
    monophasic r.
    platinum-based r.
    Pritchard intramuscular r.
    Zuspan r.

region
    breakpoint cluster r. (bcr)
    flanking r.
    hilar r.
    parietooccipital r.
    perimesencephalic r.
    Prader-Willi syndrome critical r. (PWSCR)
    regulatory r.
    sequence characterized amplified r.
    sex-determining r. (SRY)
    subependymal r.
    subpial r.
    zygomaticofrontal r.

regional
    r. analgesia
    r. block anesthesia
    r. enteritis
    r. gas exchange (R_{AW})
    r. ileitis
    r. lymphadenitis
    r. nerve block
    r. perinatal intensive care center (RPICC)
    r. wall motion abnormality

register
    high-risk r. (HRR)
    r. linkage study

registry
    cord blood r. (CBR)
    Herbst r.
    National Pediatric Trauma R. (NPTR)
    Teratogen R.

Reglan

Regonol Injection

regression
> change-point r.
> Galton law of r.
> r. of the mean
> premature luteal r.
> trophoblast in r. (TIR)
> tumor r.

regressive infantilism

regular
> R. Iletin I, II
> r. immune globulin
> r. purified pork insulin

regulated upon activation, normal T-cell expressed and secreted (RANTES)

regulation
> arginine vasopressin r.
> Baby Doe r.'s
> cellular r.
> gonadotropin r.
> menstrual cycle r.
> molecular r.
> physiologic follicular r.
> pituitary gonadotropin r.
> plasma volume r.
> prolactin r.

regulator
> autoimmune r. (AIRE)
> cystic fibrosis transmembrane r. (CFTR)
> r. gene
> Medela membrane r.

regulatory
> r. region
> r. sequence

Reguloid

regurgitant
> r. fraction
> r. murmur

regurgitate

regurgitation
> aortic r.
> effortless r.
> gastric r.
> mitral r.
> nasal r.
> physiologic r.
> pulmonic r.
> tricuspid r.

rehabilitate

rehabilitation
> r. among women with coronary artery disease (REACH)
> r. cookie swallow

Rehydralyte formula

rehydration
> rapid r.

Reichel cloacal duct

Reid sleeve

Reifenstein syndrome

Reiki

Reilly granule

reimplant
> common sheath r.

reimplantation
> extravesical ureteral r.
> r. of ureter
> ureteral trigonal r.

Reiner-Beck snare

Reiner-Knight forceps

reinforcement
> contingent r.
> negative r.
> positive r.

reinfusion
> autologous bone marrow r.

Reinke
> crystalloids of R.
> R. crystalloids

reinsemination

reinsufflated

Reissner membrane

Reis-Wertheim vaginal hysterectomy

Reiter syndrome

reject
> zero r.

rejecting

rejection
> accelerated r.
> acute r.
> allograft r.
> chronic r.
> fetal r.
> hyperacute r.

ReJuveness

relapse
> bone marrow r.
> testicular r.

relapsing
> r. fever
> r. infectious polyneuritis
> r. iridocyclitis

NOTES

relapsing *(continued)*
   r. nodular nonsuppurative
      panniculitis
related
   alcohol r. (AR)
   r. services
relation
   peer r.
relationship
   antecedent-behavior-consequence r.
   avuncular r.
   bisexual r.
   blood r.
   depth r.
   Frank-Starling r.
   gay r.
   heterosexual r.
   lesbian r.
   Poiseville-Hagen r.
   same-sex r.
   sexual r.
   spatial r.
relative
   r. afferent defect
   blood r.
   r. macroglossia
   r. osteopenia
   r. polycythemia
   r. risk
   r. shunt
   r. sterility
   r. vascular resistance (RVR)
relaxant
   muscle r.
relaxation
   pelvic r.
   pelvic girdle r. (PGR)
   pyloric sphincter r.
   r. technique
   uterine r.
   r. volume
relaxin
   intracervical purified porcine r.
   r. serum level
   vaginal recombinant human r.
release
   Acutrim Precision R.
   R. catheter
   colonoscopic r.
   complete subtalar r. (CSTR)
   counterregulatory hormone r.
   GnRH-facilitated FSH r.
   GnRH-facilitated LH r.
   growth hormone r.
   hip adduction r.
   increased renin r.
   myofascial r.
   neurotransmitter r.
   pituitary hormone r.

postganglionic acetylcholine r.
pulsatile r.
radical posteromedial and plantar r.
   (RPMPR)
Sever r.
shear stress-mediated nitric oxide r.
soft tissue r.
Relenza
reliability
Reliance urinary control insert catheter
relief
   Fleet Pain R.
ReliefBand device
religiosity
REM
   rapid eye movement
      REM latency
      REM parasomnia
      REM PolyHesive II patient return
         electrode
      REM sleep
      REM sleep behavior disorder
Remifemin Menopause tablet
remifentanil
remineralization
remission
   complete r.
   induced r.
   spontaneous r.
remnant
   branchial cleft r.
   omphalomesenteric duct r.
   tracheobronchial r.
remodeling
   bone r.
   fracture r.
remote afterloading brachytherapy
   (RAB)
removal
   extracorporeal CO_2 r. (ECOR)
   hysteroscopic r.
   surgical r.
remyelination
Renaissance spirometry system
renal
   r. acidification
   r. agenesis
   r. aminoaciduria
   r., anus, lung, polydactyly,
      hamartoblastoma (RALPH)
   r. artery stenosis
   r. biopsy
   r. blastema
   r. blood flow (RBF)
   r. calculus
   r. calyx
   r. candidiasis
   r. cell carcinoma
   r. clearance test

R

r. colic
r. cortex
r. cortex cyst
r. cortical necrosis
r. cortical nephropathy
r. cystic disease
r. duplication
r. dysfunction
r. dysgenesis
r. ectopia
r. electrolyte wasting
r. failure
r. Fanconi syndrome
r. fistula
r. function test
r. fungus ball
r. glycosuria
r. hypercalciuria
r. hyperechogenicity
r. hypertension
r. hypodysplasia
r. impairment
r. infarction
r. insufficiency
r. interstitium
r. loss
r. malrotation
r. manifestation
r. medullary carcinoma
r. medullary dysplasia
r. mesangial sclerosis-eye defects
   syndrome
r. mycetoma
r. myofibromatosis
r. obstruction
r. osteodystrophy
r. parenchyma
r. pedicle
r. pelvis
r. perfusion
r. plasma flow
r. proteinuria
r. reserve filtration capacity
   (RRFC)
r. rickets
r. salt wasting
r. scarring
r. scintigraphy
r. solute load (RSL)
r. stone
r. tract
r. transplantation

r. tuberculosis
r. tubular acidosis (RTA)
r. tubular bicarbonate wasting
r. tubular crystalluria
r. tubular epithelial cell
r. tubular Fanconi syndrome
r. tubular function
r. tubular necrosis
r. tubular pituitary syndrome
r. tubule
r. ultrasound
r. vascular resistance
r. vascular thrombosis
r. vasculitis
r. vein
r. vein thrombosis
renal-ear-anal-radial (REAR)
Rendu-Osler-Weber
   R.-O.-W. disease
   R.-O.-W. syndrome
Renese
reniform pelvis
renin
   elevated r.
   r. substrate
renin-angiotensin-aldosterone system
renin-angiotensin system (RAS)
Renografin
renogram
   MAG-3 diuretic r.
renography
   diuretic r.
renovascular
   r. hypertension
Renpenning syndrome
reossification
reossify
Reoviridae
Reovirus (type 1–3)
reoxygenation
repair
   abdominal paravaginal r.
   anterior and posterior r.
   A&P r.
   Cantwell-Ransley r.
   CDH r.
   clawhand deformity r.
   cleft palate r.
   cystocele r.
   Danus-Stanzel r.
   defect-specific r.
   delayed r.

NOTES

repair *(continued)*
    enterocele r.
    episiotomy r.
    hypospadias r.
    imperforate anus r.
    intraatrial r.
    Macer abdominal cystocele r.
    Noble-Mengert perineal r.
    Orr rectal prolapse r.
    palate r.
    paravaginal cystocele r.
    perineal r.
    Phaneuf-Graves r.
    posterior r.
    primary cleft palate r.
    Rastelli r.
    rectocele r.
    rectovaginal fascia defect r.
    Richardson paravaginal r.
    Senning r.
    Snodgrass hypospadias r.
    sphincter r.
    staged r.
    surgical r.
    Tennison-Randall r.
    transannular patch r.
    vaginal wall r.
    vesicovaginal r.
    York-Mason r.
    Zancolli clawhand deformity r.

repeat
    r. cesarean section
    r. curettage
    inter-simple sequence r.
    inverted r.
    simple sequence r.

repeated
    r. abortion
    r. complete mole
    r. partial seizure
    r. pregnancy loss (RPL)

repeat-loop excision

repellent
    insect r.

reperfusion injury

repermeabilization

repetitive
    r. DNA
    r. pregnancy loss

replacement
    cephalic r.
    esophageal r.
    estrogen r.
    fluid r.
    frozen embryo r. (FER)
    gamma globulin r.
    heart valve r.
    pancreatic enzyme r.

    PTH for osteoporotic women on estrogen r. (POWER)
    r. therapy
    volume r.

replenishment

Replens lubricant

replicate

replication
    DNA r.
    r. fork

replicon

Repliform alternative product

Replogle
    R. suction catheter
    R. sump tube

r-EPO
    recombinant human erythropoietin

repolarization

report
    Janus r.
    Walton r.

reporter

repositioning
    scapular r.

representation
    internal r.
    symbolic r.

representative section

repressed gene

repressor gene

reproduction
    assisted r.
    vegetative r.

reproductive
    r. age
    r. axis
    r. cycle
    r. disorder
    r. endocrinology
    r. endocrinology-infertility
    r. failure
    r. function
    r. genetics
    r. history
    r. liberty
    r. mortality
    r. organ
    r. performance
    r. system
    r. system development
    r. technology
    r. toxin
    r. tract
    r. tract abnormality
    r. tract embryology
    r. wastage

Repronex

reptilase time

repulsion

R

requirement
    iron r.
    mineral r.
    minimum daily r. (MDR)
    nutrient r.
    nutritional r.
    resting oxygen r.
    sodium r.
    vitamin r.
RER
    rough endoplasmic reticulum
Rescriptor
rescue
    abdominal r.
    ablative therapy with bone
      marrow r.
    r. breathing
    r. cervical cerclage
    r. dose
    r. medication
    r. surfactant
    r. therapy
    trisomic r.
research
    HIV Epidemiology R. (HER)
    International Committee for
      Contraceptive R. (ICCR)
resectability
resecting intrapartum uterine wall
resection
    abdominoperineal r.
    atretic extrahepatic bile duct r.
    bile duct r.
    bowel loop r.
    bowel segment r.
    cornual r.
    cystoscopic transurethral tumor r.
    dilated bowel loop r.
    distal dilated bowel segment r.
    duodenal r.
    en bloc r.
    endocervical r. (ECR)
    endometrial r.
    endomyometrial r. (EMR)
    extrahepatic bile duct r.
    gallbladder r.
    hysteroscopic septum r.
    laparoscopic multiple-punch r.
    laparoscopic ureterosacral
      ligament r. (LUSLR)
    laterally extended endopelvic r.
    late uterine wedge r.
    liver lobe r.
    low rectal r.
    multiple-punch r.
    ovarian wedge r.
    pancreatic head r.
    perineal r.
    posterior rectal wall r.
    pulmonary r.
    rectal wall r.
    segmental r.
    surgical r.
    Torpin cul-de-sac r.
    transcervical r.
    transsphenoidal microsurgical r.
    in utero r.
    wedge r.
resection/ablation
    outpatient endometrial r. (OPERA)
Resectisol Irrigation Solution
resectoscope
    specialized tissue aspirating r.
      (STAR)
    USA Elite System GYN rotating
      continuous flow r.
reseeding
Resercen
reserpine
reservatus
    coitus r.
reserve
    coronary flow r. (CFR)
    r. zone (RZ)
reservoir
    Camey r.
    catheter r.
    double-bubble flushing r.
    ileal r.
    Mainz pouch urinary r.
    Ommaya r.
    Pudenz r.
    sperm r.
    subcutaneous ventricular catheter r.
    ventricular r.
residential program
residua (*pl. of* residuum)
residual
    r. coarctation
    r. ductal tissue
    r. hearing
    r. ovary syndrome
    postvoid r.
    r. in situ

NOTES

residual *(continued)*
r. urine
r. vision
r. volume (RV)

residue
gastric r.
methanol extraction r. (MER)

residuum, pl. **residua**

resin
cholestyramine r.
podophyllum r.

resistance
activated protein C r. (APCR)
airway r.
androgen r.
antibiotic r.
antiretroviral r.
bromocriptine r.
dicumarol r.
differential vascular r.
fetal pulmonary vascular r.
increased vascular r.
r. index (RI)
insulin r.
intrinsic flow r. (R_{int})
lithium r.
multidrug r. (MDR)
natural r.
peripheral insulin r.
pulmonary vascular r. (PVR)
relative vascular r. (RVR)
renal vascular r.
respiratory system r. (R_{rs})
systemic vascular r. (SVR)
thyroid hormone r.
tissue insulin r.
total peripheral r. (TPR)
total pulmonary r.
vascular r.
in vitro r.

resistant
ampicillin r.
r. condyloma
drug r.
r. ovary
r. ovary syndrome
r. pneumococcus

resisted abduction

resolution
axial r.
clot r.
lateral r.

resonance
nuclear magnetic r. (NMR)

resorption
r. atelectasis
bone r.
fetal r.

osteoclast-mediated bone r.
tooth root r.

resource
R. Just for Kids with Fiber formula
R. Plus formula
r. specialist
R. Standard formula

Respa-DM

Respa-GF

Resp-EZ piezoelectric sensor

RespiGam

Respihaler
Decadron R.

Respinol-G

respiration
agonal r.'s
artificial r.
Bouchut r.
Cheyne-Stokes r.
gasping r.
grunting r.
internal r.
Kussmaul r.
paradoxical r.
percutaneous aspiration, instillation of hypertonic saline, r. (PAIR)
placental r.
sighing r.
vicarious r.

respirator
Ambu r.
BABYbird r.
Babylog 8000 r.
Bath r.
Bear r.
Bennett r.
Bird Mark 8 r.
Bourns infant r.
Bragg-Paul r.
Breeze r.
Clevedon positive pressure r.
cuirass r.
Drinker r.
Emerson r.
Engstrom r.
Gill r.
Huxley r.
mechanical r.
Med-Neb r.
Merck r.
Monaghan r.
Morch r.
Moynihan r.
negative-pressure r.
portable r.
Sanders jet r.
Stephan HF 300 r.

respiratory
- r. acidosis
- r. alkalosis
- r. arrest
- r. burst assay
- r. chamber
- r. ciliary paralysis
- r. complication
- r. compromise
- r. cycle
- r. depression
- r. distress
- r. distress syndrome (RDS)
- r. distress syndrome of the newborn
- r. drive
- r. embarrassment
- r. enteric orphan
- r. enteric orphan virus
- r. epithelium
- r. failure
- r. index score (RIS)
- r. inductive plethysmography (RIP)
- r. insufficiency
- r. movement
- r. papilloma
- r. papillomatosis
- r. pattern
- r. quotient
- r. sinus arrhythmia
- r. suction
- r. suctioning
- r. support
- r. syncytial virus (RSV, RS-virus)
- r. syncytial virus antigen
- r. syncytial virus bronchiolitis (RSVB)
- r. syncytial virus immune globulin (RSVIG, RSV-IG)
- r. syncytial virus immunoglobulin (RSVIG, RSV-IG)
- r. syncytial virus intravenous immune globulin (RSV-IGIV, RSV-IVIG)
- r. syncytial virus intravenous immunoglobulin (RSV-IGIV, RSV-IVIG)
- r. syncytial virus pneumonia
- r. system
- r. system elastance (E_{dyn})
- r. system resistance (R_{rs})
- Taiwan acute r. (TWAR)

- r. therapist
- r. therapy
- r. therapy pack
- r. toilet
- r. tract
- r. tract infection

respiratory hippus
Respirgard II nebulizer
respite care
Respitrace inductance plethysmography
Respivir
response
- abnormal r.
- acute insulin r.
- age-related pharmacodynamic r.
- allergic inflammatory r.
- amnesic r.
- anamnestic immune r.
- antibody r.
- asthmatic r.
- auditory brainstem r. (ABR, ABSR)
- auditory evoked r. (AER)
- automated auditory brainstem r. (AABR, A-ABR)
- automated brainstem auditory evoked r. (ABAER)
- Babinski r.
- baroreflex r.
- biphasic r.
- Bobath r.
- brainstem auditory evoked r. (BAER, BSAER)
- brainstem evoked r. (BSER)
- buttress r.
- characteristic emotional r.
- chronotropic r.
- clasp-knife r.
- clinical r.
- cortisol r.
- r. cost
- cremasteric r.
- CTL r.
- cytotoxic lymphocyte r.
- doll's eye r.
- early asthmatic r. (EAR)
- emotional r.
- esophago-deglutition r.
- evoked r.
- fall-away r.
- female sexual r.
- fetal inflammatory r.

NOTES

response *(continued)*
fetal startle r.
fight-and-flight r.
glabellar r.
immune r.
infantile breath-holding r.
inflammatory r.
r. inhibition
insulin r.
Koebner r.
lactation letdown r.
Landau r.
late asthmatic r. (LAR)
r. latency
local inflammatory r.
maternal immune r.
maternal inflammatory r.
maternal vascular r.
menstrual cycle hemodynamic r.
metabolic r.
Moro r.
neck r.
neuroendocrine r.
oculovestibular r.
orgasmic motor r.
parachute r.
pharmacodynamic r.
placing r.
plantar r.
postinfectious immune r.
pressor r.
pupillary light r.
pyogranulomatous r.
reflex-placing r.
Rh immune r.
righting r.
sexual r.
sound-field r.
staircase r.
startle r.
stepping r.
stress r.
sympathetic skin r.
target organ r.
thermogenic r.
thermoregulatory r.
tonic neck r.
treppe r.
vagally mediated r.
visual evoked r. (VER)
Respules
Pulmicort R.
rest
antepartum bed r.
antepartum hospital bed r.
bed r.
cystic Walthard r.
ectopic pancreatic r.
gut r.

hospitalized bed r.
r., ice, compression, elevation (RICE)
intralobar r.
Marchand r.
mesonephric r.
nephrogenic r.
PediaCare Night R.
pelvic r.
prophylactic bed r.
Walthard cell r.
wolffian r.
resting
r. anal sphincter pressure
r. calorimetry
r. energy expenditure (REE)
r. membrane potential
r. metabolic rate (RMR)
r. oxygen requirement
restless
r. legs syndrome
r. sleep
restlessness
motor r.
Restore program
Restoril
restraint
child r.
restriction
asymmetric growth r.
at-home activity r.
r. endonuclease
r. endonuclease analysis
r. enzyme
r. enzyme cutting site
fetal growth r. (FGR)
fluid r.
r. fragment
r. fragment length polymorphism (RFLP)
intrauterine growth r. (IUGR)
r. landmark genomic scanning
r. map
maternal activity r.
normotensive intrauterine growth r.
salt r.
sodium r.
symmetric growth r.
restrictive
r. breathing pattern
r. cardiomyopathy (RCM)
r. dermopathy
r. lung disease
r. respiratory disease
restructuring
rest/sleep periods
result
Surveillance, Epidemiology and End R.'s (SEER)

resumption
menstrual cycle r.
resuscitate
resuscitation
bag and mask r.
cardiopulmonary r. (CPR)
cerebral r.
fluid r.
intrauterine r.
mouth-to-mouth r.
mouth-to-nose/mouth r.
neonatal r.
newborn r.
resuscitator
Ambu infant r.
Fisher and Paykel RD1000 r.
Laerdal r.
Penlon infant r.
RD1000 r.
Resyl
RETA
rete testis aspiration
retained
r. bladder syndrome
r. fetal lung fluid (RFLF)
r. foreign body
r. hygroscopic cervical dilator
r. membrane
r. menstruation
r. myoma
r. placenta
r. placental fragment
r. products of conception (RPC)
retardate
Screening Tests for Young
Children and R.'s
Sheridan Tests for Young Children
and R.'s
retardation
alopecia-mental r. (AMR)
alopecia universalis with mental r.
alpha-thalassemia/mental r. (ATR)
American Association on
Mental R. (AAMR)
aniridia, ambiguous genitalia,
mental r. (AGR)
r., aphasia, shuffling gait, adducted
thumbs syndrome
basal ganglion disorder-mental r.
(BGMR)
Belgian type mental r.

Buenos Aires type mental r.
cataract, hypertrichosis, mental r.
(CAHMR)
Charcot-Marie-Tooth syndrome, X-
linked type II with deafness and
mental r.
congenital progressive muscular
dystrophy with mental r.
r., deafness, microgenitalism
syndrome
deafness, onychoosteodystrophy,
mental r. (DOOR)
fetal growth r.
fragile site mental r. 1 (FMR1)
fragile site mental r. 2 (FMR2)
FRAXE-associated mental r.
growth r.
r. of growth and deafness
HbH related mental r.
head-sparing intrauterine growth r.
ichthyosiform erythroderma, hair
abnormality, mental and growth r.
infantile spasms with mental r.
intrauterine growth r. (IUGR)
linear growth r.
mental r.
mild mental r.
moderate mental r.
motor-sensory neuropathy, X-linked
type II, with deafness and
mental r.
multiple exostosis-mental r.
(MEMR)
nonprogressive cerebellar disorder
with mental r.
nonspecific mental r.
peripheral dysostosis, nail
hypoplasia, mental r. (PNM)
prenatal growth r.
profound mental r.
psychomotor r.
severe mental r.
Wilms tumor, aniridia, genitourinary
malformations, mental r.
Wilms tumor, aniridia,
gonadoblastoma, mental r.
(WAGR)
X-linked alpha-thalassemia/mental r.
(ATRX)
X-linked mental r. (1-47) (MRX,
XLMR)

R

NOTES

retarded
    r. fetal growth
    specific reading r. (SRR)
rete
    r. cord
    r. cyst of ovary
    r. peg
    r. ridge elongation
    r. testis
    r. testis aspiration (RETA)
retention
    carbon dioxide r.
    r. enema
    fetal r.
    fluid r.
    ovarian r.
    r. polyp
    sodium r.
    stool r.
    r. suture
    urinary r.
Rethoré syndrome
rethrombosis
reticula (*pl. of* reticulum)
reticular
    r. dermis
    r. dysgenesis
    r. reflex myoclonus
reticulare
    magma r.
reticularis
    adrenal r.
    livedo r.
    zona r.
reticulata
    substantia nigra pars r.
reticulated
    r. hyperpigmentation
    r. pigmentation
reticulocyte count
reticulocytopenia
reticulocytosis
reticuloendothelial
    r. cell
    r. sequestration
    r. system
reticuloendotheliosis
reticulogranular pattern
reticulonodular pattern
reticulum, pl. **reticula**
    endoplasmic r. (ER)
    rough endoplasmic r. (RER)
    sarcoplasmic r.
    stellate r.
Retin-A
retina, pl. **retinae**
    commotio retinae
    dragging of r.
    dysgenesis neuroepithelialis retinae

    embryonic neural r.
    hereditary epithelial dysplasia of
      the retinae
    macula of r.
    macula retinae
    mottled r.
    neural r.
    ora serrata retinae
retinaculum, pl. **retinacula**
    peroneal r.
retinal
    r. angioma
    r. aplasia
    r. arterial narrowing and
      straightening (RANS)
    r. change
    r. detachment
    r. dysplasia
    r. edema
    r. hemorrhage
    r. infiltrate
    r. pigmentary degeneration
    r. pigmentary degeneration,
      microcephaly, mental retardation
      syndrome
    r. pigment epithelium (RPE)
    r. pseudotumor
    r. vasculitis
    r. venous dilation and tortuosity
      (RVDT)
    r. vessel telangiectasia
retinitis
    CMV r.
    gravidic r.
    indolent granular CMV r.
    neuropathy, ataxia, r. pigmentosa
      (NARP)
    r. pigmentosa
    r. pigmentosa-congenital deafness
      syndrome
    proliferative r.
    salt and pepper r.
retinoblast
retinoblastoma
    bilateral r.'s
    hereditary r.
    trilateral r.
**retinoblastoma-mental retardation
  syndrome**
retinoic
    r. acid
    r. acid embryopathy
retinoid therapy
retinol
retinol-binding protein
retinopapillitis of prematurity
retinopathy
    diabetic r.
    eclamptic r.

gravidic r.
Keith-Wagener r.
r. of newborn
nonproliferative diabetic r.
r. of prematurity (ROP)
r. punctata albescens
Purtscher r.
toxemic r. of pregnancy
retinopathy-mental retardation syndrome
retinoschisis
congenital hereditary r.
hereditary r.
juvenile X-linked r.
X-linked r.
RET protooncogene
retractile testis
retraction
accessory muscle r.
intercostal r.
nipple r.
r. ring
skin r.
subcostal r.'s
substernal r.
supraclavicular r.
r. syndrome
retractive nystagmus
retractor
Airlift balloon r.
Allport r.
Army-Navy r.
Aufricht nasal r.
Balfour r.
Berkeley-Bonney r.
bladder r.
Bookwalter r.
Breisky-Navratil r.
Brewster r.
Brown uvula r.
Cer-View lateral vaginal r.
Cottle-Neivert r.
Deaver r.
DeLee Universal r.
Desmarres r.
Ferris Smith-Sewall r.
Gelpi perineal r.
Gott malleable r.
Goulet r.
Guardian vaginal r.
Haight baby r.
Harrington r.
Heaney hysterectomy r.

Heaney-Simon r.
Iron Intern r.
Jackson right-angle r.
Kelly r.
lateral wall r.
long atraumatic r.
Luer r.
malleable r.
Murless head r.
nasal r.
r. neuropathy
O'Connor-O'Sullivan r.
Omni-Tract vaginal r.
O'Sullivan-O'Connor r.
pediatric self-retaining r.
Richardson r.
right-angle r.
Roberts thumb r.
Schuknecht r.
self-retaining r.
Senn-Dingman r.
Shambaugh r.
Sims r.
thumb r.
vaginal r.
Weitlaner r.
Wullstein r.
retractorius
nystagmus r.
retraining
bladder r.
r. diary
retransposition
arterial r.
retrieval
egg r.
oocyte r.
ovarian r.
transvaginal ultrasound-directed
oocyte r. (TUDOR)
ultrasonographically guided
oocyte r.
ultrasound-directed egg r.
retroambiguus
nucleus r.
retroauricular
retrobulbar neuritis
retrocallosal
retrocaval ureter
retrocecal hernia
retrocerebellar arachnoidal cyst
retrocervical

NOTES

retrocession
retrochiasmatic
retrocollis
retroconversion
    chemotherapeutic r.
retrodeviation
retrodisplacement
retroesophageal abscess
retroflexion, retroflection
    uterine r.
retrognathia
retrognathism
retrograde
    r. amnesia
    r. axoplasmic flow
    r. ejaculation
    r. intussusception
    r. menstrual flow
    r. menstruation
    r. pyelogram
    r. pyelography
    r. ureteral dye injection
retrolental fibroplasia (RLF)
retromammary mastitis
retroorbital lymphoma
retroperitoneal
    r. dissection
    r. drain
    r. endometriosis
    r. fetus
    r. fibrosis
    r. hematoma
    r. infection
    r. laparoscopic procedure
    r. lymphadenectomy
    r. node
    r. soft tissue
    r. soft tissue sarcoma
retroperitoneum
retropharyngeal
    r. abscess
    r. cellulitis
    r. lymph node
retroplacental
    r. hematoma
    r. hemorrhage
retroposed
retroposition
retropubic
    r. colpourethrocystopexy
    r. cystourethropexy
    r. fibrosis
    r. sling
    r. space
    r. suspension procedure
    r. urethropexy
    r. urethropexy procedure
    r. vesicourethrolysis

retrorectal
    r. space
    r. transanal pull-through
retrosternal
    r. chest pain
    r. hernia
retrotonsillar abscess
retrotorsion
retrovaginal
    r. septum
    r. space
retroversioflexion
retroversion
    femoral r.
    uterine r.
retroverted
    r. uterus
Retrovir
retroviral
    r. disease
    r. syndrome
retrovirus
retrusion
Rett
    R. disorder
    R. syndrome
rettgeri
    Providencia r.
return
    partial anomalous pulmonary
      venous r. (PAPVR)
    supracardiac total anomalous
      pulmonary venous r.
    systemic caval r.
    total anomalous pulmonary
      venous r. (TAPVR)
returning-soldier effect
Retzius
    space of R.
Reuter tube
revascularization
ReVele
revenge fantasy
reversal
    dosage-sensitive sex r. (DSS)
    gender r.
    hyperandrogenism r.
    role r.
    sex r.
    tubal r.
    vasectomy r.
reverse
    r. banding
    r. chylous syndrome
    r. dot blot hybridization
    r. dot blot sequence-specific
      oligonucleotide method
    r. FISH cytogenetic technique
    r. form McRoberts maneuver

r. last shoe
r. Marcus Gunn sign
r. nostrils
r. 3 sign
r. transcriptase
r. transcriptase inhibitor (RTI)
r. transcription
r. transcription polymerase chain reaction (RT-PCR)
r. triiodothyronine

reversed end-diastolic flow
reversible
r. biliary pseudolithiasis
r. obstructive airway
r. oligospermia
r. posterior leukoencephalopathy syndrome (RPLS)

Reversol
ReVia
review
annual r.
r. of systems (ROS)

Revised
R. Children's Manifest Anxiety Scale (RCMAS, RCMASA)
R. Trauma Score (RTS)

revised
R. Children's Manifest Anxiety Scale (RCMAS, RCMASA)
Gesell Adaptive and Personal Behavior Domain, R.
Gesell Developmental Schedules, R.
Gesell Gross Motor Domain, R.
R. Gesell Language Domain
r. Jones criteria
r. Jones criteria for diagnosis of acute rheumatic fever
R. Tests of Cognitive Ability
R. Trauma Score (RTS)

revision
Dibbell cleft lip-nasal r.
lip scar r.
shunt r.

rewarming
extracorporeal r.

Reye
R. hepatic encephalopathy
R. syndrome

Reye-like syndrome

Reynell
R. Language Development Scale (RLDS)
R. Verbal Comprehension Test

Reynolds
R. Child Depression Scale
R. number
R. suicide ideation questionnaire

RF
rheumatoid factor

RFA
right femoral artery
right frontoanterior position

RFLF
retained fetal lung fluid

RFLP
restriction fragment length polymorphism
RFLP analysis

RF-negative juvenile polyarthritis
RFP
right frontoposterior position

RF-seropositive
rFSH
recombinant follicle stimulating hormone

RFT
right frontotransverse position

rFVIIa
RGD
range-gated Doppler

R-Gene
RGH
recurrent gross hematuria

RGO
reciprocating gait orthosis

Rh
rhesus
Rh antibody
Rh antigen
Rh blood group
Rh blood group system
Rh complex
Rh D disease
Rh disease of newborn
Rh factor
Gamulin Rh
Rh hemolytic disease
Rh immune globulin (RhIg)
Rh immune response
Rh immunization
Rh immunoglobulin
Rh incompatibility
Rh isoimmune hemolytic disease

NOTES

Rh *(continued)*
    Rh isoimmunization
    Rh null cell
    Rh sensitization
rhabdoid tumor
rhabdomyoblast
rhabdomyolysis
    copper-induced r.
    hyperthermic r.
    malignant hyperthermic r.
rhabdomyoma
    cardiac r.
    fetal cardiac r.
rhabdomyosarcoma (RMS)
    r. retinoblastoma
    undifferentiated r.
rhabdosphincter
rhagas, pl. **rhagades**
    periorificial rhagades
RHAMM
    receptor for hyaluronan-mediated motility
rhamnosus
    Lactobacillus r.
RhC
    rhesus antigen C
RhCE gene
RhD
    rhesus antigen D
    RhD gene
    RhD immunoglobulin
RhE
    rhesus antigen E
rhegmatogenous detachment
rheometer
rhesus (Rh)
    r. antibody
    r. antigen
    r. antigen C (RhC)
    r. antigen D (RhD)
    r. antigen E (RhE)
    r. factor
    r. isoimmunization
    r. rotavirus tetravalent vaccine
rheumatic
    r. carditis
    r. exanthema
    r. fever
    r. heart disease
    r. pneumonia
    r. valvular heart disease
rheumatica
    polymyalgia r.
rheumaticosis
rheumatism
    desert r.
    European League Against R.
      (EULAR)
    International League Against R.

rheumatogenic
    r. strain
    r. streptococcus
rheumatoid
    r. arthritis (RA)
    r. factor (RF)
    r. granuloma
    r. nodule
    r. spondylitis
    r. vasculitis
rheumatologic disorder
rheumatology
    International League of Associations
      for R. (ILAR)
Rheumatrex Oral
rhGH
    recombinant human growth hormone
RhIg
    Rh immune globulin
rhIGF-1
    recombinant human insulin-like growth
      factor-1
Rhinall Nasal Solution
rhinencephalon
rhinitis
    allergic r.
    eosinophilic nonallergic r.
    erosive r.
    infectious r.
    r. medicamentosa
    neutrophilic r.
    nonallergenic perrenial r.
    nonallergic r.
    perennial allergic r.
    pollen-induced r.
    r. of pregnancy
    purulent r.
    seasonal allergic r.
    serosanguineous r.
    r. sicca
    syphilitic r.
    vasomotor r.
rhinobronchial reflex
rhinobronchitis
rhinocephaly
rhinocerebral
    r. infection
    r. mucormycosis
rhinoconjunctivitis
    allergic r.
Rhinocort
    R. Aqua nasal spray
    R. Turbuhaler
rhinoprobe
rhinorrhea
    CSF r.
rhinoscopy

R

rhinosinusitis
  bacterial r.
  chronic r.
Rhinosyn-DMX
Rhino Triangle brace
rhinovirus
rhizomelia syndrome
rhizomelic
  r. brachymelia
  r. chondrodysplasia
  r. chondrodysplasia punctata
  (RCDP)
  r. dwarfism
  r. limb shortening
rhizotomy
  dorsal r.
  functional posterior r.
  posterior r.
  selective dorsal r. (SDR)
  selective posterior r.
Rh-negative
  Rh-negative antibody
  blood group D variant equivalent
  to Rh-negative (Du)
  Rh-negative mother
Rh-null syndrome
rhod-2
  calcium indicator r.-2
  r.-2 imaging
rhodamine
rhodamine-auramine stain
Rhodesian trypanosomiasis
Rho(D) immune globulin
Rhodis-EC
Rhodococcus equi
RhoGAM
rhombencephalitis
rhombencephalosynapsis
rhombomere segmentation
rhonchorous cough
rhonchus, pl. **rhonchi**
Rhoprolene
Rhoprosone
Rh-positive
  Rh-p. antibody
  Rh-p. infant
  Rh-p. red cell stroma
RHS
  radial head subluxation
Rh-sensitized fetus
rhSOD
  recombinant human superoxide dismutase

rHuEPO, rHuEpo
  recombinant human erythropoietin
rhus dermatitis
rhusiopathiae
  Erysipelothrix r.
Rhus javanica
rhysodes
  Acanthamoeba r.
rhythm
  circadian r.
  diurnal r.
  escape r.
  gallop r.
  irregular r.
  junctional r.
  r. method
  r. method of contraception
rhythmic movement disorder
RI
  resistance index
RIA
  radioimmunoassay
rib
  cervical r.
  r. fracture
  r. hump
  r. notching
  r. notching sign
  r. rotation
  r. splitting
  supernumerary r.
  wavy r.
RIBA
  recombinant immunosorbent assay
ribavirin
  aerosolized r.
  intraventricular r.
Ribbing
  R. disease
  R. skeletal abnormality
ribbon
  radioactive r.'s
ribbonlike stool
rib-gap defect-micrognathia syndrome
riboflavin deficiency
ribonuclease (RNase)
ribonucleic
  r. acid (RNA)
  r. acid probe
ribonucleic acid (RNA)
ribonucleoprotein antigen
ribonucleotide

NOTES

ribosomal RNA
ribosome
ribosuria
ribotide
    succinyl aminoimidazole
      carboxamide r. (SAICAR)
RICE
    rest, ice, compression, elevation
    RICE sequence
Ricelyte
rich
    calcium r.
    Rolaids Calcium R.
Richardson
    R. paravaginal repair
    R. retractor
Richards-Rundle syndrome
Richner-Hanhart syndrome
Richner syndrome
Richter
    R. and Albrich procedure
    R. hernia
ricin
ricinus
    Ixodes r.
rickets
    familial hypophosphatemic r.
    hypophosphatemic r.
    nonnutritional r.
    nutritional r.
    oncogenous r.
    primary hypophosphatemic r.
    renal r.
    vitamin D-dependent r.
    vitamin D-resistant r.
    X-linked hypophosphatemic r.
    (XLHR)
rickettsemia
Rickettsia
    R. africae
    R. akari
    R. australis
    R. conorii
    R. felis
    R. honei
    R. japonica
    R. prowazekii
    R. rickettsii
    R. siberica
    R. typhi
rickettsial
    r. agglutination
    r. disease
    r. infection
rickettsialpox
rickettsii
    Rickettsia r.
rickettsiosis

Rid
    R. gel
    R. liquid
    R. Mousse
    R. shampoo
Rid-A-Pain
Ridaura
Ridenol
ride-on toy
ridge
    alveolar r.
    apical ectodermal r.
    cervicovaginal r.
    ectodermal r.
    genital r.
    germ r.
    gonadal r.
    hyperkeratotic r.
    mesonephric r.
    transverse r.
    urogenital r.
    wolffian r.
ridging
    metopic r.
Riechert-Mundinger stereotactic system
Riedel lobe
Rieger
    R. anomaly
    R. malformation
    R. syndrome
rifabutin
Rifadin
rifampicin
rifampin
rifamycin, rifomycin
rifapentine
    25-desacetyl r.
Rift Valley fever
RIG
    rabies immune globulin
Riga-Fede disease
right
    r. acromiodorsoposterior position
    r. anterior oblique (RAO)
    r. aortic arch (RAA)
    r. atrial hypertrophy
    r. atrial pressure
    r. axis deviation
    r. to be well-born
    Breathe R.
    r. bundle branch block (RBBB)
    r. colon pouch
    r. common carotid
    r. common carotid artery (RCCA)
    r. ductus arteriosus (RDA)
    r. femoral artery (RFA)
    r. frontoanterior position (RFA)
    r. frontoposterior position (RFP)
    r. frontotransverse position (RFT)

r. hepatectomy
r. lateral position
left to r. (L-R)
R. Light examination light
r. lower quadrant (RLQ)
r. lung-head circumference ratio
(LHR)
r. lung hypoplasia
r. mentoanterior position (RMA)
r. mentoposterior position (RMP)
r. mentotransverse position (RMT)
r. middle lobe syndrome
r. occipitoanterior position (ROA)
r. occipitoposterior position (ROP)
r. occipitoposterior presentation
r. occipitotransverse position (ROT)
r. ovarian vein syndrome
r. sacroanterior position (RSA)
r. sacroposterior position (RSP)
r. sacrotransverse position (RST)
r. scapuloanterior position (RScA)
r. scapuloposterior position (RScP)
r. sit
termination of parental r.'s
r. upper quadrant (RUQ)
r. ventricle (RV)
r. ventricular dysplasia
r. ventricular hypertrophy (RVH)
r. ventricular hypoplasia
r. ventricular infundibulum
r. ventricular outflow tract (RVOT)
r. ventricular outflow tract
obstruction (RVOTO)
r. ventricular outflow tract
reconstruction
right-angle
r.-a. retractor
r.-a. scissors
righting
head r.
r. reaction
r. reflex
r. response
right-left discrimination
right-sided
r.-s. arch, mental deficiency, facial
dysmorphism syndrome
r.-s. heart failure
r.-s. lesion
r.-s. stomach
right-to-left
r.-t.-l. shunt

r.-t.-l. shunting
r.-t.-l. shunt ratio (Qs/Qt)
rigid
r. cerebral palsy
r. clubfoot
r. cystoscopy
r. metatarsus
r. open-tube endoscope
r. perfectionism
r. spine syndrome
r. supination deformity
rigid cystoscopy
rigidity
chest wall r.
congenital articular r.
decerebrate r.
multiple articular r.
muscle r.
nuchal r.
parkinsonian r.
rigidus
hallux r.
Rigiflex balloon
rigor
RIHD
radiation-induced heart disease
rIL-2
recombinant interleukin 2
Riley-Day syndrome
Riley-Schwachman syndrome
Riley-Smith syndrome
Rimactane
rimantadine
rind
ring
amnion r.
r. applicator
Bandl r.
constriction r.
r. constriction
continence r.
contraceptive r.
division of pancreatic r.
double r.
estradiol-releasing silicone vaginal r.
Estring estradiol vaginal r.
Falope r.
r. finger
r. forceps
gestational r.
Graefenberg r.
hymenal r.

NOTES

ring *(continued)*
    Imlach r.
    Kayser-Fleischer r.
    neonatal r.
    NuvaRing vaginal contraceptive r.
    pancreatic r.
    pathologic retraction r.
    r. pessary
    phimotic r.
    physiologic retraction r.
    progestin-impregnated vaginal r.
    retraction r.
    r. sideroblast (RS)
    Silastic r.
    r. 1–22 syndrome
    trigonal r.
    T-shaped constriction r.
    tubal r.
    vascular r.
    visual tracking of red r.
    Waldeyer r.
    Wimberger r.
    Yoon r.
    zipper r.

Ringer
    heparinized lactated R.
    R. lactate
    lactated R.
    R. solution

ringworm
    beard r.
    black dot r.
    body r.
    groin r.
    nail r.
    scalp r.

Rinne test
rinse
    Nix Creme R.
    permethrin creme r.

Riopan Plus
RIP
    respiratory inductive plethysmography
RIPA
    radioimmunoprecipitation assay
ripener
    Prepidil Gel cervical r.
ripening
    Bishop score of cervical r.
    cervical r.
    spontaneous cervical r.
rippling muscle disease
RIS
    respiratory index score
risedronate
risk
    age-related r.
    r. assessment
    r. behavior
    biological r.
    direct suicide r. (DSR)
    elevated obstetric r.
    environmental r.
    established r.
    r. factor
    fetal r.
    first and second trimester
      evaluation of r. (FASTER)
    haplotype relative r. (HRR)
    high r.
    r. management
    maternal age-related r.
    neonatal mortality r. (NMR)
    prenatal r.
    recurrence r.
    relative r.
    r. stratification
    teratogenic r.

risk-benefit
    r.-b. analysis
    r.-b. ratio
risk-taking behavior
risky behavior
Risperdal
risperidone
Risser
    R. brace
    R. classification
    R. curve
    R. localizer cast
    R. sign
RIST
    radioimmunosorbent test
ristocetin
    r. cofactor
    r. cofactor activity
risus sardonicus
RITA
    radiofrequency interstitial tissue ablation
    system
Ritalin
Ritalin-SR
Rite Time
Ritgen maneuver
RIT 4385 mumps strain
ritodrine hydrochloride
ritonavir
Ritscher-Schinzel syndrome
Ritter disease
ritualism
ritualistic phenomenon
Rivotril
rizatriptan
RLDS
    Reynell Language Development Scale
RLF
    retrolental fibroplasia

RLP
  rectal linitis plastica
RLQ
  right lower quadrant
RLT
  reduced liver transplant
RMA
  right mentoanterior position
RMP
  right mentoposterior position
RMR
  resting metabolic rate
RMS
  rhabdomyosarcoma
    alveolar RMS
    embryonal RMS
    RMS Rectal
    RMS Uniserts
RMSF
  Rocky Mountain spotted fever
RMSS
  Ruvalcaba-Myhre-Smith syndrome
RMT
  right mentotransverse position
RN
  reflux neuropathy
²²²Rn
  radon-222
RNA
  ribonucleic acid
    complementary RNA
    RNA electrophoresis
    messenger RNA
    RNA nucleotidyltransferase
    packaging RNA
    poly A RNA
    RNA polymerase
    ribosomal RNA
    serum HCV RNA
    soluble RNA
    RNA splicing
    transfer RNA (tRNA)
RNA-directed DNA polymerase
RNase
  ribonuclease
ROA
  right occipitoanterior position
Robafen AC, DM
Robaxin
Robert pelvis
Roberts
  R. pseudothalidomide syndrome

  R. tetraphocomelia syndrome
  R. thumb retractor
robertsonian
  r. fusion
  r. translocation
Roberts-SC phocomelia syndrome
Robidrine
Robimycin
Robin
  R. anomalad
  R. syndrome
Robinow
  R. dwarfism
  R. mesomelic dysplasia
  R. syndrome
Robinow-Silverman-Smith syndrome
Robinow-Sorauf syndrome
Robins and Guze validation strategy
Robinul Forte
Robitussin
  R. Cough Calmers
  R. Pediatric
Robitussin-DM infant drops
Robomol
ROC
  receiver operating characteristic
  ROC XS suture fastener
Rocaltrol
Rocephin
Rochalimaea henselae
Roche
  R. Amplicor Monitor assay
  R. Diagnostics
Rocher-Sheldon syndrome
Rochester
  R. criteria
  R. HKAFO
Rochester-Ochsner forceps
Rochester-Péan forceps
rockerbottom, rocker-bottom
  r. foot
rocket dilator
Rockey-Davis incision
rocking
  body r.
Rock-Mulligan hood
Rocky
  R. Mountain spotted fever (RMSF)
  R. Mountain wood tick
rocuronium
rod
  gram-negative r.

NOTES

rod (*continued*)
- gram-positive r.'s
- Harrington r.
- hygroscopic r.
- intramedullary r.
- Küntscher r.
- r. myopathy
- nemaline r.
- pleomorphic gram-negative r.

Rodeck method
rodenticide poisoning
Rodriguez lethal acrofacial dysostosis
Roeder
- R. knot
- R. loop slipknot
- modified R.

Roenigk
- R. classification scale
- R. grade

roentgen (R)
roentgenogram
roentgenograph
roentgenographic examination
roentgenography
- chest r.

Roe v. Wade
rofecoxib
Roferon-A
Rogaine Topical
Roger
- R. forceps
- maladie de R.

rogletimide
Rohrer index
Rohr stria
Rohypnol
Rokitansky
- R. pelvis
- R. prominence
- R. protuberance
- R. tubercle

Rokitansky-Küster-Hauser syndrome
Rolaids Calcium Rich
rolandic
- r. epilepsy
- r. seizure
- r. sharp waves

role
- gender r.
- r. reversal

roll
- therapy r.

Rolland-Desbuquois syndrome
Rollator
rollerball
- r. electrode
- r. endometrial ablation (REA)
- r. technique

RollerBar electrode

rollerbar-loop-rollerbar ablation
roller-barrel electrode
RollerLoop vaporizing loop electrode
roller occlusion
rolling
- segmental r.

rollover test
ROM
- range of motion

Romaña sign
Romano-Ward long QT syndrome
Romazicon Injection
Romberg test
Rome
- R. criteria
- R. criteria for functional abdominal pain

Ronase
Rondec
- R. Drops
- R. Filmtab
- R. Syrup

Rondec-DM
Rondec-TR
rongeur
- pediatric bone r.
- Tobey ear r.

roof
- acetabular r.
- flat acetabular r.

rooftop incision
room
- r. air
- birthing r.
- delivery r.
- LDR r.
- obstetric emergency r.
- r. temperature

rooming in, rooming-in
root
- aortic r.
- broad nasal r.
- mesenteric r.
- nasal r.

rooting reflex
ROP
- retinopathy of prematurity
- right occipitoposterior position

ropelike filum terminale
rope sign
ropivacaine
- r. HCl
- r. hydrochloride

Rorschach test
ROS
- reactive oxygen species
- review of systems

rosacea
- acne r.

Rosai-Dorfman disease
rosary
    rachitic r.
    scorbutic r.
Rosch-Thurmond fallopian tube
  catheterization set
rosea
    pityriasis r.
Rosenberg Self-Esteem Scale (RSES)
Rosenmüller
    organ of R.
Rosenthal fiber
Rosenthal-Kloepfer syndrome
roseola
    r. infantum
    r. rash
roseolalike illness
rose spot
rosette
    Homer Wright r.
    mucosal r.
    r. test
rosettelike blister
Rosewater syndrome
ROSNI
    round spermatid nuclei injection
rOspA
    recombinant outer surface protein A
    rOspA Lyme disease vaccine
Ross
    R. carbohydrate-free (RCF)
    R. growth chart
    R. operation
    R. procedure
    R. pulmonary porcine valve
    R. River virus
Ro/SSA
    Ro/SSA antigen
    Ro/SSA autoantigen
Rossavik growth model
Rosselli-Gulienetti syndrome
Rossi syndrome
Ross-Konno operation
Ross-Konno-Switch operation
Rossolimo reflex
rostral
    r. direction
    r. neuropore
    r. ventromedial medulla
rostrocaudal
rostrum

ROT
    right occipitotransverse position
Rotacaps
    Ventolin R.
Rotadisk
    Flovent R.
Rotamune
rotary
    r. atlantoaxial luxation
    r. chewing
    r. subluxation
rotation
    r. and descent
    external r.
    forceps r.
    hip r.
    internal r.
    Kjelland r.
    lateral r. (LR)
    lateral hip r.
    manual r.
    medial r. (MR)
    medial hip r.
    r. movement
    neutral r.
    rib r.
    r. of spine
    trunk r.
    upward r.
rotational
    r. delivery
    r. malalignment
    r. osteotomy
rotationplasty
rotatory
    r. displacement
    r. subluxation
rotavirus
    r. enteritis
    r. gastroenteritis
    infantile diarrhea r.
    r. vaccination
    r. vaccine
Rotazyme
    R. diagnostic procedure
    R. test
rote memory
Rothmann-Makai syndrome
Rothmund syndrome
Rothmund-Thomson cancer
  predisposition syndrome
Rothmund-Werner syndrome

NOTES

Roth spot
roticulating endograsper
Roticulator 55 stapler
Rotor disease
Rotter Sentence Completion Test
rotunda
    pityriasis r.
Roubac
Rouget bulb
rough endoplasmic reticulum (RER)
rough-feeling skin
round
    r. back deformity
    r. cell tumor
    r. iliac bone
    r. ligament
    r. ligament pain
    r. ligament syndrome
    r. moon face
    r. pelvis
    r. spermatid nuclei injection
      (ROSNI)
    r. window electrocochleography
      (RWECochG)
round-back
    postural r.-b.
round-headed acrosomeless spermatozoa
roundworm
Rous sarcoma virus
Roussy-Lévy
    R.-L. disease
    R.-L. syndrome
route of delivery
routine
    r. antenatal diagnostic imaging with
      ultrasound (RADIUS)
    daily r.
    r. prenatal testing
    r. prenatal visit
    r. preoperative test
    r. screening
    r. screening cervical examination
    r. wound management
Roux-en-Y
    R.-e.-Y. anastomosis
    R.-e.-Y. choledochojejunostomy
Rovamycine
Rovsing
    R. sign
    R. test
Rowasa
    R. enema
    R. Rectal
Rowden uterine manipulator-injector
    (RUMI)
Rowland pouch
Roxanol SR
Roxicet 5/500
Roxicodone

Roxilox
roxithromycin
Royal College of General Practioners'
    Oral Contraception Study
RP
    Raynaud phenomenon
      RP with progressive sensorineural
        hearing loss
RPC
    reactive perforating collagenosis
    retained products of conception
RPD
    Pepcid RPD
RPE
    retinal pigment epithelium
RPICC
    regional perinatal intensive care center
RPL
    repeated pregnancy loss
RPLS
    reversible posterior leukoencephalopathy
      syndrome
RPM
    Raven Progressive Matrices
RPMPR
    radical posteromedial and plantar release
RPO
    reflectance pulse oximetry
      RPO oximeter
RPR
    rapid plasma reagin
      RPR titer
RPS4X
RPS4Y
RRF
    ragged red fiber
RRFC
    renal reserve filtration capacity
RRP
    recurrent respiratory papillomatosis
RS
    reactive site
    ring sideroblast
      AT3 type II PE, RS
      RS mutation
RSA
    recurrent spontaneous abortion
    right sacroanterior position
RScA
    right scapuloanterior position
RScP
    right scapuloposterior position
RSD
    reflex sympathetic dystrophy
RSE
    refractory status epilepticus
RSES
    Rosenberg Self-Esteem Scale
RSH/SLO syndrome

RSH/Smith-Lemli-Opitz
RSH syndrome
RSI
    rapid sequence intubation
RSL
    renal solute load
RSLT
    reduced-size liver transplant
RSP
    right sacroposterior position
RST
    right sacrotransverse position
RSV, RS-virus
    respiratory syncytial virus
        RSV antigen
        RSV bronchiolitis
        RSV immunoglobulin for
          intravenous administration (RSV-
          IGIV, RSV-IVIG)
        RSV monoclonal antibody
        RSV nasal wash
        RSV pneumonitis
RSV-associated wheeze
RSVB
    respiratory syncytial virus bronchiolitis
RSVIG, RSV-IG
    respiratory syncytial virus immune
      globulin
    respiratory syncytial virus
      immunoglobulin
RSV-IGIV, RSV-IVIG
    respiratory syncytial virus intravenous
      immune globulin
    respiratory syncytial virus intravenous
      immunoglobulin
    RSV immunoglobulin for intravenous
    administration
RS-virus (*var. of* RSV)
RT
    radiation therapy
RTA
    renal tubular acidosis
        distal RTA
        hyperkalemic RTA
        mineralocorticoid-deficiency RTA
        proximal RTA
        type IV RTA
RTI
    reverse transcriptase inhibitor
rt-PA
    recombinant tissue type plasminogen
    activator

RT-PCR
    reverse transcription polymerase chain
      reaction
RTS
    Revised Trauma Score
RU 486
rub
    friction r.
    pericardial friction r.
    pleural friction r.
rubber bleb nevus
rubella
    congenital r.
    r. embryopathy
    r. immune
    r. infection
    measles, mumps, r. (MMR)
    r. panencephalitis
    periconceptional r.
    r. scarlatinosa
    r. syndrome
    third disease (r.)
    r. vaccine
    r. virus
rubella-immune mother
rubella-negative mother
Rubens flap
rubeola
    r. scarlatinosa
    r. titer
Rubex
Rubin
    R. cannula
    R. maneuver
    R. test
    R. tube
Rubinstein syndrome
Rubinstein-Taybi syndrome
Rubivirus
rubor
rubra
    miliaria r.
rubrum
    tinea r.
    Trichophyton r.
ruddy
Rudiger syndrome
rudimentary
    r. testis syndrome
    r. uterine horn
    r. vagina
rudimentary-type digit

NOTES

Rud syndrome
ruga, pl. **rugae**
    rugae of vagina
    rugae vaginales
rugal fold
rugated vaginal mucosa
rugation
rugger jersey spine
rule
    10% r.
    Arey r.
    Budin r.
    four-hour r.
    Haase r.
    His r.
    informed consent disclosure r.'s
    Lossen r.
    McDonald r.
    Mittendorf-Williams r.
    Nägele r.
    r. of nines
    r. of 60s
    Ogino-Knaus r.
    Ottawa Ankle R.'s (OAR)
    r. of outlet
    seven day r.
    r. of threes
    Trauma Triage R. (TTR)
    Van Praagh loop r.
    Weinberg r.
Rumack-Matthew nomogram
rumble
    middiastolic r.
rumbling murmur
RUMI
    Rowden uterine manipulator-injector
rumination disorder
Rum-K
Rumpel-Leede phenomenon
Runeberg anemia
running
    r. imbricating stitch
    r. locked stitch
runoff
    aortic r.
runt disease
runting
rupture
    amnion r.
    angiomyolipoma r.
    aortic arch r.
    arterial r.
    cardiac r.
    esophageal r.
    follicle aspiration, sperm injection, and assisted r. (FASIAR)
    hepatic r.
    marginal sinus r.
    membrane r.

    neural tube r.
    ovarian r.
    peroneal r.
    postmembrane r.
    prelabor membrane r.
    premature amnion r.
    premature membrane r.
    premembrane r.
    prolonged r.
    splenic r.
    testicular r.
    total perineal r.
    tubal r.
    ureteral r.
    uterine r.
ruptured
    r. appendicitis
    r. bronchiole
    r. capsule
    r. cerebral aneurysm
    r. corpus luteum
    r. episiotomy
    r. globe
    r. sinus of Valsalva aneurysm
    r. symphysis pubis
    r. uterus
RUQ
    right upper quadrant
Rusch bag
Rusconi
    anus of R.
rush immunotherapy
Russell
    R. diencephalic syndrome (I, II, III)
    R. dwarf
    R. nanism
    R. sign
    R. traction
    R. viper venom time
Russell-Silver
    R.-S. dwarfism
    R.-S. dwarf syndrome
Russian
    R. spring-summer encephalitis
    R. tissue forceps
rust-colored sputum
ruthenium
Rutherfurd syndrome
Rutledge
    R. classification of extended hysterectomy
    R. lethal multiple congenital anomalies syndrome
Rutter mean score
Ruvalcaba-Myhre-Smith syndrome (RMSS)
Ruvalcaba-Myhre syndrome
Ruvalcaba-Reichert-Smith syndrome

Ruvalcaba syndrome
RV
residual volume
right ventricle
RVA
rabies vaccine, absorbed
RVC
radionuclide voiding cystography
RVDT
retinal venous dilation and tortuosity
RVH
right ventricular hypertrophy
RVOT
right ventricular outflow tract
RVOTO
right ventricular outflow tract obstruction
RVPaque cream
RVR
relative vascular resistance
RVS
recognizable viral syndrome

Rv vaccine
RWECochG
round window electrocochleography
Rx
prescription
Rx medibottle
Mission Prenatal Rx
RxFISH DNA probe and analysis system
Ryan agar
Rye classification
Ryna-C
Rynacrom
Ryna-CX
Ryna Liquid
Rynatan Pediatric
RZ
reserve zone

NOTES

S

S phase
S phase fraction

S-100 antibody

SA

sacroanterior
sinoatrial node

SAB

spontaneous abortion

Sabbagha formula

saber

S. BT blunt-tip surgical trocar
s. cut incision
s. shin
s. shin deformity

Sabin

S. OPV
S. vaccine

Sabinas brittle hair syndrome

Sabin-Feldman dye test

sabot

coeur en s.

Sabouraud medium

sabre

scleroderma en coup de s.

**Sabre FreeHand high-intensity medical
pocket light**

Sabril

sac

abnormal gestational s.
allantoic s.
aortic s.
chorionic s.
cystic s.
embryonic s.
fetal s.
gestational s. (GS)
hernia s.
intrauterine s.
Lap S.
monoamniotic s.
nasolacrimal s.
Pleatman s.
preputial s.
pseudogestational s.
pudendal s.
vitelline s.
widened thecal s.
yolk s.

SACA

Service Assessment for Children and
Adolescents

saccade

saccharate

dextroamphetamine s.

Saccharomyces

S. boulardii
S. cerevisiae

saccharopinuria

saccular

s. aneurysm
s. dilation
s. period
s. stage
s. stage of lung development

sacculation of uterus

saccus

s. anticus
s. medius
s. posticus
s. superior

sacral

s. agenesis
s. colpopexy
s. dimple
s. lymph node
s. meningomyelocele
s. nerve
s. nerve root stimulation
s. neural tube defect
s. promontory
s. reflex

sacroanterior (SA)

left s.
s. position

sacrococcygeal teratoma

sacrocolpopexy

abdominal s.
s. graft
laparoscopic s.

sacroiliac (SI)

s. dysfunction
s. joint

sacroiliitis

sacropexy

abdominal s.

sacroposterior (SP)

left s. position (LSP)
s. position
right s. position (RSP)

sacrosciatic notch

sacrosidase

sacrospinous

s. colpopexy
s. ligament
s. ligament suspension
s. vaginal vault suspension

sacrotransverse (ST)

left s. position (LST)

S

sacrotransverse *(continued)*
    s. position
    right s. position (RST)
sacrotuberous
sacrum
    hollow of s.
    hypoplastic s.
SAD
    seasonal affective disorder
    separation anxiety disorder
    source-to-axis distance
saddle
    s. block
    s. block anesthesia
    s. nose
saddleback
    s. fever
    s. temperature curve
saddlebag flap
saddle-nose deformity
S-adenosylhomocysteine (SAH)
sadness
Saenger
    S. operation
    S. ovum forceps
Saethre-Chotzen syndrome
SAFE
    sexual assault forensic evidence
    SAFE kit
Safe Tussin 30
safety
    system for thalidomide education
    and prescription s. (STEPS)
Safil synthetic absorbable surgical suture
Saf-T-Coil IUD
saginata
    Taenia s.
sagittal
    s. craniosynostosis
    s. fontanelle
    s. plane
    s. septum of rectus sheath
    s. sinus
    s. sinus thrombosis
    s. suture
    s. suture line
    s. synostosis
sagrada
    cascara s.
SAH
    S-adenosylhomocysteine
SAICAR
    succinyl aminoimidazole carboxamide ribotide
sail sign
Saint (St.)
Saizen Injection
Sakati-Nyhan syndrome

SAL
    suction-assisted lipoplasty
salaam
    s. convulsion
    infantile s.
    s. seizure
Sal-Acid Plaster
Salagen Oral
sal ammoniac
Salazopyrin
salbutamol
Saldino-Noonan
    S.-N. dwarfism
    S.-N. short rib-polydactyly
    S.-N. syndrome
Salem pump
SalEst
    S. immunoassay
    S. preterm labor test system
    S. system test
Salflex
salicylate
    choline s.
    s. intoxication
    magnesium s.
    phenyl s.
    s. poisoning
    sodium s.
    s. toxicity
salicylic
    s. acid
    s. acid ointment
    s. sugar powder
salicylism
salicylsalicylic acid
saline
    s. abortion
    s. cathartic
    s. drop test
    Dulbecco phosphate buffered s.
    extrarenal s.
    heparinized s.
    hypertonic s.
    hypotonic s.
    iced s.
    s. implant
    s. infusion sonography (SIS)
    s. infusion sonohysterography (SIS)
    isotonic s.
    s. lavage
    normal s.
    s. nose drops
    phosphate-buffered s.
    phosphate buffered s. (PBS)
    physiologic s.
    s. solution
    tris[hydroxymethyl]aminomethane-buffered s.
    s. wet smear

SalineX
saliva
salivarius
    Streptococcus s.
salivary
    s. adenitis
    s. amylase
    s. cortisol
    s. cortisol assay
    s. estriol
    s. estriol test
    s. estriol testing
    s. gland
salivation, lacrimation, urination, defecation, gastrointestinal distress, and emesis (SLUDGE)
Salk
    S. IPV
    S. vaccine
Salla disease
salmeterol
    s. powder
    s. xinafoate
Salmonella
    S. bacteria
    S. choleraesuis
    S. dublin
    S. enteritidis
    S. gastroenteritis
    S. heidelberg
    S. hirschfeldii
    S. meningitis
    S. newport
    non-typhi *S.* (NTS)
    nontyphoid *S.*
    nontyphoidal *S.*
    S. oranienburg
    S. oranienburg sepsis
    S. osteomyelitis
    S. paratyphi
    S. schottmuelleri
    S. typhi
    S. typhimurium
salmonella
salmonellosis
salmon patch
salmon-pink rash
Salmon sign
Salonen-Herva-Norio syndrome
salpingectomy
    partial s.
    postpartum partial s.

salpingemphraxis
salpinges (*pl. of* salpinx)
salpingioma
salpingitic
salpingitis
    s. after previous tubal occlusion (SPOT)
    chronic interstitial s.
    foreign body s.
    gonorrheal s.
    granulomatous s.
    s. isthmica nodosa (SIN)
    leprous s.
    nongranulomatous s.
    s. in previously occluded tubes (SPOT)
    pyogenic s.
    tuberculous s.
salpingocele
salpingocentesis
salpingocyesis
salpingography
    transcervical selective s.
salpingolysis
salpingoneostomy
salpingo-oophoritis
salpingo-oophorocele
salpingo-ovariectomy
    abdominal s.-o.
    bilateral s.-o. (BSO)
    unilateral s.-o.
salpingoovariolysis
salpingoperitonitis
salpingopexy
salpingoplasty
salpingorrhagia
salpingorrhaphy
salpingoscopy
salpingostomatomy
salpingostomy
    linear s.
salpingotomy
    abdominal s.
salpinx, pl. salpinges
salsalate
salt
    bile s.
    calcium s.
    s. craving
    s. frosting of skin
    gold s.
    guanidine s.

S

NOTES

salt *(continued)*
    inorganic mercury s.
    Pedi-Bath S.'s
    s. and pepper appearance
    s. and pepper fundus
    s. and pepper retinitis
    s. poisoning
    s. restriction
    s. wasting
Salter
    S. osteotomy
    S. procedure
Salter-Harris
    S.-H. classification
    S.-H. classification of epiphyseal
     plate injury
    S.-H. classification of fracture
    S.-H. epiphyseal fracture
    S.-H. fracture (type I–V)
salt-losing adrenogenital syndrome
  (SLAS)
salt-wasting
    s.-w. adrenogenital syndrome
    s.-w. congenital adrenal hyperplasia
     (SW-CAH)
saltwater near drowning
salutary effect
salute
    allergic s.
salvage
    s. cesarean
    s. chemotherapy
    s. intervention
    s. laparotomy
    limb s.
    s. therapy
same-sex relationship
sample
    arterial blood s. (ABS)
    blood s.
    citrate blood s.
    clean-catch midstream urine s.
    cord blood s.
    endocervical s.
    exocervical s.
    midstream urine s.
    urine s.
    venous blood s. (VBS)
sampler
    Cervex-Brush cervical cell s.
    Cordguard umbilical cord s.
    Cytobrush Plus endocervical cell s.
    SelectCells Mini endometrial s.
    Wallach Endocell endometrial
     cell s.
sampling
    axillary node s.
    biological s.
    blood s.

    capillary blood gas s.
    cerebrospinal fluid s.
    chemical s.
    chorion s.
    chorionic villus s. (CVS)
    endocervical s.
    endometrial s.
    fetal scalp blood s.
    fetal scalp platelet s.
    fetal skin s.
    hair s.
    heel capillary s.
    histologic s.
    Mucat cervical s.
    percutaneous blood s.
    percutaneous umbilical blood s.
     (PUBS)
    perimortem s.
    postmortem s.
    random s.
    scalp blood s.
    transabdominal chorionic villus s.
    transcervical chorionic villus s.
    trophoblast s.
    ultrasound-directed percutaneous
     umbilical blood s.
    umbilical blood s.
    urine s.
    venous blood s.
Sampson
    artery of S.
    S. cyst
San
    S. Joaquin fever
    S. Luis Valley syndrome
Sanchez-Cascos syndrome
Sanchez-Corona syndrome
Sanchez-Salorio syndrome
Sanders jet respirator
Sandhoff
    S. disease
    S. GM2 gangliosidosis (type I, II)
    S. syndrome
Sandifer syndrome
Sandimmune
sandle gap foot deformity
Sandoglobulin
Sandostatin LAR Depot
sandpaper rash
sandwich
    s. assay
    solid phase s.
Sanfilippo disease A, B, C, D
Sanger incision
sanguinis
    Gemella s.
sanguinolentis
    fetus s.
sanguinopurulent

Sani-Spec vaginal speculum
Sani-Supp Suppository
Sanjad-Sakati syndrome
SANS
    schedule for negative symptoms
Sansert
Santavuori
    S. disease
    muscle-eye-brain disease of S.
    S. syndrome
Santavuori-Haltia syndrome
Santulli enterostomy
SAO
    Southeast Asian ovalocytosis
SaO$_2$
    oxygen saturation
Sao Paulo MCA/MR syndrome
SAP
    surfactant-associated protein
    systolic arterial pressure
    SAP-35
SAP1
    sphingolipid activator protein-1
sap
    Prentif cavity-rim cervical s.
saphenous
    s. nerve
    s. nerve entrapment
    s. vein
    s. vein catheter insertion
saponification
Sapporo virus
saprophytic
saprophyticus
    Staphylococcus s.
SAPS
    schedule for positive symptoms
    simplified acute physiology score
saquinavir
Sarafem
SaraPem
sarcofetal pregnancy
sarcoid
    alveolar s.
sarcoid-like
sarcoidosis
    nervous system s.
    ocular s.
    subcutaneous s.
sarcolemma
sarcoma
    adenosquamous s.

alveolar soft part s.
blue-cell s.
botryoid s.
s. botryoides
Burkitt s.
cervical s.
chordoid s.
clear cell s.
embryonal s.
endometrial s.
endometrial stromal s. (ESS)
Ewing s.
extraosseous Ewing s.
granulocytic s.
heterologous uterine s.
homologous uterine s.
immunoblastic s.
Kaposi s. (KS)
Kaposi varicelliform s.
mesodermal s.
mixed mesodermal s. (MMS)
mixed müllerian s.
mixed ovarian mesodermal s.
neurogenic s.
nonrhabdomyogenic soft tissue s.
nonrhabdomyomatous s.
nonrhabdomyosarcoma soft tissue s. (NRSTS)
obesity in endometrial s.
osteogenic s.
penile Kaposi s.
penoscrotal Kaposi s.
pseudoglandular synovial s.
retroperitoneal soft tissue s.
secretory s.
soft-tissue s.
synovial s.
tenosynovial s.
testicular Kaposi s.
uterine müllerian s.
vaginal s.
vulvar s.
sarcomatous
    s. myoma degeneration
    s. tumor
sarcomere
sarcomeric filament
sarcoplasmic reticulum
Sarcoptes scabiei
sarcoptic mange
sarcosinemia
sardonic smile

NOTES

sardonicus
  risus s.
sargramostim
Sarna lotion
Sarnat
  S. encephalopathy
  S. score
SARS
  severe acute respiratory syndrome
SART
  Sexual Assault Response Team
  Society for Assisted Reproductive
    Technology
sartorial elegance
S.A.S.-500
Saskatoon
  hemoglobin M S.
SASPP
  septum pellucidum with porencephalia
    syndrome
Sassone score
**Sastid plain therapeutic shampoo and
  acne wash**
satellite
  s. DNA
  s. lesion
  s. melanocytic nevus
  s. papule
  s. pustule
satellitosis
satiety
  early s.
satisfaction
  sexual s.
sativa
  Cannabis s.
Sato syndrome
satumomab pendetite imaging agent
**saturated solution of potassium iodide
  (SSKI)**
saturation
  s. analysis
  fetal arterial oxygen s. (FS_pO_2)
  fetal oxygen s.
  O_2 s.
  oxygen s. (SaO_2)
  oxyhemoglobin s.
  postductal oxygen s.
  s. strip
  transferrin s.
satyr ear
satyriasis
Sauflon PW contact lens
Saunders
  S. disease
  S. sign
sausage digit
sausage-shaped bulla
Savage syndrome

Savant Speed-Vac drier
Save-A-Tooth
saver
  Cell S.
saw
  Gigli s.
saw-toothed flutter wave
Saxtorph maneuver
Say-Gerald syndrome
Say-Meyer syndrome
Say syndrome
SB-6 antiserum
SBE
  self-breast examination
  subacute bacterial endocarditis
    SBE prophylaxis
S-beta-thal
SBHC
  school-based health center
SBI
  serious bacterial infection
SBM
  selective broth medium
SBP
  spontaneous bacterial peritonitis
  spontaneous biliary perforation
SBPI
  sun protection behavior index
SBS
  short bowel syndrome
SBT
  serum bactericidal titer
SC
  SC disease
  hemoglobin SC
  SC phocomelia syndrome
S&C
  suction and curettage
SCA
  spinocerebellar ataxia (type 1–7)
ScA
  scapuloanterior
scabicide
scabies
  animal s.
  canine s.
  crusted s.
  human s.
  s. mite
  neonatal s.
  Norwegian s.
  s. scraping
SCAD
  short-chain acyl coenzyme A
    dehydrogenase
    SCAD deficiency
scala tympani
scalded skin syndrome (SSS)
scalding injury

scale

Abnormal Involuntary Movement S. (AIMS)
Acute Illness Observation S. (AIOS)
Alberta Infant Motor S. (AIMS)
Albert Einstein Neonatal Developmental S. (AENNS)
Anger Expression S.
anxiety-withdrawal s.
Apgar s.
Attention Deficit Disorders Evaluation S.
attrition rate s.
BAMO s.
Barnes Akathisia S. (BAS)
Bayley Mental S.
Behavioral and Emotional Rating S. (BERS)
Behavior Rating S. (BRS)
Bieri s.
Borg Perceived Exertion S.
Borg Physical Activity S.
Brazelton Neonatal Behavioral Assessment S. (BNBAS)
broad-band s.
Canadian Acute Respiratory Illness and Flu S. (CARIFS)
Capute s.
Carey Temperament S.
Cattell Infant Intelligence S.
CGI s.
Child Abuse Trauma S. (CATS)
Child and Adolescent Functional Assessment S. (CAFAS)
Childhood Autism Rating S. (CARS)
Children's Depression S.
Children's Depression Rating S.-Revised (CDRS-R)
Children's Global Assessment S. (CGAS)
Children's Manifest Anxiety S.
Clinical Adaptive Test/Clinical Linguistic and Auditory Milestone S. (CAT/CLAMS)
Clinical Linguistic and Auditory Milestone S. (CLAMS)
color analog s.
Columbia Impairment S.
Conners S.
Conners Rating S. (CRS)

Cooke-Medley Hostility S.
Cranley Maternal-Fetal Attachment S.
CRIES postoperative pain s.
depression rating s.
Depression Self-Rating S.
Disruptive Behavior Disorder S.
Dissociative Experience S. (DES)
Dyadic Adjustment S.
Dyskinesia Identification System: Condensed User S. (DISCUS)
Early Neonatal Neurobehavioral S.
Edinburgh Postnatal Depression S. (EPDS)
Einstein Neonatal Neurobehavioral Assessment S. (ENNAS)
electronic s.
ELM s.
Emotionality Activity Sociability S. (EAS)
Externalizing Behavior S.
Family Adaptability and Cohesion Evaluation S. (FACES)
Family Adaptability and Cohesion S.-III (FACES-III)
Family Environment S. (FES)
Female Sexual Distress S. (FSDS)
FLACC s.
Flint Infant Security S. (FISS)
Functional Assessment S. (FAS)
Gesell Child Development Age S. (GCDAS)
Gesell Developmental S. (GDS)
Gesell Infant S.
Glasgow Coma S. (GCS)
Graham-Rosenblith s.
gray s.
Griffith Mental Developmental S. (GMDS)
Hamilton Depression S. (HAMD)
HOME s.
HSC S.
Impact of Events S. (IES)
infant face s.
Internalizing Behavior S.
IPAT Depression S.
Kent Infant Development S. (KIDS)
Leiter International Performance S.
Likert s.
linear visual analog s.
Locus of Control S.

S

NOTES

scale *(continued)*

Maternal Attitude S. (MAS)
McCarthy Memory S.
McGrath s.
mental s.
motor s.
Multidimensional Student Life
  Satisfaction S. (MSLSS)
muscle strength grading s.
Neonatal Behavioral Assessment S.
  (NBAS)
Neonatal Infant Pain S. (NIPS)
Neurobiologic Risk S. (NBRS)
Newborn Behavior Assessment S.
  (NBAS)
NIMH global s.
Oucher s.
Parent and Teacher Conners S.
PARS s.
Peabody Developmental Motor S.
  (PDMS)
Pediatric Liver Transplant-
  Specific S. (PLTSS)
Perceived Stress S.
Piers-Harris Children's Self-
  Concept S.
Piper fatigue s.
prosocial behavior s.
Receptive-Expressive Emergent
  Language S. (REEL)
Revised Children's Manifest
  Anxiety S. (RCMAS, RCMASA)
Reynell Language Development S.
  (RLDS)
Reynolds Child Depression S.
Roenigk classification s.
Rosenberg Self-Esteem S. (RSES)
shyness s.
Simpson-Angus rating s.
sperm progression s. (0–4)
standardized observation s.
Stanford-Binet Intelligence S.
Tanner Developmental S.
Toddler Temperament S.
Toronto Alexithymia S. (TAS)
Urge Impact S. (URIS)
verbal analog pain s. (VAPS)
Vineland Adaptive Behavior S.'s
Vineland Social Maturity S.
visual analog s. (VAS)
Wechsler Memory S.
Wender Utah Rating S. (WURS)
Wong-Baker faces pain rating s.
Yale-Brown Obsessive
  Compulsive S. (YBOCS)
Yale Global Tic Severity S.
  (YGTSS)
Yale Observation S.

York Incontinence Perceptions S.
  (YIPS)

scalene muscle

scaling

brawny s.
s. bulla
keratotic s.
Organ Injury S. (OIS)
oval s.

scalloped temporalis muscle

scalloping

frontal bones s.

scalp

s. blood sampling
cutis aplasia of s.
s. electrode
s. intravenous
s. I.V.
s. laceration
s. pH
s. pH determination
s. ringworm
s. seborrheic dermatitis
s. vein
s. vein catheter
s. vein catheterization
s. vein needle

scalpel

Bowen double-bladed s.
Endo-Assist retractable s.
Harmonic s.
Shaw (I, II) s.

Scalpicin Topical

scaly dermatitis

SCAN

suspected child abuse or neglect

scan

abdominopelvic s.
abdominopelvic CT s.
bleeding s.
bone s.
CT s.
DEXA s.
double-contrast CT s.
DTPA radionuclide s.
dual-energy x-ray absorptiometry s.
expiratory s.
gallium s.
gallium-67 s.
helical s.
indium-labeled leukocyte s.
iodine 125-labeled fibrinogen s.
longitudinal s.
Meckel s.
MIBG s.
milk s.
MUGA s.
multiple gated acquisition s.
pinhole collimated s.

planar bone s.
radiofibrinogen uptake s.
radioisotope milk s.
radiolabeled white blood cell s.
radionuclide bone s.
radionuclide heart s.
red blood cell tagged s.
serial growth s.'s
spiral s.
Tc HMPAO leukocyte s.
technetium bone s.
technetium-99m bone s.
testicular flow s.
time position s.
transverse s.
ventilation/perfusion s.
V̇/Q̇ s.
xenon CT s.

Scandishake
Scanlon Assessment
scanner
Acuson 128-XP10 s.
Aloka 650 s.
Aloka SSD-720 real-time s.
BladderManager portable
ultrasound s.
EUB-405 ultrasound s.
scanning
CAT s.
CT s.
Doppler s.
duplex s.
s. electron microscopy (SEM)
gated blood pool s.
iodomethyl-norcholesterol s.
isotope s.
MEVA Probe for endovaginal s.
s. photometry
radionuclide s.
restriction landmark genomic s.
spectrophotometric s.
ultrasound s.
white cell s.
Scan ultrasound gel
Scanzoni
S. forceps
S. maneuver
S. second os
Scanzoni-Smellie maneuver
scaphocephalism
scaphocephaly

scaphoid
s. abdomen
s. fontanelle
s. pad
s. scapula
scapula, pl. scapulae
congenital elevation of the s.
scaphoid s.
scapular
s. fracture
s. repositioning
s. winging
scapularis
Ixodes s.
scapuloanterior (ScA)
left s. position (LScA)
right s. position (RScA)
scapulohumeral muscular dystrophy
scapuloperoneal dystrophy
scapuloposterior (ScP)
left s. position (LScP)
right s. position (RScP)
scapulothoracic motion
scar
depressed s.
hypertrophic s.
lower segment s.
perineal s.
s. prediction
radial s.
s. tissue
scare
vaccine-autism s.
SCARED
Screen for Child Anxiety-Related
Emotional Disorders
SCARF
skeletal abnormalities, cutis laxa,
craniostenosis, psychomotor retardation,
facial abnormalities
scarf
s. maneuver
s. sign
scarification
scarlatina antitoxin
scarlatiniform
s. eruption
s. erythema
s. rash
scarlatinosa
rubella s.
rubeola s.

NOTES

scarlet
> s. fever
> s. fever exanthem

SCARMD
> severe childhood autosomal recessive muscular dystrophy

Scarpa fascia
scarred womb
scarring
> corneal s.
> renal s.

scatoma (*var. of* fecaloma)
scattered
> s. echo
> s. scores

scattering
> Rayleigh-Tyndall s.

SCCD
> Schnyder crystalline corneal dystrophy

SCCMS
> slow-channel congenital myasthenic syndrome

SCD
> sickle cell disease

SCE
> split hand-cleft lip/palate and ectodermal dysplasia

Scepter system
SCF
> somatic cell-derived growth factor

SCFA
> short-chain fatty acid

SCFE
> slipped capital femoral epiphysis
> > acute-on-chronic SCFE
> > chronic SCFE
> > Preslip SCFE

SCH
> supracervical hysterectomy

SCHAD
> short-chain hydroxyacyl-coenzyme A dehydrogenase

Schafer syndrome
Schatz maneuver
Schauffler procedure
Schaumann body
Schauta vaginal operation
schedule
> S. for Affective Disorders and Schizophrenia for School-Age Children (K-SADS)
> S. for Affective Disorders and Schizophrenia for School-Age Children-Epidemiologic Version (K-SADS-E)
> S. for Affective Disorders and Schizophrenia for School-Age Children-Present Episode (K-SADS-P)

agglomeration s.
> Autism Diagnostic Observation S. (ADOS)
> child assessment s. (CAS)
> Gesell Developmental S.'s
> life events and difficulties s. (LEDS)
> s. for negative symptoms (SANS)
> s. for positive symptoms (SAPS)

scheduled
> s. feeding
> s. voiding

Scheibe
> S. anomaly
> S. aplasia

Scheie syndrome
schema
> TNM s.

schenckii
> *Sporothrix s.*

Scheuermann
> S. disease
> S. juvenile kyphosis

Scheuer score
Scheuthauer-Marie-Sainton syndrome
Schick
> S. sign
> S. test

Schiff test
Schilder
> S. disease
> S. encephalitis

Schiller
> S. solution
> S. test
> S. tumor

Schiller-Duvall body
Schilling test
Schimke immunoosseous dysplasia
Schimmelbusch
> S. disease
> S. syndrome

Schimmelpenning-Feuerstein-Mims syndrome
Schindler disease
Schinzel acrocallosal syndrome
Schinzel-Giedion
> S.-G. midface-retraction syndrome
> S.-G. syndrome (SGS)

SCHIP
> State Children's Health Insurance Program
> > SCHIP evaluation tool

Schirmer syndrome
schistocelia
schistocephalus
schistocormia
schistocystis
schistocyte, schizocyte

schistocytic hemolytic anemia
schistoglossia
schistomelia
schistoprosopia
Schistosoma
    S. haematobium
    S. intercalatum
    S. japonicum
    S. mansoni
    S. mekongi
schistosomal myelopathy
schistosomia
schistosomiasis
    acute s.
    cerebral s.
    chronic s.
schistosomula
schistosternia
schistothorax
schistotrachelus
schizencephaly
schizoaffective disorder
schizocyte (*var. of* schistocyte)
schizocytosis
schizoid personality disorder
schizont
schizophasia
schizophrenia
    childhood s.
    childhood-onset s. (COS)
    early-onset s. (EOS)
    very early onset s. (VEOS)
schizophrenic
schizophreniform disorder
schizotypal
schizotypy
Schlemm canal
Schlesinger solution
Schlusskoagulum
Schmid-Fraccaro syndrome
Schmidley syndrome
Schmid metaphyseal dysplasia
Schmidt-Lantermann incisure
Schmidt syndrome
Schmorl
    S. jaundice
    S. node
Schneckenbecken dysplasia
Schnyder crystalline corneal dystrophy
   (SCCD)
Schober test

Schofield weight- and height-based
  resting energy expenditure prediction
  equation
Scholz
    S. disease
    S. sclerosis
Schönlein-Henoch purpura
school
    s. avoidance
    s. failure hypothesis
    s., home, activities, depression/self-
      esteem, substance abuse, sexuality,
      safety assessment
    s. phobia
    S. Sleep Habits Survey
school-based
    s.-b. health center (SBHC)
    s.-b. intervention
schottmuelleri
    Salmonella s.
Schroeder
    S. operation
    S. tenaculum forceps
    S. tenaculum loop
    S. uterine tenaculum
    S. vulsellum forceps
Schubert uterine biopsy forceps
Schuchardt
    S. incision
    S. operation
Schuco nebulizer
Schüffner dot
Schuknecht
    S. classification
    S. classification of congenital aural
      atresia (type A–D)
    S. retractor
Schultze
    S. mechanism
    S. phantom
    S. placenta
Schwachman-Diamond syndrome
Schwachman syndrome
Schwangerschafts protein 1
Schwann cell
schwannian differentiation
schwannoma
    acoustic s.
    malignant s.
Schwartz-Jampel
    S.-J. disease
    S.-J. syndrome

S

NOTES

Schwartz-Jampel-Aberfeld syndrome
Schwartzman phenomenon
Schwartz syndrome
Schwarz measles strain
sciatic nerve
SCID
    severe combined immunodeficiency
SCIDS
SciMed-Kolobow membrane lung
scimitar syndrome
scintigram
scintigraphy
    cortical s.
    dipyridamole myocardial s.
    hepatobiliary s.
    HMPAO leukocyte s.
    nuclear s.
    radionuclide s.
    renal s.
    somatostatin receptor s.
    thyroid s.
    ventilation s.
scintillating scotoma
scintillation
scintimammography (SMM)
    s. prone breast cushion
scintography
    gallium s.
scirrhous carcinoma
scissored position
scissoring posture
scissors
    Adson ganglion s.
    Aslan endoscopic s.
    bandage s.
    Braun episiotomy s.
    curved Mayo s.
    Electroscope disposable s.
    Evershears bipolar laparoscopic s.
    fine Metzenbaum s.
    Jorgenson s.
    Lister s.
    Mayo s.
    Metzenbaum s.
    Microline Re-New II 5-mm
      modular laparoscopic s.
    right-angle s.
    Smellie s.
    Spencer stitch s.
    straight s.
    umbilical s.
    Waldman episiotomy s.
    Yankauer s.
    Z-Scissors hysterectomy s.
SCIWORA
    spinal cord injury without radiographic
      abnormality
      SCIWORA syndrome

SCJ
    squamocolumnar junction
sclera, pl. **sclerae**
    blue s.
scleral
    s. hemorrhage
    s. icterus
scleredema
    s. adultorum
    s. of Buschke
sclerema neonatorum
scleroatonic muscular dystrophy
sclerocornea
    microphthalmia, dermal aplasia, s.
      (MIDAS)
sclerocystic disease of the ovary
sclerodactyly
scleroderma
    s. en coup de sabre
    focal s.
    limited systemic s.
    linear s.
    localized s.
    progressive familial s.
    s. renal crisis
    secondary s.
    systemic s.
scleroderma-like syndrome
sclerodermatomyositis antigen
scleroembolization
    percutaneous retrograde s.
scleromyxedema
sclero-oophoritis
sclerosant
sclerose en plaque
sclerosing
    s. adenitis
    s. adenosis
    s. adenosis of breast
    s. agent
    s. cholangitis
    s. lesion
    s. osteomyelitis
    s. panencephalitis
sclerosis, pl. **scleroses**
    Ammon horn s.
    amyotrophic lateral s. (ALS)
    arterial fibrosing s.
    bone s.
    childhood progressive systemic s.
    concentric s.
    diffuse globoid body s.
    diffuse globoid cell cerebral s.
    diffuse glomerular s.
    diffuse mesangial s. (DMS)
    disseminated s.
    dominant choroidal s.
    endocardial s.
    familial centrolobal s.

focal segmental glomerular s.
globoid cell cerebral s.
glomerular s.
hippocampal s.
isolated diffuse mesangial s.
  (IDMS)
juvenile amyotrophic lateral s.
lobar s.
mantle s.
Marburg variant multiple s.
menstrual s.
mesangial s.
mesial temporal s. (MTS)
metaphysial s.
multiple s. (MS)
myelinoclastic diffuse cerebral s.
nodular cortical s.
osteopathia striata with cranial s.
ovulational s.
photothermal s.
physiologic s.
progressive systemic s.
Scholz s.
sudanophilic cerebral s.
sudanophilic diffuse s.
systemic s. (SS)
s. tuberosa
tuberous s.

sclerosis-hyalinosis
focal and segmental glomerular s.-
  h.
sclerosteosis
sclerosus
lichen s.
sclerotherapy
endoscopic s.
endoscopic variceal s. (EVS)
injection s.
sclerotic skin disease
sclerotome
SCM
split cord malformation
sternocleidomastoid
  SCM muscle
SCMC
sperm-cervical mucus contact
SCMI
single central maxillary incisor
SCN
severe chronic neutropenia
scoliometer

scoliosis
Adams test for s.
adolescent s.
adolescent idiopathic s. (AIS)
compensatory s.
congenital thoracic s.
Dwyer correction of s.
s. film
idiopathic s.
infantile idiopathic s.
juvenile idiopathic s.
mild s.
neuromuscular s.
postural s.
secondary s.
s. with dural ectasia
scombroid
s. intoxication
s. poisoning
scooter board
Scop
Transderm S.
Scopette device
scopolamine
s. methylbromide
s. poisoning
scorbutic rosary
score
abstinence s.
Apgar s.
Ashworth s.
Asthma Severity S. (ASS)
Ballard s.
Ballard Assessment S. (BAS)
Bayley Motor S.
BDI s.
Berlin s.
BIND s.
biophysical profile s.
birth weight Z s.
Bishop s.
Boix-Ochoa GER s. (BOS)
BPP s.
cervical s.
CRIB s.
Croup s.
developmental assessment s.
Downes s.
Dubowitz s.
EDIN behavioral s.
Euler and Byrne s.
externalizing s.

NOTES

S

score *(continued)*
    Ferriman-Gallwey hirsutism s.
    Glasgow Meningococcal
      Septicemia S.
    global seasonality s.
    Herson-Todd s.
    home cognitive s.
    I antigen s.
    injury severity s. (ISS)
    internalizing s.
    Johnson s. 1–10
    Kaufman Factor S.
    LOD s.
    lower triceps skinfold Z s.
    Manning s. of fetal activity
    MECA T s.
    Methods for the Epidemiology of
      Child and Adolescent Disorders s.
    Modified Injury Severity S. (MISS)
    NAS S.
    S. for Neonatal Acute Physiology
      (SNAP)
    S. for Neonatal Acute Physiology-
      Perinatal Extension (SNAP-PE)
    Neonatal Skin Assessment S.
    Neurologic and Adaptive
      Capacity S. (NACS)
    new Ballard s. (NBS)
    optimality s.
    Optimal Observation S.
    Pediatric Trauma S. (PTS)
    pelvic s.
    POMS s.
    PREM s.
    PRISM s.
    raw s.
    recovery s.
    respiratory index s. (RIS)
    Revised Trauma S. (RTS)
    Rutter mean s.
    Sarnat s.
    Sassone s.
    scattered s.'s
    Scheuer s.
    Shwachman s.
    Shwachman-Kulczycki s.
    Silverman s.
    simplified acute physiology s.
      (SAPS)
    standard deviation s. (SDS)
    Stanford-Binet s.
    T bone density s.
    Vineland standard s.'s
    WDL asthma s.
    WISC III factor s.'s
    Wood-Downes asthma s.
    Yale Optimal Observation S.
    Zatuchni-Andros s.
    Z bone density s.

scoring
    fibrosis s.
    follicular s.
SCOT
    succinyl CoA:3-oxoacid CoA transferase
      SCOT deficiency
Scotch tape slide test
scotoma, pl. **scotomata**
    facultative s.
    scintillating s.
scotopic sensitivity syndrome
Scott
    S. cannula
    S. craniodigital syndrome
Scott-Taor syndrome
Scot-Tussin DM Dough Chasers
Scotty dog sign
scout radiograph
ScP
    scapuloposterior
SC-pseudothalidomide syndrome
SCPUFA
    short-chain polyunsaturated fatty acid
scrape
    s. cytology
    s. and smear
scrapie
scraping
    conjunctival s.
    scabies s.
    skin s.
screaming
screen *(See also* screening)
    antigen s.
    S. for Child Anxiety-Related
      Emotional Disorders (SCARED)
    Glucola s.
    maternal serum triple s.
    Monospot s.
    organic acid s.
    Pap Plus HPV s.
    prenatal s.
    qualitative urine s.
    Rapid Strep s.
    serum lysosomal enzyme s.
    suicide risk s. (SRS)
    supplemental newborn s.
    TORCH s.
    toxicology s.
    triple s.
    triple-biochemical s.
    triple-marker s.
    universal bilirubin s.
    universal hearing s.
    urine toxicology s.
screener
    Algo newborn hearing s.

Oregon Adolescent Depression Project-Conduct Disorder S. (OADP-CDS)

screening
AABR hearing s.
amino acid s.
AmnioStat-FLM maturity s.
antenatal s.
antibody s.
carrier s.
colposcopic s.
s. culture
cytologic s.
Denver II s.
depression s.
developmental s.
FA s.
first trimester s.
genetic s.
hearing s.
hepatitis s.
immunologic s.
s. laboratory test
mammographic s.
s. mammography
maternal age s.
maternal serum s.
multiple marker s.
Neo-Gen s.
neonatal s.
nuchal translucency s.
prenatal s.
s. recommendation
routine s.
sickle cell s.
s. sonogram
S. Tests for Young Children and Retardates
S. Tool for Early Predictors of PTSD (STEPP)
triple-marker s.
triple serum marker s.
ultrasound s.
universal newborn hearing s. (UNHS)
uterine s.
vision s.

Screenoscope
Topcon S.

screw
cannulated s.
myoma s.

screwdriver teeth
screw-tipped intraosseous needle
scrofula
scrofulaceum
    Mycobacterium s.
scrofuloderma
scrofulosorum
lichen s.
scroll ear
scrotal
s. edema
s. hypospadias
s. mass
s. orchiopexy
s. position
s. swelling
s. testis
s. tongue
scrotum, pl. **scrota, scrotums**
bifid s.
raphe of s.
shawl s.
Scr proto-oncogene
scrub
Sklar s.
s. typhus
SCT
stem cell transplantation
Scully tumor
Scultetus binder
scurvy
hemorrhagic s.
infantile s.
scybala
SD
standard deviation
AlphaNine SD
SD disease
Profilnine SD
S/D
systolic/diastolic ratio
Gammagard S/D
Polygam S/D
S/D ratio
SDAP
single donor apheresis platelet
SDAT
senile dementia of the Alzheimer type
SDF
WinRho SDF
SDH
subdural hematoma

NOTES

SDR
  selective dorsal rhizotomy
SDS
  standard deviation score
SDYS
  Simpson dysmorphia syndrome
SE
  signed English
  status epilepticus
SEA
  seronegativity, enthesopathy, arthropathy
  spondylitis, enthesitis, arthritis
    SEA syndrome
seabather's eruption
sea-blue
  s.-b. histiocyte
  s.-b. histiocyte syndrome
Seabright bantam syndrome
seal fingers
seal-like cough
seam
  osteoid s.
  urethral s.
SeaMist
searching toe
seasonal
  s. affective disorder (SAD)
  s. allergic rhinitis
  s. asthma
  S. Pattern Assessment Questionnaire
    (SPAQ)
  s. pollinosis
Seasonale
  S. birth control pill
  S. oral contraceptive
seat
  bath s.
  belt-position booster s.
  s. belt sign
  s. belt syndrome
  Hospital Recliner s.
  Ingram bicycle s.
SEB
  staphylococcal enterotoxin B
sebaceous
  s. collar
  s. cyst
  s. duct
  s. gland
  s. gland hyperplasia
  s. gland lobule
  s. miliaria
  s. nevus
  s. nevus syndrome
sebaceum
  adenoma s.
sebaceus
  nevus s.

seborrhea
  adolescent s.
  infantile s.
seborrheic
  s. blepharitis
  s. dermatitis
  s. diaper rash
  s. eczema
  s. keratosis
seborrheic-like facies
seborrheic-looking skin lesion
Sebulex
sebum
  s. preputiale
  s. production
  s. secretion
Sebutone shampoo
seca-230 Promard wall growth chart
Sechrist neonatal ventilator
Seckel
  bird-headed dwarf of S.
  S. bird head syndrome
  S. dwarfism
  S. nanism
secobarbital
Seconal
second
  s. bicuspid
  s. branchial cleft cyst
  cycle per s. (cps)
  forced expiratory volume in 1 s.
    (FEV$_1$)
  s. heart sound
  s. impact syndrome
  S. International Standard (SIS)
  s. messenger
  S. National Incidence Study (NIS-
    2)
  s. parallel pelvic plane
  s. permanent molar
  s. primary molar
  s. stage of labor
  s. trimester
  s. trimester acute gestosis
  s. trimester termination
  s. twin
secondary
  s. abdominal pregnancy
  s. adrenal hypoplasia
  s. alopecia
  s. amenorrhea
  s. amyloidosis
  s. apnea
  s. atelectasis
  s. carnitine deficiency
  s. circular reaction
  s. closure
  s. craniosynostosis
  s. dysmenorrhea

s. dystonia
s. enuresis
s. epilepsy
s. headache
s. hematoma
s. hyperoxaluria
s. hypochondriasis
s. hypothyroidism
s. infertility
s. intention
s. localized peritonitis
s. lymphedema
s. macrodactyly
s. macular atrophy
s. microcephaly
s. moyamoya disease
s. nail dystrophy
s. nephrotic syndrome
s. osteosarcoma
s. PAP
s. phimosis
s. pneumonitis
s. polycythemia
s. prematurity prevention
s. prophylaxis
s. scleroderma
s. scoliosis
s. seizure
s. sex characteristic
s. solar urticaria
s. syphilis
s. teeth
s. tracheomalacia
s. uterine inertia
s. vesicoureteral reflux
s. vestibular dyspareunia
s. viremia

second-degree
s.-d. burn
s.-d. descent
s.-d. episiotomy
s.-d. heart block
s.-d. hypospadias
s.-d. laceration
s.-d. prolapse

second-generation progesterone
second-hand
s.-h. smoke
s.-h. smoking

second-line
s.-l. chemotherapy
s.-l. measure

second-look
S.-l. computer-aided detection system
s.-l. laparoscopy
s.-l. laparotomy
s.-l. operation

second-trimester amniocentesis
secretagogue
secrete
secretin
Secretin-Ferring Powder
secretion
abnormal cortisol s.
adrenal androgen s.
androgen s.
breast s.
cervicovaginal s.
dysregulated insulin s.
excessive acid s.
excessive insulin s.
follicular phase gonadotropin s.
FSH s.
gonadotropin s.
impaired s.
inappropriate antidiuretic hormone s.
insulin s.
luteinizing hormone s.
melatonin s.
ovarian androgen s.
oxytocin s.
persistent estrogen s.
pituitary gonadotropin s.
placental s.
progesterone s.
prolactin s.
sebum s.
steroid s.
syndrome of inappropriate antidiuretic hormone s.
vaginal s.

secretively
secretory
s. adenocarcinoma
s. carcinoma
s. diarrhea
s. disease
s. endometrium
s. IgA
s. leukocyte protease inhibitor
s. otitis media

S

NOTES

secretory *(continued)*
    s. phase
    s. sarcoma
section
    cesarean s. (C-section)
    classical cesarean s.
    cut s.
    elective cesarean s.
    emergency cesarean s.
    frozen s.
    lower segment transverse
      cesarean s. (LSTCS)
    lower segment vertical cesarean s.
      (LSVCS)
    LUST cesarean s.
    Porro cesarean s.
    postmortem cesarean s.
    primary cesarean s.
    repeat cesarean s.
    representative s.
sectioning
    clot s.
    serial s.
Sectral
secundigravida
secundina, pl. **secundinae**
secundines
secundipara
secundum
    foramen s.
    ostium s.
    septum s.
secundum-type
secure attachment
SED
    serious emotional disturbance
    spondyloepiphyseal dysplasia
      late-onset SED
sedation
    chloral hydrate s.
    conscious s.
    ketamine s.
    Observer Assessment of Alertness
      and S. (OAAS)
    pediatric s.
sedative
    s. effect
    s. poisoning
sedentary
sediment
    spun urine s.
    urinary s.
    urine s.
sedimentation rate
Sedlacková syndrome
sedlakii
    Citrobacter s.
SEE
    signed exact English

seed
    gold s.
    radioactive s.
    vitreous s.
seeding
    hematogenous s.
    single tumor with s.
    tumor s.
    vitreous s.
seeking
    food s.
Seemanová-Lesny syndrome
Seemanová syndrome (1, 2)
SEER
    Surveillance, Epidemiology and End
    Results
      SEER network
seesaw
    s. breathing
    s. nystagmus
Seessel pouch
SEF
    spectral edge frequency
segment
    chromosomal s.
    lower uterine s.
    mesodermal dysgenesis of
      anterior s.
    upper body s.
    uterine s.
segmental
    s. amyoplasia
    s. aneuploidy
    s. dystonia
    s. edema
    s. epidural analgesia
    s. hypoplasia
    s. mesangial hypercellularity
    s. neurofibromatosis
    s. resection
    s. rolling
    s. spinal instrumentation
segmentation
    rhombomere s.
segmentectomy
segmented neutrophil
segregation
    s. distortion
    postmeiotic s.
SEH
    subependymal hemorrhage
Seip-Lawrence syndrome
Seip syndrome
Seitelberger disease
Seitleis syndrome
Seitzinger
    S. device
    S. tripolar cutting forceps

seizure
absence s.
s.'s, acquired microcephaly,
  agenesis of corpus callosum
  syndrome
afebrile s.
akinetic s.
anoxic s.
apneic s.
astatic s.
atonic s.
atypical absence s.
atypical febrile s.
atypical petit mal s.
autonomic s.
benign familial neonatal s.
bicuculline-induced s.
brief tonic s.
clonic s.
complex febrile s.
complex partial s. (CPS)
s. control
convulsive s.
s. disorder
drop s.
eclamptic s.
epilepsy s.
epileptic s.
familial neonatal s.
febrile s.
fetal s.
focal motor s.
gelastic s.
generalized tonic-clonic s.
grand mal s.
hypocalcemic s.
hypoglycemic s.
hyponatremic s.
s.'s, hypotonic cerebral palsy,
  megalocornea, mental retardation
  syndrome
hysteric s.
hysterical s.
idiopathic s.
infantile monoclonic s.
infantile myoclonic s.
jackknife s.
jacksonian s.
lightning s.
local s.
localization-related epilepsy s.
major motor s.

minor motor s.
monoclonic s.
motor s.
multifocal clonic s.
myoclonic s.
myoclonic-astatic s.
neonatal s.
nonconvulsive s.
nonepileptic s.
nonphotogenic s.
partial complex s.
petit mal s.
photogenic s.
photosensitive s.
postasphyxial s.
primary generalized s.
psychogenic s.
psychomotor s.
pyridoxine-dependent s.
recurrent convulsive s.
recurrent nonconvulsive s.
reflex anoxic s.
repeated partial s.
rolandic s.
salaam s.
secondary s.
sensory s.
severe s.
simple febrile s.
simple partial s. (SPS)
subtle s.
sylvian s.
temporal lobe s.
tetanic s.
tonic s.
tonic-clonic s.
typical absence s.
versive s.
vertiginous s.
vestibular s.
vestibulogenic s.
Seldinger technique
SelectCells Mini endometrial sampler
selection
bulk s.
family s.
fecundity s.
gametic s.
insertion site s.
natural s.
prenatal s.
truncate s.

NOTES

selective
- s. abortion
- s. angiography
- s. aplasia
- s. aplasia of vermis
- s. broth medium (SBM)
- s. dorsal rhizotomy (SDR)
- s. embolization procedure
- s. estrogen receptor modulator (SERM)
- s. feticide
- s. IgA deficiency
- s. inguinal node dissection
- s. intrapartum chemoprophylaxis (SIC)
- s. mutism
- s. neuronal necrosis
- s. no-fault system
- s. photothermolysis (SPTL)
- s. posterior rhizotomy
- s. proteinuria
- s. pulmonary arteriography
- s. reading disability
- s. renal vein renin determination
- s. serotonin reuptake inhibitor (SSRI)
- s. termination
- s. transvaginal embryo reduction
- s. tubal assessment to refine reproductive therapy (STARRT)
- s. tubal occlusion procedure (STOP)
- s. tubal occlusion procedure system

Select joint
selenium sulfide
Sele-Pak
Selepen
self-breast examination (SBE)
self-catheter
- Mentor female s.-c.

self-catheterization
- clean intermittent s.-c.
- intermittent s.-c.

self-comforting behavior
self-deprecation
self-esteem
self-examination
- BD Sensability breast s.-e.
- breast s.-e. (BSE)

self-harm
- self-reported s.-h. (SRSH)

self-harming act
self-help domain
self-incompatibility
self-induced vomiting
selfing
self-injectable epinephrine
self-injurious behavior (SIB)

Self-Injury
- S.-I. Grid (SIG)
- S.-I. and Self-Restraint checklist (SISRC)

self-limited bleeding
self-loathing
self-monitoring
self-mutilating behavior
self-mutilation
- compulsive s.-m.

self-priming action
self-report
- youth s.-r. (YSR)

self-reported self-harm (SRSH)
self-retaining retractor
self-statement
- coping s.-s.

self-sterility
self-stimulation
self-test
- OvuQuick S.-t.

self-worth
sella, pl. **sellae**
- J-shaped s.
- tuberculum s.
- s. turcica

sellar enlargement
Sellheim incision
Sellick maneuver
Selsun Blue Shampoo
selvagem
- fogo s.

SEM
- scanning electron microscopy
- skin, eye, mucocutaneous
- systolic ejection murmur
- SEM infection

semantic memory
semantic-pragmatic disorder
SEMD
- spondyloepimetaphyseal dysplasia

semen
- s. analysis
- frozen s.
- s. liquefaction
- prepared s.
- viscous s.
- s. volume

SEMG
- surface electromyogram
- surface electromyography

semiallogenic
Semicid
semicircular canal
semicircularis
- linea s.

semiconservative
semidefinitive procedure

semielemental casein hydrolysate
 formula
semifluid diet
semi-Fowler position
semilithotomy position
semilobar holoprosencephaly
semilunar
 s. fold of Douglas
 s. line of rectus sheath
semimembranosus muscle
seminal
 s. fluid
 s. fluid analysis (SFA)
 s. plasma
 s. vesicle
semination
seminiferous
 s. tubule
 s. tubule dysgenesis
seminoma
 ovarian s.
semiprone position
semisolid
semisynthetic penicillin
semitendinosus muscle
Semken forceps
Semm
 S. hysterectomy
 S. Pelvi-Pneu insufflator
 S. uterine vacuum cannula
senescent red cell
Sengers
 S. cardiomyopathy
 S. mitochondrial myopathy
 S. syndrome
Sengstaken-Blakemore tube
senile
 s. dementia of the Alzheimer type
 (SDAT)
 s. urethritis
 s. vaginitis
senility
 premature s.
Senior-Loken syndrome
senna concentrate/docusate sodium
Senna-Gen
Senna X-Prep
Senn-Dingman retractor
sennetsu
 Ehrlichia s.
Senning
 S. atrial switch procedure

 S. operation
 S. repair
Senokot-S
senology
SenoScan full-field digital
 mammography system
Sensability breast self-examination aid
sensation
 genital s.
 impaired rectal s.
 integrate s.
 proprioceptive s.
 rectal s.
sense
 vibration s.
Sensenbrenner-Dorst-Owens syndrome
Sensenbrenner syndrome
SensiCare surgical glove
sensimotor induction in disturbed
 equilibrium syndrome
sensitivity
 assay s.
 chemoreceptor s.
 clitoral s.
 culture and s. (C&S)
 gluten s.
 insulin s.
 microbial s.
sensitization
 anti-Kell s.
 contact s.
 food-antigen s.
 Kell s.
 latex s.
 Rh s.
 in utero s.
sensitizer
 hypoxic cell s.
sensor
 acoustic respiratory motion s.
 (ARMS)
 anal EMG PerryMeter s.
 BreastAlert differential
 temperature s.
 differential temperature s. (DTS)
 MiniGuard CO_2 s.
 multiparameter intraarterial s.
 (MPIAS)
 Nellcor FS-10 oximeter s.
 Nellcor FS-14 oximeter s.
 Neotrend s.
 Resp-EZ piezoelectric s.

NOTES

843

Sensorcaine
Sensorcaine-MPF
Sensorimedics Horizon Metabolic Cart
sensorimotor integration
sensorineural
    s. change
    s. deafness
    s. deafness, imperforate anus,
      hypoplastic thumbs syndrome
    s. hearing impairment
    s. hearing loss (SNHL)
sensorium
    altered s.
    clouding of s.
    depressed s.
Sensormedic 3100A 8000 oscillator
sensory
    s. apraxia
    s. arthropathy
    s. deficit
    s. impairment
    s. information
    s. integration
    s. integration therapy
    s. loss
    s. nerve
    s. nerve conduction velocity
    s. neuropathy
    s. organ
    s. overload
    s. polyneuritis
    s. problem
    s. seizure
    s. stimulation
    s. threshold
sensory-motor stage
SensoScan mammography system
sentence
    five-word s.
Senter syndrome
sentinel
    s. loop
    s. lymph node
    s. lymph node biopsy
SEPA
    superficial external pudendal artery
separation
    amnion-chorion s.
    s. anxiety
    s. anxiety disorder (SAD)
    blastomere s.
    commissural s.
    decreased commissural s.
    peripartum symphysis s.
    peripheral placental s.
    physial s.
    placental s.
    premature placental s.
    sperm s.

    spontaneous placental s.
    symphysial s.
    tripus s.
    uterine scar s.
separation-reunion experience
separator
    Benson baby pylorus s.
Sephadex binding test
Sephardic Jew
Sepharose
    CNBr activated S.
Sep-Pak
Seprafilm bioresorbable membrane
sepsis, pl. **sepses**
    bacterial s.
    catheter s.
    Chlamydia s.
    early-onset s.
    Escherichia coli s.
    fulminant s.
    fungal s.
    group B streptococcal s.
    late-onset s.
    Listeria monocytogenes s.
    neonatal s.
    s. neonatorum
    nosocomial s.
    pneumococcal s.
    portal vein s.
    postanginal s.
    postoperative s.
    puerperal s.
    Salmonella oranienburg s.
    s. syndrome
    viral s.
    s. workup
sepsis-pneumonia syndrome
sepsis/shock syndrome
septa (*pl. of* septum)
septal
    s. defect
    s. deviation
    s. hypertrophy
    s. panniculitis
Septata intestinalis
septate
    s. hymen
    s. uterus
    s. vagina
septation
    aorticopulmonary s.
    cardiac s.
    internal s.
    tracheoesophageal s.
    ventricular s.
septectomy
    atrial s.
    surgical s.

septic
  s. abortion
  s. arthritis
  s. bursitis
  s. embolus
  s. encephalitis
  s. joint
  s. meningitis
  s. pelvic thrombophlebitis (SPT)
  s. pelvic vein thrombophlebitis
  s. shock
septicemia
  clostridia s.
  gonococcal s.
  meningococcal s.
  postnatal s.
  puerperal s.
  streptococcal s.
septicum
  Clostridium s.
septimetritis
septooptic-pituitary dysplasia
septophilic
septostomy
  atrial s.
  balloon s.
  balloon atrial s. (BAS)
  catheter s.
  echo-guided balloon atrial s.
  Rashkind balloon atrial s.
Septra DS
septum, pl. **septa**
  anterior nasal s.
  aortopulmonary s.
  atrioventricular s.
  conotruncal s.
  deviated s.
  enlarged cavum s.
  interventricular s.
  membranous s.
  midvaginal transverse s.
  muscular ventricular s.
  nasal s.
  orbital s.
  outlet s.
  s. pellucidum
  s. pellucidum agenesis
  s. pellucidum with porencephalia syndrome (SASPP)
  perimembranous s.
  placental septa
  s. primum

  proximal transverse s.
  pulmonary atresia with intact ventricular s. (PAIVS)
  rectovaginal s.
  retrovaginal s.
  s. secundum
  supravaginal s.
  Swiss cheese s.
  trabecular muscular s.
  tracheoesophageal s.
  transverse vaginal s.
  s. transversum
  urogenital s.
  uterine s.
  vaginal s.
  ventricular s.
  vesicovaginal s.
septuplet
sequel
  Diamox S.'s
sequela, pl. **sequelae**
  cardiovascular s.
  delayed neuropsychological s. (DNS)
  sequelae of extreme prematurity
  long-term sequelae
  neoplastic s.
  neurodevelopmental s.
  subtle neurologic s.
sequence
  amniotic band disruption s.
  autonomous replication s.
  base s.
  blepharophimosis s.
  breech deformation s.
  cephalocaudal s.
  s. characterized amplified region
  cleaved amplified polymorphic s.
  complementary s.
  consensus s.
  conserved s.
  DiGeorge malformation s.
  DNA s.
  fetal akinesia deformation s. (FADS)
  fetal brain disruption s.
  FLAIR s.
  Goldenhar s.
  HASTE s.
  insertion s.
  laterality s.
  malformation s.

NOTES

845

sequence *(continued)*
  mental retardation-overgrowth s.
  Möbius s.
  Pierre Robin s.
  Pierre Robin malformation s.
  Poland malformation s.
  Potter oligohydramnios s.
  regulatory s.
  RICE s.
  sirenomelia s.
  Sotos s.
  s. tagged microsatellite
  s. tagged site
  tandem repeat s.
  TRAP s.
  X-linked hydrocephalus-stenosis of
    aqueduct of Sylvius s.
  Y chromosome-specific DNA s.
sequencing
  chromosome s.
  gene s.
  temporal s.
  verbal s.
sequential
  s. administration
  s. delivery
  s. hormone therapy
  s. memory
  s. multiple analysis (SMA)
  s. oral contraceptive
  s. peak flow measurement
sequestered
  s. lobe
  s. lung
sequestra (*pl. of* sequestrum)
sequestration
  acute splenic s.
  bile acid s.
  bronchopulmonary s. (BPS)
  s. crisis
  extralobar s.
  fetal pulmonary s.
  intralobar pulmonary s.
  pulmonary s.
  reticuloendothelial s.
  splenic s.
sequestrative
sequestrum, pl. **sequestra**
  s. formation
  pancreatic s.
Sequoia Acuson system
sera (*pl. of* serum)
Serax
Sereen
Serentil
Serevent Diskus
serial
  s. casting
  s. digital examinations

  s. growth scans
  s. maternal serum fibrinogen
  s. neurologic examination
  s. radiograph
  s. sectioning
series
  acute abdominal s.
  eight-drugs-in-one-day treatment s.
  gastrointestinal s.
  Kell s.
  recombinant hepatitis B
    immunization s.
  treatment s.
  upper gastrointestinal s.
  S. 50 XMO fetal/maternal monitor
    with integrated fetal oxygen
    saturation monitoring
serine
  s. protease inhibitor (SERPIN)
  s. proteinase
serine-threonine . kinase
seriography
  biplane s.
serious
  s. bacterial infection (SBI)
  s. emotional disturbance (SED)
SERM
  selective estrogen receptor modulator
sermorelin acetate
seroconversion illness
seroconverting
serofibrinous pleurisy
serogroup B meningococcus
serologic
  s. test
  s. testing
  s. test for syphilis (STS)
serologic marker
serology
  C-urea s.
  nontreponemal s.
  treponemal s.
serology-negative mother
seroma
  auricular s.
  postoperative s.
Seroma-Cath system
seromuscular intestinal patch graft
Seromycin Pulvules
seronegative
  s. enthesopathy and arthropathy
    syndrome
  s. neonate
  s. spondyloarthropathy
seronegativity, enthesopathy, arthropathy
  (SEA)
Serono SR1 FSH analyzer
Serophene

seropositive
ANA s.
cytomegalovirus s.
seroprevalence
s. rate
Seroquel
seroreverter
serosa
lochia s.
peritoneal s.
vesicouterine s.
serosal
s. adhesion
s. surface
serosanguineous
s. fluid
s. rhinitis
serositis
serostatus
Serostim Injection
serotonergic
s. dysfunction
s. function
s. reuptake blockade
s. system
serotonin
s. deficiency
s. hypothesis
s. receptor antagonist
s. receptor blockade
s. reuptake blocker
s. reuptake inhibitor (SRI)
s. syndrome
s. transporter 5-HTT
serotype
serous
s. adenocarcinoma
s. carcinoma
s. cystadenocarcinoma
s. cystadenoma
s. form
s. form of tuberculous meningitis
s. otitis media
s. ovarian neoplasm
s. retinal detachment
s. tumor
serovar-specific
s.-s. IgG
s.-s. IgM
serpiginosa
elastosis perforans s.

serpiginous
s. border
s. cephalad curved physis
SERPIN
serine protease inhibitor
Serratia
S. marcescens
S. marcescens infection
Sertoli
S. cell
S. cell tumor
Sertoli-cell-only syndrome
Sertoli-Leydig
S.-L. cell
S.-L. cell tumor
sertraline
s. HCl
s. hydrochloride
serum, pl. **sera**
s. acetaminophen level
acute sera
s. albumin
s. albumin concentration
s. amino acid
s. amino acid concentration
s. aminotransferase
s. ammonia
s. amylase
s. amylase level
s. analyte
s. anticonvulsant level
s. antienterocyte antibody
antilymphocyte sera
antirabies s.
s. apolipoprotein
s. assay
s. bactericidal titer (SBT)
s. bile salt level
s. bilirubin
s. bilirubin-binding capacity
s. carotene level
s. complement
convalescent sera
convalescent s.
s. copper
s. copper level
s. cortisol level
s. digoxin level
s. enzyme-linked immunoelectrotransfer blot
s. erythropoietin
s. estrogen

NOTES

847

serum *(continued)*
    s. ferritin
    s. ferritin concentration
    fetal s.
    s. free hemoglobin
    s. glucose
    s. glutamic-oxaloacetic transferase (SGOT)
    s. glutamic-pyruvic transaminase (SGPT)
    s. HCV RNA
    s. hepatitis
    hereditary erythroblastic multinuclearity with positive acidified s. (HEMPAS)
    s. hexosaminidase A
    s. hexosaminidase assay
    s. histamine level
    s. immunoglobulin G anti-*Toxoplasma*
    s. inhibitory titer (SIT)
    s. iron
    s. ketoacid
    s. lactate dehydrogenase concentration
    s. lead level
    s. leptin
    s. leptin level
    s. lithium concentration
    s. lysosomal enzyme screen
    maternal s.
    s. melatonin concentration
    s. müllerian inhibiting substance
    s. osmolality
    s. osteocalcin
    s. parathyroid hormone
    s. PCT
    s. PHE
    postdose s.
    s. pregnancy assay cartridge
    s. procalcitonin
    s. progesterone
    s. prolactin
    s. prostaglandin
    s. protease inhibitor
    s. protein concentration
    s. sickness
    s. sickness-like reaction
    s. sickness-like syndrome
    stored sera
    s. test
    s. testosterone
    s. thyrotropin
    s. transaminase
    s. type III procollagen
    s. urea nitrogen (SUN)
    s. uric acid
    s. zinc
Serutan

service
    S. Assessment for Children and Adolescents (SACA)
    child, adolescent, and family mental health s. (CAFMHS)
    Child Protective S.'s (CPS)
    children's s.
    s. coordinator
    Crippled Children's S.'s (CCS)
    Department of Children and Family S.'s (DCFS)
    Department of Children's S.'s (DCS)
    Department of Children and Youth S.'s
    Department of Public Social S.'s (DPSS)
    Guidelines for Adolescent Preventive S.'s (GAPS)
    home care s.
    related s.'s
    support s.'s
    S. Utilization and Risk Factors (SURF)
servocontrolled
    s. homeothermy
    s. ventilation pump
Servo 900C ventilator
servomechanism
sessile polyp
SEST
    supine empty stress test
sestamibi
set
    Embryon GIFT transfer catheter s.
    Fuhrman pleural drainage s.
    haploid s.
    Health Plan Employer Data and Information S.
    H/S Elliptosphere catheter s.
    Mi-Mark endocervical curette s.
    Mi-Mark endometrial curette s.
    Neo-Sert umbilical vessel catheter insertion s.
    s. point
    Rosch-Thurmond fallopian tube catheterization s.
Setleis syndrome
Seton procedure
setting
    fire s.
setting-sun sign
seven day rule
Sever
    S. disease
    S. release
severe
    s. acute respiratory syndrome (SARS)

s. childhood autosomal recessive muscular dystrophy (SCARMD)
s. chronic neutropenia (SCN)
s. combined immunodeficiency (SCID)
s. congenital neutropenia
s. dehydration
s. gastrointestinal bleeding (SGIB)
s. growth failure
s. ketoacidosis
s. megaloblastic anemia
s. mental retardation
s. micrognathia
s. myoclonic epilepsy
s. myoclonic epilepsy in infancy (SMEI)
s. myopia
s. ovarian hyperstimulation syndrome (SOHS)
s. refractory hypoglycemia
s. respiratory compromise
s. seizure

severity
pediatric acute admission s. (PAAS)

sevoflurane

sex
s. assignment
s. cell
s. change operation
s. chromatin
chromosomal s.
s. chromosomal abnormality
s. chromosomal anomaly
s. chromosomal polysomy
s. chromosome
s. chromosome aberration
s. chromosome abnormality
s. cord
s. cord mesenchymal tumor
s. cord stromal germ cell tumor
s. cord stromal neoplasm
s. determination
endocrinologic s.
genetic s.
gonadal s.
s. hormone
s. hormone-binding globulin (SHBG)
illicit s.
morphological s.
nuclear s.

oral s.
phenotypic s.
psychological s.
s. ratio
s. reversal
social s.
s. steroid
s. steroid add-back therapy
s. steroid modulation
s. surrogate
s. therapist

sexarche
sex-conditioned gene
sex-determining region (SRY)
sex-influenced gene
sex-limited gene
sex-linked
s.-l. chromosome
s.-l. disorder
s.-l. gene
s.-l. heredity
s.-l. inheritance
s.-l. neurodegenerative disease with monilethrix

sex-related trauma
sex-specific CDC growth chart
sextuplet
sexual
s. abuse
s. activity
s. ambiguity
s. arousal
s. arousal disorder
s. asphyxia
s. assault
s. assault forensic evidence (SAFE)
S. Assault Response Team (SART)
s. assault victim
s. aversion disorder
s. contact
s. debut
s. derivation
s. desire
s. deviation
s. differentiation
s. dimorphism
s. dwarfism
s. dysfunction
s. enjoyment
s. excitement
s. function
s. habit

NOTES

sexual *(continued)*
    s. hair
    s. history
    s. infantilism
    s. initiation
    s. intercourse
    s. issue
    s. maturation
    s. maturity rating (SMR)
    s. molestation
    S. Opinion Survey
    s. orientation
    s. pain disorder
    s. pleasure
    s. practice
    s. precocity
    s. problem
    s. relationship
    s. response
    s. response curve
    s. response cycle
    s. satisfaction
    s. stimulation
    s. transmission
    s. victimization
sexuality
sexualization
    traumatic s.
sexually
    s. transmitted disease (STD)
    s. transmitted infection (STI)
SF-1
    steroidogenic factor-1
SF-36 Health Status questionnaire
SFA
    seminal fluid analysis
    subclavian flap aortoplasty
S-F Kaon
SFMS
    Smith-Fineman-Myers syndrome
SG
    Chemstrip 10 with S.
SGA
    small for gestational age
    SGA infant
    postterm SGA
    term SGA
SGAR
    spectral gradient acoustic reflectometry
SGB
    Simpson-Golabi-Behmel
SGBS
    Simpson-Golabi-Behmel syndrome
SGH
    subgaleal hematoma
SGIB
    severe gastrointestinal bleeding
SGLT1 gene

SGO
    Society of Gynecologic Oncologists
    SGO classification of cancer
SGOT
    serum glutamic-oxaloacetic transferase
SGPT
    serum glutamic-pyruvic transaminase
SGS
    Schinzel-Giedion syndrome
    short gut syndrome
SH
    sitting height
    sulfhydryl
shadow
    acoustic s.
    cardiothymic s.
    double-bubble gas s.
    heart s.
    perihilar s.
    thymic s.
shaft
    clavicular s.
shaggy heart border
shagreen
    s. patch
    s. spot
Shah permanent tube
Shah-Waardenburg syndrome
shaken
    s. baby syndrome
    s. impact syndrome
    s. infant syndrome
shake test
shaking-impact syndrome
shaking wrist
shallow
    s. acetabular fossae
    s. acetabulum
    s. orbits
    s. orbits, ptosis, coloboma, trigonocephaly, gyral malformations, mental and growth retardation syndrome
    s. ulcer
    s. ulceration
Shambaugh retractor
shampoo
    A-200 S.
    Exsel s.
    Ionil-T s.
    lindane s.
    Paratrol s.
    Polytar s.
    Pronto S.
    P&S S.
    Pyrinex Pediculicide S.
    Pyrinyl Plus S.
    R&C S.
    Rid s.

Sebutone s.
Selsun Blue S.
T/Gel s.
Tisit S.
Triple X s.
Shapleigh curette
sharing
    United Network for Organ S.
    (UNOS)
sharp
    s. curettage
    s. dissection
    s. facial features
    s. pulse
Sharplan USA ultrasonic surgical
  aspirator
sharp-wave
    s.-w. discharge
    s.-w. transient
Shauta-Aumreich procedure
Shaw (I, II) scapel
shawl
    s. scrotum
    s. scrotum syndrome
SHBG
    sex hormone-binding globulin
Shea forceps
shear
    s. fracture
    s. stress
    s. stress-mediated nitric oxide
    release
Shearer forceps
shearing
    s. of catheter
    s. force
shears
    ADC Medicut s.
    LaparoSonic coagulating s. (LCS)
shear-strain deformation
sheath
    abdominal s.
    anterior rectus s.
    Bakelite cystoscopy s.
    ERA resectoscope s.
    fibrin s.
    7 French s.
    Hemaflex s.
    Insul-Sheath vaginal speculum s.
    MicroSpan s.
    Mullins long transseptal s.
    myelin s.

optic nerve s.
posterior rectus s.
probe s.
PRO/Covers ultrasound probe s.
rectus s.
sagittal septum of rectus s.
semilunar line of rectus s.
Vimule permanent s.
Sheathes ultrasound probe cover
shedding
    asymptomatic viral s.
    s. domain
    endometrial s.
    fecal s.
    s. of nails
    s. syndrome
    vaccine strain s.
    vaccine virus s.
    viral s.
Sheehan syndrome
Sheehy syndrome
sheep cell agglutinin titer
sheepskin glove
sheet
    amniotic s.
    impervious s.
    Ioban 2 cesarean s.
sheeting
    silicon gel s.
shelf
    Blumer s.
shell
    body s.
    s. shock
    s. vial culture
shellfish poisoning
shelter
Shenton line
shepherd's
    s. crook deformity
    s. purse
Shereshevskii-Turner syndrome
Sheridan-Gardiner visual acuity cards
Sheridan Tests for Young Children
  and Retardates
SHG
    sonohysterography
Shiatsu therapeutic massage
shield
    Dalkon s.
    Fuller s.
    nipple s.

NOTES

shield *(continued)*
    plastic heat s.
    Surety S.
shield-shaped chest
shift
    biobehavioral s.
    Doppler s.
    luteoplacental s.
    midline s.
    ontogenetic s.
    paroxysmal depolarization s. (PDS)
shifting
    s. dullness
    weight s.
Shiga
    S. lipopolysaccharide
    S. toxin (Stx)
    S. toxin-producing *Escherichia coli* (STEC)
Shiga-like toxin
Shigella
    S. dysenteriae (type 1)
    S. flexneri
    S. flexneri (type 2b)
    S. sonnei
Shigella
    Shigella bacteria
    Shigella dysentery
    Shigella vaginitis
shigelloides
    Plesiomonas s.
shigellosis
Shimada
    S. criteria
    S. histology
Shimada-Chatten histology
Shimadzu
    S. IIQ ultrasound
    S. SDU-400 ultrasound
    S. ultrasound system
shin
    saber s.
    s. splint
shiner
    allergic s.
shingles
shinsplints
shipyard conjunctivitis
Shirley wound drain
Shirodkar
    S. cervical cerclage
    S. operation
    S. procedure
SHMF
    Similac Human Milk Fortifier
shock
    anaphylactic s.
    anaphylactoid s.
    bacteremic s.

    cardiogenic s.
    cardiovascular s.
    compensated s.
    cool s.
    decompensated s.
    distributive s.
    endotoxic s.
    gram-negative endotoxic s.
    gram-negative endotoxin-induced s.
    hemorrhagic s.
    hypovolemic s.
    insulin s.
    s. liver
    s. lung
    neurogenic s.
    obstructive s.
    peripheral vascular s.
    postoperative s.
    septic s.
    shell s.
    spinal s.
    s. stage
    toxic s.
    uncompensated s.
    warm s.
shoe
    s. contact dermatitis
    reverse last s.
    straight last s.
    s. wedge
shoelace technique
Shohl solution
Shokeir syndrome
Shone
    S. anomaly
    S. syndrome
Shorr stain
SHORT
    short stature, hyperextensibility of joints and/or inguinal hernia, ocular depression, Rieger anomaly, teething delay
    SHORT syndrome
short
    s. arm of chromosome (p)
    s. attention span
    s. axis
    s. beaked nose
    s. bowel syndrome (SBS)
    s. cervix
    s. course
    s. frenulum linguae
    s. gut syndrome (SGS)
    s. leg walking cast
    s. limb
    s. limb dwarfism, saddle nose, spinal alterations, metaphyseal striation syndrome
    s. maxilla

s. metacarpal bone
S. Michigan Alcoholism Screening Test (SMAST)
s. neck
s. philtrum
s. PR interval
s. process
s. process of malleus
s. rib-polydactyly syndrome (SRPS)
s. rib-polydactyly (type I, II)
s. small-bowel (SSB)
s. stature (SS)
s. stature, characteristic facies, mental retardation, macrodontia, skeletal anomalies syndrome
s. stature homeobox (SHOX)
s. stature, hyperextensibility of joints and/or inguinal hernia, ocular depression, Rieger anomaly, teething delay (SHORT)
s. stature, microcephaly, mental retardation, multiple epiphyseal dysplasia syndrome
s. stature, microcephaly, syndactyly, dysmorphic face, mental retardation syndrome
s. tandem repeat typing
s. vagina

short-acting beta-2 agonist bronchodilator
short-axis view
short-bevel 21-gauge needle
short-chain
s.-c. acyl coenzyme A dehydrogenase (SCAD)
s.-c. fatty acid (SCFA)
s.-c. hydroxyacyl-coenzyme A dehydrogenase (SCHAD)
s.-c. polyunsaturated fatty acid (SCPUFA)

shortened cervix
shortening
acromelic s.
s. dorsal wedge radial osteotomy
s. fraction
fractional s.
mesomelic s.
metacarpal s.
metatarsal s.
percent fractional s.
rhizomelic limb s.

uterosacral s.
vaginal s.

shorthand vertical mattress stitch
short-increment sensitivity index (SISI)
short-limb
s.-l. dwarfism
s.-l. dystrophy
short-rib dwarfism
short-segment stenosis
Shoshin beriberi
shot
shotgun method
shotty
s. breast
s. cervical lymphadenopathy
s. node
shoulder
s. dystocia
Little League s.
s. presentation
s. sign
s. subluxation
swimmer's s.
show
bloody s.
SHOX
short stature homeobox
SHOX gene
Shprintzen-Goldberg craniosynostosis syndrome
Shprintzen velocardiofacial syndrome
SHR
sinusoidal heart rate
SHS
Sutherland-Haan syndrome
shuddering
s. attack
s. spell
shuffling gait
Shug male contraceptive device
Shulman syndrome
shunt, shunting
absolute s.
anatomic s.
aortic-to-pulmonary s.
aortopulmonary s.
arteriovenous s.
atrial s.
atrioventricular s.
AV s.
bidirectional Glenn s.
Blalock-Taussig s.

NOTES

S

shunt *(continued)*
  s. blockage
  central s.
  Codman Accu-Flow s.
  congenital portosystemic venous s.
  Cordis-Hakim s.
  cutaneous s.
  cystoperitoneal s.
  Delta s.
  Denver hydrocephalus s.
  distal splenorenal s.
  double-bubble ventriculoperitoneal s.
  Drapanas mesocaval s.
  ductal s.
  end-to-side portocaval s.
  enterohepatic s.
  extracardiac s.
  fetoamniotic s.
  Glenn s.
  intracardiac s.
  intrapulmonary s.
  jugular s.
  Kasai peritoneal venous s.
  left-to-right s.
  LeVeen s.
  lumboperitoneal s.
  s. malfunction
  mesocaval s.
  modified Blalock-Taussig s.
  s. nephritis
  neurosurgical s.
  palliative s.
  parietal s.
  peritoneal venous s.
  pleuroamniotic s.
  portoaortal s.
  portocaval s.
  portosystemic s.
  Potts s.
  prenatal placement of
    thoracoamniotic s.
  proximal splenorenal s.
  Pudenz s.
  pulmonary s.
  relative s.
  s. revision
  right-to-left s.
  side-to-side portocaval s.
  side-to-side splenorenal s.
  single-reservoir, single-pump s.
  splenorenal s.
  subdural-peritoneal s.
  s. tap
  thoracoamniotic s.
  transjugular intrahepatic
    portosystemic s. (TIPS)
  VA s.
  ventricular s.
  ventriculoamniotic s.

  ventriculoatrial s.
  ventriculojugular s.
  ventriculoperitoneal s. (VPS)
  ventriculopleural s.
  ventriculovascular s.
  vesicoamniotic s.
  VP s.
  Warren s.
  Waterston s.
  Y s.
shunt-dependent hydrocephalus
shunted hydrocephalus
shunting
  bidirectional s.
  ductal s.
  enterohepatic s.
  intrapulmonary s.
  left-to-right s.
  right-to-left s.
  ventriculoperitoneal s.
  Y s.
shunting *(var. of* shunt)
Shur-Clens
Shur-Seal
Shur-Strip
Shute forceps
shuttle
  cortisol-cortisone s.
Shutt suture punch system
Shwachman
  S. score
  S. syndrome
Shwachman-Bodian syndrome
Shwachman-Diamond syndrome
Shwachman-Kulczycki score
Shwartzman reaction
Shy-Drager syndrome
shy-inhibited temperament
Shy-Magee syndrome
shyness scale
SI
  sacroiliac
  syncytium inducing
SIADH
  syndrome of inappropriate secretion of
  antidiuretic hormone
sialadenitis
sialadenosis
sialic
  s. acid
  s. acid storage disease
sialidase
sialidosis
sialoglycoprotein
  glomerular s.
sialogram
sialography
sialomucin
sialophorin

sialorrhea
sialuria, Finnish type
sialyl
    s. Lewis X
    s. Lewis X determinant
    s. Tn antigen
sialylated Lewis A antigen
Siamese twins
SIB
    self-injurious behavior
siberica
    Rickettsia s.
sibling oocyte
SIC
    selective intrapartum chemoprophylaxis
sicca
    s. complex
    keratitis s.
    keratoconjunctivitis s.
    rhinitis s.
    s. syndrome
sicchasia
sick
    s. euthyroid syndrome
    s. sinus node syndrome
sickle
    s. beta-thalassemia
    s. cell
    s. cell anemia
    s. cell crisis
    s. cell dactylitis
    s. cell disease (SCD)
    s. cell hemoglobin (HbS)
    s. cell-hemoglobin C, D disease
    s. cell hemoglobinopathy
    s. cell nephropathy
    s. cell preparation
    s. cell screening
    s. cell sludging
    s. cell-thalassemia disease
    s. cell trait
    s. hepatopathy
sickle-cell
    s.-c. associated hematuria
    s.-c. and beta thalassemia
Sickledex test
sicklemia
sickling
    s. crisis
    s. disorder
    intravascular s.
    red blood cell s.

sickness
    acute mountain s. (AMS)
    car s.
    falling s.
    S. Impact Profile (SIP)
    Jamaican vomiting s.
    morning s.
    motion s.
    mountain s.
    serum s.
    sleeping s.
SID
    sudden infant death
side
    s. effect
    s. lyer
    s. sitting
side-port adapter
sideroblast
    refractory anemia with ring s.'s (RARS)
    ring s. (RS)
sideroblastic anemia
siderophagic cyst
siderophilic
siderosis
    myocardial s.
side-to-end anastomosis
side-to-side
    s.-t.-s. portocaval shunt
    s.-t.-s. splenorenal shunt
sidewalls
    convergent s.
sideways walking
SIDS
    sudden infant death syndrome
    sulfoiduronate sulfatase deficiency
    near-miss SIDS
Siegel otoscope
Siegert sign
Siemens
    S. Servo 300, 900C ventilator
    S. SI 400 ultrasound
    S. Sonoline SI-400 ultrasound system
    S. Vision MRI
Siemens-Bloch pigmented dermatosis
Siemens-Elema Servo 900C ventilator
Siemerling-Creutzfeldt syndrome
Sierra-Sheldon tracheotome
SieScape imaging
sievert (Sv)

NOTES

SIFT
>transvaginal intrafallopian sperm transfer

sift
>fluid s.

SIG
>Self-Injury Grid

Siggaard-Andersen nomogram

sighing respiration

sighted
>partially s.

SigmaStat software

sigma tumor marker

sigmoid
>s. colon
>s. pouch
>s. pouch of Pratt
>s. sinus

sigmoiditis

sigmoidoscopy

sign
>3 s.
>abdominal free-fluid s.
>Ahlfeld s. (I, II)
>Alström s.
>apprehension s.
>Babinski s.
>banana s.
>Barlow s.
>Barré s.
>Battle s.
>Beccaria s.
>Biederman s.
>bilateral pyramidal tract s.'s
>blue dot s.
>Blumberg s.
>Borsieri s.
>Braxton Hicks s.
>brim s.
>Brudzinski s.
>Calkins s.
>candlestick s.
>Chadwick s.
>chandelier s.
>cherub s.
>Chvostek s.
>cock-robin s.
>Coopernail s.
>Corrigan s.
>cracked-pot s.
>cranial s.
>crenation s.
>Crowe s.
>Cullen s.
>curtsey s.
>cutoff s.
>Dalrymple s.
>Dance s.
>Danforth s.
>Darier s.

double-bleb s.
double-bubble s.
double-tract s.
dovetail s.
dragon s.
E s.
extrapyramidal s.
eye-of-the-tiger s.
fadir s.
false localizing s.
falx s.
figure-of-three s.
flag s.
fontanelle s.
Gage s.
Galeazzi s.
Gauss s.
Golden s. of S
Goodell s.
Gottron s.
Gowers s.
Granger s.
Grey Turner s.
Grisolle s.
groove s.
halo s. of hydrops
harlequin s.
Hartmann s.
Hawkins s.
Hegar s.
Hellendall s.
Hennebert s.
Hertoghe s.
Higoumenakis s.
Hoehne s.
Homans s.
Hutchinson s.
Hymenoptera s.
iliopsoas s.
Jacquemier s.
Kantor s.
Kergaradec s.
Kernig s.
Kernohan s.
Kleppinger envelope s.
Kussmaul s.
Küstner s.
Ladin s.
lambda s.
s. language
lateralizing s.
lemon s.
Lhermitte s.
localizing s.
long-tract s.
Macewen s.
Marcus Gunn s.
Marfan s.
Mayer s.

McMurray s.
meningeal s.
Metenier s.
milkmaid's s.
motor neuron s.
Munson s.
Murphy s.
Nager s.
Nelson s.
neonatal abstinence s.
Nikolsky s.
nuchal-spinal s.
obturator s.
Olshausen s.
oromotor s.
Ortolani s.
palmar-plantar s.
palpable spongy mass s.
Parinaud s.
Parrot s.
Pastia s.
pathergy s.
peritoneal s.
peroneal s.
Pinard s.
Piskacek s.
placental s.
Prehn s.
pronator s.
psoas s.
puddle s.
pyloric string s.
pyramidal tract s.
Radovici s.
Raynaud s.
reverse 3 s.
reverse Marcus Gunn s.
rib notching s.
Risser s.
Romaña s.
rope s.
Rovsing s.
Russell s.
sail s.
Salmon s.
Saunders s.
scarf s.
Schick s.
Scotty dog s.
seat belt s.
setting-sun s.
shoulder s.

Siegert s.
silk s.
Simon s.
snowman s.
soft s.
Spalding s.
square window s.
steeple s.
Stellwag s.
Sternberg s.
string s.
Tenney-Parker s.
thumb s.
Thurston Holland s.
thymic wave s.
Toriello-Carey s.
Trendelenburg s.
Tresilian s.
tripod s.
Trousseau s.
turtle s.
twin peak s.
Uhthoff s.
umbrella s.
upper motor neuron s.
Vipond s.
vital s.'s
von Fernwald s.
von Graefe s.
W s.
Wartenberg s.
water lily s.
Weill s.
Wimberger s.
Zaufal s.
SignaDRESS dressing
signal
   abnormal feedback s.
   centromeric s.
   extracellular matrix s.
   s. extraction pulse oximetry
   s. node
   peptide growth factor receptor s.
   specific growth factor s.
signaling
signed
   s. English (SE)
   s. exact English (SEE)
signet ring cell carcinoma
significance
   atypical glandular cells of
      uncertain s. (AGCUS, AGUS)

NOTES

857

significance *(continued)*
    atypical glandular cells of
      undetermined s. (AGCUS, AGUS)
    atypical squamous cells of
      undetermined s. (ASCUS)
    atypical squamous cells of
      undetermined significance/atypical
      glandular cells of undetermined s.
      (ASCUS/AGUS)
signing
Siker laryngoscope
SIL
    squamous intraepithelial lesion
Siladryl Oral
Silafed
Silapap
SIL/ASCUS lesion
Silastic
    S. band
    S. catheter
    S. cup extractor
    S. ring
    S. silo reduction of gastroschisis
    S. spring-loaded silo
    S. tube intubation
Silc extractor
silence
    electrocortical s.
silent
    s. allele
    s. amnionitis
    s. carrier
    s. celiac disease
    s. congenital CMV infection
    s. DVT
    s. fetal heart rate pattern
    s. gastroesophageal reflux
    s. gene
    s. myocarditis
    s. oscillatory pattern
    s. pelvic inflammatory disease
    s. precordium
    s. stroke
Silfedrine
    Children's S.
silhouette
    cardiac s.
silibinin
silica
silicon
    arsenic nickel s.
    s. gel sheeting
    s. rubber catheter
silicone
    s. band application
    s. catheter
    s. implant
    s. implant leakage
    s. injection

    s. microimplant
    s. plug
silicosis
Sil-K
    S.-K OB
    S.-K OB barrier
silk
    s. sign
    s. suture
    s. tie
SILL
    subischial leg length
**Sillence classification of osteogenesis
  imperfecta (type I, IA, IB, II, III,
  IV, IVA, IVB)**
silliness
    hebephrenic s.
silo
    s. decompression
    s. filler's disease
    Silastic spring-loaded s.
Silon
    S. tent
    S. wound dressing
Silphen
    S. Cough
    S. DM
Silsoft extended wear contact lens
Siltussin DM
Silvadene
silver
    s. cell
    s. fork deformity
    s. nitrate
    s. nitrate administration
    s. nitrate conjunctivitis
    s. nitrate drops
    s. nitrate eye prophylaxis
    s. nitrate solution
    s. nitrate stick
    s. stain
    s. sulfadiazine
    s. sulfadiazine cream
    s. thermal hat
    s. wire suture
Silverman
    S. and Nelles Anxiety Disorders
      Interview Schedule for Children
    S. score
Silverman-Anderson index
**Silverman-Handmaker dyssegmental
  dysplasia**
Silver-Russell
    S.-R. dwarfism
    S.-R. syndrome
Silverskiöld syndrome
silver-wire appearance
simethicone

simian
- s. B virus
- s. crease
- s. immunodeficiency virus (SIV)
- s. lines

Similac
- S.-20
- S. 2 Advance formula
- S. Alimentum Advance formula
- S. Human Milk Fortifier (SHMF)
- S. Human Milk Fortifier formula
- S. Isomil Advance 2 formula
- S. Isomil DF formula
- S. Lactose Free Advance formula
- S. Natural Care Advance formula
- S. NeoSure Advance formula
- S. PM-60/40
- S. PM 60/40 formula
- S. Special Care 20, 24, 40 formula
- S. with iron formula

similarities test
similar twins
Simkania
- S. negevensis
- S. negevensis strain Z

Simmonds
- S. disease
- S. syndrome

Simon
- S. focus
- S. position
- S. sign

Simonton technique
simple
- s. central anisocoria
- s. coarctation
- s. colloid goiter
- s. cyst
- s. ectopia lentis
- s. epispadias
- s. febrile seizure
- s. hyperplasia
- s. mastectomy
- s. meconium ileus
- s. metatarsus adductus
- s. motor tic
- s. partial seizure (SPS)
- s. phobia (SPh)
- s. pneumothorax
- s. sequence repeat

- s. squamous blepharitis
- s. syndactyly
- s. TGA
- s. ureterocele
- s. urethritis
- s. virilizing congenital adrenal hyperplasia (SV-CAH)
- s. vocal tic
- s. vulvectomy

simplex
- Dowling-Meara epidermolysis bullosa s.
- epidermolysis bullosa s.
- herpes s. (HS)
- herpetiformis epidermolysis bullosa s.
- s. infection
- Koebner epidermolysis bullosa s.
- lentigo s.
- lichen s.
- neonatal herpes s.
- nevus s.
- toxoplasmosis, other agents, rubella, cytomegalovirus, herpes s. (TORCH, ToRCH)
- Weber-Cockayne epidermolysis bullosa s.

simplified acute physiology score (SAPS)
simplistic method
Simpson
- S. dysmorphia syndrome (SDYS)
- S. dysplasia syndrome
- S. forceps
- S. uterine sound

Simpson-Angus rating scale
Simpson-Golabi-Behmel (SGB)
- S.-G.-B. fetal overgrowth syndrome
- S.-G.-B. syndrome (SGBS)

Simron
Sims
- S. curette
- S. position
- S. retractor
- S. uterine sound
- S. vaginal speculum

Sims-Huhner test
simultaneous
- s. preductal-postductal PO_2
- S. Technique for Acuity and Readiness Testing (STAR)

NOTES

S

SIMV
　　synchronized intermittent mandatory
　　　ventilation
Simview 3000
SIN
　　salpingitis isthmica nodosa
Sinai System
Sinarest 12 Hour Nasal Solution
sincipital presentation
Sindbis virus
Sinding-Larsen-Johansson syndrome
Sinding-Larsen lesion
sinensis
　　　Clonorchis s.
Sinequan Oral
Sinex Long-Acting
single
　　s. breech presentation
　　s. cell biopsy
　　s. central maxillary incisor (SCMI)
　　s. collecting system
　　s. donor apheresis platelet (SDAP)
　　s. fetal demise
　　s. footling presentation
　　s. gene defect
　　s. intrauterine death
　　s. kidney
　　s. nucleotide polymorphism
　　s. primer amplification reaction
　　s. ring-enhancing mass lesion
　　s. shot fast spin echo (SSFSE)
　　s. site BRACA
　　s. stranded conformational
　　　polymorphism
　　s. transverse palmar crease
　　s. tumor
　　s. tumor with seeding
　　s. ventricle
single-dose methotrexate therapy
single-energy photon absorptiometry
single-field hyperthermia combined with
　　radiation therapy
single-film cholangiography
single-gene
　　s.-g. abnormality
　　s.-g. disorder
single-isotope tracer technique
single-photon
　　s.-p. absorptiometry
　　s.-p. emission computed
　　　tomography (SPECT)
　　s.-p. emission tomography
single-reservoir, single-pump shunt
single-shot intravenous pyelogram
single-suture craniosynostosis
singleton
　　breech s.
　　s. breech presentation
　　s. fetus

　　s. infant
　　s. pregnancy
single-tooth tenaculum
single-twin demise
single-use diagnostic system (SUDS)
single-walled incubator
Singley forceps
Singulair
singultus
sinister
sinistrocardia
sinistrocerebral
sinistrotorsion
Sin Nombre virus
sinoatrial
　　s. block
　　s. conduction time
　　s. node (SA)
　　s. node artery
sinobronchitis
Sinografin
sinopulmonary tract infection
sinovaginal bulb
Sinubid
Sinufed
Sinumist-SR caplets
sinus
　　s. abruption
　　s. arrest
　　s. arrhythmia
　　s. bradycardia
　　branchial cleft s.
　　cavernous s.
　　cervical s.
　　complex unroofed coronary s.
　　　(CUCS)
　　coronary s.
　　s. cycle length
　　dermal s.
　　dermoid s.
　　endodermal s.
　　ethmoid s.
　　external branchial s.
　　s. fistula
　　high urogenital s.
　　s. histiocytosis
　　internal branchial s.
　　lumbosacral s.
　　marginal s.
　　maxillary s.
　　s. node dysfunction (SND)
　　s. node function
　　open dermal s.
　　paranasal s.
　　Petit s.
　　pilonidal s.
　　preauricular s.
　　s. radiogram
　　s. radiograph

sagittal s.
sigmoid s.
straight s.
superior sagittal s.
s. surgery
s. tachycardia
s. thrombophlebitis
s. thrombosis
s. tumor
unroofed coronary s.
urogenital s.
uterine s.
uteroplacental s.
Valsalva s.
s. of Valsalva
s. venosus
s. venosus defect

sinusitis
acute s.
allergic s.
anterior ethmoidal s.
bacterial s.
cavernous s.
chronic s.
idiopathic cavernous s.
invasive s.
recurrent s.

sinusoid
coronary s.
hepatic s.
lacunar s.

sinusoidal
s. channel
s. fetal heart rate
s. heart rate (SHR)
s. heart rate pattern

Sinusol-B
Sioux alarm
SIP
Sickness Impact Profile
SIPAP
social interaction and perinatal addiction
project
siphon effect
Sipple syndrome
Sippy diet
SIR
standardized incidence ratio
**Sirecust 404N neonatal monitoring
system**
sireniform fetus

sirenomelia
s. sequence
s. syndrome
sirenomelic fetus
Siri body fat percentage formula
sirolimus
SIRS
systemic inflammatory response
syndrome
SIS
saline infusion sonography
saline infusion sonohysterography
Second International Standard
SISI
short-increment sensitivity index
SISI test
SISRC
Self-Injury and Self-Restraint checklist
sister
s. chromatid
s. chromatid exchange
S. Mary Joseph nodule
Sistrunk operation
SIT
serum inhibitory titer
sit
right s.
site
antibody reaction s.
antigen binding s.
axillary vein insertion s.
binding s.
bleeding s.
episiotomy s.
fragile chromosome s. (FRA, fra)
fragile chromosome s. 1 (FRAXE1)
fragile chromosome s. 2 (FRAX2)
fragile chromosome s. E (FRAXE)
fragile chromosome s. F (FRAXF)
Luer lock s.
placental bleeding s.
s. preparation
puncture punch s.
reactive s. (RS)
restriction enzyme cutting s.
sequence tagged s.
transcription start s.
venipuncture s.
site-specific familial ovarian cancer
sitosterol
sitosterolemia

S

NOTES

sitting
>s. height (SH)
>long leg s.
>s. position
>side s.
>tailor s.

situ, in situ
>adenocarcinoma in s.
>carcinoma in s. (CIS)
>ductal carcinoma in s. (DCIS)
>in s.
>lobular carcinoma in s.
>placenta in s.
>residual in s.
>vulvar carcinoma in s.

situated learning

situs
>s. abnormality
>s. ambiguus
>s. indeterminus
>s. inversus
>s. inversus indeterminus
>s. inversus totalis
>s. inversus totalis syndrome
>s. inversus viscerum
>organ s.
>s. perversus
>s. solitus
>s. transversus
>visceral s.

sitz bath

SIV
>simian immunodeficiency virus

sivelestat

six-fingered dwarfism

sixth disease

size
>abnormal head s.
>appropriate blood pressure cuff s.
>blood pressure cuff s.
>body s.
>cardiac s.
>corpus luteum s.
>focal spot s.
>gestational sac s. (GSS)
>head s.
>infant s. (IS)
>maternal s.
>small body s.
>small head s.
>tongue s.
>tumor s.
>uterine s.

size-date discrepancy

Sjögren-Larsson syndrome

Sjögren syndrome

SK-Amitriptyline

skate flap technique

skeletal
>s. abnormalities, cutis laxa, craniostenosis, psychomotor retardation, facial abnormalities (SCARF)
>s. abnormality
>s. anomaly
>s. arthrogryposis
>s. calcium deficiency
>s. and cardiac malformations-thrombocytopenia syndrome
>cerebral, ocular, dental, auricular, s. (CODAS)
>s. defect
>s. dysplasia
>s. dysplasial, joint laxity, mental retardation syndrome
>s. dysplasia, sparse hair, dental anomalies syndrome
>s. growth
>s. infection
>s. maturation
>s. mineralization
>s. muscle biopsy
>s. muscle layer
>s. survey
>s. traction

skeleton
>gill arch s.

skeleton-skin-brain syndrome

Skene
>Bartholin, urethral, S. (BUS)
>S. duct
>S. duct opening
>S. gland

skewfoot

skier's thumb

skill
>attending s.
>basic s.
>decreased attending s.
>fine motor-adaptive s.
>gross motor s.
>Kaufman Survey of Early Academic and Language S.'s (K-SEALS)
>language s.
>meal-time s.
>motor s.
>perceptual s.
>Personal Adjustment and Role S.'s (PARS)
>personal-social s.
>thinking s.

skin
>alligator s.
>s. atrophy
>s. biopsy
>s. breakdown

s. calcification
collodion s.
congenital localized absence of s. (CLAS)
craniotubular dysplasia, growth retardation, mental retardation, ectodermal dysplasia, loose s.
crocodile s.
s. cyst
s. defect
s. discoloration
s. disease
doughy s.
dry s.
dusky s.
s. end-point titration
s., eye, mucocutaneous (SEM)
fish s.
s. flora
s. fold
gelatinous s.
s. graft
hyperextensile s.
hyperkeratotic dry s.
s. hyperlaxity
India rubber s.
s. lesion
s. mastocytosis, hearing loss, mental retardation syndrome
meconium-stained s.
mitral valve, aorta, skeleton, s. (MASS)
mottling of s.
Oxy-10 Advanced Formula for Sensitive S.
pallor of s.
parchment s.
s. penetration
s. popping
porcupine s.
s. prick test
puffy s.
s. rash
redundant s.
s. retraction
s. ridge pattern
rough-feeling s.
salt frosting of s.
s. scraping
staphylococcal scalded s.
s. staple
s. suture

s. tag
s. temperature
s. tenting
s. test conversion
s. test reactivity (STR)
s. thickening
thin vulvar s.
s. traction
s. trigger theory
vagabond s.
s. vesicle
vulvar s.
skin-covered lipomyelomeningocele
skin-eye-brain syndrome
skin-eye-mouth disease
skinfold
s. caliper technique
infarction of s.
s. thickness
skinning
s. colpectomy
s. vulvectomy
skinny-needle biopsy
skin-sparing mastectomy
skip
s. area
s. lesion
Sklar
S. aseptic germicidal cleaner
S. aseptic germicidal disinfectant
S. cream
S. foam
S. instrument polish
S. Kleen liquid
S. Kleen powder
S. lube
S. scrub
4S knot
skull
cloverleaf s.
coronal suture line of s.
s. fracture
hot cross bun s.
lacunar s.
maplike s.
natiform s.
strawberry shaped s.
sutures of s.
thickened base of s.
tower s.
West-Engstler s.

NOTES

SKY
 spectral karyotype
 spectral karyotyping
  SKY epidural pain control system
Sky-Boot stirrup system
skyline view radiograph
S/L
 A-Spas S/L
SLA
 superficial linear array
  SLA transducer
slant
 antimongoloid eye s.
 eye s.
 mongoloid s.
 palpebral s.
slapped
 s. cheek appearance
 s. cheek disease
 s. cheek rash
 s. cheek syndrome
slapping storklike gait
SLAS
 salt-losing adrenogenital syndrome
slate-gray cyanosis
Slavianski membrane
SLE
 St. Louis encephalitis
 systemic lupus erythematosus
  SLE 2000 ventilator
sleep
 active s.
 s. apnea
 s. apnea syndrome
 s. architecture
 s. attack
 s. bruxism
 s. cystogram
 s. debt
 deep s.
 delta s.
 s. disturbance
 s. efficiency
 s. epoch
 S. Guardian foam pad
 hour of s.
 s. hygiene
 indeterminate s.
 s. latency
 s. myoclonus
 narcoleptic s.
 non-REM s.
 s. paralysis
 s. pattern
 s. position
 quiet s.
 rapid eye movement s.
 REM s.
 restless s.

 s. start
 s. state
 s. study
 s. talking
 s. terror
 s. terror disorder
 transitional s.
 twilight s.
 s. with rapid eye movement
sleep-disordered
 s.-d. breathing
 s.-d. breathing syndrome
Sleepinal
sleep-induced dyskinesia
sleeping
 difficulty s.
 excessive s.
 s. habit
 s. position
 s. sickness
sleepless
 crying, requires oxygen, increased
  vital signs, expression, s.
  (CRIES)
sleeplessness
 facial expression and s.
 pressure, facial expression, s.
sleep-related headache
sleeptalking
sleep-wake transition disorder
sleepwalking disorder
sleepy infant
sleeve
 s. fracture
 s. fracture of patella
 Reid s.
SLI
 subdermal levonorgestrel implant
slick-gut syndrome
slide
 Testsimplets prestained s.
sliding
 s. hiatal hernia
 s. lock
sling
 Aldridge rectus fascia s.
 s. anomaly
 s. arm
 s. baby
 fascia lata suburethral s.
 levator s.
 Martius flap and fascial s.
 Mersilene mesh s.
 modified s.
 s. procedure
 puborectalis s.
 pulmonary artery s.
 retropubic s.
 Stratasis urethral s.

suburethral s.
two-team s.
vascular s.

slipknot
Duncan s.
Roeder loop s.
Weston s.

slipped
s. capital femoral epiphysis (SCFE)
s. epiphysis
s. upper femoral epiphysis (SUFE)

slit-lamp
s.-l. biomicroscopy
s.-l. examination

slit ventricle syndrome

SLO
Smith-Lemli-Opitz
SLO syndrome

Slo-Niacin
Slo-Phyllin Gyrocaps
Slosson Oral Reading Test-Revised (SORT-R)
Slotnick-Goldfarb syndrome
sloughed urethra syndrome
sloughing
cyclic s.
mucosal s.

slow
s. cognitive processing
S. Fe
S. Fe with folic acid
s. growth
s. rate of learning

slow-channel congenital myasthenic syndrome (SCCMS)
slowing
bilateral s.
generalized s.

Slow-Mag
slow-release sodium fluoride
Slow-Trasicor
SLUDGE
salivation, lacrimation, urination, defecation, gastrointestinal distress, and emesis

sludging
sickle cell s.

slurry
DE s.

Sly
S. disease
S. syndrome

SMA
sequential multiple analysis
spinal muscular atrophy

small
s. body size
s. bowel atresia
s. bowel biopsy
s. bowel dysmotility
s. bowel endometriosis
s. bowel enteroscopy
s. bowel injury
s. bowel intestinal polyposis
s. bowel overgrowth
s. bowel perforation
s. bowel strangulation
s. bowel transit
s. bowel transplantation
s. cell carcinoma
s. cell cleaved lymphoma
s. cell osteosarcoma
s. chromosome
s. for dates
s. for gestational age (SGA)
s. head size
s. intestine
s. intestine decompression
s. intestine stasis
s. jaw
s. left colon syndrome
s. maxillary bone
s. noncleaved cell lymphoma (SNCCL)
s. nuclear ribonucleoprotein-associated polypeptide (SNRPN)
s. patella syndrome
s. premature infant
s. round blue cell tumor of childhood
s. single copy
s. stature

smallpox vaccine
Sm antigen
SMART
surgical myomectomy as reproductive therapy

smart
street s.

SMAST
Short Michigan Alcoholism Screening Test

SMC
supernumerary marker chromosome

NOTES

S

Smead-Jones closure of peritoneum and fascia
smear
    acid-fast sputum s.
    anal Pap s.
    ASCUS s.
    blood s.
    cervical s.
    cytologic s.
    low-grade positive s.
    LSIL Pap s.
    nasal s.
    Pap s.
    Papanicolaou s.
    peripheral blood s.
    s. positive
    saline wet s.
    scrape and s.
    sputum s.
    squash and s.
    thick blood s.
    ThinPrep s.
    Tzanck s.
    vaginal irrigation s. (VIS)
    wet s.
    Wright-stained s.
smegma
    s. clitoridis
    s. embryonum
    s. preputii
SMEI
    severe myoclonic epilepsy in infancy
Smellie
    S. method
    S. scissors
Smellie-Veit method
S-methionine-labeled polypeptide
SMG22
    chromosome 22 supernumerary marker
    SMG22 syndrome
smile
    Cheshire cat s.
    sardonic s.
smiling incision
Smith
    S. pessary
    S. syndrome
Smith-Fineman-Myers syndrome (SFMS)
Smith-Hodge pessary
Smith-Lemli-Opitz (SLO)
Smith-Magenis syndrome (SMS)
Smith-McCort dwarfism
Smith-Theiler-Schachenmann syndrome
SMM
    scintimammography
SMO
    supramalleolar orthosis
smoke
    environmental tobacco s. (ETS)

    s. evacuator
    s. inhalation
    s. plume
    s. removal tube (SRT)
    second-hand s.
smokeless tobacco
smoking
    maternal s.
    prenatal s.
    second-hand s.
smooth
    s. chorion
    s. muscle
    s. muscle contraction
    s. muscle hamartoma
    s. muscle tumor
    s. philtrum
    s. tongue
SMR
    sexual maturity rating
SMS
    Smith-Magenis syndrome
SMZ-TMP
    trimethoprim-sulfamethoxazole
snakebite envenomation
SNAP
    Score for Neonatal Acute Physiology
Snaplets-FR
SNAP-PE
    Score for Neonatal Acute Physiology-
    Perinatal Extension
snapping
    s. hip
    s. knee syndrome
snapshot GRASS technique
snare
    Reiner-Beck s.
SNCCL
    small noncleaved cell lymphoma
SND
    sinus node dysfunction
Snellen
    S. acuity chart
    S. test
SNHL
    sensorineural hearing loss
sniffing
    s. position
    toluene s.
SNIPPV
    synchronized nasal intermittent positive-
    pressure ventilation
S-nitrosoglutathione
SNJ
    nevus sebaceus of Jadassohn
Sn-mesoporphyrin (SnMP)
SnMP
    Sn-mesoporphyrin
    tin mesoporphyrin

Snodgrass hypospadias repair
snoring
    habitual s. (HS)
    primary s.
snout reflex
Snow
    S. Mountain agent
    S. Mountain virus
snowflake pattern
snowman sign
snowstorm appearance
SNP
    sodium nitroprusside
SnPP
    tin protoporphyrin
Sn-protoporphyrin
SNRPN
    small nuclear ribonucleoprotein-
    associated polypeptide
snuffbox tenderness
snuffles
Snyder-Robinson syndrome (SRS)
soak
    Barrow solution s.
    Cidex s.
soap
    Alpha Keri s.
    Basis s.
    Lowila s.
    Oilatum s.
    pHisoHex s.
    TLC antiseptic s.
soap-bubble appearance
soapsuds enema
Soave abdominal pull-through procedure
sober
SOC
    surgical overhead canopy
sociability
social
    s. anxiety disorder
    s. behavior
    s. deprivation
    s. development
    s. drinking
    s. drug
    s. factor effect
    s. interaction and perinatal
    addiction project (SIPAP)
    s. isolation
    s. issue
    s. maturity
    s. milestone
    s. parents
    s. phobia
    S. Security Disability Insurance
    (SSDI)
    s. sex
    S. Support Scale for Children
    (SSSC)
    s. withdrawal
    s. worker
social-adaptive milestone
social-emotional
    s.-e. developmental area
    s.-e. domain
social-emotional learning disability
social-evaluative fear
social-occupational dysfunction
society
    American Cancer S. (ACS)
    American Fertility S. (AFS)
    American Urogynecologic S.
    S. for Assisted Reproductive
    Technology (SART)
    S. of Gynecologic Oncologists
    (SGO)
    International Continence S. (ICS)
sociobiologic
sociocultural stressor
sociodemographic data
socioeconomic status
sock
    verruca s.
socket
    dry s.
sodium (Na)
    s. acetate
    alendronate s.
    ampicillin sodium/sulbactam s.
    aqueous penicillin s.
    s. balance
    s. bicarbonate ($NaHCO_3$)
    Brevital S.
    s. bromide
    cefazolin s.
    cefoperazone s.
    cefotaxime s.
    cefoxitin s.
    ceftriaxone s.
    cefuroxime s.
    cephalothin s.
    s. channelopathy
    s. chloride (NaCl)

NOTES

sodium *(continued)*
s. citrate with citric acid
s. cromoglycate
cromolyn s.
s. cyclamate
dantrolene s.
s. diatrizoate
diclofenac s.
divalproex s.
s. docusate
docusate s.
s. equilin sulfate
ertapenem s.
estramustine phosphate s.
s. estrone sulfate
s. etidronate
s. excess
s. excretion
fluorescein s.
s. fluoride
fractional excretion of s.
heparin s.
s. hydrogen phosphate
s. hydroxide
s. hyposulfite
imipenem-cilastatin s.
s. iodide
s. iodide I-125, I-131
methicillin s.
mezlocillin s.
nafcillin s.
naproxen s.
nedocromil s.
s. nitroprusside (SNP)
nitroprusside s.
olsalazine s.
oxacillin s.
oxychlorosene s.
s. pentobarbital
Pentothal S.
s. phenylacetate
s. phenylacetate and sodium benzoate
s. phenylbutyrate
piperacillin sodium/tazobactam s.
s. polyacrylate polymer
s. polystyrene sulfonate
porfimer s.
prednisolone s.
s. requirement
s. restriction
s. retention
s. salicylate
senna concentrate/docusate s.
S. Sulamyd
tazobactam s.
s. tetradecyl sulfate
thiopental s.

s. thiosulfate
total body s.
s. valproate
s. wasting
zomepirac s.
sodium-free formula
sodium/glucose
s./g. co-transporter-1
s./g. co-transporter gene
sodomize
sodomy
Soehendra dilator
soft
s. Boston orthosis
s. cup vacuum delivery
s. hands syndrome
s. palate
s. seal catheter
s. sign
s. spot
s. tissue
s. tissue abnormality
s. tissue balancing
s. tissue ovarian neoplasm
s. tissue release
s. tissue syndactyly
S. Torque uterine catheter
Soft-Cell catheter
soft-cup extractor
softener
stool s.
Softgel
DOS S.
Vita-Plus E S.'s
softness
variable s. (VS)
Softpatch
Impress S.
SoftScan laser mammography system
soft-tissue
s.-t. density
s.-t. fat plane
s.-t. sarcoma
Soft-Wand atraumatic tissue manipulator balloon
software
BABE ultrasound report s.
EsopHogram s.
Medical Manager s.
OBG Clinical Records Manager s.
OBG LabTrack s.
SigmaStat s.
SOHS
severe ovarian hyperstimulation syndrome
Sohval-Soffer syndrome
soilage
bacterial s.

solar
    S. Beam medical examination light
    s. urticaria
Solarcaine Topical
solder
    protein s.
sole crease
Solenopsis
    S. invecta
    S. xyloni
soleus
    accessory s.
Solganal
solid
    s. food
    s. organ transplantation (SOT)
    s. phase radioimmunoassay
    s. phase sandwich
    s. rod segmental construct
    s. tumor
solid-phase
    s.-p. enzyme immunoassay
    s.-p. enzyme-linked immunospot (ELISpot)
    s.-p. enzyme-linked immunospot assay
solitarius
    nucleus tractus s.
solitary
    s. bone cyst
    s. bone lesion
    s. dilated duct
    s. kidney
    s. renal myofibromatosis
solitus
    situs s.
Solium
solium
    Taenia s.
Solomon-Fretzin-Dewald syndrome
Solomon syndrome
Solos
    S. disposable cannula
    S. disposable trocar
soluble
    s. antigen excess
    s. gas technique
    s. intercellular adhesion molecule 1
    s. RNA
    s. tumor necrosis factor receptor
Solu-Cortef Injection
Solumbra 30+ SPF fabric

Solu-Medrol Injection
Soluprick skin prick test
Solurex LA Injection
Soluspan
    Celestone S.
solute diuresis
solution
    AK-Dilate Ophthalmic S.
    AK-Nefrin Ophthalmic S.
    Alamast ophthalmic s.
    aluminum acetate s.
    Anestacon Topical S.
    arterial line flush s.
    Atrovent Inhalation S.
    Bouin s.
    Burow s.
    cardioplegic s.
    chlorhexidine s.
    clindamycin phosphate topical s.
    colloid s.
    Condylox s.
    Cornoy s.
    crystalloid s.
    Dakin antibacterial s.
    Denhardt s.
    Dey-Drop Ophthalmic S.
    Dianeal dialysis s.
    Domeboro s.
    DuraPrep surgical s.
    Duration Nasal S.
    Earle balanced salt s.
    Formula EM oral s.
    Freezone S.
    Fungoid AF Topical S.
    gum arabic rehydration s.
    Hank's balanced salt s. (HBSS)
    Hartmann s.
    hetastarch s.
    hypertonic saline s.
    Intergel irrigating s.
    iodine povidone s.
    isotonic electrolyte s.
    lacmoid staining s.
    lactated Ringer s.
    Locke s.
    Lugol iodine s.
    Melanex topical s.
    modified Ham F-10 s.
    Monsel s.
    Mucomyst s.
    Mydfrin Ophthalmic S.
    nedocromil sodium ophthalmic s.

NOTES

solution *(continued)*
- neomycin-polymycin combination otic s.
- Neo-Synephrine 12 Hour Nasal S.
- Neo-Synephrine Ophthalmic S.
- normal saline s. (NSS)
- Norvir oral s.
- Nostril Nasal S.
- Ocuflox ophthalmic s.
- oral rehydration s. (ORS)
- Orapred s.
- Pedialyte oral electrolyte maintenance s.
- phosphate-buffered saline s.
- physiologic salt s. (PSS)
- polyethylene glycol s.
- polyethylene glycol-electrolyte s.
- Polygeline colloid s.
- povidone-iodine s.
- Prefrin Ophthalmic S.
- Primsol s.
- PVP s.
- Resectisol Irrigation S.
- Rhinall Nasal S.
- Ringer s.
- saline s.
- Schiller s.
- Schlesinger s.
- Shohl s.
- silver nitrate s.
- Sinarest 12 Hour Nasal S.
- sperm viability staining s.
- tobramycin s.
- Transeptic cleansing s.
- trimethoprim HCl oral s.
- Twice-A-Day Nasal S.
- Tyrode s.
- Vigamox s.
- 4-Way Long Acting Nasal S.
- Xopenex inhalation s.
- Xylocaine Topical S.
- Zenker s.

solvent

solving
- means-end problem s. (MEPS)
- problem s.

SomaSensor

somatic
- s. cell
- s. cell-derived growth factor (SCF)
- s. chromosome
- s. complaint
- s. differentiation
- s. growth measurement
- s. hybrid
- s. mosaicism
- s. nervous system feedback loop
- s. pain
- s. sensory innervation

somatization disorder

somatoform disorder

somatoliberin

somatomammotropin
- chorionic s.

somatomedin
- s. C
- s. level

Somatom Plus computed tomography

somatopagus

somatoschisis

somatosensory
- s. aura
- s. evoked potential (SSEP)
- s. impairment

somatostatinergic

somatostatin receptor scintigraphy

somatotridymus

somatotrope

somatotropic

somatotropinoma

Somatrem growth hormone

Somatropin
- S. growth hormone
- S. of rDNA origin
- S. (rDNA origin) for injection

Somer uterine elevator

Sominex Oral

somite
- s. embryo
- s. formation

Sommer syndrome

somnambulism

somniloquy

somnolence syndrome

somnolent

Somogyi phenomenon

Somophyllin

Somophyllin-CRT

Sones catheter

Sonic Hedgehog

Sonksen-Silver visual acuity card

sonnei
- *Shigella s.*

SonoAce
- S. 6000 II ultrasound
- S. 8000 Live ultrasound

Sonoclot
- S. coagulation analyzer
- S. test

Sonoda syndrome

sonogram
- S. fetal ultrasound image card
- screening s.

sonographic
- s. abdominal circumference
- s. assessment
- s. evaluation
- s. finding

sonography
Acuson computed s.
s. blood dyscrasia
color Doppler s. (CDS)
endovaginal s.
laparoscopic s.
ovarian s.
power Doppler s.
real-time s.
saline infusion s. (SIS)
transvaginal s. (TVS)
transvaginal color Doppler s. (TV-CDS)
vaginal s.
sonohysterogram
sonohysterography (SHG)
saline infusion s. (SIS)
transvaginal s.
Sonoline
S. Prima ultrasound
Sonoline Sienna ultrasound system S.
sonolucency
sonolucent tissue
sonometer
sonomicroscopy
SonoMix ultrasound gel
Sonopsy ultrasound-guided breast biopsy system
SonoSite 180
SonoVu US aspiration needle
Soothies glycerin gel breast pad
S.O.P.
Genoptic S.O.P.
Sopher ovum forceps
sorbitol
Actidose with S.
Sorbitrate
sore
canker s.
s. throat
soreness
nipple s.
Sorensen Transpac transducer
Soriatane
sorivudine
Sorsby syndrome
sorter
fluorescence-activated cell s. (FACS)
magnetically activated cell s. (MACS)

sorting
cell s.
SORT-R
Slosson Oral Reading Test-Revised
SOS
speed of sound
SOT
solid organ transplantation
Sotos
S. cerebral gigantism
S. sequence
S. syndrome
Sotradecol
souffle
fetal s.
funic s.
funicular s.
mammary s.
placental s.
umbilical s.
uterine s.
Soules intrauterine insemination catheter
sound
abnormally wide splitting of second heart s.
active bowel s.'s
adventitious breath s.'s
ambient s.
bilabial speech s.
bowel s.'s
breath s.'s
bronchial breath s.'s
bronchovesicular breath s.'s
cracked-pot s.
cracked pot s.
decreased breath s.
fetal heart s.'s
first heart s.
first Korotkoff s.
fourth heart s.
grating s.
heart s.'s
high-pitched bowel s.'s
hyperactive bowel s.'s
hypoactive bowel s.'s
Korotkoff s.
labiodental speech s.
muffled heart s.
normoactive bowel s.'s
Pharmaseal disposable uterine s.
prominent heart s.
pulmonary s.

S

NOTES

sound *(continued)*
    second heart s.
    Simpson uterine s.
    Sims uterine s.
    speech s.
    speed of s. (SOS)
    third heart s.
    tibial speed of s.
    urethral s.
    uterine s.
    vesicular breath s.'s
    vowel s.
    Waring blender s.
sound-field response
sound-stimulated fetal movement
soup kid facies
source
    cesium s.
    dummy s.
    MX2-300 xenon quality light s.
source-to-axis distance (SAD)
source-to-skin distance (SSD)
South
    S. African genetic porphyria
    S. African tick fever
    S. American blastomycosis
Southeast Asian ovalocytosis (SAO)
Southern
    S. blot
    S. blot technique
    S. blot test
SOX9 gene
soy
    s. milk
    s. protein intolerance
Soyacal IV fat emulsion
soy-based protein isolate formula
soy-protein allergy
SP
    sacroposterior
    spastic paraplegia
    Cordran SP
SPA
    sperm penetration assay
SP-A
    surfactant protein-A
    SP-A of lungs
space
    anechoic s.
    antecubital s.
    apophysial s.
    s. blanket
    Bogros s.
    Bowman s.
    cranial s.
    dead s.
    extraembryonic celomic s. (EECS)
    intercostal s.
    intersphincteric s.

    interstitial s.
    intervillous s.
    intracranial cystic s.
    lymphovascular s.
    mechanical dead s.
    obliteration of apophyseal s.
    pararectal s.
    paravesical s.
    perivitelline s.
    pharyngeal s.
    popliteal s.
    presacral s.
    prevesical s.
    rectosacral s.
    rectovaginal s.
    retropubic s.
    retrorectal s.
    retrovaginal s.
    s. of Retzius
    s. of Retzius bleeding
    subaponeurotic cranial s.
    subchorial s.
    surgical s.
    vesicocervical s.
    vesicovaginal s.
    Virchow-Robin s.
    volume of dead s.
    yolk s.
space-occupying lesion
spacer
    dummy s.
spaciness
spacing
    third s.
Spalding sign
span
    arm s.
    attention s.
    fertilizable life s.
    liver s.
    s. of liver dullness
    poor attention s.
    short attention s.
Spangler papular dermatitis of pregnancy
Spanish fly
SPAQ
    Seasonal Pattern Assessment Questionnaire
SPARC urological sling procedure
sparfloxacin
Sparine
sparing
    brain s.
    fetal brain s.
sparse hair
spasm
    adductor s.
    arterial s.

carpopedal s.
ciliary s.
cryptogenic infantile s.
diffuse esophageal s.
esophageal s.
flexion s.
glottic s.
greeting s.
hemifacial s.
infantile s.
jackknife s.
laryngeal s.
levator ani s.
mixed infantile s.
myoclonic s.
nodding s.
symptomatic s.
tetanic s.
tubal s.
urethral s.
vascular s.
X-linked infantile s.

spasmodic
s. croup
s. dysmenorrhea
s. dysphonia
s. torticollis

spasmus nutans

spastic
s. abductor hallucis
s. ataxia
s. cerebral palsy
s. colon
s. diplegia
s. dysphonia
s. hemiparesis
s. hemiplegia
s. levator ani
s. monoplegia
s. paraparesis
s. paraplegia (SP)
s. paresis
s. quadriparesis
s. quadriplegia
s. quadriplegia, congenital ichthyosiform erythroderma, oligophrenia syndrome
s. quadriplegia, retinitis pigmentosa, mental retardation syndrome
s. spinal paralysis
s. synergy

spastica
paralysis spinalis s.
paraplegia s.

spasticity
Ashworth score of s.
bilateral s.

spatial
s. cognition
s. memory
s. orientation
s. relationship

spatula
Aylesbury s.
Ayre s.
Cytobrush s.
s. foot
Milex s.
Pap-Perfect plastic s.

SP-B
surfactant protein-B
SP-B of lungs

SP-C
surfactant protein-C
SP-C of lungs

SPEA
streptococcal exotoxin-A

spearing

Spearman-Brown prediction formula

spear tackling

special
s. education
s. needs
S. Supplemental Nutrition Program

specialist
development s.
infant development s.
mobility s.
resource s.

specialized
s. prenatal care
s. tissue aspirating resectoscope (STAR)

speciation

species
Klebsiella-Enterobacter s.
reactive oxygen s. (ROS)

species-specific antibody

specific
s. growth factor signal
s. immune globulin
s. immunotherapy
s. phobia

NOTES

S

specific *(continued)*
    s. phosphodiesterase inhibitor
    s. reading disability
    s. reading retarded (SRR)
    s. transcription factor
    s. urethritis
specificity
    assay s.
specified
    eating disorder not otherwise s. (EDNOS)
    pervasive developmental disorder not otherwise s. (PDD-NOS)
specimen
    catheter s.
    clean-catch urine s.
    forensic s.
    hemolyzed s.
    lost surgical s.
    maxillary sinus mucosal s.
    midstream urine s.
    nature of s.
    unspun catheterized urine s.
    xanthochromic s.
speckled
    s. irides
    s. lentiginous nevus
SPECT
    single-photon emission computed tomography
spectacle
    s. correction
    s. treatment
Spectazole
spectinomycin
spectophotometrical analysis
spectra *(pl. of* spectrum)
Spectra-Diasonics ultrasound
Spectra 400 extended surveillance and alert system
spectral
    s. Doppler
    s. edge frequency (SEF)
    s. gradient acoustic reflectometry (SGAR)
    s. karyotype (SKY)
    s. karyotyping (SKY)
    orthogonal polarization s. (OPS)
    s. power analysis
Spectranetics catheter
spectrin
spectrofluorometric
spectrometer
    atomic absorption s.
    Digilab FTS 40A s.
    mass s.
    Varian Spectra AA40 s.

spectrometry
    electrospray ionization mass s. (ESIMS)
    gas chromatography-mass s. (GC-MS)
    mass s. (MS)
    tandem mass s.
spectrophotometer
    narrow band s.
spectrophotometric scanning
spectrophotometry
    atomic absorption s.
    near infrared s. (NIRS, NIS)
spectroscopy
    atomic absorption s.
    gas chromatography-mass s. (GC-MS)
    infrared s.
    longitudinal proton MR s.
    magnetic resonance s. (MRS)
    medical optical s. (MOS)
    near infrared s. (NIRS, NIS)
    NMR s.
    optical s.
    proton MR s.
spectrum, pl. **spectra**
    Doppler shift spectra
    electromagnetic s.
    facioauriculovertebral s. (FAVS)
    fortification s.
    oculoauriculovertebral s. (OAVS)
Spectrum stethoscope
specula (*pl. of* speculum)
specular echo
Speculite chemiluminescent light
speculoscopy
    Pap plus s. (PPS)
speculum, pl. **specula**
    Auvard s.
    bivalve s.
    blackened s.
    Cusco s.
    duckbill s.
    ear s.
    s. examination
    Graves bivalve s.
    Halle infant nasal s.
    Holinger infant esophageal s.
    Huffman adolescent s.
    Huffman vaginal s.
    illuminated vaginal s.
    Kogan endocervical s.
    long weighted s.
    nasal s.
    Pedersen s.
    Pederson vaginal s.
    Prima Series LEEP s.
    Sani-Spec vaginal s.
    Sims vaginal s.

SRT vaginal s.
Vu-Max vaginal s.
weighted s.
s. withdrawal

Spee

curve of S.
S. embryo

speech

cued s.
s. delay
s. development
s. disorder
dysarthritic s.
dysfluent s.
hypernasal s.
hyponasal s.
s. lesson
motherese s.
parallel s.
s. pathology
pressured s.
s. problem
s. production
s. reception threshold (SRT)
s. recognition threshold (SRT)
s. sound
s. therapist
s. therapy

speech-language

s.-l. pathologist
s.-l. pathology

speechreading
speech reception threshold (SRT)
speed

s. of sound (SOS)
tibial s.

Speed-Vac
spell

A&B s.
blue s.
breath-holding s.
cyanotic breathholding s.
hypercyanotic s.
hypoxic s.
pallid breathholding s.'s
paroxysmal hypoxic s.
shuddering s.
staring s.
syncopal s.
tet s.

spelt wheat
Spemann induction

Spence

axillary tail of S.
S. axillary tail
S. and Duckett marsupialization
S. procedure

Spencer

S. probe
S. stitch scissors

sperm

acrosome-intact s.
s. agglutination test
s. allergy
anonymous donor s. (ADS)
artificial insemination with donor s.
s. aspiration
s. attrition
s. bank
s. capacitation
s. capacitation medium
s. chromatin decondensation
s. count
s. donation
donor s.
s. donor
epididymal s.
frozen s.
s. function test
s. granuloma
haploid s.
s. immobilization test
microsurgical extraction of
  ductal s. (MEDS)
motile s.
s. motility
muzzled s.
nonmotile s.
s. penetration assay (SPA)
s. progression scale (0–4)
s. reservoir
s. retrieval technique
S. Select sperm recovery system
s. separation
subzonal injection of s. (SUZI)
s. surface antibody
s. tail protein phosphorylation
s. transport
s. viability staining solution
washed s.
s. washing insemination method
  (SWIM)

Spermac stain
spermagglutination

NOTES

sperm-aster
spermatic
    s. cord
    s. venous complex
spermatid
spermatin
spermatocele
    artificial s.
spermatocide
spermatogenesis
spermatogonia
spermatotoxin
spermatozoon, pl. spermatozoa
    haploid s.
    round-headed acrosomeless
     spermatozoa
    washed spermatozoa
sperm-cervical
    s.-c. mucus contact (SCMC)
    s.-c. mucus interaction
sperm-containing cyst
sperm-counting fluid
sperm-egg adhesion
sperm-free ejaculate
spermicide
    vaginal s.
spermidine
spermine
spermiogenesis
SpermMAR mixed antiglobulin reaction test
sperm-mediated
sperm-mucus interaction
sperm-oocyte interaction
sperm-zona pellucida binding
SPh
    simple phobia
sphenocephaly
sphenoid
    s. bone
    s. dysplasia
    s. fontanelle
sphenopagus
spherical congruent hips
spherocytic
    s. HE
    s. hereditary elliptocytosis
    s. red blood cell
spherocytosis
    congenital s.
    hereditary s.
sphincter
    aganglionic s.
    AMS 800 artificial urethral s.
    anal s.
    artificial anal s.
    artificial urethral s. (AUS)
    artificial urinary s.

    s. deficiency
    esophageal s.
    external anal s.
    genitourinary s. (GUS)
    incompetent lower esophageal s.
    internal anal s.
    lower esophageal s. (LES)
    s. muscle
    s. paralysis
    patulous rectal s.
    s. repair
    s. tone
    upper esophageal s. (UES)
    urethral s.
    urinary s.
    urogenital s.
    vertiginous external anal s.
    voluntary urinary s.
sphincteric incompetence
sphincteroplasty
sphingolipid
    s. activator protein-1 (SAP1)
    s. activator protein deficiency
    s. storage disease
sphingolipidosis
    infantile cerebral s.
sphingolipodystrophy
Sphingomonas
sphingomyelin
sphingosine
sphygmomanometer
    Tycos aneroid s.
spica
    s. cast
    panty s.
    s. splint
spiculated
    s. lesion
    s. red blood cell
spider
    s. angioma
    s. bite
    black widow s.
    brown recluse s.
    s. finger
    s. nevus
    vascular s.
Spiegel
    S. criteria
    S. method
Spiegelberg criteria
Spielberger State Anxiety Inventory
Spielmeyer-Vogt
    S.-V. disease
    S.-V. neural ceroid lipofuscinosis
    S.-V. type of late infantile and
     juvenile amaurotic idiocy
spigelian hernia

spike

    benign partial epilepsy with
      centrotemporal s. (BPEC)
    centrotemporal s.
    interictal s.
    multifocal s.
    s. and wave complex

spillage

    tumor s.

spilled

    filled and s.

spilus

    nevus s.

spina

    s. bifida
    s. bifida cystica
    s. bifida occulta

spinal

    s. analgesia
    s. anesthesia
    s. angioma
    s. apoptosis
    s. arachnoiditis
    s. blockade
    s. bone loss
    s. column
    s. column closure defect
    s. compression fracture
    s. concussion
    s. cord
    s. cord compression
    s. cord dysfunction
    s. cord glioma
    s. cord injury
    s. cord injury without radiographic
      abnormality (SCIWORA)
    s. cord tethering
    s. cord tumor
    s. dysraphism
    s. epidural abscess
    s. fusion
    s. headache
    s. meningocele
    s. muscle atrophy
    s. muscular atrophy (SMA)
    s. muscular atrophy-mental
      retardation syndrome
    s. muscular atrophy, microcephaly,
      mental retardation syndrome
    s. muscular dystrophy
    s. needle
    s. neurofibromatosis

    s. osteomyelitis
    s. paralytic poliomyelitis
    s. polyneuropathy
    s. proptosis
    s. shock
    s. subarachnoid block
    s. tap
    s. tuberculosis
    s. tumor

spinal apoptosis

spinal-epidural

    combined s.-e. (CSE)

spinal proptosis

spindle

    s. cell
    s. cell epithelioid nevus
    s. cell tumor

spine

    anterior superior iliac s.
    bamboo s.
    cleft s.
    cloven s.
    curvature of s.
    dysraphia of s.
    iliac s.
    lateral curvature of s.
    posterior superior iliac s.
    rotation of s.
    rugger jersey s.
    superior iliac s.

spin-echo

    half-Fourier acquisition single-shot
      turbo s.-e. (HASTE)

Spinelli operation

Spinhaler

spinigerum

    Gnathostoma s.

spinnbarkeit

spinning-top deformity

spinocerebellar

    s. ataxia-dysmorphism syndrome
    s. ataxia (type 1–7) (SCA)
    s. degeneration
    s. degenerative disease

spinosa

    ichthyosis s.

spinothalamic sensory deficit

spinulosus

    lichen s.

spiral

    Curschmann s.
    s. electrode

NOTES

S

spiral *(continued)*
    s. endometrial artery
    s. scan
    s. tibial fracture
spiralis
    Trichinella s.
spiramycin
Spirette
    CCD S.
spirillary rat-bite fever
Spirillum minus
spirochetal infection
spirochete
spiroforme
    Clostridium s.
spirometric test
spirometry
Spironazide
spironolactone
    hydrochlorothiazide and s.
Spirozide
spit fistula
Spitz-Holter valve
Spitz nevus
splanchnic
    s. blood flow
    s. fold
    s. hypoperfusion
    s. pelvic pain
splanchnocystica
    dysencephalia s.
splanchnopathy
splanchnopleuric
splash burn
SPLATT
    split anterior tibial tendon transfer
splayfoot
spleen
    accessory s.
    fetal s.
splenectomized
splenectomy
splenic
    s. artery aneurysm
    s. flexure
    s. injury
    s. pregnancy
    s. rupture
    s. sequestration
    s. sequestration crisis
    s. sequestration syndrome
    s. tissue
    s. torsion
    s. vein
splenium, pl. **splenia**
    absent s.
    posterior s.
splenocyte
splenomegaly

splenoportography
splenorenal shunt
splenorrhaphy
splenosis
splicing
    gene s.
    RNA s.
splint
    abduction s.
    acrylic s.
    ankle stirrup s.
    clubfoot s.
    Denis Browne clubfoot s.
    Denis Browne night s.
    dorsal extension s.
    dynamic s.
    Fillauer night s.
    Frejka pillow s.
    Lorenz night s.
    malleable s.
    night s.
    opponens s.
    Orthoglass s.
    Pope night s.
    shin s.
    spica s.
    static s.
    sugar-tong s.
    talipes hobble s.
    thumb spica s.
    triangular s.
    volar s.
splinter hemorrhage
splinting
    night s.
splint/stent
    kidney internal s./s. (KISS)
split
    anterior cricoid s. (ACS)
    s. anterior tibial tendon transfer
      (SPLATT)
    s. cord malformation (SCM)
    cricoid s.
    s. flexor hallucis longus tendon
    s. foot, microphthalmia, cleft
      lip/palate-mental retardation
      syndrome
    s. hand-cleft lip/palate and
      ectodermal dysplasia (SCE)
    s. hand/foot syndrome
    s. procedure
    s. sheath catheter
    s. spinal cord malformation
      (SSCM)
split-course hyperfractionated
  radiotherapy
split-flap technique
split-foot deformity
splittable needle

split-thickness graft
splitting
> blastocyst s.
> embryo s.
> muscle s.
> rib s.

split-virus vaccine
spoke-wheel palpation
sponastrime
> spondylar changes-nasal anomaly-
> striated-metaphyses
> sponastrime dysplasia

spondylar
> s. changes-nasal anomaly-striated-
> metaphyses (sponastrime)
> s. and nasal alterations-striated
> metaphyses syndrome

spondylitis
> ankylosing s.
> s., enthesitis, arthritis (SEA)
> juvenile ankylosing s. (JAS)
> rheumatoid s.
> tuberculous s.

spondyloarthritis
spondyloarthropathy,
> pl. **spondyloarthropathies**
> ankylosing s.
> juvenile s.
> seronegative s.

spondylocostal dysplasia syndrome
spondyloepimetaphyseal
> s. dysphasia with myotonia
> s. dysplasia (SEMD)

spondyloepiphyseal
> s. dysplasia (SED)
> s. dysplasia congenita
> s. dysplasia congenita syndrome
> s. dysplasia-diabetes mellitus
> syndrome
> s. dysplasia tarda
> s. dysplasia tarda-mental retardation
> syndrome

spondylohumerofemoral hypoplasia
spondylolisthesis
spondylolysis
spondylometaepiphyseal dysplasia-extreme
> **short stature syndrome**
spondylometaphyseal
> s. dysplasia
> s. dysplasia-short limb-abnormal
> calcification syndrome
> s. dysplasia, X-linked

spondyloperipheral dysplasia
spondylothoracic
> s. dysplasia
> s. dysplasia syndrome

sponge
> absorbable gelatin s.
> s. bath
> contraceptive s.
> s. forceps
> Incert bioabsorbable s.
> intravaginal s.
> Lapwall s.
> Protectaid contraceptive s.
> Ray-Tec s.
> s. stick
> Today vaginal contraceptive s.
> vaginal s.
> Weck-cel s.

sponge-holding forceps
spongiform encephalopathy
spongioblastoma
spongiosa
> zona s.

spongiosis
> intraepidermal s.
> white matter s.

spongiosum
> corpus s.
> stratum s.

spongiosus
> status s.

spongy
> s. degeneration
> s. degeneration of infancy
> s. degeneration of white matter
> s. mass

spontaneous
> s. abortion (SAB)
> s. abortion material
> s. amputation
> s. apoptosis
> s. atrophic patch
> s. atrophic patch of prematurity
> s. bacterial peritonitis (SBP)
> s. biliary perforation (SBP)
> s. breech
> s. breech extraction
> s. cephalic delivery
> s. cervical ripening
> s. descent
> s. descent of testes
> s. evolution

NOTES

S

spontaneous *(continued)*
- s. gangrene of newborn
- s. hyperstimulation
- s. involution
- s. labor
- s. menstrual cycle
- s. miscarriage
- s. nystagmus
- s. ovulation
- s. periodic breathing
- s. placental separation
- s. pneumothorax
- s. preterm birth (SPTB)
- s. preterm delivery
- s. preterm labor with intrapartum demise
- s. remission
- s. rupture of membranes (SROM)
- s. thymic involution
- s. vaginal delivery (SVD)
- s. version
- s. vertex

spoon forceps

spoon-shaped nail

sporadic
- s. aniridia
- s. Burkitt lymphoma
- s. chromosome abnormality
- s. Creutzfeldt-Jakob disease
- s. myoglobinuria
- s. nonfamilial clear cell carcinoma

Sporanox

spore
- mold s.

Sporothrix schenckii

sporotrichoid appearance

sporotrichosis
- cutaneous s.
- extracutaneous s.

sport
- wheelchair s.

sports-related injury

sporulation enterotoxin

SPOT
- salpingitis after previous tubal occlusion
- salpingitis in previously occluded tubes

spot
- ash-leaf s.
- Bitot s.
- black s.
- blood s.
- blue s.
- blueberry muffin s.
- Brushfield s.
- café au lait s.
- cherry-red macular s.
- coast of California café au lait s.'s
- coast of Maine café au lait s.'s
- s. compression
- s. compression view
- cotton-wool s. (CWS)
- Forchheimer s.
- Fordyce s.
- Graefenberg s. (G-spot)
- hyperirritant s.
- Koplik s.
- macular cherry-red s.
- s. magnification
- mongolian s.
- pathognomonic Koplik s.
- powder burn s.
- pseudo-Roth s.'s
- rose s.
- Roth s.
- shagreen s.
- soft s.
- strawberry s.
- s. test

spotlight
- KDC-Healthdyne nonfluorescent s.

spotted
- s. fever
- s. fever group

spotting
- midcycle s.
- postcoital s.
- postdouching s.

spotty necrosis

S-pouch

spousal abuse

sprain

Spranger-Wiedemann syndrome

spray
- Astelin Nasal S.
- Atrovent Nasal S.
- butorphanol tartrate nasal s.
- CaldeCort Anti-Itch Topical S.
- DDAVP nasal s.
- desmopressin acetate nasal s.
- hair s.
- intranasal s.
- ipratropium bromide nasal s.
- Itch-X s.
- Merthiolate s.
- Miacalcin Nasal S.
- midazolam nasal s.
- mometasone furoate aqueous nasal s. (MFNS)
- Nasarel Nasal S.
- Nitrolingual Translingual S.
- Ony-Clear S.
- Rhinocort Aqua nasal s.
- sumatriptan nasal s.
- Tri-Nasal S.
- vaginal feminine s.
- Xylocaine Topical S.

SprayGel adhesive barrier system

spread
> centripetal s.
> fecal-oral s.
> halstedian concept of tumor s.
> hematogenous s.
> lymphatic s.
> transcoelomic s.
> vessel s.

spreading factor
Sprengel
> S. anomaly
> S. deformity

spring clip application
sprinkle
> Depakote s.

sprout
> syncytial s.

sprouting
> mossy fiber s.
> nerve s.

sprue
> celiac s.
> refractory s.
> tropical s.

SPS
> simple partial seizure

SPT
> septic pelvic thrombophlebitis

SPTB
> spontaneous preterm birth

SPTL
> selective photothermolysis
> SPTL vascular lesion laser

spud dissector
spun
> s. glass hair
> s. hematocrit
> s. urine
> s. urine sediment

spur
> bony s.

spuria
> melena s.
> placenta s.

spurious pregnancy
spurt
> growth s.

Spurway syndrome
sputorum
> *Campylobacter s.*
> *Pandoraea s.*

sputum, pl. **sputa**

> carbonaceous s.
> clear mucoid s.
> cloudy s.
> s. culture
> s. cytology
> s. eosinophilia
> mucoid s.
> purulent s.
> rust-colored s.
> s. smear

squalamine
squama, pl. **squama**
squamocolumnar junction (SCJ)
squamous
> s. cell
> s. cell carcinoma
> s. cell hyperplasia
> s. dysplasia
> s. epithelium
> s. intraepithelial lesion (SIL)
> s. metaplasia
> s. metaplasia of amnion

square
> s. knot
> s. matrix
> Punnett s.
> s. window
> s. window sign

squash and smear
squatting
> s. phenomenon
> s. position

squeezing
> eyelid s.

SQUIDS
> superconducting quantum interference device susceptometer

squint
> convergent s.

squirming Valsalva
S-R
> stimulus-response

SR
> Calan SR
> Cardizem SR
> Indocin SR
> Isoptin SR
> Mag-Tab SR
> Oramorph SR
> Roxanol SR

Sr.
> EpiPen Sr.

SRA Basic Reading Program
Srb syndrome
SRI
    serotonin reuptake inhibitor
        SRI automated immunoassay
          analyzer
SROM
    spontaneous rupture of membranes
SRPS
    short rib-polydactyly syndrome
SRR
    specific reading retarded
SRS
    Snyder-Robinson syndrome
    suicide risk screen
SRSH
    self-reported self-harm
SRT
    smoke removal tube
    speech reception threshold
    speech recognition threshold
        SRT vaginal speculum
SRY
    sex-determining region
SS
    short stature
    systemic sclerosis
        hemoglobin SS (HbSS)
SSB
    short small-bowel
SSCM
    split spinal cord malformation
SSCVD
    sterile, spontaneous, controlled vaginal
      delivery
SSD
    source-to-skin distance
        SSD AF
        SSD Cream
SSDI
    Social Security Disability Insurance
SSEP
    somatosensory evoked potential
SSFSE
    single shot fast spin echo
S-shaped curve
SSI
    Supplemental Security Income
SSKI
    saturated solution of potassium iodide
SSNS
    steroid-sensitive idiopathic nephrotic
      syndrome
SSPE
    subacute sclerosing panencephalitis
SSRI
    selective serotonin reuptake inhibitor

SSS
    scalded skin syndrome
        SSS syndrome
SSSC
    Social Support Scale for Children
SSSS
    staphylococcal scalded skin syndrome
SSVC
    systemic venous collateral
SSVD
    sterile, spontaneous vaginal delivery
SSW
    staggered spondaic word
ST
    sacrotransverse
    syncytiotrophoblast
        ST change
St.
    Saint
        St. Anthony's fire
        St. Clair-Thompson curette
        St. Joseph Aspirin-Free Cold
          Tablets for Children
        St. Joseph Cough Suppressant
        St. Jude Children's Research
          Hospital staging system
        St. Jude Research Hospital
        St. Louis encephalitis (SLE)
        St. Vitus dance
STA analyzer
stability
    ankle s.
    collateral ligament s.
    joint s.
stabilization
    cardiovascular s.
    hospital s.
stabilizer
    mast cell s.
stabilizing bar
stable
    s. access cannula
    s. factor
    s. microbubble test
stab wound
staccato
    s. cough
    s. voiding
staccato-like cough
Stachybotrys
    S. atra
    S. chartarum
stacked-coin appearance
Staclot test
stadiometer
    Harpenden s.
    Holtain height s.
    neonatal s.
Stadol

stage

s. A, B, C, N infection
acceptance s.
alveolar s.
anger s.
band s.
bargaining s.
canalicular s.
Carnegie s.
cleavage s.
cortical supremacy s.
decoding s.
delayed first s.
denial s.
depression s.
developmental s.
diakinesis s.
dictyate s.
germinal vesicle s.
hemolymphatic s.
hyperirritable s.
ICS bladder prolapse (s. I–III)
s. IIIc papillary tumor of low
   malignant potential
s. I–IV epithelial ovarian cancer
illocutionary s.
indifferent gonadal s.
intermediate dystonic s.
Jirasek gestation s.
s.'s of labor
leptotene s.
locutionary s.
Marshall-Tanner pubertal s. (1–5)
meningoencephalitic s.
Norwood s.
pachytene s.
perlocutionary s.
pigmentary s.
placental s.
preicteric s.
preoperational s.
prereading s.
prolapse s. I–IV
pseudoglandular s.
saccular s.
sensory-motor s.
shock s.
Tanner s.
Tanner developmental s. (1–5)
Tanner genital s. (1–5)
Tanner maturation s. (1–5)
Theiler s.

transitional reader s.
trophectoderm s.
two-part nuclear s.
zygotene s.

staged repair
Stagesic
staggered spondaic word (SSW)
staging

clinical s.
FIGO s.
genital prolapse s.
Marshall-Tanner pubertal s. (1–5)
Northway s.
surgical s.
Tanner s. (1–5)

stagnant loop syndrome
stagnation mastitis
STAI-I

State-Trait Anxiety Index-I

stain, staining

acetylcholinesterase histochemical s.
acid-fast s.
acridine orange s.
auramine-rhodamine s.
Betke s.
blood pigment s.
Brown-Hopp tissue Gram s.
Bryan-Leishman s.
calcofluor white s.
Csaba s.
DA-DAPI s.
DFA s.
Dieterle s.
eosin s.
eosin-4 s.
Feulgen s.
fluorescein s.
Giemsa s.
Golgi s.
Gomori methenamine-silver s.
Gomori trichrome s.
Gram s.
Gram-Weigert s.
Grimelius s.
Hansel s.
H&E s.
immunoperoxidase s.
India ink s.
iodine s.
Kinyoun acid-fast s.
Kinyoun carbol fuchsin s.
Kleihauer s.

S

NOTES

stain (*continued*)
    Kleihauer-Betke s.
    KOH s.
    Leder s.
    Lugol iodine s.
    Luna-Parker acid fuscin s.
    macular s.
    Masson-Fontana s.
    meconium s.
    methenamine silver s.
    modified Dieterle s.
    modified Kinyoun acid-fast s.
    modified trichrome s.
    Movat s.
    PAS s.
    Perls iron s.
    port-wine s.
    potassium chloride s.
    rhodamine-auramine s.
    Shorr s.
    silver s.
    Spermac s.
    Sudan s.
    supravital s.
    toluidine blue s.
    trichrome s.
    TUNEL s.
    Warthin-Starry silver s.
    Wayson s.
    Wright s.
    Ziehl-Neelsen s.

stained
    meconium s.

staining
    acid-Schiff s.
    corneal s.
    DFA s.
    direct immunofluorescent s.
    direct immunohistochemical s.
    endomysial s.
    meconium s.

stainless steel suture

staircase
    s. approach
    s. response

stalk
    allantoic s.
    body s.
    infundibular s.
    mesenteric s.
    narrow mesenteric s.
    yolk s.

stalking
    celery s.

Stallworth placenta

Stamey
    S. catheter
    S. modification of Pereyra
      procedure
    S. needle
    S. operation

Stamey-Malecot catheter

Stamey-Pereyra needle suspension

Stamm
    S. gastrostomy
    S. procedure

stammering
    s. bladder

stance
    Buddha s.
    horse-riding s.
    s. phase

stand
    warming s.
    s. x-ray

stand-alone pharmacotherapy

standard
    s. curve
    s. deviation (SD)
    s. deviation score (SDS)
    MapMarkers fluorescent DNA
      sizing s.
    protein s.
    Second International S. (SIS)

standardization

standardized
    s. incidence ratio (SIR)
    s. observation scale
    s. reading inventory
    s. test

stander
    prone s.

standing position

standstill
    cardiac s.

Stanford-Binet
    S.-B. Intelligence Scale
    S.-B. Intelligence Scale for
      Children
    S.-B. Intelligence Scale, 4th
      Edition
    S.-B. Intelligence Test
    S.-B. Memory Scale, 4th Edition
    S.-B. score

Stanford Diagnostic Reading Test

Stanley Way procedure

stanozolol

STAN S 21 fetal heart rate system

stapes

staphylococcal
    s. blepharitis
    s. enterotoxin B (SEB)
    s. furuncle
    s. furunculosis
    s. impetigo
    s. infection
    s. pneumonia
    s. pustulosis

s. scalded skin
s. scalded skin syndrome (SSSS)
s. scarlet fever
s. toxic shock syndrome

Staphylococcus
 S. aureus
 S. aureus molluscum
 coagulase-negative *S.*
 coagulase-positive *S.*
 S. epidermidis
 S. epidermidis folliculitis
 S. intermedius
 S. pyogenes
 S. saprophyticus

staphylococcus, pl. **staphylococci**
staple
 absorbable s.
 s. anastomosis
 s. line leak
 metallic skin s.
 skin s.
 titanium s.

stapler
 Auto Suture Multifire Endo GIA
  30 s.
 EEA s.
 Endo GIA 30 suture s.
 Endopath endoscopic articulating s.
 GIA 60, 80 s.
 GIA 80 s.
 Precise disposable skin s.
 Roticulator 55 s.
 TL-90 Ethicon s.
 30-V-3 s.
 Vista disposable skin s.

stapling
 epiphyseal s.
 gastric s.
 unilateral s.

STAR
 Simultaneous Technique for Acuity and
  Readiness Testing
 specialized tissue aspirating resectoscope
 Study of Tamoxifen and Raloxifene

StAR
 steroidogenic acute regulatory protein

star
 s. chart
 s. effect
 S. ventilator

starch malabsorption
STARFlex device

Stargardt disease
Stargate falloposcopy catheter
staring spell
Starling
 S. equation
 S. equilibrium
 S. force
 S. law of transcapillary exchange
 S. mechanism

STARRT
 selective tubal assessment to refine
  reproductive therapy
  STARRT falloposcopy system

start
 Head S.
 sleep s.

startle
 s. disease
 s. epilepsy
 s. pattern
 s. reaction
 s. reflex
 s. response

starvation
 accelerated s.
 s. ketoacidosis
 s. ketosis

stasigenesis
stasis, pl. **stases**
 bile s.
 bowel s.
 colonic s.
 gallbladder s.
 large bowel s.
 pregnancy-associated urinary s.
 small intestine s.
 urinary s.

state
 accompanying mood s.
 active and intense crying s.
 s. of alertness
 awake and active s.
 behavioral s.
 S. Children's Health Insurance
  Program (SCHIP)
 disseminated intravascular
  coagulation s.
 emotional s.
 fugue s.
 gradient recalled acquisition in the
  steady s. (GRASS)

NOTES

S

state *(continued)*
    gradient refocused acquisition in steady s. (GRASS)
    hyperammonemic s.
    hypercoagulable s.
    hypernatremic s.
    hyperosmolar s.
    hyponatremic s.
    intense emotional s.
    menstrual s.
    mood s.
    paroxysmal emotional s.
    persistent vegetative s. (PVS)
    preeclamptic s.
    preseizure s.
    Profile of Mood S.'s (POMS)
    progestational s.
    quiet and alert s.
    sleep s.
    steady s.
    transient insulinopenic s.
    uremic s.

state-of-the-art radiation

State-Trait
    S.-T. Anxiety Index-I (STAI-I)
    S.-T. Anxiety Inventory
    S.-T. Anxiety Inventory for Children

static
    s. admittance
    s. B-scanner
    s. deformity
    s. elastance (E_{st})
    s. encephalopathy
    s. immersion
    s. splint

Staticin
    O-V S.

station
    0 s.
    complete/complete/+ s.
    fetal s.

stature
    brittle hair, intellectual impairment, decreased fertility, short s. (BIDS)
    constitutional short s.
    deafness, hypogonadism, hypertrichosis, short s.
    ear, patella, short s. (EPS)
    familial short s.
    goniodysgenesis, mental retardation, short s. (GMS)
    ichthyosis, brittle hair, impaired intelligence, decreased fertility, short s. (IBIDS)
    idiopathic short s. (ISS)
    maternal s.

    non-growth hormone-deficient short s. (NGHD-SS)
    short s. (SS)
    small s.

status
    absence s.
    acid-base s.
    s. asthmaticus
    circumcision s.
    s. dysmyelinatus
    s. epilepticus (SE)
    fetal s.
    health s.
    Karnofsky performance s.
    s. loss
    s. lymphaticus
    s. marmoratus
    nonreassuring fetal s.
    paternal s.
    petit mal s.
    psychomotor s.
    socioeconomic s.
    s. spongiosus
    s. thymicolymphaticus
    s. thymicus
    visceral protein s.

statutory rape

Staudinger reaction

stavudine

S-T Cort Topical

STD
    sexually transmitted disease

steady state

steal
    s. phenomenon
    subclavian s.

stearin-lanolin cream

steatocystoma multiplex

steatohepatitis
    nonalcoholic s. (NASH)

steatorrhea
    idiopathic s.

steatosis
    liver s.
    microvesicular s.

STEC
    Shiga toxin-producing *Escherichia coli*

Steele procedure

steely-hair syndrome

steeple sign

Steiner
    S. canal
    S. electromechanical morcellator
    S. tumor

Steinert
    S. disease
    S. myotonic dystrophy
    S. syndrome

Steinfeld syndrome

Stein-Leventhal
 S.-L. syndrome
 S.-L. type of polycystic ovary
Stelazine
stellate
 s. cell
 s. ganglion ablation
 s. iris
 s. laceration
 s. mass
 s. reticulum
 s. wound
stellatoides
 Candida s.
Stellwag sign
stem
 s. cell
 s. cell assay
 s. cell bone marrow transplantation
 s. cell therapy
 s. cell transplantation (SCT)
Stemetil
stenogyria
 agenesis of corpus callosum
 with s.
stenosis, pl. **stenoses**
 acute subglottic s.
 anal s.
 anorectal s.
 antral s.
 anular s.
 aortic valve s.
 aqueductal s.
 bile duct s.
 bladder neck s.
 cervical s.
 choanal s.
 cholestasis-peripheral pulmonary s.
 chronic subglottic s.
 congenital aortic s.
 congenital esophageal s.
 congenital hypertrophic pyloric s.
 congenital nasal pyriform
 aperture s. (CNPAS)
 congenital tracheal s.
 congenital tubular s.
 critical aortic s.
 critical pulmonic s.
 discrete subaortic s. (DSS)
 duodenal s.
 esophageal s.
 s. of esophagus

 fixed s.
 hypertrophic s.
 hypertrophic pyloric s. (HPS)
 idiopathic hypertrophic subaortic s.
 (IHSS)
 infantile hypertrophic pyloric s.
 (IHPS)
 infundibular pulmonic s.
 lacrimal duct s.
 laryngeal s.
 laryngotracheal s. (LTS)
 long-segment congenital tracheal s.
 (LSCTS)
 meatal s.
 mild pulmonic s.
 mitral s.
 nasal pyriform aperture s.
 peripheral pulmonary s.
 peripheral pulmonic s.
 piriform aperture s.
 s. post intubation
 postischemic s.
 primary aqueductal s.
 pulmonary valve s.
 pulmonic s. (PS)
 pyloric s.
 renal artery s.
 short-segment s.
 subaortic s.
 subglottic s.
 supravalvular aortic s.
 supravalvular pulmonary s.
 s. of trachea
 tracheal s.
 tricuspid s.
 tubular s.
 urethral s.
 vaginal s.
 valvar aortic s.
 valvar pulmonic s.
 valvular pulmonic s.
 variable s.
 X-linked aqueductal s. (XLAS)
stenotic
 s. hymen
 s. nasolacrimal duct
Stenotrophomonas
 S. maltophilia
 S. maltophilia infection
Stensen duct
stent
 Aboulker s.

S

NOTES

stent *(continued)*
 double-J s.
 endoluminal s.
 expandable esophageal s. (EES)
 Lubri-Flex s.
 Palmaz s.
 pancreatic duct s.
 Percuflex Plus s.
 s. placement
 urinary s.
stenting
 endoluminal s.
stepdown
 s. cannula
 s. therapy
Stephan HF 300 respirator
Stephanie 8000 oscillator
Step laparoscopic trocar
stepoff
STEPP
 Screening Tool for Early Predictors of
 PTSD
stepping
 reflex s.
 s. reflex
 s. response
STEPS
 system for thalidomide education and
 prescription safety
 STEPS program
2-step testing
stepwise antiinflammatory therapy
Sterapred
stercoralis
 Strongyloides s.
stercoroma
stereoacuity
stereocolpogram
stereocolposcope
stereognosis
stereomicroscope
stereoscopic pelvimetry
stereotactic
 s. breast biopsy
 s. breast biopsy needle
 s. radiography
 s. radiosurgery
 s. thalamotomy
stereotaxis
stereotypical
 s. movement
 s. movement disorder
stereotypic behavior
stereotypy, pl. **stereotypies**
Steri-Drape 2
sterile
 s. isolation bag
 s. pus
 s. pyuria

 s. pyuria syndrome
 s. specimen trap
 s. speculum examination
 s., spontaneous, controlled vaginal
 delivery (SSCVD)
 s., spontaneous vaginal delivery
 (SSVD)
 s. vaginal examination (SVE)
 s. water gastric drip (SWGD)
sterility
 absolute s.
 adolescent s.
 one-child s.
 relative s.
sterilization
 female s.
 intermittent s.
 involuntary s.
 microlaparoscopic s.
 permanent s.
 postpartum s.
 surgical s.
 tubal s.
 voluntary s.
sterilize
Steri-Strip skin closure
sterna (*pl. of* sternum)
sternal
 s. fracture
 s. recession
Sternberg sign
sternochondral junction
sternocleidomastoid (SCM)
 s. fibroma
 s. hemorrhage
 s. muscle
sternodymus
sternomastoid
 s. foramen
 s. tumor
sternopagus
sternoschisis
sternotomy
sternoxiphopagus
sternum, pl. **sterna**
 fissure of s.
 fractured s.
steroid
 s. acne
 adrenal s.
 adrenocortical s.
 anabolic androgenic s.
 androgenic s.
 antenatal s.
 s. biosynthesis
 s. cell
 s. concentration
 s. conjugate hydrolysis
 s. contraceptive

endogenous s.
exogenous s.
gonadal s.
s. hormone
s. hormone receptor
inhaled s.
s. inhaler
17-ketogenic s.
long-acting contraceptive s.
low-dose s.'s
s. metabolism
s. metabolite
s. nucleus
ovarian s.
placental s.
s. secretion
s. secretion inhibition
sex s.
s. sulfatase
s. sulfatase deficiency
s. sulfate
systemic s.
s. therapy
s. treatment
steroid-dependent colitis
steroid-induced myopathy
steroidogenesis
adrenal s.
adrenocortical s.
fetal-placental s.
follicle s.
ovarian s.
testicular s.
steroidogenic
s. aberration
s. acute regulatory protein (StAR)
s. factor-1 (SF-1)
steroid-sensitive idiopathic nephrotic
syndrome (SSNS)
stertor
humid s.
stethoscope
Allen fetal s.
bell s.
Doptone fetal s.
MedaSonics first beat ultrasound s.
Spectrum s.
ultrasound s.
Stevens-Johnson syndrome
Stewart-Treves syndrome
STI
sexually transmitted infection

stick
arterial s.
glucose reagent s.
heel s., heelstick
silver nitrate s.
sponge s.
Universal indicator s.
Sticker disease
Stickler
S. dysplasia
S. syndrome
sties (*pl. of* sty)
stiff-baby syndrome
stiff-man syndrome
stiff neck
stiffness
lead pipe s.
stigma, pl. **stigmata**
Down stigmata
radiologic stigmata
Ulrich-Turner stigmata
stigmasterol
stigmatization
stilbestrol
Still
S. disease
S. murmur
stillbirth rate
stillborn infant
Stilling-Türk-Duane syndrome
Stillman cleft
Stilphostrol
Stimate
Stimmler syndrome
stimulant drug
stimulation
ACTH s.
cervical carcinoma s.
cranial electrical s. (CES)
direct s.
electrical s.
electrophrenic s.
endogenous estrogenic s.
endometrial s.
enterochromaffin cell s.
exogenous estrogenic s.
exogenous gonadotropin s.
fetal scalp s.
follicle maturation s.
functional electrical s.
labyrinthine s.

NOTES

stimulation *(continued)*
    laryngopharyngeal sensory s.
      (LPSS)
    nipple s.
    noncoital sexual s.
    oral s.
    ovarian s.
    ovulation s.
    oxytocic s.
    pelvic floor electrical s. (PFS)
    percutaneous Stoller afferent
      nerve s. (PerQ SANS)
    photic s.
    prolactin s.
    sacral nerve root s.
    sensory s.
    sexual s.
    sympathetic s.
    tactile s.
    s. test
    transcranial magnetic s. (TMS)
    transcutaneous electrical nerve s.
      (TENS)
    vagal nerve s.
    vestibular s.
    vibratory acoustic s. (VAS)
    vibroacoustic s. (VAS)
    visual s.
stimulator
    adrenergic s.
    alpha-adrenergic s.
    hematopoietic system s.
    Innova pelvic floor s.
    long-acting thyroid s. (LATS)
    luteinization s.
stimulus, pl. **stimuli**
    amblyogenic s.
    antigenic s.
    click s.
    congenital amblyogenic s.
    high-intensity click s.
    neonatal amblyogenic s.
    nociceptive s.
    tactile s.
stimulus-response (S-R)
sting
    hornet s.
stinging insect allergy
Sting procedure
stippled epiphysis
stippling
    basophilic s.
    bone s.
    corneal s.
    s. of epiphyses
stirrup
    Allen laparoscopic s.'s
    candy-cane s.'s
    hanging s.

    high s.'s
    Lloyd-Davies s.'s
stitch
    s. abscess
    baseball s.
    imbricated s.
    inverting baseball s.
    McCall s.
    running imbricating s.
    running locked s.
    shorthand vertical mattress s.
STNR
    symmetrical tonic neck reflex
Stocco dos Santos syndrome
stockinette
    s. cap
    impervious s.
stocking
    antiembolism s.
    elastic s.
    Juzo-Hostess two-way stretch
      compression s.
    leg-compression s.
    pneumatic compression s.
    TED s.
stocking-glove sensory loss
Stock-Spielmeyer-Vogt syndrome
Stokes-Adams
    S.-A. attack
    S.-A. syndrome
Stoll syndrome
Stolte forceps
stoma, pl. **stomas, stomata**
    ileal s.
stomach
    s. ache
    s. bubble
    s. cancer metastasis
    herniated s.
    infarction of herniated s.
    leather-bottle s.
    right-sided s.
Stomahesive
stomas (*pl. of* stoma)
stomata (*pl. of* stoma)
stomatitis
    angular s.
    aphthous s.
    fusospirillary gangrenous s.
    gangrenous s.
    herpes s.
    herpetic s.
    recurrent aphthous s.
    vesiculoulcerative s.
    Vincent s.
stomatocyte
stomatocytosis
    hereditary s.
stomatomy

stomatoschisis
stomatotomy
stomocephalus
stone
    cholesterol s.
    cystine s.
    s. debris
    hemolysis-derived black pigment s.
    kidney s.
    pigment s.
    renal s.
    struvite s.
    uric acid s.
    womb s.
stool
    acholic s.
    s. antigen test
    s. colonization
    s. culture for O&P
    currant jelly s.
    electron microscopy of s.
    s. examination
    greasy s.
    grossly bloody s.
    guaiac-negative s.
    guaiac-positive s.
    heme-negative s.
    heme-positive s.
    s. impaction
    s. loss
    milk s.
    pale s.
    pea soup s.
    s. porphyrin
    s. retention
    ribbonlike s.
    s. softener
    transition s.
    s. withholding
stooling
stool-reducing substance
STOP
    selective tubal occlusion procedure
    STOP nonsurgical permanent
      contraception device
stopcock
    three-way s.
stop codon
STOP-ROP
    Supplemental Therapeutic Oxygen for
    Prethreshold Retinopathy of Prematurity
    STOP-ROP trial

storage
    abnormal glucosylceramide s.
    s. disease
    s. disorder
STORCH, ToRCHS
    syphilis, toxoplasmosis, other agents, rubella, cytomegalovirus, herpes simplex virus
    toxoplasmosis, rubella, cytomegalovirus, herpes simplex, syphilis
    STORCH test
stored sera
storiform-pleomorphic histologic subtype
stork bite
storm
    affective s.
    thyroid s.
Stormby brush
story-stem
    new MacArthur emotion s.-s.'s
Storz
    S. disposable cannula
    S. disposable trocar
    S. endoscope
    S. infant bronchoscope
    S. laparoscope
Stoxil
STR
    skin test reactivity
    STR typing
strabismic amblyopia
strabismus
    comitant s.
    constant s.
    s. convergens alternans
    convergent s.
    divergent s.
    incomitant s.
    intermittent s.
    nonparalytic s.
    paralytic s.
    s. syndrome
straddle injury
straddling atrioventricular valve
straight
    s. back syndrome
    s. catheter test
    s. last shoe
    s. scissors
    s. sinus

NOTES

straightening
retinal arterial narrowing and s. (RANS)
Straight-In surgical system
straight-leg immobilizer
strain
compression-rarefaction s.
s. down
Enders Edmonston measles s.
impetigo s.
Jeryl Lynn mumps s.
macrophage-tropic s.
M-tropic s.
non-syncytium-inducing s.
NSI s.
Oka s.
RA27/3 rubella s.
recombinant inbred s.
rheumatogenic s.
RIT 4385 mumps s.
Schwarz measles s.
Simkania negevensis s. Z
T-cell-tropic syncytium-inducing s.
T-trophic SI s.
strait
inferior s.
superior s.
strand
antisense s.
stranger
s. anxiety
s. reaction
strangulated hernia
strangulating obstruction
strangulation
clitoral s.
small bowel s.
stranguria
strangury
S-transferase
glutathione S.-t.
strap
figure-of-eight clavicle s.
Montgomery s.
strapping
figure-of-eight s.
Strassman
S. metroplasty
S. operation
S. technique
transverse fundal incision of S.
strata (*pl. of* stratum)
Stratasis urethral sling
StrataSorb dressing
strategy
maladaptive coping s.
Robins and Guze validation s.
stratification
risk s.

stratified squamous epithelium
Stratton-Parker syndrome
stratum, pl. **strata**
s. basale
s. compactum
s. corneum
s. functionale
s. spongiosum
Strauss method
strawberry
s. appearance
s. cervix
s. hemangioma
s. mark
s. nevus
s. patch
s. shaped skull
s. spot
s. tongue
streak
gonadal s.
s. gonads
intraabdominal s.
marbled hypopigmented s.
nonfunctional s.
primitive s.
streaking
perihilar s.
streaky infiltrate
streblodactyly
street
Great Ormond S. (GOS)
s. smart
Streeter
S. band
S. dysplasia
S. horizon
Strema
strength
Allerest Headache S.
Allerest Maximum S.
Anbesol Maximum S.
Biotin Forte Extra S.
Clocort Maximum S.
double s. (XX)
Kaopectate Maximum S.
Orajel Maximum S.
Tums Extra S.
Tylenol Extra S.
Vanceril Double S.
strep
s. breath
s. throat
Streptase
streptavidin peroxidase
Streptex rapid strep test
Streptobacillus moniliformis
streptococcal
s. antibody

s. antigen panel
s. bacteremia
s. cellulitis
s. exotoxin-A (SPEA)
s. gangrene
s. group
s. infection
s. meningitis
s. pharyngitis
s. pneumonia
s. pyoderma
s. septicemia
s. tonsillitis
s. tonsillopharyngitis
s. toxic shock syndrome
s. vaginitis
streptococci (*pl. of* streptococcus)
streptococcosis
Streptococcus
    S. agalactiae
    S. aureus
    S. bacteria
    beta-hemolytic *S.*
    S. bovis
    S. constellates
    S. milleri
    S. mitis
    S. mutans
    S. pneumonia
    S. pneumoniae
    S. pyogenes
    S. salivarius
    S. viridans
streptococcus, pl. **streptococci**
anaerobic s.
beta-hemolytic s.
fecal streptococci
group A s.
group A beta-hemolytic s. (GABHS)
group B s. (GBS)
group C s.
group D s.
group G s.
pediatric autoimmune neuropsychiatric disorders associated with s. (PANDAS)
s. rapid antigen detection test
rheumatogenic s.
viridans s.
streptogramin

streptokinase factor
streptokinase-urokinase
Streptomyces griseus
streptomycin
streptozocin
streptozocin-induced diabetes
Streptozyme test
stress
adrenocortical s.
antepartum s.
behavioral s.
clastogenic s.
cold s.
end-systolic s. (ESS)
end-systolic wall s.
s. erythrocytosis
s. erythropoiesis
s. fracture
s. incontinence
s. incontinence de novo
s. injury
life s.
maternal s.
neonatal s.
s. neonate
oxidative s.
s. oximetry
postmenstrual s.
psychological s.
s. reaction
s. reaction in exenteration
s. response
shear s.
s. test
thermal s.
s. urinary incontinence (SUI)
s. view radiograph
visual analog scale for s.
stress-associated ulcer
stressed fetus
stress-induced syncope
stressor
sociocultural s.
stress-related peptic ulcer disease
stretch
s. mark
s. syncope
stretched
s. penile length
s. phallic length

NOTES

stretching
    bladder s.
    brachial plexus s.
stria, pl. **striae**
    abdominal s.
    striae atrophicae
    striae cutis distensae
    striae gravidarum
    Haab s.
    Langhans s.
    Rohr s.
    s. vascularis
    Wickham s.
striata
    osteopathia s.
striatal toe
striate
    s. body
    s. hyperkeratosis
striated circular muscle
striation
    dense s.
    hyperostosis generalisata with s.
    longitudinal dense s.
    transverse dense s.
    vertical s.
striatothalamic junction
striatum
striatus
    lichen s.
stricto
    Borrelia burgdorferi sensu s.
stricture
    colonic s.
    esophageal s.
    midureteral s.
stricturoplasty
stride
stridor
    audible s.
    biphasic s.
    congenital laryngeal s.
    expiratory s.
    inspiratory s.
    laryngeal s.
    postextubation s.
stridulous breathing
strike
    heel s.
string
    egg on a s.
    s. phlebitis
    s. sign
Stringer technique
strip
    ColorpHast Indicator S.'s
    Cover-Strip wound closure s.
    Dextrostix reagent s.
    DiaScreen reagent s.

    fascial s.
    fetal monitoring s.
    leucocyte detection s.
    lung s.
    Mersilene fascial s.
    pHydrion s.
    polypropylene fascial s.
    QuickVue UrinChek 10+ urine
     test s.
    reagent s.
    saturation s.
    s. test
stripe
    endometrial s.
    thickened endometrial s.
stripping
    apical pleural s.
    capsular s.
    membrane s.
    periosteal s.
    s. of pleura
Stroganoff method
stroke
    mitochondrial encephalopathy, lactic
     acidosis, s.
    perinatal s.
    prenatal s.
    silent s.
strokelike episode
stroma, pl. **stromata**
    cellular desmoplastic s.
    cervical s.
    endometrial s.
    fibromuscular cervical s.
    fibromyxoid s.
    gonadal s.
    malignant mesenchymal s.
    ovarian s.
    Rh-positive red cell s.
    uterine endolymphatic s.
    uterine endometrial s.
    uterine epithelial s.
stromal
    s. adenomyosis
    s. cell
    s. development
    s. endometriosis
    s. hyperplasia
    s. hyperthecosis
    s. luteoma
    s. microinvasion
    s. tumor
stromal-epithelial interaction
stromata (*pl. of* stroma)
stromatosis
stromelysin
strong virilization
Strongyloides stercoralis
strongyloidiasis

strongyloidosis
strontium bromide
Stroop test
strophocephaly
strophulus
structural
    s. airway change
    s. anomaly
    s. brain defect
    s. gene
    s. heart defect
    s. integration
structure
    appendiceal s.
    erectile s.
    genetic fine s.
    hypoechoic s.
    limbic s.
    peripheral airway s.
Strudwick syndrome
struma, pl. **strumae**
    s. ovarii
strumal carcinoid of ovary
Strumpell-Lorrain disease
struvite stone
strychnine poisoning
STS
    serologic test for syphilis
    STS deficiency
ST-segment
    ST-s. abnormality
    ST-s. elevation
ST-T wave abnormality
Stuart
    S. factor
    S. index
    S. Prenatal vitamins
StuartNatal
Stuart-Prower factor
stub thumb
stuck
    s. twin gestation
    s. twin phenomenon
    s. twins
    s. twin syndrome
studding
    peritoneal s.
study
    acoustic stimulation s.
    acute-phase serum s.
    barium s.
    biochemical s.

Bogalusa Heart S. (BHS)
breath hydrogen s.
CASH s.
child behavioral s. (CBS)
Childhood Cancer Survivor S.
chromosomal s.
ciliary function s.
clinical cohort s.
coagulation s.
cohort s.
Collaborative Perinatal S. (CPS)
cytogenetic s.
cytologic s.
Diabetes in Early Pregnancy S.
Diagnostic Interview for Genetic S.
  (DIGS)
DONALD s.
Doppler flow s.
double-blind s.
Dunedin longitudinal s.
electroencephalographic sleep s.
embryonic organ culture s.
epidemiologic s.
fetal blood s.
gene s.
genetic s.
heart and estrogen/progestin
  replacement s. (HERS)
HER S.
histopathological s.
HOPE-ROP s.
immunofluorescence s.
immunologic s.
Iowa Women's Health S.
large-volume blood s.
longitudinal s.
low birth weight-maternal
  employment s. (LBW-MES)
MacArthur Longitudinal Twin S.
MECA s.
methodology s.
mineral balance s.
molecular genetic s.
Multicenter AIDS Cohort S.
  (MACS)
National Acute Spinal Cord
  Injury S.
nerve conduction s.
neuroimaging s.
neuroradiographic s.
North American Collaborative
  Crohn Disease S. (NCCDS)

S

NOTES

study *(continued)*
  Oxford Family Planning Association Contraceptive S.
  PEPI s.
  Persutte and Lenke s.
  placebo-controlled s.
  postmortem s.
  Preterm Prediction S.
  quadruple-contrast s.
  radioisotopic reperfusion and excretion s.
  register linkage s.
  Royal College of General Practioners' Oral Contraception S.
  Second National Incidence S. (NIS-2)
  sleep s.
  S. of Tamoxifen and Raloxifene (STAR)
  tissue s.
  transesophageal electrophysiologic s.
  videofluoroscopic swallowing s. (VFSS)
  videourodynamic s.
  water-deprivation s.
  Women and Infants Transmission S. (WITS)
  Women's HOPE s.
  women's interagency HIV s. (WIHS)
  women's intervention nutrition s. (WINS)
stuff
  Numby S.
stump
  appendiceal s.
  cervical s.
  inverted appendiceal s.
  rectal s.
  umbilical s.
stun
  cardiac s.
stunned myocardium
stunning
  myocardial s.
stunted
  s. embryo
  s. fetus
stunting
  growth s.
stupor
stuporous
Sturge-Kalischer-Weber syndrome
Sturge-Weber
  S.-W. angiomatosis
  S.-W. anomalad
  S.-W. disease
  S.-W. syndrome (SWS)

Sturge-Weber-Dimitri syndrome
Sturge-Weber-Krabbe syndrome
Sturmdorf
  S. hemostatic suture
  S. operation
stuttering
  medication-induced s.
  neurogenic s.
Stüve-Wiedemann (SW)
  S.-W. syndrome (SWS)
Stx
  Shiga toxin
sty, stye, pl. **styes, sties**
style
  learning s.
stylomastoid foramen
stylopodium
stype
subacute
  s. anterior uveitis
  s. bacterial endocarditis (SBE)
  s. combined degeneration
  s. encephalitis
  s. fetal hypoxia
  s. myeloopticoneuropathy
  s. necrotizing encephalomyopathy
  s. necrotizing encephalopathy
  s. neuritis
  s. neuronopathic Gaucher disease
  s. osteomyelitis
  s. sclerosing panencephalitis (SSPE)
  s. thyroiditis
  s. tracheitis
subaortic
  s. conus
  s. hypertrophic cardiomyopathy
  s. lymph node
  s. membrane
  s. stenosis
  s. stenosis-short stature syndrome
subaponeurotic cranial space
subarachnoid
  s. analgesia
  s. block
  s. bolt
  s. hemorrhage
subareolar
  s. abscess
  s. duct papillomatosis
  s. tissue
subaverage intelligence
subcapsular
  s. cyst
  s. hepatic hematoma
  s. hepatic hemorrhage
subchorial
  s. lake
  s. space

subchorionic
- s. hematoma
- s. hemorrhage

subclavian
- s. artery
- s. artery defect
- s. flap aortoplasty (SFA)
- s. steal

subclinical hypothyroidism
subconjunctival hemorrhage
subcoronal hypospadias
subcortical
- s. band heterotopia
- s. laminar heterotopia

subcostal
- s. incision
- s. retractions
- s. view

subcutanea
- lipogranulomatosis s.

subcutaneous
- s. calcification
- s. catheter tunnel formation
- s. desferrioxamine therapy
- s. emphysema
- s. fat necrosis
- s. granuloma annulare
- s. mastectomy
- s. neurofibroma
- s. nodule
- s. sarcoidosis
- s. suspensory ligament
- s. tunnel
- s. ventricular catheter reservoir

subcutaneum
subdermal
- s. contraceptive system
- s. implant
- s. levonorgestrel implant (SLI)

subdiaphragmatic air
subdural
- s. abscess
- s. effusion
- s. empyema
- s. hematoma (SDH)
- s. hemorrhage
- s. puncture
- s. tap

subdural-peritoneal shunt
subendocardial
subendometrial myoma

subependymal
- s. bleeding
- s. cryptic angioma
- s. germinal matrix hemorrhage
- s. germinolysis
- s. hemorrhage (SEH)
- s. heterotopia
- s. region
- s. tuber

subepidermal
- s. blister
- s. keratin cyst

subfecundity
subfertility
subfibulare
- os s.

subfragment-1
subgaleal
- s. hematoma (SGH)
- s. hemorrhage

subglottic
- s. edema
- s. erosion
- s. stenosis

subhyaloid hemorrhage
subiculum
subinvolution
subischial leg length (SILL)
subitum
subjective probability
sublamina densa
sublethal gene
Sublimaze Injection
sublingual
- s. gland
- s. hematoma
- Nitrostat S.
- s. onychomycosis
- s. thyroid

subluxating patella
subluxation
- atlantoaxial rotary s.
- cervical spine s.
- s. dislocation
- habitual shoulder s.
- radial head s. (RHS)
- rotary s.
- rotatory s.
- shoulder s.

subluxed hip
submammary mastitis
submaxillary gland

S

NOTES

submental
    s. hematoma
    s. lymphadenitis
    s. lymphadenopathy
submentovertex view
submersion
    iced saline s.
    s. injury
submetacentric chromosome
submucosa
submucosal
    s. arterial malformation
    s. mass
    s. myoma
    s. plexus
    s. urethral augmentation
submucous
    s. cleft
    s. cleft palate
    s. fibroid
    s. leiomyoma
    s. myoma
subnormal
    s. growth velocity
    s. temperature
subnormality
    mental s.
suboccipital craniectomy
suboccipitobregmatic diameter
suboptimal surgery
suborbital edema
subpannicular area
subpectoral implant
subperiosteal
    s. abscess
    s. aspiration
subphrenic
    s. abscess
    s. gas collection
subpial region
subpleural
    s. bleb
    s. reticulonodular pattern
subpulmonic area
Sub-Q-Set
subretinal
    s. exudate
    s. fluid
subsalicylate
    bismuth s.
subscale
subscapular skinfold thickness
subsegmental atelectasis
subseptate uterus
subsequent fertility
subserosal
    s. nodule
    s. pedunculated myoma

subserous
    s. fascia
    s. fibroid
    s. myoma
subset
substance
    s. abuse
    illegal s.
    müllerian inhibiting s. (MIS)
    s. P immune reactivity
    s. P pain neurotransmitter
    reducing s.
    serum müllerian inhibiting s.
    stool-reducing s.
    thiobarbituric acid-reacting s.
     (TBARS)
    urine-reducing s.
    s. use disorder (SUD)
    vasoactive s.
    s. X
substance-induced psychotic disorder
substantia
    s. gelatinosa
    s. nigra
    s. nigra pars reticulata
    s. propria
substernal retraction
substitute
    s. care
    Oxygent temporary blood s.
    perflubron emulsion temporary
     blood s.
    PolyHeme blood s.
substrate
    renin s.
subsyndromal depressive symptom
subtalar facet
subtest
    Digit Span S.
subthalamicum
    corpus s.
subtilis
    Bacillus s.
subtle
    s. neurologic sequela
    s. seizure
subtotal hysterectomy
subtrigonal injection
subtype
    myxoid histopathologic s.
    storiform-pleomorphic histologic s.
subungual
    s. exostosis
    s. fibroma
    s. oncychomycosis
subunit
    beta s.
    inhibin s.
    inhibin-A s.

subureteric Teflon injection
suburethral
    s. diverticulitis
    s. sling
subvalvular
subxiphoid
subzonal
    s. injection (SUZI)
    s. injection of sperm (SUZI)
    s. insemination (SUZI)
    s. insertion (SUZI)
succedaneum
    caput s.
succenturiate placenta
successful pregnancy
succimer
succinate
    s. dehydrogenase
    hydrocortisone sodium s.
    sumatriptan s.
succinyl
    s. aminoimidazole carboxamide
      ribotide (SAICAR)
    s. CoA:3-ketoacid CoA transferase
    s. CoA:3-oxoacid CoA transferase
      (SCOT)
succinylcholine
succinylsulfathiazole
succumb
suck
    poor s.
    weak s.
sucking
    s. blister
    s. cushion
    nonnutritive s.
    s. pad
    s. reflex
suckle
suckling reflex
Sucraid
sucralfate
sucrase-isomaltase deficiency
Sucrets
    S. Cough Calmers
    S. Sore Throat
sucrose
    concentrated oral s.
    s. gradient
    s. hemolysis test
    s. pacifier
sucrose-free formula

sucrosuria
suction
    airway s.
    bulb s.
    s. catheter
    s. and curettage (S&C)
    s. curette
    s., dilation, and curettage
    s. drainage
    nasopharyngeal s.
    open endotracheal s.
    s. pump
    respiratory s.
    Tis-u-Trap endometrial s.
    Trach Care s.
    Vabra s.
    vacuum s.
    wall s.
suction-assisted lipoplasty (SAL)
suctioning
    bulb s.
    chest s.
    closed endotracheal tube s.
    DeLee s.
    nasopharyngeal s.
    open endotracheal s.
    respiratory s.
    tracheal s.
suction-irrigator
    Nezhat-Dorsey s.-i.
suctorial pad
SUD
    substance use disorder
    sudden unexpected death
Sudafed 12 Hour
sudamen, pl. **sudamina**
    miliary sudamina
sudanophilic
    s. cerebral sclerosis
    s. diffuse sclerosis
    s. leukodystrophy
Sudan stain
sudden
    s. infant death (SID)
    s. infant death syndrome (SIDS)
    s. infant death unexplained by
      history
    s. intrauterine unexplained death
    s. unexpected death (SUD)
Sudeck atrophy
sudomotor dysfunction
sudoral miliaria

S

NOTES

Sudrin
SUDS
single-use diagnostic system
SUDS HIV-1 antibody test
SUFE
slipped upper femoral epiphysis
Sufenta Injection
sufentanil
s. citrate
sufficient
pancreas s. (PS)
s. quantity
quantity not s. (QNS)
suffocation
infant s.
mechanical s.
suffusion
conjunctival s.
sugar
blood s.
s. diabetes
fasting blood s.
s. intoxication
low blood s.
mannose-type s.
sugar-dipped pacifier
Sugarman
S. brachydactyly
S. syndrome
sugar-tong splint
Sugiura procedure
SUI
stress urinary incontinence
suicidal ideation
suicidality
suicide
attempted s.
s. gene
s. gene therapy
hospitalized attempted s. (HAS)
s. risk screen (SRS)
suis
Brucella s.
Herpesvirus s.
suit
MAST s.
Sulamyd
Sodium S.
sulbactam
ampicillin and s.
sulconazole
sulcus, pl. **sulci**
coronal s.
Harrison s.
Sulf-10
sulfa
sulfabenzamide
sulfacarbamide
sulfacetamide

sulfachlorpyridazine
sulfacytine
sulfadiazine
silver s.
sulfadimethoxine
sulfadimidine
sulfadoxine and pyrimethamine
sulfaethidole
sulfafurazole, sulphafurazole
sulfaguanidine
Sulfair
sulfalene
sulfamerazine
sulfameter
sulfamethazine
sulfamethizole
Sulfamethoprim
sulfamethoxazole
sulfamethoxazole/phenazopyridine hydrochloride
sulfamethoxazole and trimethoprim
sulfamethoxydiazine
sulfamethoxypyridazine
Sulfamylon cream
sulfaphenazole
sulfapyridine
sulfasalazine
sulfatase
iduronate s. (IDS)
steroid s.
sulfate
amikacin s.
amphetamine s.
anhydrous magnesium s.
atropine s.
bleomycin s.
chondroitin s.
dehydroepiandrosterone s. (DHEAS)
dehydroisoandrosterone s.
dermatan s.
dextran s.
dextrin s.
dextroamphetamine s.
DHEA s.
ephedrine s.
estrone s.
ferric s.
ferrous s. ($FeSO_4$)
gentamicin s.
heparan s.
hexoprenaline s.
hydrazine s.
hydroxychloroquine s.
hyoscyamine s.
keratan s.
magnesium s. ($MgSO_4$)
metaproterenol s.
morphine s.
neomycin s.

netilmicin s.
piperazine estrone s.
Plaquenil S.
polymyxin B s.
protamine s.
quinine s.
sodium equilin s.
sodium estrone s.
sodium tetradecyl s.
steroid s.
terbutaline s.
trimethoprim s.
vincristine s.
zinc s.
sulfathiazole
sulfathiourea
sulfatide
sulfatidosis
juvenile s.
Sulfatrim DS
Sulfa-Trip
sulfaturia
keratan s.
sulfhydryl (SH)
sulfide
selenium s.
sulfisomidine
sulfisoxazole
**sulfisoxazole/phenazopyridine
  hydrochloride**
sulfite oxidase deficiency
Sulfizole
**sulfoiduronate sulfatase deficiency
  (SIDS)**
sulfonamide
sulfonate
2-mercaptoethane s. (mesna)
sodium polystyrene s.
sulfonylurea
sulfotransferase
estrogen s.
sulfoxide
dimethyl s. (DMSO)
sulfur
s. dioxide
s. granule
s. and salicylic acid
sulfur-deficient brittle hair syndrome
sulindac
sulphafurazole (*var. of* sulfafurazole)
sulpiride
sulprostone

Sultrin
sum
Sumacal formula
sumatriptan
s. nasal spray
s. succinate
summation gallop
Sumycin Oral
SUN
serum urea nitrogen
sunburn
blistering s.
sunburst appearance
sunflower
s. cataract
s. oil challenge test
sunken anterior fontanelle
Sunlight Omnisense ultrasound
Sunna circumcision
Sunnex Tri-Star lamp
sunny-side up delivery
sun protection behavior index (SBPI)
sunrise view
sun-seeking pattern
sunset eyes
sunsetting eyes
sunstroke
super
s. blue light
s. female
s. syringe
superabsorbent
superactivity
phosphoribosylpyrophosphate
  synthetase s.
PRPP synthetase s.
**superconducting quantum interference
  device susceptometer (SQUIDS)**
superfamily
transforming growth factor B s.
superfecundation
superfetation
superficial
s. circumflex iliac artery
s. compartment
s. compartment of vulva
s. ectopic testis
s. epigastric artery
s. external pudendal artery (SEPA)
s. linear array (SLA)
s. necrosis
s. onychomycosis

S

NOTES

superficial *(continued)*
    s. spreading melanoma
    s. thrombophlebitis
    s. thrombus
    s. transverse perineal muscle
superfluous
superimposed
    s. eclampsia
    s. preeclampsia
superimpregnation
superinfection
superinvolution
superior
    s. epigastric artery
    s. fascia
    s. iliac crest
    s. iliac spine
    s. laryngeal nerve
    s. mediastinal syndrome
    s. mesenteric angiogram
    s. mesenteric artery
    s. mesenteric artery syndrome
    s. mesenteric plexus
    s. mesenteric vein
    s. oblique muscle
    s. olivary nucleus
    s. olive
    s. ramus
    saccus s.
    s. sagittal sinus
    s. strait
    s. vena cava (SVC)
    s. vena caval syndrome
    s. vena cava syndrome
    s. venous system
    s. vesical fissure
superlactation
supernatant
    amniotic fluid s.
supernumerary
    s. breast
    s. chromosome
    s. digit
    s. kidney
    s. mamma
    s. marker chromosome (SMC)
    s. nipple
    s. ovary
    s. placenta
    s. proboscis
    s. rib
superovulation induction
superoxide
    s. dismutase-1
    s. radical
supersaturation of bile
SuperVent
supervoltage radiation
supinate

supination
    passive s.
supine
    s. empty stress test (SEST)
    s. hypotensive syndrome
    s. length
    s. pressor test
    s. sleep position
Suplena formula
supplement, supplementation
    Aminosyn-PF s.
    Boost nutritional s.
    calcium s.
    dietary s.
    EleCare nutritional s.
    enzyme s.
    Fer-In-Sol s.
    infant dietary s.
    iron s.
    Lactaid Ultra lactase enzyme s.
    magnesium s.
    NeoSure nutritional s.
    nutritional s.
    Pediatrician infant dietary s.
    phosphate s.
    potassium s.
    vitamin s.
    zinc s.
supplemental
    s. newborn screen
    s. oxygen
    S. Security Income (SSI)
    S. Therapeutic Oxygen for Prethreshold Retinopathy of Prematurity (STOP-ROP)
supplementary
    s. gene
    s. menstruation
supplementation *(var. of* supplement)
supply
    arterial s.
    iodine s.
    milk s.
    musculofascial s.
support
    advanced cardiac life s. (ACLS)
    advanced life s. (ALS)
    advanced pediatric life s. (APLS)
    advanced trauma life s. (ATLS)
    basic life s. (BLS)
    s. catheter
    extensive s.
    extracorporeal life s. (ECLS)
    s. group
    Gynemesh PS polypropylene mesh s.
    inotropic s.
    intermittent s.
    limited s.

luteal phase s.
medial longitudinal arch s.
Multidimensional Scale of
  Perceived Social S. (MSPSS)
neonatal adjuvant life s. (NALS)
s. network
noninvasive respiratory s.
nutritional s.
pediatric advanced life s. (PALS)
pervasive s.
psychosocial s.
s. reflex
respiratory s.
s. services
s. trust
urethral s.
urethrovesical angle s.
vaginal vault s.
ventilator s.
ventilatory s.
supportive
s. care
s. group therapy
s. psychotherapy
suppository
Anusol-HC S.
AVC s.
bisacodyl s.
Cort-Dome High Potency S.
Dilaudid S.
glycerin s.
intravaginal s.
Monistat 3 vaginal s.
paracetamol s.
prostaglandin s.
Prostin E2 Vaginal S.
rectal s.
Sani-Supp S.
Terazol vaginal s.
triple sulfa s.
vaginal s.
Supprelin
suppressant
St. Joseph Cough S.
suppressed menstruation
suppression
adrenal s.
antibody-mediated immune s.
  (AMIS)
bone marrow s.
s. burst

endogenous gonadotropin activity s.
estradiol s.
fetal parathyroid s.
gonadal steroid s.
immunologic s.
pituitary gonadotropin s.
prolactin s.
testosterone s.
Suppress lozenges
suppressor
s. gene
s. T cell
Supprettes
Aquachloral S.
suppurate
suppurating sinus tract
suppuration
intracranial s.
joint s.
pulmonary s.
suppurativa
hidradenitis s.
hydradenitis s.
vulvar hidradenitis s.
suppurative
s. appendicitis
s. arthritis
s. bursitis
s. cholangitis
s. infection
s. labyrinthitis
s. lymphadenitis
s. mastitis
s. mediastinitis
s. otitis media
s. parotitis
s. phlebitis
s. pneumonia
s. thyroiditis
suprabasal blister
suprabulbar paresis
supracardiac total anomalous pulmonary venous return
supracervical hysterectomy (SCH)
supraciliary tap
supraclavicular
s. indrawing
s. retraction
supracondylar
s. humeral fracture
supracristal ventricular septal defect

NOTES

supraglottic
   s. aperture
   s. web
supraglottitis
supralevator
   s. abscess
   s. imperforate anus
supramalleolar orthosis (SMO)
supranormal scrotal position
supranuclear palsy
supraorbital nerve block
suprapineal recess
suprapubic
   s. aspiration of urine
   s. bladder aspiration
   s. catheter
   s. cystostomy
   s. cystotomy
   s. discomfort
   s. fat pad
   s. mass
   5-mm s. trocar
   s. pain
   s. pressure
   s. stab wound
   s. urethrovesical suspension
    operation
suprasellar
   s. arachnoid cyst
   s. meningioma
suprasternal
   s. notch
   s. notch thrill
   s. view
supratentorial
   s. anaplastic ependymoma
   s. white matter
supratip nasal tip deformity
supraumbilical incision
supravaginalis
   portio s.
supravaginal septum
supravalvular
   s. aortic stenosis
   s. pulmonary stenosis
supraventricular
   s. tachyarrhythmia (SVT)
   s. tachycardia (SVT)
   s. tachydysrhythmia
supraventricularis
   crista s.
Supravital
supravital
   s. stain
   s. stain test
Suprax
sural nerve biopsy
SureCell
   S. Chlamydia Test kit

   S. Herpes (HSV) Test
   S. rapid test kit for pregnancy
SurePress
   S. dressing
   S. wrap
SureSite dressing
767 SureTemp 4 oral thermometer
Surety Shield
SURF
   Service Utilization and Risk Factors
surface
   adaptive s.
   amniotic-chorionic s.
   s. antigen
   s. antigen (subtype ayw1–ayw4)
   antimesenteric s.
   decreased mucosal s.
   denuded s.
   s. electromyogram (SEMG)
   s. electromyography (SEMG)
   s. epithelium
   s. epithelium vascular channel
   external s.
   s. furrowing
   s. furrowing of tongue
   s. immunoglobulin
   s. irradiation
   lingual s.
   serosal s.
   s. tension
surfactant
   s. administration
   beractant s.
   bovine s.
   bovine lavage extract s. (BLES)
   s. deficiency syndrome
   exogenous s.
   heterologous s.
   homologous s.
   Human Surf s.
   Infasurf s.
   s. lavage
   porcine s.
   s. protein-A (SP-A)
   s. protein-B (SP-B)
   s. protein-C (SP-C)
   s. protein deficiency
   pulmonary s.
   s. replacement therapy
   s. replacement trial
   rescue s.
   Survanta s.
   synthetic s.
surfactant-associated
   s.-a. protein (SAP)
   s.-a. protein C enhancer
surfactant-deficient lung
Surfak
Sur-Fast needle

Surfaxin
    dilute S.
surge
    estrogen s.
    LH s.
    midcycle s.
    postnatal gonadotropin s.
    preovulatory LH s.
    TSH s.
surgeon
    pediatric s.
    pelvic reconstruction s.
surgeon's knot
surgery
    ablative s.
    antivesicuoreteral reflux s.
    bladder neck s.
    bypass s.
    conservative s.
    corrective s.
    cytoreductive s.
    definitive s.
    emergency s.
    endoscopic sinus s.
    extirpative s.
    extraocular muscle s.
    feminizing s.
    fetal s.
    gamma knife s.
    gastric reduction s.
    hysteroscopic s.
    inferior turbinate s.
    intraabdominal s.
    laser s.
    lung s.
    muscle s.
    open heart s.
    orthognathic s.
    palliative s.
    pediatric lung s.
    pelvic-floor s.
    pelvic reconstructive s.
    peripheral ablative s.
    prenatal s.
    previous transfundal uterine s.
    primary cytoreductive s.
    pull-through s.
    radical s.
    radioreceptor-guided s.
    reconstructive pelvic s.
    sinus s.
    suboptimal s.
    thoracic s.
    tubal reconstruction s.
    vaginal s.
    video-assisted thoracic s. (VATS)
    video-assisted thoracoscopic s. (VATS)
    zero gravity s.
surgical
    s. asplenia
    s. containment
    s. correction
    s. cricothyrotomy
    s. debulking
    s. disruption
    s. emergency
    s. enucleation
    s. evacuation
    s. hemostasis
    s. infection
    s. management
    s. mastoiditis
    s. myomectomy as reproductive therapy (SMART)
    s. neonate
    S. Nu-Knit
    s. oophorectomy
    s. overhead canopy (SOC)
    s. pleurodesis
    s. removal
    s. repair
    s. resection
    s. scarlet fever
    s. septectomy
    s. space
    s. staging
    s. sterilization
    s. sterilization procedure
    s. tape occlusion
    s. termination
    s. weight loss
surgically-induced abortion
Surgicel
Surgicenter 40 CO_2 laser
surgicopathologic staging system
Surgidac suture
Surgilase 55W laser
Surgilene
Surgin hemorrhage occluder pin
Surgi-Prep
Surgiview laparoscope
Surmontil
surrender posture

NOTES

surrogacy
>gestational s.
>traditional s.

surrogate
>gestational s.
>s. gestational motherhood
>s. mother
>sex s.

Survanta surfactant
surveillance
>antepartum fetal s.
>s. colonoscopy
>developmental s.
>S., Epidemiology and End Results (SEER)
>fetal s.
>immunologic s.
>maternal s.
>nutritional s.
>posttreatment s.
>s. technique
>s. tracheal aspirate
>ultrasound s.

survey
>Juvenile Wellness and Health S. (JWHS)
>Kids Eating Disorder S. (KEDS)
>National Ambulatory Medical Care S. (NAMCS)
>National Educational Longitudinal S. (NELS)
>National Health Interview S. (NHIS)
>National Health and Nutrition Examination S. (NHANES)
>National Hospital Discharge S. (NIDS)
>National Maternal and Infant Health S.
>School Sleep Habits S.
>Sexual Opinion S.
>skeletal s.
>youth risk behavioral s. (YRBS)

survival
>actuarial s.
>allograft s.
>decreased red blood cell s.
>disease-free s. (DFS)
>event-free s. (EFS)
>life table s.
>long-term s.
>s. rate

survivor guilt
susceptibility
>genetic s.
>s. hypothesis

susceptible

susceptometer
>superconducting quantum interference device s. (SQUIDS)

Susp
>Megacillin S.

suspected
>s. child abuse or neglect (SCAN)
>s. pituitary adenoma

suspension
>Aldridge-Studdefort urethral s.
>Alexander-Adams uterine s.
>Baldy-Webster uterine s.
>bladder neck s.
>budesonide inhalation s. (BIS)
>Children's Motrin S.
>Ciprodex otic s.
>Coffey s.
>Cortisporin Ophthalmic S.
>Cortisporin Otic S.
>Cortisporin-TC Otic S.
>Curosurf intratracheal s.
>DisperMox oral s.
>endoscopic bladder neck s. (EBNS)
>Gilliam-Doleris uterine s.
>Gittes urethral s.
>high uterosacral ligament s.
>horizontal s.
>iliococcygeus fascia s.
>Infasurf intratracheal s.
>inhalation s.
>Michigan four-wall sacrospinous s.
>minimal-incision pubovaginal s.
>needle s.
>Olshausen s.
>Omnicef oral s.
>orciprenaline oral s.
>paravaginal s.
>Pereyra needle s.
>protamine insulin zinc s.
>Raz bladder neck s.
>sacrospinous ligament s.
>sacrospinous vaginal vault s.
>Stamey-Pereyra needle s.
>transvaginal bladder neck s.
>uterine s.
>uterosacral ligament s.
>vaginal vault s.
>ventral s.
>Yachia incisionless bladder s.

suspensory
>s. ligament laxity
>s. ligament of ovary
>s. ligaments of Cooper
>s. sling operation

Sustacal Plus formula
Sustagen formula
sustained
>s. autonomic hypoarousal

s. clonus
s. ventricular tachycardia
sustained-release
s.-r. albuterol
s.-r. theophylline
Sustiva
Sutherland-Haan syndrome (SHS)
Sutherland procedure
Sutilains Ointment
sutural calcification
suture
absorbable s.
apposition of skull s.
Caprosyn monofilament s.
catgut s.
coated Vicryl Rapide s.
continuous running monofilament s.
coronal s.
cranial s.
Dexon II s.
Dexon Plus s.
DG Softgut s.
Endoloop s.
Ethibond polybutilate-coated
polyester s.
frontal s.
Gambee s.
s. grasper forceps
gut s.
interrupted s.
inverted subcuticular s.
Investa s.
Kelly s.
s. ligated
s. material
Maxon delayed-absorbable s.
Mersilene s.
Monocryl s.
nasofrontal s.
overriding of s.'s
s. penile laceration
perianal s.
permanent s.
polyglactic acid s.
polyglactin 910 s.
polyglycol s.
polyglyconate s.
Polysorb s.
premature closure of coronal s.
Prolene s.
purse-string s.
retention s.

Safil synthetic absorbable
surgical s.
sagittal s.
silk s.
silver wire s.
skin s.
s.'s of skull
stainless steel s.
Sturmdorf hemostatic s.
Surgidac s.
Vicryl Rapide s.
wide cranial s.
suture-ligation
suture-ligature
Suture-Mate
suxamethonium
SUZI
subzonal injection
subzonal injection of sperm
subzonal insemination
subzonal insertion
Sv
sievert
SVC
superior vena cava
SV-CAH
simple virilizing congenital adrenal
hyperplasia
SVD
spontaneous vaginal delivery
SVE
sterile vaginal examination
SVR
systemic vascular resistance
SVT
supraventricular tachyarrhythmia
supraventricular tachycardia
fetal reentrant SVT
SW
Stüve-Wiedemann
swab
calcium alginate s.
cotton-tipped s.
s. examination
nasal s.
nasopharyngeal s.
Puritan s.
rectal s.
s. test
throat s.
umbilical s.

NOTES

swallow
    barium s.
    modified barium s. (MBS)
    s. reflex
    rehabilitation cookie s.
    s. syncope
swallowed
    s. blood syndrome
    s. maternal blood
swallowing
    air s.
    s. difficulty
    fetal s.
    s. reflex
Swan-Ganz catheter
sway
    lateral shoulder s.
swayback
SW-CAH
    salt-wasting congenital adrenal
    hyperplasia
sweat
    s. chloride
    s. chloride concentration
    s. chloride determination
    s. chloride iontophoresis
    s. chloride level
    s. chloride test
    s. duct
    s. gland
    night s.
    s. testing
sweating
    anhidrotic s.
    eccrine s.
    excessive s.
    hypohidrotic s.
    nocturnal s.
sweaty feet syndrome
Swedish
    S. national growth chart
    S. porphyria
Sween Cream
sweep
    s. gas
    s. the pelvis
    The Cell S.
sweetened pacifier
Sweet syndrome
swelling
    brain s.
    cerebral s.
    diffuse brain s. (DBS)
    focal axonal s.
    global brain s.
    hydrocephalic brain s.
    hypoosmotic s. (HOS)
    labioscrotal s.
    scrotal s.

Swenson pull-through procedure
SWGD
    sterile water gastric drip
Swift disease
SWIM
    sperm washing insemination method
Swim-Ear water drying aid
swimmer's
    s. ear
    s. itch
    s. shoulder
swimming
    s. movement
    s. pool granuloma
    s. position
    s. reflex
swim-up technique
swine-flu influenza vaccine
swinging
    blanket s.
    s. flashlight test
Swiss
    S. cheese endometrium
    S. cheese hyperplasia
    S. cheese septum
switch
    adaptive s.
    genetic s.
    s. operation
    venous s.
swivel-arm system
swivel walker
swollen
    s. glomerular tuft
    s. joint
swordfish test
SWS
    Sturge-Weber syndrome
    Stüve-Wiedemann syndrome
Swyer-James-Macleod syndrome
Swyer-James syndrome
Swyer syndrome
SX-T
    Proplex SX-T
sycosis barbae
Sydenham
    S. chorea
    S. chorea criteria
Sydney
    S. crease
    S. line
Syed-Neblett dedicated vulvar plastic template
Syllact
sylvatic typhus
sylvian
    s. aqueduct syndrome
    s. epilepsy
    s. seizure

Sylvius
    aqueduct of S.
    hydrocephalus due to congenital
      stenosis of aqueduct of S.
      (HSAS, HYCX)
Symadine
symbiotic psychosis
symblepharon
symbolic representation
symbrachydactyly
Syme amputation
symmelia
symmetric
    s. communicating uterus
    s. demyelination
    s. growth restriction
    s. IUGR
    s. progressive erythrokeratodermia
symmetrical
    s. conjoined twins
    s. movement
    s. tonic neck reflex (STNR)
symmetros
    duplicitas s.
sympathectomy, sympathetectomy
    presacral s.
sympathetic
    s. adrenergic function
    s. blockade
    s. chain
    s. ganglion
    s. innervation
    s. nervous system
    s. skin response
    s. stimulation
    s. tissue
sympatholytic drop
sympathomimetic amine
sympathovagal
symphalangism
symphyseotome (*var. of* symphysiotome)
symphyseotomy (*var. of* symphysiotomy)
symphyses
symphyses (*pl. of* symphysis)
symphysial
    s. separation
    s. wall
symphysiotome, symphyseotome
symphysiotomy, symphyseotomy
symphysis, pl. **symphyses**
    pubic s.

    s. pubis
    s. pubis diastasis
symphysis-fundus height
symphysodactyly
sympodia
symptom
    B s.'s
    Bristol Female Lower Urinary
      Tract S.'s (BFLUTS)
    s. contagion
    depressive s.
    dissociative s.
    duration of s.'s
    intrusion s.
    neurovegetative functioning or s.
    obstructive s.
    paraneoplastic s.
    pathognomonic s.
    PIH s.
    postmenopausal urogenital s.
    posttraumatic signs or s.'s (PTSS)
    pregnancy-induced hypertension s.
    premenstrual s.'s
    prodromal s.
    refractory depressive s.
    schedule for negative s.'s (SANS)
    schedule for positive s.'s (SAPS)
    subsyndromal depressive s.
    tic s.
    Uhthoff s.
    vegetative s.
    vertiginous s.
symptomatic
    s. chronic empyema
    s. dystonia
    s. epilepsy
    s. infection
    s. porphyria
    s. primary immunodeficiency
      disorder
    s. progressive hydrocephalus
    s. spasm
    s. status epilepticus
symptomatica
    porphyria cutanea tarda s.
symptomatology
symptom-giving PGR
symptothermal method
symptothermic contraceptive method
sympus
Synacort Topical
synactive theory

S

NOTES

synadelphus
synagiosis
Synagis
Synalar Topical
Synalgos-DC
synangiosis
    encephaloduroarterial s.
synapse
synapsis
synaptic pruning
synaptogenesis
synaptonemal complex
synaptophysin
Synarel
syncephalus
    s. asymmetros
    craniothoracopagus s.
syncheilia
synchondrosis disruption
synchondrotomy
synchronic
synchronized
    s. DC cardioversion
    s. intermittent mandatory ventilation
      (SIMV)
    s. nasal intermittent positive-
      pressure ventilation (SNIPPV)
synchronized intermittent mandatory
  ventilation (SIMV)
synchronous breathing
synchronously
syncinesis (*var. of* synkinesis)
synclitic
synclitism
syncopal
    s. episode
    s. spell
syncope
    adolescent stretch s.
    arrhythmogenic s.
    cardiac s.
    cerebral s.
    cough s.
    hair groomer's s.
    hysterical s.
    infantile s.
    micturition s.
    neurally mediated s. (NMS)
    neurocardiogenic s.
    neuropsychiatric s.
    orthostatic s.
    reflex s.
    stress-induced s.
    stretch s.
    swallow s.
    vasopressor s.
    vasovagal s.
syncytia (*pl. of* syncytium)
syncytia

syncytial
    s. bud
    s. cell
    s. knot
    s. sprout
syncytiotrophoblast (ST)
    malignant s.
syncytiotrophoblastic tumor giant cell
syncytium, pl. **syncytia**
    s. inducing (SI)
syndactylism
syndactylization
syndactyly
    s., cataracts, mental retardation
      syndrome
    Cenani-Lenz s.
    complex s.
    digit s.
    s., microcephaly, mental retardation
      syndrome
    simple s.
    soft tissue s.
    toe s.
syndactyly-anophthalmos syndrome
syndesis
syndesmosis, pl. **syndesmoses**
    tibiofibular s.
syndet cleaning bar
syndrome (*See also* disease)
    AAA s.
    AADH s.
    Aagenaes s.
    Aarskog s.
    Aarskog-Scott s. (ASS)
    Aase s.
    Aase-Smith s.
    Abderhalden-Fanconi s.
    abdominal compartment s. (ACS)
    abdominal muscle deficiency s.
    abdominal musculature aplasia s.
    abducted thumbs s.
    Aberfeld s.
    ablepharon-macrostomia s. (AMS)
    absence of abdominal muscle s.
    absent pulmonary valve s.
    abstinence s.
    Abt-Letterer-Siwe s.
    abuse dwarfism s.
    Accutane dysmorphic s.
    ACD mental retardation s.
    ACF s.
    achalasia-microcephaly s.
    Achard s.
    Achard-Thiers s.
    achondrogenesis s.
    achondroplasia s.
    acid aspiration s.
    acquired immune deficiency s.
      (AIDS)

acquired immunodeficiency s. (AIDS)
acquired inflammatory Brown s.
acral-renal-mandibular s.
acrocallosal s. (ACS)
acrodysgenital s.
acrodysostosis s.
acrodysplasia-dysostosis s.
acrofacial dysostosis with postaxial defects s.
acromegaloid-cutis verticis gyrata-leukoma s.
acroosteolysis s.
acrorenal s.
acrorenomandibular s.
acrorenoocular s.
acute aseptic meningitis s.
acute chest s. (ACS)
s. of acute hemiplegia
acute meningoencephalitis s.
acute radiation s.
acute respiratory distress s. (ARDS)
acute retroviral s.
acute traumatic compartment s.
acute urethral s.
Adair-Dighton s.
Adams-Oliver s.
Adams-Stokes s.
Addison disease-cerebral sclerosis s.
Addison disease-spastic paraplegia s.
addisonian s.
Addison-Schilder s.
adducted thumb-clubfoot s.
adducted thumbs s.
adducted thumbs-mental retardation s.
Adie chronic pupillary s.
adiposogenital s.
ADR s.
adrenal virilizing s.
adrenocortical atrophy-cerebral sclerosis s.
adrenogenital syndrome (AGS)
adult-onset polyglandular s.
adult respiratory distress s. (ARDS)
AEC s.
AFA s.
afebrile pneumonia s.
AFFN dysostosis s. 1

agenesis of corpus callosum-mental retardation-osseous lesions s.
aglossia-adactylia s.
agonadism, mental retardation, short stature, retarded bone age s.
AGR s.
agyria-pachygyria s.
Aicardi s.
Aicardi-Goutières s.
air leak s.
airway obstruction s.
Alagille s.
Alagille-Watson s. (AWS)
Alajouanine s.
Albers-Schönberg s.
albinism-deafness s.
Albright s.
ALCAPA s.
aldosteronism-normal blood pressure s.
Aldred s.
Aldrich s.
Ale-Calo s.
Alexander s.
Alice in Wonderland s.
Allan-Herndon s.
Allan-Herndon-Dudley s. (AHDS)
Allemann s.
Allen-Masters s.
Allgrove s.
alopecia, anosmia, deafness, hypogonadism s.
alopecia, contracture, dwarfism, mental retardation s.
alopecia, epilepsy, oligophrenia s.
alopecia, mental retardation, epilepsy, microcephaly s.
Alpers s.
Alport s.
Alström s.
Alström-Hallgren s.
Ambras s.
AMC s.
ameloonychohypohidrotic s.
amenorrhea-galactorrhea s.
aminopterin embryopathy s.
aminopterin-like embryopathy s.
Amish brittle hair s.
amniotic band s.
amniotic banding s.
amniotic fluid embolism s.
amniotic fluid embolus s.

NOTES

syndrome *(continued)*

amniotic infection s.
amotivational s.
AMR s.
anal-ear-renal-radial malfunction s.
Andermann s.
Andersen s.
Anderson s.
Andogsky s.
androgen insensitivity s.
androgen resistance s.
anemia s.
Angelman s.
angiomatosis-oculo-orbito-thalamo-
  encephalic s.
angioosteohypertrophy s.
aniridia, cerebellar ataxia-
  oligophrenia s.
aniridia, Wilms tumor
  association s.
aniridia, Wilms tumor,
  gonadoblastoma s.
ankyloblepharon, ectodermal
  dysplasia, clefting s.
ankyloglossia superior s.
anomalous left coronary artery
  from pulmonary artery s.
anophthalmia, hand-foot defects,
  mental retardation s.
anophthalmia-limb anomalies s.
anophthalmia-syndactyly s.
anophthalmia-Waardenburg s.
anorectal s.
anterior chamber cleavage s.
anterior chamber dysgenesis s.
anterior cord s.
anticonvulsant hypersensitivity s.
antiphospholipid s. (APS)
antiphospholipid antibody s.
Antley-Bixler s.
anus-hand-ear s.
aortic arch anomaly, peculiar
  facies, mental retardation s.
aortic stenosis, corneal clouding,
  growth and mental retardation s.
Apak s.
Apert s.
Apert-Crouzon s.
aplastic abdominal muscle s.
Appelt-Gerkin-Lenz s.
apraxia-ataxia-mental deficiency s.
apraxia-oculomotor contracture-
  muscle atrophy s.
aprosencephaly s.
aprosencephaly-atelencephaly s.
Arakawa s.
ARCS s.
Argonz-Del Castillo s.

arhinia, choanal atresia,
  microphthalmia s.
Arkless-Graham s.
Arnold-Chiari s.
arteriomesenteric duodenal
  compression s.
arthritis-dermatitis s.
arthrochalasis multiplex congenita
  Ehlers-Danlos s.
arthrogryposis, ectodermal dysplasia,
  cleft lip/palate developmental
  delay s.
Arts s.
ASB s.
Ascher s.
aseptic meningitis s.
Asherman s.
Asperger s. (AS)
asphyxiating thoracic dysplasia s.
asphyxiating thoracodystrophy s.
aspiration s.
asplenia s.
asymmetric short stature s.
ataxia-deafness s.
ataxia, myoclonic encephalopathy,
  macular degeneration, recurrent
  infections s.
ataxia-telangiectasia s.
atelencephalic s.
Atkin-Flaitz s.
Atkin-Flaitz-Patil s.
ATRX s.
atypical hemolytic uremia s.
Austin s.
autism, dementia, ataxia, loss of
  purposeful hand use s.
autism-fragile X s. (AFRAX)
autistic s.
auto-brewery s.
autoimmune lymphoproliferative s.
  (ALPS)
autoimmune polyendocrine s.
autoimmune polyglandular s.
autosomal dominant
  macrocephaly s.
autosomal dominant Opitz s.
  (ADOS)
autosomal recessive ocular Ehlers-
  Danlos s.
AWTA s.
Axenfeld s.
Axenfeld-Rieger s.
Babinski-Fröhlich s.
baby bottle s.
bacterial overgrowth s.
Ballantyne-Runge s.
Ballantyne-Smith s.
Baller-Gerold s. (BGS)
Ballinger-Wallace s.

Bamforth s.
Banki s.
Bannayan s.
Bannayan-Riley-Ruvalcaba s. (BRRS)
Bannayan-Zonana s. (BZS)
Bannwarth s.
Banti s.
Baraitser-Burn s.
Baraitser-Winter s.
Barber-Say s.
Bardet-Biedl s. (BBS)
bare lymphocyte s.
Barlow s.
Bart s.
Barth s.
Bartholin-Patau s.
Bartsocaas-Papas s.
Bartter s. (BS)
basal cell nevus s. (BCNS)
Bassen-Kornzweig s.
battered buttock s.
battered child s.
battered fetus s.
battered wife s.
Bazex s.
Bazex-Dupré-Christol s.
BBB s.
BCD s.
BD s.
Beare s.
Beare-Stevenson cutis gyrata s.
Beckwith s.
Beckwith-Wiedemann s. (BWS)
Beemer-Langer s.
Beemer lethal malformation s.
Begeer s.
Behçet s.
Behr s.
Benjamin s.
Berardinelli s.
Berardinelli-Seip s.
Berardinelli-Seip-Lawrence s.
Berdon s.
Bergia s.
Berlin breakage s.
Bernard-Soulier s.
Berry s.
Berry-Kravis and Israel s.
Berry-Treacher Collins s.
Bertini s.
Beuren s.

BGMR s.
Bianchine-Lewis s.
Bickers-Adams s.
BIDS s.
Bielschowsky s.
Biemond s. 1, 2
Biglieri s.
bile-plug s.
Binder s.
binge eating s.
biopsychosocial s.
bird-headed dwarf s.
birdlike face s.
bitemporal forceps marks s.
Bixler s.
Björnstad s.
Blackfan-Diamond s.
black locks with albinism and deafness s. (BADS)
bladder outlet s.
Bland-Garland-White s.
blepharocheilodontic s.
blepharonasofacial malformation s.
blepharophimosis, ptosis, epicanthus inversus s. (BPEIS)
blepharophimosis, ptosis, epicanthus inversus, primary amenorrhea s.
blepharophimosis, ptosis, syndactyly, short stature s.
blepharoptosis, blepharophimosis, epicanthus inversus, telecanthus s.
blind loop s.
Blizzard s.
Bloch-Siemens s.
Bloch-Sulzberger s.
Bloodgood s.
Bloom s.
Blount s.
blue baby s.
blueberry muffin s.
blue diaper s.
blue dome s.
blue histiocyte s.
blue rubber bleb nevus s. (BRBNS)
bobble-head doll s.
BOD s.
Bodian-Schwachman s.
Bohring s.
Bonneau s.
Bonnet-Dechaume-Blanc s.
Bonnevie-Ullrich s.

S

NOTES

syndrome *(continued)*

Boom s.
boomerang s.
BOR s.
Börjeson s.
Börjeson-Forssman-Lehmann s.
(BFLS)
Bosma Henkin Christiansen s.
Bourneville s.
Bourneville-Pringle s.
Bowen-Conradi s.
Bowen Hutterite s.
Brachmann-Cornelia de Lange s.
(BCDLS)
brachycephaly, deafness, cataract,
microstomia, mental retardation s.
brachydactyly-distal
symphalangism s.
brachydactyly, dwarfism, hearing
loss, microcephaly, mental
retardation s.
brachydactyly, mesomelia, mental
retardation, aortic dilation, mitral
valve prolapse, characteristic
facies s.
brachydactyly, nystagmus, cerebellar
ataxia s.
brachymesomelia-renal s.
brachymetacarpalia, cataract,
mesiodens s.
brachymorphism, onychodysplasia,
dysphalangism s.
bradycardia-tachycardia s.
Brailsford s.
brain-death s.
branchial arch s.
branchial clefts-lip pseudocleft s.
branchiooculofacial s. (BOFS)
branchiootic s.
Brandt s.
breast/ovarian familial cancer s.
Brentano s.
Brett s.
Briard-Evans s.
bright thalamus s.
Brissaud s.
brittle hair-mental deficit s.
broad ligament tear s.
broad thumb-hallux s.
broad thumb-mental retardation s.
bronze baby s.
Brooks s.
Brooks-Wisniewski-Brown s.
brown baby s.
Brown-Séquard s.
Brown superior oblique tendon
sheath s.
Brown vertical retraction s.
Brown-Vialetto-Van Laere s.

Bruck-de Lange s.
Brugada s.
Brunner s.
Brusa-Toricelli s.
Brushfield-Wyatt s.
BSG s.
bubbly lung s.
Budd-Chiari s.
bulldog s.
burning vulva s.
Burn-McKeown s.
Buschke-Ollendorf s.
Byler s.
C s.
3C s.
Caffey pseudo-Hurler s.
Caffey-Silverman s.
Caffey-Smyth-Roske s.
CAHMR s.
Calabro s.
Calvé-Legg-Perthes s.
CAMAK s.
CAMFAK s.
camptomelic s.
Camurati-Englemann s.
cancer family s.
cancer predisposition s.
Cantrell s.
Cantú s.
capillary leak s. (CLS)
carbohydrate-deficient
glycoprotein s. (type I, II)
(CDGS)
carcinoid s.
cardiac, abnormal facies, thymic
hypoplasia, cleft palate,
hypocalcemia s. (CATCH)
cardiac-limb s.
cardiocranial s.
cardiofacial s.
cardiogenital s.
cardiovascular/central nervous
system s.
cardiovertebral s.
Carey-Fineman-Ziter s.
Carmi s.
Carnevale s.
Carney s.
Caroli s.
Carpenter s.
Cast s.
cataract, ataxia, deafness,
retardation s.
cataract-dental s.
cataract, mental retardation,
hypogonadism s.
cataract, motor system disorder,
short stature, learning difficulty,
skeletal abnormalities s.

cataract-oligophrenia s.
catatonic s.
CATCH 22 s.
Catel-Manzke s.
cat eye s. (CES)
cat's cry s.
cat's eye s. (CES)
cat's urine s.
cauda equina s.
caudal appendage, short terminal phalanges, deafness, cryptorchidism, mental retardation s.
caudal dysplasia s.
caudal regression s. (CRS)
cavernous sinus s.
cavum septum pellucidum, cavum vergae, macrocephaly, seizures, mental retardation s.
Cayler cardiofacial s.
CCC s.
celiac s.
central anticholinergic s. (CAS)
central cord s.
central hypoventilation s.
central nervous system/cardiovascular s.
centromeric instability-immunodeficiency s.
cephalopolysyndactyly s.
s. of cerebral atrophy
cerebral dysfunction s.
cerebral malformations, seizures, hypertrichosis, overlapping fingers s.
cerebral palsy, hypotonic seizures, megalocornea s.
cerebroarthrodigital s.
cerebrocostomandibular s. (CCMS)
cerebrohepatorenal s. (CHRS)
cerebrooculomuscular s. (COMS)
cerebrooculonasal s.
cerebroosteonephrosis s.
CFA s.
CFC s.
Chanarin-Dorfman s.
Chapple s.
Char s.
characteristic face, hypogenitalism, hypotonia, pachygyria s.
Charcot-Marie-Tooth s. (CMTS)
Charcot-Marie-Tooth-Hoffmann s.

Charcot-Marie-Tooth s. X-linked recessive type II
CHARGE s.
Charlevois-Saguenay s.
Cheadle s.
Chédiak-Higashi s.
Chemke s.
Cheney s.
cherry-red spot myoclonus s.
cherubism, gingival fibromatosis, epilepsy, mental deficiency s.
chest s.
Chiari-Arnold s.
Chiari-Frommel s.
Chilaiditi s.
CHILD s.
CHIME s.
Chinese restaurant s.
cholestasis, pigmentary retinopathy, cleft palate s.
cholestatic s.
chondrodysplasia-pseudohermaphrodism s.
chondroectodermal dysplasia-like s.
chorioretinal anomalies, corpus callosum agenesis, infantile spasms s.
Chotzen s.
Christian s. (1. 2)
Christian-Andrews-Conneally-Muller s.
Christian-Opitz s.
Christ-Siemens-Touraine s.
chromosomal breakage-immunodeficiency s.
chromosome diploid/tetraploid mixoploidy s.
chromosome GI deletion s.
chromosome 9 inversion s.
chromosome 1–22 monosomy s.
chromosome 1p–22p deletion s.
chromosome 1q–22q deletion s.
chromosome 1q–22q duplication s.
chromosome 1q–22q tetrasomy s.
chromosome 1q–22q triplication s.
chromosome 8 recombinant s.
chromosome 1–22 ring s.
chromosome tetraploidy s.
chromosome triploidy s.
chromosome 1–22 trisomy s.
chromosome 14 uniparental disomy s.

NOTES

syndrome *(continued)*

chromosome X autosome translocation s.
chromosome X fragility s.
chromosome X inversion s.
chromosome XO s.
chromosome Xp21 deletion s.
chromosome Xp22 deletion s.
chromosome Xq deletion s.
chromosome Xq duplication s.
chromosome XXX s.
chromosome 47,XXX s.
chromosome XXXXX s.
chromosome XXXXY s.
chromosome XXY s.
chromosome Y;18 translocation s.
chronic aspiration s.
chronic biopsychosocial s.
chronic compartment s.
chronic fatigue s. (CFS)
chronic pupillary s.
Chudley s. (1, 2)
Chudley-Lowry-Hoar s.
Churg-Strauss s.
chylomicronemia s.
Cianchetti s.
circumferential skin creases-psychomotor retardation s.
Clarke-Hadfield s.
clasped thumbs-mental retardation s.
cleavage s.
clefting, ocular anterior chamber defect, lid anomalies s.
cleft lip, cleft palate, lobster claw deformity s.
cleft palate, diaphragmatic hernia, coarse facies, acral hypoplasia s.
cleft palate, microcephaly, large ears, short stature s.
cleidocranial dysplasia s.
cleidorhizomelic s.
Clifford s.
climacteric s.
clitoris tourniquet s. (CTS)
clomiphene-resistant polycystic ovary s.
Clouston s.
cloverleaf skull s.
clumsy child s.
COACH s.
Cobb s.
Cockayne s. (A, B)
cocktail party s.
CODAS s.
COD-MD s.
Coffin s. (1, 2)
Coffin-Lowry s.
Coffin-Siris s.
Coffin-Siris-Wegienka s.

COFS s.
Cogan s.
Cohen s.
Cole s.
Cole-Carpenter s.
Cole-Hughes macrocephaly-mental retardation s.
Cole-Rauschkolb-Toomey s.
coloboma-anal atresia s.
coloboma, clefting, mental retardation s.
coloboma cleft lip/palate-mental retardation s.
coloboma, mental retardation, hypogonadism, obesity s.
coloboma, microphthalmos, hearing loss, hematuria, cleft lip/palate s.
coloboma, obesity, hypogenitalism, mental retardation s.
compartment s.
compensatory antiinflammatory s.
complete androgen insensitivity s. (CAIS)
complete androgen resistance s.
complete DiGeorge s.
complete feminizing testes s.
complex regional pain s. (CRPS)
concussion s.
congenital acromicria s.
congenital anemia s.
congenital anosmia-hypogonadotropic hypogonadism s.
congenital arthromyodysplastic s.
congenital bone marrow failure s.
congenital cataracts, sensorineural deafness, Down syndrome facial appearance, short stature, mental retardation s.
congenital central hypoventilation s. (CCHS)
congenital clasped thumbs-mental retardation s.
congenital emphysema, cryptorchidism, penoscrotal web, deafness, mental retardation s.
congenital Guillain-Barré s.
congenital heart defect s.
congenital high airway obstruction s. (CHAOS)
congenital hydantoin s.
congenital hypertrichosis-osteochondrodysplasia-cardiomegaly s.
congenital hypocupremia s.
congenital hypothyroidism s.
congenital ichthyosis-mental retardation-spasticity s.
congenital ichthyosis-trichodystrophy s.

congenital LCMV s.
congenital long QT s.
congenital microcephaly, hiatus hernia, nephrotic s.
congenital muscular hypertrophy-cerebral s.
congenital nephrotic s.
congenital pseudohydrocephalic progeroid s.
congenital rubella s. (CRS)
congenital thrombocytopenia, Robin sequence, agenesis of corpus callosum, distinctive facies, developmental delay s.
congenital varicella s.
congenital warfarin s.
congestive cardiomyopathy-hypergonadotropic hypogonadism s.
conjunctivitis-otitis s.
Conn s.
conotruncal anomaly face s. (CTAF)
conotruncal facial s.
Conradi s.
Conradi-Hünermann s.
constriction band s.
constrictive pericarditis-dwarfism s.
contiguous gene deletion s.
contractural arachnodactyly s.
contracture, muscle atrophy, oculomotor apraxia s.
conus medullaris s.
Cooks s.
Cooper s.
Cornelia de Lange s. (CDLS)
corpus callosum agenesis, chorioretinal abnormality s.
corpus callosum agenesis, chorioretinopathy, infantile spasms s.
corpus callosum agenesis, facial anomalies, salaam seizures s.
corpus luteum deficiency s.
Costello s.
coumarin s.
Cowchock s.
Cowchock-Fischbeck s.
Cowden s.
coxoauricular s.
CPLS s.
Crandall ectodermal dysplasia s.

Crane-Heise s.
cranial sclerosis, osteopathia striata, macrocephaly s.
cranioacrofacial s.
craniocarpotarsal s.
craniocerebellocardiac s.
craniofacial anomalies, polysyndactyly s.
craniofacial, deafness, hand s.
craniofacial dysmorphism, absent corpus callosum, iris colobomas, connective tissue dysplasia s.
craniofacial dysmorphism-polysyndactyly s.
craniofrontonasal s. (CNFS)
cranioorodigital s.
craniosynostosis, arachnodactyly, abdominal hernia s.
craniosynostosis, arthrogryposis, cleft palate s.
craniosynostosis, ataxia, trigeminal anesthesia, parietal anesthesia and pons, vermis fusion s.
craniosynostosis-lid anomalies s.
craniosynostosis-radial aplasia s.
craniosynostotic s.
CRASH s.
CREST s.
cretinism-muscular hypertrophy s.
Creutzfeldt-Jakob s.
cri-du-chat s.
Crigler-Najjar s. (type I, II)
Crisponi s.
s. of crocodile tears
Crome s.
Cronkhite-Canada s.
crooked fingers s.
Cross s.
Cross-McKusick-Breen s.
Crouzon s.
CRST s.
crying cat s.
cryptomicrotia-brachydactyly s.
cryptophthalmos s.
cryptophthalmos-syndactyly s.
CSW s.
Curran s.
Curry-Jones s.
Curtis s.
Cushing s.
cushingoid s.

S

NOTES

syndrome *(continued)*

cutis verticis gyrata, thyroid aplasia, mental retardation s.

cyclic vomiting s.

Cypress facial neuromusculoskeletal s.

cytomegaly s.

dancing eye s.

Dandy-Walker s. (DWS)

Dandy-Walker-like s.

Dandy-Walker malformation-basal ganglia disease-seizures s.

Danlos s.

Darrow-Gamble s.

Davidenkow s.

David-O'Callaghan s.

dead fetus s.

deafness-craniofacial s.

deafness-nephritis s.

Deal s.

Debré-Sémélaigne s.

De Crecchio s.

defective abdominal wall s.

de Grouchy s. 1, 2

Dejerine-Klumpke s.

Dejerine-Sottas s.

de Lange s.

de Lange s. 1, 2

delay s.

delayed sleep phase s. (DSPS)

del Castillo s.

deletion 1–22 s.

deletion 1p–22p s.

deletion 1q–22q s.

deletion Xp21 s.

deletion Xp22 s.

deletion Xq s.

Delleman s.

Demons-Meigs s.

de Morsier s.

de Morsier-Gauthier s.

dengue shock s.

Dennie-Marfan s.

Denys-Drash s.

depressor anguli oris muscle hypoplasia s.

dermotrichic s.

Derry s.

De Sanctis-Cacchione s.

Desbuquois s.

Desmons s.

de Toni-Fanconi s.

de Toni-Fanconi-Debré acute s.

De Vaal s.

developmental delay-multiple strawberry nevi s.

dextrocardia/situs inversus s.

diabetes-deafness s.

diabetes mellitus, mental retardation, lipodystrophy, dysmorphic traits s.

Diamond-Blackfan s.

diaper s.

diaphragmatic hernia, abnormal face, distal limb anomalies s.

diaphragmatic hernia, distal digital hypoplasia s.

diaphragmatic hernia, exophthalmos, hypertelorism s.

diaphragmatic hernia, myopia, deafness s.

diarrhea-associated hemolytic uremic s.

diarrhea-malnutrition s.

Dickinson s.

DIDMO s.

DIDMOAD s.

diencephalic s. (DS)

DiFerrante s.

diffuse mesangial sclerosis-ocular abnormalities s.

DiGeorge microdeletion s.

Dighton-Adair s.

digital anomalies, short palpebral fissures, atresia of esophagus or duodenum s.

digitoorofacial s. (I–V)

digitooropalatal s.

digitorenocerebral s. (DRC)

Dilantin s.

DiSala s.

disequilibrium s.

dislocated elbow, bowed tibiae, scoliosis, deafness, cataract, microcephaly, mental retardation s.

distal arthrogryposis, hypopituitarism, mental retardation, facial anomalies s.

distal arthrogryposis, mental retardation, characteristic facies s.

distal intestinal obstruction s. (DIOS)

distal limb deficiency-mental retardation s.

distal transverse limb defects, mental retardation, spasticity s.

disturbed equilibrium s.

disuse s.

Donahue s.

Donohue s.

DOOR s.

double cortex s.

Down s.

Drash s.

dry eye s.

Duane retraction s.

Dubin-Johnson s.
Dubowitz s.
Duchenne s.
Duchenne-Griesinger s.
dumping s.
Duncan s.
duplication-deficiency s.
duplication 1p–22p s.
duplication 1q–22q s.
duplication Xq s.
dup (10p)/del (10q) s.
dup (1p)–(22p) s.
dup (9q)/del(9p) s.
dup (1q)–(22q) s.
dup (Xq) s.
dwarf s.
dwarfism, congenital medullary
   stenosis s.
dwarfism, ichthyosiform
   erythroderma, mental deficiency s.
dwarfism, onychodysplasia s.
dwarfism, pericarditis s.
dwarfism, polydactyly, dysplastic
   nails s.
Dyggve-Melchior-Clausen s.
Dyke-Davidoff s.
dyscephaly, congenital cataract,
   hypotrichosis s.
dysequilibrium s. (DES)
dysfibronectinemic Ehlers-Danlos s.
dysgenesis s.
dysmaturity s.
dysmorphic s.
dysmotile cilia s.
dysmotility s.
dysostotic idiocy, gargoylism,
   lipochondrodystrophy s.
dysplasia s.
dysplastic nevus s.
dystocia-dystrophia s.
dystonia-deafness s.
dystrophia retinae-dysacousis s.
dysuria-pyuria s.
dysuria-sterile pyuria s.
Eagle-Barrett s.
early-onset diabetes mellitus-
   epiphyseal dysplasia s.
early-onset Parkinsonism-mental
   retardation s.
Eastman-Bixler s.
Eaton-Lambert myasthenic s.
ecchymotic Ehlers-Danlos s.

ectodermal dysplasia, cleft lip and
   palate, hand and foot deformity,
   mental retardation s.
ectodermal dysplasia, cleft lip and
   palate, mental retardation,
   syndactyly s. (I, II)
ectodermal dysplasia, mental
   retardation, syndactyly s.
ectrodactyly-cleft lip/palate s.
ectrodactyly, ectodermal dysplasia
   and cleft lip/palate s.
ectrodactyly, mandibulofacial
   dysostosis s.
ectrodactyly, spastic paraplegia-,
   ental retardation s.
Eddowes s.
Edinburgh malformation s.
Edwards s.
Edwards-Gale s.
EEC s.
Ehlers-Danlos s. (EDS)
Eisenmenger s.
Elejalde s.
elfin facies hypercalcemia s.
Ellis-Sheldon s.
Ellis-van Creveld s.
ElSahy-Waters s.
embryofetal alcohol s. (EFAS)
embryonic testicular regression s.
Emery-Dreifuss s.
EMG s.
empty scrotum s.
empty sella s.
encephalotrigeminal s.
endovascular hemolytic-uremic s.
Engman s.
enterocolitis s.
eosinophilia-myalgia s.
epicomus s.
epidermal nevus s.
epileptic s.
epiphyseal s.
epiphyseal dysplasia, microcephaly,
   nystagmus s.
epiphyseal dysplasia, short stature,
   microcephaly, nystagmus s.
episodic dyscontrol s.
EPS s.
Erb s.
Erb-Charcot s.
Erb-Goldflam s.
Erlacher-Blount s.

S

NOTES

syndrome *(continued)*

Eronen s.
Escalante s.
Escobar s.
ethmocephaly s.
euthyroid sick s.
Evans s.
extended rubella s.
extraordinary urinary frequency s.
extrapyramidal-pyramidal s.
eye defects-diffuse renal mesangial
 sclerosis s.
facet s.
facial-digital-genital s.
facial dysmorphia s.
facial dysplasia, hyperextensibility
 of joints, clinodactyly, growth
 retardation, mental retardation s.
faciocardiorenal s.
faciocerebroskeletocardiac s.
faciodigitogenital s.
faciogenital s.
Fadhil s.
FAE s.
Fairbank-Keats s.
Fallot s.
familial aortic ectasia s.
familial ataxia-hypogonadism s.
familial atypical multiple mole
 melanoma s.
familial cardiac myxoma s.
familial chylomicronemia s.
familial congenital alopecia, mental
 retardation, epilepsy, unusual
 EEG s.
familial endocrine-neuroectodermal
 abnormalities s.
familial insomnia s.
familial macroglossia-omphalocele s.
familial polysyndactyly-craniofacial
 anomalies s.
familial pterygium s.
familial pyridoxine-dependency s.
familial third and fourth pharyngeal
 pouch s.
familial Turner s.
Fanconi-Albertini Zellweger s.
Fanconi-Bickel s.
Fanconi pancytopenia s.
Fanconi-Petrassi s.
Fanconi-Prader s.
Fanconi-Schlesinger s.
Farber s.
fast channel s.
fatigue s.
FCS s.
Feingold s.
Feinmesser-Zelig s.
Felty s.

female pseudo-Turner s.
feminization s.
feminizing testes s.
femoral-facial s.
fetal Accutane s.
fetal akinesia s.
fetal alcohol s. (FAS)
fetal aminopterin s.
fetal aminopterin-like s.
fetal anticoagulant s.
fetal aspiration s.
fetal cocaine s.
fetal Dilantin s.
fetal distress s.
fetal dysmaturity s.
fetal face s.
fetal facies s.
fetal gigantism, renal hamartoma,
 nephroblastomatosis s.
fetal hydantoin s. (FHS)
fetal inflammatory response s.
fetal isotretinoin s.
fetal methotrexate s.
fetal nutritional deprivation s.
fetal overgrowth s.
fetal paramethadione-
 trimethadione s.
fetal phenytoin s.
fetal rubella s.
fetal tobacco s.
fetal transfusion s.
fetal trimethadione s.
fetal valproate s. (FVS)
fetal varicella s. (FVS)
fetal warfarin s.
fetofetal transfusion s.
Feuerstein-Mims s.
Fèvre-Languepin s.
FFU s.
FG s.
FHUF s.
fibrinogen-fibrin conversion s.
fifth digit s.
Filippi s.
Fine-Lubinsky s.
first and second branchial arch s.
Fishman s.
Fitz-Hugh-Curtis s.
Fitzsimmons s.
Floating-Harbor s. (FHS)
floppy infant s.
flulike s.
FOAR s.
focal dermal hypoplasia s.
follicular atrophoderma, basal cell
 carcinoma s.
follicular atrophoderma, basocellular
 proliferation, hypotrichosis s.
Fontaine s.

food-induced enterocolitis s.
Forbes-Albright s.
formiminotransferase deficiency s.
Fountain s.
four-day s.
FPO s.
fragile X s. (FRAX, FXS)
fragile X mental retardation s.
fragile Xq s.
Franceschetti s.
Franceschetti-Goldenhar s.
Franceschetti-Jadassohn s.
Franceschetti-Klein s.
Franceschetti-Zwahlen s.
Franceschetti-Zwahlen-Klein s.
Francois dyscephalic s.
Fraser s.
Fraser-Francois s.
Fraser-like s.
fra(X) s.
FRAXq27 s.
FRAX28 s.
Freeman-Sheldon s.
frequency dysuria s.
Fried s.
Friend s.
Fritsch s.
Fritsch-Asherman s.
Fröhlich s.
frontodigital s.
Fryns s. (1–3)
Fryns-Moerman s.
Fryns-van den Berghe s.
FTT s.
Fuhrmann s.
Fukuyama s.
Fuller Albright s. 1
functional prepuberal castrate s.
Funston s.
G s.
Gaillard s.
galactorrhea-amenorrhea s.
Galloway s.
Galloway-Mowat s.
Gamble-Darrow s.
Garcia-Lurie s.
Gardner s.
Gardner-Silengo-Wachtel s.
Gareis-Mason s.
Gasser s.
gastrointestinal s.
gender dysphoria s.

Genée-Wiedemann s.
generalized hypertrichosis terminalis-
gingival hyperplasia s.
generalized hypotonia, congenital
hydronephrosis, characteristic
face s.
genetic s.
genital anomaly-cardiomyopathy s.
genital ulcer s.
genitopalatocardiac s.
Genoa s.
Gerhardt s.
German s.
Gerstmann s.
Gerstmann-Sträussler-Scheinker s.
Gianotti-Crosti s.
giant platelet s.
Gilbert s.
Gilbert-Dreyfus s.
Gilbert-Lereboullet s.
Gilles de la Tourette s.
Gillespie s.
gingival fibromatosis, hypertrichosis,
cherubism, mental retardation,
epilepsy s.
gingival fibromatosis, hypertrichosis,
mental retardation, epilepsy s.
gingival hyperplasia, hirsutism,
convulsions s.
gingival hypertrophy-corneal
dystrophy s.
Gitelman s.
Glanzmann s.
Glanzmann-Riniker s.
glossopalatine ankylosis s.
gloves and socks s.
glutaric aciduria s. (type I, II)
GMS s.
goiter-deafness s.
Golabi-Ito-Hall s.
Golabi-Rosen s. (GRS)
Goldberg s.
Goldenhar-Gorlin s.
Goldenhar microphthalmia s.
Goldston s.
Goltz s.
Goltz-Gorlin s.
Goltz-Peterson-Gorlin-Ravitz s.
GOMBO s.
Gomez and López-Hernández s.
gonadal agenesis s.
gonadal dysgenesis s.

S

NOTES

syndrome *(continued)*

gonadal failure, short stature, mitral valve prolapse, mental retardation s.

gonadotropin-resistant ovary s.

goniodysgenesis, mental retardation, short stature s.

Goodman s.

Goodpasture s.

Gordon s.

Gorlin s. (1, 2)

Gorlin-Goltz s.

Gorlin-Psaume s.

Gougerot-Carteaud s.

Gradenigo s.

Graefe-Usher s.

Graham s.

granddad s.

Grant s.

gravis type Ehlers-Danlos s.

gray baby s.

gray platelet s.

Greig s.

Griscelli s.

Grisel s.

growth failure-pericardial constriction s.

growth retardation, small and puffy hands, eczema s.

Grubben s.

Gruber s.

grunting baby s.

Guerin-Stein s.

Guillain-Barré s. (GBS)

Guillain-Barré-Landry s.

Gurrieri s.

Gustavson s.

HAIR-AN s.

hair-brain s.

Hajdu-Cheney s.

Hakim s.

Hakim-Adams s.

Halban s.

Halbrecht s.

Hall s. (1, 2)

Hallermann s.

Hallermann-Streiff s.

Hallermann-Streiff-François s.

Hallervorden-Spatz s.

Hallopeau-Siemens s.

Hall-Pallister s.

Hall-Riggs s.

Halpern s.

hamartoneoplastic s.

hamartopolydactyly s.

Hamel s.

Hamman-Rich s.

hand-foot s.

hand-foot-genital s.

hand-foot-mouth s.

hand-foot-uterus s.

Hand-Schüller-Christian s.

Hanhart s.

hantavirus cardiopulmonary s. (HCPS)

hantavirus pulmonary s.

happy puppet s.

HARD s.

HARD+/-E s.

Hardikar s.

HARP s.

Harrod s.

Hart s.

Haw River s.

Hay-Wells s.

HbH disease-mental retardation s.

hearing loss, mental deficiency, growth retardation, clubbed digits, EEG abnormalities s.

hearing-loss–nephritis s.

heart defect s.

heart-hand s.

Heerfordt s.

Heiner s.

HELLP s.

hemangioma-thrombocytopenia s.

hemangiomatous branchial clefts/lip pseudocleft s.

hematophagocytic s.

hematopoietic s.

hematuria, dysuria s. (HDS)

hematuria, nephropathy, deafness s.

hemignathia and microtia s.

hemoglobin Bart hydrops fetalis s.

hemolysis, elevated liver enzymes, low platelet count s.

hemolytic uremic s. (HUS)

hemophagocytic s.

hemorrhagic fever with renal s. (HFRS)

hemorrhagic shock s.

hemorrhagic shock and encephalopathy s. (HSES)

Hennekam lymphangiectasia-lymphedema s.

hepatic copper overload s.

hepatic ductular hypoplasia-multiple malformations s.

hepatitis B arthritis-dermatitis s.

hepatofacioneurocardiovertebral s.

hepatopulmonary s. (HPS)

hepatorenal s.

hepatotoxic s.

hereditary benign intraepithelial dyskeratosis s.

hereditary blepharophimosis, ptosis, epicanthus inversus s.

hereditary dysplastic nevus s.

hereditary hematuria s.
hereditary nephritis deafness,
  abnormal thrombogenesis s.
Hermansky-Pudlak s.
Hernandez s.
heterotaxia s.
heterotaxy s.
HHH s.
HHHO s.
hiatus hernia, microcephaly,
  nephrosis s.
high airway obstruction s.
Hinman s.
Hirschsprung disease, microcephaly,
  mental retardation, characteristic
  facies s.
hirsutism, skeletal dysplasia, mental
  retardation s.
HMC s.
H2O s.
Holt-Oram s.
Holzgreve s.
Hootnick-Holmes s.
Hopkins s.
Horner s.
Hoyeraal-Hreidarsson s. (HHS)
Hughes s.
Hünermann-Happle s.
Hunter s.
Hunter-Fraser s.
Hunter-MacMurray s.
Hunter-McAlpine craniosynostosis s.
Hurler s.
Hurler-like s.
Hurler-Pfaundler s.
Hurler-Scheie s.
Hurst s.
Hutchinson s.
Hutchinson-Gilford s.
hyaline membrane s.
hydantoin s.
Hyde-Forster s.
hydrocephalus-cerebellar agenesis s.
hydrocephalus, skeletal anomalies,
  mental disturbances s.
hydrolethalus s.
hydronephrocolpos,
  postaxialpolydactyly, congenital
  heart disease s.
17-hydroxylase deficiency s.
21-hydroxylase deficiency s.

hyperammonemia, hyperornithinemia,
  homocitrullinuria s.
hyperammonemic s.
hyperandrogenemic chronic
  anovulation s.
hyperandrogenism, insulin resistance,
  acanthosis nigricans s.
hypercalcemia elfin-facies s.
hypercalcemia, peculiar facies,
  supravalvular aortic stenosis s.
hypercalcemia/Williams-Beuren s.
hypereosinophilic s.
hyper-IgD s.
hyper-IgE s.
hyper-IgM s.
hyperimmunoglobulin E s.
hyperinsulinism hyperammonemia s.
hyperkinetic child s.
hyperlucent lung s.
hypermobile Ehlers-Danlos s.
hypermobility s.
hyperphosphaturic s.
hyperplastic right heart s.
hyperprostaglandin E_2 s.
hyperprostaglandinuric tubular s.
hypertelorism-hypospadias s.
hypertelorism, microtia, clefting s.
hypertrichosis, coarse face,
  brachydactyly, obesity, mental
  retardation s.
hyperventilation s.
hyperviscosity s.
hypocalcemia, dwarfism, cortical
  thickening s.
hypocalcemia and microdeletion
  22q11 s.
hypochondroplasia s.
hypocomplementemic urticarial
  vasculitis s. (HUVS)
hypogenital dystrophy with diabetic
  tendency s.
hypoglossia-hypodactyly s.
hypogonadism-anosmia s.
hypogonadotropic hypogonadism,
  mental retardation,
  microphthalmia s.
hypohidrotic ectodermal dysplasia,
  hypothyroidism, agenesis of
  corpus callosum s.
hypomelia, hypotrichosis, facial
  hemangioma s.

S

NOTES

syndrome *(continued)*

hypoparathyroidism, stature, mental retardation, seizures s.

hypopituitary s.

hypoplasia, endocrine disturbances, tracheostenosis s.

hypoplastic congenital anemia s.

hypoplastic left heart s. (HLHS)

hypoplastic right heart s. (HRHS)

hypospadias-dysphagia s.

hypospadias-mental retardation s.

hypothalamic hamartoblastoma s.

hypothalamic hamartoblastoma, hypopituitarism, imperforate anus, postaxial polydactyly s.

hypothyroidism s.

hypothyroid-large muscle s.

hypotonia, hypopigmentia, hypogonadism, obesity s.

hypotonia, hypopigmentia, hypogonadism, obesity s.

hypotonia, obesity, hypogonadism, mental retardation s.

hypotonia, obesity, prominent incisors s.

hypoventilation s.

IADH s.

IBIDS s.

ICE s.

ICF s.

ichthyosis, alopecia, ectropion, mental retardation s.

ichthyosis, characteristic appearance, mental retardation s.

ichthyosis, cheek, eyebrow s.

ichthyosis, hypogonadism, mental retardation, epilepsy s.

ichthyosis, male hypogonadism s.

ichthyosis, mental retardation, dwarfism, renal impairment s.

ichthyosis, mental retardation, epilepsy, hypogonadism s.

ichthyosis, oligophrenia, epilepsy s.

ichthyosis, spastic neurologic disorder, oligophrenia s.

ichthyosis, split hair, aminoaciduria s.

ichthyosis with keratitis and deafness s.

Idaho s.

idiopathic hemolytic uremia s.

idiopathic hypercalcemia-supravalvular aortic stenosis s.

idiopathic infantile hypercalcemia s.

idiopathic long Q-T s.

idiopathic minimal lesion nephrotic s. (IMLNS)

idiopathic nephrotic s. (INS)

idiopathic primary renal hematuric proteinuric s.

idiopathic respiratory distress s. (IRDS)

idiopathic steroid-resistant proteinuria/nephrotic s.

IFAP s.

IgE s.

iliotibial band friction s.

Illum s.

Imerslünd s.

Imerslünd-Grasbeck s.

immotile cilia s.

immunodeficiency, centromeric heterochromatin instability, facial anomalies s.

impingement s.

s. of inappropriate antidiuretic hormone secretion

s. of inappropriate secretion of antidiuretic hormone (SIADH)

incontinentia pigmenti s.

infancy-onset diabetes mellitus, multiple epiphyseal dysplasia s.

infantile bilateral striatal necrosis s. (IBSN)

infantile optic atrophy-ataxia s.

infantile respiratory distress s.

infantile spasms, hypsarrhythmia, mental retardation s.

infantile tremor s.

infant respiratory distress s. (IRDS)

infection-associated hemophagocytic s. (IAHS)

inflammatory Brown s.

influenza-like s.

inherited hemolytic uremia s.

insensitive ovary s.

insomnia s.

inspissated bile s.

inspissated milk s.

insulin-resistant diabetes, acanthosis nigricans, hypogonadism, pigmentary retinopathy, deafness, mental retardation s.

intestinal lymphangiectasia, lymphedema, mental retardation s.

intraepithelial dyskeratosis s.

intrauterine growth retardation, microcephaly, mental retardation s.

intrauterine parabiotic s.

inversion 9 s.

inversion duplication (15) chromosome s.

inversion duplication (8p) s.

Ionasescu s.

iris, coloboma, ptosis,
hypertelorism, mental
retardation s.
irritable bowel s. (IBS)
Isaac s.
Isaac-Merton s.
isochromosome 10p s.
isochromosome 12p s.
isolated autosomal dominant s.
isotretinoin dysmorphic s.
isotretinoin teratogenic s.
Ito s.
Ivemark s.
Jabs s.
Jackson-Weiss s. (JWS)
Jacob s.
Jacobsen s.
Jacobsen-Brodwall s.
Jadassohn-Lewandowski s.
Jaeken s.
Jaffe-Campanacci s.
Jaffe-Lichtenstein s.
Jahnke s.
Jakob-Creutzfeldt s.
Jaksch s.
James s.
Jancar s.
Jansen s.
Jansky-Bielschowsky s.
Janus s.
Janz s.
Jarcho-Levin s.
jaw cysts, basal cell tumors,
skeletal anomalies s.
JC s.
Jensen s.
Jervell and Lange-Nielsen long
QT s.
Jessner-Cole s.
Jeune s.
Job s.
Johanson-Blizzard s.
Johnson-McMillin s.
Johnson neuroectodermal s.
Joseph s.
Josephs-Diamond-Blackfan s.
Joubert s.
Joubert-Boltshauser s.
Juberg-Hayward s.
Juberg-Holt s.
Juberg-Marsidi s. (JMS)
jumping Frenchmen of Maine s.

Junius-Kuhnt s.
juvenile cataract, cerebellar atrophy,
mental retardation, myopathy s.
juvenile hyperuricemia s.
juxtaglomerular hyperplasia s.
Kabuki s. (KS)
Kabuki makeup s. (KMS)
Kalischer s.
Kallmann s.
Kallmann-de Morsier s.
Kanner s.
Kaplan s.
Kapur-Toriello s.
Kartagener s.
Kasabach-Merritt s.
Kaufman-McKusick s.
Kaufman oculocerebrofacial s.
Kaveggia s.
Kawasaki s. (KS)
Kaznelson s.
KBG s.
Kearns-Sayre s. (KSS)
Keipert s.
Keller s.
Kelley-Seegmiller s.
Kelly s.
Kenny s.
Kenny-Caffey s.
Kenny-Linarelli s.
Kenny-Linarelli-Caffey s.
keratosis palmaris et plantaris-
corneal dystrophy s.
keratosis palmoplantaris-corneal
dystrophy s.
ketoaciduria-mental deficiency s.
Keutel s. (1, 2)
KID s.
Killian s.
Kimmelstiel-Wilson s.
kinky-hair s.
Kinsbourne s.
KIO s.
kleeblattschädel s.
Kleine-Levin s.
Klein-Waardenburg s.
Klinefelter s.
Klinefelter-Reifenstein s.
Klinefelter-Reifenstein-Albright s.
Klippel-Feil s.
Klippel-Trenaunay s.
Klippel-Trenaunay-Parkes-Weber s.
Klippel-Trenaunay-Weber s.

S

NOTES

syndrome *(continued)*

Kloepfer s.
Klotz s.
Klüver-Bucy s.
Kniest s.
Kobberling-Dunnigan s.
Koby s.
Kocher-Debré-Sémélaigne s.
Koerber-Salus-Elschnig s.
Kosenow-Sinios s.
Kostmann s.
Kowarski s.
Krabbe s.
Kramer s.
Krause s.
Krause-Kivlin s.
Krause-van Schooneveld-Kivlin s.
Laband s.
lacrimoauriculodentodigital s.
Ladd s.
LAMB s.
Lambert s.
Lambert-Eaton s.
Lambotte s.
Landau-Kleffner s. (LKS)
Landing s.
Landry-Guillain-Barré s.
Lange-Nielsen s.
Langer s.
Langer-Giedion s.
Langer-Petersen-Spranger s.
Langer-Saldino s.
Laron s.
Larsen s.
laryngeal atresia s.
late embryonic testicular
  regression s.
late luteal phase s.
late-onset local junctional
  epidermolysis bullosa-mental
  retardation s.
Laugier-Hunziker s.
Launois s.
Launois-Cléret s.
Laurence-Moon s.
Laurence-Moon-Biedl s.
Laurence-Moon-Biedl-Bardet s.
  (LMBBS)
Lawford s.
Lawrence s.
Lawrence-Seip s.
lazy bladder s.
lazy leukocyte s.
LCMV s.
Leigh s.
Leiner s.
Lejeune s.
Lemierre s.
Lemli-Opitz s.

Lennox s.
Lennox-Gastaut s.
lentigines (multiple),
  electrocardiographic abnormalities,
  ocular hypertelorism, pulmonary
  stenosis, abnormalities of
  genitalia, retardation of growth,
  and deafness (sensorineural) s.
Lenz dysmorphogenic s.
Lenz-Majewski s.
Lenz microphthalmia s.
LEOPARD s.
Leri s.
Leri-Weill s.
Leroy s.
Leschke s.
Lesch-Nyhan s. (LNS)
lethal multiple pterygium s.
leukoencephalopathy s.
leukoerythroblastic s.
levator ani s.
Levin s.
Levy-Hollister s.
lexical-syntactic s. (LSS)
Lhermitte-Duclos s.
LHON s.
Liddle s.
Li-Fraumeni cancer s.
Lightwood-Albright s.
Lignac s.
limb abnormality s.
limb girdle s. (LGS)
limp infant s.
linear nevus sebaceus s.
linear sebaceous nevus s.
Lin-Gettig s.
lipodystrophy-acromegaloid
  gigantism s.
lip-palate s.
lip pseudocleft-hemangiomatous
  branchial cyst s.
Lison s.
LMB s.
Lobstein s.
lobster-claw with ectodermal
  defects s.
lobulation-polydactyly s.
Löffler s.
Löfgren s.
long Q-T s. (LQTS)
Lorain-Lévi s.
Louis-Bar s.
low cardiac output s.
Lowe s. (LS)
Lowe oculocerebrorenal s.
Lowe-Terry-MacLachlan s.
Lown-Ganong-Levine s.
Lowry s.
Lowry-Maclean s.

Lowry-Wood s. (LWS)
low-sodium s.
low T3 s.
Lub s.
Lucey-Driscoll s.
Lujan-Fryns s.
lupus anticoagulant s.
lupus-like s.
lupus obstetric s.
luteinized unruptured follicle s.
  (LUFS)
Lutembacher s.
Lyell s.
lymphoproliferative s.
Lynch s.
lysine malabsorption s.
3M s.
MacDermot-Winter s.
Machado-Joseph s.
Macleod s.
macrocephaly, cutis marmorata,
  telangiectatica congenita s.
macrocephaly, facial abnormalities,
  disproportionate tall stature,
  mental retardation s.
macrocephaly-hamartomas s.
macrocephaly, hypertelorism, short
  limbs, hearing loss, developmental
  delay s.
macrocephaly, multiple lipomas,
  hemangiomata s.
macrocephaly, pseudoepithelioma,
  multiple hemangiomas s.
macroglossia-omphalocele s.
macroglossia-omphalocele-
  visceromegaly s.
macrophage activation s. (MAS)
macrosomia-mental retardation s.
Maestre de San Juan-Kallmann-de
  Morsier s.
Mafucci s.
Majewski s.
malabsorption s.
malalignment s.
male pseudohermaphroditism,
  persistent müllerian structures,
  mental retardation s.
male Turner s.
malformation s.
Mallory-Weiss s.
Malouf s.
Malpuech facial clefting s.

mandibulofacial dysostosis with
  epibulbar dermoids s.
mandibulofacial dysostosis with
  limb malformations s.
Marañón s.
Marden-Walker s.
Marfan s.
marfanoid craniosynostosis s.
marfanoid habitus, mental
  retardation s.
marfanoid habitus, microcephaly,
  glomerulonephritis s.
Marie s.
Marie-Sainton s.
Marinesco-Garland s.
Marinesco-Sjögren s.
Marinesco-Sjögren-Garland s.
Marinesco-Sjögren-like s.
marker X s.
Maroteaux-Lamy s.
Maroteaux-Malamut s.
Marshall s.
Marshall-Smith s. (MSS)
Martin-Bell s. (MBS)
Martin-Bell-Renpenning s.
Martsolf s.
marX s.
MASA s.
masquerade s.
Masters-Allen s.
maternal Bernard-Soulier s.
maternal deprivation s.
maternal hydrops s.
Mauriac s.
Mayer-Rokitansky-Küster-Hauser s.
McCune-Albright s.
McDonough s.
McKusick-Kaufman s.
McLeod s.
Meadows s.
Meckel s.
Meckel-Gruber s.
meconium aspiration s. (MAS)
meconium blockage s.
meconium plug s.
medial collateral ligament s.
medial snapping hip s.
median cleft upper lip, mental
  retardation, pugilistic facies s.
median facial cleft s.
s. of median longitudinal fasciculus
megacystis-megaureter s.

S

NOTES

syndrome *(continued)*

megacystis, microcolon, intestinal hypoperistalsis s.

megalencephaly, cranial sclerosis, osteopathia striata s.

megalocornea, developmental retardation, dysmorphic s.

megalocornea, macrocephaly, mental and motor retardation s. (MMMM)

megalocornea-mental retardation s. (MMR)

Meier-Gorlin s.

Meigs s.

Meigs-Kass s.

Meinecke-Peper s.

MELAS s.

Melkersson s.

Melkersson-Rosenthal s.

Melnick-Fraser s.

Melnick-Needles s.

MEMR s.

mendelian s.

Mendelson s.

Mendenhall s.

Mengert shock s.

Ménière s.

meningoencephalitis s.

meningovascular s.

Menkes s.

Menkes-Kaplan s.

Menkes kinky hair s. (MKHS)

menopausal s.

mental deficiency, spasticity, congenital ichthyosis s.

mental and growth retardation-amblyopia s.

mental and physical retardation, speech disorders, peculiar facies s.

mental retardation-absent nails of hallux and pollex s.

mental retardation-adducted thumbs s.

mental retardation, ataxia, hypotonia, hypogonadism, retinal dystrophy s.

mental retardation, blepharonasofacial abnormalities, hand malformations s.

mental retardation-clasped thumb s.

mental retardation, coarse face, microcephaly, epilepsy, skeletal abnormalities s.

mental retardation, coarse facies, epilepsy, joint contracture s.

mental retardation, congenital contracture, low fingertip arches s.

mental retardation-distal arthrogryposis s.

mental retardation, dysmorphism, cerebral atrophy s.

mental retardation, dystonic movements, ataxia, seizures s.

mental retardation, epilepsy, short stature, skeletal dysplasia s.

mental retardation, facial anomalies, hypopituitarism, distal arthrogryposis s.

mental retardation, gynecomastia, obesity s.

mental retardation, hearing impairment, distinctive facies, skeletal anomalies s.

mental retardation, hip luxation, G6PD variant s.

mental retardation, macroorchidism s.

mental retardation, microcephaly, blepharochalasis s.

mental retardation, mitral valve prolapse, characteristic face s.

mental retardation, optic atrophy, deafness, seizures s.

mental retardation-overgrowth s.

mental retardation, pre- and postnatal overgrowth, remarkable face, acanthosis nigricans s.

mental retardation-psoriasis s.

mental retardation, retinopathy, microcephaly s.

mental retardation, scapuloperoneal muscular dystrophy, lethal cardiomyopathy s.

mental retardation, short stature, hypertelorism s.

mental retardation, short stature, obesity, hypogonadism s.

mental retardation, skeletal dysplasia, abducens palsy s. (MRSD)

mental retardation-sparse hair s.

mental retardation, spasticity, distal transverse limb defects s.

mental retardation, spastic paraplegia, palmoplantar hyperkeratosis s.

mental retardation, typical facies, aortic stenosis s.

MERRF s.

mesiodens-cataracts s.

mesoaxial hexadactyly-cardiac malformation s.

mesomelic dwarfism-small genitalia s.

metabolic acidosis s.

metabolic s. X

methionine malabsorption s.
Meyer-Schwickerath and Weyers s.
Michelin-tire baby s.
Michels s.
microangiopathic hemolytic
 uremic s.
microcephalic primordial dwarfism-
 cataracts s.
microcephaly-calcification of
 cerebral white matter s.
microcephaly-cardiomyopathy s.
microcephaly-chorioretinopathy s.
microcephaly-deafness s.
microcephaly-digital anomalies s.
microcephaly, hiatus hernia,
 nephrotic s.
microcephaly, hypergonadotropic
 hypogonadism, short stature s.
microcephaly, infantile spasm,
 psychomotor retardation,
 nephrotic s.
microcephaly, mental retardation,
 cataract, hypogonadism s.
microcephaly, mental retardation,
 retinopathy s.
microcephaly, microphthalmia,
 ectrodactyly, prognathism s.
 (MMEP)
microcephaly, mild developmental
 delay, short stature, distinctive
 face s.
microcephaly, mild mental
 retardation, short stature, skeletal
 anomalies s.
microcephaly, muscular build,
 rhizomelia-cataracts s.
microcephaly, oculo-digito-
 esophageal, duodenal s. (MODED)
microcephaly, sparse hair, mental
 retardation, seizures s.
microcephaly-spastic diplegia s.
microdeletion s.
microdontia, microcephaly, short
 stature s.
micrognathia-glossoptosis s.
microphthalmia-mental deficiency s.
microtia, absent patellae,
 micrognathia s.
MIDAS s.
midfetal testicular regression s.
midline cleft s.
Miescher s.

Mietens s.
Mietens-Weber s.
migraine s.
Mikity-Wilson s.
Mikulicz s.
Miles s.
Miles-Carpenter s. (MCS)
milk-alkali s.
Miller s.
Miller-Dieker s.
Miller-Dieker lissencephaly s.
 (MDLS)
Miller-Fisher variant of Guillain-
 Barré s.
MIMyCA s.
minimal change nephrotic s.
 (MCNS)
minimal lesion nephrotic s.
 (MLNS)
Minkowski-Chauffard s.
Minot-von Willebrand s.
Mirhosseini-Holmes-Walton s.
mirror s.
MISHAP s.
mitis type Ehlers-Danlos s.
mixed antiinflammatory s. (MARS)
mixed sclerosing bone dysplasia,
 small stature, seizures, mental
 retardation s.
MLASA s.
MMEP s.
MMIH s.
MMT s. (MMT)
MNBCC s.
Möbius s.
Mohr s.
Mohr-Claussen s.
Mohr-Tranebjaerg s. (MTS)
Mollica s.
Mollica-Pavone-Anterer s.
MOMO s.
MOMX s.
mononucleosis-type s.
monosomy 7 s.
monosomy G s.
Montefiore s.
Moore-Federman s.
Morgagni-Adams-Stokes s.
Morgagni-Turner s.
Morgagni-Turner-Albright s.
morning glory s.
Morquio s.

NOTES

syndrome *(continued)*

Morquio-Brailsford s.
Morquio-Ullrich s.
mosaic tetrasomy 8p s.
mosaic Turner s.
moyamoya s.
Moynahan alopecia s.
Moynihan s.
MSN s.
mucocutaneous lymph node s.
  (MCLS, MLNS)
mucosal neuroma s.
Müller s.
multiorgan dysfunction s. (MODS)
multiple basal cell carcinoma
  syndrome multiple basal cell
  nevus s.
multiple basal cell nevoid s.
s. of multiple endocrine neoplasia
multiple epiphyseal dysplasia-early
  onset diabetes mellitus s. (MED-
  IDDM)
multiple epiphyseal dysplasia
  tarda s.
multiple hamartoma s.
multiple lentigines s.
multiple neuroma s.
multiple nevoid-basal cell
  carcinoma s.
multiple nevoid, basal cell
  epithelioma, jaw cysts, bifid
  rib s.
multiple organ dysfunction s.
  (MODS)
multiple pterygium s.
multiple synostoses s.
multiple X s.
Mulvihill-Smith s.
Münchausen s.
MURCS s.
muscle atrophy-contracture-
  oculomuscle apraxia s.
muscle-eye-brain s. (MEBS)
muscular hypertrophy s.
musculoskeletal pain s. (MSPS)
Mutchinick s.
myasthenia-like s.
myasthenic s.
myelodysplastic s. (MDS)
myeloproliferative s.
Myhre s.
myocardial steal s.
myoclonus s.
myofascial pain s. (MPS II, MPS,
  MPS VII)
myopathic limb-girdle s.
myopathy-myxedema s.
mystery s.
myxedema-myotonic dystrophy s.

Naegeli s.
Nager s.
Nager-de Reynier s.
nail-patella s.
Najjar s.
NAME s.
Nance-Horan s. (NHS)
nanism-constrictive pericarditis s.
narcotic withdrawal s.
NARP s.
nasal hypoplasia, peripheral
  dysostosis, mental retardation s.
Navajo brainstem s.
near-miss sudden infant death s.
Neill-Dingwall s.
Nelson s.
neonatal abstinence s. (NAS)
neonatal Bartter s. (NBS)
neonatal Guillain-Barré s.
neonatal hepatitis s.
neonatal lupus s.
neonatal Marfan s.
neonatal myasthenic s.
neonatal progeroid s.
neonatal pseudohydrocephalic
  progeroid s.
neonatal small left colon s.
nephrosis-microcephaly s.
nephrosis, microcephaly, hiatus
  hernia s.
nephrosis-neural dysmigration s.
nephrosis-neuronal dysmigration s.
nephrotic s.
Netherton s.
Nettleship s.
Neuhauser s.
Neu-Laxova s. (NLS)
neurocutaneous melanosis s.
neurofaciodigitorenal s.
neurofibromatosis-Noonan s. (NF-
  NS, NFNS)
neuroichthyosis-hypogonadism s.
neuroleptic malignant s. (NMS)
neurological disease s.
neuromuscular scoliosis s.
neurotrichocutaneous s.
Nevo s.
nevoid basal cell carcinoma s.
  (NBCCS, NBS)
nevoid basal cell epithelioma, jaw
  cysts, bifid rib s.
newborn narcotic withdrawal s.
newborn respiratory distress s.
Nezelof s.
NFDR s.
nigricans s.
nigricans-hyperinsulinemia s.
Niikawa-Kuroki s.
Nijmegen breakage s. (NBS)

Noack s.
nonautoimmune myasthenic s.
noncleft median face s.
nongenetic s.
nonnarcotic abstinence s.
Nonne-Milroy-Meige s.
nonprogressive hypoplastic s.
nonprogressive motor impairment s.
nonsalt-losing adrenogenital s.
Noonan s.
Noonan-Ehmke s.
Noonan-like giant cell lesion s.
 (NLGCLS)
Norman-Landing s.
Norman-Roberts lissencephaly s.
Norman-Wood s.
Norrie s.
Norrie-Warburg s.
nutritional deprivation s.
OAV s.
obesity-hypotonia s.
obesity-hypoventilation s.
obesity, short stature, mental
 deficiency, hypogonadism,
 micropenis, finger contracture,
 cleft lip-palate s.
Obrinsky s.
obstruction s.
obstructive sleep apnea s. (OSAS)
OCC s.
occipital horn s.
Ochoa s.
OCR s.
OCRL s.
ocular coloboma-imperforate anus s.
oculoauriculofrontonasal s.
oculocerebral hypopigmentation s.
oculocerebrofacial s.
oculodental s.
oculodentodigital s.
oculogenitolaryngeal s.
oculomandibulodyscephaly-
 hypotrichosis s.
oculopalatoskeletal s.
ODD s.
ODED s.
odontogenic keratocytosis-skeletal
 anomalies s.
OFD s., type I–IV, VI–IX
Ohdo blepharophimosis s.
Ohtahara s.
olfactogenital s.

oligoasthenoteratozoospermia s.
 (OATS)
oligophrenia-ichthyosis s.
oligoteratoasthenozoospermia s.
Oliver s.
Oliver-McFarlane s.
Ollier s.
Ollier-Klippel-Trenaunay-Weber s.
Omenn s.
OMF s.
omphalocele-cleft palate s.
Onat s.
Ondine-Hirschsprung s.
onychodystrophy-congenital
 deafness s.
OPD s.
opercular s.
ophthalmoacromelic s.
Opitz BBBG s.
Opitz-Christian s.
Opitz-Frias s.
Opitz G/BBB s.
Opitz-Kaveggia s.
Opitz trigonocephaly s.
Oppenheim s.
s. of opsoclonus-myoclonus
optic atrophy-ataxia s.
oral allergy s.
Orbeli s.
organic hyperkinetic s.
organic mental s.
organoid nevus s.
orocraniodigital s.
orodigitofacial s.
orogenital s.
oromandibuloauricular s.
oromandibulootic s.
orthostatic tachycardia s.
Osebold-Remondini s.
Osgood-Schlatter s.
Osler-Weber s.
Osler-Weber-Rendu s. (OWRS)
ossified ear cartilages, mental
 deficiency, muscle wasting, bony
 changes s.
osteogenesis imperfecta congenita s.
osteogenesis imperfecta, optic
 atrophy, retinopathy, developmental
 delay s.
osteohypertrophic varicose s.
osteopathia striata, deafness, cranial
 osteopetrosis s.

NOTES

syndrome *(continued)*

osteopathia striata, macrocephaly, cranial sclerosis s.
osteopenia, sparse hair, mental retardation s.
osteoporosis-pseudoglioma s. (OPS)
Ostrum-Furst s.
otitis-conjunctivitis s.
otofaciocervical s.
otomandibular s.
otopalatodigital s.
otosclerosis s.
otospongiosis s.
Otto s.
ovarian dysgenesis-sensorineural deafness s.
ovarian hyperstimulation s. (OHSS)
ovarian remnant s.
ovarian short stature s.
ovarian vein s.
overdistention s.
overdose s.
overgrowth s.
overtraining s.
overuse s.
4p s.
5p s.
9p s.
pachyonychia congenita s.
Pagon s.
Pai s.
Paine s.
Palant cleft palate s.
palatal-digital-oral s.
Pallister-Hall s.
Pallister-Killian s.
Pallister mosaic s.
Pallister W s.
pancreatic insufficiency s.
pancytopenia s.
Papillon-Léage-Psaume s.
Papillon-Lefèvre s.
paramethadione s.
paraneoplastic s.
Parenti-Fraccaro s.
parietal foramina, brachymicrocephaly, mental retardation s.
Parinaud oculoglandular s.
Parkes Weber-Dimitri s.
Parrot s.
Parry-Romberg s.
partial DiGeorge s.
partial trisomy 10q s.
Partington-Anderson s.
Partington X-linked mental retardation s. (PRTS)
Pashayan s.
Pashayan-Pruzansky s.

Passos-Bueno s.
Patau s.
patellofemoral pain s. (PFPS)
patellofemoral stress s.
Patterson pseudoleprechaunism s.
Patterson-Stevenson-Fontaine s.
Pearson marrow-pancreas s.
pediatric acquired immunodeficiency s.
PEHO s.
Pelletier-Leisti s.
Pellizzi s.
pelvic congestion s.
pelvic venous congestion s.
Pena-Shokeir s. (I, II)
Pendred s.
pentasomy X s.
penta-X s.
PEO s.
Pepper s.
Perheentupa s.
pericardial constriction-growth failure s.
perisylvian s.
Perlman nephroblastomatosis s.
Perrault s.
persistent müllerian duct s.
Peters anomaly, corneal clouding, growth and mental retardation s.
Peters anomaly-short limb dwarfism s.
Peters-plus s.
Pettigrew s. (PGS)
Peutz-Jeghers s.
Pfaundler-Hurler s.
Pfeiffer s.
PHACE s.
pharyngeal pouch s.
Phocas s.
phocomelia s.
phonologic-syntactic s.
PHS s.
physiologic addiction/abstinence s.
pickwickian s.
PIE s.
Pierre Robin s.
pigmentary retinopathy, hypogonadism, mental retardation, nerve deafness, glucose intolerance s.
pink diaper s.
Pirie s.
piriformis s.
Pitt s.
Pitt-Rogers-Danks s. (PRDS)
placental dysfunction s.
placental hemangioma s.
placental transfusion s.
Plott s.

POEMS s.
pointer s.
Poland s.
poliomyelitis-like s.
Pollitt s.
polycystic ovarian s. (PCOS)
polycystic ovary s. (PCOS, POS)
polycythemia-hyperviscosity s.
polydactyly-chondrodystrophy s.
polydactyly-craniofacial anomalies s.
polydactyly-craniofacial
  dysmorphism s.
polydactyly-imperforate anus s.
polydactyly, imperforate anus,
  vertebral anomalies s.
polyglandular s.
polyglandular autoimmune s.
polyneuropathy-cataract-deafness s.
polyposis s.
polysplenia s.
polysyndactyly-dyscrania s.
polysyndactyly-peculiar skull s.
polysynostoses s.
Pompe s.
popliteal pterygium s.
popliteal web s.
Porak-Durante s.
porencephaly, cerebellar hypoplasia,
  internal malformations s.
Porteous s.
POSSUM database of genetic s.'s
postabortal s.
postanoxic dystonic s.
postaxial acrofacial dysostosis s.
  (POADS)
postcoartectomy s.
postconcussion s.
postembolization s.
posterior leukoencephalopathy s.
postexchange transfusion s.
postgastroenteritis malabsorption s.
postirradiation s.
postmaturity s.
postmenopausal palpable ovary s.
postpartum hemolytic uremic s.
postpartum pituitary necrosis s.
postperfusion s.
postpericardiotomy s. (PPS)
postphlebitic s. (PPS)
postpolio s.
postrubella s.
postscabetic s.

posttraumatic stress s.
posttubal ligation s.
postural orthostatic tachycardia s.
  (POTS)
postvagotomy dumping s.
Potter s.
PPO s.
Prader-Labhart-Willi s.
Prader-Labhart-Willi-Fanconi s.
Prader-Willi s. (PWS)
Prader-Willi habitus, osteopenia,
  camptodactyly s.
Prader-Willi habitus, osteoporosis,
  hand contracture s.
precordial catch s.
preexcitation s.
preleukemic s.
premenstrual s. (PMS)
premenstrual salivary s.
premenstrual tension s.
Prieto s. (PRS)
primary antiphospholipid antibody s.
primary empty sella s.
primary hyperuricemia s.
primary nephrotic s.
Primrose s.
progeria s.
progeria-like s.
progeroid short stature-pigmented
  nevi s.
prolapse-gastropathy s. (PGS)
prolonged QT s.
prominent incisors-obesity-
  hypotonia s.
proteiform s.
Proteus s. (PS)
Proud s.
prune belly s.
pseudoachondroplasia s.
pseudoaminopterin s.
pseudoappendicular s.
pseudo-Hurler s.
pseudoprogeria s.
pseudothalidomide s.
pseudotoxoplasmosis s.
pseudotrisomy 13 s.
pseudo-Turner s.
pseudo-Ullrich-Turner s.
pseudo-Wernicke s.
pterygium colli, mental retardation,
  digital anomalies s.

NOTES

syndrome *(continued)*

ptosis, downslanting palpebral fissures, hypertelorism, seizures, mental retardation s.
pug nose-peripheral dysostosis s.
pulmonary dysmaturity s.
pulmonary infiltrate with eosinophilia s.
pulmonic stenosis-café-au-lait spots s.
pupillary s.
puppetlike s.
purple toes s.
Purtilo s.
pyknodysostosis s.
Pyle s.
pyridoxine-dependency s.
22q11.2 deletion s.
Quan-Smith s.
quintuple-X s.
Rabson-Mendenhall s.
radial aplasia-thrombocytopenia s.
radial ray defects, triangular face, telecanthus, sparse hair, dwarfism, mental retardation s.
radial-renal s.
radiation s.
radio-reno-ocular s.
radioulnar synostosis, developmental retardation, hypotonia s.
radioulnar synostosis, short stature, microcephaly, scoliosis, mental retardation s.
Raine s.
RALPH s.
Rambam-Hasharon s.
Ramon s.
Ramsay Hunt s. (I–III)
rancid butter s.
rape trauma s.
Rapp-Hodgkin ectodermal dysplasia s.
Rasmussen s.
Raynaud s.
RCDP s.
REAR s.
rec 8 s.
recessive deafness-onychodystrophy s.
recessive enhanced S-cone s.
recessive Usher s.
recognizable viral s. (RVS)
recombinant chromosome 8 s.
recurrent hemolytic uremia s.
Reed s.
Refetoff s.
Refsum s.
Regenbogen-Donnai s.
Reifenstein s.

Reiter s.
renal Fanconi s.
renal mesangial sclerosis-eye defects s.
renal tubular Fanconi s.
renal tubular pituitary s.
Rendu-Osler-Weber s.
Renpenning s.
residual ovary s.
resistant ovary s.
respiratory distress s. (RDS)
restless legs s.
retained bladder s.
retardation, aphasia, shuffling gait, adducted thumbs s.
retardation, deafness, microgenitalism s.
Rethoré s.
retinal pigmentary degeneration, microcephaly, mental retardation s.
retinitis pigmentosa-congenital deafness s.
retinoblastoma-mental retardation s.
retinopathy-mental retardation s.
retraction s.
retroviral s.
Rett s.
reverse chylous s.
reversible posterior leukoencephalopathy s. (RPLS)
Reye s.
Reye-like s.
rhizomelia s.
Rh-null s.
rib-gap defect-micrognathia s.
Richards-Rundle s.
Richner s.
Richner-Hanhart s.
Rieger s.
right middle lobe s.
right ovarian vein s.
right-sided arch, mental deficiency, facial dysmorphism s.
rigid spine s.
Riley-Day s.
Riley-Schwachman s.
Riley-Smith s.
ring 1–22 s.
Ritscher-Schinzel s.
Roberts pseudothalidomide s.
Roberts-SC phocomelia s.
Roberts tetraphocomelia s.
Robin s.
Robinow s.
Robinow-Silverman-Smith s.
Robinow-Sorauf s.
Rocher-Sheldon s.
Rokitansky-Küster-Hauser s.

Rolland-Desbuquois s.
Romano-Ward long QT s.
Rosenthal-Kloepfer s.
Rosewater s.
Rosselli-Gulienetti s.
Rossi s.
Rothmann-Makai s.
Rothmund s.
Rothmund-Thomson s.
Rothmund-Thomson cancer
  predisposition s.
round ligament s.
Roussy-Lévy s.
RSH s.
RSH/SLO s.
rubella s.
Rubinstein s.
Rubinstein-Taybi s.
Rud s.
Rudiger s.
rudimentary testis s.
Russell diencephalic s. (I, II, III)
Russell-Silver dwarf s.
Rutherfurd s.
Rutledge lethal multiple congenital
  anomalies s.
Ruvalcaba s.
Ruvalcaba-Myhre s.
Ruvalcaba-Myhre-Smith s. (RMSS)
Ruvalcaba-Reichert-Smith s.
Sabinas brittle hair s.
Saethre-Chotzen s.
Sakati-Nyhan s.
Saldino-Noonan s.
Salonen-Herva-Norio s.
salt-losing adrenogenital s. (SLAS)
salt-wasting adrenogenital s.
Sanchez-Cascos s.
Sanchez-Corona s.
Sanchez-Salorio s.
Sandhoff s.
Sandifer s.
Sanjad-Sakati s.
San Luis Valley s.
Santavuori s.
Santavuori-Haltia s.
Sao Paulo MCA/MR s.
Sato s.
Savage s.
Say s.
Say-Gerald s.
Say-Meyer s.

scalded skin s. (SSS)
Schafer s.
Scheie s.
Scheuthauer-Marie-Sainton s.
Schimmelbusch s.
Schimmelpenning-Feuerstein-Mims s.
Schinzel acrocallosal s.
Schinzel-Giedion s. (SGS)
Schinzel-Giedion midface-
  retraction s.
Schirmer s.
Schmid-Fraccaro s.
Schmidley s.
Schmidt s.
Schwachman s.
Schwachman-Diamond s.
Schwartz s.
Schwartz-Jampel s.
Schwartz-Jampel-Aberfeld s.
scimitar s.
SCIWORA s.
scleroderma-like s.
scotopic sensitivity s.
Scott craniodigital s.
Scott-Taor s.
SC phocomelia s.
SC-pseudothalidomide s.
SEA s.
sea-blue histiocyte s.
Seabright bantam s.
seat belt s.
sebaceous nevus s.
Seckel bird head s.
secondary nephrotic s.
second impact s.
Sedlacková s.
Seemanová s. (1, 2)
Seemanová-Lesny s.
Seip s.
Seip-Lawrence s.
Seitleis s.
seizures, acquired microcephaly,
  agenesis of corpus callosum s.
seizures, hypotonic cerebral palsy,
  megalocornea, mental
  retardation s.
Sengers s.
Senior-Loken s.
Sensenbrenner s.
Sensenbrenner-Dorst-Owens s.
sensimotor induction in disturbed
  equilibrium s.

NOTES

syndrome *(continued)*

sensorineural deafness, imperforate anus, hypoplastic thumbs s.

Senter s.

sepsis s.

sepsis-pneumonia s.

sepsis/shock s.

septum pellucidum with porencephalia s. (SASPP)

seronegative enthesopathy and arthropathy s.

serotonin s.

Sertoli-cell-only s.

serum sickness-like s.

Setleis s.

severe acute respiratory s. (SARS)

severe ovarian hyperstimulation s. (SOHS)

Shah-Waardenburg s.

shaken baby s.

shaken impact s.

shaken infant s.

shaking-impact s.

shallow orbits, ptosis, coloboma, trigonocephaly, gyral malformations, mental and growth retardation s.

shawl scrotum s.

shedding s.

Sheehan s.

Sheehy s.

Shereshevskii-Turner s.

Shokeir s.

Shone s.

SHORT s.

short bowel s. (SBS)

short gut s. (SGS)

short limb dwarfism, saddle nose, spinal alterations, metaphyseal striation s.

short rib-polydactyly s. (SRPS)

short stature, characteristic facies, mental retardation, macrodontia, skeletal anomalies s.

short stature, microcephaly, mental retardation, multiple epiphyseal dysplasia s.

short stature, microcephaly, syndactyly, dysmorphic face, mental retardation s.

Shprintzen-Goldberg craniosynostosis s.

Shprintzen velocardiofacial s.

Shulman s.

Shwachman s.

Shwachman-Bodian s.

Shwachman-Diamond s.

Shy-Drager s.

Shy-Magee s.

sicca s.

sick euthyroid s.

sick sinus node s.

Siemerling-Creutzfeldt s.

Silver s.

Silver-Russell s.

Silverskiöld s.

Simmonds s.

Simpson dysmorphia s. (SDYS)

Simpson dysplasia s.

Simpson-Golabi-Behmel s. (SGBS)

Simpson-Golabi-Behmel fetal overgrowth s.

Sinding-Larsen-Johansson s.

Sipple s.

sirenomelia s.

situs inversus totalis s.

Sjögren s.

Sjögren-Larsson s.

skeletal and cardiac malformations-thrombocytopenia s.

skeletal dysplasial, joint laxity, mental retardation s.

skeletal dysplasia, sparse hair, dental anomalies s.

skeleton-skin-brain s.

skin-eye-brain s.

skin mastocytosis, hearing loss, mental retardation s.

slapped cheek s.

sleep apnea s.

sleep-disordered breathing s.

slick-gut s.

slit ventricle s.

SLO s.

Slotnick-Goldfarb s.

sloughed urethra s.

slow-channel congenital myasthenic s. (SCCMS)

Sly s.

small left colon s.

small patella s.

SMG22 s.

Smith s.

Smith-Fineman-Myers s. (SFMS)

Smith-Magenis s. (SMS)

Smith-Theiler-Schachenmann s.

snapping knee s.

Snyder-Robinson s. (SRS)

soft hands s.

Sohval-Soffer s.

Solomon s.

Solomon-Fretzin-Dewald s.

Sommer s.

somnolence s.

Sonoda s.

Sorsby s.

Sotos s.

spastic quadriplegia, congenital ichthyosiform erythroderma, oligophrenia s.

spastic quadriplegia, retinitis pigmentosa, mental retardation s.

spinal muscular atrophy-mental retardation s.

spinal muscular atrophy, microcephaly, mental retardation s.

spinocerebellar ataxia-dysmorphism s.

splenic sequestration s.

split foot, microphthalmia, cleft lip/palate-mental retardation s.

split hand/foot s.

spondylar and nasal alterations-striated metaphyses s.

spondylocostal dysplasia s.

spondyloepiphyseal dysplasia congenita s.

spondyloepiphyseal dysplasia-diabetes mellitus s.

spondyloepiphyseal dysplasia tarda-mental retardation s.

spondylometaepiphyseal dysplasia-extreme short stature s.

spondylometaphyseal dysplasia-short limb-abnormal calcification s.

spondylothoracic dysplasia s.

Spranger-Wiedemann s.

Spurway s.

Srb s.

SSS s.

stagnant loop s.

staphylococcal scalded skin s. (SSSS)

staphylococcal toxic shock s.

steely-hair s.

Steinert s.

Steinfeld s.

Stein-Leventhal s.

sterile pyuria s.

steroid-sensitive idiopathic nephrotic s. (SSNS)

Stevens-Johnson s.

Stewart-Treves s.

Stickler s.

stiff-baby s.

stiff-man s.

Stilling-Türk-Duane s.

Stimmler s.

Stocco dos Santos s.

Stock-Spielmeyer-Vogt s.

Stokes-Adams s.

Stoll s.

strabismus s.

straight back s.

Stratton-Parker s.

streptococcal toxic shock s.

Strudwick s.

stuck twin s.

Sturge-Kalischer-Weber s.

Sturge-Weber s. (SWS)

Sturge-Weber-Dimitri s.

Sturge-Weber-Krabbe s.

Stüve-Wiedemann s. (SWS)

subaortic stenosis-short stature s.

sudden infant death s. (SIDS)

Sugarman s.

sulfur-deficient brittle hair s.

superior mediastinal s.

superior mesenteric artery s.

superior vena cava s.

superior vena caval s.

supine hypotensive s.

surfactant deficiency s.

Sutherland-Haan s. (SHS)

swallowed blood s.

sweaty feet s.

Sweet s.

Swyer s.

Swyer-James s.

Swyer-James-Macleod s.

sylvian aqueduct s.

s. of symmetric parasagittal parietooccipital polymicrogyria

syndactyly-anophthalmos s.

syndactyly, cataracts, mental retardation s.

syndactyly, microcephaly, mental retardation s.

systemic inflammatory response s. (SIRS)

systemic vasculitis s.

tachy-brady s.

Takao s.

TAR s.

Tariverdian s.

tarsal-carpal coalition s.

Taussig-Bing s.

Tay s.

Taybi s.

Taybi-Linder s.

S

NOTES

syndrome *(continued)*

Teebi s.
telecanthus-hypospadias s.
Temtamy s.
teratogenic s.
ter Haar s.
Terry s.
Teschler-Nicola and Killian s.
testicular feminization s.
tethered cord s.
tetra amelia s.
tetrahydrofolate-methyltransferase
deficiency s.
tetralogy of Fallot s.
tetraphocomelia-cleft lip-palate s.
tetraploidy s.
tetrasomy 15p s.
tetra-X s.
thalidomide teratogenicity s.
Thal intermedia-like s.
thanatophoric dysplasia s.
Thiemann s.
third and fourth pharyngeal
pouch s.
thoracic compression s.
thrombocytopenia with absent
radius s.
thymic aplasia s.
thymic and parathyroid agenesis s.
thyrohypophysial s.
tibial aplasia-ectrodactyly s.
Tietze s.
tin ear s.
tired housewife s.
Tolosa-Hunt s.
tooth anomalies, skeletal dysplasia,
sparse hair s.
tooth and nail s.
TORCH s.
Toriello s. (1, 2)
Toriello-Carey s.
Torsten Sjögren s.
Tourette s.
Townes s.
Townes-Brocks s.
toxemia s.
toxemic shock s.
toxic oil s.
toxic shock s. (TSS)
toxoplasmosis, rubella,
cytomegalovirus, herpes simplex s.
tracheal agenesis s.
tracheoesophageal fistula, esophageal
atresia, multiple congenital
anomaly s.
Tranebjaerg s. (1, 2)
transfusion s.
transient myeloproliferative s.
transient neonatal myasthenic s.

transient respiratory distress s.
(TRDS)
translocation Down s.
TRAP s.
trapezoidocephaly-synostosis s.
traumatic compartment s.
Treacher Collins s.
Treacher Collins-Franceschetti s.
tremor s.
trichodental dysplasia, microcephaly,
mental retardation s.
trichodentoosseous s.
trichorhinophalangeal s.
trichorrhexis nodosa s.
trichothiodystrophy-congenital
ichthyosis s.
trichothiodystrophy-neurocutaneous s.
trichothiodystrophy-xeroderma
pigmentosum s.
Trichuris dysentery s.
Tridione s.
trigonocephaly s.
trilateral retinoblastoma s.
trimethadione s.
triple X s.
triploidy s.
trip 15q s.
trismus-pseudocamptodactyly s.
trisomy 1–22 s.
trisomy C,D,E,G s.
trisomy 18-like s.
trisomy 1p–22p s.
trisomy 1q–22q s.
Troyer s. (TS)
tuberous sclerosis s.
tubular stenosis, hypocalcemia,
convulsions, dwarfism s.
tubulopathy of Lowe s.
tumor lysis s.
Turcot s.
Turner-Albright s.
Turner-Kieser s.
Turner-like s.
Turner mosaic s.
Turner XO s.
twin-peak s.
twin-to-twin transfusion s. (TTS,
TTTS)
t Y;18 s.
tyrosinemia, palmar and plantar
keratosis, ocular keratitis s.
Ullrich-Bonnevie s.
Ullrich-Feichtiger s.
Ullrich and Fremerey-Dohna s.
Ullrich-Noonan s.
Ullrich-Turner s.
ulnar hypoplasia, club feet, mental
retardation s.
ulnar-mammary s.

umbilical cord s.
s. of uncal herniation
uncombable hair s.
unilateral fibular aplastic s.
universal joint s.
Unna-Thost s.
unstable bladder s.
unusual facies, mental retardation,
  intrauterine growth retardation s.
Unverricht-Lundborg s.
upper airways resistance s. (UARS)
upper motor neuron s.
Urban s.
Urban-Rogers-Meyer s.
uremic s.
urethral s.
urgency s.
urgency-frequency s.
urofacial s.
Usher s. (US)
uterine hernia s.
uveal coloboma, cleft lip/palate,
  mental retardation s.
uveomeningoencephalitic s.
uveoparotid fever s.
VACTERL association with
  hydrocephalus s.
VACTERL-H s.
valproic acid s.
Van Buchem s.
van den Bosch s.
van der Hoeve s.
van der Woude s.
Van Haldergem s.
vanishing testes s.
vanishing testicle s.
vanishing twin s.
Van Maldergem s.
Váradi s.
Váradi-Papp s.
varicella s.
vascular ring s.
vasculitis s.
VATER s.
velocardiofacial s. (VCFS)
Verner-Morrison s.
viral s.
Virchow-Seckel s.
visceromegaly s.
viscous s.
vitamin B_6 dependence s.
Vles s.

Vogt s.
Vogt-Koyanagi s.
Vogt-Koyanagi-Harada s.
Vohwinkel s.
von Hippel-Lindau s.
von Willebrand s.
Voorhoeve s.
vulnerable child s.
vulvar vestibulitis s. (VVS)
VURD s.
W s.
Waardenburg-Klein s.
Waardenburg recessive
  anophthalmia s.
Waelsch s.
Wagner s.
WAGR s.
Waisman s.
Waisman-Laxova s.
Walker-Clodius s.
Walker lissencephaly s.
Walker-Warburg s.
Walton s.
Warburg s.
warfarin s.
Waring blender s.
Warkany s. 1, 2
wasting s.
Waterhouse-Friderichsen s.
Watson s.
Watson-Alagille s.
Watson-Miller s.
Weaver s.
Weaver-Smith s. (WSS)
Weaver-Williams s.
Weber s.
Weber-Christian s.
Weber-Dimitri s.
Weill-Marchesani s.
Weismann-Netter s.
Weissenbacher-Zweymuller s.
Werdnig-Hoffmann s.
Wermer s.
Werner s.
Wernicke s.
Wernicke-Korsakoff s.
West s.
wet brain s.
wet lung s.
Weyers oligodactyly s.
Whelan s.
Whipple s.

NOTES

syndrome *(continued)*

whistling face s.

whistling face-windmill vane hand s.

WIC s.

Wieacker s.

Wieacker-Wolff s.

Wiedemann s.

Wiedemann-Beckwith s.

Wiedemann-Beckwith-Combs s.

Wiedemann-Rautenstrauch s. (WR)

Wildervanck s.

Wildervanck-Smith s.

Wilkins s.

Willebrand-Jurgens s.

Williams s. (WS)

Williams-Barratt s.

Williams-Beuren s.

Williams-Campbell s.

Wilms tumor, aniridia gonadoblastoma, mental retardation s.

Wilson-Mikity s.

Wilson-Turner s. (WTS)

Winchester s.

Winter s.

Wisconsin s.

Wiskott-Aldrich s. (WAS)

Wittwer s.

Wohlfart-Kugelberg-Welander s.

Wolcott-Rallison s.

Wolf s.

Wolff mental retardation s.

Wolff-Parkinson-White s.

Wolf-Hirschhorn s.

Wolfram s.

Woods s.

Worster-Drought s.

wrinkly skin s. (WSS)

Wyburn-Mason s.

s. X

45,X s.

XK s.

XK-aprosencephaly s.

X-linked cataract-dental s.

X-linked congenital cataracts-microcornea s.

X-linked dominant s.

X-linked dysplasia-gigantism s. (DGSX)

X-linked Ehlers-Danlos s.

X-linked Hurler s.

X-linked lymphoproliferative s.

X-linked mental deficiency-megalotestes s.

X-linked mental handicap-retinitis pigmentosa s.

X-linked mental retardation s. 1–6 (MRXS1–6)

X-linked mental retardation-aphasia s. (MRXA)

X-linked mental retardation-blindness-deafness-multiple congenital anomalies s.

X-linked mental retardation-fragile site s. 2

X-linked mental retardation-growth hormone deficiency s.

X-linked mental retardation-hypogenitalism-cerebral anomaly s.

X-linked mental retardation-marfanoid habitus s.

X-linked mental retardation, microphthalmia, microcornea, cataract, hypogenitalism, mental retardation-spasticity s.

X-linked mental retardation-psoriasis s.

X-linked mental retardation-spastic diplegia s.

X-linked mental retardation, thin habitus, osteoporosis, kyphoscoliosis s.

X-linked mental retardation with fragile X s.

X-linked Opitz s. (XLOS)

X-linked recessive deafness s.

X-linked recessive skeletal Ehlers-Danlos s.

X-linked seizures, acquired micrencephaly, agenesis of corpus callosum s.

X-linked severe combined immunodeficiency s.

XO s.

Xq+ s.

Xq- s.

Xq Klinefelter s.

XX male s.

46,XX male s.

XXX s.

47,XXX s.

XXXX s.

XXXXX s.

XXXXY s.

49, XXXXY s.

XXY s.

47,XXY s.

XYY s.

yellow nail s.

yellow vernix s.

Young s.

Young-Hughes s.

Young-Madders s.

Yunis-Varon s.

YY s.

Zellweger cerebrohepatorenal s.

Zerres s.

Ziehen-Oppenheim s.
Zimmermann-Laband s. (ZLS)
Zinsser s.
Zinsser-Cole-Engman s.
Zinsser-Engman-Cole s.
Ziprokowski-Margolis s.
Zlotogora-Ogür s.
Zollinger-Ellison s.
Zollino s.
Zunich s.
Zwahlen s.

syndromic
s. cleft
s. craniosynostosis
s. paucity

synechia, pl. **synechiae**
anterior s.
cleft palate-lateral s. (CPLS)
intrauterine s.
posterior s.
s. vulvae

Synemol Topical
synencephalocele
Synercid
synergism
synergistic gangrene
synergy
spastic s.

synesthesia
Synevac vacuum curettage system
Synflex
syngamy
syngeneic
s. bone marrow transplantation
s. stem cell
s. tissue

syngnathia congenita
syngraft
synkinesia
mouth-and-hand s.

synkinesis, syncinesis
Syn-Minocycline
synophthalmia
Synophylate
synorchidism
synoscheos
synostosis, pl. **synostoses**
coronal s.
cranial s.
humeroradial s.
lambdoid s.
multiple synostoses

s. multiplex
premature suture s.
radioulnar s.
sagittal s.
tribasilar s.
unilambdoid s.

synovectomy
synovial
s. biopsy
s. fluid
s. fluid analysis
s. hypertrophy
s. joint
s. sarcoma

synoviocyte
fibroblastoid s.

synovioma
synovitis
monoarticular s.
plant thorn s.
toxic s.
transient monoarticular s.
villonodular s.

synovium
Synphasic
Synsorb Pk
syntax
syntenic gene
synteny
synthase
cystathionine s.
methionine s.
prostaglandin endoperoxide s.
pyloric nitric oxide s.

synthesis, pl. **syntheses**
bile acid s.
cholesterol s.
decidual prolactin s.
estrogen s.
inborn error of bile acid s.
ovarian estrogen s.
progesterone s.
thyroxine s.
tissue s.

synthesize
synthesizer
voice s.

synthetase
carbamoyl phosphate s. (CPS)
endothelial nitric oxide s.
holocarboxylase s.

S

NOTES

synthetase *(continued)*
    N-acetylglutamate s.
    6-pyruvoyl tetrahydropteridine s.
synthetic
    s. conjugated estrogen
    s. DNA
    s. gliadin peptide
    s. prostaglandin E_1
    s. pterin
    s. surfactant
    s. suture material
Synthroid
    S. Injection
    S. Oral
syphilis
    biological false-positive serologic
      test for s. (BF-STS)
    congenital s.
    early congenital s.
    endemic s.
    s. hereditaria tarda
    late congenital s.
    latent s.
    latent-stage s.
    parenchymatous congenital s.
    primary s.
    secondary s.
    serologic test for s. (STS)
    tertiary s.
    s., toxoplasmosis, other agents,
      rubella, cytomegalovirus, herpes
      simplex virus (STORCH,
      ToRCHS)
    toxoplasmosis, rubella,
      cytomegalovirus, herpes
      simplex, s. (STORCH, ToRCHS)
syphilitic
    s. infection
    s. keratitis
    s. meningitis
    s. pemphigus
    s. phlebitis
    s. rhinitis
syphilotherapy
Syprine
Syracol-CF
syringe
    Asepto s.
    Auto S.
    bulb s.
    s. feeding
    Luer Lok s.
    super s.
    tuberculin s.
syringes *(pl. of* syrinx)
syringobulbia
syringocele
syringocystadenoma papilliferum
syringohydromyelia

syringoma
    eruptive s.
syringomeningocele
syringomyelia
    familial lumbosacral s.
syringomyelic cavity
syringomyelocele
syringopleural drainage
syringosubarachnoid drainage
syrinx, pl. **syringes**
syrup
    Bromfed S.
    Claritin s.
    Decofed S.
    s. of ipecac
    ipecac s.
    Karo s.
    Promethazine VC Plain S.
    Rondec S.
    Tusstat S.
    Versed s.
    Zyrtec s.
Sysmex NE8000 cell counter
system
    Abbott LifeCare PCA Plus II
      infusion s.
    ABI model 373, 377 sequencing
      gel s.
    ABI model 377 sequencing gel s.
    ABO blood group s.
    adnexal adhesion classification s.
    AEGIS sonography management s.
    Affirm VP microbial
      identification s.
    Affymetrix GeneChip s.
    AFS adhesion scoring s.
    Aggregate Neurobehavioral Student
      Health & Education Review S.
    AI 5200 S Open Color Doppler
      imaging s.
    Aladdin Infant Flow S.
    Aloka SD ultrasound s.
    alternative s.
    Androderm Transdermal S.
    Ann Arbor Staging S.
    Apgar scoring s.
    Apogee 800 ultrasound s.
    AquaSens FMS 1000 Fluid
      Monitoring S.
    ascending reticular activating s.
      (ARAS)
    ASG s.
    AspenVac smoke evacuation s.
    ATL HDI 3000 ultrasound s.
    Aurora MR breast imaging s.
    AutoCyte S.
    autonomic nervous s. (ANS)
    AutoPap 300 QC s.
    Autoread centrifuge hematology s.

Auto Suture ABBI s.
Aviva mammography s.
BABE OB ultrasound reporting s.
Baby CareLink s.
Bactec blood-culturing s.
Bair Hugger patient warming s.
Balloon Therapy S.
basolateral membrane transport s.
BDProbeTec ET s.
behavior contract s.
17beta-E2 transdermal drug-delivery s.
Bethesda classification s.
Bethesda II s.
bicarbonate-carbonic acid s.
Biliblanket Plus phototherapy s.
Biogel Reveal puncture indication s.
BioMerieux Vitek s.
Bishop pelvic scoring s.
Bishop Prelabor Scoring S.
breast leakage inhibitor s. (BLIS)
Breslow microstaging s.
bursa-dependent s.
CADD-Prizm pain control s.
Capasee diagnostic ultrasound s.
cardiovascular s.
CatsEye digital camera s.
CDE blood group s.
Cell Recovery S. (CRS)
central nervous s. (CNS)
centrencephalic s.
cerebellar-vestibular s.
Cineloop image review ultrasound s.
circulatory s.
Clark microstaging s.
Climara estradiol transdermal s.
ColorMate TLc BiliTest S.
Companion 318 Nasal CPAP S.
Conceptus fallopian tube catheterization s.
continuous distention irrigation s. (CDIS)
cotyledon perfusion s.
Cre/loxP s.
CRYOcare cryoablation s.
Cryomedics electrosurgery s.
CrystalEyes endoscopic video s.
CS-5 cryosurgical s.
cytochrome *b* s.
Diastat Rectal Delivery S.

digestive s.
digital mammography s.
Dolphin hysteroscopic fluid management s.
dopaminergic s.
double collecting s.
drainage s.
drooping lily appearance of lower collecting s.
Duffy s.
dynamic optical breast imaging s. (DOBI)
Dynamite mattress s.
dysfunctional voiding scoring s. (DVSS)
Eccocee ultrasound s.
Eklund positioning s.
electroshield monitoring s.
embryonic branchial s.
EMLA disc topical anesthetic adhesive s.
EnAbl thermal ablation s.
Endermologie LPG s.
endocrine s.
Endotek urodynamics s.
ENTec coblator plasma s.
Entree II trocar and cannula s.
Entree Plus trocar and cannula s.
EntriStar Gastrostomy S.
Esclim estradiol transdermal s.
Esclim transderm s.
Estraderm transdermal s.
estradiol transdermal s.
EUB-405 ultrasound s.
Exact-Touch Saccomanno Pap smear collection s.
extrapyramidal nervous s.
EZ-EM Bio-Gun automated biopsy s.
Ferriman-Gallwey hirsutism scoring s.
fibrinolytic and clotting s.
FoamCare cleansing s.
Force GSU argon-enhanced electrosurgery s.
GE Senographe 2000D digital mammography s.
Glucometer Elite diabetes care s.
Gordon diagnostic s. (GDS)
Guardian DNA s.
Gynecare Thermachoice uterine balloon therapy s.

NOTES

system *(continued)*

HabitEX smoking cessation s.
Halo Sleep S.
haversian s.
hematopoietic s.
HemoCue blood glucose s.
HemoCue blood hemoglobin s.
Her Option uterine cryoablation therapy s.
His-Purkinje s.
Histofreezer cryosurgical s.
Hitachi EUB 405 imaging s.
Hitachi UB 420 digital ultrasound s.
humoral immune s.
Hydro ThermAblator endometrial ablation s.
hypothalamic-pituitary s.
Illumina Pro Series CO_2 surgical laser s.
iLook 15 handheld ultrasound s.
image recording s.
Imelab vascular diagnostic s.
Imexlab vascular diagnostic s.
immune s.
Infant Flow nCPAP s.
In-Fast bone screw s.
Innova electrotherapy s.
Innova feminine incontinence treatment s.
INOvent delivery s.
International Neuroblastoma Staging S. (INSS)
International Staging S.
intrauterine contraceptive progesterone s. (ICPS)
JustVision diagnostic ultrasound s.
Kagan staging s.
kallikrein-kinin s.
KOH colpotomizer s.
Lact-Aid nursing trainer s.
Lancefield streptococcal typing s.
Laparolift s.
LATCH s.
limbic GABAergic s.
Lone Star retractor s.
lower collecting s.
Lumex PT fiberoptic cystometry s.
lymphatic s.
lymphoreticular s.
male reproductive s.
Mammex TR computer-aided mammography diagnosis s.
Mammomat C3 mammography s.
MammoReader computer-aided detection s.
MammoScan digital imaging s.
Mammotest breast biopsy s.
Mammotome breast biopsy s.

Maturna bra s.
McAllister grading s.
MEMS 6 TrackCap Monitor medication monitoring s.
MicroLap Gold s.
MicroSpan microhysterescopy s.
MiniMed continuous glucose monitoring s.
mini Vidas automated immunoassay s.
mitochondrial glycine cleavage s.
Mityvac vacuum delivery s.
molecular adsorbent recirculating s. (MARS)
motion artifact rejection s. (MARS)
musculoskeletal s.
Nellcor N-400/FS s.
NeoCure cryoablation s.
Neonatal Abstinence Scoring S. (NASS)
neonatal facial coding s. (NFCS)
Neotrend s.
nervous s.
neuroendocrine s.
NexPill SmartCap medication monitoring s.
noradrenergic s.
Norplant s.
Nottingham breast cancer grading s.
NovaSure impedance-controlled endometrial ablation s.
OpenGene automated DNA sequencing s.
opsonization s.
OPUS immunoassay s.
OraSure oral HIV-1 antibody testing s.
orthogonal lead s.
OsteoView 2000 s.
Ovation falloposcopy s.
PadKit sample collection s.
PalmVue s.
PapNet automated cervical cystology s.
PapNet testing s.
Pap-Perfect supply s.
parasympathetic nervous s.
Performa Acoustic Imaging s.
Performa diagnostic ultrasound imaging s.
PerQ SANS s.
POPQ staging s.
portal s.
Pregnancy Risk Assessment Monitoring S. (PRAMS)
press-in bone anchor s.
primer pair s.

Priscilla White classification of diabetes in pregnancy s. (class A, A1, A2, B, C, D, F, R, H, T)
probe s.
prognostic scoring s.
prorenin-renin-angiotensin s.
ProTime microcoagulation s.
Puregene DNA extraction s.
Quips genetic imaging s.
radiofrequency interstitial tissue ablation s. (RITA)
Redi+Wash cleansing s.
Renaissance spirometry s.
renin-angiotensin s. (RAS)
renin-angiotensin-aldosterone s.
reproductive s.
respiratory s.
reticuloendothelial s.
review of s.'s (ROS)
Rh blood group s.
Riechert-Mundinger stereotactic s.
RxFISH DNA probe and analysis s.
SalEst preterm labor test s.
Scepter s.
Second-Look computer-aided detection s.
selective no-fault s.
selective tubal occlusion procedure s.
SenoScan full-field digital mammography s.
SensoScan mammography s.
Sequoia Acuson s.
Seroma-Cath s.
serotonergic s.
Shimadzu ultrasound s.
Shutt suture punch s.
Siemens Sonoline SI-400 ultrasound s.
Sinai S.
single collecting s.
single-use diagnostic s. (SUDS)
Sirecust 404N neonatal monitoring s.
Sky-Boot stirrup s.
SKY epidural pain control s.
SoftScan laser mammography s.
Sonopsy ultrasound-guided breast biopsy s.

Spectra 400 extended surveillance and alert s.
Sperm Select sperm recovery s.
SprayGel adhesive barrier s.
STAN S 21 fetal heart rate s.
STARRT falloposcopy s.
St. Jude Children's Research Hospital staging s.
Straight-In surgical s.
subdermal contraceptive s.
superior venous s.
surgicopathologic staging s.
swivel-arm s.
sympathetic nervous s.
Synevac vacuum curettage s.
Technos ultrasound s.
Teratogen Information S. (TERIS)
Testoderm Transdermal S.
s. for thalidomide education and prescription safety (STEPS)
Thermachoice uterine balloon therapy s.
thermal balloon s.
ThermoChem-HT s.
TLX alloantigen s.
transdermal therapeutic s. (TTS)
TroGARD electrosurgical blunt trocar s.
1.5 T superconductive s.
T-TAC s.
Tylok high-tension cerclage cabling s.
UD-2000 urodynamic measurement s.
Ultramark ultrasound s.
underwater drainage s.
UPS 2020 ambulatory measurement s.
urinary s.
Urocyte diagnostic cytometry s.
UroVive s.
Vaccine Adverse Events Reporting S. (VAERS)
Vacutainer s.
Valleylab REM s.
Valley Vac smoke evacuation s.
Vesica press-in suture anchor s.
VestaBlate s.
Vidas automated immunoassay s.
Vidas immunoanalysis testing s.
visual magnocellular s.
Vivelle-Dot estradiol transdermal s.

S

NOTES

system *(continued)*
    Wallaby Phototherapy S.
    WAVE nucleic acid fragment
      analysis s.
systematicus
    nevus pigmentosus s.
systematisata
    melanoblastosis cutis linearis
      sive s.
systemic
    s. arteriovenous fistula
    s. azole therapy
    s. behavior family therapy
    s. candidiasis
    s. carnitine deficiency
    s. caval return
    s. fatty acid deficiency
    s. flow
    s. illness
    s. inflammatory response syndrome
    (SIRS)
    s. juvenile chronic arthritis
    s. lupus erythematosus (SLE)
    s. manifestation
    s. mastocytosis

    s. outflow obstruction
    s. scleroderma
    s. sclerosis (SS)
    s. side effect
    s. steroid
    s. vascular resistance (SVR)
    s. vasculitis
    s. vasculitis syndrome
    s. venous collateral (SSVC)
systemic-active nonspecific
  immunotherapy
systemic-onset juvenile rheumatoid
  arthritis
systole
systolic
    s. arterial pressure (SAP)
    s. blood pressure
    s. component
    s. continuous murmur
    s. ejection murmur (SEM)
    s. overload
    s. overload pattern
systolic/diastolic ratio (S/D)
Syva test

T

T band
T bone density score
T cell
T connector
T extension
T helper
T lymphocyte
T protein
T strain mycoplasma

T2

diiodothyronine

T3

triiodothyronine

T4

thyroxine

t

t. Y;18 syndrome

TA

Takayasu arteritis
therapeutic abortion
thoracoabdominal

T&A

tonsillectomy and adenoidectomy

¹⁸²Ta

tantalum-182

TAA

tumor-associated antigen

TAB

therapeutic abortion

tab

Apo-Doxy T.'s
Meda T.

Tabb crura tissue forceps

tabes

t. dorsalis
t. infantum
juvenile t.
t. mesenterica

tabetic neurosyphilis

table

Bayley-Pinneau t.
contingency t.
cross t.
cystoscopy t.
height t.

tablet

Actifed Allergy T.
Allerest Children's T.'s
Aviane-28 t.
Benadryl Decongestant Allergy T.
Bextra t.
bisacodyl t.
Bromfed T.
Cenestin t.

Coricidin T.'s
Coricidin-D T.'s
Cryselle t.
Cyclessa t.
Dexone T.
Enpresse t.
Focalin t.
Hexadrol T.
Histalet Forte T.
hormonal pregnancy test t.
Levlite t.
Materna T.'s
Metadate ER t.'s
Methitest t.
Mircette t.
Mylocel t.
NatalCare Plus film-coated t.
NataTab CFe film-coated t.
NataTab FA film-coated t.
NataTab Rx film-coated t.
Prenate GT delayed-release gel-
coated t.
Remifemin Menopause t.
Trivora-28 t.
Veltane T.

tabula rasa

TAC

tetracaine, adrenaline, cocaine
transient aplastic crisis

Tac-3 Injection

tache noir

tachyarrhythmia

atrial t.
supraventricular t. (SVT)

tachyarrhythmia-bradyarrhythmia (tachy-brady)

tachy-brady

tachyarrhythmia-bradyarrhythmia
tachy-brady syndrome

tachycardia

aberrant supraventricular t.
accelerated junctional ectopic t.
atrial t.
atrioventricular nodal reentrant t.
(AVNRT)
atrioventricular reciprocating t.
(AVRT)
automatic atrial t.
AV nodal reentry t.
baseline fetal t.
chaotic atrial t.
congenital paroxysmal atrial t.
ectopic atrial t.
fetal t.
junctional t.

T

tachycardia *(continued)*
    junctional ectopic t. (JET)
    maternal t.
    multifocal atrial t.
    narrow complex supraventricular t.
    nodal t.
    nonsustained ventricular t.
    paraventricular t.
    paroxysmal t.
    paroxysmal atrial t. (PAT)
    persistent t.
    postural t.
    reentrant supraventricular t.
    sinus t.
    supraventricular t. (SVT)
    sustained ventricular t.
    ventricular t.
    wide complex t.
tachydysrhythmia
    supraventricular t.
tachygastria
tachyphylaxis
tachypnea
    transient t.
tachypneic
tachysystole
    uterine t.
tacker
    Origin T.
tackling
    spear t.
tacrolimus
tactile
    t. defensiveness
    t. discrimination
    t. fever
    t. fremitus
    t. hallucination
    t. sensory monitoring
    t. stimulation
    t. stimulus
    t. temperature
Taenia
    T. saginata
    T. solium
taeniasis
TAF
    tracheobronchial aspirate fluid
    tumor angiogenesis factor
tag
    cutaneous t.
    expressed sequence t.
    hymenal t.
    perianal skin t.
    preauricular t.
    skin t.
Tagamet-HB
Tago diagnostic kit

TAH
    total abdominal hysterectomy
tail
    axillary t.
    t. bud
    Spence axillary t.
tailgut
tailor sitting
Taiwan acute respiratory (TWAR)
Takao syndrome
Takayasu
    T. arteritis (TA)
    T. disease
TAL
    tendo Achillis lengthening
talar
    t. decancellation
    t. dome fracture
    t. to first metatarsal angle
    t. tilt test
talc
talcum powder
tali (*pl. of* talus)
talipes
    t. calcaneovalgus
    t. calcaneovarus
    t. calcaneus
    t. cavovalgus
    t. cavus
    t. equinovalgus
    t. equinovarus (TEV)
    t. equinovarus deformity
    t. equinus
    t. hobble splint
    t. planovalgus
    t. planus
    t. valgus
    t. varus
talipomanus
talk
    receptor cross t.
talking
    sleep t.
talocalcaneal (TC)
    t. angle (TCA)
    t. bar
    t. fusion
talus, pl. **tali**
    congenital vertical t.
    vertical t.
Talwin NX
Tambocor
TAME
    tosylarginine methyl ester
Tamm-Horsfall
    T.-H. mucoprotein
    T.-H. protein
Tamofen
Tamone

tamoxifen
    t. citrate
    Cytoxan, methotrexate, fluorouracil,
      prednisone, t. (CMFPT)
tampon
    nasal t.
    t. test
    vaginal t.
tamponade
    balloon t.
    cardiac t.
    gastroesophageal balloon t.
    pericardial t.
tandem
    T. Icon II hCG
    t. mass spectrometry
    t.-repeat
    t. repeat sequence
    t. walking
Tandem-R Ostase osteoporosis test
tangential breast field
Tangier disease
tangle
Tanner
    T. classification (1–5)
    T. Developmental Scale
    T. developmental stage (1–5)
    T. genital stage (1–5)
    T. maturation stage (1–5)
    T. sex maturity rating
    T. stage
    T. stages of development (1–5)
    T. staging (1–5)
    T. staging of genital development
      (1–5)
Tanner-Whitehouse
    T.-W. bone age reference value
    T.-W. II bone/age determination
      method
tan papilloma
tantalum
    t.-182 (^{182}Ta)
tantrum
    temper t.
tanycyte
TAP
    transport-associated protein
    transvaginal amniotic puncture
    trypsin activation peptide
tap
    bladder t.
    infant subdural t.

    lung t.
    percutaneous lung t.
    peritoneal t.
    shunt t.
    spinal t.
    subdural t.
    supraciliary t.
    ventricular t.
    VP shunt t.
    wet t.
Tapanol
Tapar
Tapazole
tape
    Broselow t.
    glucose oxidase test t.
    lap t.
    Medipore H soft cloth surgical t.
    tension-free vaginal t. (TVT)
    twill t.
tapering cytoplasmic process
tapetoretinal degeneration
tapeworm
    pork t.
taping
    buddy t.
tapir
    levre de t.
    t. mouth
tapiroid
TAPVC
    total anomalous pulmonary venous
      connection
TAPVR
    total anomalous pulmonary venous return
Taq **I enzyme**
TAR
    thrombocytopenia absent radius
    TAR syndrome
tar
    Aqua T.
    coal t.
    DHS T.
tarda
    chondrodystrophia congenita t.
    Edwardsiella t.
    hypophosphatasia t.
    lymphedema t.
    osteopetrosis t.
    porphyria cutanea t.
    spondyloepiphyseal dysplasia t.

T

NOTES

tardive
    t. dyskinesia
    t. dystonia
target
    t. cell
    t. lesion
    t. organ response
targeted
    t. ultrasonographic examination
    t. ultrasound
targeting
    gene t.
targetoid lesion
Tariverdian syndrome
Tarkowski method
Tarnier axis-traction forceps
Taro-Ampicillin
Taro-Cloxacillin
Taro-Sone
tarry cyst
tarsal
    t. coalition
    t. navicular osteochondritis
    t. plate
tarsal-carpal coalition syndrome
tarsalis
    Culex t.
tarsi (*pl. of* tarsus)
tarsometatarsal mobilization
tarsorrhaphy
tarsus, pl. **tarsi**
tartrate
    butorphanol t.
    ergotamine t.
    metoprolol t.
    zolpidem t.
Tarui disease
TAS
    Toronto Alexithymia Scale
task
    Continuous Performance T.
    t. load
    Paired Associate Learning T.
      (PALT)
    phoneme segmentation t.
    phonemic awareness t.
taste
    t. bud
    impaired t.
TAS/TVS
    transabdominal/transvaginal ultrasound
TAT
    tetanus antitoxin
    tray agglutination test
    tyrosine aminotransferase
TATD
    tyrosine aminotransferase deficiency
taurine
taurodontism

Taussig-Bing
    T.-B. anomaly
    T.-B. disease
    T.-B. syndrome
tautomenial
taxis
    bipolar t.
Taxol
Taxotere
Taybi-Linder syndrome
Taybi syndrome
Taylor dispersion
Tay-Sachs
    T.-S. disease
    T.-S. disease with visceral
      involvement
Tay syndrome
tazarotene
Tazicef
Tazidime
tazobactam
    piperacillin and t.
    t. sodium
TB
    tuberculosis
TBARS
    thiobarbituric acid-reacting substance
TBE
    tick-borne encephalitis
TBG
    thyroid-binding globulin
    thyroxine-binding globulin
      TBG deficiency
      TBG excess
TBI
    total body irradiation
    traumatic brain injury
TBK
    total body potassium
TBLC
    term birth, living child
TBMD
    thin basement membrane disease
TBP
    thyroxine-binding protein
TBSA
    total body surface area
      TBSA burned
TBW
    total body water
TC
    talocalcaneal
    transcobalamin (I, II) deficiency
TC7 adhesion barrier
TCA
    talocalcaneal angle
    trichloroacetic acid
    tricyclic antidepressant

TcB
  transcutaneous bilirubin
TCC
  transcatheter closure
TCD
  transcranial Doppler
TCE
  trichloroethanol
T-cell
  T-c. activation defect
  T-c. antibody induction therapy
  T-c. depletion
  T-c. dysfunction
  T-c. lymphoma
  T-c. subset
  T-c. trophic (T-trophic, T-tropic)
T-cell-depleted
  T.-c.-d. graft
  T.-c.-d. haploidentical bone marrow stem cell
T-cell-mediated disease
T-cell-tropic syncytium-inducing strain
Tc HMPAO
  technetium hexamethylpropyleneamine oxime
    Tc HMPAO leukocyte scan
TCI
  T. OcuLook saliva ovulation tester kit
  T. OvuLook ovulation tester
TCIFTT
  transcervical intrafallopian tube transfer
tCpO$_2$
  transcutaneous partial pressure of oxygen
TCT coagulation test
TD
  Tourette disorder
  traveler's diarrhea
T.D.
  Diamine T.
Td
  tetanus and diphtheria
    Td toxoid vaccine
TdaP-IPV vaccine
TdaP vaccine
TDEE
  total daily energy expenditure
T/Derm
  Neutrogena T.
TDF
  testis-determining factor

TDI
  therapeutic donor insemination
  tissue Doppler imaging
Td-IPV vaccine
TDLU
  terminal ductal lobular unit
  terminal duct lobular unit
TDT
  transmission disequilibrium test
TDxFLM Assay
TDxFLx Assay
tdy gene
TE
  thromboembolic event
tea
  herbal t.
TEACCH
  treatment and education of autistic and related communications handicapped children
    Project TEACCH
teacher
  infant t.
  T. Rating Form (TRF)
  T. Report Form (TRF)
team
  interdisciplinary t.
  multidisciplinary t.
  Patient Outcomes Research T. (PORT)
  Sexual Assault Response T. (SART)
  transdisciplinary t.
tear
  absent t.'s
  t. film
  Mallory-Weiss t. (MWT)
  meniscus t.
  no t.'s
  t. overflow
  syndrome of crocodile t.'s
tear-drop vesicle
T4/ebp-1
  thyroid-specific enhancer binding protein-1
Tebrazid
TEC
  transient erythroblastopenia of childhood
technetium
  t. bone scan
  t. hexamethylpropyleneamine oxime (Tc HMPAO)

NOTES

technetium-labeled red blood cell
technetium-99m
    t. bone scan
    t. pertechnetate
technical artifact
technique (*See also* surgery, procedure,
    operation)
        agar gel precipitation t.
        agar immunoprecipitin t.
        automated radiometric t.
        Ayre spatula-Zelsmyr Cytobrush t.
        balloon catheter t.
        Ball pelvimetry t.
        Barlow mitral regurgitation repair t.
        Beverly-Douglas lip-tongue
            adhesion t.
        biofeedback t.
        brain imaging t.
        Brockenbrough transseptal
            catheterization t.
        Brown-Wickham urethral pressure
            profilometry t.
        Bruhat t.
        buccal feeding t.
        capillary isoelectric focusing t.
        catheter-in-a-catheter t.
        catheter-over-needle t.
        catheter-over-wire t.
        clean-catch t.
        clip t.
        clonogenic t.
        cobalt-60 moving strip t.
        Cobb measurement t.
        Cohen transtrigonal t.
        Colcher-Sussman x-ray pelvimetry t.
        contraceptive t.
        Counsellor-Flor modification of
            McIndoe t.
        dead space t.
        2-diameter pocket t.
        Döderlein hysterectomy t.
        dot-blot t.
        double-catheter t.
        double-freeze t.
        Dufourmentel transposition flap t.
        Dyban oocyte fixation t.
        Eklund mammography t.
        enzyme-multiplication
            immunoassay t. (EMIT)
        enzyme-multiplied immunoassay t.
            (EMIT)
        evoked potential t.
        ex utero intrapartum t. (EXIT)
        ferning t.
        fetal assessment t.
        fetal surveillance t.
        Gittes bladder suspension t.
        Glenn-Anderson ureteric reflux
            repair t.

Goebell-Frangenheim-Stoeckel
    urethrovesical suspension t.
Gomco circumcision t.
gracilis flap t.
GRASS MRI t.
Hamou t.
Heaney vaginal vault closure t.
hemisection uterine morcellation t.
hold t.
hook traction t.
hybridoma t.
hyperglycemic clamp t.
hyperinsulinemic-euglycemic
    clamp t.
immune monitoring t.
immune separation t.
immunoperoxidase t.
insemination swim-up t.
intraluminal electrical impedance t.
Jones and Jones wedge t.
Kety-Schmidt cerebral blood flow
    measurement t.
Kidde cannula t.
Kleihauer fetomaternal hemorrhage
    estimation t.
labial traction t.
Lapides vesicourethropexy t.
Lazarus-Nelson closed peritoneal
    lavage t.
Leboyer episiotomy t.
Lich-Gregoire t.
Lich vesicoureteral reflux repair t.
Limberg flap t.
loss-of-resistance t.
marsupialization t.
M-FISH cytogenetic t.
minimally invasive surgical t.
    (MIST)
Mitrofanoff continent urinary
    diversion t.
Miyazaki t.
modified Pomeroy tubal ligation t.
molecular genetic t.
multicolor FISH cytogenetic t.
multipuncture t.
Mustard TGA t.
myofascial release t.
NAA t.
Nuss concave chest correction t.
Ortolani congenital hip
    dislocation t.
oscillometric t.
pants-over-vest t.
Parkland Hospital t.
Percoll sperm preparation t.
percutaneous multipuncture t.
percutaneous Seldinger t.
Politano-Leadbetter
    ureteroneocystostomy t.

Pomeroy tubal ligation t.
pull-through t.
recombinant DNA t.
relaxation t.
reverse FISH cytogenetic t.
rollerball t.
Seldinger t.
shoelace t.
Simonton t.
single-isotope tracer t.
skate flap t.
skinfold caliper t.
snapshot GRASS t.
soluble gas t.
Southern blot t.
sperm retrieval t.
split-flap t.
Strassman t.
Stringer t.
surveillance t.
swim-up t.
thorascopic t.
three-point t.
Tompkins median bivalving t.
toothbrush culture t.
tripod fixation t.
tubal ligation band t.
tube insertion t.
U t.
Wallace t.

technology
assisted reproductive t. (ART)
assistive t. (AT)
genetic engineering t.
recombinant DNA t.
reproductive t.
Society for Assisted
Reproductive T. (SART)
t. transfer
ultrasound t.

Technos ultrasound system
tectal brainstem glioma
tectocephaly
tectocerebellar dysraphia
tectum
mesencephalic t.

TED
thromboembolic disease
TED stocking

teddy-bear gait
TEE
transesophageal echocardiography

Teebi syndrome
Teejel
teenager
Problem-Oriented Screening
Instrument for T.'s (POSIT)

Teen-Tot Clinic
teeth
baby t.
conical t.
crowded t.
deciduous t.
Fournier t.
Hutchinson t.
hypoplastic t.
mental retardation, congenital heart
disease, blepharophimosis,
blepharoptosis, hypoplastic t.
milk t.
missing t.
Moon t.
natal t.
neonatal t.
peglike t.
permanent t.
pitted t.
precocious t.
predeciduous t.
primary t.
screwdriver t.
secondary t.
X-linked cataract with
hutchinsonian t.

teething
Babee T.

TEF
thermic effect of food
tracheoesophageal fistula
transesophageal fistula

Teflon-coated wire
Teflon periurethral injection
tegmen, pl. **tegmina**
tegmentum, pl. **tegmenta**
Tegretol
Tegretol-XR
Tegrin-HC Topical
teicoplanin
Teilum tumor
telangiectasia
ataxia t.
calcinosis, Raynaud phenomenon,
esophageal dysmotility,
sclerodactyly, t. (CREST)

T

NOTES

953

telangiectasia *(continued)*
>calcinosis, Raynaud phenomenon, sclerodactyly, t. (CRST)
>flat red-black t.
>hemorrhagic t.
>hereditary hemorrhagic t. (HHT)
>intestinal t.
>t. macularis eruptiva perstans
>nail bed t.
>nail fold t.
>oculocutaneous t.
>raised red-black t.
>red-black t.
>retinal vessel t.

telangiectasis
>conjunctival t.
>cutaneous t.

telangiectatic
>t. granuloma
>t. nevus
>t. osteosarcoma

telangiectatica
>cutis marmorata t.

telecanthus
telecanthus-hypospadias syndrome
telecardiology
telefetal monitoring
telemammography
telemedicine
telemetry
telencephalic
>t. neuroepithelium
>t. subependymal germinal matrix

teleologic theory
telepsychiatry
teleradiology
teleroentgenogram
telescopy
>percutaneous suprapubic t.

teletherapy
television epilepsy
TeLinde operation
telocentric chromosome
telogen
>t. effluvium
>t. phase

telomere
telophase
TEM
>therapeutic electromembrane
>transanal endoscopic microsurgery
>transmission electron microscopy

temazepam
Temovate
Temp-a-dot thermometer
temperament
>shy-inhibited t.

temperature
>absolute t.
>ambient t.
>artificial t.
>aseptic t.
>aural t.
>axillary t.
>basal body t. (BBT)
>body t.
>core t.
>critical t.
>t. dysregulation
>ephemeral t.
>erratic t.
>eruptive t.
>maximum t. (T-max)
>normal t.
>oral t.
>t. pattern
>rectal t.
>room t.
>skin t.
>subnormal t.
>tactile t.
>tympanic t.

temperature-controlled isolette
temper tantrum
template
>Syed-Neblett dedicated vulvar plastic t.

temporal
>t. balding
>t. lobe
>t. lobe epilepsy
>t. lobe seizure
>t. sequencing

temporale
>planum t.

temporalis muscle
temporary diverting colostomy
temporomandibular
>t. joint (TMJ)
>t. joint dysfunction

temporospatial pattern
Tempra
Temtamy syndrome
TEN
>titanium elastic nailing
>toxic epidermal necrolysis

tenacious
tenaculum, pl. **tenacula**
>Braun-Schroeder single-tooth t.
>cervical t.
>double-tooth t.
>Emmett cervical t.
>t. hook
>t. hook loop
>Jacobs t.
>Schroeder uterine t.
>single-tooth t.
>uterine t.

Tenckhoff catheter
tendency
    familial t.
    prothrombic t.
tender enthesis
tenderness
    abdominal t.
    cervical motion t. (CMT)
    costovertebral angle t. (CVAT)
    CVA t.
    epigastric t.
    fundal t.
    joint line t.
    lower abdominal t.
    pelvic t.
    point t.
    point of maximum t. (PMT)
    rebound t.
    snuffbox t.
Tender-Touch
    T.-T. extractor
    T.-T. vacuum birthing cup
tendineae, pl. tendineae
    chordae tendinea
tendineus
    arcus t.
tendinitis, tendonitis
    patellar t.
    triceps t.
tendinous arch
tendo
    t. Achillis
    t. Achillis lengthening (TAL)
tendon
    Achilles t.
    bowstringing of t.
    calcaneal t.
    conjoined t.
    fat flexor hallucis longus t.
    flexor hallucis longus t.
    t. forceps
    t. lengthening
    peroneus brevis t.
    peroneus longus t.
    split flexor hallucis longus t.
    t. stretch reflex
    t. transfer
    t. xanthoma
tendon-bone interface
tendonitis (*var. of* tendinitis)
tenesmus
    perimenstrual t.

Tenex
teniposide
Tenney-Parker sign
tennis elbow
Tennison-Randall repair
tenosynovial sarcoma
tenosynovioma
tenosynovitis
tenosynovitis-dermatitis
tenotomy
    percutaneous adductor t.
TENS
    transcutaneous electrical nerve stimulation
tense
    t. ascites
    t. blister
    t. lobule
Tensilon test
tension
    t. cyst
    end-tidal CO_2 t.
    t. headache
    t. hydrothorax
    t. myalgia
    t. pneumocephalus
    t. pneumothorax
    postmenstrual t. (PMT)
    premenstrual t.
    surface t.
    vaginal tape t.
tension-discharging phenomenon
tension-free
    t.-f. vaginal tape (TVT)
    t.-f. vaginal tape procedure
tensor fasciae latae (TFL)
tent
    CAM t.
    face t.
    intracervical t.
    laminaria t.
    mist t.
    oxygen t.
    Silon t.
tenting
    skin t.
tentorial
    t. laceration
    t. margin
    t. opening
tentorium
Tenuate

NOTES

tenuis
  Dirofilaria t.
tenuous
Tenzel calipers
TEOAE
  transient evoked otoacoustic emission
  TEOAE testing
tepid
teras, pl. **terata**
teratism
teratoblastoma
teratocarcinoma
teratogen
  environmental t.
  t. exposure
  T. Information System (TERIS)
  T. Registry
teratogenesis
teratogenic
  t. agent
  t. effect
  t. exposure
  t. medication
  t. outcome
  t. properties
  t. risk
  t. syndrome
teratogenicity
teratogen-induced malformation
teratoid tumor
teratologic dislocation
teratology
teratoma, pl. **teratomata**
  atypical t.
  benign cystic t. (BCT)
  benign cystic ovarian t.
  cervical t.
  cystic t.
  germ cell t.
  immature t. (grade 0–3)
  immature ovarian t.
  malignant ovarian t.
  mature t.
  mature cystic t.
  mature cystic ovarian t.
  mediastinal t.
  ovarian cystic t.
  ovarian embryonal t.
  pediatric ovarian t.
  sacrococcygeal t.
teratophobia
teratospermia
teratotoxicity
teratozoospermia
Terazol
  T. Vaginal
  T. 3, 7 vaginal cream
  T. vaginal suppository
terbinafine

terbutaline
  caffeine t.
  t. sulfate
terconazole
teres
  ligamentum t.
terfenadine
Terfluzine
ter Haar syndrome
TERIS
  Teratogen Information System
term
  t. AGA
  t. birth, living child (TBLC)
  t. delivery
  full t. (FT)
  t. gestation
  t. infant
  t. infants, premature infants, abortions, living children (TPAL)
  t. LGA
  t. pregnancy
  t. SGA
Term-Guard
terminal
  t. blush
  t. blush formation
  t. bronchiole
  t. cardiotocogram
  t. choledochus
  t. complement component
  t. complement component deficiency
  t. deletion
  t. deoxyribonucleotidyl transferase-mediated biotin-16-dUTP nick-end labeling (TUNEL)
  t. ductal lobular unit (TDLU)
  t. duct lobular unit (TDLU)
  t. hair
  t. heating method
  t. ileitis
  t. lung differentiation
  t. maturation
  t. motor latency
  t. neosalpingostomy
  t. saccular period
  t. transverse acheiria defect
  t. transverse limb defect
terminale
  filum t.
  ossiculum t.
  ropelike filum t.
terminalis
  lamina t.
terminate
termination
  t. codon
  elective t.

first trimester t.
medical t.
t. of parental rights
pregnancy t.
second trimester t.
selective t.
surgical t.
terminus
vaginal t.
Terramycin I.M. Injection
terreus
Aspergillus t.
terror
night t.
sleep t.
terrorizing
Terry
T. questionnaire
T. syndrome
Terson disease
tertiary
t. care center
t. closure
t. hypothyroidism
t. prevention
t. referral hospital
t. syphilis
TESA
testicular sperm aspiration
Teschler-Nicola and Killian syndrome
TESE
testicular sperm extraction
Teslac
Tessier craniofacial operation
TEST
tubal embryo stage transfer
test (*See also* testing)
Accu-Chek t.
AccuStat hCG pregnancy t.
acid elution t.
acidified serum lysis t.
acoustic reflex t.
acoustic stimulation t. (AST)
ACTH stimulation t.
activated partial thromboplastin time
coagulation t.
Adams forward-bending t.
Affirm VPIII t.
agglutination inhibition t.
air leak t.
Alcohol Use Disorders
Identification T. (AUDIT)

Allen-Doisy t.
Allen picture t.
alternate-cover t.
alternating breath t. (ABT)
ambulatory uterine contraction t.
Amiel-Tison t.
amine t.
AmnioStat-FLM t.
AneuVysion Assay prenatal
genetic t.
anterior drawer t.
antigen detection t.
antiglobulin t.
antitreponemal t.
Apley compression t.
apprehension t.
APT-Downey t.
APTT coagulation t.
arginine-insulin stimulation t.
arginine-insulin tolerance t.
arginine tolerance t. (ATT)
Aschheim-Zondek t.
automated reagin t. (ART)
BAER t.
Ballard t.
Barlow hip dysplasia t.
Barlow and Ortolani t.
BD t.
Bender Visual Motor Gestalt T.
Benton Visual Retention T.
Berens 3-character t.
Bernstein t.
Betke-Kleihauer t.
BH_4 loading t.
Biocept-G pregnancy t.
Biocept-5 pregnancy t.
BioStar Strep A OIA t.
bitterling pregnancy t.
bladder muscle stress t.
bladder neck elevation t.
block design t.
blood-type t.
Bonney blue stress incontinence t.
Boston Naming T.
bovine mucus penetration t.
BRACA mutation t.
branching snowflake t.
Bratton-Marshall t.
breast stimulation contraction t.
(BSCT)
breath H_2 t.
breath hydrogen excretion t.

NOTES

957

test *(continued)*
    Breslow-Day t.
    Brodie-Trendelenburg t.
    bronchial challenge t.
    Brouha t.
    Bruckner pupillary light reflex t.
    Bruininks-Oseretsky t.
    BTA stat t.
    bubble stability t.
    Burt Word Reading T.
    CAGE t.
    cAMP t.
    cancer antigen 125 t.
    Candida skin t.
    caramel t.
    carbon-14 t.
    carbon-13 urea breath t.
    Cattell Infant Intelligence T.
    CF t.
    Children of Alcoholics
      Screening T. (CAST)
    Children's Depression Inventory t.
    Children's Eating Attitudes T.
      (ChEAT)
    Chlamydiazyme t.
    chlortetracycline fluorescence t.
    chromosome breakage t.
    Clearview hCG pregnancy t.
    Clinical Adaptive T. (CAT)
    clomiphene citrate challenge t.
      (CCCT, C3T)
    coagulation t.
    cocaine t.
    Colaris genetic susceptibility t.
    Collins t.
    Color Trails T.
    complement t.
    complementation t.
    complement fixation t.
    Concise Plus hCG urine t.
    continuous performance t. (CPT)
    contraction stress t. (CST)
    Coombs t.
    corneal light reflex t.
    Corner-Allen t.
    Corsi block tapping t.
    Cortrosyn stimulation t.
    cosyntropin stimulation t.
    cotton swab t.
    cough t.
    cover t.
    cover-uncover eye t.
    criterion-referenced t.
    C-urea breath t.
    cyclic adenosine monophosphate t.
    cytochrome oxidase t.
    DAP t.
    deferoxamine challenge t.

    dehydroepiandrosterone sulfate
      loading t.
    Denver Developmental Screening T.
      (DDST)
    Denver Developmental Screening T.
      II
    dexamethasone suppression t.
    DFA t.
    Dick t.
    DIF t.
    differential agglutination t.
    Digene Hybrid Capture II HPV T.
    diiodothyronine t.
    dipstick t.
    direct antiglobulin t. (DAT)
    direct Coombs t.
    DNA probe t.
    dot-blot HPV hybridization t.
    dot ELISA t.
    Draw-a-Person T.
    Duncan t.
    dye decolorization t.
    dye disappearance t.
    Eagle t.
    early pregnancy t. (EPT)
    Eastern blot t.
    Eating Attitudes T.
    edrophonium t.
    Einstein screening t.
    Elek t.
    ELISA t.
    ELISpot t.
    enzyme-linked antiglobulin t.
    epicutaneous t.
    estrogen-progestin t.
    E-tegrity t.
    Expressive One-Word Picture
      Vocabulary T.
    factor V Leiden mutation t.
    Fact Plus Pro pregnancy t.
    family-based t.
    Farber t.
    Farr t.
    FAST blood t.
    fern t.
    ferric chloride t.
    ferritin level t.
    fetal acoustic stimulation t.
    fetal activity t.
    fetal fibronectin t.
    fetal surveillance t.
    Fibrindex t.
    figure-of-four t.
    finger-nose-finger t.
    finger-tapping t.
    fingertip number writing t.
    finger-to-nose t.
    five-hop t.
    five-hour glucose tolerance t.

FLM t.
fluorescein-conjugated monoclonal antibody t.
fluorescein treponema antibody t.
fluorescence actin staining t.
fluorescence spot t.
fluorescent antimembrane antibody t. (FAMA)
foam stability t. (FST)
food challenge t.
Fortel ovulation t.
forward-bending t.
four-site skinfold t.
Franklin-Dukes t.
Free Running Asthma T. (FRAST)
Frei t.
Friberg microsurgical agglutination t.
Friedman-Lapham t.
Friedman rabbit t.
fructose intolerance t.
FTA t.
galactose breath t.
Gardner Expressive One-Word Vocabulary T.-Revised
gelatin agglutination t.
GeneAmp PCR t.
genetic t.
Gen-Probe amplified CT t.
geometric design t.
germ tube t.
Gesell Preschool T.
Gesell School Readiness T.
Gilmore Oral Reading T. (GORT)
glucose challenge t.
glucose tolerance t. (GTT)
Goldmann perimeter visual field t.
gonadotropin agonist stimulation t. (GAST)
Gonozyme t.
Goodenough-Harris Drawing T.
Gordon Distractibility T.
granulocyte immunofluorescence t. (GIFT)
Gravindex t.
Gray Oral Reading T. (GORT)
Gray Oral Reading T.-Revised (GORT-R)
growth hormone stimulation t. (GHST)
guaiac t.
Guthrie t.

HABA binding t.
hair bulb incubation t.
halo t.
hanging-drop t.
HealthCheck One-Step One Minute pregnancy t.
heel-to-shin t.
Heller t.
hemagglutination t.
hemagglutination treponemal t. (HATT)
Hematest t.
Hemoccult II t.
HemoCue glucose t.
HemoCue hemoglobin t.
hemoglobin S solubility t.
HEMPAS t.
heparan sulfate urine t.
heparin challenge t.
Heritage Panel genetic screening t.
Herp-Check t.
heterophil t.
Hinton t.
hip rotation t.
Hirschberg corneal reflex t.
Hirschberg light reflex t.
HIV t.
HIVAGEN t.
Hogben t.
home pregnancy t.
homocysteine loading t.
1-hour glucose challenge t.
Huhner t.
Huhner-Sims t.
Human Figure Drawing T.
human ovum fertilization t.
hydrogen breath t.
Hypan t.
hyperoxia t.
hyperventilation provocative t.
ICD-p24 t.
Icon serum pregnancy t.
Icon strep B t.
Icon urine pregnancy t.
IDI-Strep B t.
IFA t.
IgA AGA t.
IgA HIV antibody t.
IgG-IFA t.
IgM-IFA t.
IgM indirect fluorescent antibody t.
IHA t.

T

NOTES

test *(continued)*

    immunobead t. (IBT)
    immunofluorescent *Chlamydia* t.
    immunologic pregnancy t.
    impingement t.
    India ink t.
    Indiclor t.
    indirect Coombs t.
    inhibin t.
    insulin sensitivity t.
    insulin tolerance t.
    intelligence t.
    intradermal t.
    inversion stress tilt t.
    ischemic exercise t.
    Isojima t.
    IVA visual consistency t.
    Jadassohn t.
    Kahn t.
    Kapeller-Adler t.
    Kell t.
    Kibrick t.
    Kibrick-Isojima infertility t.
    Kinyoun acid-fast staining t.
    Kleihauer t.
    Kleihauer-Betke t.
    Kodak hCG serum t.
    Kodak SureCell Chlamydia T.
    Kodak SureCell hCG-Urine T.
    Kodak SureCell Herpes (HSV) T.
    Kodak SureCell LCH in-office
      pregnancy t.
    Kodak SureCell Strep A t.
    KOH t.
    Kolmer t.
    Korotkoff t.
    Kremer penetration t.
    Kupperman menopausal distress t.
    Kurzrok-Miller t.
    Kurzrok-Ratner t.
    Kveim t.
    KW t.
    laboratory t.
    Lachman t.
    lactose breath hydrogen t.
    lactose tolerance t.
    Landau t.
    Lange t.
    latex agglutination inhibition t.
      (LAIT)
    latex fixation t.
    latex particle agglutination t.
    LCx Probe System t.
    leak-point pressure t.
    Letter-R intelligence t.
    leucine tolerance t.
    leukocyte histamine release t.
    levothyroxine t.
    LH color t.

    Liddle t.
    limulus lysate t.
    t. of linkage disequilibrium
    liver function t.'s
    Locke-Wallace Marital
      Adjustment t.
    Lumadex-FSI t.
    Lundh t.
    lysis t.
    lysoPC diagnostic ovarian cancer t.
    Macherey-Nagel strep t.
    Mantoux tuberculin skin t.
    MAR t.
    Marchetti t.
    Marshall t.
    Matritech NMP22 bladder cancer t.
    Mazzini t.
    McCaman-Robins t.
    McMurray t.
    McNemar t.
    mental arithmetic t.
    metabolic t.
    methemoglobin reduction t.
    Metopirone t.
    metyrapone t.
    Micral urine dipstick t.
    microhemagglutination t.
    microimmunofluorescence t.
    microscopic agglutination t. (MAT)
    MicroTrak t.
    MIF t.
    Miraluma t.
    monoclonal antibody
      coagglutination t.
    Monospot t.
    Monosticon Dri-Dot t.
    Montenegro skin t.
    mucin clot t.
    Multiple Sleep Latency T. (MSLT)
    multipuncture t. (MPT)
    MultiVysion PB assay t.
    muscle enzyme t.
    NAA t.
    nappy t.
    NBT dye t.
    newborn genetic screening t.
    nipple stimulation t.
    Nitrazine t.
    nitrite urine t.
    nitroblue tetrazolium dye
      reduction t.
    nitrogen washout t.
    Noguchi t.
    nongamma Coombs t.
    noninvasive t.
    nonstress t. (NST)
    nontreponemal t.
    norm-referenced t.
    Northern blot t.

N-telopeptide t.
NTx t.
OAE t.
object assembly t.
Ogita t.
Omniprobe t.
OncoScint t.
one-hour glucose tolerance t.
Optochin t.
oral glucose challenge t. (OGCT)
oral glucose tolerance t. (OGTT)
OraSure oral HIV t.
O'Riain wrinkle t.
orthostatic t.
Ortolani t.
osmotic fragility t.
OsteoGram bone density t.
Osteomark NTx serum t.
Osteosal t.
Otis-Lennon Intelligence T.
OvuKIT t.
OvuQuick Self-T.
oxytocin challenge t. (OCT)
oxytocin stress t.
PACE-2C DNA probe t.
paced auditory serial addition t.
T. PackChlamydia test
pad t.
PapNet t.
passive head-up tilt t.
Pathfinder DFA t.
Paul-Bunnell antibody t.
Paul-Bunnell-Davidsohn t.
PCR t.
Peabody Picture Vocabulary T. (PPVT)
Peabody Picture Vocabulary T.-Revised (PPVT-R)
Penetrak t.
phenolsulfonphthalein t.
phenylketonuria t.
picture completion t.
pinhole t.
PKU t.
plasmacrit t.
platelet function t.
poor man's clot t.
Porges-Meier t.
postcoital t. (PCT)
postvoid residual urine t.
Prechtl t.
Precise pregnancy t.

predictive value of t.
pregnancy t.
prick t.
Profile viral probe t.
progesterone challenge t.
prone extension t.
prothrombin time coagulation t.
provocation t.
provocative stress t.
PSA t.
psychometric t.
PT coagulation t.
pulmonary function t. (PFT)
QTest Strep t.
Quality of Upper Extremities T. (QUEST)
quantitative intradermal skin t.
quantitative sudomotor axon-reflex t.
Queckenstedt t.
Quick t.
QuickVue *Chlamydia* t.
QuickVue In-Line One-Step Strep A t.
QuickVue one-step hCG-Combo pregnancy t.
QuickVue One-Step hCG-urine t.
QuickVue One-Step *H. pylori* t.
Quidel group B strep t.
QuikPac-II OneStep hCG pregnancy t.
radioallergosorbent t. (RAST)
radioimmunosorbent t. (RIST)
rapid antigen detection t.
rapid plasma reagin card t.
rapid slide t.
rapid strep t.
red glass t.
red reflex t.
reflex HPV t.
renal clearance t.
renal function t.
Reynell Verbal Comprehension T.
Rinne t.
rollover t.
Romberg t.
Rorschach t.
rosette t.
Rotazyme t.
Rotter Sentence Completion T.
routine preoperative t.
Rovsing t.

NOTES

test *(continued)*
  Rubin t.
  Sabin-Feldman dye t.
  SalEst system t.
  saline drop t.
  salivary estriol t.
  Schick t.
  Schiff t.
  Schiller t.
  Schilling t.
  Schober t.
  Scotch tape slide t.
  screening laboratory t.
  Sephadex binding t.
  serologic t.
  serum t.
  shake t.
  Short Michigan Alcoholism
    Screening T. (SMAST)
  Sickledex t.
  similarities t.
  Sims-Huhner t.
  SISI t.
  skin prick t.
  Slosson Oral Reading T.-Revised
    (SORT-R)
  Snellen t.
  Soluprick skin prick t.
  Sonoclot t.
  Southern blot t.
  sperm agglutination t.
  sperm function t.
  sperm immobilization t.
  SpermMAR mixed antiglobulin
    reaction t.
  spirometric t.
  spot t.
  stable microbubble t.
  Staclot t.
  standardized t.
  Stanford-Binet Intelligence T.
  Stanford Diagnostic Reading T.
  stimulation t.
  stool antigen t.
  STORCH t.
  straight catheter t.
  Streptex rapid strep t.
  streptococcus rapid antigen
    detection t.
  Streptozyme t.
  stress t.
  strip t.
  Stroop t.
  sucrose hemolysis t.
  SUDS HIV-1 antibody t.
  sunflower oil challenge t.
  supine empty stress t. (SEST)
  supine pressor t.
  supravital stain t.

  SureCell Herpes (HSV) T.
  swab t.
  sweat chloride t.
  swinging flashlight t.
  swordfish t.
  Syva t.
  talar tilt t.
  tampon t.
  Tandem-R Ostase osteoporosis t.
  TCT coagulation t.
  Tensilon t.
  Test PackChlamydia t.
  tetraiodothyronine t.
  Thayer-Martin gonorrhea t.
  therapeutic pulmonary function t.
  ThinPrep Pap t.
  Thorn t.
  thrombin clot t.
  thrombin clotting time
    coagulation t.
  Thrombostat platelet function t.
  Thrombo-Wellco t.
  thrombus precursor protein t.
  thymol turbidity t.
  thyroid function t. (TFT)
  thyrotropin-releasing hormone
    stimulation t.
  thyroxine t.
  tilt t.
  tilt-table t.
  tine t.
  tissue thromboplastin-inhibition t.
  Titmus stereoacuity t.
  TOH t.
  TOL t.
  toluidine blue t.
  TPI t.
  TpP t.
  Trail Making T.
  transglutaminase antibody t.
  transmission disequilibrium t. (TDT)
  transmission/disequilibrium t.
  tray agglutination t. (TAT)
  Trendelenburg t.
  Treponema pallidum
    immobilization t.
  triiodothyronine t.
  triple screen t.
  triple swab t.
  tuberculin t.
  tuberculin skin t. (TST)
  Tuttle t.
  Tzanck t.
  UCG-Slide T.
  Uniprobe t.
  urea breath t. (UBT)
  Uri-Check t.
  urinary concentration t.
  urinary dipstick t.

urine CIE t.
urine ferric chloride t.
urine latex t.
Uriscreen urine t.
Urispec GPA t.
Urispec 9-Way t.
vaginal cornification t.
vaginal mucification t.
van den Bergh t.
T. of Variables of Attention (TOVA)
t. of variables of attention deficit disorder
VDRL t.
Venning-Brown t.
ViraPap HPV DNA t.
ViraType t.
visual-motor integration t.
visual-perceptual t.
vocabulary t.
Vysis PathVysion genomic disease management t.
Wada t.
Wampole t.
Wasserman t.
water t.
Watson-Schwartz t.
Weber t.
Wepman Auditory Discrimination T.
Western blot t.
wet mount t.
wheat sperm agglutination t.
whiff amine t.
Whitaker t.
Wide Range Achievement T.-Revised (WRAT-R)
Wide Range Assessment of Memory and Learning T.
Wisconsin Card Sorting T. (WCST)
withdrawal bleeding t.
Woodcock-Johnson reading t.
WRAML t.
Xenopus t.
Ziehl-Neelsen t.
zona-free hamster egg penetration t.
ZstatFlu t.

test/assay
Berkson-Gage t.

tester
TCI OvuLook ovulation t.
testes (*pl. of* testis)
testicle
undescended t.
testicular
t. absence
t. appendage
t. appendage torsion
t. atrophy
t. attachment
t. cancer
t. descent
t. differentiation
t. dislocation
t. dysfunction
t. dysgenesis
t. feminization
t. feminization syndrome
t. flow scan
t. growth
t. hematoma
t. hypertrophy
t. Kaposi sarcoma
t. leukemia
t. neoplasm
t. pull-down
t. relapse
t. rupture
t. sperm aspiration (TESA)
t. sperm extraction (TESE)
t. steroidogenesis
t. tumor
t. volume
testing (*See also* test)
airway reactivity t.
ambulatory t.
antenatal t.
antepartum fetal t.
antimicrobial susceptibility t.
audiological t.
audiometric t.
breath t.
bronchial provocation t.
carrier t.
couple t.
cranial nerve t.
dexamethasone suppression t. (DST)
DNA t.
DNA-based t.
dynamic exercise t.
fecal occult blood t. (FOBT)

T

NOTES

testing *(continued)*
    fetal maturity t.
    fetal surveillance t.
    FP blood lead t.
    genetic t.
    inhalation bronchial challenge t.
    Institute of Personality and
      Ability T. (IPAT)
    invasive t.
    laryngopharyngeal sensory
      stimulation t.
    ligase chain reaction t.
    LPSS t.
    manual muscle t.
    methacholine provocation t.
    muscle t.
    mutation t.
    nonreassuring fetal t.
    OAE t.
    oral glucose tolerance t. (OGTT)
    outpatient fetal nonstress t.
    PapNet t.
    paracoccidioidin skin t.
    postcoital t.
    provocative bronchial challenge t.
    pulmonary function t.
    rapid filter t.
    rectal compliance t.
    routine prenatal t.
    salivary estriol t.
    serologic t.
    Simultaneous Technique for Acuity
      and Readiness T. (STAR)
    2-step t.
    sweat t.
    TEOAE t.
    thermoregulatory sweat t.
    thyrotropin t.
    tuberculin t.
    upright tilt-table t.
    urodynamics t.
    Weil-Felix antibody t.
testis, pl. **testes**
    absent testes
    acquired ascending undescended t.
    adenocarcinoma of infantile t.
    anular t.
    appendix t.
    canalicular t.
    contralateral hypertrophy of testes
    cryptorchid t.
    t. determination
    dislocated t.
    testes down
    dysgenetic t.
    ectopic t.
    endocrine nonfunctional t.
    femoral t.
    gonadotropin-resistant t.

    hidden t.
    high annular t.
    high scrotal t.
    intraabdominal t.
    maldescensus t.
    t. migration defect
    nonpalpable t.
    perineal t.
    prepenile t.
    rete t.
    retractile t.
    scrotal t.
    spontaneous descent of testes
    superficial ectopic t.
    torsion of t.
    transverse scrotal t.
    true undescended t.
    t. tumor
    undescended t.
    vanished testes
    t. within superficial inguinal pouch
      of Denis Browne
    yolk sac tumor of t.
testis-determining factor (TDF)
testitoxicosis
Testoderm
    T. Transdermal System
    T. TTS
    T. with Adhesive
test-of-cure culture
testolactone
testosterone
    bound t.
    circulating t.
    t. cypionate
    t. enanthate
    ethinyl t.
    free t.
    t. index
    non-sex hormone-binding globulin
      bound t.
    plasma t.
    serum t.
    t. suppression
    topical t.
    total t.
testosterone/dihydrotestosterone ratio
testosterone-estrogen-binding globulin
testosterone-secreting adrenal adenoma
testotoxicosis
Testred
Testsimplets prestained slide
test-tube baby
TET
    tubal embryo transfer
tet
    tetralogy of Fallot
      tet spell

tetani
    Clostridium t.
tetania
    t. gravidarum
    t. neonatorum
tetanic
    t. seizure
    t. spasm
    t. uterine contraction
    t. uterus
tetanism
tetanospasmin
tetanus
    t. antiserum
    t. antitoxin (TAT)
    cephalic t.
    t. and diphtheria (Td)
    diphtheria, pertussis, t. (DPT)
    t. and diphtheria toxoids vaccine
    generalized t.
    t. immune globulin
    t. immunoglobulin (TIG)
    neonatal t.
    t. neonatorum
    t. neurotoxin
    postpartum t.
    t. prophylaxis
    puerperal t.
    t. toxin
    t. toxoid (TT)
    t. toxoid booster
    t. toxoid and diphtheria
    t. toxoid and diphtheria vaccine
    uterine t.
tetanus-diphtheria immunization
tetany
    hypocalcemic t.
    hypomagnesemic t.
    infantile t.
    neonatal t.
    t. of vitamin D deficiency
tethered
    t. catheter
    t. conus medullaris
    t. cord syndrome
    t. spinal cord
tethering
    spinal cord t.
tetra amelia syndrome
tetrabenazine
tetrabrachius

tetracaine
    t., adrenaline, cocaine (TAC)
    lidocaine, epinephrine, t. (LET)
tetrachirus
tetrachloride
    carbon t.
tetracycline
    t. analog
    t. hydrochloride
    t. pleurodesis
    prophylactic t.
tetracycline-induced esophagitis
Tetracyn
tetrad
tetradactyly
tetraethyl lead
tetrahydrobiopterin
    t. cofactor (BH_4)
    t. deficiency
tetrahydrocannabinol, 9-
  tetrahydrocannabinol (THC)
tetrahydrocortisol
tetrahydrofolate (THF)
tetrahydrofolate-methyltransferase
  deficiency syndrome
tetrahydrozoline
tetraiodothyronine test
tetralogy
    t. of Fallot (tet, TF, TOF)
    t. of Fallot syndrome
tetramastia
tetramelus
tetramonodactyly
tetranitrate
    erythrityl t.
    pentaerythritol t.
tetranophthalmos
tetraotus
tetraparesis
tetraphocomelia-cleft lip-palate syndrome
tetraplegia
    flaccid t.
tetraploid
    t. distribution
    t. embryo
tetraploidy syndrome
tetrascelus
tetrasomy
    chromosome 8p mosaic t.
    partial t. 10p
    t. 15p syndrome
    t. 21q

T

NOTES

tetravalent
tetra-X
  t.-X chromosomal aberration
  t.-X syndrome
tetrazolium
  t. dye assay
  nitroblue t. (NBT)
tetrodotoxin poisoning
TEV
  talipes equinovarus
TEWL
  transepidermal water loss
Texas Scottish Rite Hospital (TSRH)
Texidor twinge
TF
  tetralogy of Fallot
Tf
  transferrin
TFA
  thigh-foot angle
tFA
  trans fatty acid
TFCC
  triangular fibrocartilaginous complex
TFL
  tensor fasciae latae
TFM
  total fat mass
TFP
  trifunctional protein deficiency
TFPI
  tissue factor pathway inhibitor
TfR
  transferrin receptor
TFT
  thyroid function test
TFX catheter stylet
TG
  transglutaminase
TGA
  transposition of great arteries
    isolated TGA
    simple TGA
TGEF
  transabdominal thin-gauge
  embryofetoscopy
T/Gel shampoo
T-Gesic
TGF
  transforming growth factor
TGF-1
  transforming growth factor 1
TGF alpha
  transforming growth factor alpha
TGFA polymorphism
TGF beta
  transforming growth factor beta

TGV
  thoracic gas volume
  transposition of great vessels
TH
  total hydroperoxide
Thal
  T. fundoplication
  T. intermedia-like syndrome
thalamostriatal artery
thalamostriate vasculopathy (TSV)
thalamotomy
  stereotactic t.
thalamus
thalassemia
  alpha t.
  beta t.
  t. facies
  hemoglobin S t. (HbS-Thal)
  homozygous t.
  t. intermedia
  Lepore t.
  t. major
  t. minor
  sickle-cell and beta t.
  t. trait
  transfusion-dependent t.
thalassemic patient
thalidomide
  t. embryopathy
  fetal t.
  t. teratogenicity syndrome
thallium
  t. imaging
  t. intoxication
  t. poisoning
thallium-201
THAM
  tromethamine
thanatophoric
  t. dwarfism
  t. dysplasia
  t. dysplasia syndrome
thawing
  embryo t.
Thayer-Martin
  T.-M. agar
  T.-M. gonorrhea test
  T.-M. medium
THC
  tetrahydrocannabinol
the
  T. Cell Sweep
  T. Female Condom
  T. Injury Prevention Program
  (TIPP)
theca
  t. cell tumor
  t. externa
  t. interna

lumbar t.
t. lutein cell
t. lutein cyst
theca-granulosa cell cooperativity
thecal interstitial cell
thecoma
luteinized t.
ovarian t.
Theiler stage
thelarche
idiopathic premature t.
premature t.
theleplasty
theloncus
thelorrhagia
T-helper cell
thenar
Theo-24
Theochron
Theolair
Theon
theophyllinate
choline t.
theophylline
t. level
sustained-release t.
t. toxicity
theory
birth trauma t.
clonal selection t.
crowding t.
endorphin, dopamine, and
prostaglandin t.
Freud t.
ganglion trigger t.
gate-control t.
grandmother t.
implantation t.
Lamarck t.
t. of mind
operant conditioning t.
pulsion t.
skin trigger t.
synactive t.
teleologic t.
traction t.
Trivers-Willard t.
Thera-Flur
Thera-Flur-N
TheraGym exercise ball
therapeutic
t. abortion (TA, TAB)

t. anticoagulation
t. blood level
t. donor insemination (TDI)
t. electromembrane (TEM)
t. heparinization
t. insemination
t. insemination, husband (THI, TIH)
t. option
t. pulmonary function test
t. pulmonary lavage
t. touch
t. window
therapeutics
biofield t.
therapist
respiratory t.
sex t.
speech t.
vision t.
therapy
add-back t.
adjuvant chemoradiation t.
aerosol t.
afterload reduction t.
aldosterone replacement t.
alkali t.
alternative t.
ambulatory anticoagulation t.
amnioinfusion t.
animal-assisted t. (AAT)
antenatal corticosteroid t.
antepartum steroid t.
antiangiogenic t.
antibacterial t.
antibiotic infusion t.
antibody induction t.
antibody replacement t.
anticoagulation t.
anticysticercal t.
anti-D t.
antidepressant t.
antiemetic t.
antifungal drug t.
antihelminthic t.
antihypertensive t.
antiinflammatory t.
antileukemic t.
antimicrobial t.
antioxidant t.
antiparasitic drug t.
antiplatelet t.

NOTES

therapy *(continued)*

antipyretic t.
antiretroviral t.
antithyroid drug t.
antituberculous t.
antiviral t.
axillary irradiation t.
azole t.
balloon heating t.
behavioral t.
behavioral family systems t. (BFST)
belly bath t.
BEP t.
biofeedback t.
bisphosphonate t.
blood component t.
Bobath physical t.
bolus fluid t.
breast conservation t. (BCT)
breast-conserving t. (BCT)
breast-preserving t.
broad-spectrum antibiotic t.
bromocriptine t.
budesonide t.
butyrate t.
caffeine t.
cancer t.
chelation t.
chest physical t. (CPT)
chest wall radiation t.
cognitive t.
cognitive behavioral t. (CBT)
combined hormone t. (CHT)
conservative t.
constraint-induced movement t.
corticosteroid t.
deficit t.
desferrioxamine t.
dexamethasone t.
dinitrochlorobenzene t.
directly observed t. (DOT)
DNCB t.
drainage, irrigation, fibrinolytic t. (DRIFT)
ego-oriented individual t. (EOIT)
electroconvulsive t. (ECT)
electrolyte t.
electroshock t.
embolization t.
empiric t.
endocavitary radiation t.
enterostomal t.
enzyme replacement t.
eradication t.
estrogen add-back t. (EABT)
estrogen-progestin replacement t.
estrogen replacement t. (ERT)
exogenous surfactant t.

extended field irradiation t.
external beam radiation t.
external radiation t.
external x-ray t.
ex vivo liver-directed gene t.
eye salvage t.
family t.
fetal drug t.
fibrinolytic t.
flashlamp-pulsed laser t.
fluid replacement t.
frappage t.
Functional Assessment of Cancer T. (FACT)
gene t.
genetic t.
glucocorticosteroid t.
gold t.
group problem-solving t.
helmet-molding t.
higher-dose t.
highly active antiretroviral t. (HAART)
home antibiotic infusion t.
hormonal antineoplastic t.
hormone t.
hormone replacement t. (HRT)
HS-tk gene t.
human gene t.
humidification t.
hyperbaric oxygen t. (HOBT)
hyperfractionated radiation t.
immunosuppressive t.
induction t.
inotropic t.
interactive play t.
interferon t.
internal radiation t.
InterStim t.
interstitial t.
intracisternal t.
intralesional steroid t.
intraperitoneal radiation t.
intravenous fluid t.
intraventricular fibrinolytic t.
iodide t.
I.V. anti-D t.
laser t.
LH-RH agonist t.
light t.
ʟ-thyroxine t.
Lupron add-back t.
macrolide t.
maintenance t.
massage t.
maternal blood clot patch t.
megavitamin t.
menopausal estrogen replacement t.
milieu t.

mist t.
monoclonal antibody t.
multidrug t. (MDT)
multisystemic t. (MST)
myoblast transfer t.
natural hormone replacement t.
neoadjuvant hormonal t. (NHT)
neurodevelopment t. (NDT)
neutron t.
nicotine patch t.
occupational t. (OT)
octreotide t.
oral contraceptive t. (OCT)
oral hormone replacement t.
oral rehydration t. (ORT)
orthomolecular t.
oxygen t.
pancreatic enzyme replacement t.
   (PERT)
parenteral fluid t.
patterning t.
percussion t.
percutaneous t.
permission, limited information,
   specific suggestions and
   intensive t. (PLISSIT)
phenytoin t.
photodynamic t.
physical t. (PT)
play t.
polyvalent immunoglobulin t.
postmenopausal estrogen
   replacement t.
progestational t.
progestogen support t.
prophylactic antibiotic t.
psychodynamic t.
pulse steroid t.
quadrantectomy, axillary dissection,
   radiation t. (QUART)
radiation t. (RT)
radical surgical t.
radioiodine ablative t.
recombinant enzyme replacement t.
replacement t.
rescue t.
respiratory t.
retinoid t.
t. roll
salvage t.
selective tubal assessment to refine
   reproductive t. (STARRT)

sensory integration t.
sequential hormone t.
sex steroid add-back t.
single-dose methotrexate t.
single-field hyperthermia combined
   with radiation t.
speech t.
stem cell t.
stepdown t.
stepwise antiinflammatory t.
steroid t.
subcutaneous desferrioxamine t.
suicide gene t.
supportive group t.
surfactant replacement t.
surgical myomectomy as
   reproductive t. (SMART)
systemic azole t.
systemic behavior family t.
T-cell antibody induction t.
Thermachoice uterine balloon t.
thiamin t.
thrombolytic t.
tocolytic t.
transdermal hormone replacement t.
transdermal nicotine replacement t.
transfusion t.
triple-drug t.
uterine balloon t. (UBT)
in utero stem cell t.
vaginal estrogen t.
vasopressin t.
vision t.
vitamin t.
in vivo gene t.
xanthochromia t.
x-ray t.
zinc t.
Theratope vaccine
Therex
ThermAblator
Thermachoice
   T. uterine balloon therapy
   T. uterine balloon therapy system
Therma Jaw hot urologic forceps
thermal
   t. balloon ablation
   t. balloon system
   t. burn
   t. gel gradient electrophoresis
   t. hat
   t. homeostasis

NOTES

thermal *(continued)*
 t. injury
 t. neutral environment
 t. stress
Thermasonic gel warmer
Thermazene
thermic effect of food (TEF)
thermistor
 nasal tip t.
 t. thermometer
ThermoChem-HT system
thermodilution
 t. method
 pulmonary artery t.
thermodynamic
thermogenesis
 brown fat nonshivering t.
 nonexercise activity t.
thermogenic response
thermography
thermolability
 MTHFR t.
thermometer
 basal body t.
 Braun tympanic t.
 LighTouch Neonate t.
 Ototemp 3000 t.
 Philips SensorTouch temple t.
 767 SureTemp 4 oral t.
 Temp-a-dot t.
 thermistor t.
 Thermoscan Pro-1-Instant t.
 Thermoscan tympanic instant t.
thermoplasty
 balloon t.
thermoregulation
thermoregulatory
 t. response
 t. sweat testing
Thermoscan
 T. Pro-1-Instant thermometer
 T. tympanic instant thermometer
thermotherapy
Theroxide Wash
theta dimeric protein
thetaiotaomicron
 Bacteroides t.
THF
 tetrahydrofolate
THI
 therapeutic insemination, husband
 transient hypogammaglobulinemia of
 infancy
thiabendazole
thiacetazone
thiamin
 t. deficiency
 t. hypovitaminemia
 t. therapy

thiaminase
thiamin-response sideroblastic anemia
thiazide diuretic
thick
 t. blood smear
 t. neck
thickened
 t. base
 t. base of skull
 t. endometrial stripe
thickening
 bronchial wall t.
 bronchiolar t.
 decidual mural t.
 fusiform nerve t.
 intimal t.
 nerve t.
 nodular nerve t.
 nuchal pad t.
 pial t.
 skin t.
 vaginal t.
thickness
 endometrial t.
 fetal neck fold t.
 fetal nuchal translucency t.
 nuchal translucency t. (NTT)
 placental t.
 skinfold t.
 subscapular skinfold t.
 triceps skinfold t. (TSF)
Thiemann
 T. disease
 T. syndrome
Thiersch-Duplay urethroplasty
Thiersch operation
thiethylperazine
thigh-foot
 t.-f. angle (TFA)
 t.-f. axis
thigh-leg angle (TLA)
thimerosal-free vaccine
thin
 t. basement membrane disease
 (TBMD)
 t. basement membrane nephropathy
 t. vaginal mucosa
 t. vulvar skin
thinking
 abstract t.
 auditory integration t. (AIT)
 t. skill
thin-layer chromatography (TLC)
thinned dermis
thinness
 drive for t.
ThinPrep
 T. Pap test

T. processor
T. smear
THINsite dressing
thiobarbituric acid-reacting substance (TBARS)
thioctic acid
thiocyanate
thioglycollate broth medium
thioguanine
thiomalate
gold sodium t.
thiopental sodium
Thioplex
thiopropazate
thiopurine methyltransferase (TPMT)
thioridazine hydrochloride
thiosulfate
t. lotion
sodium t.
Thiosulfil
thiotepa
thiothixene
thiphenamil hydrochloride
third
t. disease
t. disease (rubella)
t. and fourth pharyngeal pouch syndrome
t. heart sound
t. parallel pelvic plane
t. permanent molar
t. space loss
t. spacing
t. spacing of fluid
t. stage of labor
t. trimester
t. trimester bleeding
t. trimester measurement
t. ventricle fenestration
third-degree
t.-d. AV block
t.-d. burn
t.-d. defect
t.-d. descent
t.-d. episiotomy
t.-d. hypospadias
t.-d. laceration
third-degree prolapse
third-generation progesterone
third-line measure
THL
true histiocytic lymphoma

thlipsencephalus
Thomas
T. curette
T. heel
Thomas-Gaylor biopsy forceps
Thomsen
T. disease
T. myotonia congenita
Thomsen-Friedenreich
T.-F. antigen
T.-F. antigen assay
thonzonium
thoracentesis
needle t.
thoracic
t. aortogram
t. asphyxiant dystrophy
t. cavity
t. clamp
t. compression syndrome
t. duct drainage
t. duct ligation
t. gas volume (TGV)
t. kyphosis
t. spine fracture
t. surgery
t. trauma
t. wall excursion
thoracic-pelvic-phalangeal dystrophy
thoracoabdominal (TA)
t. ectopia cordis
thoracoamniotic shunt
thoracoceloschisis
thoracodelphus, thoradelphus
thoracodidymus
thoracogastrodidymus
thoracogastroschisis
thoracolumbar
t. gibbus
t. kyphosis
t. kyphotic curvature
t. rachischisis
t. sympathetic nerve
thoracolumbosacral orthosis (TLSO)
thoracomelus
thoracopagus twins
thoracoparacephalus
thoracoplasty
thoracoschisis
thoracoscope
thoracoscopic pleural débridement
thoracoscopy

T

NOTES

thoracostomy
    tube t.
    t. tube
thoracotomy
    closed t.
thoradelphus (*var. of* thoracodelphus)
thorascopic technique
thorax
    Amazon t.
    t. compression
    great vessel of t.
    milk lines of t.
Thorazine
Thorn test
thought
    t. action fusion
    t. disorder
    t. disturbance
threadworm infestation
thready pulse
threatened
    t. abortion
    t. miscarriage
three
    Pediatric Examination at T. (PEET)
three-day
    t.-d. fever
    t.-d. measles
three-dimensional
    t.-d. ultrasonography
    t.-d. ultrasound
    t.-d. videoendoscope
three-point
    t.-p. position
    t.-p. technique
three-quarter strength formula
three-stage Norwood-Fontan procedure
three-vessel cord
three-way stopcock
threonine
threshold
    high pain t.
    low sensory t.
    pain t.
    phenotypic t.
    sensory t.
    speech reception t. (SRT)
    speech recognition t. (SRT)
    t. trait
thrill
    diastolic t.
    presystolic t.
    suprasternal notch t.
thrive
    failure to t. (FTT)
    nonorganic failure to t. (NOFT, NOFTT)
throat
    t. clearing

    eyes, ears, nose, t. (EENT)
    sore t.
    strep t.
    Sucrets Sore T.
    t. swab
thrombasthenia
    Glanzmann t.
    t. of Glanzmann and Naegeli
thrombectomy
thrombi (*pl. of* thrombus)
thrombin
    t. clot test
    t. clotting time
    t. clotting time coagulation test
    t. receptor-activating peptide (TRAP)
    topical t.
thrombocyte
thrombocythemia
    essential t. (ET)
    primary t. (PT)
thrombocytopenia
    t. absent radii
    t. absent radius (TAR)
    alloimmune t.
    autoimmune t.
    congenital amegakaryocytic t.
    consumptive t.
    familial dominant t.
    fetal t.
    fetomaternal alloimmune t. (FMAIT)
    gestational t.
    heparin–induced t. (HIT)
    immune t.
    immune-mediated t.
    isoimmune fetal t.
    maternal t.
    megakaryocytic t.
    neonatal alloimmune t.
    neonatal autoimmune t.
    neonatal isoimmune t.
    transfusion-induced t.
    t. with absent radius syndrome
    X-linked t.
thrombocytopenic purpura
thrombocytosis
thromboembolic
    t. complication
    t. disease (TED)
    t. event (TE)
thromboembolism
    idiopathic venous t.
    pulmonary t.
    venous t. (VTE)
Thrombogen
thrombohemolytic disease
thrombolytic therapy
thrombomodulin

thrombopenia
thrombophilia
    factor V Leiden t.
    familial t.
    genetic t.
    hereditary t.
thrombophlebitis
    cortical t.
    deep vein t.
    diffuse cortical t.
    pelvic vein t.
    peripheral t.
    septic pelvic t. (SPT)
    septic pelvic vein t.
    sinus t.
    superficial t.
    venous sinus t.
thromboplastin
    plasma t.
thrombopoiesis
thrombopoietin (TPO)
thromboprophylaxis
thrombosis, pl. **thromboses**
    anal t.
    arterial t.
    cavernosal artery t.
    cavernous sinus t.
    cerebral t.
    coronary t.
    decidual fibrin t.
    deep vein t. (DVT)
    deep venous t. (DVT)
    dural sinus t.
    dural venous t.
    external anal t.
    intracranial venous sinus t.
    jugular vein t.
    lateral sinus t.
    maternal cortical vein t.
    multiorgan t.
    mural t.
    ovarian vein t. (OVT)
    pelvic ovarian vein t. (POVT)
    placental t.
    pregnancy-associated t.
    purulent venous t.
    renal vascular t.
    renal vein t.
    sagittal sinus t.
    sinus t.
    vacular t.

    vascular t.
    venous sinus t.
thrombospondin
Thrombostat platelet function test
thrombotic
    t. endocarditis
    t. microangiopathy (TMA)
    t. phlegmasia
    t. purpura
    t. thrombocytopenic purpura (TTP)
Thrombo-Wellco test
thromboxane
    t. A2
    t. dominance
thrombus, pl. **thrombi**
    chorionic vessel t.
    endocardial t.
    fibrin t.
    intramural t.
    t. precursor protein (TpP)
    t. precursor protein test
    superficial t.
thrush
    oral t.
    plaque of t.
    t. pneumonia
thrust
    jaw t.
    manual t.
    tongue t.
thumb
    broad t.
    congenital clasped t.'s
    deafness, imperforate anus, hypoplastic t.'s
    floating t.
    gamekeeper's t.
    hitchhiker's t.
    t. hyperabduction
    hypoplastic t.
    indwelling t.
    mental retardation, aphasia, shuffling gait, adducted t. (MASA)
    t. in palm deformity
    t. retractor
    t. sign
    skier's t.
    t. spica cast
    t. spica splint
    stub t.
    triphalangeal t.

NOTES

thumbing
    cortical t.
thumbsucking
thump
    precordial t.
Thurston Holland sign
thymectomy
    neonatal t.
thymic
    t. agenesis
    t. alymphoplasia
    t. aphasia
    t. aplasia
    t. aplasia syndrome
    t. asthma
    t. dysplasia
    t. hypoplasia
    t. hypoplasia anomaly
    t. lymphocyte antigen (TL)
    t. and parathyroid agenesis
      syndrome
    t. shadow
    t. wave sign
thymic-dependent deficiency
thymic-parathyroid aplasia
thymidine analog NRTI
thymine nucleotide
thymocyte
thymol turbidity test
thymoma
thymopoietin
thymosin
thymus
    t. gland
    t. hyperplasia
    t. primordium
    t. transplantation
Thyrel TRH
thyroarytenoid muscle
thyroglobulin
thyroglossal
    t. duct
    t. duct cyst
    t. duct cyst excision
thyrohypophysial syndrome
thyroid
    t. aplasia
    t. autoantibody
    t. cancer
    t. carcinoma
    t. crisis
    t. deficiency
    t. disease
    t. dysfunction
    ectopic t.
    t. function
    t. function test (TFT)
    t. gland
    t. gland dysfunction

    t. gland malformation
    t. hormone
    t. hormone resistance
    t. hormone unresponsiveness
    hypothalamic, pituitary, t. (HTP)
    t. index
    t. Lahey clamp
    t. neoplasia
    t. nodule
    t. ophthalmopathy
    t. and pituitary agenesis
    t. scintigraphy
    t. storm
    sublingual t.
    t. transcription factor-1 (TTF-1)
thyroid-binding
    t.-b. globulin (TBG)
    t.-b. globulin deficiency
thyroidectomy
thyroiditis
    acute suppurative t.
    autoimmune t.
    chronic lymphocytic t.
    Hashimoto t.
    lymphocytic t.
    postpartum t.
    postviral subacute t.
    subacute t.
    suppurative t.
thyroid-related ophthalmopathy (TRO)
thyroid-specific enhancer binding
    protein-1 (T4/ebp-1)
thyroid-stimulating
    t.-s. hormone (TSH)
    t.-s. hormone assay
    t.-s. immunoglobulin
Thyrolar
thyrotoxic crisis
thyrotoxicosis
    gestational t.
    neonatal t.
thyrotrope
thyrotropic, thyrotrophic
    t. hormone
thyrotropin
    chorionic t.
    t. deficiency
    neonatal t.
    t. releasing hormone (TRH)
    serum t.
    t. testing
thyrotropin-secreting pituitary adenoma
thyroxine, thyroxin (T4)
    free t.
    t. synthesis
    t. test
thyroxine-binding
    t.-b. globulin (TBG)

t.-b. globulin deficiency
t.-b. protein (TBP)
TIA
transient ischemic attack
tiagabine
Tiamol
Tiazac
TIBC
total iron-binding capacity
tibia, pl. **tibiae**
congenital longitudinal deficiency
of t.
congenital pseudoarthrosis of t.
osteochondrosis deformans tibiae
posteromedial bow of t.
pseudoarthrosis of t.
t. vara
tibial
t. aplasia-ectrodactyly syndrome
t. bowing
childhood accidental spiral t.
(CAST)
t. epiphysis
t. film
t. hemimelia
t. metaphysis
t. pseudoarthrosis
t. shaft fracture
t. speed
t. speed of sound
t. stress fracture
t. torsion
t. tubercle
t. valgus osteotomy
t. version
tibiofibular syndesmosis
tibolone
tic
chronic t.
complex motor t.
complex vocal t.
cough t.
t. disorder
maladie des t.'s
motor t.
multiple t.'s
psychogenic cough t.
simple motor t.
simple vocal t.
t. symptom
vocal t.
Ticar

ticarcillin
t. clavulanate
t. and clavulanate potassium
t. disodium
ticarcillin/clavulanic acid
Tice BCG
tick
t. bite
deer t.
dog t.
t. fever
Lone Star t.
t. paralysis
Rocky Mountain wood t.
wood t.
tick-borne
t.-b. encephalitis (TBE)
t.-b. infection
t.-b. relapsing fever
t.-b. typhus
ticlopidine
ticonazole
TID
tubal inflammatory damage
tidal
t. breathing
t. liquid ventilation (TLV)
t. volume (TV, VT)
tide mark dermatitis
tie
silk t.
Tietze syndrome
TIG
tetanus immunoglobulin
Tigan
T. Injection
T. Rectal
tight heel cord
tightness
idiopathic heel-cord t.
TIH
therapeutic insemination, husband
Tilade Inhalation Aerosol
Tillaux
T. disease
fracture of T.
T. fracture
tilt
head t.
head-up t. (HUT)
lateral head t.
pelvic t.

NOTES

T

tilt *(continued)*

  t. test
  ulnar t.
tilted disc
tilt-table test
tiludronate
time

  activated clotting t. (ACT)
  activated partial thromboplastin t. (APTT)
  bleeding t.
  capillary filling t.
  capillary refill t.
  cell generation t.
  circulation t.
  doubling t.
  euglobulin clot lysis t. (ECLT)
  euglobulin lysis t. (ELT)
  gastric emptying t.
  inspiration t. (I-time)
  inspiratory t. (IT)
  isovolumic relaxation t. (IVRT)
  Ivy bleeding t.
  kaolin clotting t.
  Lee-White clotting t.
  orocecal transit t.
  partial thromboplastin t. (PTT)
  t. position scan
  prothrombin t. (pro-time, PT)
  recovery t.
  reptilase t.
  Rite T.
  Russell viper venom t.
  sinoatrial conduction t.
  thrombin clotting t.
timed

  t. endometrial biopsy
  t. intercourse
Timentin
time-of-flight and absorbance (TOFA)
time-out
timer

  Apgar t.
time-resolved fluoroimmunoassay
timing

  coital t.
Timolide
timolol maleate
Timoptic Ophthalmic
Timoptic-XE Ophthalmic
timothy grass
tin

  t. ear syndrome
  t. mesoporphyrin (SnMP)
  t. protoporphyrin (SnPP)
Tinactin
tincture

  alcoholic t.

  t. of iodine
  opium t.
T-independent antigen
tinea

  t. capitis
  t. corporis
  t. corpus
  t. cruris
  t. gladiatorum
  t. incognito
  t. manuum
  t. nigra palmaris
  t. pedis
  t. profunda
  t. rubrum
  t. unguium
  t. versicolor
tine test
tinidazole
tinnitus
tinted
TINU

  tubulointerstitial nephritis
tioconazole 6.5% ointment
TIP

  tubularized incised plate
tip

  bulbous nasal t.
  Corometrics Gold Quik Connect Spiral electrode t.
  Frazier suction t.
  needle t.
  nonfrosted t.
TIPP

  The Injury Prevention Program
TIPS

  transjugular intrahepatic portosystemic shunt
tiptoeing
TIR

  trophoblast in regression
tired housewife syndrome
Tischler cervical biopsy forceps
Tischler-Morgan

  T.-M. biopsy punch
  T.-M. uterine biopsy forceps
Tisit

  T. Blue Gel
  T. Liquid
  T. Shampoo
tissue

  accessory ovarian t.
  t. activator-induced fibrinolysis
  adipose t.
  anechoic t.
  t. anoxia
  attenuating t.
  breast biopsy t.

bronchus-associated lymphoid t. (BALT)
t. catabolism
choriodecidual t.
conductive t.
t. confirmation
connective t.
contused t.
t. culture-grown attenuated virus
t. Doppler imaging (TDI)
echogenic t.
ectopic endometrial t.
ectopic ovarian t.
embryonic t.
endometriotic t.
epipericardial connective t.
erectile t.
t. expander
t. expansion vaginoplasty
t. factor
t. factor pathway inhibitor (TFPI)
fibroareolar t.
fibrous connective t.
fibrovascular t.
t. forceps
fragile t.
gastrointestinal-associated
  lymphoid t. (GALT)
glandular t.
granulation t.
gut-associated lymphoid t. (GALT)
t. homogeneity
hyperplastic lymphoid t.
hypertrophied t.
t. inhibitors of metalloproteinase
t. insulin resistance
intestine-associated lymphoid t.
  (IALT)
intralobular connective t.
larynx-associated lymphoid t.
  (LALT)
t. link floating ball
t. loss
lymphoid t.
maternal t.
mucosa-associated lymphoid t.
  (MALT)
nasopharyngeal-associated
  lymphoid t. (NALT)
t. necrosis
neovascular t.
neural crest t.

paravaginal soft t.
pelvic connective t.
perilobular connective t.
persistent trophoblastic t.
t. pH monitoring
placental trophoblastic t.
t. plasminogen activator (t-PA)
t. regeneration
residual ductal t.
retroperitoneal soft t.
scar t.
soft t.
sonolucent t.
t. specific imaging
splenic t.
t. study
subareolar t.
sympathetic t.
syngeneic t.
t. synthesis
t. thromboplastin-inhibition test
t. tolerance to radiation
t. transglutaminase (tTG)
t. transplant
trophoblastic t.
t. typing
xenogeneic t.

tissue-specific antibody
Tis-u-Trap endometrial suction
titanium
  t. elastic nail
  t. elastic nailing (TEN)
  t. staple

titer
  ADB t.
  AH t.
  ANCA t.
  anti-DNase B t.
  antihyaluronidase t.
  antimycoplasma t.
  t. of anti-ragweed IgE antibody
  anti-Rho(D) t.
  ASO t.
  Forssman t.
  geometric mean t. (GMT)
  HI t.
  IgG antibody t.
  IgM antibody t.
  maternal t.
  non-*Treponema* t.
  RPR t.
  rubeola t.

NOTES

T

titer *(continued)*
    serum bactericidal t. (SBT)
    serum inhibitory t. (SIT)
    sheep cell agglutinin t.
    TORCH t.
    viral t.
    virus t.
Titmus stereoacuity test
Titralac Plus Liquid
titrate
titration
    skin end-point t.
titubation
    head t.
TKO
TL
    thymic lymphocyte antigen
    tubal ligation
TL-90 Ethicon stapler
TLA
    thigh-leg angle
TLC
    thin-layer chromatography
    total lung capacity
        TLC antiseptic soap
TLSO
    thoracolumbosacral orthosis
TLV
    tidal liquid ventilation
    total liquid ventilation
TLX alloantigen system
TMA
    thrombotic microangiopathy
    transcription-mediated amplification
    transmalleolar axis angle
        TMA assay
T-max
    maximum temperature
TMD
    transient myeloproliferative disorder
TMES
    transient marrow edema syndrome of the hip
TMJ
    temporomandibular joint
TMP-SMX
    trimethoprim-sulfamethoxazole
TMS
    transcranial magnetic stimulation
TND
    transient neonatal diabetes
TNDM
    transient neonatal diabetes mellitus
TNF
    tumor necrosis factor
TNF-alpha
    tumor necrosis factor alpha
        TNF-alpha converting enzyme

TNM
    tumor, node, metastases
        TNM classification
        TNM nomenclature
        TNM schema
TNR
    tonic neck reflex
TnT
    troponin T
T&O
    tubes and ovaries
TOA
    tuboovarian abscess
to-and-fro
    t.-a.-f. flow
    t.-a.-f. murmur
TOAPOT
    tuboovarian abscess after previous tubal occlusion
toast
    bananas, rice, applesauce, tea, t. (BRATT)
    bananas, rice cereal, applesauce, t. (BRAT)
tobacco
    smokeless t.
Tobey ear rongeur
TOBI
    tobramycin solution for inhalation
Tobin index
TobraDex
tobramycin
    t. solution
    t. solution for inhalation (TOBI)
Tobrex Ophthalmic
TOC
    tuboovarian complex
tococardiography
tocodynagraph
tocodynamometer
tocodynamometry
tocograph
tocography
tocology
tocolysis
    acute t.
    prenatal t.
tocolytic
    t. agent
    t. drug
    t. therapy
tocometer
tocopherol deficiency
tocophobia
tocotransducer
Today vaginal contraceptive sponge
Todd
    T. paralysis
    T. paresis

Todd-Hewitt broth
toddler-age nodulocystic acne
toddler's
> t. diarrhea
> t. fracture

Toddler Temperament Scale
toe
> adducted great t.
> broad t.
> catheter t.'s
> clubbing of fingers and t.'s
> curly t.
> floating great t.
> t. grasp
> great t.
> hammer t.
> mallet t.
> overlapping t.
> overriding t.
> pigeon t.
> searching t.
> striatal t.
> t. syndactyly
> t. walking

toeing
> t. in
> t. out

toe-in gait
toenail
> ingrown t.

toe-off
toe-out gait
Toesen
toe-walking
TOF
> tetralogy of Fallot
> tracheoesophageal fistula

TOFA
> time-of-flight and absorbance

Togaviridae
togavirus
TOH
> Tower of Hanoi
> TOH test

toilet
> pulmonary t.
> respiratory t.
> t. training

toileting problem
Toitu MT-810 cardiographic monitor
Tokos monitor

TOL
> Tower of London
> TOL test

Tolamide
tolazamide
tolazoline hydrochloride
tolbutamide
Toldt
Tolectin DS
tolerance
> antigen t.
> carbohydrate t.
> glucose t.
> immunologic t.
> impaired glucose t. (IGT)
> radiation t.

Tolerex formula
tolfenamic acid
Tolinase
tolmetin
tolnaftate
Tolosa-Hunt syndrome
tolterodine
toluene sniffing
toluidine
> t. blue
> t. blue stain
> t. blue test

Tolu-Sed DM
tomaculous neuropathy
Tom Jones closure
tomogram
tomographic
> computerized t. (CT)

tomography
> automated computerized axial t. (ACAT)
> computed t. (CT)
> computed axial t. (CAT)
> delayed-phase computed t.
> electron-beam computed t. (EBCT)
> focused computed t.
> high-resolution chest computed t.
> high-resolution computed t. (HRCT)
> hypocycloidal t.
> optical t.
> positron emission t. (PET)
> quantitative computed t. (QCT)
> single-photon emission t.
> single-photon emission computed t. (SPECT)
> Somatom Plus computed t.

NOTES

Tompkins
    T. median bivalving technique
    T. metroplasty
    T. procedure
tone
    anal sphincter t.
    bronchomotor t.
    decreased anal t.
    decreased sphincter t.
    detrusor t.
    fetal t.
    flaccid t.
    flexor t.
    fluctuating t.
    high t.
    low muscle t.
    muscle t.
    parasympathetic t.
    poor muscle t.
    pulmonary vascular t.
    sphincter t.
    uterine t.
    vagal t.
    vascular t.
tongs
    Gardner-Wells t.
tongue
    t. biting
    black hairy t.
    chameleon t.
    t. crib
    crocodile t.
    darting t.
    t. depressor
    t. fasciculation
    fern leaf t.
    fissured t.
    free t.
    geographic t.
    hairy t.
    hypoplastic t.
    large t.
    protruding t.
    t. protrusion reflex
    raspberry t.
    red strawberry t.
    scrotal t.
    t. size
    smooth t.
    strawberry t.
    surface furrowing of t.
    t. thrust
    white strawberry t.
tongue-lip adhesion
tongue-tied
tonic
    t. downgaze
    t. labyrinthine reflex
    t. neck pattern

    t. neck reflex (TNR)
    t. neck response
    t. seizure
tonic-clonic
    t.-c. convulsion
    t.-c. movements
    t.-c. seizure
    t.-c. seizure activity
tonicoclonic seizure activity
Tonnis hip dysplasia procedure
tonoclonic
tonometry
    gastric t.
    gut t.
tonsil
    cerebellar t.'s
    palatine t.
tonsillar
    t. edema
    t. exudate
tonsillectomy and adenoidectomy (T&A)
tonsillitis
    acute exudative t.
    acute follicular t.
    adenoviral t.
    exudative t.
    follicular t.
    streptococcal t.
    white t.
tonsillopharyngeal exudate
tonsillopharyngitis
    streptococcal t.
tonsurans
    Trichophyton t.
tonus
    baseline t.
    uterine t.
tool
    Adolescent and Pediatric Pain T.
    (APPT)
    SCHIP evaluation t.
too-soft voice
tooth
    t. anomalies, skeletal dysplasia,
    sparse hair syndrome
    t. bud
    canine t.
    t. decay
    dystrophic t.
    t. loss
    t. and nail syndrome
    t. placement
    t. root resorption
    wisdom t.
toothbrush culture technique
Topamax
Topaz-UPS
Topcon Screenoscope

topectomy
tophus, pl. **tophi**
   urate tophi
Topicaine
topical
   Achromycin T.
   Aclovate T.
   Acticort T.
   Aeroseb-HC T.
   Ala-Cort T.
   Ala-Scalp T.
   Alphatrex T.
   Anusol HC-1 T.
   Anusol HC-2.5% T.
   Aristocort T.
   Aristocort A T.
   A/T/S T.
   Baciguent T.
   Benadryl T.
   Betatrex T.
   CaldeCort T.
   Caldesene T.
   Canesten T.
   Carmol-HC T.
   Cetacort T.
   Cloderm T.
   CortaGel T.
   Cortaid Maximum Strength T.
   Cortaid with Aloe T.
   Cort-Dome T.
   Cortef Feminine Itch T.
   Cortizone-5, -10 T.
   Cruex T.
   Cyclocort T.
   Delcort T.
   Dermacort T.
   Dermarest Dricort T.
   Derma-Smoothe/FS T.
   Dermolate T.
   Dermtex HC with Aloe T.
   DesOwen T.
   Diprolene AF T.
   Diprosone T.
   Efudex T.
   Eldecort T.
   Eurax T.
   Exelderm T.
   Fluoroplex T.
   Gynecort T.
   Hi-Cor-1.0, -2.5 T.
   Hycort T.
   Hydrocort T.
   Hydro-Tex T.
   Hytone T.
   t. imidazole
   t. iodine application
   Kenalog T.
   LactiCare-HC T.
   Lanacort T.
   Locoid T.
   Lotrimin T.
   Maxivate T.
   MetroGel T.
   Micatin T.
   Monistat-Derm T.
   Mycitracin T.
   Mycogen II T.
   Mycolog-II T.
   Mytrex F T.
   N.G.T. T.
   t. nitroglycerin
   Nutracort T.
   Orabase HCA T.
   Ovide T.
   Oxistat T.
   Pedi-Dri T.
   Pedi-Pro T.
   Penecort T.
   t. podophyllin
   Polysporin T.
   Rogaine T.
   Scalpicin T.
   Solarcaine T.
   S-T Cort T.
   Synacort T.
   Synalar T.
   Synemol T.
   Tegrin-HC T.
   t. testosterone
   t. thrombin
   t. treatment
   Triacet T.
   Tridesilon T.
   Triple Antibiotic T.
   U-Cort T.
   Undoguent T.
   Uticort T.
   Vitec T.
   Vytone T.
   Westcort T.
Topicort
   T. cream
   T. ointment
Topicort-LP

NOTES

Topilene
topiramate
Topisone
topographic cervical
topography
    perisulcal t.
topoisomerase-1 inhibitor
Toposar Injection
topotecan hydrochloride
Topsyn
Toradol
    T. Injection
    T. Oral
TORCH, ToRCH
    toxoplasmosis, other agents, rubella,
    cytomegalovirus, herpes simplex
    TORCH infection
    TORCH screen
    TORCH syndrome
    TORCH titer
ToRCHS (var. of STORCH)
toremifene citrate
Toriello-Carey
    T.-C. sign
    T.-C. syndrome
Toriello syndrome (1, 2)
Torkildsen procedure
Toronto
    T. Alexithymia Scale (TAS)
    T. parapodium
torovirus
torpedo
Torpin cul-de-sac resection
Torpin-Waters-McCall culdoplasty
torque depressor
torr
torrential pulmonary flow
torsade de pointes
torsemide
torsion
    adnexal t.
    appendage t.
    t. of appendix
    appendix testis t.
    cord t.
    t. dystonia
    external femoral t.
    external tibial t.
    femoral t.
    t. of gut
    internal femoral t.
    internal tibial t.
    intravaginal testicular t.
    lateral femoral t. (LFT)
    lateral tibial t. (LTT)
    medial femoral t. (MFT)
    medial tibial t. (MTT)
    ovarian t.
    t. of ovary

    penile t.
    splenic t.
    testicular appendage t.
    t. of testis
    tibial t.
torsional
    t. alignment
    t. deformity
    t. profile
torso presentation
Torsten Sjögren syndrome
torti
    pili t.
torticollis
    acquired t.
    acute t.
    benign paroxysmal t.
    congenital muscular t.
    idiopathic t.
    infantile muscular t.
    juvenile muscular t.
    muscular t.
    neonatal t.
    paroxysmal t.
    spasmodic t.
tortuosity
    retinal venous dilation and t.
    (RVDT)
tortuous capillary
Torulopsis glabrata
torulosis
torus fracture
tosylarginine
    t. methyl ester (TAME)
    t. methyl ester esterase
total
    t. abdominal hysterectomy (TAH)
    t. anomalous pulmonary venous
    connection (TAPVC)
    t. anomalous pulmonary venous
    return (TAPVR)
    t. ascertainment
    t. bilirubin
    t. body iron
    t. body iron content
    t. body irradiation (TBI)
    t. body potassium (TBK)
    t. body sodium
    t. body surface area (TBSA)
    t. body water (TBW)
    t. breech extraction
    t. cavopulmonary anastomosis
    t. cavopulmonary connection
    t. colonic aganglionosis
    t. colpectomy
    t. communication
    t. daily energy expenditure (TDEE)
    T. Eclipse moisturizing skin lotion
    t. energy expenditure

t. fat mass (TFM)
t. hemispherectomy
t. hemolytic complement
t. hepatectomy
t. hydroperoxide (TH)
t. iron-binding capacity (TIBC)
t. liquid ventilation (TLV)
t. lung capacity (TLC)
t. magnesium
t. mastectomy
t. mixing lesion
t. muscle paralysis
t. oxyhemoglobin
t. parenteral nutrition (TPN)
t. parenteral nutrition-associated cholestasis
t. pelvic exenteration
t. perineal rupture
t. peripheral parenteral nutrition (TPPN)
t. peripheral resistance (TPR)
t. placenta previa
t. previa
t. pulmonary resistance
t. quality management (TQM)
t. serum bilirubin (TSB)
t. testosterone
t. testosterone index
t. vaginal vault prolapse
t. villous atrophy
t. weight gain

totalis
alopecia universalis t.
rachischisis t.
situs inversus t.
totipotent cell
totipotential cell
toto
in t.
touch
t. imprint
therapeutic t.
Tourette
T. disease
T. disorder (TD)
Gilles de la T.
T. syndrome
tourniquet
hair t.
Touro Ex

TOVA
Test of Variables of Attention
TOVA ADD/ADHD assessment
Towako method
towel
t. clip
DisCide disinfecting t.
tower
T. of Hanoi (TOH)
T. of London (TOL)
t. skull
Townes-Brocks syndrome
Townes syndrome
Townsend
T. biopsy punch
T. endocervical biopsy curette
toxemia, toxicemia
florid t.
preeclamptic t. (PET)
t. of pregnancy
t. syndrome
toxemic
t. rash of pregnancy
t. retinopathy of pregnancy
t. shock syndrome
toxic
t. alopecia
t. appearance
t. cascade
t. dynamics
t. epidermal necrolysis (TEN)
t. erythema
t. hepatitis
t. ingestion
t. megacolon
t. myocarditis
t. neuropathy
t. oil syndrome
t. shock
t. shock syndrome (TSS)
t. shock syndrome toxin-1 (TSST-1)
t. synovitis
toxicemia (*var. of* toxemia)
toxicity
acetaminophen t.
alkali t.
aluminum t.
bismuth t.
bone marrow t.
carbon monoxide t.
chronic cyanide t.

NOTES

toxicity *(continued)*
    citrate t.
    cognitive t.
    cyanide t.
    iron t.
    lidocaine t.
    methylmercury t.
    oxygen t.
    phosphate t.
    salicylate t.
    theophylline t.
    zinc t.
    t. zone
toxicokinetics
toxicologic analysis
toxicology screen
toxicosis
    copper t.
    idiopathic copper t.
toxicum
    erythema neonatorum t.
toxidrome
toxin
    albumin-bound t.
    bacterial t.
    botulinum t.
    botulinum t. A (BTA)
    botulism t.
    clostridial t.
    Clostridium botulinum type A t.
    diphtheria t. (DT)
    environmental t.
    epidermolytic t.
    epsilon t.
    t. exposure
    pertussis t. (PT)
    reproductive t.
    Shiga t. (Stx)
    Shiga-like t.
    tetanus t.
toxin-1
    toxic shock syndrome t.-1 (TSST-1)
toxin-induced scarlet fever exanthem
Toxocara
    T. canis
    T. cati
toxocariasis
toxoid
    pertussis t. (PT)
    pneumococcal conjugate diphtheria t. (PncD)
    tetanus t. (TT)
Toxoplasma
    T. antigen
    T. encephalitis
    T. gondii
    T. lymphadenopathy
Toxoplasma gondii

toxoplasmic
    t. chorioretinitis
    t. encephalitis
toxoplasmosis
    congenital t.
    fetal t.
    ocular t.
    t., other agents, rubella, cytomegalovirus, herpes
    t., other agents, rubella, cytomegalovirus, herpes simplex (TORCH, ToRCH)
    t., other agents, rubella, cytomegalovirus, herpes simplex virus
    t., rubella, cytomegalovirus, herpes simplex syndrome
    t., rubella, cytomegalovirus, herpes simplex, syphilis (STORCH, ToRCHS)
toy
    ride-on t.
t-PA
    tissue plasminogen activator
TPAL
    term infants, premature infants, abortions, living children
TPC
    tympanocentesis
TPHA
    Treponema pallidum hemagglutination
T-Phyl
TPI
    Treponema pallidum immobilization
    triose phosphate isomerase
    TPI deficiency
    TPI test
TPMT
    thiopurine methyltransferase
    TPMT deficiency
TPN
    total parenteral nutrition
TPO
    thrombopoietin
    plasma TPO
TPP
    tubal perfusion pressure
TpP
    thrombus precursor protein
    TpP test
TPPN
    total peripheral parenteral nutrition
TPR
    total peripheral resistance
TQM
    total quality management
TRA
    traumatic rupture of thoracic aorta
trabecular muscular septum

trabeculate
trabeculodysgenesis
trabeculotomy
Trace-4
trace metal
tracer
  radioactive t.
Trach Care suction
trachea
  blind t.
  stenosis of t.
tracheal
  t. agenesis syndrome
  t. aspirate
  t. atresia
  t. catheter
  t. compression
  t. intubation
  t. lavage
  t. occlusion
  t. stenosis
  t. suctioning
  t. tube
  t. tumor
  t. web
tracheal-aspirate culture
tracheitis
  acute t.
  bacterial t.
  subacute t.
trachelectomy
  radical vaginal t.
trachelitis
trachelobregmatic diameter
trachelopanus
trachelopexia, trachelopexy
tracheloplasty
  ex utero intrapartum t. (EXIT)
trachelorrhaphy
tracheloschisis
trachelotomy
tracheobronchial
  t. aspirate
  t. aspirate fluid (TAF)
  t. compression
  t. obstruction
  t. remnant
  t. trauma
  t. tree
  t. tree injury
tracheobronchitis
tracheobronchomalacia

tracheobronchomegaly
tracheocutaneous fistula
tracheoesophageal
  t. atresia
  t. fistula (TEF, TOF)
  t. fistula, esophageal atresia,
    multiple congenital anomaly
    syndrome
  t. septation
  t. septum
tracheolaryngomalacia
tracheomalacia
  intrathoracic t.
  primary t.
  secondary t.
tracheostomy
  flap t.
  percutaneous t.
  t. tube
  t. tube flange
tracheotome
  Sierra-Sheldon t.
tracheotomy
trachoma inclusion conjunctivitis (TRIC)
trachomatis
  Chlamydia t. (CT)
tracing
  lead t.
  NST t.
track
  bear t.'s
tracker
  Breath T.
tracking
  J t.
  visual t.
Tracrium
tract
  aerodigestive t.
  brainstem auditory t.
  dermal sinus t.
  dermoid sinus t.
  endomesenchymal t.
  extrahepatic biliary t.
  extrapyramidal t.
  female reproductive t.
  gastrointestinal t.
  genital outflow t.
  genitourinary t.
  gooseneck deformity of left
    ventricular outflow t.
  intestinal t.

T

NOTES

tract *(continued)*
    left ventricular outflow t. (LVOT)
    Lissauer t.
    lower genital t.
    lower respiratory t.
    mesolimbic dopamine t.
    narrow pulmonary outflow t. (NPOT)
    nerve t.
    nigrostriatal t.
    outflow t.
    patch unroofing of outflow t.
    pin t.
    proximal outflow t.
    pyramidal t.
    renal t.
    reproductive t.
    respiratory t.
    right ventricular outflow t. (RVOT)
    suppurating sinus t.
    upper respiratory t.
    urinary t.
    urogenital t.
    ventricular outflow t.

traction
    90/90 t.
    t. alopecia
    t. apophysitis
    t. apophysitis of medial epicondyle
    t. atrophy
    axial t.
    axis t.
    Bryant t.
    45-degree skin t.
    distal femoral skeletal t.
    t. enterocele
    halo t.
    t. injury
    Russell t.
    skeletal t.
    skin t.
    t. theory
    t. treatment

tractional retinal detachment
traditional surrogacy
traffic-light diet
tragus, pl. **tragi**
    accessory t.

TRAIDS
    transfusion-related AIDS
Trail Making Test
training
    auditory t.
    auditory integration t. (AIT)
    forced bowel t.
    Lovaas t.
    parent effectiveness t. (PET)
    toilet t.

trait
    autosomal dominant t.
    autosomal recessive t.
    cytoplasmic t.
    dominant lethal t.
    familial t.
    galtonian t.
    hereditary t.
    mendelian t.
    multifactorial t.
    penetrant t.
    recessive t.
    sickle cell t.
    thalassemia t.
    threshold t.
    X-linked t.

TRALI
    transfusion-associated lung injury
TRAM
    transverse rectus abdominis
    myocutaneous
    TRAM flap
TRAMP
    transverse rectus abdominis
    musculoperitoneal
    TRAMP flap
TRAMPE
    trichorhinophalangeal multiple exostoses
trampoline
Trandate
Tranebjaerg syndrome (1, 2)
tranexamic acid
tranquilizer drug
transabdominal
    t. amnioinfusion
    t. cervicoisthmic cerclage
    t. chorionic villus sampling
    t. needle transfer
    t. thin-gauge embryofetoscopy (TGEF)
    t. transducer
    t. ultrasonography
    t. ultrasound
    t. urethrolysis
    t. uterine electromyography
transabdominal/transvaginal ultrasound (TAS/TVS)
transalar sphenoidal encephalocele
transaminase
    alanine t. (ALT)
    aspartate t. (AST)
    elevated t.
    glutamic-pyruvic t.
    hepatic t.
    serum t.
    serum glutamic-pyruvic t. (SGPT)
transanal
    t. endoscopic microsurgery (TEM)
    t. rectal biopsy

transanimation
transannular patch repair
transcapillary
    t. fluid
    t. fluid balance
transcarbamylase
    ornithine t. (OTC)
transcarotid balloon valvuloplasty
transcatheter
    t. closure (TCC)
    t. coil embolization
    t. uterine artery embolization
transcelomic (*var. of* transcoelomic)
transcephalic impedance
transcervical
    t. balloon tuboplasty
    t. chorionic villus sampling
    t. division
    t. Foley catheter
    t. intrafallopian tube transfer (TCIFTT)
    t. resection
    t. selective salpingography
    t. tubal access
    t. tubal access catheter (T-TAC)
    t. ultrasound
transcobalamin (I, II) deficiency (TC)
transcoelomic, transcelomic
    t. spread
transcortin
transcranial
    t. Doppler (TCD)
    t. Doppler ultrasonography
    t. magnetic stimulation (TMS)
transcript
    X inactive, specific t. (XIST)
transcriptase
    reverse t.
transcription
    gene t.
    helix-loop-helix t.
    reverse t.
    t. start site
transcriptionally active human papillomavirus
transcription-mediated
    t.-m. amplification (TMA)
    t.-m. amplification assay
transcutaneous
    t. bilirubin (TcB)
    t. blood gas monitor
    t. blood gas monitoring

    t. electrical nerve stimulation (TENS)
    t. jaundice meter
    t. measurement
    t. neurolysis
    t. oximetry
    t. oxygen tension monitoring
    t. partial pressure of oxygen ($tCpO_2$)
transcystoscopically
transdermal
    t. administration
    Alora T.
    Catapres-TTS T.
    Duragesic T.
    Esclim T.
    Estraderm T.
    t. estrogen
    t. fentanyl patch
    t. glyceryl trinitrate patch
    t. hormone replacement therapy
    t. medication patch
    t. nicotine replacement therapy
    t. therapeutic system (TTS)
    Vivelle T.
Transderm-Nitro Patch
Transderm Scop
transdiaphragmatic
transdisciplinary team
transducer
    anular-array t.
    blood pressure t.
    endovaginal t.
    Oxisensor t.
    pressure t.
    SLA t.
    Sorensen Transpac t.
    transabdominal t.
    ultrasound t.
    Voluson sector t.
transducer-tipped catheter
transduction
transection
    complete cord t.
    cord t.
    esophageal t.
    lower esophageal t.
    multiple subpial t. (MST)
transepidermal water loss (TEWL)
Transeptic cleansing solution
transesophageal
    t. echocardiography (TEE)

NOTES

transesophageal *(continued)*
    t. electrophysiologic study
    t. fistula (TEF)
trans fatty acid (tFA)
transfection
transfer
    anterior tibialis t.
    antibody transplacental t.
    blastocyst t.
    direct oocyte t. (DOT)
    direct oocyte sperm t. (DOST)
    donor oocyte t.
    embryo t. (ET)
    embryo intrafallopian t. (EIFT)
    embryo thawing with t.
    t. factor
    frozen-thawed embryo t.
    gamete intrafallopian t. (GIFT)
    gas t.
    gene t.
    intrafallopian t.
    linear energy t.
    t. medium
    peritoneal oocyte sperm t. (POST)
    placental t.
    placental oxygen t.
    pronucleate stage embryo t.
      (PROST)
    pronucleate stage tubal t. (PROST)
    t. ribonucleic acid (tRNA)
    t. RNA (tRNA)
    split anterior tibial tendon t.
      (SPLATT)
    technology t.
    tendon t.
    transabdominal needle t.
    transcervical intrafallopian tube t.
      (TCIFTT)
    transplacental allergen t.
    transvaginal intrafallopian sperm t.
      (SIFT)
    tubal embryo t. (TET)
    tubal embryo stage t. (TEST)
    in vitro fertilization-embryo t.
      (IVF-ET)
    zygote intrafallopian t. (ZIFT)
transferase
    t. deficient galactosemia
    gamma glutamyl t. (GGT)
    glucuronyl t.
    serum glutamic-oxaloacetic t.
      (SGOT)
    succinyl CoA:3-ketoacid CoA t.
    succinyl CoA:3-oxoacid CoA t.
      (SCOT)
transferrin (Tf)
    t. receptor (TfR)
    t. saturation

transformation
    malignant t.
    t. zone (TZ)
transforming
    t. growth factor (TGF)
    t. growth factor 1 (TGF-1)
    t. growth factor alpha (TGF alpha)
    t. growth factor B
    t. growth factor beta (TGF beta)
    t. growth factor B superfamily
transfusion
    acute intrapartum t.
    acute perinatal t.
    antenatal fetofetal t.
    autologous blood t.
    blood t.
    t. controversy
    cryoprecipitate t.
    double-volume exchange t.
    erythrocyte t.
    exchange t. (EXT)
    fetal t.
    fetofetal t.
    fetomaternal t. (FMT)
    fetoplacental t.
    gamma-irradiated cellular
      products t.
    granulocyte t.
    HLA-matched platelet t.
    intrapartum fetoplacental t.
    intraperitoneal blood t.
    intraperitoneal fetal t.
    intrauterine intraperitoneal fetal t.
    intrauterine maternofetal t.
    intravascular t.
    late complication of t.
    leukocyte t.
    massive t.
    maternofetal t.
    neutrophil t.
    packed RBC t.
    packed red blood cell t.
    partial exchange t.
    percutaneous fetal t.
    placental t.
    placentofetal t. (PFT)
    plasma t.
    platelet t.
    prophylactic red-cell t.
    t. reaction
    red blood cell t.
    t. syndrome
    t. therapy
    t. transmitted (TT)
    t. transmitted virus
    twin-to-twin t.
    twin-twin t.
    umbilical cord t.

umbilical vein packed red blood
cell t.
umbilical vein platelet t.
whole blood t.
transfusion-associated
t.-a. cytomegalovirus
t.-a. lung injury (TRALI)
transfusion-dependent thalassemia
transfusion-induced
t.-i. hemosiderosis
t.-i. thrombocytopenia
transfusion-related AIDS (TRAIDS)
transgastric window
transgene
transgenerational analysis
transgenesis
mammalian t.
transgenic organism
transglutaminase (TG)
t. antibody
t. antibody test
t. deficiency
tissue t. (tTG)
trans-Golgi network
transgradiens
transgrediens
keratoderma palmoplantaris t.
transgrow bottle
transient
t. amblyopia
t. aplastic crisis (TAC)
t. bilirubin encephalopathy
t. bullous dermolysis of the
newborn
t. candidemia
t. cerebellar ataxia
t. congenital hypothyroidism
t. cortical blindness
t. dystonia
t. dystonic posturing
t. erythroblastopenia
t. erythroblastopenia of childhood
(TEC)
t. erythroid hypoplasia
t. evoked otoacoustic emission
(TEOAE)
t. familial neonatal
hyperbilirubinemia
t. fetal distress
t. hematuria
t. hemianopia

t. hyperammonemia
t. hypertension
t. hypertension of pregnancy
t. hyperthyrotropinemia
t. hypogammaglobulinemia
t. hypogammaglobulinemia of
infancy (THI)
t. hypoglycemia
t. hypothyroxinemia
t. hypotonia
t. insulinopenic state
t. ischemic attack (TIA)
t. keratitis
t. marrow edema syndrome of the
hip (TMES)
t. monoarticular synovitis
t. mutism
t. myeloproliferative disorder
(TMD)
t. myeloproliferative syndrome
t. neonatal cystinuria
t. neonatal diabetes (TND)
t. neonatal diabetes mellitus
(TNDM)
t. neonatal myasthenia
t. neonatal myasthenia gravis
t. neonatal myasthenic syndrome
t. neonatal pustular melanosis
t. neutropenia
t. oliguria
t. opsoclonus
t. pharyngeal muscle dysfunction
t. protein intolerance
t. proteinuria
t. quadriplegia
t. respiratory acidosis
t. respiratory distress syndrome
(TRDS)
sharp-wave t.
t. tachypnea
t. tachypnea of newborn (TTN)
t. tic disorder
t. tyrosinemia
t. tyrosinemia of newborn
t. vasospasm
transiliac lengthening osteotomy
transilluminate
transillumination
blood vessel t.
t. of head
vessel t.

NOTES

989

transit
>abnormal t.
>small bowel t.

transition
>fetal-neonatal t.
>fetal-to-neonatal t.
>t. plan
>t. stool

transitional
>t. cell tumor
>t. reader stage
>t. sleep

transitory
>t. fever
>t. fever of newborn
>t. hydrocele

transjugular intrahepatic portosystemic shunt (TIPS)

translabial ultrasound

translation
>anterior t.
>nick t.

translevator imperforate anus

translocation
>autosome t.
>bacterial t.
>balanced t.
>t. carrier
>centric fusion t.
>chromosomal t.
>t. of chromosome 22
>de novo balanced t.
>t. Down syndrome
>jumping t.
>mosaic t.
>reciprocal t.
>robertsonian t.
>t. trisomy 21
>unbalanced t.
>X 19 t.
>X-autosome t.

translucency
>nuchal t.

transmalleolar
>t. axis
>t. axis angle (TMA)

transmembrane
>t. conductance regulator gene
>t. conductance regulatory protein
>t. glycoprotein gp41

transmesenteric hernia

transmigration
>ovular t.

transmissible spongiform encephalopathy (TSE)

transmission
>t. disequilibrium
>t. disequilibrium test (TDT)
>t. electron microscopy (TEM)

horizontal t.
>maternal-fetal t.
>t. medium
>mother-infant t.
>perinatal t.
>pressure t.
>sexual t.
>vertical HIV t.
>viral t.

transmission/disequilibrium test

transmitted
>transfusion t. (TT)

transmucosal midazolam

transmural inflammation

transnasal administration

Transorbent dressing

transparenchymal needle puncture

transparency mode

transparent bulla

transpeptidase
>gamma glutamyl t.
>glutamyl t. (GTP)

transpericardial echocardiography

transperineal
>t. implant
>t. ultrasonography
>t. ultrasound

transperitoneal cesarean

transplacental
>t. allergen transfer
>t. hemorrhage
>t. infection
>t. passage

transplant
>autologous ovarian t.
>bone marrow t. (BMT)
>t. coronary artery disease
>fetal tissue t.
>fetus-to-fetus t.
>haploidentical bone marrow t.
>heart t.
>liver t.
>organ t.
>t. patient
>placental tissue t.
>reduced liver t. (RLT)
>reduced-size liver t. (RSLT)
>tissue t.

transplantation
>allogenic bone marrow t.
>allogenic stem cell t.
>t. antigen
>autologous bone marrow t.
>autologous stem cell t.
>auxiliary orthotopic liver t.
>bone marrow t. (BMT)
>cardiac t.
>cord blood t. (CBT)
>cord stem cell marrow t.

double-lung t.
fetal stem cell t.
heart t.
hematopoietic stem cell t.
hepatic t.
heterotopic liver t.
high-dose chemotherapy with
    autologous bone marrow t.
    (HDC-ABMT)
t. immunology
International Society for Heart T.
    (ISHT)
intestinal t.
kidney t.
liver t.
lung t.
marrow t.
organ t.
orthotopic heart t.
orthotopic liver t. (OLTx)
partial auxiliary orthotopic liver t.
peripheral stem cell t.
pituitary gland t.
renal t.
small bowel t.
solid organ t. (SOT)
stem cell t. (SCT)
stem cell bone marrow t.
syngeneic bone marrow t.
thymus t.
umbilical cord blood t.
in utero t.

transport
bus t.
t. disorder
egg t.
fixed-wing t.
t. medium
neonatal t.
ovum t.
sperm t.

transport-associated protein (TAP)
transporter
carbohydrate homeostasis t.
glucose t. (GLUT)
transposable element
transposase
transposed adnexa
transposition
aortopulmonary t.
arterial t.
complete t.

t. of great arteries (TGA)
t. of great vessels (TGV)
lateral ovarian t.
muscle t.
t. of ovary
penoscrotal t.
physiologically corrected t.
t. of viscera
transposon
transpulmonary pressure
transpyloric
t. enteral feeding
t. tube feeding
t. tube insertion
transrectal
t. approach
t. probe
t. surgical treatment
t. ultrasound (TRUS)
transsexual
transsexualism
transsphenoidal
t. microsurgical resection
t. operation
transtelephonic monitoring (TTM)
transtentorial herniation
transthoracic echocardiography
transthyretin (TTR)
transtracheal
t. aspiration
t. catheter
t. ventilation
**transtubular potassium concentration
gradient (TTKG)**
transudate
mucosal t.
vaginal t.
transudation
vaginal t.
transudative pleural effusion
**transumbilical breast augmentation
(TUBA)**
transurethral
t. ablation
t. ablation of valve
t. catheter
t. collagen injection
t. electrocautery
t. marsupialization
t. self-detachable balloon
transvaginal
t. amniotic puncture (TAP)

NOTES

transvaginal *(continued)*
    t. bladder neck suspension
    t. color Doppler sonography (TV-CDS)
    t. cone
    t. fine-needle biopsy
    t. implant
    t. intrafallopian sperm transfer (SIFT)
    t. sacrospinous colpopexy
    t. sonography (TVS)
    t. sonohysterography
    t. transducer probe
    t. treatment
    t. tubal catheterization
    t. ultrasonography
    t. ultrasound (TVU, TV-UST)
    t. ultrasound-directed oocyte retrieval (TUDOR)
    t. ultrasound-guided urethral reconstruction
    t. urethrolysis
transvalensis
    Nocardia t.
transvascular
transvenous
    t. coil embolization
    t. pacing
transversalis fascia
transversal nasal crease
Trans-Ver-Sal Transdermal Patch
transverse
    t. arch hypoplasia
    t. arrest
    t. cervical ligament
    t. colon
    t. dense striation
    t. diameter
    t. fetal lie
    t. fracture
    t. fundal incision of Strassman
    t. hemimelia
    t. lie presentation
    t. loop colostomy
    lower uterine segment t. (LUST)
    t. myelitis
    t. nail groove
    occiput t. (OT)
    t. oval pelvis
    t. plication
    t. rectus abdominis musculoperitoneal (TRAMP)
    t. rectus abdominis myocutaneous (TRAM)
    t. ridge
    t. scan
    t. scrotal testis
    t. skin incision
    t. vaginal septum

transversion
transversum
    septum t.
transversus
    t. abdominis muscle
    situs t.
Tranxene
tranylcypromine
TRAP
    thrombin receptor-activating peptide
    twin reversed arterial perfusion
    TRAP sequence
    TRAP syndrome
trap
    filtered specimen t.
    Luekens t.
    sterile specimen t.
TRAP-activated neonatal platelet
trapezoidocephaly-synostosis syndrome
trapped ovum
trapping
    air t.
    ion t.
    platelet t.
Trasicor
trastuzumab
Trasylol
trauma, pl. **traumata, traumas**
    abdominal t.
    acoustic t.
    American Association for the Surgery of T. (AAST)
    birth t.
    blunt cardiac t.
    blunt chest t.
    cardiac t.
    central nervous system t.
    chest t.
    childhood genital t.
    closed head t. (CHT)
    corneal t.
    craniocerebral t.
    dehydration, poisoning, t. (DPT)
    dental t.
    diaphragmatic t.
    fetal t.
    Focused Assessment by Sonography for T. (FAST)
    forceps birth t.
    genital tract t.
    gluteal t.
    head t.
    lap-belt t.
    maternal t.
    penetrating t.
    perinatal t.
    perineal t.
    psychological t.

T. Score and Injury Severity Score
Analysis (TRISS)
sex-related t.
T. Symptom Checklist for Children
(TSCC)
thoracic t.
tracheobronchial t.
T. Triage Rule (TTR)
TraumaCal formula
trauma-related acute pelvic hemorrhage
traumas (*pl. of* trauma)
traumata (*pl. of* trauma)
traumatic
t. alopecia
t. amenorrhea
t. amputation
t. aortic disruption
t. aortic injuries in children
t. birth injury
t. bowing
t. brain injury (TBI)
t. compartment syndrome
t. delivery
t. dissection
t. glaucoma
t. hematoma
t. hemobilia
t. hyphema
t. idiocy
t. imagery
t. labyrinthitis
t. pneumothorax
t. rupture of thoracic aorta (TRA)
t. sexualization
t. vaginitis
Travamine
Travamulsion IV fat emulsion
traveler's diarrhea (TD)
tray
t. agglutination test (TAT)
EZ-EM PercuSet amniocentesis t.
HSG t.
Unimar HSG t.
trazodone
TRDS
transient respiratory distress syndrome
Treacher
T. Collins-Franceschetti syndrome
T. Collins mandibulofacial
dysostosis
T. Collins syndrome
treadmill

treatment
add-back t.
adjunctive t.
allergy t.
ambulatory antibiotic t.
antenatal corticosteroid t. (ANS)
antenatal phenobarbital t.
antibiotic t.
anticonvulsant t.
anti-D globulin t.
antiinflammatory t.
antimanic t.
antimicrobial t.
ART t.
biologic t.
brace t.
continuous/combined t.
corticosteroid t.
domestic violence t.
double diaper t.
Early and Periodic Screening,
Diagnosis, and T. (EPSDT)
t. and education of autistic and
related communications
handicapped children (TEACCH)
empiric t.
exogenous thyroxine t.
ex utero intrapartum t. (EXIT)
t. failure
gonadal hormone t.
hormonal t.
hyperbaric oxygen t.
immunomodulatory t.
infertility t.
laparoscopic t.
laser t.
local t.
mutagenic t.
neurodevelopmental t.
Otovent negative pressure t.
Pacis BCG bladder cancer t.
pharmacologic t.
phase advance t.
phase delay t.
P32 intraperitoneal t.
pityriasis rotunda t.
postexposure t. (PET)
prenatal t.
preventive allergy t. (PAT)
prophylactic t.
rape t.
t. recommendation

NOTES

treatment *(continued)*
    t. series
    spectacle t.
    steroid t.
    topical t.
    traction t.
    transrectal surgical t.
    transvaginal t.
    updraft t.
    ureteral surgical t.
    zidovudine t.
treatment-associated pregnancy
treatment-independent pregnancy
treatment-refractory depression
treatment-resistant proteinuria
Trecator-SC
tree
    bronchial t.
    extrahepatic biliary t.
    t. pollen
    tracheobronchial t.
trefoil pelvis
Treitz
    ligament of T.
trembling
    hereditary chin t.
tremor
    coarse t.
    essential t.
    familial t.
    hereditary t.
    intention t.
    primary writing t.
    t. syndrome
tremulousness
trench
    t. fever
    t. mouth
Trendelenburg
    T. gait
    T. limp
    T. position
    T. sign
    T. test
Trental
trephination
    nail t.
trephine, trepan
Treponema
    T. carateum
    T. pallidum
    T. pallidum antibody
    T. pallidum antigen
    T. pallidum hemagglutination (TPHA)
    T. pallidum immobilization (TPI)
    T. pallidum immobilization test
    T. pertenue
treponemal serology

treponematosis
treppe response
Tresilian sign
tretinoin
Trevor disease
Trexan
TRF
    Teacher Rating Form
    Teacher Report Form
TRH
    thyrotropin releasing hormone
    Thyrel TRH
Triacet Topical
triacetyloleandomycin
triad
    AGR t.
    aspirin t.
    atopic t.
    Beck t.
    Charcot t.
    Currarino t.
    Cushing t.
    female athlete t. (FAT)
    t. of head tilt disorder
    Hutchinson t.
triage
trial
    Bernoulli t.
    breast cancer prevention t. (BCPT)
    Canadian Crohn Relapse Prevention T.
    cervical incompetence prevention randomized cerclage t. (CIPRACT)
    chemotherapy phase t.
    diabetes control and complications t. (DCCT)
    Diabetes Prevention T.
    digital mammographic imaging screening t. (DMIST)
    t. forceps
    high-frequency ventilation t. (HIFT)
    labor t.
    promotion of breastfeeding intervention t. (PROBIT)
    RADIUS t.
    STOP-ROP t.
    surfactant replacement t.
    voiding t.
    WAVE t.
Triam-A Injection
triamcinolone
    t. acetonide
    t. acetonide ointment
    t. hexacetonide
Triam Forte Injection
Triaminic
    T. AM Decongestant Formula
    T. Oral Infant Drops

triamterene
triangle
> Burger t.
> Codman t.
> Einthoven t.
> femoral t.
> Hesselbach t.
> inguinal t.
> Kiesselbach t.
> Petit lumbar t.
> posterior t.
> pubic t.
> Ward t.

triangular
> t. facies
> t. fibrocartilaginous complex (TFCC)
> t. ligament
> t. splint
> t. uterus
> t. vaginal patch sling procedure

triatriatum
> cor t.

Triaz benzoyl peroxide pad
triazolam
Triazole
Triban
tribasilar synostosis
tribrachius
TRIC
> trachoma inclusion conjunctivitis

tricephalus
triceps
> t. reflex
> t. skinfold thickness (TSF)
> t. tendinitis

tricheiria
trichilemmal cyst
trichilemmoma
Trichinella spiralis
trichinosis
trichiura
> *Trichuris* t.

Trichlorex
trichlormethiazide
trichloroacetic acid (TCA)
trichloroethanol (TCE)
trichloroethylene
2,4,5-trichlorophenoxyacetic acid
trichobezoar
trichodental dysplasia, microcephaly, mental retardation syndrome

trichodentoosseous syndrome
trichodysplasia
> hereditary t.

trichoepithelioma
trichomegaly
> eyelash t.

trichomonad
trichomonal
> t. infection
> t. vaginitis

Trichomonas
> *T.* infection
> *T. vaginalis*
> *T. vaginalis* vaginitis

trichomoniasis
trichophagia
trichophagy
Trichophyton
> *T. mentagrophytes*
> *T. rubrum*
> *T. tonsurans*

trichopoliodystrophy
trichorhinophalangeal
> t. multiple exostoses (TRAMPE)
> t. multiple exostosis dysplasia
> t. syndrome

trichorino-auriculophalangeal multiple exostoses dysplasia
trichorionic
trichorrhexis
> t. blastysis
> t. invaginata
> t. nodosa
> t. nodosa syndrome

trichoschisis
Trichosporon beigelii
trichosporonosis
trichothiodystrophy 2 (TTD 2)
trichothiodystrophy-congenital ichthyosis syndrome
trichothiodystrophy-neurocutaneous syndrome
trichothiodystrophy-xeroderma pigmentosum syndrome
trichotillomania
trichrome stain
trichuriasis
Trichuris
> *T.* dysentery syndrome
> *T. trichiura*

Tricosal

NOTES

tricuspid
 t. atresia
 t. insufficiency
 t. regurgitation
 t. stenosis
 t. valve
Tri-Cyclen
 Ortho T.-C.
tricyclic antidepressant (TCA)
tridactylism
Tridesilon Topical
tridihexethyl chloride
Tridione syndrome
tridymus
triencephalus
triene-to-tetraene ratio
trientine
triethanolamine polypeptide oleate-condensate
triethnic
triethylene tetramine dihydrochloride
triethylenethiophosphoramide
trifluoperazine hydrochloride
trifluorothymidine
triflupromazine hydrochloride
trifluridine
trifunctional protein deficiency (TFP)
trigeminal
 t. herpes zoster
 t. nerve
 t. nerve distribution
trigemino-encephalo-angiomatosis
trigger
 t. digit
 environmental t.
 t. phenomenon
 t. point
triglyceride
 t. hyperlipidemia
 medium-chain t. (MCT)
 milk t.
 t. storage disease
triglycine
 mercaptoacetyl t.
trigonal
 t. hypertrophy
 t. plate
 t. ring
 t. urothelium
trigone
 urinary t.
trigonitis
 pseudomembranous t.
trigonocephaly syndrome
trigonum
 os t.
Trihexane
trihexose
 ceramide t.

Trihexy
trihexyphenidyl
TriHIBit vaccine
trihydrate
 ampicillin t.
trihydroxycoprostanic acidemia
Tri-Immunol vaccine
triiniodymus
triiodothyronine (T3)
 free t.
 reverse t.
 t. test
Tri-K
Trikacide
trilaminar
 t. blastoderm
 t. embryonic disc
trilateral
 t. retinoblastoma
 t. retinoblastoma syndrome
trileaflet aortic valve
Tri-Levlen contraceptive pill
trilineage development
Trilisate
triloba
 placenta t.
trilogy
 Fallot t.
 t. of Fallot
trilostane
Trilucent breast
trimegestone
trimeprazine
trimester
 first t.
 second t.
 third t.
trimethadione
 t. embryopathy
 t. syndrome
trimethaphan camsylate
trimethoprim
 cotrimoxazole t.
 t. HCl oral solution
 t. sulfate
trimethoprim-sulfamethoxazole (SMZ-TMP, TMP-SMX)
 t.-s. prophylaxis
trimethylaminuria
trimipramine
Trimstat
Trinalin
Tri-Nasal Spray
trinitrate
 glyceryl t. (GTN)
Tri-Norinyl
Trinsicon
trinucleotide repeat expansion mutation
triocephalus

triodurin
triopathy
triophthalmos
triose
- t. phosphate isomerase (TPI)
- t. phosphate isomerase deficiency

Triostat Injection
triotus
tripartita
- placenta t.

Tripedia vaccine
tripelennamine hydrochloride
tripe palm
triphalangeal thumb
triphasic
- t. oral contraceptive
- t. pattern blastemal cell

Triphasil contraceptive pill
triphenylethylene selective estrogen receptor modulator
triphosphatase
- adenosine t. (ATPase)

triphosphate
- adenosine t. (ATP)
- deoxynucleotide t.
- digoxigenin-labeled deoxyuridine t.
- guanosine t. (GTP)
- lead t.

5′-triphosphate
triplane fracture
triple
- T. Antibiotic Topical
- t. arthrodesis
- t. bromide
- t. diapers
- t. dye
- T. Paste
- T. Paste ointment
- t. screen
- t. screen test
- t. serum marker screening
- t. sulfa cream
- t. sulfa suppository
- t. swab test
- T. X Liquid
- T. X shampoo
- t. X syndrome

triple-biochemical screen
triple-drug therapy
triplegia
triple H (*var. of* HHH)

triple-lumen
- t.-l. catheter
- t.-l. tube

triple-marker
- t.-m. screen
- t.-m. screening

triplet pregnancy
triple-X, triplo-X
- t.-X chromosomal aberration
- t.-X female

triplication
- ureteral t.

triploid
- t. embryo
- t. fetus
- t. preembryo

triploidy
- placental mosaicism for t.
- t. syndrome

triplo-X (*var. of* triple-X)
tripod
- t. fixation technique
- t. position
- t. sign

tripodia
tripoding
tripod-supporting position
trip 15q syndrome
triprolidine
- t. hydrochloride
- t. and pseudoephedrine

Triptil
TripTone caplets
triptorelin
tripus
- t. conjoined twins
- ischiopagus t. separation
- ischiopagus t. twins
- t. limb
- t. separation

triradius
- distal t.

trisalicylate
- choline magnesium t.

trisegmentectomy
triseriatus
- *Aedes* t.

tris[hydroxymethyl]aminomethane-buffered saline
trismus
- t. nascentium

NOTES

T

trismus *(continued)*
    t. neonatorum
    persistent t.
trismus-pseudocamptodactyly syndrome
trisomic
    t. fetus
    t. rescue
trisomy
    t. 1–22
    autosomal t.
    t. C,D,E,G syndrome
    chromosome 1–22 t.
    chromosome 1p–22p t.
    chromosome 1q–22q t.
    chromosome Xq t.
    t. 18-like syndrome
    mosaic t. 14
    t. 8 mosaicism
    nondisjunction t. 21
    partial t. 1p–22p
    t. 1p–22p syndrome
    t. 1q–22q syndrome
    t. 1–22 syndrome
    translocation t. 21
    t. X
    X t.
    t. Xq
trisphosphate
    inositol t.
TRISS
    Trauma Score and Injury Severity Score
    Analysis
TriStar trocar
Trisulfa
trisulfapyrimidine
Trisulfa-S
Trivagizole 3 vaginal cream
trivalent live cold-adapted influenza
    vaccine (CAIV-T)
Trivers-Willard theory
Tri-Vi-Flor vitamins
Tri-Vi-Sol vitamins
Trivora-28 tablet
TRIzol
    TRIzol reagent
    TRIzol RNA extractor
trizygotic
tRNA
    transfer ribonucleic acid
    transfer RNA
TRO
    thyroid-related ophthalmopathy
Trobicin
trocar
    Bluntport disposable t.
    Cabot t.
    Circon-ACMI t.
    Core Dynamics disposable t.
    Dexide disposable t.

    Endopath bladeless t.
    Endopath TriStar t.
    Ethicon disposable t.
    t. guide
    t. hernia
    t. implantation metastasis
    Jarit disposable t.
    laparoscopic t.
    Marlow disposable t.
    5-mm suprapubic t.
    Olympus disposable t.
    Origin t.
    Saber BT blunt-tip surgical t.
    t. site ecchymosis
    Solos disposable t.
    Step laparoscopic t.
    Storz disposable t.
    TriStar t.
    Visiport optical t.
    Weck disposable t.
    Wisap disposable t.
    Wolf disposable t.
    Ximed disposable t.
trochanter
    greater t.
troche
    Cepacol Anesthetic T.
    clotrimazole t.
trochlear
    t. nerve
    t. nerve palsy
trochocephaly
TroGARD electrosurgical blunt trocar
    system
troglitazone
troleandomycin
trombiculiasis
tromethamine (THAM)
    carboprost t.
    dinoprost t.
    fosfomycin t.
    ketorolac t.
    lodoxamide t.
Tronolane
TrophAmine hyperalimentation
trophectoderm
    t. biopsy
    t. stage
trophic
    t. feed
    T-cell t. (T-trophic, T-tropic)
trophoblast
    extravillous t.
    intermediate t. (IT)
    t. in regression (TIR)
    t. sampling
trophoblastic
    t. cell
    t. embolus

t. invasion
t. neoplasia
t. neoplastic disease
t. pseudotumor
t. tissue
t. tumor
trophospongia
trophotropism
trophozoite
tropic
t. hormone
macrophage t.
tropica
Leishmania t.
Tropicacyl
tropical
t. ataxic neuropathy
t. bubo
t. pyomyositis
Quinsana Plus T.
t. spastic paraparesis (TSP)
t. spastic paraparesis/HTLV-I associated myelopathy (TSP/HAM)
t. sprue
tropicalis
Candida t.
tropicamide
tropism
tropoelastin
tropomodulin
troponin
t. C
cardiac t. T
t. I
t. I level
t. T (TnT)
trough
peak and t.
t. tacrolimus level
trousers
antishock t.
military antishock t. (MAST)
Trousseau sign
trovafloxacin
Trovan/Zithromax Compliance Pak
Troyer syndrome (TS)
true
t. accessory breast
t. conjugate
t. hermaphroditism
t. histiocytic lymphoma (THL)
t. incontinence

t. labor
t. macroglossia
t. pelvis
t. precocious puberty
t. precocity
t. twins
t. undescended testis
t. uterine inertia
t. vertigo
trumpet
t. cannula
Iowa t.
truncal
t. acne
t. asymmetry
t. ataxia
t. incurvation reflex
t. obesity
t. rash
truncate selection
truncation
uterine positioning via ligament investment fixation t. (UPLIFT)
truncus
t. arteriosus
t. arteriosus communis
trunk
t. control
t. presentation
pulmonary arterial t.
t. rotation
TRUS
transrectal ultrasound
trust
support t.
Tru-Trax
TruZone PFM
Trypanosoma
T. brucei
T. cruzi
trypanosomal chancre
trypanosome
trypanosomiasis
African t.
American t.
cerebral t.
Cruz t.
Gambian t.
Rhodesian t.
trypsin activation peptide (TAP)
trypsinization

T

NOTES

trypsinogen
 immunoreactive t. (IRT)
tryptase
tryptophan
 t. ethylester
 t. malabsorption
tryptophanuria
tryptorelin
TS
 Troyer syndrome
TSB
 total serum bilirubin
TSC
 tuberous sclerosis complex
TSCC
 Trauma Symptom Checklist for Children
TSE
 transmissible spongiform encephalopathy
tsetse fly
TSF
 triceps skinfold thickness
TSH
 thyroid-stimulating hormone
  TSH surge
T-shaped
 T-s. constriction ring
 T-s. uterus
TSP
 tropical spastic paraparesis
TSP/HAM
 tropical spastic paraparesis/HTLV-I
 associated myelopathy
TSRH
 Texas Scottish Rite Hospital
  TSRH crosslink
  TSRH instrumentation
TSS
 toxic shock syndrome
TSST-1
 toxic shock syndrome toxin-1
TST
 tuberculin skin test
TSTA
 tumor-specific transplantation antigen
T-Stat
1.5 T superconductive system
tsutsugamushi
 t. fever
 Orientia t.
TSV
 thalamostriate vasculopathy
TT
 tetanus toxoid
 transfusion transmitted
  TT virus (TTV)
T-TAC
 transcervical tubal access catheter
  T-TAC system

TTD 2
 trichothiodystrophy 2
TTF-1
 thyroid transcription factor-1
tTG
 tissue transglutaminase
TTKG
 transtubular potassium concentration
 gradient
T1–T10 lymphocyte
TTM
 transtelephonic monitoring
TTN
 transient tachypnea of newborn
TTP
 thrombotic thrombocytopenic purpura
TTR
 transthyretin
 Trauma Triage Rule
T-trophic, T-tropic
 T-cell trophic
  T-trophic SI strain
TTS
 transdermal therapeutic system
 twin-to-twin transfusion syndrome
  Estraderm TTS
  TTS fentanyl
  Testoderm TTS
TTTS
 twin-to-twin transfusion syndrome
T-tube cholangiogram
T-tubules
TTV
 TT virus
TUBA
 transumbilical breast augmentation
tubage
tubal
 t. abortion
 t. banding
 t. colic
 t. damage
 t. distortion
 t. diverticulum
 t. dysmenorrhea
 t. embryo stage transfer (TEST)
 t. embryo transfer (TET)
 t. endometriosis
 t. endometrium
 t. factor
 t. factor infertility
 t. gestation
 t. inflammatory damage (TID)
 t. insufflation
 t. ligation (TL)
 t. ligation band technique
 t. mass
 t. metaplasia
 t. microsurgery

t. obstruction
t. occlusion
t. ostium
t. patency
t. perfusion pressure (TPP)
t. pregnancy
t. recanalization
t. reconstruction surgery
t. reversal
t. ring
t. rupture
t. spasm
t. sterilization
tubatorsion (*var. of* tubotorsion)
tube
bilateral myringotomy t.'s (BMT)
bronchial t.
Cantor t.
chest t.
Cole endotracheal t.
Cole orotracheal t.
t. connector
cuffed endotracheal t.
cuffed ET t.
dislodged t.
Dobbhoff nasogastric feeding t.
double-focus t.
ear ventilation t.
embryonic neural t.
endotracheal t.
EntriStar Skin Level T.
ET t.
eustachian t.
fallopian t.
t. feed
feeding t.
fimbriated end of fallopian t.
Foley t.
follicle aspiration t.
gastrointestinal t.
gastrostomy t.
infundibulum of fallopian t.
t. insertion technique
Keofeed t.
knuckle of t.
laser office ventilation of ears with
  insertion of t.'s (LOVE IT)
Linton t.
Malecot t.
Miller-Abbott t.
molybdenum rotating anode x-
  ray t.

Moss t.
myringotomy t.
nasogastric t. (NGT)
nasojejunal t.
neural t.
NG t.
NJ t.
OG t.
oral gastric t.
t.'s and ovaries (T&O)
PE t.
Pedi PEG t.
PEG t.
percutaneous endoscopic
  gastrostomy t.
Pezzer t.
t. placement
polyethylene feeding t.
t. position
pressure equalization t. (PET)
pus t.
Replogle sump t.
Reuter t.
Rubin t.
salpingitis in previously
  occluded t.'s (SPOT)
Sengstaken-Blakemore t.
Shah permanent t.
smoke removal t. (SRT)
thoracostomy t.
t. thoracostomy
tracheal t.
tracheostomy t.
triple-lumen t.
tympanostomy t.
uncuffed endotracheal t.
uterine t.
ventilation t.
tubectomy
tuber
cortical t.
cryptic t.
subependymal t.
tubercle
choroid t.
genital t.
Ghon t.
Montgomery t.
Morgagni t.
Müller t.
pubic t.

NOTES

T

tubercle *(continued)*
    Rokitansky t.
    tibial t.
tuberculid
    papulonecrotic t.
tuberculin
    t. skin test (TST)
    t. syringe
    t. test
    t. testing
tuberculoid
    borderline t.
    t. leprosy
tuberculoma
    infratentorial t.
tuberculoprotein
tuberculosis (TB)
    abdominal t.
    bovine t.
    cavitary t.
    congenital t.
    cutaneous t.
    disseminated t.
    drug-resistant t.
    endobronchial t.
    endometrial t.
    extrapulmonary t.
    extrathoracic t.
    gastrointestinal t.
    genital t.
    hematogenous primary t.
    infectious pulmonary t.
    intrathoracic t.
    miliary t.
    multidrug-resistant t. (MDR-TB)
    mycobacteria other than t. (MOTT)
    Mycobacterium t.
    orificial t.
    t. papulonecrotica
    pediatric t.
    pelvic t.
    primary pulmonary t.
    progressive primary pulmonary t.
    pulmonary t.
    reactivation t.
    renal t.
    spinal t.
    t. verrucosa cutis
    visceral t.
tuberculous
    t. abscess
    t. adenitis
    t. cervical lymphadenitis
    t. chancre
    t. colitis
    t. dactylitis
    t. enteritis
    t. gumma
    t. keratoconjunctivitis

    t. meningitis
    t. osteomyelitis
    t. peritonitis
    t. pleural effusion
    t. pneumonia
    t. salpingitis
    t. spinal arachnoiditis
    t. spondylitis
tuberculum sella
tuberosa
    sclerosis t.
tuberosity
    bicipital t.
tuberous
    t. breast abnormality
    t. mole
    t. sclerosis
    t. sclerosis complex (TSC)
    t. sclerosis syndrome
    t. subchorial hematoma of the
        decidua
Tubex
Tubigrip bandage
tubing
    blow-by through t.
    Mini-Med t.
    pressure-separator t.
tuboabdominal pregnancy
tubocornual
    t. anastomosis
    t. microsurgery
    t. reanastomosis
tubocurarine chloride
tuboendometrial cell
tuboovarian
    t. abscess (TOA)
    t. abscess after previous tubal
        occlusion (TOAPOT)
    t. complex (TOC)
    t. pregnancy
    t. varicocele
tuboovaritis
tuboplasty
    balloon t.
    transcervical balloon t.
    ultrasound-guided transcervical t.
    ultrasound transcervical t.
tubotorsion, tubatorsion
tubouterine
    t. implantation
    t. pregnancy
tubovaginal fistula
tubular
    t. atrophy
    t. bone
    t. breathing
    t. cancer
    t. carcinoma
    t. disruption

t. dysgenesis
t. hypoplasia
t. interstitial fibrosis
t. necrosis
t. proteinuria
t. stenosis
t. stenosis, hypocalcemia,
  convulsions, dwarfism syndrome
tubularization
in situ t.
tubularized incised plate (TIP)
tubule
anular t.
convoluted t.
mesonephric t.
proximal convoluted t.
renal t.
seminiferous t.
tubuloglomerular feedback
tubulointerstitial
t. disease
t. lesion
t. nephritis (TINU)
tubulopathy
hypokalemic salt-losing t.
t. of Lowe syndrome
proximal t.
tuck
Tucker-McLane forceps
Tucker-McLane-Luikart forceps
TUDOR
transvaginal ultrasound-directed oocyte
  retrieval
tuft
central gliotic t.
digital t.
distal t.
epithelial t.
gliotic t.
glomerular t.
t. of hair
swollen glomerular t.
tugging at ears
tularemia
glandular t.
oculoglandular t.
oropharyngeal t.
pneumonic t.
pulmonary t.
t. (type A, B)
typhoidal t.

ulceroglandular t.
t. vaccine
tularensis
Francisella t.
tumbling E chart
tumescence
physiologic t.
tumescent absorbent bandage
tumor
adenomatoid oviduct t.
adnexal t.
adrenal cell rest t.
adult granulosa cell t. (AGCT)
androgen-producing t.
t. angiogenesis factor (TAF)
angiomatoid t.
t. antigen
t. antigenicity
t. ascites
Askin t.
atypical teratoid t.
atypical teratoid/rhabdoid t.
autochthonous t.
autonomic nerve t.
benign t.
bladder t.
t. blush
bone t.
borderline epithelial ovarian t.
brain t.
Brenner t.
t. burden
carcinoid t.
central primitive neuroectodermal t.
  (cPNET)
cerebellar t.
cervical cord t.
cervical stump t.
clear cell t.
CNS t.
colorectal t.
craniofacial t.
t. debulking
debulking of t.
desmoid t.
desmoplastic small round cell t.
  (DSRCT)
dumbbell t.
embryonal t.
endocervical sinus t.
endodermal sinus t. (EST)
endometrial t.

NOTES

T

tumor *(continued)*
endometrioid epithelial cell t.
epithelial liver t.
epithelial serous t.
epithelial stromal t.
Ewing t.
extragonadal germ cell t.
extranodal t.
extrapelvic solid t.
extrarenal rhabdoid t.
eyelid t.
feminizing adrenal t.
fibrovascular t.
Frantz t.
functioning t.
gastrointestinal autonomic nerve t.
  (GANT)
genital tract t.
germ cell testicular t.
germinal cell t.
gestational trophoblastic t. (GTT)
Glazunov t.
glomus t.
glycoprotein-producing t.
gonadal stromal cell t.
gonadal stromal ovarian t.
t. grading
granulosa cell t.
granulosa-stromal cell t.
granulosa-theca cell t.
hairlike t.
hemispheric t.
hilar cell t.
hilus cell t.
hormone-secreting t.
hypothalamic t.
t. immunology
t. immunotherapy
infratentorial t.
insulin-secreting pancreatic t.
intracranial t.
intraocular t.
intrapulmonary t.
intrinsic t.
islet cell t.
juvenile granulosa cell t. (JGCT)
juxtaglomerular cell t. (JGCT)
Koenen t.
Krukenberg t.
Leydig cell t.
lipid cell ovarian t.
lipoid ovarian t.
liver t.
t. lysis syndrome
malignant brain t.
malignant epithelial t.
malignant extrarenal rhabdoid t.
malignant germ cell t.
malignant mesodermal t.

malignant mixed müllerian t.
  (MMMT)
malignant nerve sheath t.
malignant ovarian germ cell t.
t. marker
t. mass
mediastinal t.
mesodermal t.
mesonephroid t.
metastatic gynecologic t.
midline craniofacial t.
mixed germ cell t.
mixed mesodermal t.
mixed müllerian t. (MMT)
mixed uterine t.
monodermal t.
mucinous t.
mulberry t.
müllerian t.
t. necrosis
t. necrosis factor (TNF)
t. necrosis factor alpha (TNF-alpha)
nerve sheath t.
neural crest t.
neuroectodermal t.
neurogenic t.
t., node, metastases (TNM)
nonalpha cell t.
nondysgerminomatous germ cell t.
nonfunctional pituitary t.
nonhematogenous t.
nonsecreting pituitary t.
null cell t.
optic nerve t.
optic pathway t.
orbital t.
ovarian malignant germ cell t.
pancreatic t.
paratesticular t.
parovarian t.
pelvic t.
periaqueductal t.
peripheral neuroectodermal t.
peripheral primitive
  neuroectodermal t. (PPNET)
persistent postmolar gestational
  trophoblastic t.
phyllodes t.
piloid t.
pineal t.
pituitary gland t.
placental site t.
placental site trophoblastic t.
  (PSTT)
pleomorphic spindle cell t.
polypoid epithelial t.
pontine t.
posterior fossa t.

postmolar persistent gestational trophoblastic t.
Pott puffy t.
pregnancy t.
prepuberal testicular t. (PPTT)
primary intraocular t.
primary tracheal t.
primitive neuroectodermal t. (PNET)
t. progression
pseudomucinous t.
Purkinje cell t.
radioresistant yolk sac t.
Recklinghausen t.
t. regression
rhabdoid t.
round cell t.
sarcomatous t.
Schiller t.
Scully t.
t. seeding
serous t.
Sertoli cell t.
Sertoli-Leydig cell t.
sex cord mesenchymal t.
sex cord stromal germ cell t.
single t.
sinus t.
t. size
smooth muscle t.
solid t.
t. spillage
spinal t.
spinal cord t.
spindle cell t.
Steiner t.
sternomastoid t.
stromal t.
t. suppression gene
t. suppressor gene
Teilum t.
teratoid t.
testicular t.
testis t.
theca cell t.
tracheal t.
transitional cell t.
trophoblastic t.
ulcerative t.
uterine corpus t.
ventricular t.
virilizing adrenal t.

vitelline t.
Wilms t. (stage I–V)
yolk sac t.
tumor-associated antigen (TAA)
tumor-cloning assay
tumorigenesis
tumorigenicity
tumor-limiting factor
tumorous hyperprolactinemia
tumor-specific transplantation antigen (TSTA)
Tums Extra Strength
TUNEL
    terminal deoxyribonucleotidyl transferase-mediated biotin-16-dUTP nick-end labeling
    TUNEL assay
    TUNEL stain
tungiasis
tunica
    t. albuginea
    t. vaginalis
tunnel
    intracardiac t.
    lateral atrial t. (LAT)
    subcutaneous t.
    t. vision
tunneled CVL
tunnel-view radiography
Tuohy spinal needle
turbidity
Turbinaire
    Decadron T.
    Dexacort Phosphate T.
turbinate
    t. bone
    nasal t.
Turbuhaler
    budesonide T.
    Pulmicort T.
    Rhinocort T.
turbulence
turbulent airflow
turcica
    sella t.
Turco posteromedial release of clubfoot
Turcot syndrome
turgescence
turgescent
turgor
Turner
    T. mosaic

NOTES

T

Turner *(continued)*
    T. mosaicism
    T. mosaic syndrome
    T. phenotype
    T. phenotype with normal
      karyotype
    T. syndrome in female with X
      chromosome
    T. XO syndrome
Turner-Albright syndrome
Turner-Kieser syndrome
Turner-like syndrome
Turner-Warwick urethroplasty
turning
    contralateral head t. (CHT)
turnover
    bone t.
    iron t.
turricephaly
turtle sign
Tuss-DM
Tussin
    Safe T. 30
Tussi-Organidin DM NR
Tusstat Syrup
Tuttle test
TV
    tidal volume
TV-CDS
    transvaginal color Doppler sonography
TVS
    transvaginal sonography
TVT
    tension-free vaginal tape
TVU
    transvaginal ultrasound
TV-UST
    transvaginal ultrasound
TWAR
    Taiwan acute respiratory
      TWAR agent
T-wave
    T-w. abnormality
    T-w. axis
    T-w. inversion
Tween 80
twenty-nail dystrophy
Twice-A-Day Nasal Solution
twilight sleep
Twilite Oral
twill tape
twin
    allantoidoangiopagous t.'s
    asymmetrical conjoined t.'s
    binovular t.'s
    t. birth
    t. birth weight discordance
    breech-first t.
    concordant t.'s

conjoined t.'s
t. delivery
t. demise
diamniotic t.'s
dicephalic t.'s
dichorionic t.'s
dichorionic-diamniotic t.'s
diovular t.'s
discordant t.'s
dissimilar t.'s
dizygotic t.
donor t.
enzygotic t.
equal conjoined t.'s
false heteroovular t.'s
fraternal t.'s
t. gestation
growth-discordant t.'s
heterologous t.'s
heteroovular t.
identical t.'s
impacted t.'s
incomplete conjoined t.'s
janiceps t.'s
locked t.'s
locking t.'s
membranous t.'s
t. method
monoamniotic t.'s
monochorial t.'s
monochorionic t.'s
monochorionic-diamniotic t.'s
monovular t.'s
monozygotic t.'s
omphaloangiopagous t.'s
one-egg t.'s
parabolic t.'s
t. peak sign
perfused t.'s
t. placenta
t. pregnancy
pump t.'s
recipient t.
t. reversed arterial perfusion
  (TRAP)
second t.
Siamese t.'s
similar t.'s
stuck t.'s
symmetrical conjoined t.'s
thoracopagus t.'s
tripus conjoined t.'s
true t.'s
two-egg t.'s
unequal conjoined t.'s
uniovular t.'s
unlike t.'s
vanishing t.
xiphoomphaloischiopagus tripus t.'s

twinge
   Texidor t.
twinning
   cardiac t.
twin-peak syndrome
twin-to-twin
   t.-t.-t. transfusion
   t.-t.-t. transfusion reaction
twin-to-twin transfusion syndrome (TTS, TTTS)
twin-twin transfusion
twisted
   t. hair
   t. neck
twister cable
twitch
twitching
   arrhythmic t.
TwoCal HN formula
two-cell
   t.-c. embryo
   t.-c. mechanism
   t.-c. zygote
two-dimensional echocardiogram
two-egg twins
two-hit hypothesis
two-part nuclear stage
two-point discrimination
two-stage arterial switch operation
two-team sling
two-vessel cord
Tycos aneroid sphygmomanometer
Tygon catheter
Tylenol
   T. and Codeine Elixir
   T. Cold, Children's
   T. Extra Strength
   T. With Codeine No. 2, 3, 4
Tylok high-tension cerclage cabling system
tylosis ciliaris
Tylox
tympani
   chorda t.
   scala t.
tympanic
   t. membrane
   t. membrane compliance
   t. membrane perforation
   t. temperature
tympanites
   uterine t.

tympanitic abdomen
tympanocentesis (TPC)
tympanogram
tympanomastoid suture line
tympanometer
tympanometric
   t. gradient
   t. width
tympanometry
   impedance t.
tympanosclerosis
tympanosquamous suture line
tympanostomy tube
tympanum
tympany
Ty-Pap
type
   accelerated skeletal maturation, Marshall-Smith t.
   t. A IL-8 receptor
   alpha-thalassemia/mental retardation syndrome, deletion t. (ATR1, ATR-16)
   alpha-thalassemia/mental retardation syndrome, nondeletion t. (ATR2, ATR, nondeletion)
   Amsterdam t.
   axonal t.
   Babesia WA1 t.
   Batten-Bielschowsky t.
   t. B IL-8 receptor
   blood t. A, AB, B, O
   breech t.
   Caldwell-Moloy pelvis t.'s
   clinical t.
   dementia of the Alzheimer t. (DAT)
   t. 1, 2 diabetes mellitus
   D-mosaic blood t.
   dominantly hyperactive impulsive t.
   Du variant blood t.
   epidermolysis bullosa, macular t. (EBM)
   facial clefting syndrome, Gypsy t.
   gangliosidosis GM1 juvenile t.
   generalized gangliosidosis GM1 adult t.
   t. 7 glycogenosis
   hereditary bullous skin dystrophy, macular t.
   t. I collagen C-telopeptide
   t. I, II AT3 deficiency

T

NOTES

type *(continued)*
 t. II pneumocyte
 t. II pneumonocyte
 t. IV RTA
 MALT t.
 mating t.
 normal female sex chromosome t.
  (XX)
 normal male sex chromosome t.
  (XY)
 t. 16 papillomavirus
 peroneal muscular atrophy,
  axonal t.
 Pi t.
 protease inhibitor t.
 senile dementia of the
  Alzheimer t. (SDAT)
 sialuria, Finnish t.
 wave t.
 wild t.
typhi
 Rickettsia t.
 Salmonella t.
typhimurium
 Salmonella t.
typhlitis
typhoid
 t. autoantibody
 t. fever
 t. vaccine
typhoidal tularemia
typhus
 t. fever
 flying squirrel t.
 t. group
 louse-borne t.
 murine t.
 North Asian tick t.
 Queensland tick t.
 recrudescent t.
 scrub t.
 sylvatic t.
 tick-borne t.
typical
 t. absence epilepsy
 t. absence seizure
 t. measles

typing
 blood t.
 DNA t.
 HLA t.
 newborn platelet antigen t.
 short tandem repeat t.
 STR t.
 tissue t.
typus
 t. degenerativus amstelodamensis
 t. edinburgensis
Tyrode solution
tyropanoate sodium
tyrosinase-negative oculocutaneous
 albinism
tyrosinase-positive oculocutaneous
 albinism
tyrosine
 t. aminotransferase (TAT)
 t. aminotransferase deficiency
  (TATD)
 t. kinase
 t. kinase receptor
 t. phosphatase
 t. transaminase deficiency
tyrosinemia
 hepatorenal t.
 hereditary t.
 oculocutaneous t.
 Oregon-type t.
 t., palmar and plantar keratosis,
  ocular keratitis syndrome
 transient t.
 t. (type 1, 2)
tyrosinosis
 oculocutaneous t.
 t. (type 1, 2)
Tyzine Nasal
TZ
 transformation zone
Tzanck
 T. prep
 T. smear
 T. test

UA
    umbilical artery
    urinalysis
UAC
    umbilical artery catheter
UAE
    uterine artery embolization
UAL
    umbilical artery line
UALTE
    unexplained apparent life-threatening
        event
UAO
    urine acid output
UARS
    upper airways resistance syndrome
UBE3A gene
UBT
    urea breath test
    uterine balloon therapy
UCAC
    uterine cornual access catheter
Ucephan Oral
UCG
    urinary chorionic gonadotropin
UCG-Slide Test
Uchida
    U. fimbriectomy
    U. method
    U. procedure
    U. tubal ligation
UCI
    umbilical coiling index
        PPROM UCI
U-Cort
    U-C. cream
    U-C. Topical
UDI
    urinary diagnostic index
    Urinary Distress Inventory
    Urogenital Distress Inventory
UDP
    uridine diphosphate
UDP-galactose-4-epimerase (GALE)
**UD-2000 urodynamic measurement
    system**
UE
    upper extremity
uE3
    unconjugated estriol
U elevator
UEP
    urinary excretion of protein
UES
    upper esophageal sphincter

UF
    ultrafiltration
        hydraulic UF
        osmotic UF
        rapid UF
U/F
        Fulvicin U/F
UFE
    uterine fibroid embolization
UGA
    urogenital atrophy
u-hFSH
    urinary-derived human follicle-
        stimulating hormone
Uhl anomaly
Uhthoff
        U. sign
        U. symptom
UI
    uteroplacental insufficiency
U/L
    upper body segment to lower body
        segment ratio
ulcer
        aphthous u.
        chancroid u.
        corneal u.
        decubitus u.
        duodenal u.
        genital aphthous u.
        herpetiform aphthous u.
        herpetiform corneal u.
        Hunner u.
        idiopathic u.
        jejunal u.
        kissing u.
        Lipschütz u.
        mucocutaneous u.
        oral aphthous u.
        peptic u.
        recurrent genital aphthous u.
        shallow u.
        stress-associated u.
        vaginal u.
ulcera (*pl. of* ulcus)
ulcerans
        Mycobacterium u.
ulceration
        aphthous u.
        corneal u.
        digital u.
        esophageal u.
        genital u.
        nasal u.
        oral u.

U

ulceration *(continued)*
    penile u.
    perianastomotic u.
    shallow u.
ulcerative
    u. blepharitis
    u. colitis
    u. tumor
    u. vulvitis
ulceroglandular
    u. disease
    u. tularemia
ulcus, pl. **ulcera**
    u. vulvae acutum
ULE
    unilateral laterothoracic exanthem
ulegyria
uLH
    urinary luteinizing hormone
ulinastatin
Ullrich
    U. disease
    U. and Fremerey-Dohna syndrome
Ullrich-Bonnevie syndrome
Ullrich-Feichtiger syndrome
Ullrich-Noonan syndrome
Ullrich-Turner syndrome
ulna
ulnar
    u. clubhand
    u. collateral ligament
    u. hypoplasia, club feet, mental
      retardation syndrome
    u. nerve block
    u. neuropathy
    u. palmar grasp
    u. styloid fracture
    u. tilt
ulnar-mammary syndrome
Ulrich-Turner stigmata
ULR-LA
ultra
    Prenate U.
Ultracef
ultrafast
    u. magnetic resonance imaging
    u. MRI
ultrafiltrate
ultrafiltration (UF)
    u. membrane
    u. virus clearance
Ultrafort prenatal vitamins
Ultramark ultrasound system
ultrasensitive assay
ultrasonic
    u. cephalometry
    u. egg recovery
    u. endovaginal finding
    u. fetometry

ultrasonogram
ultrasonographic
    u. assessment
    u. determination
    u. diagnosis
    u. guidance
ultrasonographically guided oocyte
  retrieval
ultrasonography
    color Doppler u.
    compression u.
    cranial u.
    diagnostic u.
    Doppler u.
    endoanal u.
    endovaginal u.
    graded compression u.
    gray-scale u.
    hepatobiliary u.
    high-resolution u.
    intravascular u.
    level III u.
    obstetric u.
    real-time u.
    three-dimensional u.
    transabdominal u.
    transcranial Doppler u.
    transperineal u.
    transvaginal u.
    umbilical artery Doppler u.
ultrasonohysterography
ultrasonologist
ultrasound
    abdominal u.
    Acuson 128 Doppler u.
    Acuson 128XP u.
    Acuson 128XP-10 u.
    Advantage u.
    Aloka 650 CL u.
    Aloka OB/GYN u.
    A-mode u.
    Ansaldo AU560 u.
    antenatal u.
    u. assessment
    ATL Ultramark 4,8,9 u.
    BABE u.
    B-mode u.
    Cineloop U.
    cranial u.
    3D u.
    u. diagnosis
    digital u.
    Doppler u.
    duplex u.
    dynamic image on u.
    Elscint ESI-3000 u.
    endoanal u.
    Endosound endoscopic u.
    endovaginal u. (EVUS)

fetal u.
u. fetometry
GE RT 3200 Advantage II u.
u. guidance
HDI 3000 u.
head u.
high-resolution u.
Hitachi EUB 420 digital u.
intracoronary u.
intravascular u. (IVUS)
Maggi disposable biopsy needle
  guide for u.
M-mode u.
noncontact u.
obstetric u.
pancreatic u.
pelvic u.
Performa u.
Pie Medical u.
prenatal u.
ProSound SSD-5500 u.
pulsed Doppler u.
pulsed-wave u.
quantitative u. (QUS)
real-time imaging on u.
renal u.
routine antenatal diagnostic imaging
  with u. (RADIUS)
u. scanning
u. screening
Shimadzu IIQ u.
Shimadzu SDU-400 u.
Siemens SI 400 u.
SonoAce 6000 II u.
SonoAce 8000 Live u.
Sonoline Prima u.
Spectra-Diasonics u.
u. stethoscope
Sunlight Omnisense u.
u. surveillance
targeted u.
u. technology
three-dimensional u.
transabdominal u.
transabdominal/transvaginal u.
  (TAS/TVS)
transcervical u.
u. transcervical tuboplasty
u. transducer
translabial u.
transperineal u.
transrectal u. (TRUS)

transvaginal u. (TVU, TV-UST)
vaginal probe u.
volumetric bladder u.
ultrasound-directed
  u.-d. egg retrieval
  u.-d. percutaneous umbilical blood
    sampling
**ultrasound-guided transcervical
tuboplasty**
Ultravate
ultraviolet (UV)
  u. A, B
  u. light
  psoralen and u. A (PUVA)
Ultra-Vue amniocentesis needle
umbilical
  u. anomaly
  u. arterial EDV
  u. arterial pH
  u. artery (UA)
  u. artery catheter (UAC)
  u. artery catheterization
  u. artery Doppler ultrasonography
  u. artery Doppler velocimetry
  u. artery line (UAL)
  u. artery pulsatility index to
    middle cerebral artery pulsatility
    index ratio
  u. artery waveform notching
    abnormality
  u. blood flow
  u. blood sampling
  u. cardiovascular circulation
  u. clamp
  u. coiling index (UCI)
  u. cord
  u. cord accident
  u. cord anomaly
  u. cord blood bank
  u. cord blood transplantation
  u. cord hematoma
  u. cord insertion
  u. cord leptin
  u. cord mass
  u. cord prolapse
  u. cord syndrome
  u. cord transfusion
  u. cyst
  u. Doppler flow velocity
  u. fistula
  u. fold
  u. fungus

U

NOTES

umbilical *(continued)*
- u. granuloma
- u. hernia
- u. ligament
- u. line
- 10-mm u. port
- u. polyp
- u. presentation
- u. scissors
- u. souffle
- u. stump
- u. swab
- u. vein
- u. vein catheter (UVC)
- u. vein catheterization
- u. vein packed red blood cell transfusion
- u. vein platelet transfusion
- u. vein varix
- u. velocity ratio
- u. venous catheter (UVC)
- u. venous flow
- u. venous line (UVL)
- u. venous plasma amino acid
- u. vessel
- u. vessel catheter

umbilicalis
- arteritis u.

umbilication of lesion

umbilicoplacental vessel

umbilicoplasty

umbilicus
- furrowlike u.
- u. reconstruction

Umbilicutter

umbrella
- Bard PDA U.
- u. device
- u. sign
- vascular u.

Unasyn

unavoidable hemorrhage

unbalanced
- u. AV canal defect
- u. translocation

unborn child

unbound iron

uncalcified
- u. bacterial plaque
- u. bone matrix

uncal herniation

uncinate fit

uncombable hair syndrome

uncompensated
- u. hydrocephalus
- u. shock

uncomplicated
- u. hernia
- u. measles

unconjugated
- u. bilirubin
- u. estriol (E3, uE3)
- u. estriol level
- u. hyperbilirubinemia

unconjugated estriol (E3, uE3)

uncuffed endotracheal tube

undecapeptide

undecylenic
- u. acid
- u. acid ointment

underdeveloped
- u. chin
- u. mandible

underdevelopment
- face u.
- middle third of face u.

underdose

underfeeding

underinflation

underlying disease

undernourished

undernourishment
- maternal u.

undernutrition

underperfusion
- uterine u.

undervascularity
- pulmonary u.

underwater
- u. delivery
- u. drainage system
- u. weighing

Underwood disease

undescended
- u. testicle
- u. testis

undifferentiated
- u. gonad
- u. rhabdomyosarcoma

Undoguent Topical

Undritz anomaly

undulant fever

unemancipated

unequal
- u. aeration
- u. conjoined twins
- u. visual input

unestrogenized vaginal mucosa

unexplained
- u. apparent life-threatening event (UALTE)
- u. fever
- u. infertility
- u. jaundice
- u. recurrent miscarriage

unfavorable cervix

unfractionated heparin

UNG
    uracil-N-glycosylase
ungual
unguium
    tinea u.
UNHS
    universal newborn hearing screening
UNHSP
    universal newborn hearing screening
    program
Uni-Ace
unicameral bone cyst
Unicare breast pump
unicellular
unicentric
unicollis
    uterus bicornis u.
unicommisural
unicornis
    uterus u.
unicornuate uterus
unicorn uterus
unidentified bright object
unifactorial disorder
unifocal clonic movement
unilambdoid synostosis
unilateral
    u. bar
    u. congenital ptosis
    u. cryptorchidism
    u. facial microsomia
    u. fibular aplastic syndrome
    u. flank mass
    u. hearing impairment
    u. hemimegalencephaly
    u. hyperlucent lung
    u. hypoplastic pectoral muscle
    u. intrauterine facial necrosis
    u. laterothoracic exanthem (ULE)
    u. lower lip paralysis
    u. mandibulofacial dysostosis
    u. megalencephaly
    u. microtia
    u. mydriasis
    u. neonatal hydronephrosis
    u. occipital plagiocephaly
    u. optic neuritis
    u. optokinetic nystagmus
    u. partial facial paralysis
    u. renal agenesis
    u. salpingo-oophorectomy

    u. stapling
    u. ureteral obstruction (UUO)
unilocular
    u. cystic ovarian mass
    u. ovarian cyst
Unimar
    U. HSG tray
    U. Pipelle
uninhibited bladder
uninterrupted estrogen
union
    delayed u.
uniovular twins
uniparental disomy (UPD)
Unipath
Uniphyl
Uniplant
unipolar
    u. depression
    u. electrode
Uniprobe test
Uniserts
    acetaminophen U.
    bisacodyl U.
    Hemril-HC U.
    RMS U.
Unisom
unit
    Alexander u.
    antenatal testing u.
    antepartum u.
    Bethesda u.
    BiliBed phototherapy u.
    bone collagen equivalent u. (BCE)
    Bovie u.
    bubble isolation u.
    calf compression u.
    colony-forming u. (CFU)
    dentoalveolar u.
    fetal-placental u.
    Flowtron DVT prophylaxis u.
    human *neu* u. (HNU)
    immunizing u. (IU)
    u. inheritance
    intensive special care u. (ISCU)
    International U. (IU)
    lipase u.
    Log-a-Rhythm Signal Acquisition u.
    maternal-fetal medicine u. (MFMU)
    maternal-placental u.
    maternal-placental-fetal u.
    nem (breast milk nutritional u.)

U

NOTES

unit *(continued)*
    neonatal intensive care u. (NICU)
    newborn intensive care u. (NBICU)
    newborn special care u. (NBSCU)
    Nytone enuretic control u.
    Orthotic Research and Locomotor
        Assessment U. (ORLAU)
    pediatric intensive care u. (PICU)
    pediatric sedation u. (PSU)
    pilosebaceous u.
    plaque-forming u. (pfu)
    terminal ductal lobular u. (TDLU)
    terminal duct lobular u. (TDLU)
United
    U. Network for Organ Sharing
        (UNOS)
    U. States Preventive Services Task
        Force (USPSTF)
    U. States Preventive Services Task
        Force (USPSTF)
Unitensen
units-erythroid
    burst-forming u.-e. (BFU-E)
univariate
univentricular
universal
    u. bilirubin screen
    u. hearing screen
    U. indicator stick
    u. joint syndrome
    u. newborn hearing screening
        (UNHS)
    u. newborn hearing screening
        program (UNHSP)
    u. nose of childhood
    U. vaginal probe
universale
    pterygium u.
universalis
    alopecia u.
    neurinomatosis u.
unlike twins
unmalleable
Unna
    U. mark
    U. nevus
Unna-Thost syndrome
unopposed estrogen
UNOS
    United Network for Organ Sharing
unpaired chromosome
unpasteurized milk product
unplanned pregnancy
unrecognized
    u. apnea
    u. pregnancy
unregulated catabolism

unresponsive
    alertness, response to voice,
        response to pain, u. (AVPU)
unresponsiveness
    ACTH u.
    immunologic u.
    thyroid hormone u.
unrestrictive ventricular septal defect
unroofed coronary sinus
unroofing
    endoscopic u.
    patch u.
unruptured tubal gestation
unsaturated
    u. fat
    u. linolenic acid
    u. phosphatidylcholine
unspun
    u. catheterized urine specimen
    u. urine
unstable
    u. bladder
    u. bladder of childhood
    u. bladder syndrome
    u. fetal presentation
    u. hemoglobin
    u. lie
unusual
    u. facies, mental retardation,
        intrauterine growth retardation
        syndrome
    u. hunger
Unverricht disease
Unverricht-Lundborg
    U.-L. disease
    U.-L. syndrome
UOAC
    uterine ostial access catheter
up
    pinked up
u-PA
    urokinase plasminogen activator
upbeat nystagmus
UPD
    uniparental disomy
updraft treatment
UPJ
    ureteropelvic junction
    UPJ obstruction
UPLIFT
    uterine positioning via ligament
        investment fixation truncation
    UPLIFT procedure
upper
    u. airway noise
    u. airway sleep-disordered breathing
    u. airways resistance syndrome
        (UARS)
    u. body segment

u. body segment to lower body
    segment ratio (U/L)
u. contractile portion of uterus
u. esophageal sphincter (UES)
u. extremity (UE)
u. gastrointestinal
u. gastrointestinal series
u. genital tract infection
u. GI lesion
u. humeral epiphysis
u. limb amelia
u. limb deficiency
u. motor neuron disease
u. motor neuron sign
u. motor neuron syndrome
u. respiratory illness
u. respiratory infection (URI)
u. respiratory tract
u. respiratory tract infection
    (URTI)
u. urinary tract infection

UPPP
uvulopalatopharyngoplasty
upregulation
upright
u. abdominal radiograph
u. chest film
u. tilt-table testing
upsaliensis
Campylobacter u.
**UPS 2020 ambulatory measurement
system**
UPSC
uterine papillary serous carcinoma
upside-down ptosis
upslanting palpebral fissure
upstairs-downstairs heart
upstream
upstroke
uptake
bone mineral u.
maximum oxygen u. (VO$_2$max)
minute oxygen u.
radioactive u.
upward
u. gaze
u. gaze weakness
u. rotation
urachal
u. cyst
u. fistula

urachus
obliterated u.
patent u.
persistent u.
Uracid
Uracil
uracil-N-glycosylase (UNG)
uranoschisis
uranostaphyloschisis
urate
u. calculus
u. clearance
u. crystal
u. nephropathy
u. tophi
Urbach-Wiethe disease
Urban
U. operation
U. syndrome
Urban-Rogers-Meyer syndrome
urea
u. breath test (UBT)
u. clearance
u. cycle
u. cycle disease
u. cycle disorder
u. cycle enzyme defect
u. nitrogen
u. plaster
urealyticum
Ureaplasma u.
Ureaphil
Ureaplasma
U. culture
U. urealyticum
Urecholine
ureidopenicillin
uremia
uremic
u. encephalopathy
u. state
u. syndrome
ureter
atretic u.
double u.
duplicated u.
ectopic u.
u. fistula
ileal u.
partially duplicated u.
reimplantation of u.
retrocaval u.

U

NOTES

ureteral
- u. course
- u. duplication
- u. dysmenorrhea
- u. ectopia
- u. injury
- u. jet
- u. node
- u. obstruction
- u. patency
- u. peristalsis
- u. rupture
- u. surgical treatment
- u. trigonal reimplantation
- u. triplication
- u. valve

ureteric bud
ureterocalycostomy
ureterocele
- ectopic u.
- prolapsed ectopic u.
- simple u.

ureterocervical
ureterocystoplasty
- augmentation u.

ureteroileostomy
- Bricker u.

ureteroneocystostomy
- Glen Anderson u.
- Politano-Leadbetter u.

ureteropelvic junction (UPJ)
ureteropyelocaliectasis
ureteropyeloscope
- Karl Storz flexible u.

ureteropyelostomy
ureterosigmoidostomy
ureterostomy
- cutaneous u.

ureterotubal anastomosis
ureteroureteral anastomosis
ureteroureterostomy
ureterouterine
ureterovaginal fistula
ureterovesical
- u. junction (UVJ)
- u. obstruction
- u. reflux

ureterovesicoplasty
- Leadbetter-Politano u.

urethra, pl. **urethrae**
- bulbus urethrae
- compressor u.
- dilated posterior u.
- drain-pipe u.
- fusiform dilation of u.
- imperforate u.
- lead pipe u.
- low-pressure u.
- penile u.

- pipestem u.
- posterior u.
- proximal u.

urethral
- u. advancement and glanuloplasty
- u. angle
- u. atresia
- u. candle
- u. caruncle
- u. catheterization
- u. closure pressure
- u. coaptation
- u. detachment
- u. discharge
- u. diverticulectomy
- u. diverticulum
- u. duplication
- u. elongation
- u. epithelium
- u. function
- u. gland
- u. hypermobility
- u. lumen
- u. meatus
- u. opening
- u. plate
- u. plate division
- u. pressure cough profile
- u. pressure profile
- u. pressure profilometry
- u. prolapse
- u. seam
- u. sound
- u. spasm
- u. sphincter
- u. stenosis
- u. support
- u. syndrome
- u. valve

urethralis
- habenula u.

urethritis
- anterior u.
- chlamydial u.
- follicular u.
- gonococcal u.
- granular u.
- nongonococcal u.
- nonspecific u. (NSU)
- u. petrificans
- posterior u.
- senile u.
- simple u.
- specific u.
- u. venerea

urethrocele
urethrocutaneous fistula
urethrocystometry
urethrocystoscopy

urethrography
    positive pressure u.
urethrolysis
    transabdominal u.
    transvaginal u.
urethropexy
    Burch retropubic u.
    retropubic u.
urethroplasty
    Badenoch u.
    Thiersch-Duplay u.
    Turner-Warwick u.
urethroscopy
urethrotome
urethrotomy
    direct vision internal u. (DVIU)
urethrotrigonitis
urethrovaginal
    u. fistula
    u. sphincter muscle
urethrovesical
    u. angle
    u. angle support
Urex
urge
    U. Impact Scale (URIS)
    u. incontinence
urgency
    u. syndrome
    urinary u.
urgency-frequency syndrome
URI
    upper respiratory infection
uric
    u. acid
    u. acid infarction
    u. acid lithiasis
    u. acid nephrolithiasis
    u. acid stone
Uri-Check test
uricosuria
Uricult culture
uridine diphosphate (UDP)
Uridon
uridyltransferase
    galactose-1-phosphate u. (GALT)
urinalysis (UA)
    bagged u.
    clean-catch u.
    enhanced u.
urinary
    u. beta-core fragment

u. bladder
u. bladder dysfunction
u. calculus
u. cast
u. catheter
u. catheterization
u. chorionic gonadotropin (UCG)
u. concentrating capacity
u. concentrating defect
u. concentration test
u. conduit
u. copper
u. coproporphyrin
u. coproporphyrin I
u. diagnostic index (UDI)
u. diary
u. dipstick test
U. Distress Inventory (UDI)
u. diversion
u. diverticulum
u. excreted melatonin
u. excretion
u. excretion of protein (UEP)
u. exertional incontinence
u. fistula
u. free cortisol
u. free progesterone
u. frequency
u. glucose
u. glycosaminoglycan
u. iodine
u. lactate:creatinine ratio
u. luteinizing hormone (uLH)
u. menopausal gonadotropin
u. mucopolysaccharide pattern
u. orotic acid
u. outlet obstruction
u. ovulation detection kit
u. ovulation predictor kit
u. potassium wasting
u. pterin
u. reflux
u. retention
u. sediment
u. sphincter
u. stasis
u. stent
u. steroid conjugate
u. stress incontinence
u. system
u. tract
u. tract abnormality

U

NOTES

urinary *(continued)*
  u. tract anomaly
  u. tract dilation
  u. tract disorder
  u. tract dysplasia
  u. tract endometriosis
  u. tract infection (UTI)
  u. tract malformation
  u. tract obstruction
  u. trigone
  u. trypsin inhibitor
  u. unidiversion procedure
  u. urgency
urinary-derived human follicle-stimulating hormone (u-hFSH)
urination
  fetal u.
urine
  u. acid output (UAO)
  u. CIE test
  Coke-colored u.
  cola-colored u.
  concentrated u.
  u. culture
  u. cytology
  dark u.
  delirium, infection, atrophic urethritis/vaginitis, pharmaceuticals, psychological, excess u.
  dilute u.
  u. dipstick
  u. ferric chloride test
  fetal u.
  u. flow
  u. ketoacid
  u. latex test
  u. leakage
  u. ligase chain reaction
  malodorous u.
  maple syrup u.
  u. mucopolysaccharide
  u. organic acid
  u. output
  persistent alkaline u.
  residual u.
  u. sample
  u. sampling
  u. sediment
  spun u.
  suprapubic aspiration of u.
  u. toxicology screen
  unspun u.
  u. vanillylmandelic acid
  vin rosé-colored u.
urine-reducing substance
uriniferous breath
urinoma
URIS
  Urge Impact Scale

Uriscreen urine test
Urispas
Urispec
  U. GPA test
  U. 9-Way test
Uristat
Uri-Three urine culture kit
Uri-Two petri dish
urobilinogen excretion
urobilinogenuria
urobilinoid
urocanase deficiency
urocanic
  u. acid
  u. aciduria
Urocit-K
Urocyte diagnostic cytometry system
urocytogram
urodynamic
urodynamically
urodynamics testing
uroepithelium
urofacial syndrome
uroflowmetry
urofollitropin
  u. for injection
  u. for injection, purified
urogenital
  u. atrophy (UGA)
  u. congenital anomaly
  u. diaphragm
  U. Distress Inventory (UDI)
  u. epithelium
  u. fistula
  u. fold
  u. hiatus
  u. ridge
  u. septum
  u. sinus
  u. sphincter
  u. tract
urogenitogram
urogenitography
Urogesic
urogram
  excretory u.
  intravenous u. (IVU)
urography
  intravenous u. (IVU)
  intravenous excretory u.
  magnetic resonance u. (MRU)
urogynecologic
urogynecologist
urogynecology
urokinase
  u. plasminogen activator (u-PA)
Uro-KP-Neutral
Urolene Blue Oral
urolithiasis

urologic
    u. history
    u. problem
urological
    u. evaluation
    u. injury
urologist
urology
Uro-Mag capsule
uropathogen
uropathy
    bilateral u.
    fetal u.
    lower obstructive u. (LOU)
    obstructive u.
urorectal
urosepsis
urothelium
    trigonal u.
UroVive system
Urozide
ursi
    uva u.
Urso
ursodeoxycholic acid
ursodiol
URTI
    upper respiratory tract infection
urticaria
    acquired u.
    acute u.
    cholinergic u.
    chronic idiopathic u.
    cold u.
    cutaneous u.
    idiopathic u.
    papular u.
    u. pigmentosa
    pressure u.
    primary acquired u.
    secondary solar u.
    solar u.
urticarial
    u. papule
    u. raised lesion
urticate
urtication
US
    Usher syndrome
    US 1005 uroflow meter
USA Elite System GYN rotating continuous flow resectoscope

use
    compassionate u.
    conservative drug u.
    illicit drug u.
    intravaginal foreign body u.
    intravenous drug u. (IDU)
    maternal cocaine u.
    Maternal Interview of Substance U. (MISU)
    oral contraceptive u.
    prophylactic aspirin u.
    rape kit u.
U-shaped
    U.-s. deceleration
    U.-s. vestibulectomy
Usher syndrome (US)
USPSTF
    United States Preventive Services Task Force
U technique
uterectomy
uteri (*gen. and pl. of* uterus)
uterine
    u. abnormality
    u. absence
    u. access
    u. action
    u. activity
    u. activity alteration
    u. activity monitor
    u. agenesis
    u. angiosarcoma
    u. anomaly
    u. arteriovenous malformation
    u. artery
    u. artery embolization (UAE)
    u. artery hemodynamic adaptation
    u. artery ligation
    u. artery pseudoaneurysm
    u. atony
    u. balloon therapy (UBT)
    u. ballottement
    u. blood flow
    u. calculus
    u. carcinosarcoma
    u. cast
    u. cavity
    u. chondrosarcoma
    u. colic
    u. compression
    u. contractile agent
    u. contractility

NOTES

U

uterine *(continued)*
- u. contraction
- u. coring
- u. cornu
- u. cornual access catheter (UCAC)
- u. corpus
- u. corpus carcinoma
- u. corpus tumor
- u. cough
- u. cramping
- u. cry
- u. curette
- u. decompression
- u. displacement
- u. dysfunction
- u. dysmenorrhea
- u. elevator
- u. endolymphatic stroma
- u. endometrial stroma
- u. enlargement
- u. epithelial stroma
- u. epithelium
- u. evacuator
- u. evaluation
- U. Explora Curette endometrial sampling device
- u. exteriorization
- u. factor
- u. fibroid
- u. fibroid carneous degeneration
- u. fibroid embolization (UFE)
- u. fibroid red degeneration
- u. fibromyoma
- u. flora
- u. fragmentation
- u. gland
- u. hematoma
- u. hemodynamics
- u. hemorrhage
- u. hernia syndrome
- u. horn
- u. hyperstimulation
- u. hypertonus
- u. hypotonia
- u. incarceration
- u. incision
- u. inertia
- u. infection
- u. insufficiency
- u. inversion
- u. lateral fusion defect
- u. leiomyomata
- u. lysosome level
- u. malposition
- u. manipulator
- u. mass
- u. massage
- u. milk
- u. morcellation
- u. müllerian sarcoma
- u. myoma
- u. myometrium
- u. necrosis
- u. neoplasm
- u. ostial access catheter (UOAC)
- u. outflow obstruction
- u. packing
- u. papillary serous carcinoma (UPSC)
- u. pathology
- u. perforation
- u. position
- u. positioning via ligament investment fixation truncation (UPLIFT)
- u. pregnancy
- u. prolapse
- u. pyomyoma
- u. quiescence
- u. reconstruction
- u. relaxation
- u. retroflexion
- u. retroversion
- u. rupture
- u. sarcoma metastasis
- u. scar dehiscence
- u. scar separation
- u. screening
- u. segment
- u. septum
- u. sinus
- u. size
- u. souffle
- u. sound
- u. suspension
- u. tachysystole
- u. tenaculum
- u. tenaculum forceps
- u. tetanus
- u. tone
- u. tonus
- u. tube
- u. tympanites
- u. underperfusion
- u. vein
- u. vessel
- u. window formation
- u. withdrawal bleeding

uterinus
- vagitus u.

uterismus
uteritis
utero
- fetal death in u. (FDIU)
- fetal demise in u.
- fetal version in u.
- in u. (IU)
- in u. sensitization

uteroabdominal pregnancy
Uterobrush endometrial sample collector
uterocystostomy
uterofixation
uterolith
uterometer
uteroovarian
    u. circulation
    u. ligament
    u. varicocele
uteroperitoneal fistula
uteropexy
uteroplacental
    u. apoplexy
    u. blood flow
    u. circulation
    u. insufficiency (UI)
    u. perfusion
    u. sinus
    u. vessel
uteroplasty
uterosacral
    u. complex
    u. ligament
    u. ligament pedicle
    u. ligament suspension
    u. nerve ablation
    u. nerve ligation
    u. nodularity
    u. shortening
uterosalpingography
uteroscope
uteroscopy
uterotomy
uterotonic
uterotonin
uterotubal junction (UTJ)
uterotubography
uterovaginal
    u. canal
    u. primordium
    u. prolapse
uterus, gen. and pl. uteri
    u. acollis
    adnexa uteri
    anomalous u.
    arcuate u.
    u. arcuatus
    AV/AF u.
    benign nonprolapsed u.
    u. bicornis
    u. bicornis unicollis

bicornuate u.
bifid u.
u. bifidus
biforate u.
u. biforis
u. bilocularis
bipartite u.
u. bipartitus
bivalving of the u.
boggy u.
capped u.
communicating u.
cordiform u.
u. cordiformis
corpus of u.
Couvelaire u.
Credé maneuver of u.
u. didelphys
double u.
double-mouthed u.
u. duplex
duplex u.
duplicate u.
gravid u.
heart-shaped u.
hourglass u.
hypoplastic u.
impacted u.
incarcerated gravid u.
incudiform u.
u. incudiformis
large-for-dates u.
leiomyoma uteri
midposition u.
myoma uteri
myoma uteri
one-horned u.
u. parvicollis
pear-shaped u.
placenta, ovary, u. (POU)
prolapsed u.
retroverted u.
ruptured u.
sacculation of u.
septate u.
u. septus
subseptate u.
u. subseptus
symmetric communicating u.
tetanic u.
triangular u.
u. triangularis

NOTES

U

uterus *(continued)*
    T-shaped u.
    unicorn u.
    u. unicornis
    unicornuate u.
    upper contractile portion of u.
UTI
    urinary tract infection
        febrile UTI
Uticort Topical
UTJ
    uterotubal junction
Utrata forceps
utricle
    prostatic u.
utriculoplasty
utriculovaginal pouch
utterance
    mean length of u. (MLU)
UUO
    unilateral ureteral obstruction
UV
    ultraviolet
uva ursi

UVC
    umbilical vein catheter
    umbilical venous catheter
uveal coloboma, cleft lip/palate, mental retardation syndrome
uveitis
    acute anterior u.
    posterior u.
    subacute anterior u.
uveokeratitis
uveomeningitic disease
uveomeningoencephalitic syndrome
uveoparotid
    u. fever
    u. fever syndrome
UVJ
    ureterovesical junction
        UVJ obstruction
UVL
    umbilical venous line
uvula, pl. **uvuli**
    bifid u.
uvulitis
uvulopalatopharyngoplasty (UPPP)

V
    venous
    ventral
    volt
        V code rational problems
        V line
V33W Endocavity probe
30-V-3 stapler
VA
    venoarterial
    ventriculoatrial
        VA shunt
VAA
    verbal-auditory agnosia
Vabra
        V. aspiration
        V. cannula
        V. catheter
        V. cervical aspirator
        V. suction
        V. suction curette
VAC
    vincristine, actinomycin D,
      cyclophosphamide
VACA
    valvuloplasty and angioplasty of
      congenital anomalies
vaccination (*See also* vaccine)
    rotavirus v.
    varicella v.
    v. varicella
    yellow fever 17D v.
vaccinatum
    eczema v.
vaccine
    Acel-Imune v.
    acellular pertussis v.
    ActHIB v.
    V. Adverse Events Reporting
      System (VAERS)
    aP v.
    autogenous v.
    bacille Calmette-Guérin v.
    bacillus Calmette-Guérin v.
    BCG v.
    Certiva v.
    chickenpox v.
    cholera v.
    cold-adapted influenza v. (CAIV)
    cold-adapted intranasal influenza v.
    Comvax v.
    conjugate pneumococcal v.
    diphtheria, tetanus, acellular
      pertussis v. (DTPa)

diphtheria, tetanus, pertussis v.
  (DTP)
diphtheria, tetanus toxoid, acellular
  pertussis v.
diphtheria, tetanus toxoids, whole-
  cell pertussis v.
DTP v.
Edmonston-Zagreb measles v.
Engerix-B hepatitis B v.
enhanced inactivated polio v.
  (eIPV)
Escherichia coli v.
five-component v.
FluMist v.
GBS v.
Haemophilus influenzae type b
  conjugate v.
Haemophilus pertussis v. (HPV)
Havrix v.
hepatitis A v. (HAV)
hepatitis B v. (HBV)
hepatitis B oligosaccharide-
  CRM197 v. (HbOC)
Hib conjugate v.
Hib polysaccharide v.
HibTITER v.
human diploid cell v.
human diploid cell rabies v.
  (HDCV)
inactivated polio v.
inactivated poliomyelitis v.
inactivated poliovirus v. (IPV)
inactivated virus v.
Infanrix v.
influenza v.
intranasal live influenza v.
IPOL poliovirus v.
IPV v.
killed virus v.
live-attenuated virus v.
live poliovirus v.
live-virus v.
Lyme disease v.
measles v.
MenCon v.
meningococcal conjugate v.
meningococcal polysaccharide v.
  (MENps)
MENps v.
mercury-free v.
MMR II v.
mumps v.
nonvalent pneumococcal
  conjugate v. (PnCV)
Oka strain varicella v.

V

vaccine *(continued)*
OPV v.
oral attenuated *Salmonella typhi* v.
oral polio v. (OPV)
oral poliovirus v. (OPV)
Orimune poliovirus v.
OvaRex v.
O-Vax v.
PCEC v.
Pediatrix v.
PedvaxHIB v.
pentavalent v.
PFP v.
plague v.
PncD v.
PNCRM7 v.
PncT v.
pneumococcal conjugate v.
pneumococcal polysaccharide v.
pneumococcal protein conjugate v.
pneumococcal 7-valent conjugate v.
  (PCV7)
poliovirus v.
polyvalent pneumococcal v.
Prevnar pneumococcal v.
protein-conjugated v.
rabies v.
recombinant hepatitis B v.
rhesus rotavirus tetravalent v.
rOspA Lyme disease v.
rotavirus v.
rubella v.
Rv v.
Sabin v.
V. Safety Datalink (VSD)
Salk v.
smallpox v.
split-virus v.
v. strain shedding
swine-flu influenza v.
TdaP v.
TdaP-IPV v.
Td-IPV v.
Td toxoid v.
tetanus and diphtheria toxoids v.
tetanus toxoid and diphtheria v.
Theratope v.
thimerosal-free v.
TriHIBit v.
Tri-Immunol v.
Tripedia v.
trivalent live cold-adapted
  influenza v. (CAIV-T)
tularemia v.
typhoid v.
7-valent pneumococcal conjugate v.
Vaqta v.
varicella-zoster virus v.
Varivax v.

v. virus shedding
7VPnC v.
VZV v.
whole-cell diphtheria-tetanus-
  pertussis v.
whole-cell DTP v.
whole-virus v.
yellow fever v.
vaccine-acquired poliovirus
vaccine-associated
v.-a. paralytic polio (VAPP)
v.-a. paralytic poliomyelitis (VAPP)
v.-a. pneumonia
vaccine-autism scare
vaccinia
v. virus
v. of vulva
vacciniforme
hydroa v.
Vaccinium macrocarpon
vache
coitus la v.
VACTERL
vertebral anomalies, anal atresia, cardiac
  defects, tracheoesophageal fistula, renal
  anomalies, limb anomalies
    VACTERL association
    VACTERL association with
      hydrocephalus syndrome
VACTERL-H syndrome
Vacu-Irrigator
Vozzle V.-I.
vacular thrombosis
vacuo
hydrocephalus ex v.
vacuolar myelopathy
vacuolated
vacuolation
vacuole
vacuolization
double v.
duodenal v.
Vacurette
Berkeley V.
Vacutainer
EDTA-anticoagulated V.
V. system
vacuum
v. aspiration
v. aspirator
v. cannula
v. clitoral therapy device
v. cup
v. curettage
Egnell v.
v. extraction
v. extraction delivery
v. extractor
v. extractor delivery

v. pressure
v. suction
vacuum-assisted delivery
VAD
    vitamin A deficiency
VAERS
    Vaccine Adverse Events Reporting
    System
vagabond skin
vagal
    v. activity
    v. inhibition
    v. maneuver
    v. nerve stimulation
    v. reaction
    v. tone
vagally mediated response
Vagifem
vagina
    anterior v.
    apex of v.
    artificial v.
    atretic v.
    blind v.
    blind-ending v.
    bulbus vestibuli v.'s
    bulb of vestibule of v.
    distal v.
    dry v.
    duplicated v.
    exstrophic v.
    imperforate v.
    neutral pH of v.
    posterior v.
    prepubescent v.
    rudimentary v.
    rugae of v.
    septate v.
    short v.
vaginae
    adenosis v.
    melanosis v.
vaginal
    v. absence
    v. acidification
    v. adenosis
    v. administration
    v. advancement
    v. agenesis
    v. anomaly
    v. apex
    v. artery

v. atresia
v. atrophy
v. birth after cesarean (VBAC)
v. birth after cesarean trial of
    labor (VBAC-TOL)
v. birth after myomectomy
v. bleeding
v. breech delivery
v. bulb
v. cancer
v. candidiasis
v. candidosis
v. candle
Canesten V.
v. carcinoma
v. celiotomy
v. cellular maturation
v. clear cell adenocarcinoma
v. colonization
v. condom
v. cone
v. contraceptive
v. contraceptive film (VCF)
v. cornification test
v. cream
v. cuff
v. cuff adhesion
v. cystourethropexy
v. cytology
v. decompression
v. dilator
v. dimple
v. discharge
v. disinfection
v. douche
v. drainage
v. dysmenorrhea
v. dysontogenetic cyst
v. ectopic anus
v. embryonic cyst
v. epithelial abnormality
v. estrogen therapy
v. eversion
v. evisceration
v. examination
v. extension
v. feminine spray
v. flora
v. fluid arborization
v. fluid ferning
v. fluid neutrophil defensins
v. foreign body

NOTES

V

vaginal *(continued)*
    v. fornix
    v. GIFT
    Gyne-Lotrimin V.
    v. hand
    v. hematoma
    v. hood
    v. hysterectomy
    v. hysterotomy
    v. inclusion cyst
    v. infection
    v. injury
    v. interruption of pregnancy with dilatation and curettage (VIP-DAC)
    v. intraepithelial neoplasia (VAIN)
    v. introitus
    v. irrigation smear (VIS)
    v. laceration
    v. lithotomy
    v. lubricant
    v. lubrication
    v. microflora
    v. misoprostol
    v. moisture
    Monistat V.
    v. morcellation
    v. mucification test
    v. mucosa
    v. myomectomy
    v. narrowing
    v. neurofibroma
    v. neurofibromatosis
    Ogen V.
    v. opening
    Ortho-Dienestrol V.
    v. outlet
    v. pack
    v. packing
    v. palpation
    v. parity
    v. perineorrhaphy
    v. pessary
    v. pH
    v. plate
    v. pouch
    v. probe ultrasound
    v. prolapse prosthesis
    v. prostaglandin
    v. receptivity
    v. recombinant human relaxin
    v. retractor
    v. ring contraception
    v. sarcoma
    v. secretion
    v. septum
    v. shortening
    v. smear intermediate cell
    v. smear parabasal cell

    v. smear superficial cell
    v. soft tissue dystocia
    v. sonography
    v. speculum loop
    v. spermicide
    v. sponge
    v. squamous metaplasia
    v. stenosis
    v. stump prolapse
    v. suppository
    v. surgery
    v. switch operation
    v. tampon
    v. tape tension
    Terazol V.
    v. terminus
    v. thickening
    v. transudate
    v. transudation
    v. tubal procedure
    v. ulcer
    Vagistat-1 V.
    v. vault
    v. vault prolapse
    v. vault support
    v. vault suspension
    v. venous plexus
    v. wall
    v. wall flap
    v. wall repair
    v. wall sling procedure
    v. wash
    v. window
    v. yeast
vaginales
    rugae v.
vaginalis
    Corynebacterium v.
    Gardnerella v.
    Haemophilus v.
    obliterated processus v.
    portio v.
    processus v.
    Trichomonas v.
    tunica v.
vaginally parous
vaginam
    per v.
vaginapexy
vaginectomy
vaginismus, vaginism
    posterior v.
vaginitis, pl. **vaginitides**
    v. adhesiva
    adhesive v.
    amebic v.
    atrophic v.
    bacterial v.
    candidal v.

chemical v.
chlamydial v.
Corynebacterium v.
v. cystica
cytolytic v.
desquamative inflammatory v.
v. emphysematosa
Gardnerella v.
Haemophilus v.
Mobiluncus v.
Mobiluncus mulieris
monilial v.
nonspecific v.
pinworm v.
recurrent v.
senile v.
v. senilis
Shigella v.
streptococcal v.
traumatic v.
trichomonal v.
Trichomonas vaginalis v.
yeast v.
vaginocele
vaginodynia
vaginofixation
vaginogram
vaginography
vaginohysterectomy
vaginometer
vaginomycosis
vaginopathy
vaginoperineoplasty
vaginoperineorraphy
vaginoperineotomy
vaginopexy
Norman Miller v.
vaginoplasty
Fenton v.
tissue expansion v.
vaginoscope
Cameron-Myers v.
Huffman v.
vaginoscopy
pediatric v.
vaginosis
anaerobic v.
bacterial v. (BV)
mycotic v.
vaginotomy
anterior v.
Vagisil intimate moisturizer

Vagistat-1 Vaginal
Vagi-TEST
vagitus uterinus
vagotomy
vagotonia
vagotonic
v. bradycardia
v. maneuver
vagus nerve
VAIN
vaginal intraepithelial neoplasia
valacyclovir
v. HCl
v. hydrochloride
valdecoxib
Valentine position
7-valent pneumococcal conjugate vaccine
valerate
betamethasone v.
estradiol v.
hydrocortisone v.
valerian root
Valertest No. 1
valga
coxa v.
valgum
genu v.
physiologic genu v.
valgus
cubitus v.
forefoot v.
hallux v.
heel v.
hindfoot v.
obligatory heel v.
v. osteotomy
rearfoot v.
talipes v.
VALI
ventilatory-associated lung injury
valine
Valium
V. Injection
V. Oral
vallecula, pl. **valleculae**
Valle hysteroscope
Valley
V. fever
V. Vac smoke evacuation system
Valleylab
V. ball electrode

NOTES

Valleylab *(continued)*
  V. Force IC electrosurgical
    generator
  V. loop electrode
  V. pencil
  V. REM system
Valorin
valproate
  sodium v.
valproic
  v. acid
  v. acid embryopathy
  v. acid syndrome
valrubicin
Valsalva
  V. maneuver
  V. sinus
  sinus of V.
  squirming V.
Valstar
Valtchev uterine manipulator
Valtrex
value
  acid-base v.
  adaptive v.
  Astrup blood gas v.
  baseline v.
  complement v.
  fetal blood v.
  maturation v.
  Tanner-Whitehouse bone age
    reference v.
valvar
  v. aortic stenosis
  v. pulmonic stenosis
valve
  v. ablation
  aortic v.
  atrioventricular v.
  bicuspid aortic v.
  bleed-back v.
  double-orifice mitral v.
  Heyer-Schulte v.
  Jatene v.
  mitral v.
  neoaortic v.
  v. obstruction
  one-way v.
  parachute mitral v.
  pop-off v.
  porcine v.
  posterior urethral v. (PUV)
  v. prolapse
  pulmonary porcine v.
  pulmonic v.
  Ross pulmonary porcine v.
  Spitz-Holter v.
  straddling atrioventricular v.

  transurethral ablation of v.
  tricuspid v.
  trileaflet aortic v.
  ureteral v.
  urethral v.
  3-way Hans Rudolph v.
valvectomy
valvotomy
  aortic v.
  balloon v.
valvular
  v. heart disease
  v. insufficiency
  v. prosthesis
  v. pulmonic stenosis
valvulitis
  murmur of v.
valvuloplasty
  v. and angioplasty of congenital
    anomalies (VACA)
  balloon pulmonary v.
  transcarotid balloon v.
valvulotomy
  balloon v.
  v. procedure
VAMP
  vincristine, actinomycin D, methotrexate,
  prednisone
    VAMP chemotherapy
van
  v. Bogaert disease
  V. Buchem syndrome
  v. den Bergh reaction
  v. den Bergh test
  v. den Bosch syndrome
  v. der Hoeve syndrome
  v. der Woude syndrome
  V. Haldergem syndrome
  V. Maldergem syndrome
  v. Ness procedure
  V. Praagh classification of truncus
    arteriosus
  V. Praagh loop rule
Vancaillie uterine cannula
Vancenase
  V. AQ
  V. Nasal Inhaler
Vanceril
  V. Double Strength
  V. Oral Inhaler
Vancocin
  V. Injection
  V. Oral
Vancoled Injection
vancomycin
  v. hydrochloride
  v. intermediate resistant
    Staphylococcus aureus (VISA)

vancomycin-resistant
> v.-r. enterococcus (VRE)
> v.-r. *Staphylococcus aureus* (VRSA)

Vanicream

vanillylmandelic acid (VMA)

Vaniqa

vanished testes

vanishing
> v. bile duct
> v. fetus
> v. testes syndrome
> v. testicle syndrome
> v. twin
> v. twin syndrome

Vanquin

Vantin

VAP
> ventilator-associated pneumonia

vapocauterization

vapocoolant

Vapo-Iso

vaporization
> bipolar v.
> endometrial v.
> laser v.

vaporizer
> cool-mist v.
> water v.

Vaporole
> Amyl Nitrate V.

vapor poisoning

VAPP
> vaccine-associated paralytic polio
> vaccine-associated paralytic poliomyelitis

VAPS
> verbal analog pain scale

Vaqta vaccine

vara
> adolescent tibia v.
> coxa v.
> idiopathic tibia v.
> infantile tibia v.
> juvenile tibia v.
> tibia v.

Váradi-Papp syndrome

Váradi syndrome

variabilis
> *Dermacentor v.*
> erythrokeratodermia v.

variability
> baseline v. of fetal heart rate
> beat-to-beat v.

fetal heart rate v.
heart rate v. (HRV)
interpretation v.

variable
> v. deceleration
> v. obstruction
> v. softness (VS)
> v. stenosis

variance
> additive genetic v.
> dominance v.
> environmental v.
> genetic v.
> phenotypic v.
> v. ratio

Varian Spectra AA40 spectrometer

variant
> albopapuloid epidermolysis
>   bullosa v.
> deafness-causing allele v.
> v. hemoglobin
> Hurler v.
> hyperammonemia v.
> hyperinsulinism with
>   hyperammonemia v.
> Klinefelter v.
> Landau-Kleffner syndrome v.
> migraine v.
> papillary v.
> Pasini v.
> petit mal v.

variation
> continuous v.

varicella
> breakthrough v.
> v. bullosa
> bullous v.
> disseminated v.
> v. encephalitis
> v. gangrenosa
> v. immunization
> v. infection
> v. inoculata
> neonatal v.
> v. pneumonia
> v. pneumonitis
> pustular v.
> v. pustulosa
> v. syndrome
> vaccination v.
> v. vaccination

V

NOTES

varicella-zoster
    v.-z. encephalomyelitis
    v.-z. immune globulin (VZIG)
    v.-z. immunoglobulin (VZIG)
    v.-z. virus (VZV)
    v.-z. virus infection
    v.-z. virus vaccine
varicelliform
varices (*pl. of* varix)
varicocele
    ovarian v.
    tuboovarian v.
    uteroovarian v.
varicocelectomy
varicosity
    vulvar v.
variegata
    porphyria v.
variegate porphyria (VP)
variety
variola virus
varioliform
Varivax vaccine
varix, pl. **varices**
    gelatinous v.
    umbilical vein v.
    vulvar v.
varum
    developmental genu v.
    genu v.
    physiologic genu v.
    pseudo-genu v.
varus
    v. clubfoot
    congenital metatarsus v.
    cubitus v.
    dynamic pes v.
    forefoot v.
    metatarsus v.
    metatarsus primus v.
    v. osteotomy
    rearfoot v.
    talipes v.
VAS
    vibratory acoustic stimulation
    vibroacoustic stimulation
    visual analog scale
vas, pl. **vasa**
    v. deferens
    v. deferens aplasia
    vasa nervorum
    vasa previa (VP)
    vasa vasorum
vasal
Vas-Cath catheter
vascular
    v. anomaly
    v. bed
    v. birthmark
    v. calcification
    v. cell adhesion molecule (VCAM)
    v. channel
    v. clip applier
    v. communication
    v. complication
    v. congestion
    v. disease
    v. endothelial growth factor (VEGF)
    v. endothelium
    v. engorgement
    v. headache
    v. injury
    v. leiomyoma
    v. malformation
    v. metastasis
    v. myelopathy
    v. neoplasm
    v. nevus
    v. parabiosis
    v. permeability
    v. permeability factor
    v. proliferative lesion
    v. reactivity
    v. resistance
    v. ring
    v. ring syndrome
    v. sling
    v. spasm
    v. spider
    v. thrombosis
    v. tone
    v. umbrella
vascularis
    stria v.
vascularization
    chorionic v.
vascularized appendix
vasculature
    atypical v.
    v. flow pattern
vasculitic
    v. erythema
    v. skin lesion
vasculitis
    asthma with v.
    v. of childhood
    Churg-Strauss v.
    cutaneous v.
    dermal v.
    disseminated granulomatous v.
    epididymal vessel v.
    fetal v.
    granulomatous v.
    gut v.
    hypersensitivity v.
    immune complex v.
    immune complex-mediated v.

leukocytoclastic v.
lymphocytic v.
necrotizing granulomatous v.
occlusive v.
ovarian v.
renal v.
retinal v.
rheumatoid v.
v. syndrome
systemic v.
vasculogenesis
vasculopathy
fetal thrombotic v. (FTV)
noncalcific v.
proliferative v.
thalamostriate v. (TSV)
vasectomy reversal
Vaseline-impregnated gauze
vasitis
vasoactive
v. intestinal peptide (VIP)
v. intestinal polypeptide (VIP)
v. prostaglandin
v. substance
VasoClear Ophthalmic
vasocongestion
vasoconstriction
hypoxic v.
vasoconstrictor
Vasodilan
vasodilation
pulmonary v.
vasodilator cream
vasogenic edema
vasomotor
v. flush
v. rhinitis
vasoocclusion
vasoocclusive
v. crisis
v. episode
vasopathy
calcific v.
vasopressin
v. analog
arginine v. (AVP)
v. infusion
placental v.
v. therapy
vasopressor syncope
vasoregulation

vasorum
vasa v.
Vasospan
vasospasm
cerebral v.
coronary v.
transient v.
Vasotec
V. I.V.
V. Oral
vasotocin
arginine v.
vasovagal
v. faint
v. reflex apnea
v. syncope
vasovasostomy
vastus
v. lateralis
v. lateralis muscle
v. medialis
VATER
vertebral (defects), (imperforate) anus,
tracheoesophageal (fistula), radial and
renal (dysplasia)
VATER complex
hydrocephalus with features of
VATER
VATER syndrome
Vater
ampulla of V.
papilla of V.
VATS
video-assisted thoracic surgery
video-assisted thoracoscopic surgery
vault
v. cap
v. prolapse
rectal v.
vaginal v.
vaulting
VBAC
vaginal birth after cesarean
VBAC-TOL
vaginal birth after cesarean trial of labor
VBG
venous blood gas
VBM
vertebral bone mass
vBMD
volumetric bone mineral density

V

NOTES

VBP
vinblastine, bleomycin, cisplatin
VBS
venous blood sample
VC
vital capacity
Phenergan VC
VCA
viral capsid antigen
VCAM
vascular cell adhesion molecule
V-Cath catheter
VCD
vocal cord dysfunction
VCF
vaginal contraceptive film
VCFS
velocardiofacial syndrome
VCP
vincristine, cyclophosphamide, and
prednisone
VCU
videocystourethrography
VCU examination
VCUG
vesicoureterogram
voiding cystourethrogram
voiding cystourethrograph
voiding cystourethrography
VD
venereal disease
VDR
vitamin D receptor
VDRL
Venereal Disease Research Laboratory
CSF VDRL
VDRL test
VE
volume of expired gas
Vecchietti
V. method
V. operation
vectis
vector
cloning v.
vecuronium
v. bromide
Veda-scope
VEE
Venezuelan equine encephalitis
Veetids
vegan
vegetable
cruciferous v.
v. oil fat-based formula
vegetans
pyoderma v.
vegetarian diet
vegetarianism

vegetation
nonbacterial thrombotic v. (NBTV)
vegetative
v. reproduction
v. symptom
VEGF
vascular endothelial growth factor
vehicle
all-terrain v. (ATV)
PAB-equipped v.
Veillonella
V. atypica
V. dispar
V. parvula
vein
anomalous pulmonary v.
antecubital v.
axillary v.
azygos v.
bridging v.
cardinal v.
cephalic v.
v. compression
dilated v.
dilated collateral v.
v. flap
v. of Galen
v. of Galen aneurysm
v. of Galen malformation
greater saphenous v.
hypogastric v.
iliac v.
inferior mesenteric v.
innominate v.
internal jugular v.
jugular v.
left renal v.
left vertical v.
main renal v.
maternal cortical v.
mesenteric v.
obliterated v.
v. obstruction
ovarian v.
persistent right umbilical v.
pulmonary v.
renal v.
saphenous v.
scalp v.
splenic v.
superior mesenteric v.
umbilical v.
uterine v.
Veingard dressing
vela (*pl. of* velum)
velamen, pl. **velamina**
v. vulvae
velamentosa
placenta v.

velamentous
- v. cord insertion
- v. insertion of cord
- v. placenta
- v. vessel

velamina (*pl. of* velamen)

vellus
- v. hair
- v. hypertrichosis

velocardiofacial syndrome (VCFS)

velocimetry
- Doppler v.
- fetal aortic Doppler v.
- fetal arterial v.
- umbilical artery Doppler v.

velocity
- bone quantitative ultrasound v.
- cerebral blood flow v. (CBFV)
- end-diastolic v. (EDV)
- growth v. (GV)
- head growth v.
- height v. (HV)
- linear growth v.
- nerve conduction v. (NCV)
- peak growth v.
- sensory nerve conduction v.
- subnormal growth v.
- umbilical Doppler flow v.

velofacial hypoplasia

velopharyngeal incompetence (VPI)

Velosef

Velosulin Human

Velpeau bandage

Veltane Tablet

velum, pl. **vela**

vena
- v. cava
- v. caval filter
- v. caval interruption

venenata
- dermatitis v.

venereal
- v. bubo
- v. collar
- v. disease (VD)
- V. Disease Research Laboratory (VDRL)
- v. lymphogranuloma
- v. wart

venereology

venereum
- lymphogranuloma v. (LGV)

veneris
- mons v.

Venezuelan equine encephalitis (VEE)

Venilon human immunoglobulin

venipuncture
- external jugular v.
- v. site

venlafaxine
- v. HCl
- v. hydrochloride

Venning-Brown test

venoarterial (VA)
- v. cannulation

venodilation

Venodyne pneumatic compressive device

Venoglobulin

Venoglobulin-S

venogram

venography
- ascending v.
- contrast v.
- full v.
- hepatic wedged v.
- limited v.
- radionuclide v.

venom
- Hymenoptera v.

venoocclusive disease (VOD)

venosus
- ductus v.
- patent ductus v.
- sinus v.

venous (V)
- v. angioma
- v. bleb
- v. blood gas (VBG)
- v. blood sample (VBS)
- v. blood sampling
- v. catheter
- v. collateral
- v. engorgement
- v. flow
- v. hum
- v. lake
- v. line
- v. malformation (VM)
- v. obstruction
- v. occlusion plethysmography
- v. oozing
- v. pH
- v. pooling
- v. pressure

NOTES

venous *(continued)*
    v. sinus thrombophlebitis
    v. sinus thrombosis
    v. switch
    v. thromboembolism (VTE)
venovenous (VV)
    v. cannulation
    v. ECMO
venter propendens
vent gleet
ventilation
    alveolar v.
    assist control v.
    assisted v. (AV)
    bag and mask v.
    BVM v.
    controlled mechanical v. (CMV)
    endotracheal intubation and
      mechanical v. (EI/MV)
    hand v.
    HFJ v.
    HFO v.
    HFPP v.
    high-frequency v. (HFV)
    high-frequency jet v. (HFJV)
    high-frequency oscillatory v.
      (HFOV)
    high-frequency positive-pressure v.
      (HFPPV)
    intermittent mandatory v. (IMV)
    intermittent mechanical v. (IMV)
    intermittent positive pressure v.
      (IPPV)
    intratracheal pulmonary v. (ITPV)
    inverse ratio v. (IRV)
    jet v.
    liquid v. (LV)
    liquid-assisted high-frequency
      oscillatory v. (LA-HFOV)
    v. by mask
    mask and bag v.
    mechanical v.
    noninvasive motion v. (NIMV)
    oscillatory v.
    partial liquid v. (PLV)
    patient-triggered v.
    positive-pressure v. (PPV)
    pressure support v.
    pulmonary v.
    v. scintigraphy
    synchronized intermittent
      mandatory v. (SIMV)
    synchronized nasal intermittent
      positive-pressure v. (SNIPPV)
    tidal liquid v. (TLV)
    total liquid v. (TLV)
    transtracheal v.
    v. tube
    volume-controlled v.

ventilation/perfusion
    v./p. imbalance
    v./p. mismatch
    v./p. quotient
    v./p. ratio ($\dot{V}/\dot{Q}$)
    v./p. scan
ventilator
    Amsterdam infant v.
    BABYbird II v.
    Bear Cub infant v.
    Bennett PR-2 v.
    Bourns LS104-150 infant v.
    Breeze v.
    CPAP v.
    extrathoracic v.
    Healthdyne v.
    HFJ v.
    HFO v.
    HFPP v.
    high-frequency v.
    high-oscillation v.
    humidification v.
    infant Star high-frequency v.
    jet v.
    nebulization v.
    Newport Wave v.
    noninvasive extrathoracic v. (NEV)
    PEEP v.
    Porta-Lung noninvasive
      extrathoracic v.
    pressure-cycled v.
    pressure-preset v.
    Pulmo-Aid v.
    Sechrist neonatal v.
    Servo 900C v.
    Siemens-Elema Servo 900C v.
    Siemens Servo 300, 900C v.
    SLE 2000 v.
    Star v.
    v. support
    Vix infant v.
    volume-limited v.
    Wave v.
ventilator-associated pneumonia (VAP)
ventilator-induced lung injury (VILI)
ventilatory
    v. drive
    v. failure
    v. support
**ventilatory-associated lung injury
  (VALI)**
Ventolin
    V. Nebules
    V. Rotacaps
ventral (V)
    v. hernia
    v. mesentery
    v. pancreatic anlage
    v. suspension

v. wall
v. wall defect
ventricle
v.'s to atrium
common-inlet single right v.
dilation of v.
double-inlet left v.
double-inlet right v.
double-outlet v.
double-outlet right v. (DORV)
hyperdynamic v.
hypoplastic left v.
isolated double outlet right v.
left v. (LV)
v.'s to peritoneal cavity (VP)
right v. (RV)
single v.
ventricular
v. afterload
v. aneurysm
v. assist device
v. bypass
v. catheter
v. dysplasia
v. dysrhythmia
v. filling
v. fluid
v. function
v. hypertrophy
v. inversion
left v. (LV)
v. outflow obstruction
v. outflow tract
v. outflow tract reconstruction
v. peritoneal (VP)
v. preload
v. premature contraction (VPC)
v. premature depolarization
v. puncture
v. reservoir
v. response rate
v. septal defect (VSD)
v. septal defect patch closure
v. septation
v. septum
v. shunt
v. shunt procedure
v. tachycardia
v. tap
v. tumor
ventriculitis
gram-negative v.

ventriculoamniotic shunt
ventriculoarterial
ventriculoatrial (VA)
v. shunt
ventriculocisternostomy
ventriculography
ventriculojugular shunt
ventriculomegaly
bilateral cerebral v.
cerebral v.
fetal v.
nonprogressive v.
posthemorrhagic v. (PHVM)
ventriculoperitoneal (VP)
v. shunt (VPS)
v. shunting
ventriculopleural shunt
ventriculoseptal defect (VSD)
ventriculovascular shunt
ventrogluteal
ventroposterior (VP)
ventrosuspension
Venturi mask
venule
Venus
collar of V.
VEOS
very early onset schizophrenia
VEP
visual evoked potential
VEP acuity
flash VEP
VER
visual evoked response
vera
placenta accreta v.
polycythemia rubra v.
verapamil
Veratrum **alkaloid**
verbal
v. abuse
v. analog pain scale (VAPS)
v. fluency
v. sequencing
verbal-auditory agnosia (VAA)
verbalize
verbally assaultive
Verelan
Veress needle
vergae
cavum v.

NOTES

verge
    anal v.
Veriloid
vermicularis
    Enterobius v.
vermiculation
vermiform
    v. appendix
    v. lesion
vermilion border of lip
vermis
    agenesis of cerebellar v.
    cerebellar v.
    v. cerebelli
    v. hypoplasia
    hypoplasia of v.
    hypoplastic superior cerebellar v.
    partial agenesis of v.
    selective aplasia of v.
Vermont-Oxford Neonatal Database
Vermox
vernal conjunctivitis
Verner-Morrison syndrome
vernix
    v. caseosa
    v. membrane
Vero cell
vero cytotoxin
verotoxin
verruca, pl. **verrucae**
    mosaic v.
    v. peruana
    v. plana
    v. plantaris
    v. sock
    v. vulgaris
Verruca-Freeze
verruciformis
    epidermodysplasia v.
verrucous
    v. carcinoma
    v. endocarditis
    v. papule
    v. plaque
    v. streaky epidermal nevus
VersaLab APM2 portable antepartum monitor
VersaLap
Versed syrup
Versenate
    Calcium Disodium V.
versicolor
    pityriasis v.
    tinea v.
version
    bimanual v.
    bipolar v.
    Braxton Hicks v.

California Verbal Learning Test-Children's V.
    cephalic v.
    combined v.
    external v.
    external cephalic v. (ECV)
    Hicks v.
    internal podalic v.
    pelvic v.
    podalic v.
    postural v.
    Potter v.
    Schedule for Affective Disorders and Schizophrenia for School-Age Children-Epidemiologic V. (K-SADS-E)
    spontaneous v.
    tibial v.
    Wigand v.
    Wright v.
versive seizure
vertebra, pl. **vertebrae**
    apical v.
    biconcave v.
    block v.
    butterfly vertebrae
    cleft vertebrae
    codfish v.
    fishmouth v.
    v. plana
    wedge v.
vertebral
    v. anomalies, anal atresia, cardiac defects, tracheoesophageal fistula, renal anomalies, limb anomalies (VACTERL)
    v. arch defect
    v. artery
    v. artery compression
    v. body
    v. bone loss
    v. bone mass (VBM)
    v. column
    v. column defect
    v. compression fracture
    v. (defects), (imperforate) anus, tracheoesophageal (fistula), radial and renal (dysplasia) (VATER)
    v. fracture
    v. laminar arch
    v. microfracture
    v. osteomyelitis
vertebrodidymus
vertex, pl. **vertices**
    v. delivery
    external cephalic version and spontaneous v.
    instrumental v.
    v. position

v. potential
v. presentation
spontaneous v.
vertex-breech twin presentation
vertex-nonvertex pair
vertex-transverse twin presentation
vertex-vertex pair
vertical
  v. gaze palsy
  v. HIV transmission
  v. hymen
  v. incision
  v. lie
  v. muscle
  v. nystagmus
  v. pocket depth
  v. striation
  v. talus
vertically
  v. acquired infection
  v. infected
vertices (*pl. of* vertex)
verticillata
  cornea v.
vertiginous
  v. condition
  v. external anal sphincter
  v. seizure
  v. symptom
vertigo
  benign paroxysmal v. (BPV)
  epidemic v.
  Ménière v.
  paroxysmal v.
  peripheral v.
  true v.
very
  v. cold water near drowning
  v. early onset schizophrenia
    (VEOS)
  v. long chain acyl-CoA
    dehydrogenase (VLCAD)
  v. long chain fatty acid (VLCFA)
  v. low birth weight (VLBW)
  v. low birth weight child
  v. low birth weight infant
  v. low density lipoprotein (VLDL)
Vesica
  V. press-in suture anchor system
  V. sling kit
vesical neck

vesicle
  brain v.
  chorionic v.
  football-shaped v.
  germinal v.
  graafian v.
  nabothian v.
  seminal v.
  skin v.
  tear-drop v.
vesicoamniotic shunt
vesicobullous
  v. disorder
  v. eruption
  v. skin lesion
vesicocele
vesicocentesis
vesicocervical space
vesicocutaneous fistula
vesicofixation
vesicomyectomy
vesicomyotomy
vesicopustular lesion
vesicostomy
  cutaneous v.
vesicotomy
vesicoureteral reflux (grade 1–4) (VUR)
vesicoureteric reflux (grade 1–4) (VUR)
vesicoureterogram (VCUG)
vesicourethral
  v. canal
  v. primordial
vesicourethrolysis
  retropubic v.
vesicouterine
  v. fistula
  v. serosa
vesicovaginal
  v. fistula
  v. repair
  v. septum
  v. space
vesicovaginorectal
  v. fistula
vesicular
  v. breath sounds
  v. exanthem
  v. mole
  v. palmar lesion
  v. skin lesion
  v. stomatitis virus (VSV)

NOTES

V

vesiculation
    intraepidermal v.
vesiculopapular eruption
vesiculopustular dermatitis
vesiculoulcerative
    v. lesion
    v. stomatitis
vespid allergy
vessel
    afferent v.
    blood v.
    brachiocephalic v.
    chorioallantoic v.
    chorioangiopagus placental v.
    complete transposition of great v.'s
    corkscrew conjunctival blood v.
    dilated optic v.
    engorged v.
    fetoscopic laser occlusion of
      chorioangiopagus v.'s (FLOC)
    ghost v.
    great v.
    hairpin v.
    infundibulopelvic v.
    v. injury
    iris v.
    laser photocoagulation of the
      communicating v.'s (LPCV)
    v. obliteration
    v. ostium
    ovarian v.
    palliation of great v.'s
    v. spread
    v. transillumination
    transposition of great v.'s (TGV)
    umbilical v.
    umbilicoplacental v.
    uterine v.
    uteroplacental v.
    velamentous v.
vest
    E-Z-On V.
VestaBlate system
vestibular
    v. adenitis
    v. anus
    v. apparatus
    v. board
    v. bulb
    v. cyst
    v. damage
    v. duct
    v. dyspareunia
    v. fistula
    v. gland
    v. input
    v. nerve
    v. neuronitis
    v. nystagmus

    v. seizure
    v. stimulation
vestibule
vestibulectomy
    U-shaped v.
    Woodruff v.
vestibulitis
    vulvar v.
vestibulocochlear nerve
vestibulodynia
vestibulogenic
    v. epilepsy
    v. seizure
vestibulovaginal bulb
vestigial
VFSS
    videofluoroscopic swallowing study
viability
    fetal v.
viable
    v. endometrial cell
    v. fetus
    v. infant
vial
    Nickerson BiGGY v.'s
Viasorb dressing
Vibracare
Vibramycin
Vibra-Tabs
vibration sense
vibrator
vibratory
    v. acoustic stimulation (VAS)
    v. murmur
Vibrio
    V. cholerae
    V. fetus
    V. parahaemolyticus
    V. vulnificus
vibriocidal antibody
vibroacoustic-induced fetal movement
vibroacoustic stimulation (VAS)
vibrotactile hearing aid
vicarious
    v. menstruation
    v. respiration
Vicks
    V. Children's NyQuil
    V. Formula 44
    V. Formula 440
    V. Formula 44 Pediatric
    V. Pediatric 44E, 44M
Vicodin ES
Vicryl Rapide suture
victim
    sexual assault v.
victimization
    physical v.
    sexual v.

Victor Gomel method
vidarabine
Vidas
    V. automated immunoassay system
    V. Estradiol II assay kit
    V. immunoanalysis testing system
    V. varicella zoster assay
Vi-Daylin vitamins
video
    v. camera
    v. electroencephalography
    v. game epilepsy
    v. monitoring
video-assisted
    v.-a. thoracic surgery (VATS)
    v.-a. thoracoscopic surgery (VATS)
videocystourethrography (VCU)
videoendoscope
    three-dimensional v.
videofluoroscopic swallowing study (VFSS)
videofluoroscopy
    modified barium swallow with v.
videolaparoscope
Video Overlay Method
videoradiography
videosomnography
videourodynamic study
Videx Oral
Vi-Drape bowel bag
vietnamiensis
    Burkholderia v.
view
    anteroposterior v.
    apical four-chamber v.
    axillary v.
    calcaneal v.
    Caldwell v.
    comparison v.
    craniocaudal v.
    exaggerated craniocaudal v.
    field of v.
    four-chamber v.
    frogleg v.
    Harris v.
    jug handle v.
    lateral oblique v.
    lateromedial oblique v.
    long-axis v.
    medial oblique v.
    mediolateral v.

    Merchant v.
    mortise v.
    Neer v.
    oblique v.
    occipitomental v.
    open-mouth v.
    Panorex v.
    parasternal short-axis v.
    pulmonary artery/ductus v.
    short-axis v.
    spot compression v.
    subcostal v.
    submentovertex v.
    sunrise v.
    suprasternal v.
    Waters v.
vigabatrin
Vigamox solution
vigilance
    generalized v.
Vignal cell
vigorous infant
VILI
    ventilator-induced lung injury
villi (*pl. of* villus)
villitis
    focal v.
villoglandular configuration
villonodular synovitis
villositis
villous
    v. atrophy
    v. atrophy of jejunum
    v. chorion
    v. edema
    v. placenta
villus, pl. **villi**
    anchoring v.
    arachnoid v.
    chorionic villi
    flattened v.
    hydropic chorionic v.
    hydropic placental v.
    placental v.
vimentin
    v. gene
    v. protein
Vim-Silverman needle
Vimule
    V. cap
    V. permanent sheath

NOTES

V

VIN
vulvar intraepithelial neoplasia
VIN (grade 1–3)
vinblastine
v., bleomycin, cisplatin (VBP)
cisplatin, methotrexate, v. (CMV)
methotrexate, cisplatin, v. (MCV)
Vinca alkaloid
Vincasar PFS
Vincent
V. angina
V. gingivitis
V. infection
V. stomatitis
vincristine
v., actinomycin D,
cyclophosphamide (VAC)
v., actinomycin D, methotrexate,
prednisone (VAMP)
v., cyclophosphamide, and
prednisone (VCP)
v. and dexamethasone
v. sulfate
vinegar douching
Vineland
V. Adaptive Behavior Scales
V. Adaptive Behavior Scales,
Survey Form
V. Social Maturity Scale
V. standard scores
vin rosé-colored urine
vinyl chloride
Viokase
violaceous
v. eruption
v. erythema
v. hue
v. lesion
v. polygonal papule
violence
domestic v.
violent rage
violet
crystal v.
gentian v.
viomycin
Vioxx
VIP
vasoactive intestinal peptide
vasoactive intestinal polypeptide
voluntary interruption of pregnancy
VIP-DAC
vaginal interruption of pregnancy with
dilatation and curettage
Vipond sign
viprynium
Vira-A Ophthalmic
Viracept

viral
v. arthritis
v. capsid antigen (VCA)
cellular v.
v. cerebellitis
v. conjunctivitis
v. culturing
v. DNA polymerase
v. encephalitis
v. enteritis
v. esophagitis
v. exanthem
v. gastroenteritis
v. hepatitis
v. laryngitis
v. laryngotracheobronchitis
v. load
v. lower respiratory illness (VLRI)
v. meningitis
v. meningoencephalitis
v. myelitis
v. myocarditis
v. necrotizing bronchiolitis
v. pharyngitis
v. pneumonia
v. pneumonitis
v. prodrome
v. sepsis
v. shedding
v. syndrome
v. thymidine kinase
v. titer
v. transmission
v. upper respiratory tract infection
Viramune
ViraPap HPV DNA test
ViraType
V. HPV DNA typing assay
V. probe
V. test
Virazole Aerosol
Virchow
pneumonia alba of V.
Virchow-Robin space
Virchow-Seckel syndrome
viremia
plasma v.
secondary v.
viremic phase
Viresolve ultrafiltration membrane
virgin
virginal
v. breast hypertrophy
v. hymen
v. introitus
Virginia needle
virginity
viridans
v. enterococcus

Streptococcus v.
v. streptococcus
virilescence
virilism
adrenal v.
virilization
external v.
strong v.
virilizing
v. adenoma
v. adrenal tumor
v. 3 alpha-androstanediol
glucuronide
v. ovarian mass
Virilon capsule
virion
intranuclear v.
virologic assay
virology
Viroptic Ophthalmic
virtual
v. bronchoscopy
v. labor monitor (VLM)
virulence
virulent bubo
viruria
virus
acquired immunodeficiency
syndrome-related v. (ARV)
antibody to hepatitis A v. (anti-
HAV)
arthropod-borne v.
Borna disease v.
chickenpox v.
chikungunya v.
v. clearance
Congo v.
cultivable v.
dengue v.
Dobrava v.
ECHO v.
Epstein-Barr v. (EBV)
fecal shedding of v.
GB v. C (GBV-C)
Hantaan v.
hepatitis A v. (HAV)
hepatitis B v. (HBV)
hepatitis C v. (HCV, HVC)
hepatitis D v. (HDV)
hepatitis E v. (HEV)
hepatitis F v. (HFV)
hepatitis G v. (HGV)

hepatotropic v.
herpes v.
herpes simplex v. (HSV)
herpes simplex v. 1 (HSV1, HSV-
1)
herpes simplex v. 2 (HSV2, HSV-
2)
herpes zoster v. (HZV)
horizontal transmission of v.
human immunodeficiency v. (HIV)
human immunodeficiency v.-1
(HIV-1)
human T-cell leukemia v. (HTLV)
human T-cell leukemia v. type I,
II, III
human T-cell lymphotropic v. type
I (HTLV-I)
human T-cell lymphotropic v. type
II (HTLV-II)
influenza v.
Inoue-Melnick v.
Japanese B encephalitis v.
JC v.
Junin v.
LAC v.
Lassa v.
live-attenuated v.
lymphadenopathy-associated v.
(LAV)
lymphocytic choriomeningitis v.
(LCMV)
Machupo v.
Marburg v.
Mayaro v.
measles v.
molluscum contagiosum v. (MCV)
monkey polyoma v.
Montgomery County v.
mumps v.
non-A, non-B hepatotropic v.
non-syncytium-inducing variant of
AIDS v.
Norwalk v.
Norwalk-like v.
Ockelbo v.
Omsk v.
o'nyong-nyong v.
papillomavirus, polyoma virus,
simian virus 40 vacuolating v.
(PAPOVA)
parainfluenza v. (PIV)
parainfluenza v. (type 1–4)

NOTES

virus *(continued)*
    Pogosta v.
    recurrent Japanese encephalitis v.
    respiratory enteric orphan v.
    respiratory syncytial v. (RSV, RS-virus)
    Ross River v.
    Rous sarcoma v.
    rubella v.
    Sapporo v.
    simian B v.
    simian immunodeficiency v. (SIV)
    Sindbis v.
    Sin Nombre v.
    Snow Mountain v.
    syphilis, toxoplasmosis, other agents, rubella, cytomegalovirus, herpes simplex v. (STORCH, ToRCHS)
    tissue culture-grown attenuated v.
    v. titer
    toxoplasmosis, other agents, rubella, cytomegalovirus, herpes simplex v.
    transfusion transmitted v.
    TT v. (TTV)
    vaccinia v.
    varicella-zoster v. (VZV)
    variola v.
    vesicular stomatitis v. (VSV)
    visna v.
    West Nile v.
    wild v.
    wild-type measles v.
virus-induced epithelial damage
virus-neutralizing antibody (VNA)
VIS
    vaginal irrigation smear
VISA
    vancomycin intermediate resistant *Staphylococcus aureus*
viscera (*pl. of* viscus)
visceral
    v. abscess
    v. cleft
    v. cranium
    v. heterotaxy
    v. larva migrans
    v. leishmaniasis
    v. myopathy
    v. pain
    v. pericardiectomy
    v. peritoneum
    v. protein status
    v. situs
    v. tuberculosis
viscerale
    cranium v.
visceroatrial situs inversus

visceromegaly syndrome
viscerosensory aura
viscerum
    situs inversus v.
viscid
viscoelastic
viscosity
viscosus
    Actinomyces v.
viscous
    v. fluid
    v. semen
    v. syndrome
viscus, pl. **viscera**
    herniated viscera
    hollow viscera
    inversion of viscera
    perforated v.
    transposition of viscera
    in utero reduction of herniated viscera
visible
    v. cortical mantle
    v. peristalsis
Visicath
Visine
    V. Extra Ophthalmic
    V. L.R. Ophthalmic
vision
    20/20 v.
    binocular v.
    blurred v.
    color v.
    cortical v.
    distance v.
    field of v.
    impaired v.
    low v.
    near v.
    peripheral v.
    residual v.
    v. screening
    v. therapist
    v. therapy
    tunnel v.
Visiport optical trocar
visit
    health maintenance v.
    postpartum v.
    preconception v.
    routine prenatal v.
visna virus
Vista disposable skin stapler
Vistaril
    V. Injection
    V. Oral
Vistide
visual
    v. acuity

v. analog scale (VAS)
v. analog scale for stress
v. aura
v. change
v. cortex
v. development
v. disturbance
v. evoked potential (VEP)
v. evoked response (VER)
v. field
v. field defect
v. learner
v. loss
v. magnocellular system
v. pathway
v. phobic hallucination
v. reflex epilepsy
v. regard
v. reinforcement audiometry (VRA)
v. response audiometry (VRA)
v. sequential memory
v. spatial memory
v. stimulation
v. tracking
v. tracking of red ring
v. training exercise

visualization
indirect v.

visual-motor
v.-m. coordination
v.-m. integration (VMI)
v.-m. integration test

visual-perceptual test
visuomotor integration (VMI)
visuoperceptual/simultaneous information processing
visuospatial
visuscope
Vitabee 6, 12
Vita-C
VitaGuard
V. 1000 event recorder
V. monitor

vital
v. capacity (VC)
V. High Nitrogen formula
v. signs

vitamin
v. A
v. A deficiency (VAD)
v. A, D intoxication
v. B_6

v. B_{12}
B complex v.'s
v. B complex
v. B_{12} deficiency
v. B_6 dependence syndrome
v. B_{12} level
Bronson chewable prenatal v.'s
v. C
v. C deficiency
v. C drops
v. D
v. D-binding protein
v. D deficiency
v. D dependence
v. D-dependent rickets
v. D receptor (VDR)
v. D-resistant rickets
v. E
v. E deficiency
Fer-In-Sol v.'s
v. K
v. K deficiency
v. K-dependent serine protease
v. K prophylaxis
Materna prenatal v.
v. metabolism
Poly-Vi-Flor v.'s
Poly-Vi-Sol v.'s
v. requirement
Stuart Prenatal v.'s
v. supplement
v. therapy
Tri-Vi-Flor v.'s
Tri-Vi-Sol v.'s
Ultrafort prenatal v.'s
Vi-Daylin v.'s

Vitaneed formula
Vita-Plus E Softgels
Vitec Topical
Vite E Cream
vitelliform degeneration
vitelline
v. cord
v. duct
v. duct cyst
v. fistula
v. membrane
v. sac
v. tumor

vitellinum
mesoblastoma v.

NOTES

vitellointestinal
    v. cyst
    v. duct
vitiligo
    dermal v.
Vitrasert
vitrectomy
vitreoretinopathy
    familial exudative v. (FEV)
vitreous
    v. band
    v. body
    v. chamber
    v. humor
    persistent hyperplastic primary v.
      (PHPV)
    v. seed
    v. seeding
vitro
    in v. fertilization (IVF)
    in v.
vitronectin
Vivactil
vivax
    Plasmodium v.
Vivelle-Dot estradiol transdermal system
Vivelle Transdermal
Vivigen diagnostics
viviparity
viviparous
vivo
    ex v.
    in v.
Vivol
Vivonex
    V. Pediatric
    V. Pediatric formula
    V. Plus formula
    V. Ten formula
Vix infant ventilator
VK
    Apo-Pen VK
V$_{Leiden}$
    factor V^{Leiden}
V-Lax
VLBW
    very low birth weight
    VLBW infant
VLCAD
    very long chain acyl-CoA dehydrogenase
VLCFA
    very long chain fatty acid
VLDL
    very low density lipoprotein
Vles syndrome
VLM
    virtual labor monitor
VLRI
    viral lower respiratory illness

VM
    venous malformation
VMA
    vanillylmandelic acid
VMI
    visual-motor integration
    visuomotor integration
VNA
    virus-neutralizing antibody
Vo$_2$
    oxygen consumption per minute
vocabulary
    v. test
vocal
    v. cord
    v. cord dysfunction (VCD)
    v. cord paralysis
    v. fremitus
    v. nodule
    v. play
    v. tic
vocalization
    irregular stereotyped v.
vocalize
VOD
    venoocclusive disease
Vogt
    V. cephalodactyly
    V. syndrome
Vogt-Koyanagi-Harada syndrome
Vogt-Koyanagi syndrome
Vogt-Spielmeyer disease
Vohwinkel syndrome
voice
    v. disorder
    high-pitched v.
    hoarse v.
    hot potato v.
    v. inflection
    nasal v.
    v. synthesizer
    too-soft v.
voiceless cry
voiceprint
void
    flow v.
Void-Ease urine collection bag
voiding
    v. cystography
    v. cystourethrogram (VCUG)
    v. cystourethrograph (VCUG)
    v. cystourethrography (VCUG)
    v. diary
    v. dysfunction
    dysfunctional v.
    v. pattern
    scheduled v.
    staccato v.
    v. trial

volar
    v. angulation
    v. ganglion
    v. hyperhidrosis
    v. splint
volatile
    v. acid
    v. anesthetic
volitional movement
Volkmann
    V. deformity
    V. disease
    V. ischemic contracture
Volmax
Volpe method
volt (V)
    electron v. (eV)
    megaelectron v. (MeV)
voltage
voltage-dependent calcium channel
Voltaren
    V. Ophthalmic
    V. Oral
Voltaren-XR Oral
Voltolini disease
volume
    amniotic fluid v. (AFV)
    blood v.
    cerebral blood v. (CBV)
    constant tidal v.
    v. contraction
    v. of dead space
    end-diastolic v. (EDV)
    end-expiratory lung v. (EELV)
    end-systolic v. (ESV)
    v. expander
    v. expansion
    expiratory flow v.
    expiratory reserve v. (ERV)
    v. of expired gas (VE)
    extracellular v. (ECV)
    fetal blood v.
    fetoplacental blood v.
    v. flow
    forced expiratory v. (FEV)
    gastric residual v. (GRV)
    inspiratory reserve v. (IRV)
    intracranial v.
    intrauterine v.
    intravascular v.
    v. load
    lung v.

    maternal plasma v.
    mean corpuscular v. (MCV)
    mean platelet v. (MPV)
    minute ventilatory v.
    neonatal blood v.
    v. overload
    v. percent of cream in milk (CRCT)
    plasma v.
    red blood cell v.
    relaxation v.
    v. replacement
    residual v. (RV)
    semen v.
    testicular v.
    thoracic gas v. (TGV)
    tidal v. (TV, VT)
volume-controlled ventilation
volume-limited ventilator
volumetric
    v. bladder ultrasound
    v. bone density
    v. bone mineral density (vBMD)
voluntary
    v. coughing
    v. interruption of pregnancy (VIP)
    v. sterilization
    v. urinary sphincter
Voluson sector transducer
volutrauma
volvulus
    gastric v.
    intestinal v.
    v. malrotation
    malrotation with midgut v.
    mesenteroaxial v.
    midgut v.
    neonatal midgut v.
    v. neonatorum
    Onchocerca v.
    organoaxial v.
VO₂max
    maximum oxygen uptake
vomer
vomerian groove
vomiting
    bilious v.
    cyclic v.
    nausea and v. (N/V)
    nonbilious v.
    pernicious v.

NOTES

vomiting *(continued)*
    postoperative nausea and v.
    (PONV)
    v. of pregnancy
    projectile v.
    self-induced v.
vomitus
    bilious v.
von
    von Fernwald sign
    von Gierke glycogenosis
    von Gierke glycogen storage
    disease
    von Graefe sign
    von Hippel-Lindau disease
    von Hippel-Lindau syndrome
    von Jaksch anemia
    von Meyenburg complex
    von Recklinghausen disease
    von Recklinghausen
    neurofibromatosis
    von Willebrand disease (type IIB,
    III)
    von Willebrand factor (vWF)
    von Willebrand factor antigen
    von Willebrand panel
    von Willebrand syndrome
Voorhees bag
Voorhoeve
    V. dyschondroplasia
    V. syndrome
vorozole
VoSol
    V. HC otic
    V. otic
vowel sound
voyeurism
Vozzle Vacu-Irrigator
VP
    variegate porphyria
    vasa previa
    ventricles to peritoneal cavity
    ventricular peritoneal
    ventriculoperitoneal
    ventroposterior
    VP shunt
    VP shunt tap
VPC
    ventricular premature contraction
VPI
    velopharyngeal incompetence
7VPnC vaccine
VPS
    ventriculoperitoneal shunt
V/Q
    ventilation/perfusion ratio
    $\dot{V}/\dot{Q}$ matching
    $\dot{V}/\dot{Q}$ mismatch
    $\dot{V}/\dot{Q}$ scan

VRA
    visual reinforcement audiometry
    visual response audiometry
VRE
    vancomycin-resistant enterococcus
Vrolik disease
VRSA
    vancomycin-resistant *Staphylococcus*
    aureus
VS
    variable softness
VSD
    Vaccine Safety Datalink
    ventricular septal defect
    ventriculoseptal defect
    perimembranous VSD
VSV
    vesicular stomatitis virus
VT
    tidal volume
VTE
    venous thromboembolism
vu
    déjà vu
    jamais vu
vulgaris
    acne v.
    ichthyosis v.
    lupus v.
    neonatal pemphigus v.
    pemphigus v.
    psoriasis v.
    verruca v.
vulnerable child syndrome
vulnificus
    Vibrio v.
Vulpe Assessment Battery
vulsellum clamp
vulva, gen. and pl. **vulvae**
    anterior labial arteries of v.
    autoimmune disease of the v.
    Camper fascia of v.
    erythrasma of v.
    leukoderma of v.
    lichen sclerosis of v.
    melanosis vulvae
    molluscum contagiosum of the v.
    noma vulvae
    Paget disease of v.
    pigmentation disorder of v.
    superficial compartment of v.
    synechia vulvae
    vaccinia of v.
vulvar
    v. adenocystic adenocarcinoma
    v. adenoid cystic adenocarcinoma
    v. adenosquamous carcinoma
    v. algesiometer
    v. angiokeratoma

v. apocrine cystadenoma
v. apocrine hydrocystoma
v. atrophy
v. atypia
v. biopsy
v. carcinoma in situ
v. colposcopy
v. condyloma
v. congenital dysplastic angiopathy
v. dermatosis
v. dystrophy
v. edema
v. endometriosis
v. fibroma
v. hemangioma
v. hematoma
v. hidradenitis suppurativa
v. hypopigmentation
v. inclusion cyst
v. infection
v. intercourse
v. intraepithelial neoplasia (VIN)
v. lipoma
v. lymph node
v. malignancy
v. melanoma
v. neoplasm
v. neurofibroma
v. nevomelanocytic nevus
v. papillomatosis
v. pigmented lesion
v. pruritus
v. psoriasis
v. sarcoma
v. seborrheic dermatitis
v. skin
v. squamous hyperplasia
v. varicosity
v. varix
v. vestibulitis
v. vestibulitis syndrome (VVS)
v. wart

vulvectomy
Basset radical v.
Parry-Jones v.
partial v.
radical v.
simple v.
skinning v.
vulvismus
vulvitis
adhesive v.

allergic v.
chronic atrophic v.
chronic hypertrophic v.
creamy v.
cyclic v.
erosive v.
focal v.
follicular v.
leukoplakic v.
plasma cell v.
ulcerative v.
Zoon v.
v. of Zoon
vulvodynia
cyclic v.
dysesthetic v.
essential v.
idiopathic v.
vulvoplasty
vulvovaginal
v. anus
v. burning
v. candidiasis (VVC)
v. carcinoma
v. cystectomy
v. disorder
v. erythema
v. inflammation
v. itching
v. lesion
v. outlet
v. pouch
v. pouch of Williams
v. premenarchal infection
vulvovaginitis
adolescent v.
candidal v.
chemical v.
contact v.
cyclic v.
irritative v.
nonspecific v.
premenarchal v.
vulvovaginoplasty
Williams v.
Vu-Max vaginal speculum
Vumon
VUR
vesicoureteral reflux (grade 1–4)
vesicoureteric reflux (grade 1–4)

NOTES

VURD
posterior urethral valves, unilateral reflux, renal dysplasia
VURD syndrome

VV
venovenous

VVC
vulvovaginal candidiasis

VVS
vulvar vestibulitis syndrome

V.V.S.

vWF
von Willebrand factor
vWF antigen

VX-478

Vysis PathVysion genomic disease management test

Vytone
V. Topical

VZIG
varicella-zoster immune globulin
varicella-zoster immunoglobulin

VZV
varicella-zoster virus
VZV vaccine

VZV-specific IgM antibody

W

W chromosome
W position of legs
W sign
W sitting position
W syndrome

Waardenburg-Klein syndrome
Waardenburg recessive anophthalmia syndrome
Wachendorf membrane
Wada test
waddling gait
Wade

Roe v. W.

Wadia elevator
WADIC

Wing Autistic Disorder Interview Checklist

Waelsch syndrome
wafer

Fiberall W.

Wagner syndrome
WAGR

Wilms tumor, aniridia, gonadoblastoma, mental retardation
WAGR syndrome

WAI

Weinberger Adjustment Inventory

Waisman-Laxova syndrome
Waisman syndrome
waist

narrow mediastinal w.

waist:hip ratio (WHR)
waiter tip posture
waitlist control
Walcher position
Waldenström

W. disease
W. macroglobinemia

Waldeyer

fossa of W.
germinal epithelium of W.
W. layer
W. preurethral ligament
W. ring

Waldman episiotomy scissors
Waldmann disease
walk

bear w.

walker

W. chart
W. lissencephaly syndrome
Maddacrawler w.
ORLAU swivel w.
swivel w.

Walker-Clodius syndrome
Walker-Warburg

W.-W. malformation
W.-W. syndrome

walking

automatic w.
chromosome w.
w. epidural anesthetic
idiopathic toe w. (ITW)
w. reflex
sideways w.
tandem w.
toe w.

wall

abdominal w.
anterior abdominal w.
anterior thoracic w.
anterolateral free w. (ALFW)
bladder w.
cystic w.
lateral pelvic w.
opposing w.
pelvic side w.
resecting intrapartum uterine w.
w. suction
symphysial w.
vaginal w.
ventral w.

wallaby

W. Phototherapy System
w. pouch

Wallace

W. catheter
W. technique

Wallach

W. Endocell collection device
W. Endocell endometrial cell sampler
W. LL100 cryosurgical cryogun

Wallach-Papette disposable cervical cell collector
wallerian degeneration
walleye
walnut-shaped bladder
Walt Disney dwarfism
Walthard

W. cell rest
W. nest

Walther dilator
Walton

W. report
W. syndrome

W

WAMBA
Wise areola mastopexy breast augmentation
WAMBA procedure
Wampole test
wandering
w. atrial pacemaker
w. ovary
Wangensteen needle holder
Warburg syndrome
Wardill four-flap method
Wardill-Kilner advancement flap method
Ward-Mayo vaginal hysterectomy
Ward triangle
Ware Short Form-35
warfarin
w. embryopathy
w. syndrome
Warfilone
Waring
W. blender sound
W. blender syndrome
Warkany syndrome 1, 2
warm
w. antibody
w. autoantibody
w. shock
w. water near drowning
warmer
Ecowarm gel w.
Kreiselman infant w.
Ohio w.
overhead w.
radiant w.
Thermasonic gel w.
warming stand
Warren
W. flap
W. shunt
wart
anogenital w.
brain w.
common w.
exophytic w.
filiform w.
flat w.
genital w.
laryngeal w.
mucous membrane w.
periungual w.
plantar w.
venereal w.
vulvar w.
water w.
Wartenberg sign
Warthin-Starry silver stain
warty dyskeratoma

WAS
Wiskott-Aldrich syndrome
wash
Benzac AC, W W.
gastric w.
hexachlorophene w.
nasal w.
nasopharyngeal w.
Oxy 10 W.
RSV nasal w.
Sastid plain therapeutic shampoo and acne w.
Theroxide W.
vaginal w.
washed
w. intrauterine insemination
w. sperm
w. spermatozoa
washer
Gravlee jet w.
washing
cytologic w.
gastric w.
peritoneal w.
preputial w.'s
washout
antral w.
nitrogen w.
w. pyelogram
wasp allergy
Wassel classification
Wasserman test
wastage
early pregnancy w.
fetal w.
pregnancy w.
reproductive w.
wasting
bicarbonate w.
cerebral salt w. (CSW)
phosphate w.
renal electrolyte w.
renal salt w.
renal tubular bicarbonate w.
salt w.
sodium w.
w. syndrome
urinary potassium w.
water
w. aerobics
bag of w.'s (BOW)
w. bottle appearance
centimeter of w. (cmH$_2$O)
w. deficit calculation
dextrose in w.
w. enema
w. excretion
extravascular lung w. (EVLW)
false w.'s

w. intoxication
w. lily sign
w. loss
w. metabolism
w. on brain
w. pacifier
w. test
total body w. (TBW)
w. vaporizer
w. wart
water-deprivation study
waterhammer effect
Waterhouse-Friderichsen syndrome
water-perfused manometry catheter
Waters
W. operation
W. view
waterseal drainage
watershed
w. distribution
w. lesion
w. zone
water-soluble contrast enema
Waterston
W. aortopulmonary anastomosis
W. shunt
W. shunt procedure
Waterston-Cooley procedure
watery diarrhea
Watson
W. capsule
W. method
W. syndrome
Watson-Alagille syndrome
Watson-Miller syndrome
Watson-Schwartz test
WAVE
women's angiographic vitamins and
estrogen
WAVE nucleic acid fragment
analysis system
WAVE trial
wave
brain w.
w. change
delta w.
fibrillatory w.
fluid w.
flutter w.
gastric peristaltic w.
jugular venous A w.
Mayer w.

Osborne w.
peristaltic w.
pulsed electromagnetic w.
rolandic sharp w.'s
saw-toothed flutter w.
w. type
W. ventilator
waveform
aortic blood flow velocity w.
arterial w.
discordant artery flow velocity w.
Doppler flow-velocity w.
flow velocity w.
wavy rib
3-way Hans Rudolph valve
4-Way Long Acting Nasal Solution
Way operation
Wayson stain
WBC
white blood cell
WBI
whole-bowel irrigation
WBN
well-baby nursery
WCC
well-child care
wcp
whole chromosome paint
WCST
Wisconsin Card Sorting Test
WDL
Wood-Downes-Lecks
WDL asthma score
WE
Wernicke encephalopathy
weak
w. cry
w. suck
weakness
collagen w.
girdle w.
homolateral w.
hypotonic w.
postictal w.
proximal pattern w.
upward gaze w.
wean and feed protocol
weaning brash
wearing position
Weaver-Smith syndrome (WSS)
Weaver syndrome
Weaver-Williams syndrome

NOTES

W

web
　　w. cerclage
　　esophageal w.
　　gastric w.
　　interdigital w.
　　intraluminal w.
　　laryngeal w.
　　supraglottic w.
　　tracheal w.
　　windsock w.
webbed
　　w. fingers
　　w. neck
　　w. penis
webbing
Webb-McCall peak
Weber
　　W. syndrome
　　W. test
Weber-Christian syndrome
Weber-Cockayne epidermolysis bullosa simplex
Weber-Dimitri syndrome
Webril bandage
webspace
Webster operation
Wechsler
　　W. Adult Intelligence Scale, 3rd Edition
　　W. Intelligence Scale for Children (WISC)
　　W. Intelligence Scale for Children III
　　W. Intelligence Scale for Children-Revised (WISC-R)
　　W. Intelligence Scale, 3rd Edition
　　W. Memory Scale
　　W. Preschool and Primary Scale of Intelligence (WPPSI)
　　W. Preschool and Primary Scale of Intelligence-Revised (WPPSI-R)
Weck
　　W. disposable cannula
　　W. disposable trocar
Weck-cel sponge
wedge
　　w. osteotomy
　　pulmonary artery w. (PAW)
　　w. resection
　　shoe w.
　　w. vertebra
wedge-shaped platform
wedging
WEE
　　Western equine encephalitis
WeeFIM
　　Functional Independence Measure for Children

week
　　pill-free w.
weekend drug holiday
weeping
　　w. dermatitis
　　w. lesion
　　w. willow
Weerda laparoscope
Wegener granulomatosis (WG)
Wegner disease
Weibel-Palade body
weighing
　　underwater w.
weight
　　birth w. (BW)
　　body w.
　　chest wall w.
　　critical body w.
　　dry w.
　　estimated fetal w. (EFW)
　　extremely low birth w. (ELBW)
　　fetal w.
　　w. gain
　　w. loss
　　low birth w. (LBW)
　　low molecular w. (LMW)
　　maternal w.
　　mean birth w.
　　w. molecular w. (HMW)
　　percent of ideal body w. (%IBW)
　　placental w.
　　w. reduction
　　refusal to bear w.
　　w. shifting
　　very low birth w. (VLBW)
　　w. Z-score
weight for age (WFA)
weightbearing bone
weighted speculum
weight/height (W/H)
　　w./h. index
weight-lifter blackout
Weil disease (leptospirosis)
Weil-Felix
　　W.-F. antibody testing
　　W.-F. reaction
Weill
　　W. disease (polyosteochondritis)
　　W. sign
Weill-Marchesani syndrome
Weinberger Adjustment Inventory (WAI)
Weinberg rule
Weismann-Netter syndrome
Weissenbacher-Zweymuller syndrome
Weitlaner retractor
Welch
　　W. Allyn AudioPath Platform hearing acuity instrument

W. Allyn AudioScope
W. Allyn SureSight eye chart
welfare
well-baby nursery (WBN)
well-being
fetal w.-b.
maternal w.-b.
well-born
right to be w.-b.
Wellbutrin
well-child care (WCC)
well-circumscribed carcinoma
well-defined mass
well engaged in pelvis
well-hydrated baby
well-oxygenated
w.-o. baby
w.-o. infant
well-perfused baby
welt
Wenckebach
W. block
W. phenomena
Wender Utah Rating Scale (WURS)
Wepman Auditory Discrimination Test
Werdnig-Hoffmann
W.-H. disease (type I–III)
W.-H. disorder
W.-H. muscular atrophy
W.-H. paralysis
W.-H. syndrome
werkmanii
Citrobacter w.
Werlhof disease
Wermer syndrome
werneckii
Exophiala w.
Werner syndrome
Wernicke
W. aphasia
W. area
W. disease
W. encephalopathy (WE)
W. syndrome
Wernicke-Korsakoff syndrome
Wertheim operation
Wertheim-Schauta operation
Wessel colic
West
W. Haven-Yale Multidimensional
Pain Inventory
W. Nile fever

W. Nile virus
W. syndrome
Westcort Topical
West-Engstler skull
westermani
Paragonimus w.
Western
W. blot
W. blot test
W. equine encephalitis (WEE)
W. immunoblot
Weston
W. knot
W. slipknot
Westrim-I, -LA
wet
w. brain syndrome
w. burp
w. drowning
w. lung disease
w. lung syndrome
w. mount
w. mount test
w. nurse
w. prep
w. preparation
w. purpura
w. rale
w. smear
w. tap
wetting defect of cornea
Weyers oligodactyly syndrome
WFA
weight for age
WG
Wegener granulomatosis
W/H
weight/height
W/H index
Wharton jelly
wheal
w. and flare reaction
punctate w.
wheat
spelt w.
w. sperm agglutination test
Wheaton Pavlik harness
wheelchair sport
wheeze, wheezing
high-pitched w.
monophonic w.
nonmusical w.

NOTES

wheeze (*continued*)
    polyphonic w.
    RSV-associated w.
wheezer
    happy w.
    nonatopic w.
wheezy bronchitis
Whelan syndrome
whey
    hydrolyzed w.
whiff
    w. amine test
whiplash injury
Whipple
    W. disease
    W. procedure
    W. syndrome
whipworm
whispered pectoriloquy
whistle-tip catheter
whistling
    w. face syndrome
    w. face-windmill vane hand
    syndrome
Whitaker test
white
    w. blood cell (WBC)
    w. blood cell count
    w. blood cell lysosomal enzyme
    analysis
    w. cell scanning
    W. classification
    w. coat effect
    w. coat hypertension
    w. dermographism
    w. epithelium
    w. forelock
    w. grape juice
    w. infarction
    w. leg
    w. matter
    w. matter damage (WMD)
    w. matter degeneration
    w. matter lucency
    w. matter necrosis
    w. matter pallor
    w. matter spongiosis
    w. papule
    w. plaque
    w. pseudomembranous material
    w. pupil
    w. pupillary reflex
    w. retinal infiltrate
    w. scleral hue
    w. sponge nevus
    w. strawberry tongue
    w. superficial onychomycosis
    w. tonsillitis
whitehead

white-out
white-yellow plaque
Whitfield ointment
whitlow
    herpetic w.
Whitten medium
Whittingham medium
WHO
    World Health Organization
    WHO formula
whole
    w. abdominal radiation
    w. blood
    w. blood transfusion
    w. chromosome paint (wcp)
    w. chromosome 1-22 paint
    w. chromosome X, Y paint
whole-abdomen irradiation
whole-body irradiation
whole-bowel irrigation (WBI)
whole-cell
    w.-c. diphtheria-tetanus-pertussis
    vaccine
    w.-c. DTP vaccine
whole-pelvis irradiation
whole-virus vaccine
Wholey balloon occlusion catheter
Whoo Noz
whoop
    inspiratory w.
whooping cough
whorl
    hair w.
whorled macular hyperpigmentation
WHR
    waist:hip ratio
WI-38 cell
Wiberg
    center edge angle of W.
WIC
    women, infants, children
    WIC syndrome
wick
    gauze w.
Wickham stria
wide
    w. complex tachycardia
    w. cranial suture
    w. excision
    w. plane
    w. pulse pressure
    W. Range Achievement Test-
    Revised (WRAT-R)
    w. range assessment of memory
    and learning (WRAML)
wide-based shuffling gait
wide-field myringotomy
widely spaced eyes

widened
- w. growth plate
- w. metaphysis
- w. symphysis pubis
- w. thecal sac

widening
- mediastinal w.

width
- cardiac w.
- chest w.
- funnel w.
- maximal cardiac w.
- maximal chest w.
- pulse w.
- tympanometric w.

Wieacker syndrome
Wieacker-Wolff syndrome
Wiedemann-Beckwith-Combs syndrome
Wiedemann-Beckwith syndrome
Wiedemann-Rautenstrauch syndrome (WR)
Wiedemann syndrome
Wigand
- W. maneuver
- W. version

Wigraine
WIHS
- women's interagency HIV study

wild
- w. type
- w. virus

Wildermuth ear
Wildervanck-Smith syndrome
Wildervanck syndrome
wild-type
- w.-t. allele
- w.-t. gene
- w.-t. measles virus

Wilkie disease
Wilkins
- W. disease
- W. syndrome

Willebrand-Jurgens syndrome
Willett
- W. clamp
- W. forceps

Williams
- W. disease
- W. syndrome (WS)
- vulvovaginal pouch of W.
- W. vulvovaginoplasty

Williams-Barratt syndrome

Williams-Beuren syndrome
Williams-Campbell syndrome
Willis
- circle of W.

willow
- weeping w.

Willy Meyer mastectomy
Wilms
- W. tumor, aniridia, genitourinary malformations, mental retardation
- W. tumor, aniridia, gonadoblastoma, mental retardation (WAGR)
- W. tumor, aniridia gonadoblastoma, mental retardation syndrome
- W. tumor (stage I–V)
- W. tumor suppression gene

Wilson disease
wilsonian
Wilson-Mikity syndrome
Wilson-Turner syndrome (WTS)
Wimberger
- W. ring
- W. sign

Winchester syndrome
Winckel disease
window
- aortopulmonary w.
- middle meatus nasal antral w.
- nasal antral w.
- w. operation
- oval w.
- w. period
- square w.
- therapeutic w.
- transgastric w.
- vaginal w.

windpipe
windsock web
windswept deformity
Wing Autistic Disorder Interview Checklist (WADIC)
wing-beating appearance
winging
- scapular w.

wink
- anal w.

Winkler body
Winkler-Waldeyer
- closing ring of W.-W.

WinRho
- W. DS
- W. SDF

W

NOTES

WINS
women's intervention nutrition study
Winston cervical clamp
Winter
W. glans-cavernosal procedure
W. placental forceps
W. syndrome
Wintrobe index
wipe
disposable w.
povidone-iodine w.
wiping
front-to-back w.
wire
electrosurgical w.
3F thermistor w.
iridium w.
Kirschner w. (K-wire)
lead w.
Teflon-coated w.
Wirsung
main duct of W.
Wisap
W. disposable cannula
W. disposable trocar
WISC
Wechsler Intelligence Scale for Children
WISC III
WISC III factor scores
Wisconsin
W. Card Sorting Test (WCST)
W. syndrome
WISC-R
Wechsler Intelligence Scale for Children-Revised
wisdom tooth
WISE
women's ischemia syndrome evaluation
Wise areola mastopexy breast augmentation (WAMBA)
WISH
Wistar Institute Susan Hayflick
WISH cell
Wiskott-Aldrich syndrome (WAS)
wispy hair
Wistar Institute Susan Hayflick (WISH)
witch's milk
withdrawal
w. bleeding
w. bleeding test
w. dyskinesia
estrogen w.
maternal estrogen w.
w. position
social w.
speculum w.
withdrawal-like activity
withdrawn behavior

withholding
stool w.
within-the-infant depressive disorder
Witness
Jehovah's W.
WITS
Women and Infants Transmission Study
Wittner biopsy punch
Wittwer syndrome
WMD
white matter damage
Wohlfart-Kugelberg-Welander syndrome
Wolcott-Rallison syndrome
Wolf
W. disposable cannula
W. disposable trocar
W. laparoscope
W. syndrome
Wolf-Castroviejo needle holder
Wolfe classification of breast cancer
wolffian
w. duct
w. duct carcinoma
w. remnant cyst
w. rest
w. ridge
Wolff mental retardation syndrome
Wolff-Parkinson-White syndrome
Wolf-Hirschhorn syndrome
Wolfram syndrome
Wolfring lacrimal accessory gland
Wolf-Veress needle
Wolman disease
Wolraich questionnaire
woman
amenorrheic w.
androgenized w.
battered w.
eumenorrheic w.
euprolactinemic w.
formula-feeding w.
hirsute w.
hypoestrogenic w.
hypogonadal w.
hypomenorrheic w.
infertile w.
lactating w.
nulliparous w.
parous w.
perimenopausal w.
postmenopausal w.
womb
falling of the w.
scarred w.
w. stone
women
w., infants, children (WIC)
W. and Infants Transmission Study (WITS)

women-held antenatal record
Women's
> W. Choice condom
> W. HOPE
> W. HOPE study

women's
> w. angiographic vitamins and
>   estrogen (WAVE)
> w. interagency HIV study (WIHS)
> w. intervention nutrition study
>   (WINS)
> w. ischemia syndrome evaluation
>   (WISE)

Wong-Baker faces pain rating scale
wood
> W. light
> w. tick
> W. ultraviolet lamp

Woodcock-Johnson
> W.-J. Psychoeducational Battery
> W.-J. reading test
> W.-J. Tests of Achievement

Wood-Downes asthma score
Wood-Downes-Lecks (WDL)
Woodruff vestibulectomy
Woods
> W. corkscrew maneuver
> W. syndrome

woolly
> w. hair disease
> w. hair nevus

word
> W. Bartholin gland catheter
> W. bladder catheter
> number of different w.'s (NDW)
> staggered spondaic w. (SSW)

work
> w. of breathing
> w. factor
> parent guidance w.

worker
> healthcare w. (HCW)
> social w.

Working Group on Asthma and
** Pregnancy**
workup
> malabsorption w.
> preconceptual w.
> pregnancy w.
> sepsis w.

world
> W. Association for Infant Mental
>   Health
> fantasy/make-believe w.
> W. Health Organization (WHO)

worm
wormian bones
worried facial appearance
Worster-Drought syndrome
wort
> mother w.

wound
> w. botulism
> w. breakdown
> w. dehiscence
> w. infection
> perforating w.
> stab w.
> stellate w.
> suprapubic stab w.

woven bone
WPPSI
> Wechsler Preschool and Primary Scale of
>   Intelligence

WPPSI-R
> Wechsler Preschool and Primary Scale of
>   Intelligence-Revised

WR
> Wiedemann-Rautenstrauch syndrome

WRAML
> wide range assessment of memory and
>   learning
> WRAML test

Wramsby hypothesis
wrap
> CircPlus compression w./dressing
> mummy w.
> SurePress w.

WRAT-R
> Wide Range Achievement Test-Revised

wrestling
Wright
> W. peak flow meter
> W. stain
> W. version

Wright-stained smear
wringing
> hand w.

wrinkly skin syndrome (WSS)
wrist
> gymnast's w.
> shaking w.

NOTES

W

wristwatch
    QT-Watch messaging w.
writer's cramp
writhing
written consent
wrongful
    w. birth
    w. birth and life
    w. conception
wry
wryneck, wry neck
wryneck deformity
WS
    Williams syndrome

WSS
    Weaver-Smith syndrome
    wrinkly skin syndrome
W-stapled urinary reservoir procedure
WTS
    Wilson-Turner syndrome
Wullstein retractor
WURS
    Wender Utah Rating Scale
Wyanoids
Wyburn-Mason syndrome
Wycillin

X

X chromatin
X chromosome
X chromosome aneuploidy
X inactivation
X inactivation center (XIC)
X inactive, specific transcript (XIST)
X 19 translocation
X trisomy
X zone

45,X

45,X karyotype
45,X syndrome

45,X/46,XY mosaicism

XA

chromosome XA

Xa

X-acto knife

Xanar 20 Ambulase CO₂ laser

Xanax

xanthan/guar combination

xanthelasma

xanthine oxidase deficiency

xanthinuria, xanthiuria

xanthochromia therapy

xanthochromic

x. CSF
x. fluid
x. specimen

xanthogranuloma

juvenile x. (JXG)

xanthogranulomatous

x. infiltrate
x. pyelonephritis

xanthoma

Achilles tendon x.
eruptive x.
palmar x.
x. striata palmaris
tendon x.

xanthomatosis

cerebrotendinous x.
primary x.

Xanthomonas maltophilia

xanthopsia

xanthosis cutis

xanthous

xanthurenic

x. acid
x. aciduria

X-autosome translocation

X-chromosome abnormality

Xe

xenon

xenogamy

xenogeneic

x. antibody
x. tissue

xenograft

xenon (Xe)

x. arc
x. clearance
x. CT scan

xenopi

Mycobacterium x.

Xenopus test

xeroderma pigmentosum

xerodermic idiocy

xerography

xeromammography

xeromenia

xerophthalmia

xerosis

x. conjunctiva
x. cornea

xerostomia

XIC

X inactivation center

Ximed

X. disposable cannula
X. disposable trocar

xinafoate

salmeterol x.

xiphisternum

xiphoid

bifid x.

xiphoomphaloischiopagus tripus twins

xiphopagus

XIST

X inactive, specific transcript

XK-aprosencephaly syndrome

XK syndrome

XL

Ditropan XL
Procardia XL

XLA

X-linked agammaglobulinemia

XLAS

X-linked aqueductal stenosis

XLCM

X-linked cardiomyopathy
X-linked dilated cardiomyopathy

XLD

X-linked dominant

XLHN

X-linked hypercalciuric nephrolithiasis

XLHR

X-linked hypophosphatemic rickets

X

X-linked

X-l. adrenoleukodystrophy

X-l. agammaglobulinemia (XLA)

X-l. alpha-thalassemia/mental retardation (ATRX)

X-l. aqueductal stenosis (XLAS)

X-l. cardiomyopathy (XLCM)

X-l. cardioskeletal myopathy

X-l. cardioskeletal myopathy and neutropenia

X-l. cataract-dental syndrome

X-l. cataract with hutchinsonian teeth

X-l. centronuclear myopathy

X-l. cerebellar ataxia (CLA)

X-l. cerebral hypoplasia/hydrocephalus

X-l. chronic granulomatous disease

X-l. congenital cataracts-microcornea syndrome

X-l. congenital glycerol kinase deficiency

X-l. congenital recessive muscle hypotrophy with central nuclei

X-l. dilated cardiomyopathy (XLCM)

X-l. dominant (XLD)

X-l. dominant condition

X-l. dominant disease

X-l. dominant disorder

X-l. dominant inheritance

X-l. dominant syndrome

X-l. dyskeratosis congenita

X-l. dysplasia-gigantism syndrome (DGSX)

X-l. Ehlers-Danlos syndrome

X-l. gene

X-l. heredity

X-l. Hurler syndrome

X-l. hydrocephalus

X-l. hydrocephalus-stenosis of aqueduct of Sylvius sequence

X-l. hypercalciuric nephrolithiasis (XLHN)

X-l. hypogammaglobulinemia

X-l. hypophosphatemia

X-l. hypophosphatemic rickets (XLHR)

X-l. ichthyosis

X-l. immunodeficiency with hyper IgM

X-l. infantile spasm

X-l. lymphoproliferative syndrome

X-l. mental deficiency-megalotestes syndrome

X-l. mental handicap-retinitis pigmentosa syndrome

X-l. mental retardation (1-47) (MRX, XLMR)

X-l. mental retardation-aphasia syndrome (MRXA)

X-l. mental-retardation-bilateral clasp thumb anomaly

X-l. mental retardation-blindness-deafness-multiple congenital anomalies syndrome

X-l. mental retardation-fragile site syndrome 2

X-l. mental retardation-growth hormone deficiency syndrome

X-l. mental retardation-hypogenitalism-cerebral anomaly syndrome

X-l. mental retardation-marfanoid habitus syndrome

X-l. mental retardation, microphthalmia, microcornea, cataract, hypogenitalism, mental retardation-spasticity syndrome

X-l. mental retardation/multiple congenital anomaly (XLMR/MCA)

X-l. mental retardation-psoriasis syndrome

X-l. mental retardation-seizures-acquired microcephaly-agenesis of corpus callosum

X-l. mental retardation-spastic diplegia syndrome

X-l. mental retardation syndrome 1–6 (MRXS1–6)

X-l. mental retardation, thin habitus, osteoporosis, kyphoscoliosis syndrome

X-l. mental retardation with fragile X syndrome

X-l. monoamine oxidase deficiency

X-l. myotubular myopathy (MTMX, XLMTM)

X-l. OPCA

X-l. Opitz syndrome (XLOS)

X-l. phenomenon

X-l. primary hyperuricemia

X-l. pyridoxine-responsive sideroblastic anemia

X-l. recessive (XLR)

X-l. recessive centronuclear myopathy

X-l. recessive condition

X-l. recessive deafness syndrome

X-l. recessive disease

X-l. recessive disorder

X-l. recessive dysgenesis

X-l. recessive inheritance

X-l. recessive muscular dystrophy

X-l. recessive myotubular myopathy

X-l. recessive nephrolithiasis

X-l. recessive skeletal Ehlers-Danlos syndrome

X-l. recessive-type diabetes insipidus

X-l. retinoschisis

X-l. seizures, acquired micrencephaly, agenesis of corpus callosum syndrome

X-l. severe combined immunodeficiency (X-SCID)

X-l. severe combined immunodeficiency syndrome spondylometaphyseal dysplasia, X-l.

X-l. thrombocytopenia

X-l. trait

X-l. uric aciduria enzyme defect

XLMR

X-linked mental retardation (1-47)

XLMR/MCA

X-linked mental retardation/multiple congenital anomaly

XLMTM

X-linked myotubular myopathy

XLOS

X-linked Opitz syndrome

XLR

X-linked recessive

XO

XO chromosome

XO chromosome anomaly

XO karyotype

XO syndrome

XomaZyme-H65

Xopenex inhalation solution

Xp deletion

X-Prep

X-P. Liquid

Senna X-P.

Xq

isochromosome Xq

Xq Klinefelter syndrome

monosomy Xq

partial trisomy Xq

trisomy Xq

Xq- syndrome

Xq+ syndrome

XR

Dilacor XR

x-ray

x-r. absorptiometry

chest x-r. (CXR)

dual-energy x-r.

Lauenstein pelvic x-r.

x-r. mammogram

x-r. mammography

x-r. pelvimetry

stand x-r.

x-r. therapy

X-SCID

X-linked severe combined immunodeficiency

X-tra

AFP X-tra

XX

double strength

normal female sex chromosome type

XX chromosome

XX hermaphroditism

XX karyotype

XX male syndrome

XX and XY Turner phenotype

46,XX

46,XX karyotype

46,XX male

46,XX male syndrome

47,XX karyotype

XX-type gonadal dysgenesis

XXX

XXX karyotype

mosaicism for XXX

XXX syndrome

47,XXX

47,XXX syndrome

XXXX syndrome

XXXXX syndrome

XXXXY

XXXXY aneuploidy

XXXXY syndrome

XXY

XXY karyotype

XXY male

XXY syndrome

47,XXY

47,XXY karyotype

47,XXY syndrome

69,XXY

XY

normal male sex chromosome type

XY gonadal dysgenesis

XY karyotype

46,XY

46,XY karyotype

46,XY/47,XY karyotype

47,XY karyotype

xylitol

NOTES

Xylocaine
    X. HCl I.V. Injection for Cardiac Arrhythmias
    X. jelly
    X. Oral
    X. Topical Ointment
    X. Topical Solution
    X. Topical Spray
    X. With Epinephrine
xylometazoline
xyloni
    Solenopsis x.

Xylo-Pfan
xylose lysine deaminase agar
xylosoxidans
    Achromobacter x.
    Alcaligenes x.
xylulose dehydrogenase deficiency
XYY
    XYY male
    XYY syndrome
X-zone

Y

Y chromatin
Y chromosome
Y chromosome-specific DNA
sequence
Y connector
Y incision
Y linkage
Y shunt
Y shunting

YAC

yeast artificial chromosome

Yachia incisionless bladder suspension

YAG

yttrium-aluminum-garnet
YAG laser
YAG pellet

Yale

Y. Global Tic Severity Scale
(YGTSS)
Y. Observation Scale
Y. Optimal Observation Score

**Yale-Brown Obsessive Compulsive Scale
(YBOCS)**

Yang-Monti ileovesicostomy

Yankauer

Y. catheter
Y. curette
Y. scissors

YAPA

young adult psychiatric assessment

Yasmin

yaws

YBOCS

Yale-Brown Obsessive Compulsive Scale

y-cystathionase deficiency

year

y. of birth (YOB)
y. 7 conduct disorder
postnatal y.

yeast

y. artificial chromosome (YAC)
bismuth sulfite, glucose, glycine, y.
(BiGGY)
y. infection
Pityrosporum y.
vaginal y.
y. vaginitis

Yellen clamp

yellow

y. fever
y. fever 17D vaccination
y. fever vaccine
y. jacket
y. jacket allergy
y. nail
y. nail syndrome
y. OCA
y. retinal infiltrate
y. vernix syndrome

yellow-green pallor

Yeoman forceps

Yersinia

Y. arthritis
Y. enterocolitica
Y. pestis
Y. pseudotuberculosis

yersinial infection

yersiniosis

yes protooncogene

yew

English y.
Pacific y.

YGTSS

Yale Global Tic Severity Scale

YIPS

York Incontinence Perceptions Scale

Y-linked

Y.-l. character
Y.-l. gene
Y.-l. inheritance

YOB

year of birth

Yocon

Yodoxin

yogurt douche

Yohimex

yolk

accessory y.
y. cell
formative y.
y. membrane
y. sac
y. sac carcinoma
y. sac tumor
y. sac tumor of testis
y. space
y. stalk

Yom Kippur effect

Yoon ring

**York Incontinence Perceptions Scale
(YIPS)**

York-Mason repair

young

y. adult psychiatric assessment
(YAPA)
maturity-onset diabetes of the y.
(MODY)

youngae

Citrobacter y.

Young-Dees-Leadbetter bladder neck reconstruction
Young-Hughes syndrome
Young-Madders syndrome
Young syndrome
youth
> GLB y.'s
> Great Smoky Mountains Study of Y. (GSMS)
> maturity-onset diabetes of y. (MODY)
> y. risk behavioral survey (YRBS)
> y. self-report (YSR)

Y-plasty
Yq
> AZFa region of Yq
> AZFb region of Yq
> AZFc region of Yq

YRBS
> youth risk behavioral survey

YSI neonatal temperature probe
Y-specific DNA amplification
YSR
> youth self-report

yttrium-aluminum-garnet (YAG)
> y.-a.-g. laser

Yunis-Varon syndrome
Yuzpe
> Y. contraceptive method
> Y. regimen of combined oral contraceptives for emergency contraception

YY syndrome

Z

Z allele
Z band
Z bone density score
Z degree of contraction
Z foot
Z sampler endometrial sampling device

zafirlukast
Zagam
zalcitabine (ddC)
zanamivir
Zancolli clawhand deformity repair
Zanosar
Zantac 75
zaprinast
Zarontin
Zaroxolyn
Zatuchni-Andros score
Zaufal sign
Zavanelli maneuver
Z-Clamp hysterectomy forceps
ZD

zona drilling

Z' degree of contraction
Zeasorb-AF Powder
Zeasorb powder
zebra body
Zeis

Z. gland
pilosebaceous gland of Z.

Zeiss colposcope
Zellweger

Z. cerebrohepatorenal syndrome
Z. disease

Zelsmyr Cytobrush
Zemplar
Zemuron
Zenapax
Zenate
Zenker solution
Zephrex LA
Zeppelin clamp
Zerit
zero

z. end-expiratory pressure
z. gravity surgery
z. reject
Z. to Three children's mental health diagnostic classification

zero-voltage baseline
Zerres syndrome
Zestril
Zetar
Ziagen

zidovudine

z. monotherapy
z. treatment

Ziehen-Oppenheim syndrome
Ziehl-Neelsen

Z.-N. stain
Z.-N. test

ZIFT

zygote intrafallopian transfer

ZIG

zoster immune globulin

zigzagplasty
Zilactin-B Medicated
zileuton
Zimmermann-Laband syndrome (ZLS)
Zinacef Injection
Zinaderm
zinc

z. deficiency
z. oxide
z. oxide ointment
z. oxide paste
z. peroxide
z. poisoning
z. protoporphyrin (ZnPP)
z. protoporphyrin to heme ratio (ZnPP/H)
serum z.
z. stearate powder
z. sulfate
z. supplement
z. therapy
z. toxicity

Zinca-Pak
Zincate
zinc-dependent enzyme
zinc-free

z.-f. plastic bag
z.-f. plastic-lined diaper
z.-f. plastic specimen cup

Z-incision
Zincofax
Zinecard
Zinnanti uterine manipulator-injector (ZUMI)
Zinsser

Z. disease
Z. syndrome

Zinsser-Cole-Engman syndrome
Zinsser-Engman-Cole syndrome
ZIPP

Zoladex in premenopausal patients

zipper ring
ziprasidone
Ziprokowski-Margolis syndrome

Z

Zithromax
Zixoryn
Zlotogora-Ogür syndrome
ZLS
Zimmermann-Laband syndrome
ZM-1 coloscope
ZnPP
zinc protoporphyrin
ZnPP/H
zinc protoporphyrin to heme ratio
Zofran ODT
Zoladex
Z. Implant
Z. in premenopausal patients (ZIPP)
zoledronate
Zollinger-Ellison syndrome
Zollino syndrome
Zoloft
zolpidem tartrate
zomepirac sodium
zona, pl. **zonae**
z. basalis
z. compacta
z. drilling (ZD)
z. fasciculata
z. functionalis
z. glomerulosa
z. pellucida (ZP)
z. protein
z. reaction
z. reticularis
z. spongiosa
zona-free hamster egg penetration test
zonal aganglionosis
Zonalon Topical Cream
zonary placenta
zone
Barnes z.
basement membrane z. (BMZ)
beta-hCG discriminatory z.
cervical transformation z.
chemoreceptor trigger z. (CTZ)
echo-free z.
extranodal marginal z.
germinal z.
growth z.
hypertrophic z. (HZ)
hypertrophic growth z.
interthreshold z.
ipsilon z.
large loop excision of transformation z. (LLETZ)
loop excision of the transformation z. (LETZ)
marginal z.
needle excision of the transformation z.
normal transformation z.

null z.
z. of preparatory calcification (ZPC)
proliferative z. (PZ)
reserve z. (RZ)
toxicity z.
transformation z. (TZ)
watershed z.
X z.
Zone-A Forte
zonoskeleton
zonula, pl. **zonulae**
z. adherens
z. occludens
zonular cataract
zoogonous
zoogony
Zoomscope colposcope
Zoon
Z. erythroplasia
vulvitis of Z.
Z. vulvitis
zoonotic infection
zoosperm
zoster
herpes z.
z. immune globulin (ZIG)
z. myelitis
trigeminal herpes z.
zosteriform
z. lentiginous nevus
z. lesion
Zostrix-HP
Zosyn
Zovia
Zovirax
ZP
zona pellucida
ZPC
zone of preparatory calcification
Z-plasty
four-flap Z-p.
Z″ degree of contraction
Z-Sampler endometrial suction curette
Z-Scissors hysterectomy scissors
Z-score
BMI Z-s.
height velocity Z-s.
weight Z-s.
Z-shaped duodenum
ZstatFlu test
Z-stitch
Zuckerkandl organ
zuclopenthixol
ZUMI
Zinnanti uterine manipulator-injector
Zunich syndrome
Zuska disease
Zuspan regimen

Zwahlen syndrome
Zwanck pessary
Zyderm
Zydone
Zyflo
zygodactyly
zygoma
zygomatic
    z. arch
    z. bone
    z. head
    z. head of quadratus labii
        superioris muscle
zygomaticofrontal region
zygomaticomaxillary fracture
zygomycosis
zygopodium
zygosity

zygosyndactyly
zygote
    frozen z.
    z. intrafallopian transfer (ZIFT)
    two-cell z.
zygotene
    z. phase of meiosis
    z. stage
Zyklomat infusion pump
Zyloprim
zymase
zymogen
    coagulation factor z.
Zynergy Zolution catheter
Zyplast
Zyrtec syrup
ZZ male

NOTES

Appendix 1
Anatomical Illustrations

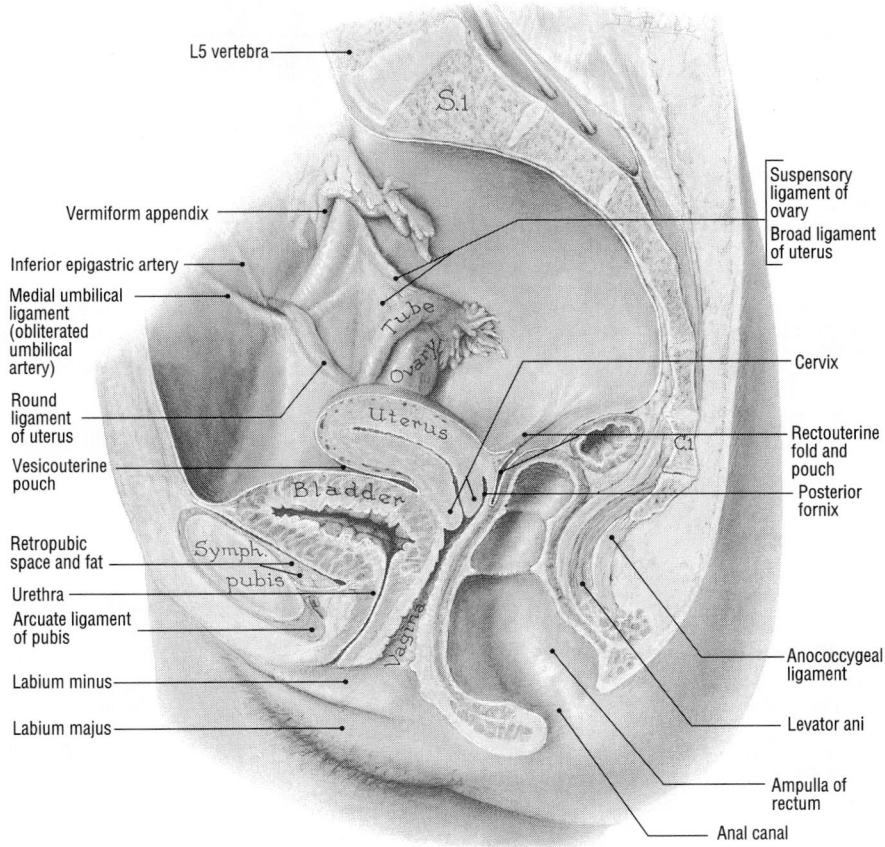

Figure 1. Female pelvis, median section.

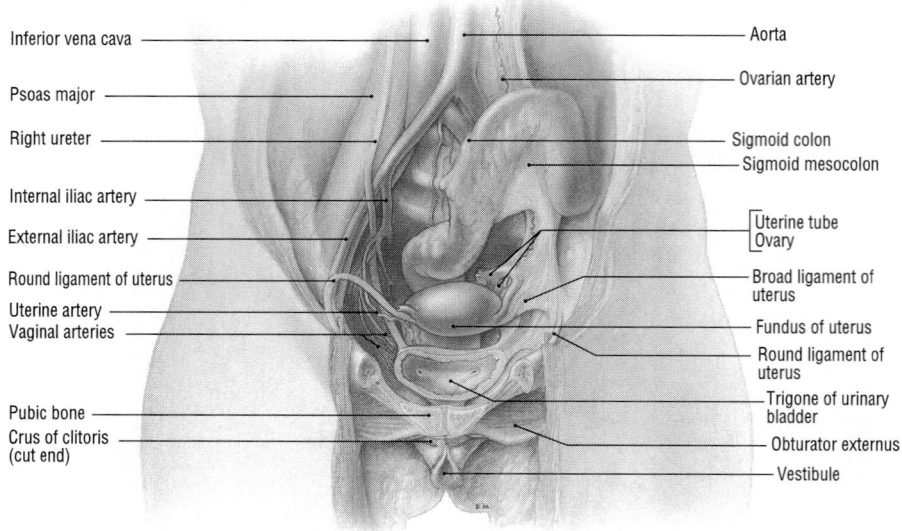

Figure 2. Female genital organs, anteroposterior view.

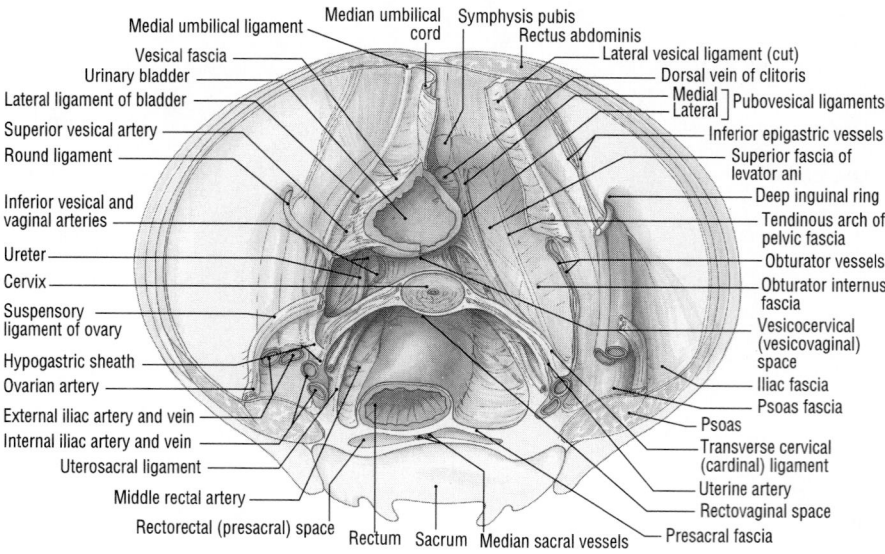

Figure 3. Pelvic fascia and the supporting mechanism of the cervix and upper vagina, superior view.

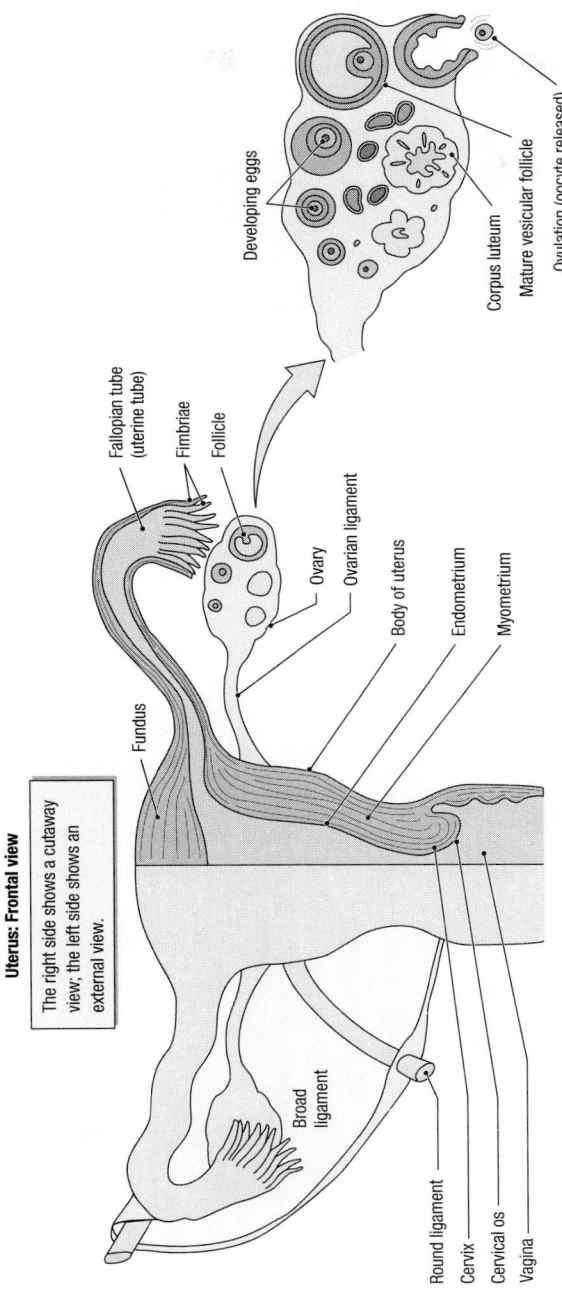

Uterus: Frontal view

The right side shows a cutaway view; the left side shows an external view.

Fallopian tube (uterine tube)

Fimbriae

Follicle

Fundus

Ovary

Ovarian ligament

Body of uterus

Endometrium

Myometrium

Broad ligament

Round ligament

Cervix

Cervical os

Vagina

Developing eggs

Corpus luteum

Mature vesicular follicle

Ovulation (oocyte released)

Figure 4. Female reproductive system.

Appendix 1

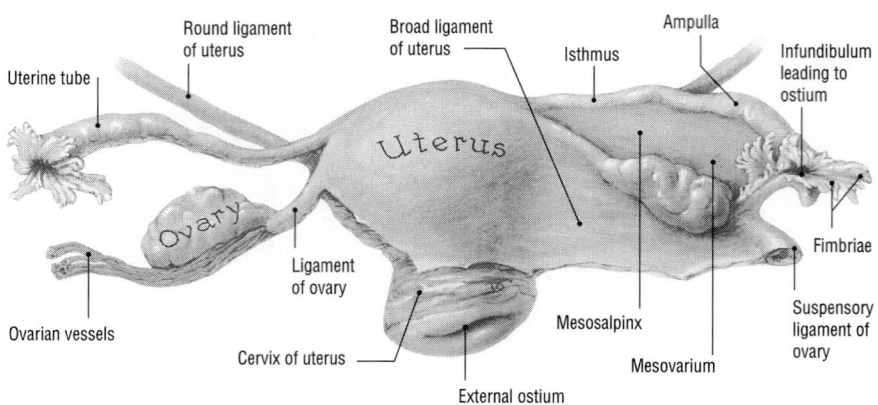

Figure 5. Uterus and adnexa, posterior view.

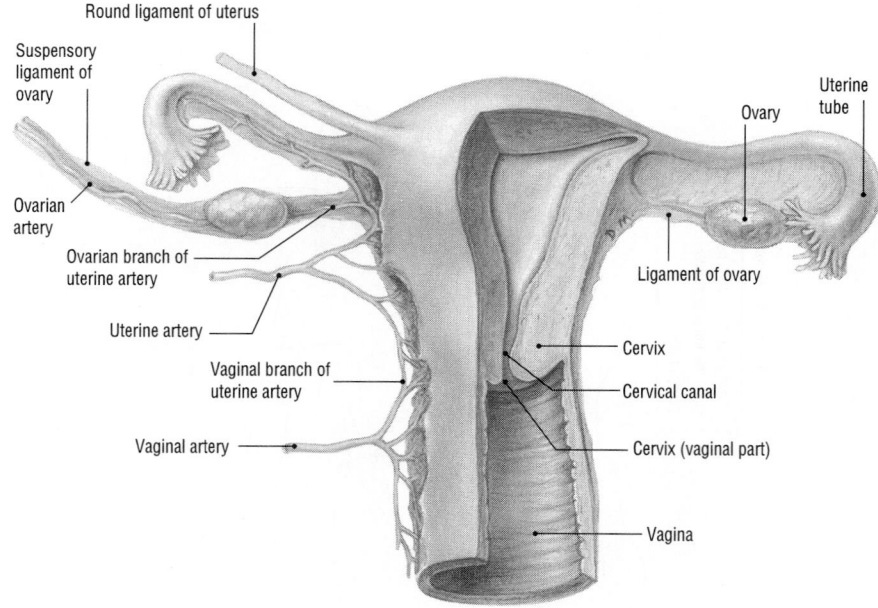

Figure 6. Blood supply to uterus and adnexa.

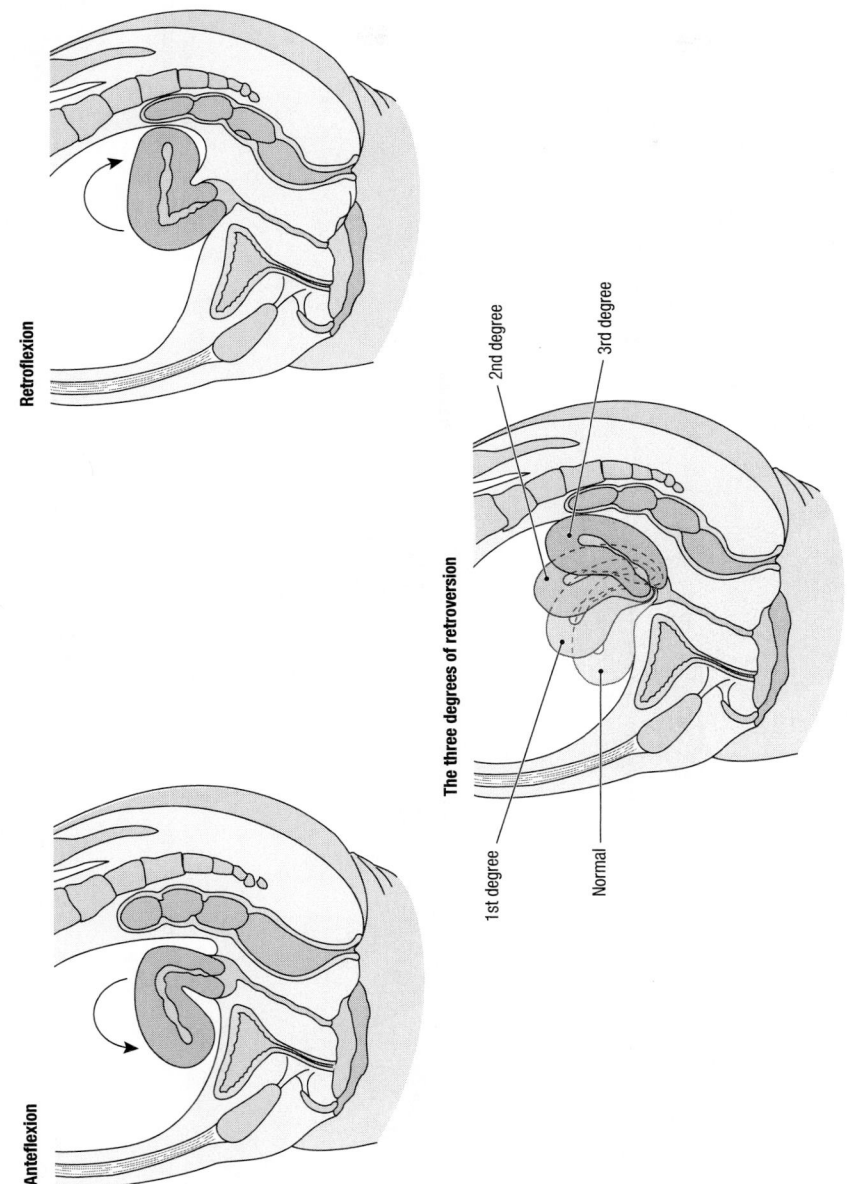

Figure 7. Displacements of the uterus.

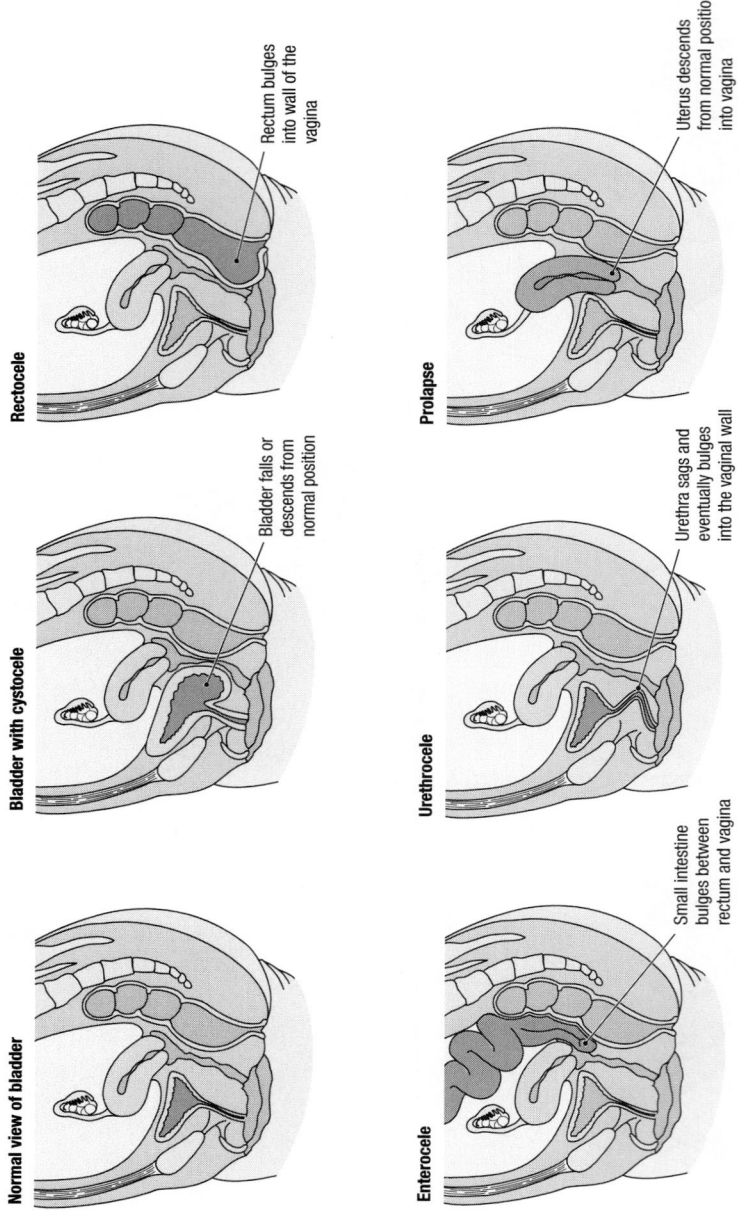

Figure 8. Pelvic floor relaxation.

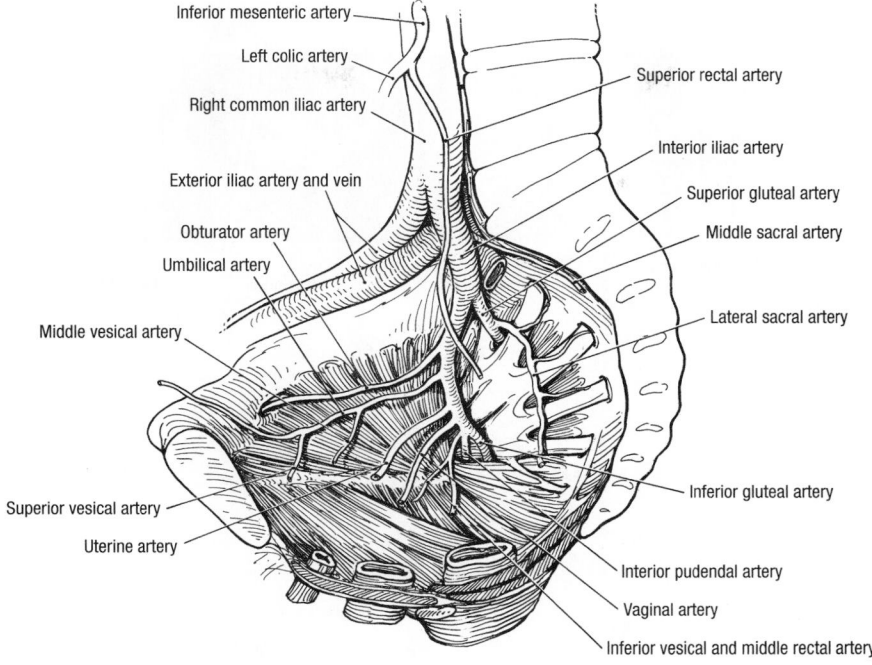

Figure 9. Pelvis, blood supply. Sagittal view of the pelvis with viscera removed, showing position of major arteries.

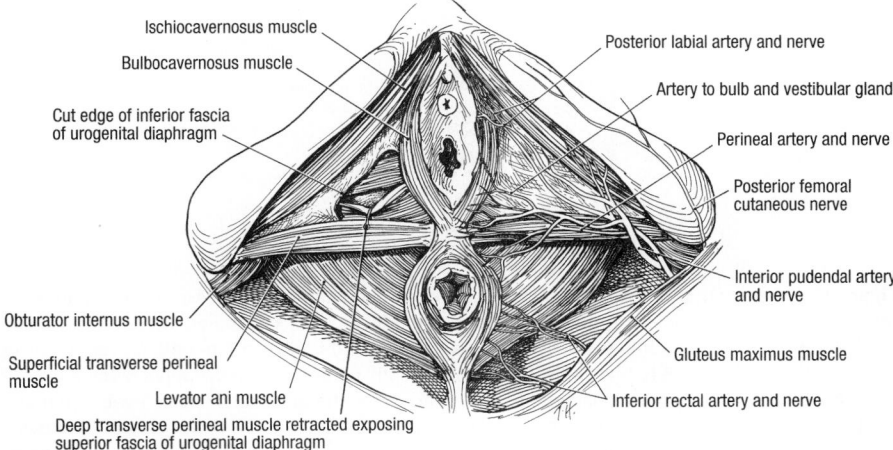

Figure 10. Perineum, superficial compartment. View from below of the superficial perineal compartment, displaying arteries, nerves, muscles and fascia of the urogenital diaphragm.

Appendix 1

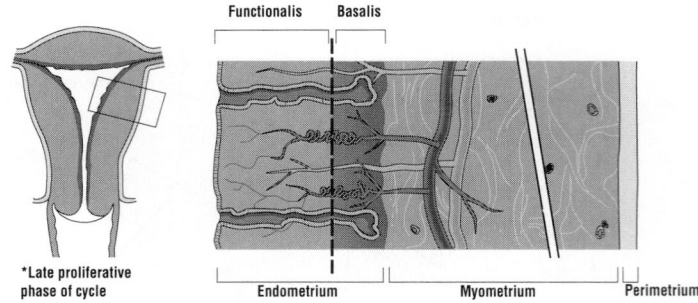

Figure 11.   Layers of uterus.

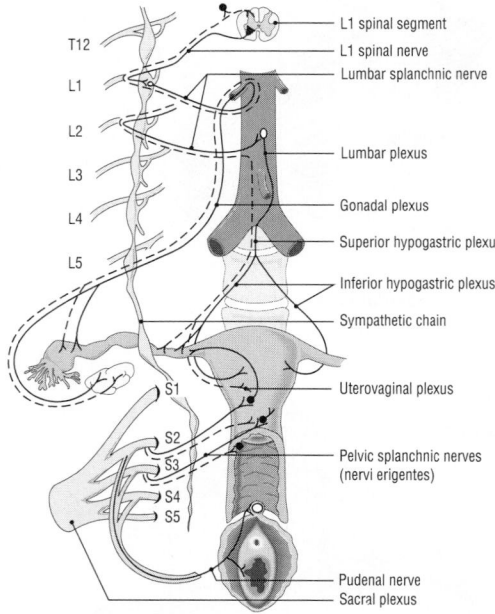

Figure 12.   Innervation of the female reproductive tract and genitalia. The sympathetic pathways arise from the lower thoracic and upper lumbar spinal levels (black triangle). There are no white rami below L2. These reach the aortic plexus via thoracic and lumbar splanchnic nerves. Synapse occurs in the aortic plexus (white circles). The postsynaptic neurons reach the pelvic viscera via hypogastric plexuses. The parasympathetic pathways arise from the midsacral spinal levels and reach the pelvic viscera via the splanchnic nerves. Synapse occurs in the walls of the viscera (white circles). Visceral afferent fibers (dashed) from the pelvic viscera travel specifically along either one or the other automatic pathways, have their cell bodies in the dorsal root ganglia, and produce specific patterns of referred pain. The pudendal nerve provides somatic innervation to and from the perineum.

A8

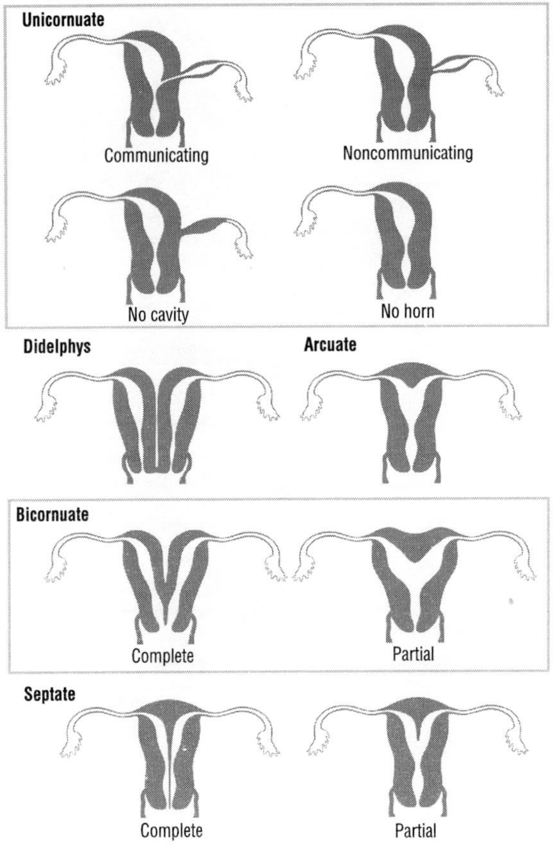

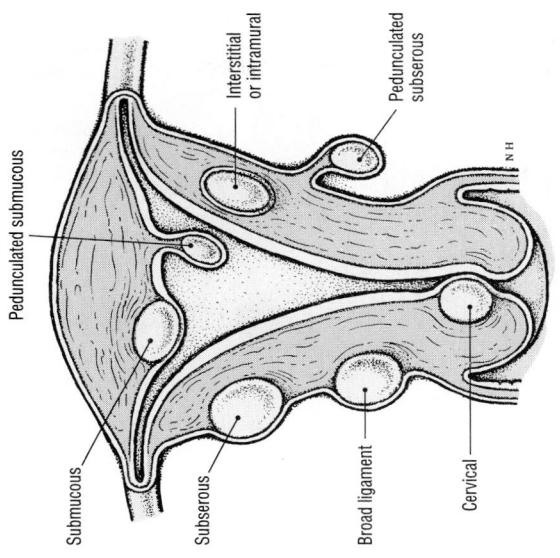

Figure 14. Location of fibroids.

Peducnulated submucous

Submucous

Subserous

Broad ligament

Cervical

Interstitial or intramural

Pedunculated subserous

Unicornuate

Communicating

Noncommunicating

No cavity

No horn

Arcuate

Didelphys

Bicornuate

Complete

Partial

Septate

Complete

Partial

Figure 13. Developmental anomalies of the uterus.

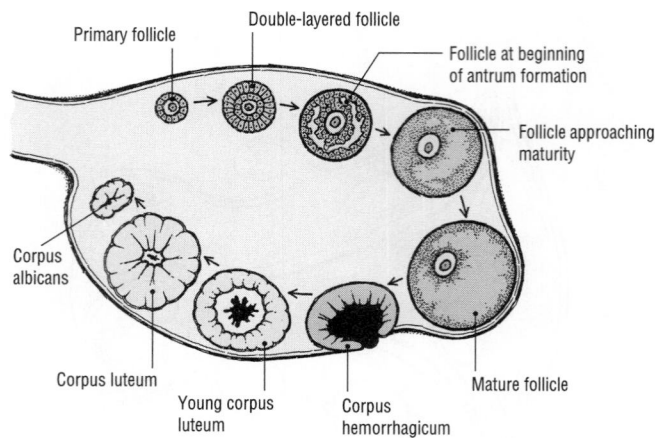

Figure 15. Ovulation.

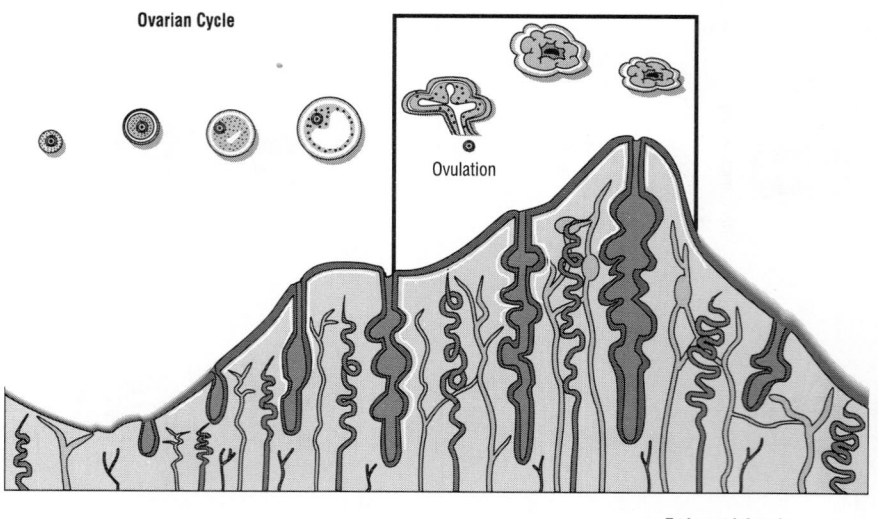

Figure 16. Menstrual cycle.

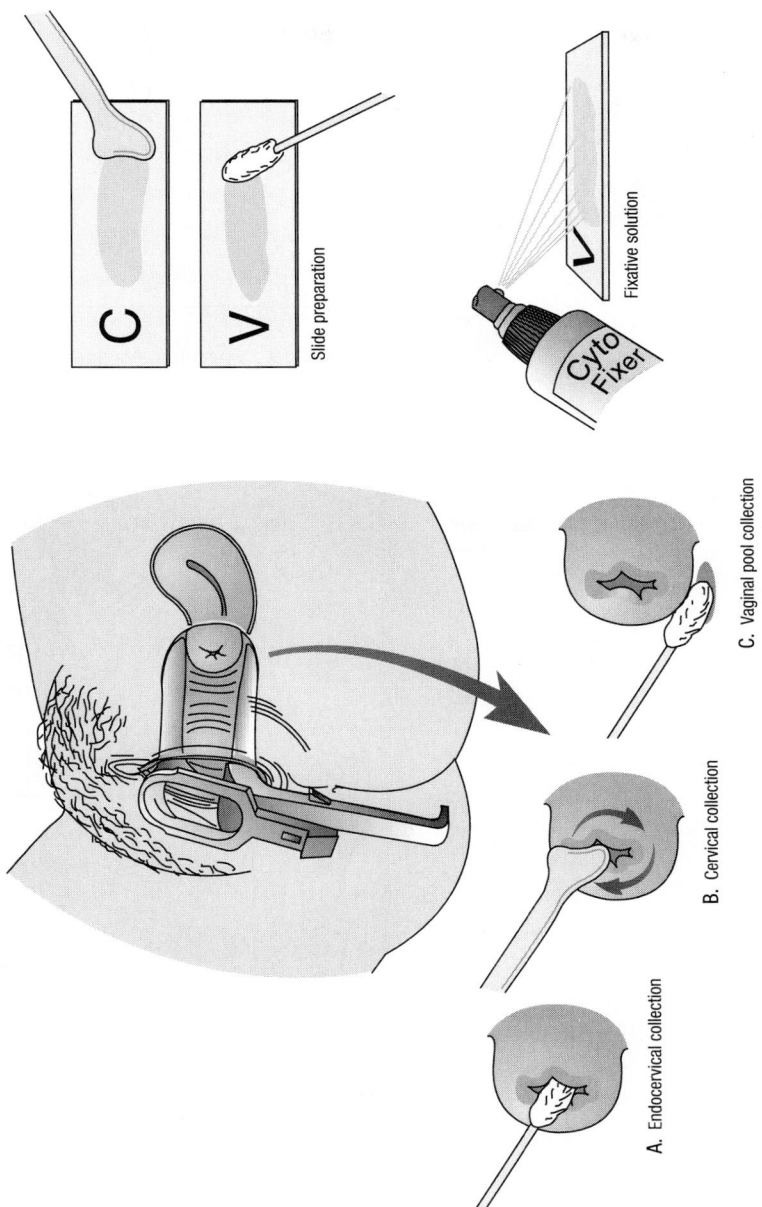

Slide preparation

C

V

Fixative solution

V

Cyto Fixer

A. Endocervical collection

B. Cervical collection

C. Vaginal pool collection

Figure 17. Obtaining a Pap smear. (A) Specimen taken from endocervix; (B) Specimen taken from cervix; (C) Specimen taken from vaginal pool.

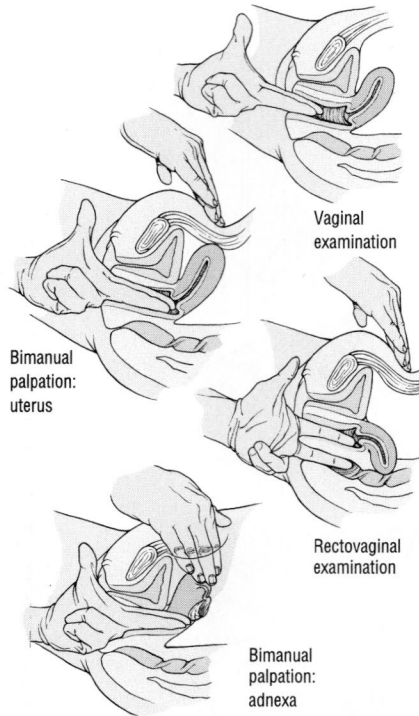

Figure 18. Pelvic examination.

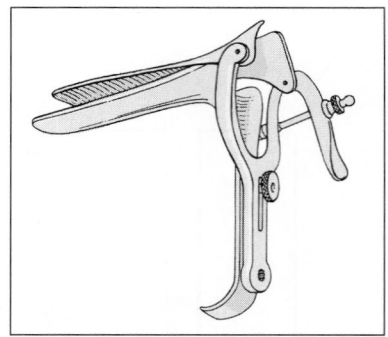

Figure 19. Speculum. Vaginal duckbill.

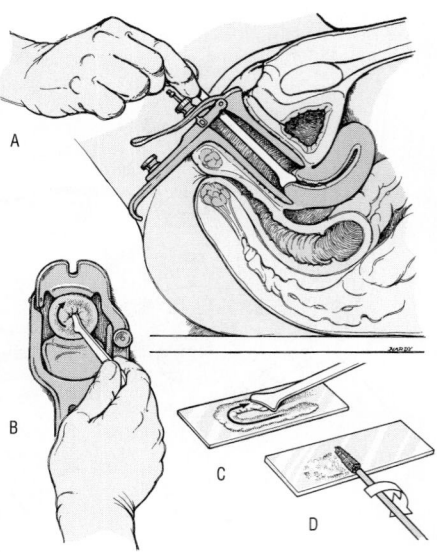

Figure 20. Pap smear. (A) Speculum in place and Ayre spatula in position at cervical os; (B) Tip of spatula placed in the cervical os and rotated 360 degrees; (C) Cellular material clinging to spatula is then smeared smoothly on glass slide, which is promptly placed in fixative solution; (D) Cytobrush is rotated in cervical os and rolled onto glass slide.

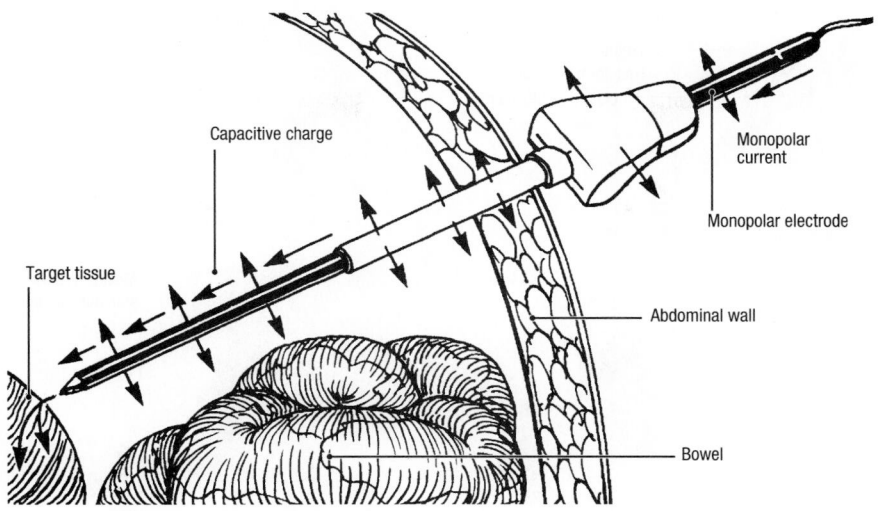

Figure 21. Laparoscopy, current diversion, step 1. The activated unipolar laparoscopic electrode develops a surrounding electromagnetic charge, capable of completing the circuit in a nearby conductor.

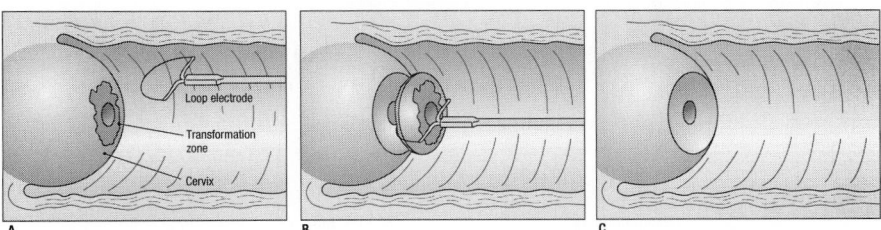

Figure 22. Loop electrosurgical excision procedure (LEEP) or large loop excision of the transformation zone (LLETZ). (A) electrode approach; (B) Removal of transformation zone; (C) Excision site (region between endocervix and ectocervix).

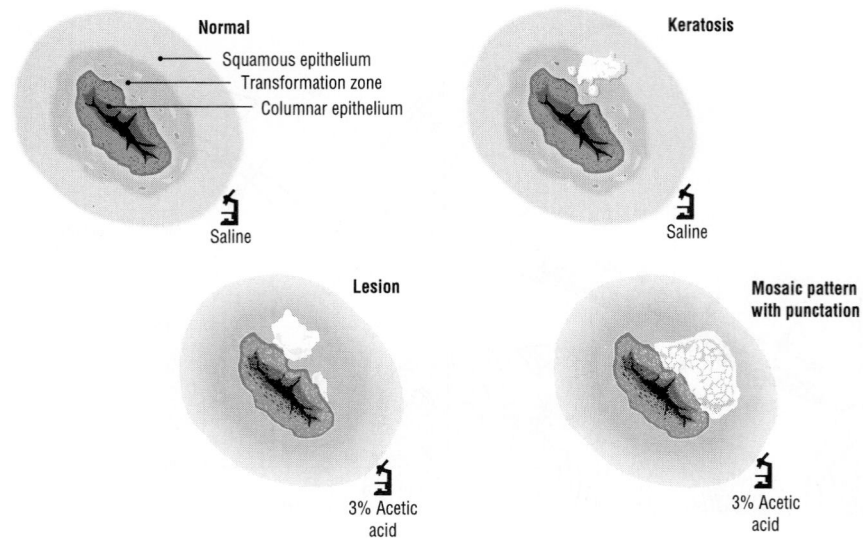

Figure 23. Colposcopy findings.

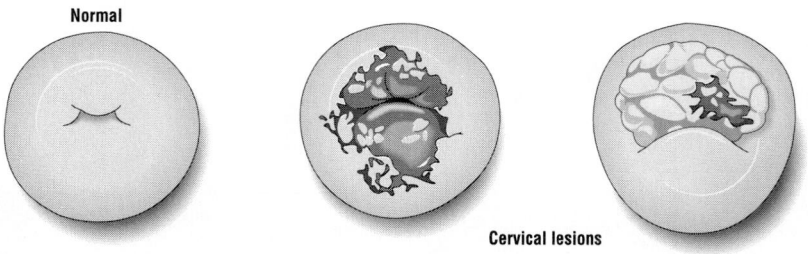

Figure 24. Cervical lesions.

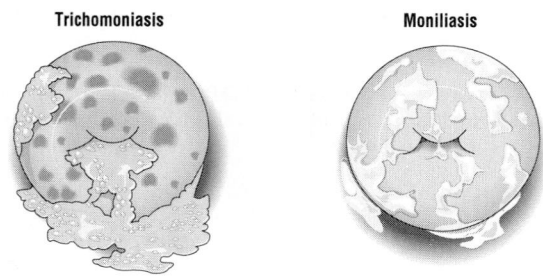

Figure 25. Vaginitis.

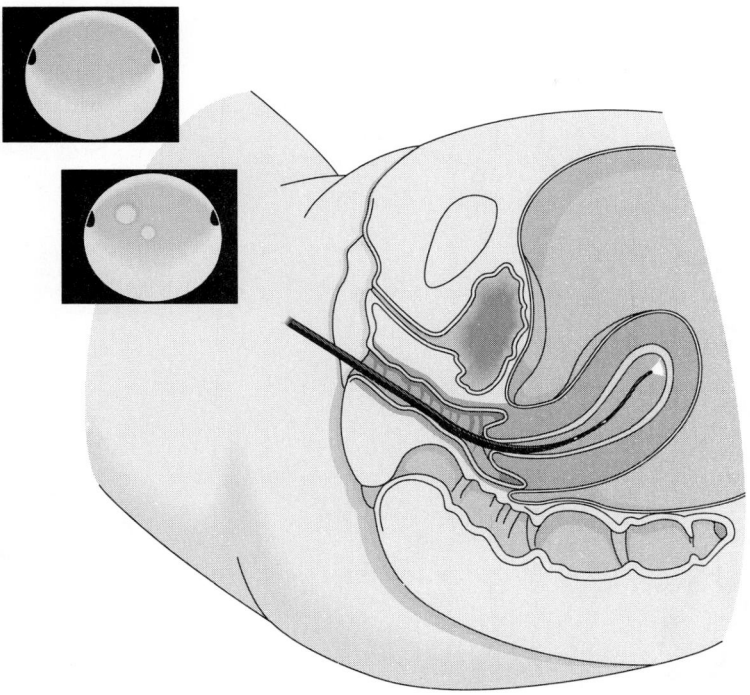

Figure 26. Hysteroscopy.

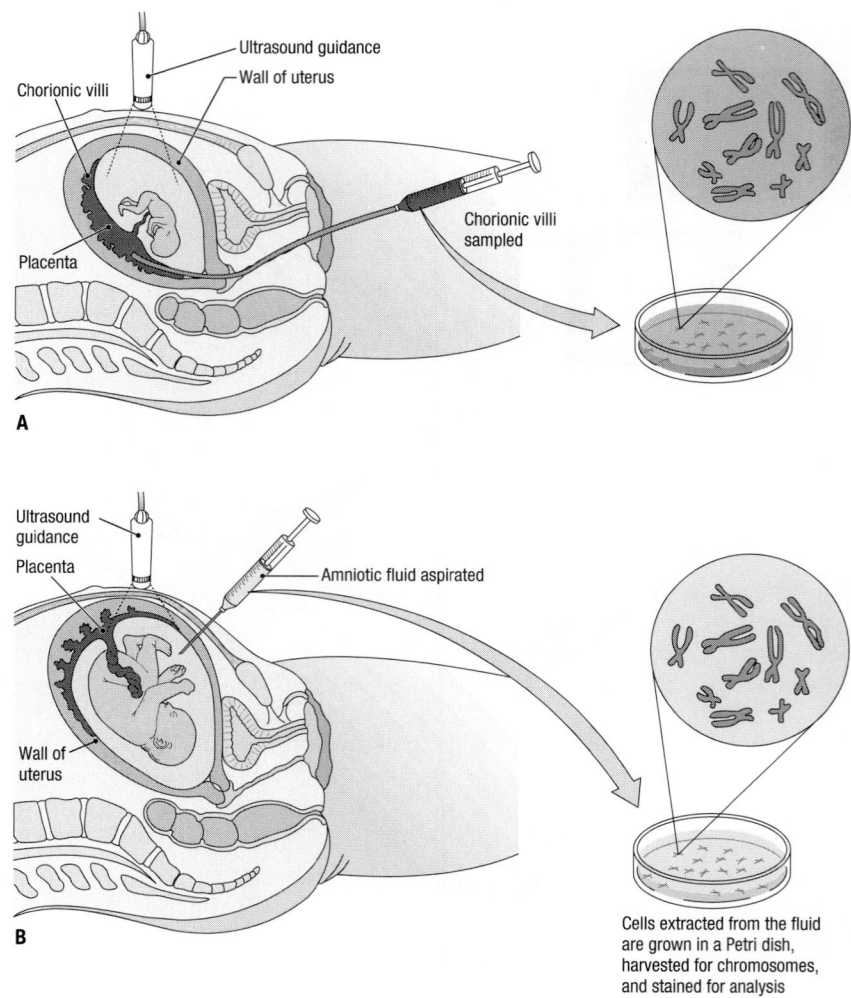

Figure 27. (A) Chorionic villus sampling (9 to 11 weeks); (B) Amniocentesis (15 to 18 weeks).

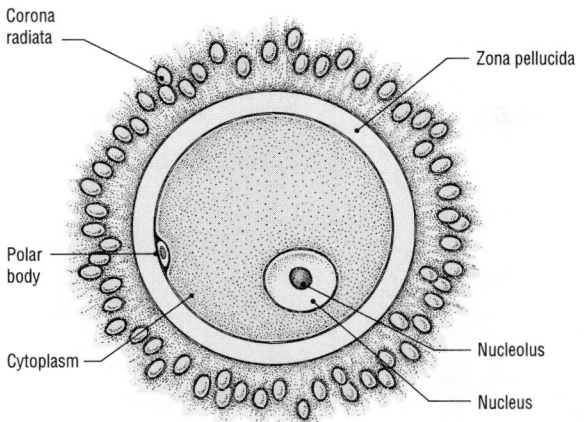

Figure 28. Mature oocyte (ovum).

Figure 29. Morula.

Figure 30. Blastula, hemisected.

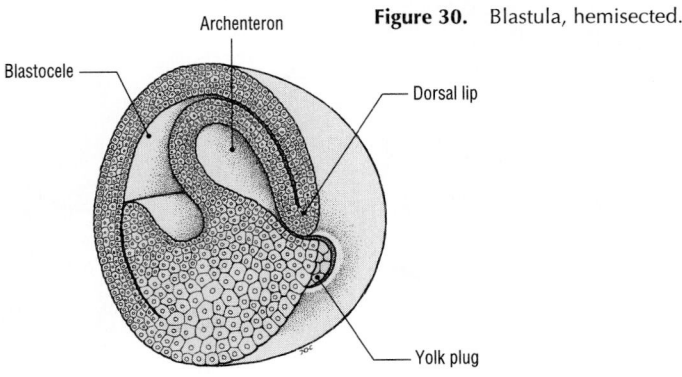

Figure 31. Gastrula.

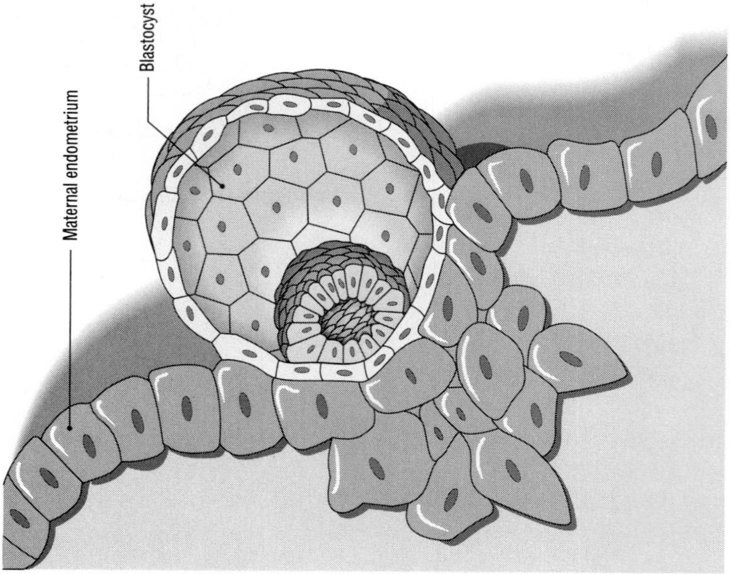

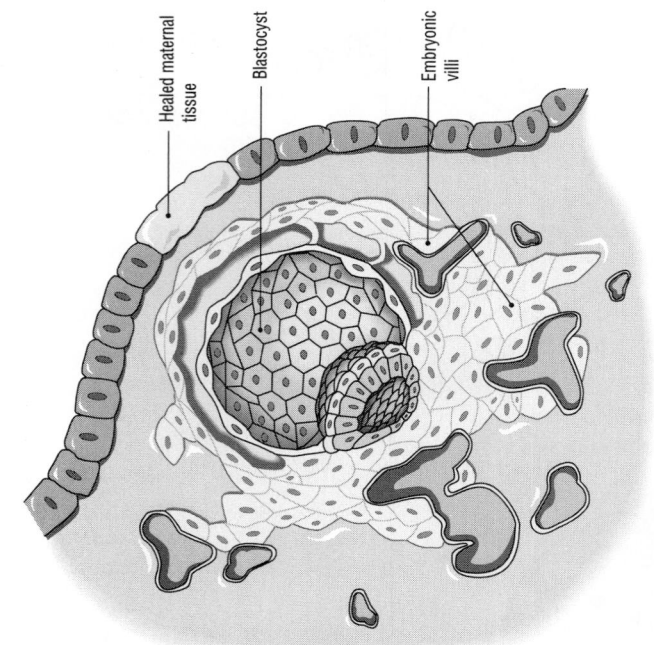

Figure 33. Second state of implantation.

Healed maternal tissue

Blastocyst

Embryonic villi

Maternal endometrium

Blastocyst

Figure 32. First stage of implantation.

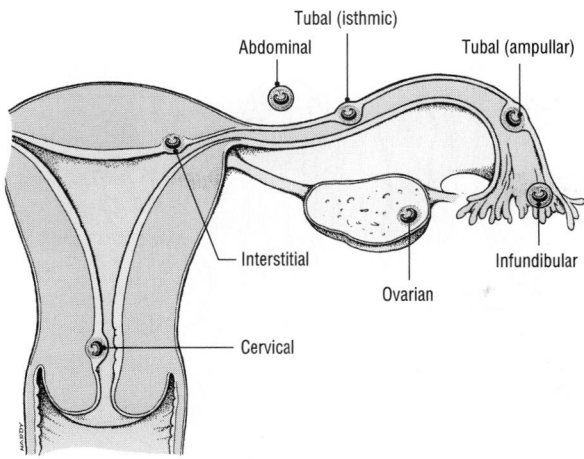

Figure 34. Sites of ectopic pregnancy.

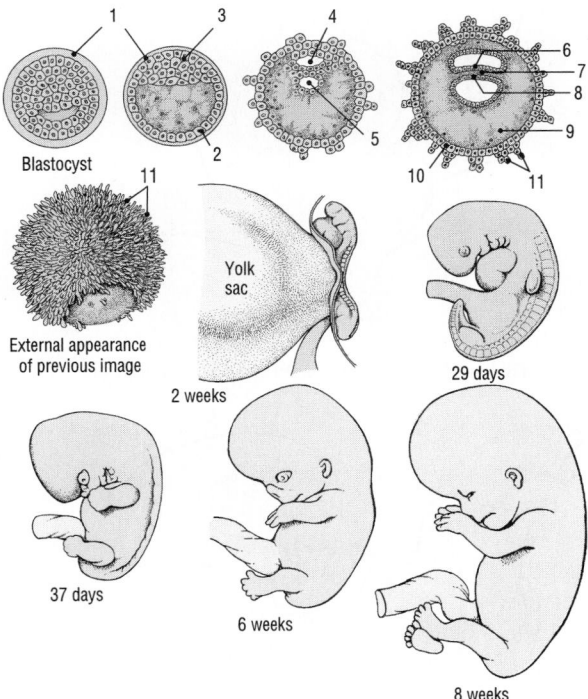

Figure 35. Development; from blastocyst to fetus. (1) zona pellucida; (2) trophectoderm; (3) inner cell mass; (4) amniotic cavity; (5) yolk sac; (6) ectoderm; (7) mesoderm; (8) entoderm; (9) mesoderm; (10) trophectoderm; (11) chorionic villi.

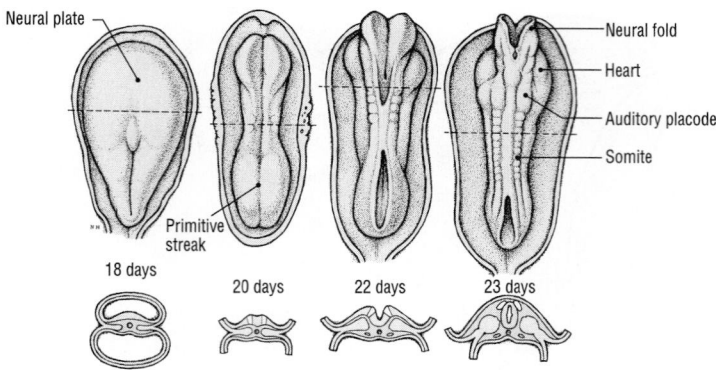

Figure 36. Blastoderm. Top, dorsal views. Bottom, cross-sectional views.

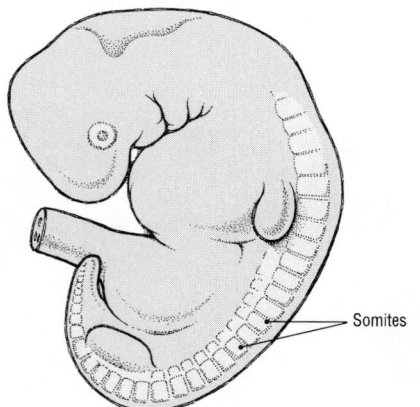

Figure 37. Somites in a 29-day human embryo.

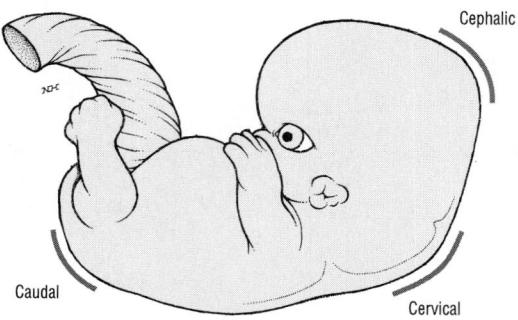

Figure 38. Flexures seen in a 6-week-old embryo.

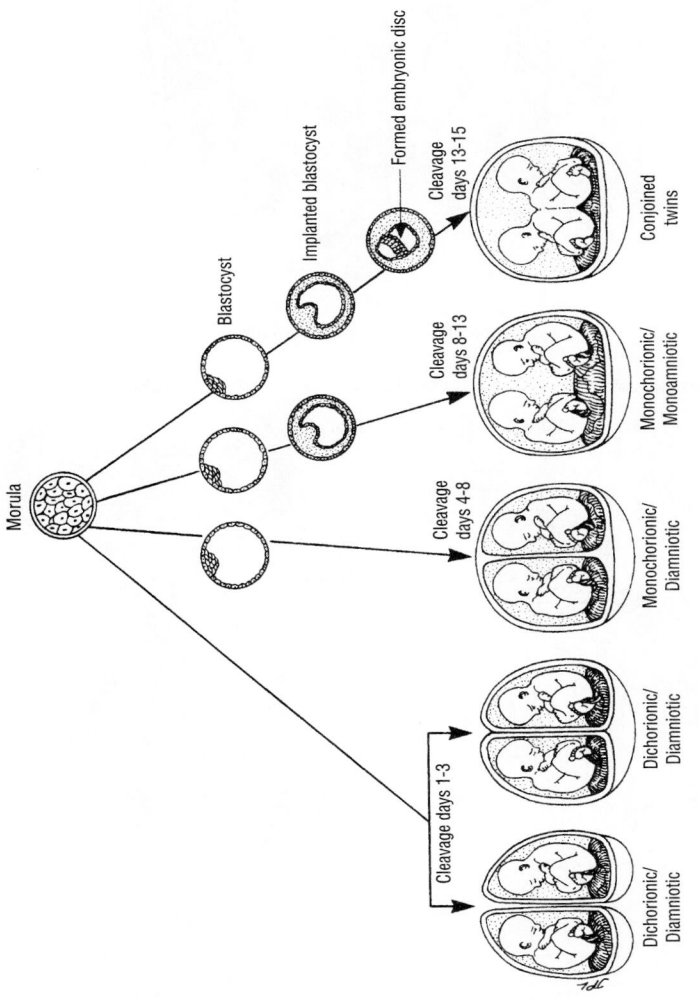

Figure 39. Genesis of identical (monozygotic) twins.

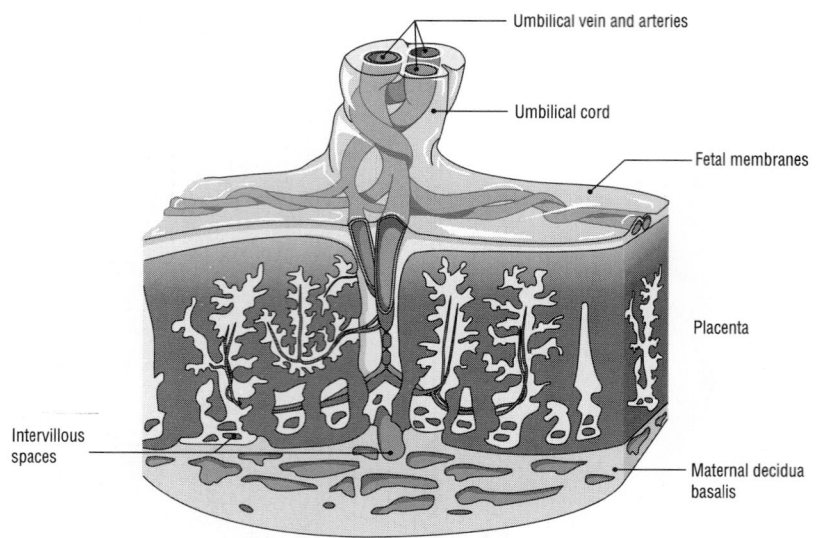

Figure 40. Placental circulation.

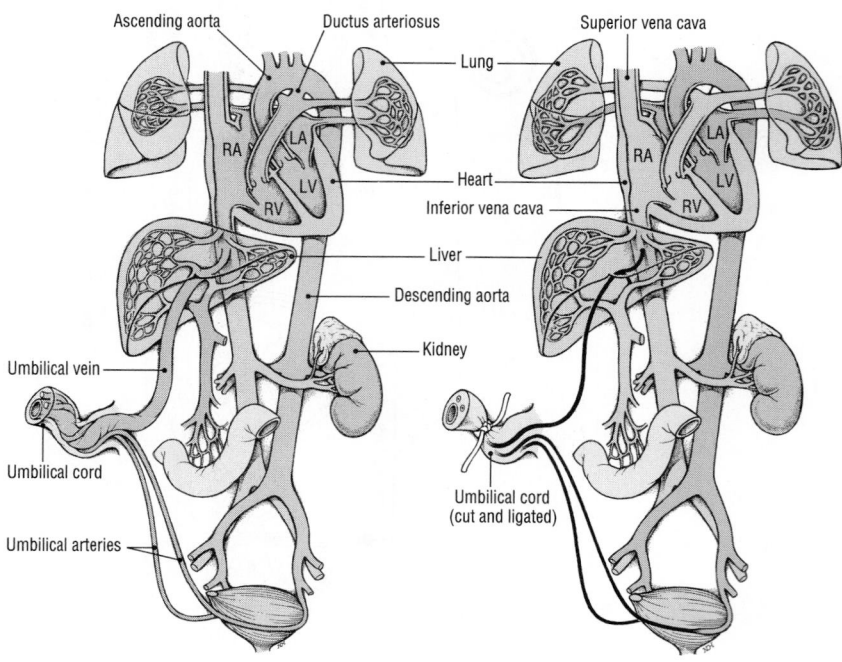

Figure 41. Fetal circulation. Left, during pregnancy, oxygen diffuses from the maternal circulation to the fetal circulation in the placenta; oxygenated blood returns to the fetus through the umbilical vein. Right, after birth, umbilical cord is cut and blood is oxygenated as it passes through the lungs. RA indicates right atrium; LA, left atrium; LV, left ventricle; and RV, right ventricle.

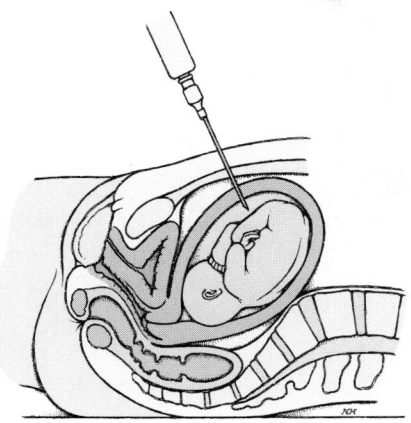

Figure 42. Amniocentesis.

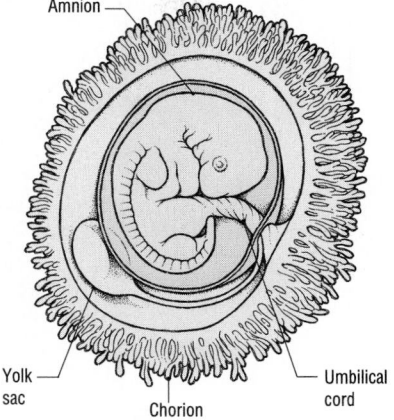

Figure 43. Amnion and related structures showing 5-week embryo.

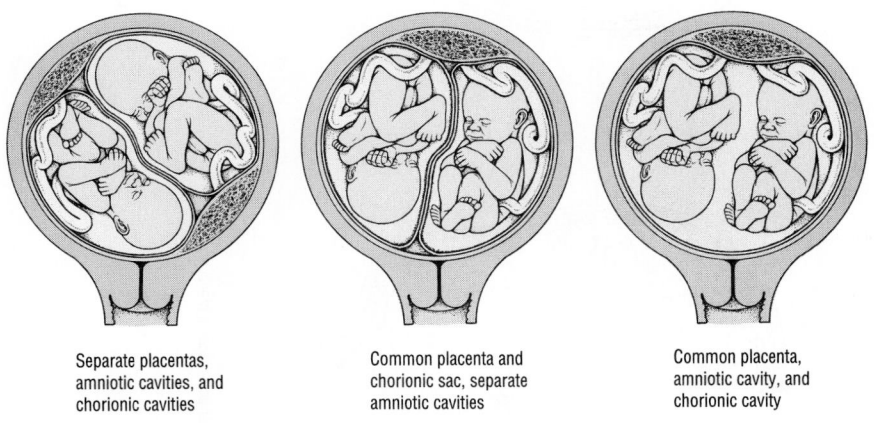

Separate placentas, amniotic cavities, and chorionic cavities

Common placenta and chorionic sac, separate amniotic cavities

Common placenta, amniotic cavity, and chorionic cavity

Figure 44. Twins. Schematic diagrams showing the possible relations of the fetal membranes in monozygotic twins.

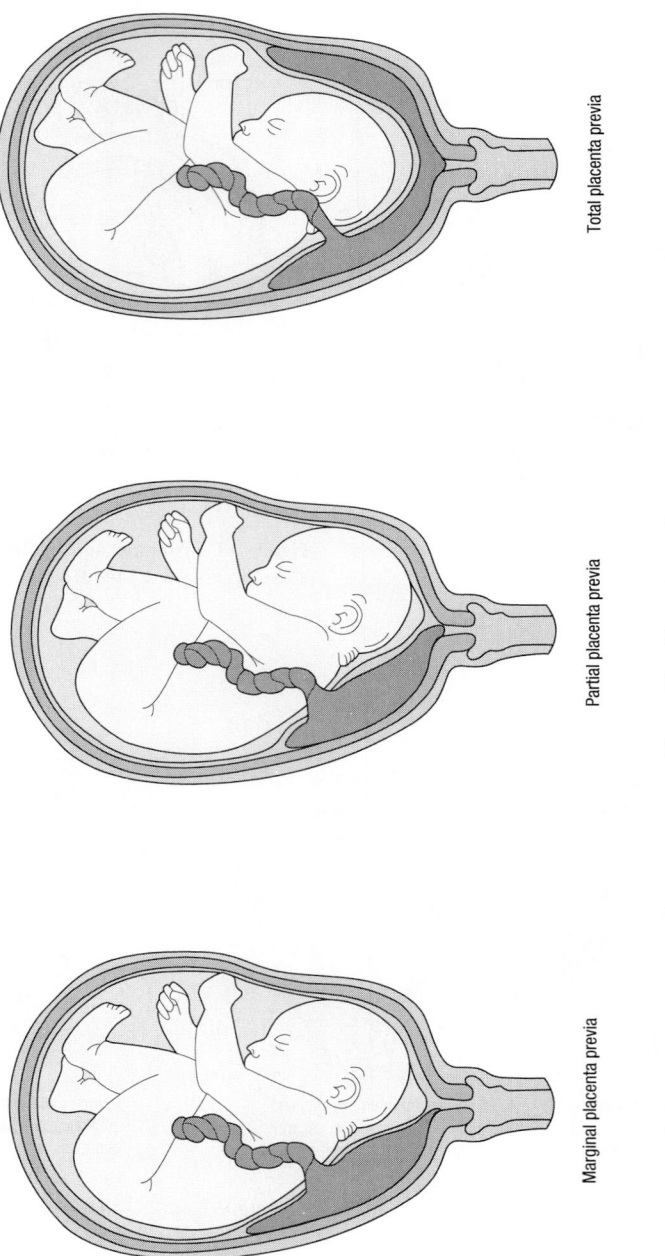

Total placenta previa

Partial placenta previa

Marginal placenta previa

Figure 45. Placenta previa.

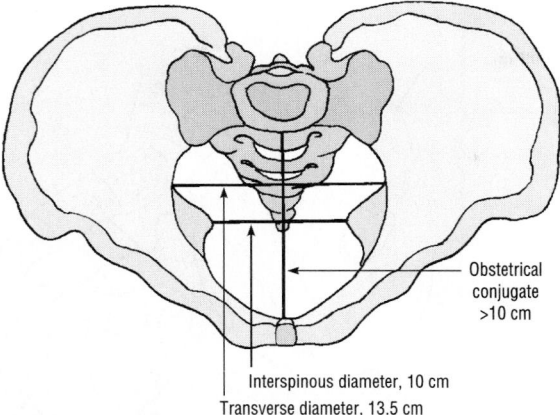

Figure 46. Pelvic diameters. Superior view of female pelvis, indicating normal distances between structures.

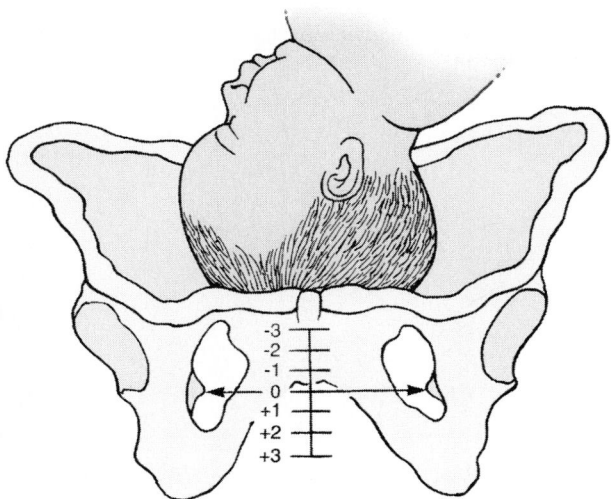

Figure 47. Presentation, vertex, station estimation. Estimation of station by traditional three-station system. Station is estimated by palpation of the bony segment of the presenting part during a vaginal examination and determining the distance from the plane of the ischial spines.

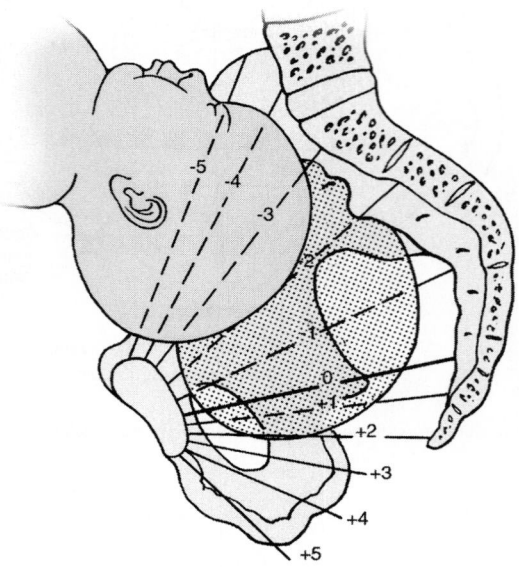

Figure 48. Presentation, vertex, station estimation. Illustration shows the estimation of station by current ACOG centimeter system.

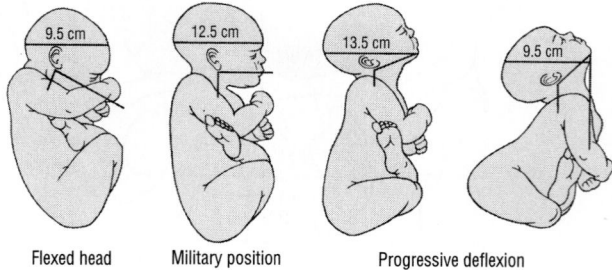

Flexed head   Military position   Progressive deflexion

Figure 49. Presentation, breech, cranial diameters. Importance of cranial flexion is emphasized by noting the increased diameters presented to the birth canal with progressive deflexion.

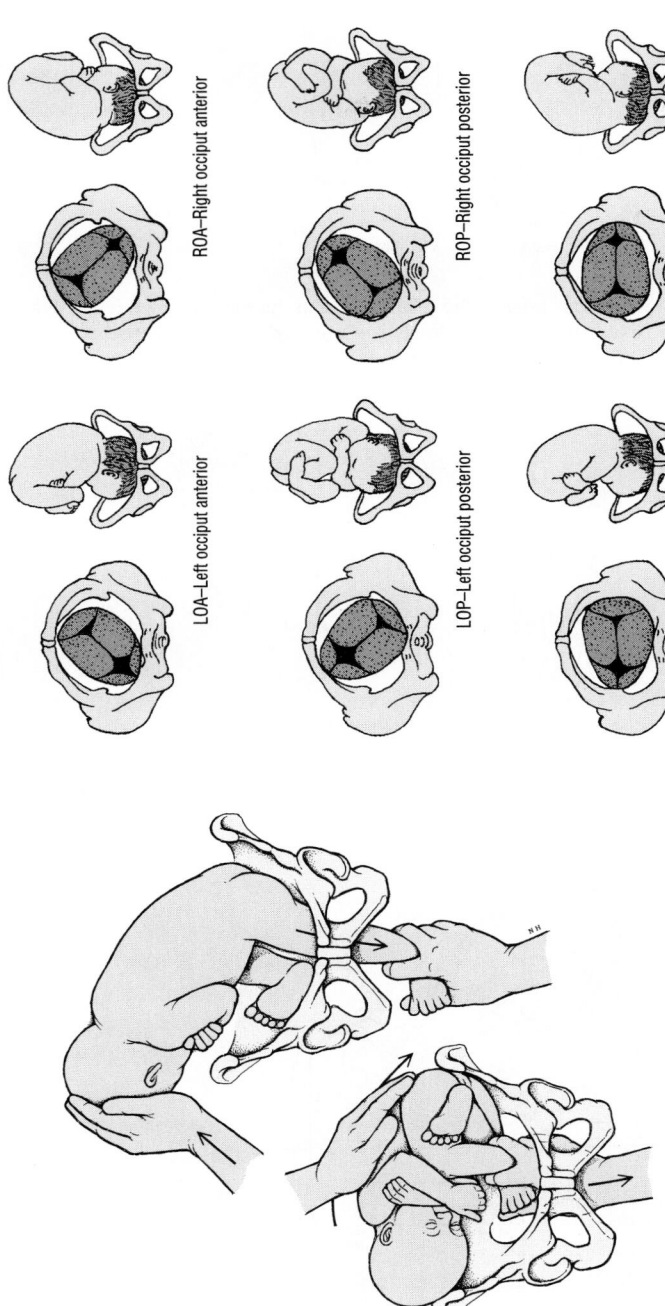

ROA–Right occiput anterior

ROP–Right occiput posterior

ROT–Right occiput transverse

LOA–Left occiput anterior

LOP–Left occiput posterior

LOT–Left occiput transverse

Figure 51. Vertex presentation. Fetal head positions within the pelvic girdle in a vertex presentation.

Figure 50. Internal podalic version. Conversion from dorsoposterior transverse lie to breech. Left, obstetrician's right hand grasps fetal foot within uterus while left hand applies pressure externally to rotate breech toward pelvic inlet. Right, obstetrician maneuvers fetus into longitudinal orientation by applying traction to foot while externally directing head into fundus, so that delivery can proceed as in breech presentation.

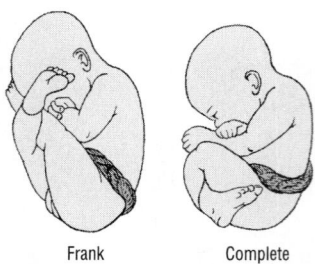

Frank   Complete

Figure 52. Full breech presentations refer to the relationships at the hip and knee joints. Frank breech: both hip joints are flexed, and both knee joints are extended. Complete breech: both hip joints and knee joints are flexed.

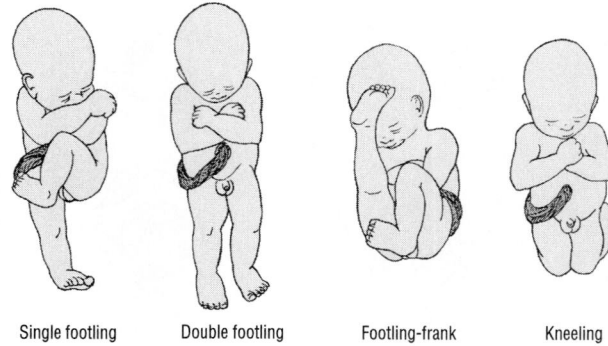

Single footling   Double footling   Footling-frank   Kneeling

Figure 53. Varieties of incomplete breech presentations refer to incomplete flexion at either the hip or knee joints.

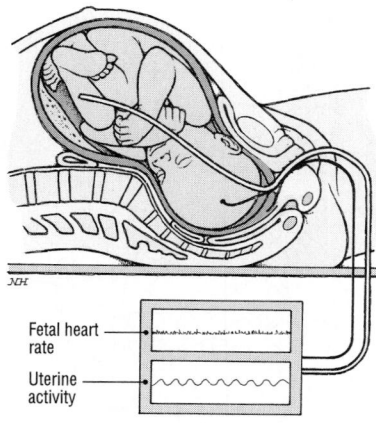

Fetal heart rate

Uterine activity

Figure 54. Electronic fetal monitoring.

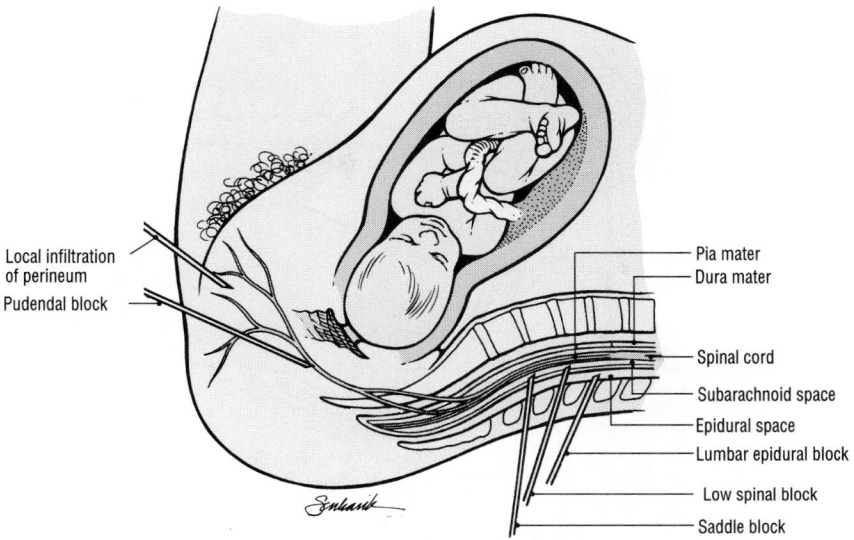

Local infiltration of perineum

Pudendal block

Pia mater
Dura mater

Spinal cord
Subarachnoid space
Epidural space
Lumbar epidural block
Low spinal block
Saddle block

Figure 55. Regional anesthesia for childbirth. Sites of injection.

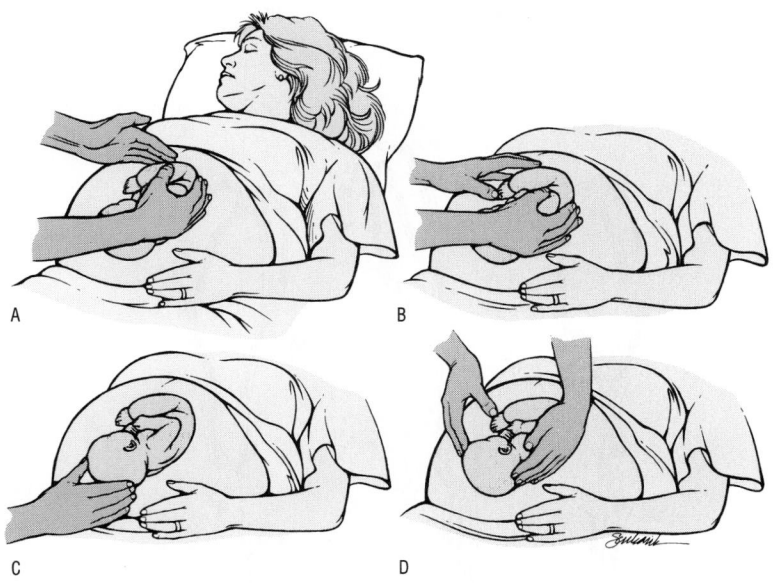

A

B

C

D

Figure 56. Leopold maneuvers. (A) First maneuver, palpate superior surface of fundus; (B) Second maneuver, palpate sides of uterus to determine which direction fetal back is facing; (C) Third maneuver, palpate to discover what is at inlet of pelvis; (D) Fourth maneuver, assuming fetus has been found to be in cephalic presentation, fetal attitude should then be determined (degree of flexion).

A29

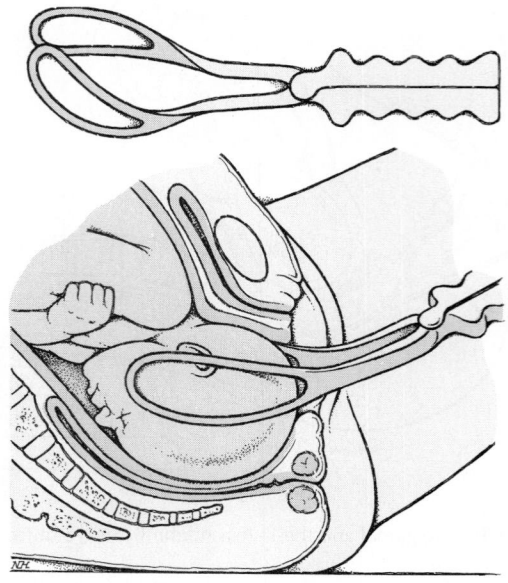

Figure 57. Obstetrical forceps.

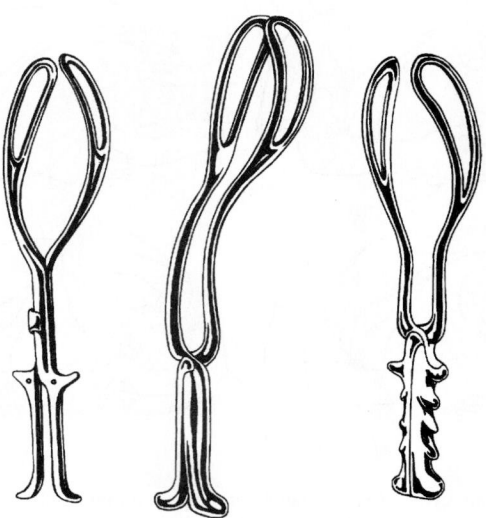

Figure 58. Obstetrical forceps. Left, Kjelland. Middle, Piper. Right, Simpson.

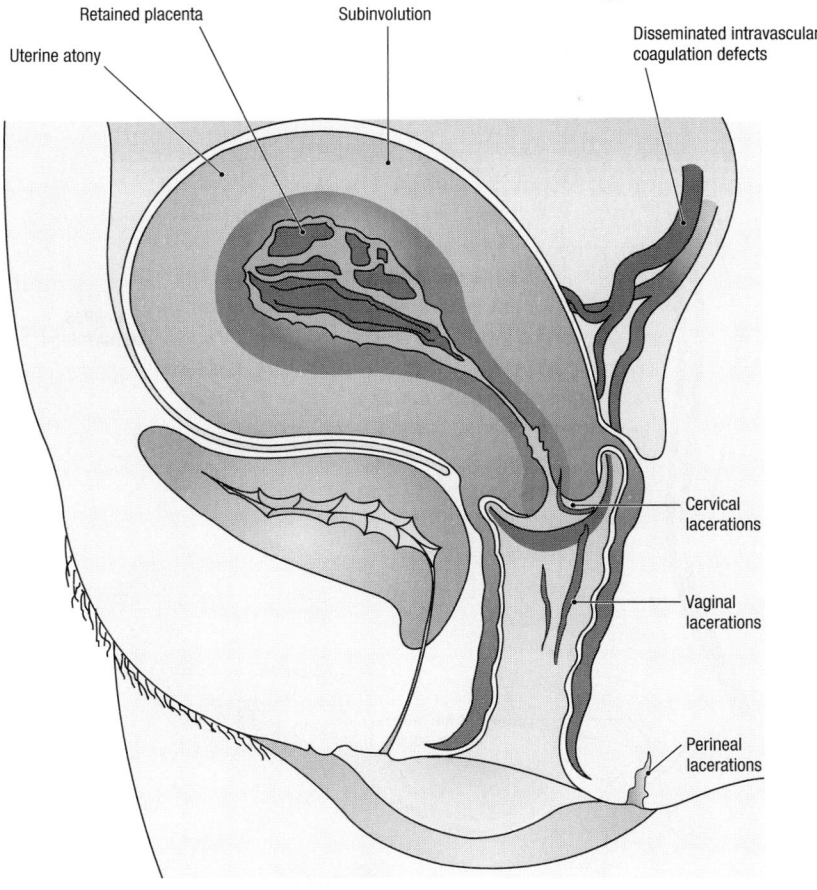

Uterine atony

Retained placenta

Subinvolution

Disseminated intravascular coagulation defects

Cervical lacerations

Vaginal lacerations

Perineal lacerations

Figure 59.   Common causes of postpartum hemorrhage.

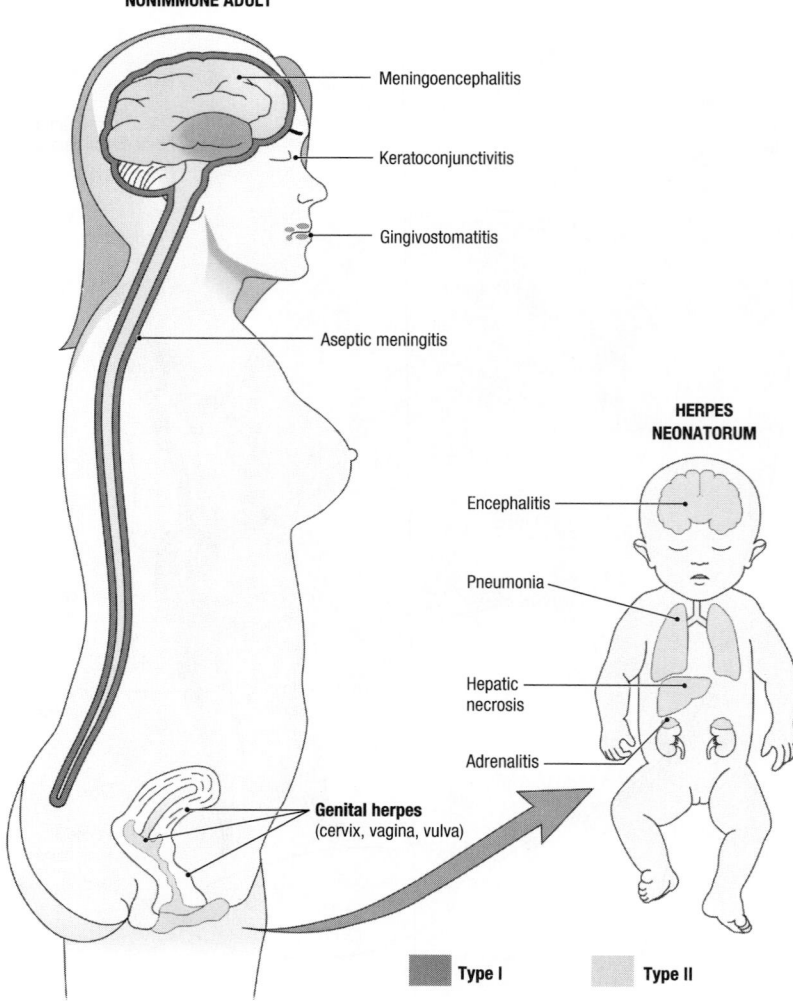

Figure 60. Herpesvirus infections. Herpes simplex virus type 1 infects a nonimmune adult, causing gingivostomatitis ("fever blister" or "cold sore"), keratoconjunctivitis, meningoencephalitis, and aseptic spinal meningitis. Herpes simplex virus type 2 infects the genitalia of a nonimmune adult, involving the cervix, vagina, and vulva. Herpes simplex virus type 2 infects the fetus as it passes through the birth canal of an infected mother. The infant's lack of a mature immune system results in disseminated infection with herpes simplex virus type 1. The infection is often fatal, involving lung, liver, adrenal glands, and central nervous system.

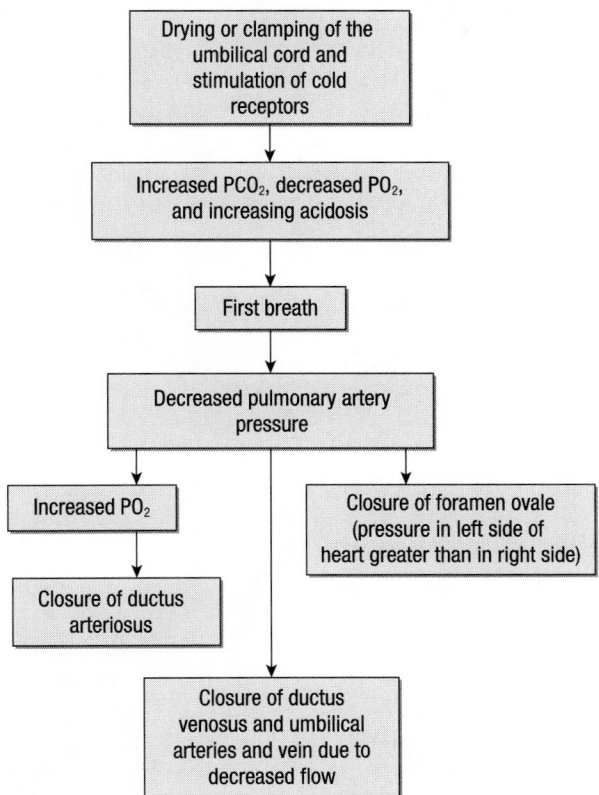

Figure 61. Circulatory events at birth.

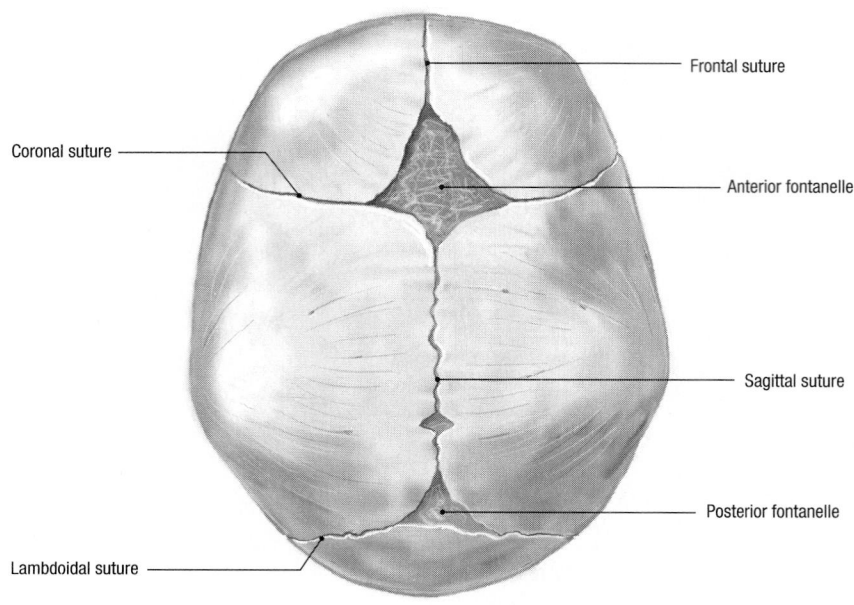

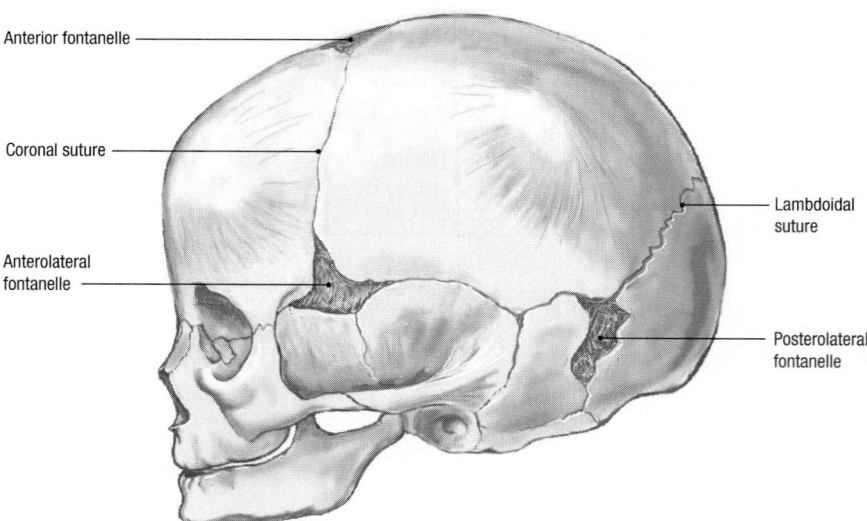

Figure 62. Newborn skull. Top, Superior view. Bottom, Lateral view.

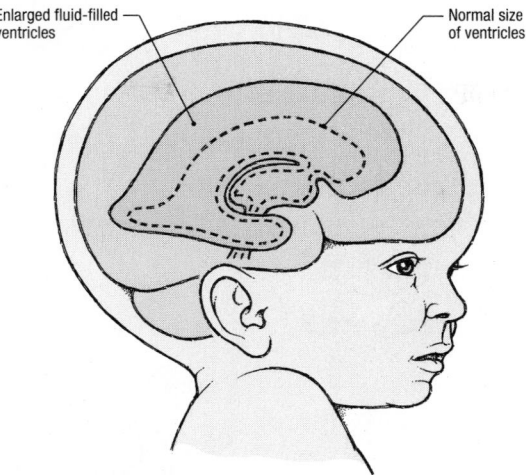

Enlarged fluid-filled ventricles

Normal size of ventricles

Figure 63. Hydrocephalus.

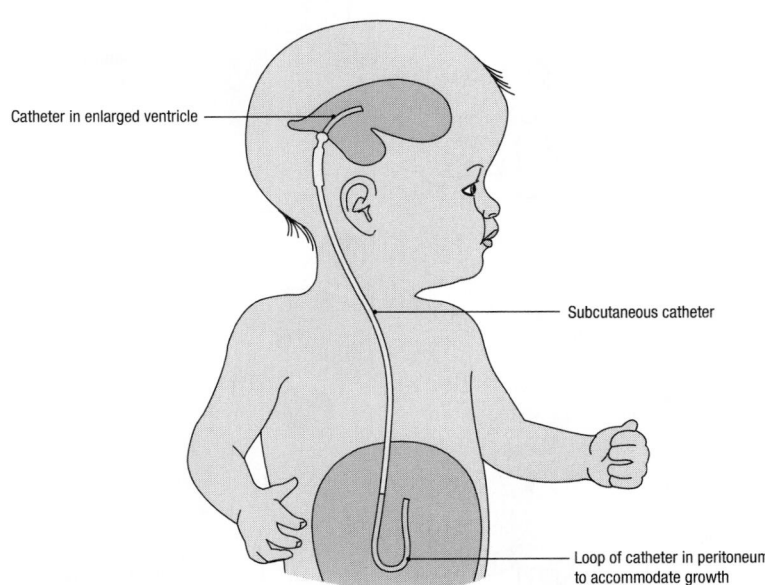

Catheter in enlarged ventricle

Subcutaneous catheter

Loop of catheter in peritoneum to accommodate growth

Figure 64. Image of infant with ventriculoperitoneal shunt in place. The shunt removes excess cerebrospinal fluid from the ventricles and shunts it to the peritoneum. A one-way valve is present in the tubing behind the ear.

A35

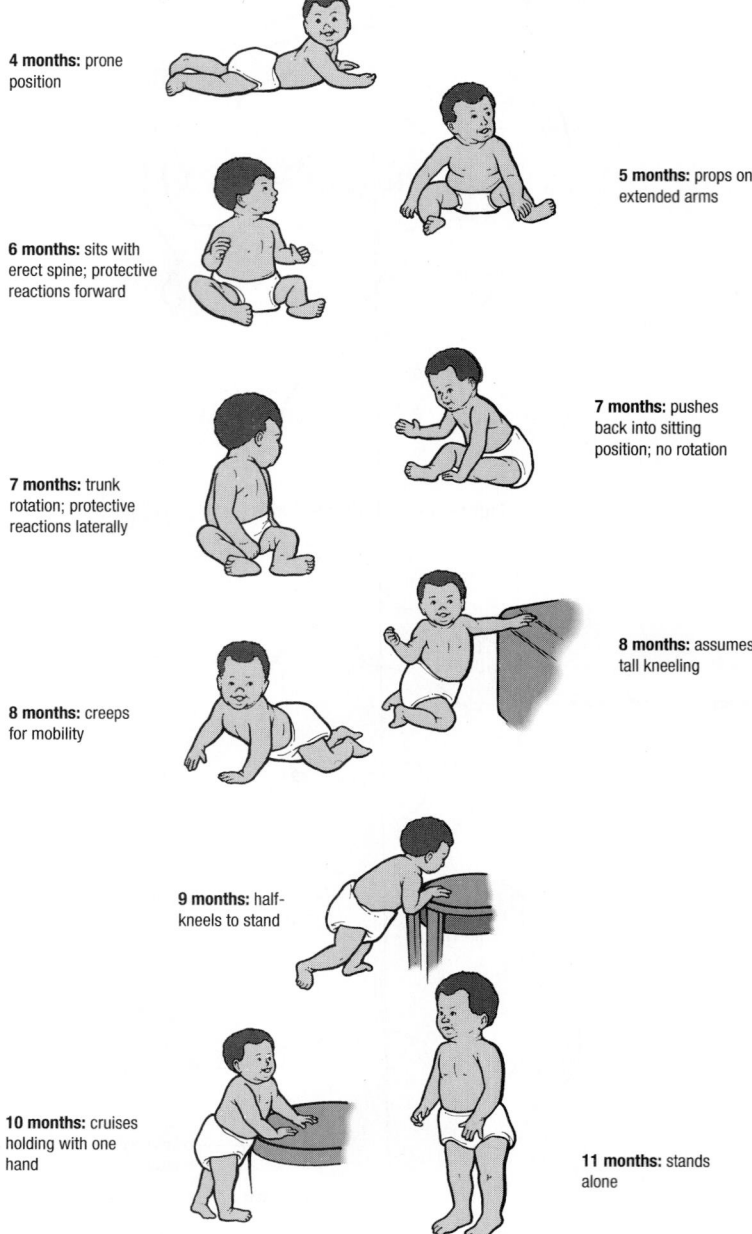

4 months: prone position

5 months: props on extended arms

6 months: sits with erect spine; protective reactions forward

7 months: pushes back into sitting position; no rotation

7 months: trunk rotation; protective reactions laterally

8 months: assumes tall kneeling

8 months: creeps for mobility

9 months: half-kneels to stand

10 months: cruises holding with one hand

11 months: stands alone

Figure 65. Developmental milestones.

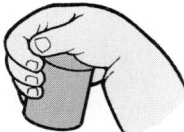

5 months: palmar grasp: fingers on top surface of object press it into center of palm; thumb abducted

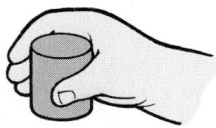

6 months: radial-palmar grasp: fingers on far side of object press it against opposed thumb and radial side of palm

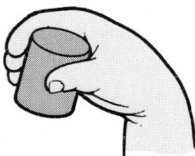

7 months: inferior-scissors grasp: raking into palm with abducted, totally flexed thumb and all flexed fingers, **or** raking object into palm with abducted, totally flexed thumb and 2 partly extended fingers

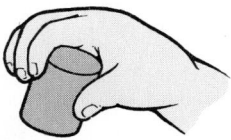

7 months: radial-palmar grasp: wrist straight

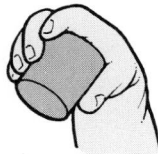

8 months: scissors grasp: between thumb and side of curled index finger, distal thumb joint slightly flexed; proximal thumb joint extended

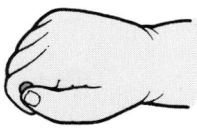

8 months: radial-digital grasp: object held with opposed thumb and fingertips, space visible between

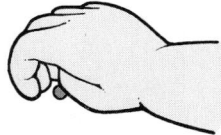

9 months: inferior-pincer grasp: between ventral surfaces of thumb and index finger, distal thumb joint extended; beginning thumb opposition

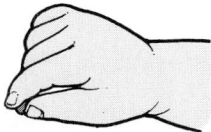

9 months: radial-digital grasp: wrist extended

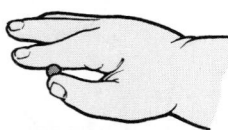

10 months: pincer grasp: between distal pads of thumb and index finger, distal thumb slightly flexed; thumb opposed

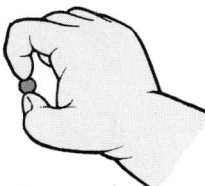

12 months: fine pincer grasp: between fingertips or fingernails; distal thumb joint flexed

Figure 66. Pinch and grasp patterns.

Appendix 1

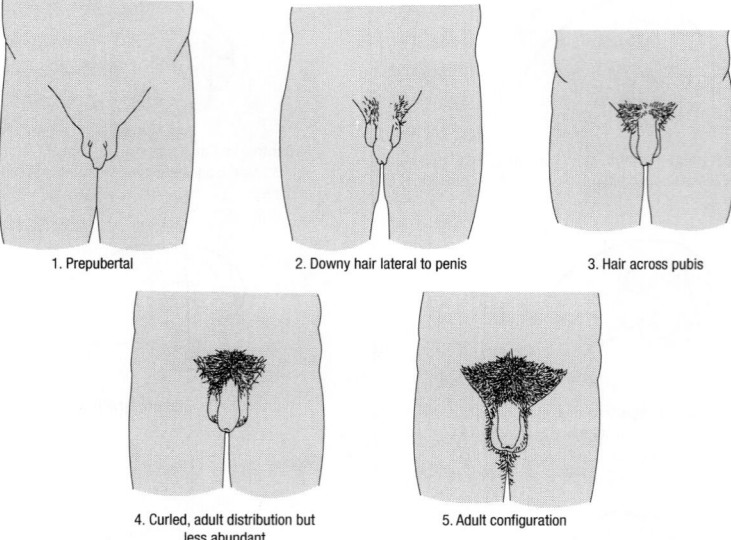

Figure 67. Tanner stages in the male. Rating 1–5.

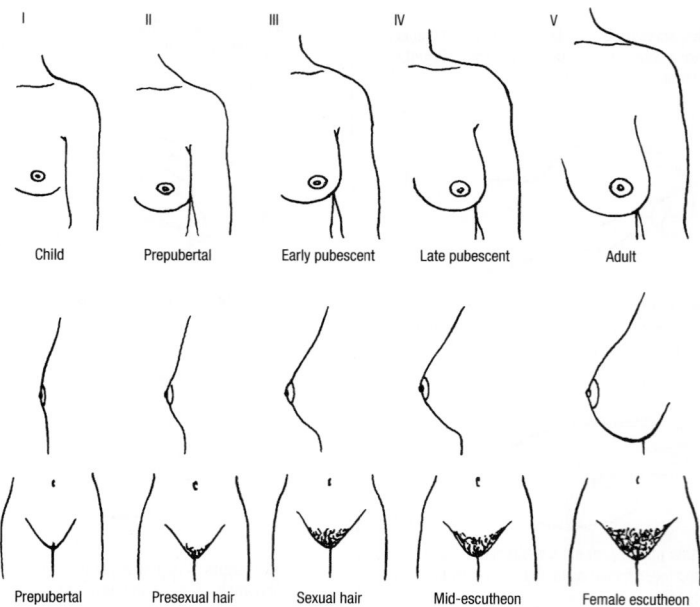

Figure 68. Tanner stages in the female. Rating I–V.

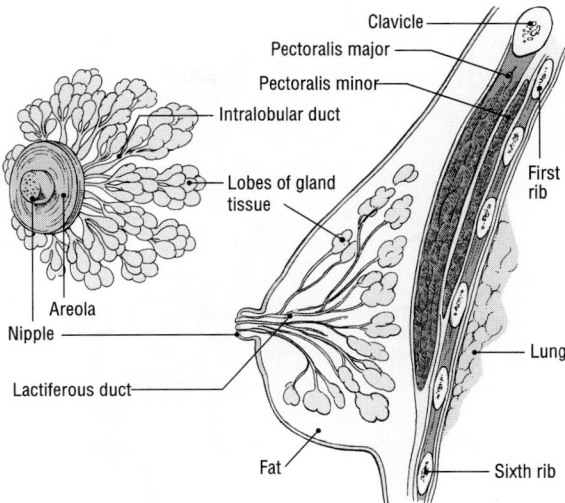

Figure 69. Breast. Glandular tissue and ducts of the mammary gland.

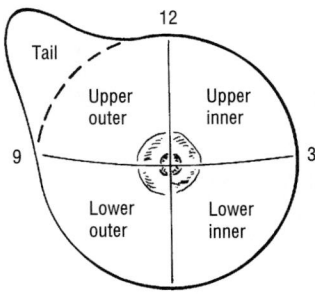

Figure 70. Breast. Schematic of breast as clock with nipple at center to assist reference.

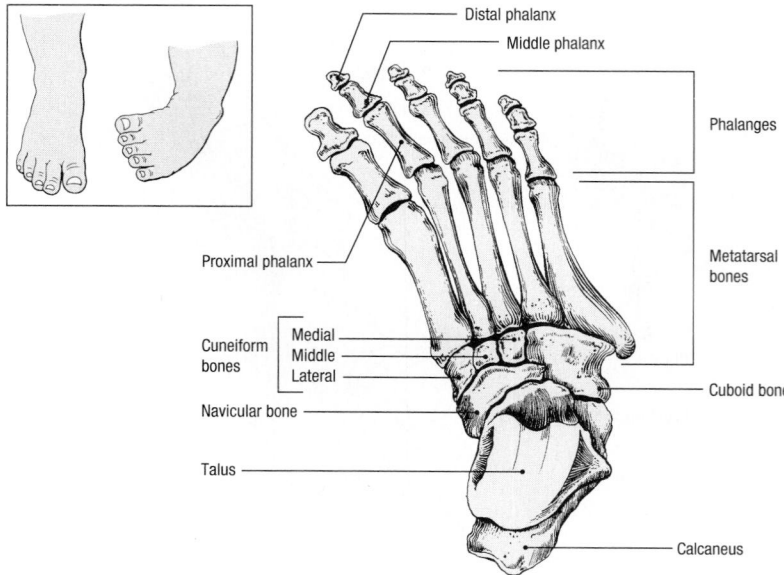

Figure 71. Clubfoot. Bones in a clubfoot deformity; note tarsal navicular moved medial to talus, talus is forced laterally, which in turn has pushed calcaneus into varus and equinus. Anterior view of a child's two feet, the left of which is clubbed (inset).

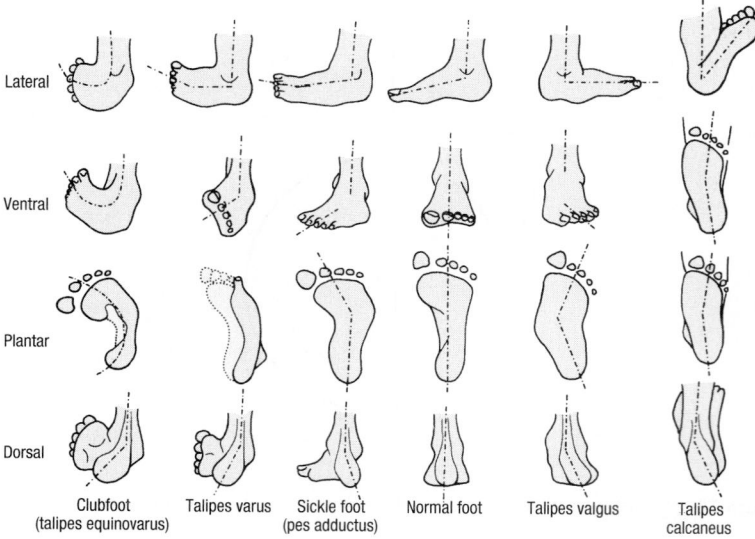

Figure 72. Foot deformities.

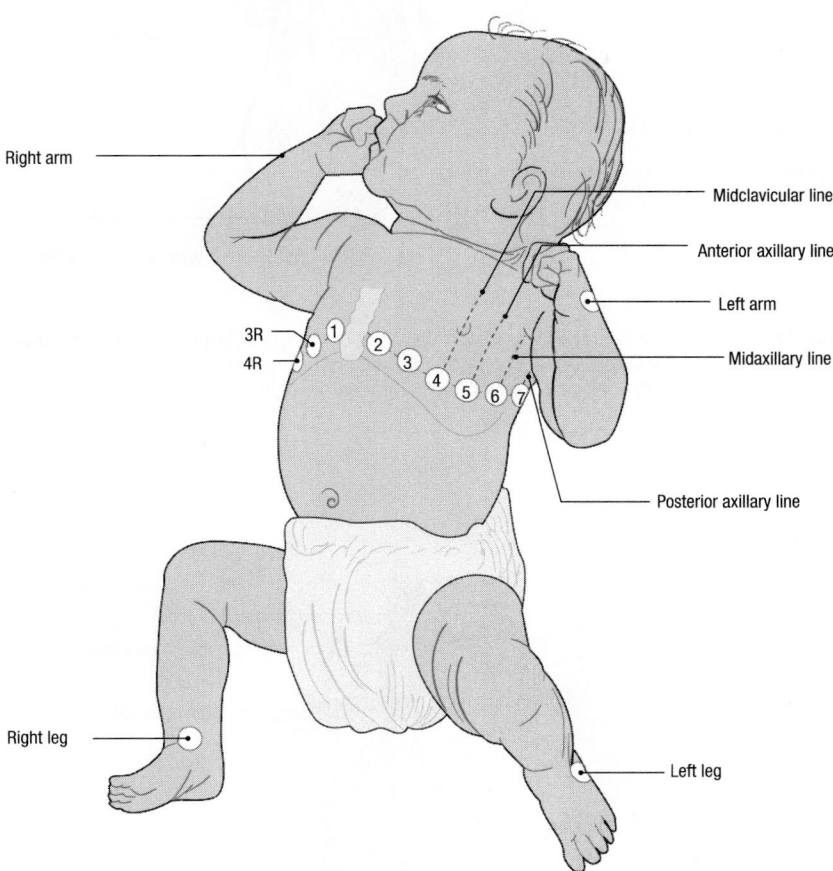

Right arm

Midclavicular line

Anterior axillary line

Left arm

3R

4R

Midaxillary line

Posterior axillary line

Right leg

Left leg

Figure 73. Electrocardiogram (ECG) lead placement.

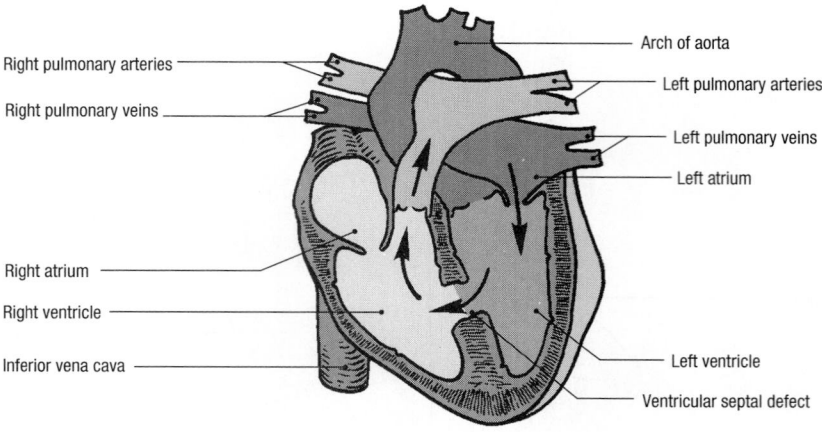

Figure 74. Auscultation, ventricular septal defect (VSD). VSD is so large there is no pressure between the ventricles. Flow is dependent on systemic and pulmonary arterial resistance. If pulmonary vascular resistance (PVR) is less than systemic (SVR), a left-to-right shunt occurs.

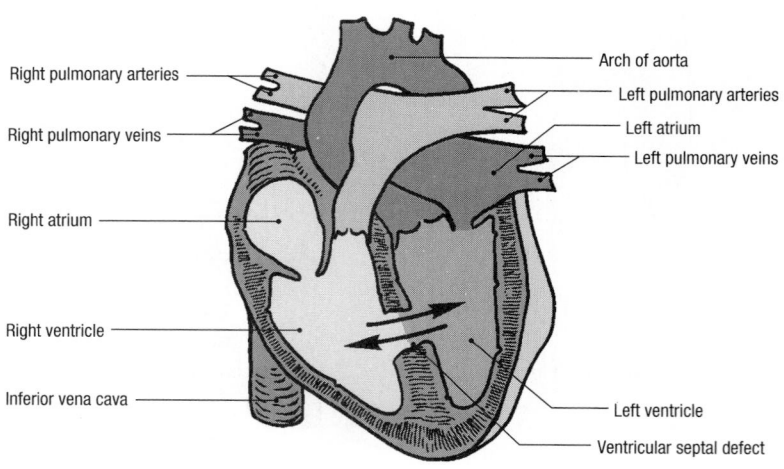

Figure 75. Auscultation, ventricular septal defect. When pulmonary vascular resistance is equal to or greater than systemic in the presence of a large ventricular septal defect, a murmur may not be detected due to low shunt volume. A loud single second sound is heard as aortic and pulmonary closures occur.

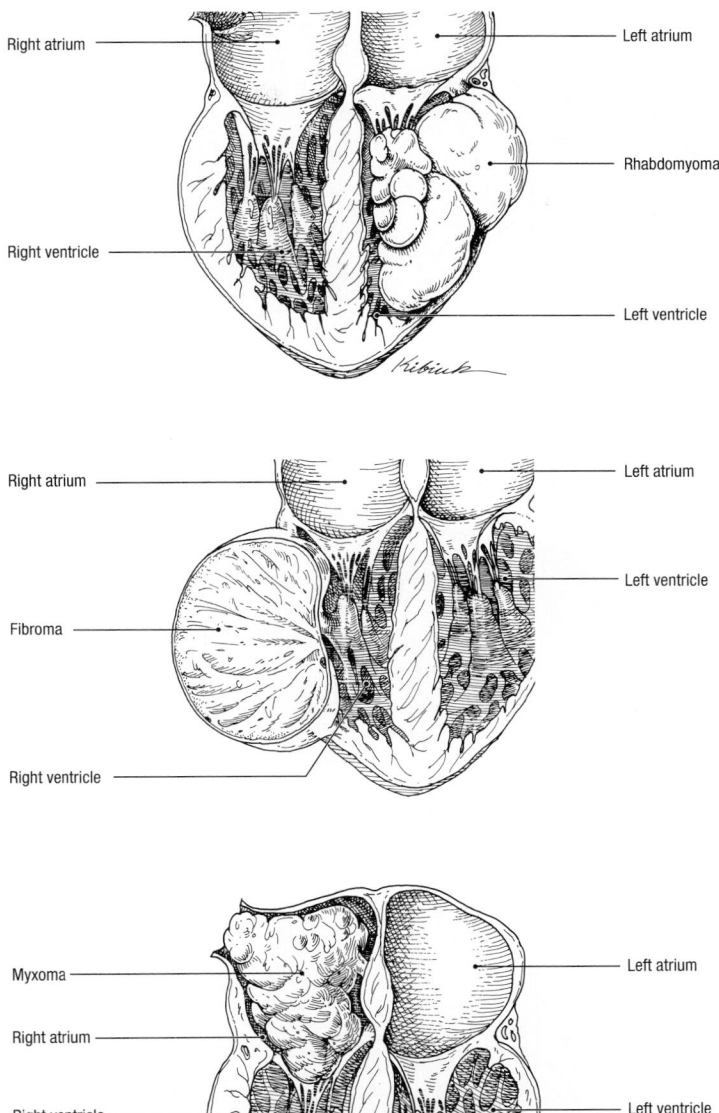

Right atrium — — Left atrium

— Rhabdomyoma

Right ventricle —

— Left ventricle

Right atrium — — Left atrium

— Left ventricle

Fibroma —

Right ventricle —

Myxoma — — Left atrium

Right atrium —

Right ventricle — — Left ventricle

Figure 76. Cardiac tumors in children. Primary cardiac tumors in children appear to be associated with familial syndromes with autosomal dominant inheritance. Rhabdomyoma is the most common benign tumor and is derived from striated muscle elements. It is located within the wall of the myocardium (top). The fibroma is a solitary ventricular structure derived from fibrous connective tissue. It occurs in children under 10 years of age (middle). The myxoma arises from the lining of the atrium and resembles a polyp. It is a benign tumor (bottom).

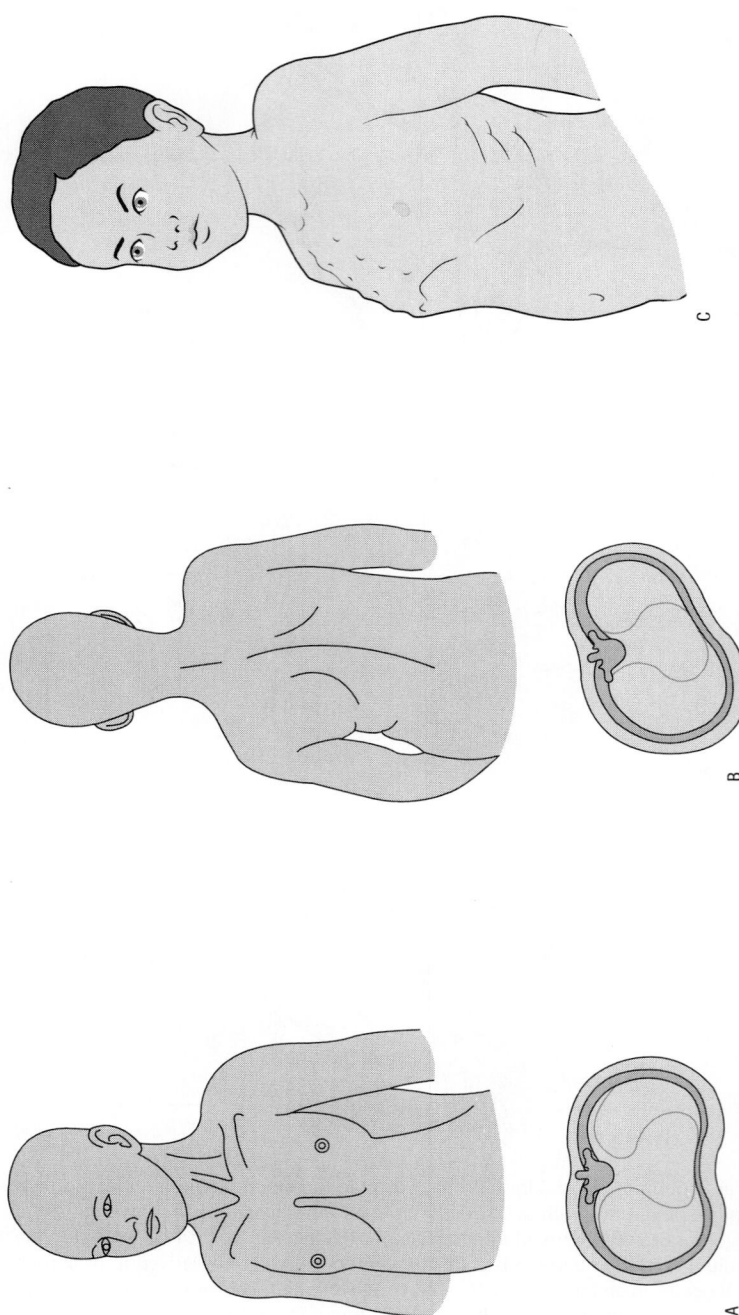

Figure 77. Thoracic deformities. (A) Anterior and transverse view of male child with pectus excavatum (funnel chest); (B) Posterior and transverse view of male child with thoracic kyphoscoliosis; (C) Anteroposterior view of male child with pectus carinatum (pigeon chest). Note the protruding thoracic cage.

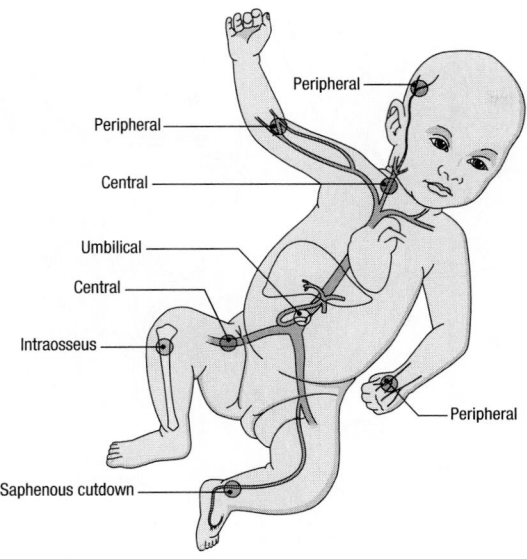

Figure 78. Pediatric IV sites: peripheral, umbilical, central, intraosseus, and saphenous cutdown.

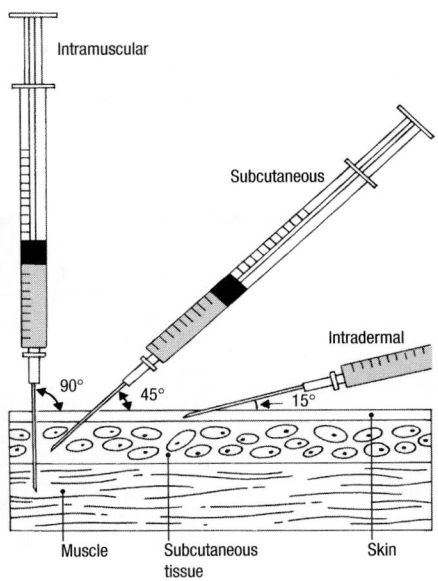

Figure 79. Angles of insertion of injection.

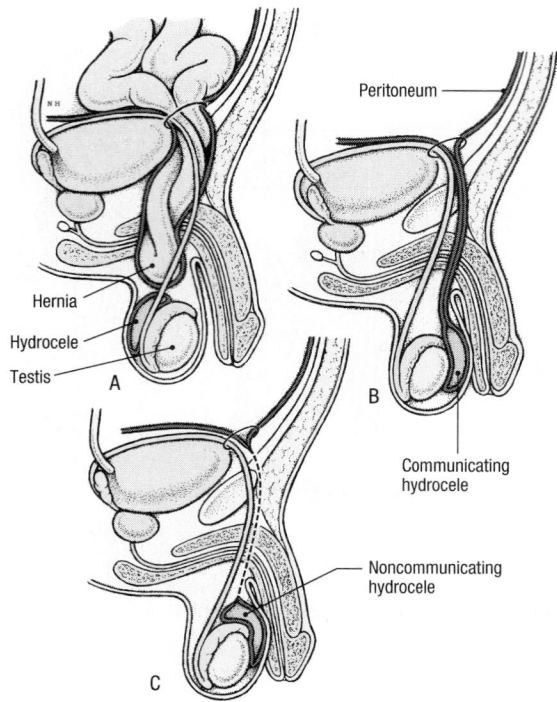

Figure 80. Types of hydroceles (peritoneum shown in dark gray). (A) Hydrocele with indirect inguinal hernia; (B) Communicating hydrocele; (C) Noncommunicating hydrocele.

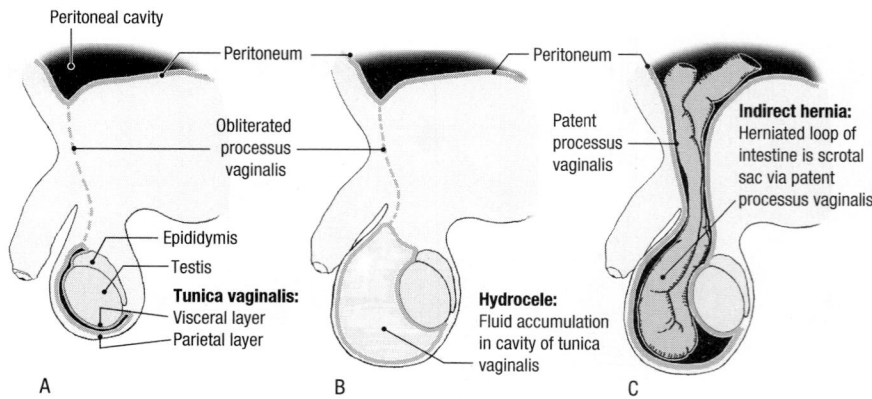

Figure 81. Processus vaginalis and tunica vaginalis. (A) Normal anatomy; (B) Hydrocele; (C) Indirect hernia.

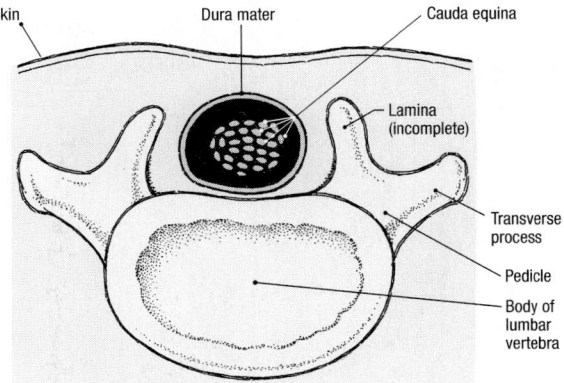

Figure 82. Spina bifida occulta.

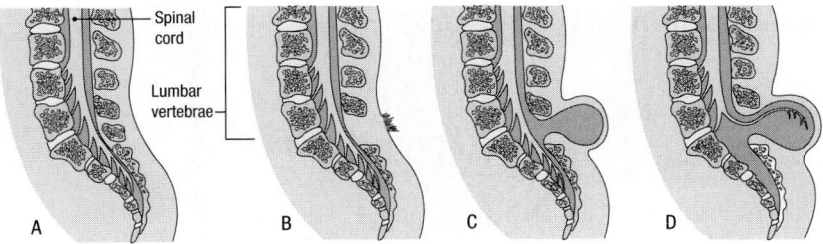

Figure 83. Four degrees of spinal cord anomalies. (A) Normal spinal cord; (B) Spina bifida occulta; (C) Meningocele; (D) Myelomeningocele.

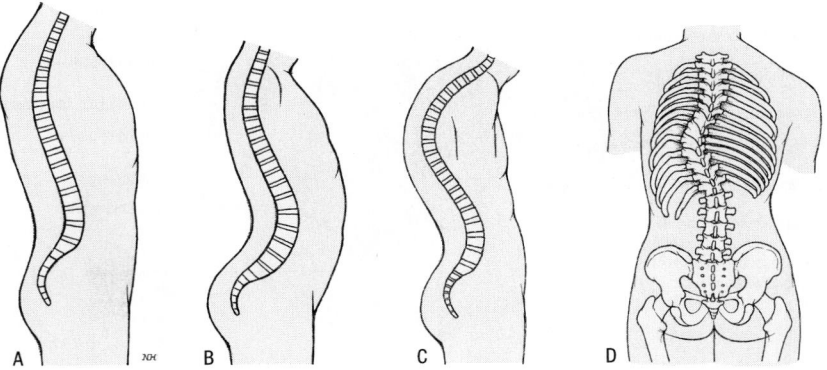

Figure 84. Spinal curvatures. (A) Normal; (B) Lordosis; (C) Kyphosis; (D) Scoliosis.

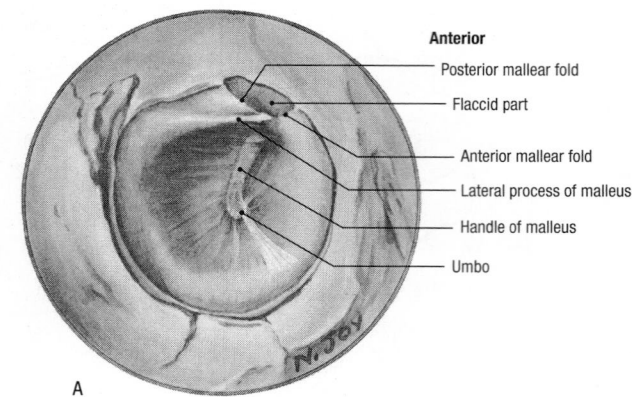

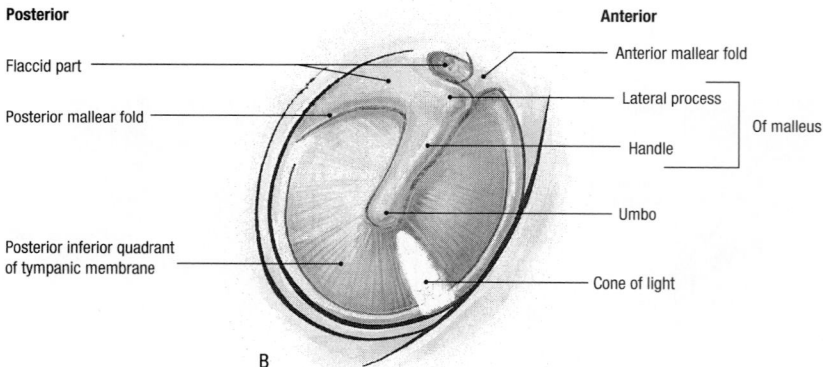

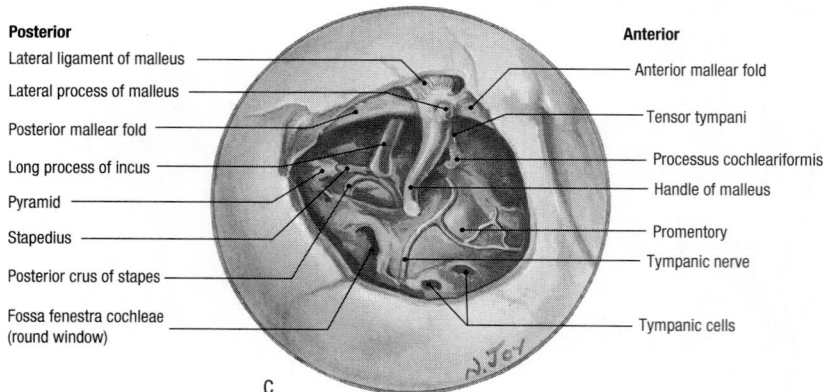

Figure 85. Tympanic membrane. (A) Lateral view; (B) Auriscopic view; (C) Tympanic membrane removed, inferolateral view.

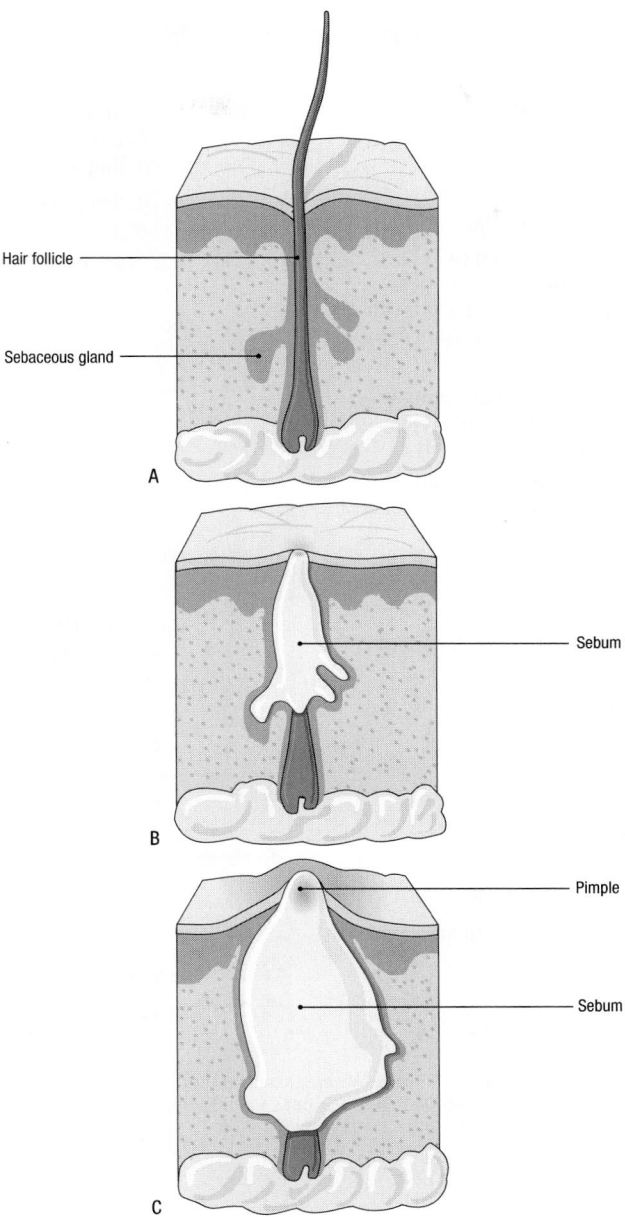

Figure 86. Acne formation. (A) Hair follicle and sebaceous gland; (B) First stage in acne develop-ment; follicle becomes blocked, sebum begins to fill follicle cavity; (C) Inflamed pustule and pim-ple; follicle is blocked, sebum has filled and expanded follicle cavity.

Appendix 2
Genetic Symbols

□ male

○ female

◇ sex unspecified

□○ normal individuals

■●◆ affected individual (with ≥ 2 conditions, the symbol is partitioned and shaded with different fill defined in a key or legend)

⑤⑤◇ multiple individuals, number known (number of siblings written inside symbol)

ⁿⓃ◇ multiple individuals, number unknown ("n" used in place of specific number)

□○ mating

□○ consanguinity

(+) uncommon or uncertain mode of inheritance

parents and offspring, in generations

□○ dizygotic twins

□○ monozygotic twins

④③ number of children of sex indicated

(□)(○) adopted individuals

□○ individual died without leaving offspring

□○ no issue

■● affected individuals

■● proband or propositus (first affected family member coming to medical attention)

examined professionally · normal for trait

not examined · dubiously reported to have trait

not examined · reliably reported to have trait

■◐ heterozygotes for autosomal recessive

⊙ carrier of sex-linked recessive

◻∅ death

SB 28wk   SB 30wk   SB 34wk   stillbirth (SB)

P   P 20wk   P
LMP 7/1/94   pregnancy (P); gestational age and karotype (if known) below symbol

□○ consultand (individual seeking genetic counseling/testing)

△ male   △ female   △ ECT   spontaneous abortion (SAB); ECT below symbol indicates ectopic pregnancy

▲ male   ▲ female   ▲ 16wk   affected SAB (gestational age, if known, below symbol, and key or legend used to define shading)

△ male   △ female   termination of pregnancy (TOP)

▲ male   ▲ female   affected TOP (key or legend used to define shading)

Source: Genetic symbols are public domain. We credit and gratefully acknowledge the *American Journal of Human Genetics* (56:746–747, 1995) as our source for these symbols.

A50

Appendix 3
Normal Lab Values

Tests	Conventional Units	SI Units
acetone		
serum		
qualitative	negative	negative
quantitative	0.3–2.0 mg/dL	0.05–0.34 mmol/L
*alanine aminotransferase (ALT, SGPT), serum		
males	13–40 U/L (37°C)	0.22–0.68 μkat/L (37°C)
females	10–28 U/L (37°C)	0.17–0.48 μkat/L (37°C)
albumin		
serum		
adult	3.5–5.2 g/dL	35–52 g/L
urine		
qualitative	negative	negative
quantitative	50–80 mg/24 h.	50–80 mg/24 h.
CSF	10–30 mg/dL	100–300 mg/dL
alpha-1-antitrypsin, serum	78–200 mg/dL	0.78–200 g/L
alpha-fetoprotein (AFP), serum	< 15 ng/mL	< 15 μg/L
ammonia		
plasma (Hep)	9–33 μmol/L	9–33 μmol/L
*amylase		
serum	27–131 U/L	0.46–2.23 μkat/L
bilirubin		
serum		
adult		
conjugated	0.0–0.3 mg/dL	0–5 μmol/L
unconjugated	0.1–1.1 mg/dL	1.7–1.9 μmol/L
delta	0–0.2 mg/dL	0–3 μmol/L
total	0.2–1.3 mg/L	3–22 μmol/L
*bilirubin		
serum		
neonates		
conjugated	0–0.6 mg/dL	0–10 μmol/L
unconjugated	0.6–10.5 mg/dL	10–180 μmol/L
total	1.5–12 mg/dL	1.7–180 μmol/L
CA 125, serum	< 35 U/mL	< 35 kU/L
CA 19–9, serum	< 37 U/mL	< 37 kU/L
calcium, serum	8.6–10.0 mg/dL (slightly higher in children)	2.15–2.50 mmol/L (slightly higher in children)

continued

Tests	Conventional Units	SI Units
carbon dioxide (PCO_2), blood arterial	males 35–48 mmHg females 32–45 mmHg	4.66–6.38 kPa 4.26–5.99 kPa
carotene, serum	10–85 μg/dL	0.19–1.58 μmol/L
catecholamines, urine		
dopamine	65–400 μg/24 h.	425–2610 nmol/24 h.
epinephrine	0–20 μg/24 h.	0–109 nmol/24 h.
norepinephrine	15–80 μg/24 h.	89–473 nmol/24 h.
CEA, serum, smokers	< 5.0 ng/mL	< 5.0 μg/L
*cell counts, adult		
RBC males	4.7–6.1×10^6/μL	4.7–6.1×10^{12}/L
females	4.2–5.4×10^6/μL	4.2–5.4×10^{12}/L
leukocytes		
total	4.8–10.8×10^3/μL	4.8–10.8×10^6/L
platelets	130–400×10^3/μL	1340–400×10^9/L
reticulocytes	0.5–1.5% red cells	0.005–0.015 of RBC
cells, CSF	0–10 lymphocytes /mm3 0 RBC/ mm3	0–10 lymphocytes /mm3 0 RBC/ mm3
chloride		
serum or plasma	98–107 mmol/L	98–107 mmol/L
cholesterol, serum		
adult desirable	< 200 mg/dL	< 5.2 mmol/L
borderline	200–239 mg/dL	5.2–6.2 mmol/L
high risk	≥240 mg/dL	≥6.2 mmol/L
cholinesterase, serum	4.9–11.9 U/mL	4.9–11.9 kU/L
chorionic gonadotropin, intact serum or plasma		
males/nonpregnant females	< 5.0 mIU/mL	< 5.0 IU/L
pregnant females	varies with gestational age	
urine, qualitative		
males/nonpregnant females	negative	negative
pregnant females	positive	positive
coagulation tests antithrombin III		
(synthetic substrate)	80–120% of normal	0.8–1.2 of normal
bleeding time (Duke)	0–6 min	0–6 min
bleeding time (Ivy)	1–6 min	1–6 min
bleeding time (template)	2.3–9.5 min	2.3–9.5 min
clot retraction, qualitative	50–100% in 2 h.	0.5–1.0/2 h.
complement components		
total hemolytic complement activity, plasma	75–160 U/mL	75–160 kU/L
total complement decay	10–20%	fraction decay rate: 0.10–0.20
rate (functional), plasma	deficiency: > 50%	> 0.50

continued

Tests	Conventional Units	SI Units
C1q, serum	14.9–22.1 mg/dL	149–221 mg/L
C1r, serum	2.5–10.0 mg/dL	25–100 mg/L
C1s (C1 esterase), serum	5.0–10.0 mg/dL	50–100 mg/L
C2, serum	1.6–3.6 mg/dL	16–36 mg/L
C3, serum	90–180 mg/dL	0.9–1.8 g/L
C4, serum	10–40 mg/dL	0.1–0.4 mg/L
C5, serum	5.5–11.3 mg/dL	55–113 mg/L
C6, serum	17.9–23.9 mg/dL	179–239 mg/L
C7, serum	2.7–7.4 mg/dL	27–74 mg/L
C8, serum	4.9–10.6 mg/dL	49–106 mg/L
C9, serum	3.3–9.5 mg/dL	33–95 mg/L
Coombs test		
direct	negative	negative
indirect	negative	negative
copper		
serum		
males	70–140 μg/dL	11–22μmol/L
females	80–155 μg/dL	13–24μmol/L
cortisol, serum		
plasma (Hep, EDTA, Ox)		
8 a.m.	5–23 μg/dL	138–635 nmol/L
4 p.m.	3–16 μg/dL	83–441 nmol/L
C-reactive protein, serum	< 0.5 mg/dL	< 5 mg/L
creatine kinase (CK)		
serum		
males	15–105 U/L (30°C)	0.26–1.79 μkat/L (30°C)
females	10–80 U/L (30°C)	0.17–1.36 μkat/L (30°C)
*creatinine		
serum or plasma, adult		
males	0.7–1.3 mg/dL	62–115 μmol/L
females	0.6–1.1 mg/dL	53–97 μmol/L
cryoglobulins, serum	0	0
dehydroepiandrosterone		
(DHEA), serum		
males	180–1250 ng/dL	6.2–43.3 nmol/L
females	130–980 ng/dL	4.5–34.0 nmol/L
dehydroepiandrosterone sulfate		
(DHEAS), serum or plasma		
males	59–452 μg/mL	1.6–12.2 μmol/L
females		
premenopausal	12–379 μg/mL	0.8–10.2 μmol/L
postmenopausal	30–260 μg/mL	0.8–7.1 μmol/L
delta aminolevulinic acid,		
urine	1.3–7.0 mg/24 h.	10–53 μmol/24 h.

continued

Appendix 3

Tests	Conventional Units	SI Units
estradiol, serum		
adult males	10–50 pg/mL	37–184 pmol/L
adult females	varies with menstrual cycle	
ferritin, serum		
males	20–150 ng/mL	20–250 µg/L
females	10–120 ng/mL	10–120 µg/L
*fibrinogen, plasma (NaCit)	200–400 mg/dL	2–4 g/L
follicle-stimulating hormone (FSH), serum and plasma		
males	1.4–15.4 mIU/mL	1.4–15.4 IU/L
females		
follicular phase	1–10 mIU/mL	1–10 IU/L
mid cycle	6–17 mIU/mL	6–17 IU/L
luteal phase	1–9 mIU/mL	1–9 IU/L
postmenopausal	19–100 mIU/mL	19–100 IU/L
gamma-glutamyltransferase (GGT), serum		
males	2–30 U/L (37°C)	0.03–0.51 µkat/L (37°C)
females	1–24 U/L (37°C)	0.02–0.41 µkat/L (37°C)
glucose (fasting)		
blood	65–95 mg/dL	3.5–5.3 mmol/L
plasma or serum	74–106 mg/dL	4.1–5.9 mmol/L
glucose, urine		
quantitative	< 500 mg/24 h.	< 2.8 mmol/24 h.
qualitative	negative	negative
glucose, CSF	40–70 mg/dL	2.2–3.9 mmol/L
glucose-6-phosphate dehydrogenase (G6PD) in erythrocytes,	12.1 ± 2.1 U/g Hb (SD)	0.78 ± 0.13 mU/mol Hb
whole blood	351 ± 60.6 U/10^{12} RBC	0.35 ± 0.06 nU/RBC
(ACD, EDTA, or Hep)	4.11 ± 0.71 U/mL RBC	4.11 ± 0.71 kU/L RBC
haptoglobin, serum	30–200 mg/dL	0.3–2.0 g/L
hematocrit		
males	42–52%	0.42–0.52
females	37–47%	0.37–0.47
newborns	53–65%	0.53–0.65
children (varies with age)	30–43%	0.30–0.43
hemoglobin (Hb)		
males	14.0–18.0 g/dL	2.17–2.79 mmol/L
females	12.0–16.0 g/dL	1.86–2.48 mmol/L
newborn	17.0–23.0 g/dL	2.64–3.57 mmol/L
children (varies with age)	11.2–16.5 g/dL	1.74–2.56 mmol/L
hemoglobin, fetal	≥1 y old: < 2% of total Hb	≥1 y old: < 0.02% of total Hb

continued

Tests	Conventional Units	SI Units
hemoglobin electrophoresis whole blood (EDTA, Cit, or Hep)		
HbA	> 95%	> 0.95 Hb fraction
HbA2	1.5–3.7%	0.015–0.37 Hb fraction
HbF	< 2%	< 0.02 Hb fraction
immunoglobulins, serum		
IgG	700–1600 mg/dL	7–16 g/L
IgA	70–400 mg/dL	0.7–4.0 g/L
IgM	40–230 mg/dL	0.42.3 g/L
IgD	0–8 mg/dL	0–80 mg/L
IgE	3–423 mg/dL	3–423 kIU/L
immunoglobulin G (IgG)		
CSF	0.5–6.1 mg/dL	0.5–6.1 g/L
*iron, serum		
males	65–175 μg/dL	11.6–31.3 μmol/L
females	50–170 μg/dL	9.0–30.4 μmol/L
iron binding capacity, serum		
total (TIBC)	250–425 μg/dL	44.8–71.6 μmol/L
*lactate dehydrogenase (LDH)		
newborn	290–775 U/L	4.9–13.2 μkat/L
neonate	545–2000 U/L	9.3–34 μkat/L
infant	180–430 U/L	3.1–7.3 μkat/L
child	110–295 U/L	1.9–5 μkat/L
adult	100–190 U/L	1.7–3.2 μkat/L
> 60 y	110–210 U/L	1.9–3.6 μkat/L
lead, whole blood (Hep)	< 25 μg/dL	< 1.2 μmol/L
lecithin-sphingomyelin	2.0–5.0 indicates	same
(L/S) ratio, amniotic fluid	probable fetal lung maturity; < 3.5 in diabetics	
luteinizing hormone (LH), serum or plasma		
males	1.24–7.8 mIU/mL	1.24–7.8 IU/L
females		
follicular phase	1.68–15.0 mIU/mL	1.68–15.0 IU/L
mid-cycle peak	21.9–56.6 mIU/mL	21.9–56.6 IU/L
luteal phase	0.61–16.3 mIU/mL	0.61–16.3 IU/L
postmenopausal	14.2–52.5 mIU/mL	14.2–52.5 IU/L
*lipase, serum	23–300 U/L (37°C)	0.39–5.1 μkat/L (37°C)
magnesium		
serum	1.3–2.1 mEq/L	0.65–1.07 mmol/L
	1.6–2.6 mg/dL	16–26 mg/L
mean corpuscular hemoglobin (MCH)	27–31 pg	0.42–0.48 fmol

continued

Tests	Conventional Units	SI Units
mean corpuscular hemoglobin concentration (MCHC)	33–37 g/dL	330–370 g/L
mean corpuscular volume (MCV)		
males	80–94 μm^3	80–94 fL
females	81–99 μm^3	81–99 fL
metanephrine, total, urine	0.1–1.6 mg/24 h.	0.5–8.1 μmol/24 h.
5'-nucleotidase, serum	2–17 U/L	0.034–0.29 μkat/L
osmolality, urine	50–1200 mOsm/kg water	50–1200 mmol/kg water
oxygen, blood tension		
pO2 arterial and capillary	83–108 mmHg	11.1–14.4 kPa
partial thromboplastin time		
activated (APTT)	< 35 sec	< 35 sec
pH		
blood, arterial	7.35–7.45	7.35–7.45
urine	4.6–8.0 (depends on diet)	same
partial thromboplastin time, activated (aPTT)	< 35 sec	< 35 sec
phosphatidylglycerol (PG), amniotic fluid		
fetal lung immaturity	absent	absent
fetal lung maturity	present	present
porphobilinogen, urine		
qualitative	negative	negative
quantitative	< 2.0 mg/24 h.	< 9 μmol/24 h.
porphyrins, urine		
coproporphyrin	34–230 μg/24 h.	52–351 nmol/24 h.
uroporphyrin	27–52 μg/24 h.	32–63 nmol/24 h.
potassium		
serum		
premature		
cord	5.0–10.2 mmol/L	5.0–10.2 mmol/L
48 h.	3.0–6.0 mmol/L	3.0–6.0 mmol/L
newborn cord	5.6–12.0 mmol/L	5.6–12.0 mmol/L
newborn	3.7–5.9 mmol/L	3.7–5.9 mmol/L
infant	4.1–5.3 mmol/L	4.1–5.3 mmol/L
child	3.4–4.7 mmol/L	3.4–4.7 mmol/L
adult	3.5–5.1 mmol/L	3.5–5.1 mmol/L
progesterone, serum		
adult males	13–97 ng/dL	0.4–31 nmol/L
adult females		
follicular phase	15–70 ng/dL	0.5–2.2 nmol/L

continued

Tests	Conventional Units	SI Units
luteal phase	200–2500 ng/dL	6.4–79.5 nmol/L
pregnancy	varies with gestational week	
*protein, serum		
total	6.4–8.3 g/dL	64–83 g/L
urine		
qualitative	negative	negative
quantitative	50–80 mg/24 h.	50–80 mg/24 h.
	(at rest)	(at rest)
CSF, total	8–32 mg/dL	80–320 mg/dL
*prothrombin time (PT)	12–14 sec	12–14 sec
protoporphyrin, total, WB	< 60 μg/dL	< 600 μg/L
sedimentation rate		
Wintrobe		
males	0–10 mm in 1 h.	0–10 mm/h
females	0–20 mm in 1 h.	0–20 mm/h
Westergren		
males	0–15 mm in 1 h.	0–15 mm/h
females	0–20 mm in 1 h.	0–20 mm/h
sodium		
serum or plasma (Hep)		
premature		
cord	116–140mmol/L	116–140 mmol/L
48 h.	128–148 mmol/L	128–148 mmol/L
newborn, cord	126–166 mmol/L	126–166 mmol/L
newborn	133–146 mmol/L	133–146 mmol/L
infant	139–146 mmol/L	139–146 mmol/L
child	138–145 mmol/L	138–145 mmol/L
adult	136–145 mmol/L	136–145 mmol/L
specific gravity, urine	1.002–1.030	1.002–1.030
transferrin, serum		
newborn	130–275 mg/dL	1.3–2.75 g/L
adult	212–360 mg/dL	2.12–3.60 g/L
> 60 y	190–375 mg/dL	1.9–3.75 g/L
triglycerides, serum, fasting		
desirable	< 250 mg/dL	< 2.83 mmol/L
urea nitrogen, serum	6–20 mg/dL	2.1–7.1 mmol Urea/L
*uric acid		
serum, enzymatic		
males	4.5–8.0 mg/dL	0.27–0.47 mmol/L
females	2.5–6.2 mg/dL	0.15–0.37 mmol/L
child	2.0–5.5 mg/dL	0.12–0.32 mmol/L
urobilinogen, urine	0.1–0.8 Ehrlich unit/2 h.	0.1–0.8 Ehrlich unit/2 h.
	0.5–4.0 mg/24 h.	0.5–4.0 mg/24 h.

continued

Appendix 3

Tests	Conventional Units	SI Units
vanillylmandelic acid (VMA),urine (4-hydroxy-3-methoxymandelic acid	1.4–6.5 mg/24 h.	7–33 μmol/d
viscosity, serum	1.00–1.24 cP	1.00–1.24 cP
vitamin B_{12}, serum	110–800 pg/mL	81–590 pmol/L

* Test values are method dependent.
Abbreviations: CSF indicates cerebrospinal fluid; EDTA, ethylenediaminetetraacetic acid; Hep, heparin; Ox, oxalate; and RBC, red blood cell(s).

Appendix 4
Biophysical Profile Scoring: Technique and Interpretation

Biophysical variable	Normal (score = 2)	Abnormal (score = 0)
Fetal breathing movements	≥ 1 episode of ≥ 30 sec. in 30 min. ≥ 3 discrete body-limb movements in 30 min. (episodes of active continuous movement considered)	Absent or no episode of ≥ 30 min. ≤ 2 episodes of body-limb movements in 30 min. as single movement
Fetal tone	≥ 1 episode of active extension with return to flexion of fetal limb(s) or trunk Opening and closing of hand considered normal tone	Either slow extension with return to partial flexion movement of limb(s) in full extension or absent fetal movement
Reactive fetal heart rate	≥ 2 episodes of acceleration of ≥ 15 bpm and of >15 sec. associated with fetal movement in 20 min.	> 2 episodes of acceleration fetal heart rate or acceleration of > 15 bpm in 20 min.
Qualitative amniotic fluid volume	≥ 1 pocket of fluid measuring 2 cm in vertical axis	Either no pockets or largest pocket > 2 cm in vertical axis
Nonstress test	Reactive	Nonreactive

From Reece EA, Hobbins JC, eds. Medicine of the Fetus and Mother, Second Edition. Philadelphia: Lippincott-Raven Publishers, 1999.

Appendix 5
Sample Reports and Dictation

ACUTE SCROTAL PAIN EMERGENCY ROOM REPORT

CHIEF COMPLAINT: This 8-year-old Hispanic male was awakened from sleep by severe, unremitting scrotal pain, which has been present for approximately 3 hours. He denies trauma to the area and has had no fever, chills, nausea, vomiting, hesitancy or blood on urination. He states that nothing he does makes the pain better.

PHYSICAL EXAMINATION: Young male in obvious distress. Vital signs are normal. Exam is limited to the genitalia. The penis is normal in appearance, and there is no urethral discharge. The right hemiscrotum is edematous and erythematous. There is marked tenderness on palpation; the right testicle has a transverse lie. The right cremasteric reflex is absent. The left hemiscrotum and testicle are normal to exam.

LABORATORY DATA: Stat complete blood count and urinalysis are within normal limits. Ultrasound of the scrotum reveals blood flow to be absent to the right testicle and epididymis. No mass is noted. Normal blood flow is demonstrated to the left testicle.

PLAN: The patient has been admitted to the pediatric floor and will be seen in emergent urologic consultation within the hour.

DIAGNOSIS: Probable testicular torsion; bell clapper deformity.

ADENOTONSILLECTOMY

PREOPERATIVE DIAGNOSES: Chronic tonsillitis and obstructive adenoids.

POSTOPERATIVE DIAGNOSES: Chronic tonsillitis and obstructive adenoids.

PROCEDURE PERFORMED: Adenotonsillectomy.

ANESTHESIA: General endotracheal.

BLOOD LOSS: Approximately 10 mL.

INDICATIONS FOR PROCEDURE: The patient is an 8-year-old Hispanic male who has had repeated bouts of tonsillitis that have caused him to miss a considerable amount of school. His tonsils are kissing and cryptic. His adenoids are also enlarged, causing him to be a mouth breather and to snore when he is asleep.

DESCRIPTION OF PROCEDURE: The patient was placed in the Rose position with a shoulder roll, and general endotracheal anesthesia was administered. A McIvor mouth gag with a slotted tongue depressor was placed in the oral cavity and suspended from a Mayo stand. A red rubber catheter was used to retract the soft palate.

The adenoids were adequately visualized and removed with adenoid curette. The nasopharynx was packed. Bovie electrocautery was used to remove each tonsil without incident, dissecting between the superior constrictor muscle and tonsillar capsule. Suction cautery was used to ensure hemostasis was achieved. The airway was carefully suctioned free of debris. The mouth gag was released, and the area was once again checked for bleeding points. There were none. The patient was taken to the recovery room in good condition.

BILATERAL LAPAROSCOPIC TUBAL LIGATION

DESCRIPTION OF PROCEDURE: After successful induction of general anesthesia, the patient was placed in the lithotomy position. Abdomen, perineum, and vagina were prepped and draped in a routine fashion. The urinary bladder was catheterized with a Foley catheter and emptied.

Pelvic examination was performed. Vulva and vagina appeared multiparous, cervix regular. Uterus was normal size. Adnexa were not palpable.

The weighted Sims speculum was inserted. The cervix was grasped with the single-toothed tenaculum. The uterine cavity was sounded to 10-cm and was regular. The cervix was dilated to Hegar #4 and a HUMI cannula was inserted and the abdomen prepared for laparoscopy.

A small cut was made in the center of the umbilicus, passed the Veress needle, and introduced 3 liters of carbon dioxide. The incision was extended and the trocar was passed. Through the trocar, the laparoscope was passed with both tubes identified; they were normal. Both ovaries were normal. Cul-de-sac was normal.

An anterior puncture was performed, and a 5-mm trocar was introduced. Through the trocar, the bipolar forceps were passed. The right tube was grasped in the center and this segment cauterized. Grasping proximally next to it, another segment was cauterized. There was whitish-yellowish tissue typical for completely burned tube. The same procedure was completed on the other side. The scissors were then passed, and the tubes were cut on each side and the ends again coagulated. There was no bleeding.

The anesthesiologist was instructed to give 2 g of Cefotan. The pneumoperitoneum and instruments were removed under direct vision. The skin was closed with 3-0 Dexon and the HUMI removed.

Bilateral Tubal Ligation, Modified Pomeroy Method

Preoperative Diagnosis: Elective sterilization by tubal ligation.

Postoperative Diagnosis: Elective sterilization by tubal ligation.

Procedure Performed: Pomeroy bilateral tubal ligation.

Estimated Blood Loss: Negligible.

Indications for Procedure: The patient and her husband have 4 healthy children and desire now to take steps to assure there will be no further pregnancies. They have been counseled regarding alternative measures of birth control, surgical risks, and their choice is to proceed with bilateral tubal ligation. Consent forms were obtained.

Description of Procedure: Under spinal anesthesia, the patient was placed in the supine position and prepped and draped in a sterile manner. An infraumbilical incision was made with sharp dissection and carried through layers of the abdominal wall. The peritoneum was entered and extended. Care was taken to avoid the bowel.

The right tube was brought through the incision and a modified Pomeroy tubal ligation was performed with 0 plain ties. Knuckles of tube were excised, and good hemostasis was noted. The left tube was then delivered through the incision and ligated in the same manner. Good hemostasis was noted. Both tubes were then returned to their appropriate anatomical position in the abdominal cavity. Both specimens were sent to pathology.

The fascia was closed with 0 Vicryl suture in a running fashion. The skin was closed with 3-0 Vicryl in a running fashion. A sterile dressing was applied.

The patient was taken to the day surgery recovery area in satisfactory condition.

Dilatation And Curettage

Preoperative Diagnosis: Irregular vaginal bleeding after spontaneous abortion.

Postoperative Diagnosis: Retained products of conception after spontaneous abortion.

PROCEDURE PERFORMED: Dilatation and curettage with removal of retained products of conception following spontaneous abortion.

ESTIMATED BLOOD LOSS: Minimal.

DESCRIPTION OF PROCEDURE: After transportation to the surgical suite, the patient was placed in the supine position on the operating table. Adequate general anesthesia was administered, and she was prepped and draped in the usual sterile fashion. She was then placed in the dorsal lithotomy position for dilatation and curettage.

A weighted speculum was placed into the vagina. The cervix was then grasped with a double-tooth tenaculum. The cervix sounded to 8 cm and admitted a 7-mm suction curette. Products of conception were evacuated without difficulty, followed by sharp curette.

Instruments were removed and the patient was once again placed in the supine position. Instrument counts were correct x2.

The patient tolerated the procedure well. She was returned to the recovery area in good condition.

ECTOPIC PREGNANCY DISCHARGE SUMMARY

HISTORY OF PRESENT ILLNESS: The patient is a 37-year-old female, G4, P2, AB1, who presented with 12 weeks of amenorrhea and persistent vaginal spotting for 3 to 4 days. Pregnancy test was positive. She was referred for sonogram, which revealed a normal uterine cavity; however, there was a dilated cervical canal and a live gestation of approximately 12 weeks. Therefore, the patient was diagnosed with cervical ectopic pregnancy.

HOSPITAL COURSE: The patient was started on methotrexate therapy. This was followed by transvaginal intracardiac instillation of potassium chloride to cause fetal demise. A Doppler scan confirmed fetal demise, with continuing endometrial hypervascularity around the ectopic gestational sac. She, therefore, underwent uterine artery embolization and dilatation and curettage with evacuation of products of conception, which she tolerated well. Examination by pathology confirmed the ectopic pregnancy diagnosis.

DISPOSITION: The patient is released to home on the day after dilatation and curettage. She will be seen in the office in 2 weeks, sooner if needed.

DIAGNOSIS: Cervical ectopic pregnancy.

PROCEDURES: Uterine artery embolization; dilatation and curettage.

ENDOMETRIAL CANCER HISTORY & PHYSICAL

HISTORY OF PRESENT ILLNESS: The patient is a 65-year-old Hispanic female, gravida 4, para 4, who was hospitalized in June 1998 for treatment of endometrial adenocarcinoma that was discovered while she was on tamoxifen. Her oncologic history began in 1993 when she underwent lumpectomy and axillary dissection for a tumor of the left breast. Pathology revealed a grade 3 infiltrating duct carcinoma of the right breast, with 2 of 13 lymph nodes positive for involvement. Dosage of hormonal receptors was performed and revealed strong staining for estrogen receptors and for progesterone receptors. The patient was postmenopausal and received radiotherapy as adjuvant therapy. She also received 20 mg of tamoxifen daily. This hormonal treatment was planned to continue for 5 years.

Before the breast surgery, she underwent complete gynecological examination, including Pap smear and vaginal ultrasound. The ultrasound revealed thick mucosa and a possible polyp. Operative hysteroscopy was performed with removal of an endometrial polyp. Pathology reported this to be a benign proliferative polyp without atypia.

The patient was followed annually with complete gynecological examinations, including vaginal ultrasounds which were normal until her most recent one this past month. Vaginal ultrasound at that time revealed endometrial thickening of 11 mm, an increase of 6 mm since last year. The ultrasound also revealed bilateral adnexal cysts, the right a heterogeneous cyst measuring 20 x 15 mm, the left a homogeneous cyst measuring 75 x 30 mm.

The patient is admitted now for vaginal hysterectomy with bilateral salpingo-oophorectomy.

PAST MEDICAL HISTORY: The patient has had an appendectomy and tonsillectomy, both in the remote past. She has been remarkably healthy otherwise.

ALLERGIES: She is allergic to no known medicines.

MEDICATIONS: In addition to tamoxifen, she takes a multivitamin each day.

FAMILY HISTORY: The patient is a widow. She lives with her youngest daughter and her family. She is a retired school teacher.

SOCIAL HISTORY: She does not smoke and indulges in an occasional glass of wine.

PHYSICAL EXAMINATION: HEENT: Without abnormality or lesion. NECK: Without swelling or nodules. Good range of motion. CHEST: Lungs are clear to auscultation and percussion, without rales or rhonchi. No bruits are heard. Heart is regular in rate and rhythm, without gallop or murmur. BREASTS: Normal appearing, soft, no masses are felt. ABDOMEN: Soft, flat, normal bowel sounds. No tenderness. EXTREMITIES: Normal. GENITALIA: Deferred. See attached office notes. NEUROLOGIC: Deferred.

PLAN: The patient will undergo vaginal hysterectomy and bilateral salpingo-oophorectomy tomorrow morning.

GENETICS CONSULTATION: ANGELMAN SYNDROME

HISTORY OF PRESENT ILLNESS: The child was born vaginally after a full-term, uncomplicated pregnancy. He presents now with postnatal onset microcephaly, global development milestone delay, and speech impairment that were observed when he was approximately 12 months old. Feeding problems also occurred, which included drooling, gagging, and choking. Family history is negative for neurologic problems or developmental delays.

PHYSICAL EXAMINATION: Abnormal physical findings included a head circumference that is less than 2nd percentile for his age. Height and weight are in the 45th and 25th percentile, respectively. He is distractible and hyperactive and frequently smiles and laughs. He has very pale blue eyes, and his hair is quite pale in color. On neurologic exam he demonstrates involuntary hand movements, a wide-based gait, and dystonically up-going toes.

IMAGING STUDIES: An MRI of the brain revealed incomplete myelination in the periventricular white matter, and an increased T2 signal bilaterally in the putamen, white and gray matter of the medial temporal lobe, static.

EEG revealed posterior slowing on the left and rhythmic delta runs in the left posterior region, as well as background slowing for his age.

DIAGNOSTIC STUDIES: Initial diagnostic studies failed to detect the 3 common defects that are responsible for Angelman syndrome on chromosome 15. Further studies that included sequence analysis revealed a previously unreported variant in the exon 9 of the UBE3A gene, which confirms the diagnosis of Angelman syndrome.

HENOCH-SCHÖNLEIN CONSULTATION

REASON FOR CONSULTATION: This 5-1/2-year-old white male is referred to this office because of the recent onset of joint pain and a rash over his lower extremities. He also complains of itchiness of his ears bilaterally and colicky abdominal pain. He is also recovering from a recent bout of upper respiratory infection.

PHYSICAL EXAMINATION: At consultation, the patient was not in distress but did appear to be somewhat uncomfortable. His temperature was slightly elevated at 100; the rest of the vital signs were within normal range. There were erythematous lesions on both ears with slight edema of the pinnae. There was a macular eruption, nonblanching, on the buttocks and lower extremities. He complained of knee and ankle joint pain, though the joints were not warm or erythematous. The feet were slightly edematous. Because a copy of his complete physical examination accompanied him, we did not repeat examination of other systems.

PAST MEDICAL HISTORY: According to the parents, this child's past medical history is unremarkable. There is no history of serious illness, hospitalizations, or surgeries.

FAMILY HISTORY: The family history is also unremarkable.

IMPRESSION AND PLAN: The findings here are consistent with Henoch-Schönlein purpura. His parents were advised to stop all medications. He should be monitored closely for any sign of renal complication. If his abdominal and joint discomforts do not start to diminish on their own in a few days, he may start a trial of corticosteroid therapy. Most symptoms in these cases resolve on their own within 4 weeks.

HYPOPITUITARISM IN INFANT HISTORY & PHYSICAL

CHIEF COMPLAINT: Persistent hypoglycemia, physiologic hyperbilirubinemia, abnormally small penis.

HISTORY OF PRESENT ILLNESS: The patient is a 10-day-old white male, born at gestational age of 39 weeks by date and 30 weeks by examination. His birth weight was 6 pounds 14 ounces (75th percentile), and his length was 20-1/2 inches (50th percentile). Apgar scores were 2, 4, and 6 at one, three, and eight minutes, respectively. He was given 100% oxygen because of duskiness, poor cry response, and difficulty breathing. He responded well. He was noted to have an extra digit on his right hand, and there was molding of the head. At birth his blood sugar was 26 mg/dL.

The infant was transferred to the neonatal intensive care unit, where oxygen supplementation was continued. Blood sugars continued to be low in the 30s, with the infant feeding well and remaining asymptomatic.

The infant was jaundiced and became mottled by 4 days old. We began phototherapy, and breast milk was withheld. A septic workup was done. Sugars were in the 60s post feeding and dropped into the low 30s at 3 to 4 hours after feedings.

FAMILY HISTORY: Father is 30 years old and has type 2 diabetes. Mother is 27, recently diagnosed with breast cancer, doing well post lumpectomy. There are no siblings. There is a positive history of type 2 diabetes in the maternal grandmother and aunt. Paternal grandmother and grandfather are deceased from automobile accident.

PHYSICAL EXAMINATION: GENERAL: His appearance is that of a moderately jaundiced infant. Today his weight is 7 pounds 2 ounces. VITAL SIGNS: Temperature 98.7, pulse 120, respirations 28. HEENT: The anterior and posterior fontanelles are slightly enlarged and soft. HEART: Regular rate and rhythm. No murmur is heard. LUNGS: Clear. ABDOMEN: Soft, with normal active bowel sounds. GENITOURINARY: The penis is small, measuring 2.6 cm, nondistended. The testes are descended bilaterally. NEUROLOGIC: The baby has strong suck, gag, and Moro reflexes.

DIAGNOSES: Hypoglycemia, hyperbilirubinemia, small penis. Rule out hypopituitarism.

PLAN: Will order labs, bilirubin, cortisol, growth hormone, thyroid-stimulating hormone (TSH) level, serum insulin, white blood count, blood cultures, and total testosterone. We will also obtain a magnetic resonance imaging (MRI) of the brain.

HYSTERECTOMY DISCHARGE SUMMARY

HISTORY OF PRESENT ILLNESS: The patient is a gravida 2, para 2 female who was noted on pelvic examination to have an enlarged pelvic mass. Vaginal ultrasound revealed an enlarged fibromyoma with a complex mass posterior to the uterus. She was admitted for exploratory laparotomy, total abdominal hysterectomy, and bilateral salpingo-oophorectomy.

PHYSICAL EXAMINATION: The patient's general physical examination on admission was within normal limits. Pelvic examination revealed an irregular enlarged uterus, 15 x 10 x 8 cm in dimension, with no definite adnexal mass palpable.

LABORATORY DATA: Preoperative laboratory tests included CBC, SMA-16, chest X-ray, and EKG, all of which were essentially normal with the exception of a cholesterol level of 270.

HOSPITAL COURSE: On the day of admission, the patient was taken to the operating room where exploratory laparotomy was performed, confirming an enlarged uterine fibromyoma. A dilatation and curettage and frozen section were performed. Pathology reported benign endometrium. Total abdominal hysterectomy and bilateral salpingo-oophorectomy were performed without complication.

The patient's postoperative course was essentially unremarkable. She remained afebrile throughout her hospital stay. The incision was healing well, her appetite was good, and there was normal return of bowel function so she was discharged on the 4th postoperative day in good condition. Staples were left intact and will be removed 4 days post discharge in the office.

DISCHARGE DIAGNOSES: Enlarged uterine fibromyoma and uterine adenomyosis, status post total abdominal hysterectomy and bilateral salpingo-oophorectomy.

INFANT WITH INTRAUTERINE AND NEONATAL COMPLICATIONS DISCHARGE SUMMARY

NEONATAL HISTORY: This female infant was delivered by cesarean section because of abnormalities found on fetal monitoring. Her mother is a 30-year-old, gravida 3, para 2 woman at 33 weeks' gestation at the time of delivery. Anti-Kell antibodies were detected during mother's previous pregnancy. Titers remained at 1:128 during this pregnancy. At 26 weeks' gestation, hydrops with moderate ascites was demonstrated on ultrasound. Subsequent serological testing was negative for toxoplasmosis, lues, parvovirus, hepatitis B, and rubella. Cordocentesis was done and revealed severe anemia, with hemoglobin of 56. The patient subsequently underwent 4 intrauterine transfusions, with resolution of the hydrops.

After delivery, her Apgar scores were 7, 8, and 9 at one, four, and ten minutes, respectively. Birth weight was in the 90th percentile at 2840 g. The infant developed tachypnea with mild respiratory distress, and this responded well to transient oxygen. Her skin was pale, with several bluish-red lesions on her torso, consistent with blueberry muffin spots. The liver was mildly enlarged but the spleen was normal.

LABORATORY DATA: Hemoglobin was 75 without evidence of hemolysis. Bilirubin was stable. Direct Coombs test was negative. Hematopoiesis was suppressed, with reticulocyte count of 0.3%. There were no peripheral erythroblasts. However, erythropoietin concentration in the umbilical cord blood was very high with 3240 units per liter, with normal being 5 to 25 units per liter. There was also thrombocytopenia and leukopenia. Cytomegalovirus cultures of her urine were negative. No pathology was revealed on ultrasound studies of the brain and abdomen.

HOSPITAL COURSE: The patient was given 1 transfusion of packed red blood cells, and the thrombocytopenia and leukopenia resolved spontaneously. The blueberry muffin spots also resolved spontaneously.

She was discharged in excellent condition 1 week after delivery, feeding well, without further problems. She will be seen by her pediatrician in a week.

DISCHARGE DIAGNOSES: 1. Hemolytic disease of the newborn, resolved.
2. Blueberry muffin spots, resolved.

INFERTILITY REFERRAL LETTER

REASON FOR CONSULTATION: This 32-year-old woman is referred for consultation because of infertility.

HISTORY: The patient has been married since age 22 and has had unprotected intercourse since age 26. According to her history, she has had irregular menstrual cycles since discontinuing birth control pills (Norinyl). The cycles occur every 27 days to 48 days. Temperature charts reveal an ovulatory pattern in approximately one-fourth of the charts. Before practicing birth control, her periods were regular, every 29 days.

The patient reports that she has never experienced dysmenorrhea or endometriosis, nor is there a family history of infertility or menstrual irregularities with her mother or female siblings. Hysterosalpingogram revealed normal patency of the fallopian tubes bilaterally.

PHYSICAL EXAMINATION: Her physical examination is normal throughout. She is conscious about her health and strives to maintain a balanced diet and a routine exercise program. Her weight has remained steady at 110 pounds for the past 5 years.

STUDIES: Her husband's semen analysis reveals a normal count, motility, and morphology. She and her husband have appropriately timed intercourse.

PLAN: The patient and her husband are eager to have a child and wish to proceed with further studies.

LAPAROSCOPIC UTERINE SUSPENSION

PREOPERATIVE DIAGNOSIS: Uterine prolapse.

POSTOPERATIVE DIAGNOSIS: Uterine prolapse.

PROCEDURE PERFORMED: Laparoscopic uterine suspension.

ESTIMATED BLOOD LOSS: Negligible.

DESCRIPTION OF PROCEDURE: The patient was brought to the operating suite and placed in the supine position on the operating table. General anesthesia was administered, and she was prepped and draped in the usual sterile manner.

A speculum was introduced into the vagina, and the anterior lip of the cervix was grasped with a single-toothed tenaculum. A uterine manipulator was then placed into the uterine cavity, and the bladder was emptied with a straight catheter.

An infraumbilical incision was made, and a laparoscopic trocar and sheath were introduced through it. By placing the laparoscope into the abdomen, the intraperitoneal position was confirmed. Separate suprapubic incisions were made, and assisting trocars and sheaths were introduced. After this, the pelvis was inspected. No abnormal findings were observed.

Plication was performed of the round ligament of the left side of the uterus, and small incisions above and lateral to the pubic symphysis were made bilaterally. Local anesthesia was injected into the incision sites to determine the exact incision sites.

A MetraPass suture passer with Ethicon suture was passed through the abdominal wall into the lateral portion of the round ligament. It was then threaded through the round ligament toward the uterus. The suture passer exited the ligament approximately 1 cm from the uterus. A grasper held the suture as the passer was withdrawn. A 2nd pass was made in the same manner. After this a fascial bridge was developed and the suture was tagged. The same procedure was done on the right.

The uterine manipulator was then removed. Sutures were tied without excess tension, and the uterus was positioned more anteriorly. Suture knots were buried beneath fascia.

Sponge and instrument counts were correct x3. Incisions were closed with 4-0 Vicryl subcuticular sutures, and Steri-Strips were applied over the wounds.

The patient tolerated the procedure well and was transported to the recovery area in good condition.

NEWBORN HISTORY & PHYSICAL EXAMINATION

HISTORY OF PRESENT ILLNESS: This infant, weight 3980 g, was born to a 22-year-old, gravida 1, para 0 Hispanic female at 39 weeks by dates, 41 weeks by Dubowitz exam. The mother did not receive prenatal care until late in her pregnancy, beginning at approximately 28 weeks. An ultrasound at that time revealed a large for gestational age, single intrauterine pregnancy.

Prenatal laboratory results include blood type O negative, negative RPR, negative HIV, gonorrhea, and Chlamydia, normal Pap smear, and urine culture was negative. She was given RhoGAM.

Prenatal vitamins were the only medications taken during her pregnancy. Of note was an elevated 1-hour Glucola test of 160. The fasting blood sugar was 84, 1-hour glucose 130, and 3-hour glucose was 100. She received dietary counseling but no other intervention.

Onset of labor was spontaneous, with the first stage lasting 9 hours, the second stage 2 hours, and the third stage 5 minutes. Spontaneous rupture of membranes occurred 3 hours before delivery, with clear amniotic fluid. The baby was delivered without anesthesia. The intact placenta appeared normal.

PHYSICAL EXAMINATION: The baby was resuscitated with drying, suction, and blow-by oxygen. Apgar scores were 7 at one minute and 9 at five minutes. Footprints were taken and shown to mother, and the baby was then taken to the level I nursery for care. GENERAL: Alert, vigorous newborn in no distress. SKIN: Warm, dry, well perfused. No lesions noted. HEAD: There is some caput over the crown. Anterior and posterior fontanelles are soft and flat; sutures are mobile. FACE: Symmetric, normal in appearance. EYES: Red reflex x2, sclerae clear, normal in overall appearance. EARS: Symmetrical, normal in appearance and position. No abnormalities noted. NOSE: Nares symmetrical; septum intact and midline. MOUTH: Hard and soft palates intact; tongue and uvula midline. Lips are normal in appearance. CHEST AND LUNGS: Normal shape. No retractions. Breath sounds clear bilaterally. No wheezes, rhonchi, or rales. HEART: Normal S1 and S2. No S3 or S4. Regular rate and rhythm; no murmurs heard. No rubs, heaves, or thrills. Peripheral pulses are 2+ and symmetrical. ABDOMEN: Soft, good bowel sounds present. Liver is 1 cm below the left costal margin. Spleen is not felt. BACK: Spine is midline. GENITOURINARY: Normal female genitalia, with no vaginal discharge. The anus is midline and patent. MUSCULOSKELETAL: She is moving all extremities without difficulty. There are no hip clicks bilaterally. NEUROLOGIC: Good suck, grasp, and Moro reflexes. Toes are up-going bilaterally.

IMPRESSION: Large for gestational age newborn female; hypoglycemia.

TREATMENT PLAN: Heel-stick glucose was 30 at 1 hour of life. She was fed 1 ounce of formula per os, with repeat glucose of 28. Baby received hepatitis B vaccine. She was given erythromycin ophthalmic ointment in both eyes and vitamin K. We will give baby glucose until glucose levels stay consistently above 40. We will check it every 2 hours.

PEDIATRIC NEUROBLASTOMA DISCHARGE SUMMARY

HISTORY OF PRESENT ILLNESS: The patient is a 20-month-old white male who was admitted with the chief complaint of recurrent opsoclonus and myoclonus. Six months before admission the patient had an MRI of the brain, which revealed no abnormalities. A whole-body CT scan was also negative. The symptoms improved but returned over time and worsened.

PHYSICAL EXAMINATION: The patient is an otherwise healthy child.

IMAGING STUDIES: On admission, the patient underwent a CT scan of his abdomen and pelvis. This revealed a midline presacral mass. MRI demonstrated invasion of the mass into the lowest sacral neural foramina on the left side. Bone scan was subsequently negative for metastases.

HOSPITAL COURSE: The patient was taken to surgery where pathological findings on transrectal biopsy confirmed our suspicion of neuroblastoma. Pathology reported positive lymph node involvement.

DISCHARGE PLAN: The patient will receive several cycles of chemotherapy in the next 2 months. If the size of the tumor is adequately decreased, we will schedule surgery to remove the tumor via posterior transsacral approach.

DIAGNOSIS: Neuroblastoma with metastatic spread to upper sacral lymph nodes.

PEDIATRIC PULMONOLOGY DISCHARGE SUMMARY

HISTORY OF PRESENT ILLNESS: The patient is a 5-year-old boy with Down syndrome. He was admitted for evaluation of an abnormal chest x-ray and complaints of wheezing and intermittent difficulty breathing.

PAST MEDICAL AND SURGICAL HISTORY: He was delivered at 36 weeks' gestation by cesarean section and weighed 4 pounds 2 ounces. The neonatal period was without respiratory problems. He was hospitalized at 9 months of age with bronchiolitis.

Surgical history includes bilateral myringotomy, with placement of polyethylene tubes and adenotonsillectomy at 1-1/2 years of age.

He was hospitalized last year with Mycoplasma pneumoniae. Treatment at that time included supplemental oxygen. Chest x-ray was improved at discharge, but follow-up x-rays at 3-month intervals revealed hyperinflation of the lungs and interstitial markings consistent with emphysema.

FAMILY HISTORY: His father died at 42 of myocardial infarction. His mother is 40 and well. There are 2 siblings, ages 10 and 7, who are in good health.

PHYSICAL EXAMINATION: HEENT: The patient has facial features consistent with Down syndrome. CHEST: Wheezing is heard bilaterally. The AP diameter is slightly increased, and he has a mild pectus deformity. The heart reveals a normal rate and rhythm, with a grade 1/6 to 2/6 systolic murmur. ABDOMEN: Normal to palpation. NEUROLOGIC: There is developmental delay and hypotonia.

LABORATORY DATA AND IMAGING STUDIES: Laboratory values were normal, including CBC, ESR, and IgE. Chest x-ray revealed the above-noted interstitial markings and hyperinflation. Chest CT revealed numerous bilateral bullae.

HOSPITAL COURSE: Oxygen saturation remained normal through his hospitalization. The patient gradually became asymptomatic, with improved chest x-ray.

DISCHARGE PLAN: The patient is discharged with albuterol p.r.n. Mother will bring him to the office in 1 week for follow-up. There are no diet or activity restrictions.

POSTPARTUM OVARIAN VEIN THROMBOSIS DISCHARGE SUMMARY

HISTORY OF PRESENT ILLNESS: The patient is a 25-year-old Hispanic female, G1, P2. The patient experienced a normal vaginal delivery of twins at 28 weeks' gestation. Approximately 4 hours after delivery she experienced pain in the right iliac fossa and right loin area, and she spiked a temperature to 103 degrees Fahrenheit. She complained of nausea but there was no vomiting. On exam there was exquisite tenderness in the right iliac fossa but no mass was felt.

HOSPITAL COURSE: An abdominal ultrasound was done and was normal. White blood count was elevated. The diagnosis of acute appendicitis was made, and she was taken to the operating suite where she underwent exploratory laparotomy. At surgery, the appendix was found to be normal. There was an inflamed retroperitoneal mass extending from the right side of the pelvis to the right lumbar area.

Postoperatively, a contrast-enhanced CT scan revealed thrombosis of the right ovarian vein extending into the inferior vena cava. This finding was confirmed on MRI.

She was treated for 10 days with intravenous heparin, amoxicillin, gentamicin, and metronidazole. The pain and fever subsequently resolved, and she was discharged on warfarin.

FOLLOW-UP: She is to be followed up in 3 days in the office, or sooner if there is need.

PRIMARY LOW-FLAP CESAREAN SECTION

DESCRIPTION OF PROCEDURE: The patient was taken to the operating room. After adequate spinal anesthesia, she was prepped and draped in the usual manner for cesarean section.

A Pfannenstiel incision was made taken down to the level of the rectus fascia. The fascia was incised and the incision was extended. The peritoneal cavity was bluntly entered and the incision was extended. The bladder flap was created and a bladder blade was placed.

A low transverse incision was made into the uterus. The vertex was elevated and noted to be in direct occiput posterior. The nasopharynx and oropharynx were suctioned, and the delivery of the infant was completed. The cord was clamped and cut, and the baby was handed to the pediatricians in attendance.

The infant received Apgar scores of 9 at one minute and 10 at five minutes. The placenta was delivered. The uterus was delivered through the incision. The incision was closed with 2 layers of 1-0 chromic suture, the first in a locking fashion and the second imbricating the first. Hemostasis was noted.

The abdomen was thoroughly irrigated and suctioned of all irrigation and blood clots. The bladder flap was closed with a running suture of 2-0 chromic. The uterus was returned to the abdominal cavity. The parietal peritoneum was closed with a running layer of 2-0 chromic suture. The fascia was closed with 0 Dexon suture. The skin was closed with skin staples.

TOTAL ABDOMINAL HYSTERECTOMY WITH BILATERAL SALPINGO-OOPHORECTOMY

DESCRIPTION OF PROCEDURE: Under satisfactory general anesthesia, Foley catheter was inserted in a sterile manner. The vagina was prepped with Betadine, the abdomen shaved as well as the pubic hair, and the patient was prepped and draped for a Pfannenstiel incision. This was carried down through the skin, the subcutaneous tissue. The fascia was incised transversely. The rectus muscles were separated and the peritoneum entered in a vertical manner. O'Sullivan-O'Connor retractor was utilized. Four laparotomy pads were placed at the pelvic brim to retract the bowel out of the pelvis and also to put a laparotomy pad under each blade of the retractor.

Visualization of the pelvis showed a normal-looking small uterus, normal tubes and ovaries. The round ligaments were bilaterally clamped, cut and suture ligated. The infundibulopelvic ligaments were bilaterally clamped, cut and suture ligated. The uterine blood vessels were bilaterally clamped, cut and suture ligated. A 0 Vicryl was used throughout the case. Approximately 4 bites were necessary on either side of the cervix to go down and take the cardinal ligament and paracervical tissue to reach the vaginal vault. The ligament was clamped, cut and suture ligated bilaterally.

On reaching the vaginal vault, the vagina was entered anteriorly and the specimen removed by cutting circumferentially about the cervix. The specimen thus consisted of uterus, cervix, tubes, and ovaries.

Angled sutures were placed bilaterally, incorporating the posterior vaginal mucosa, the anterior vaginal mucosa, and the cardinal ligament stump. The hemostatic running locking suture was then placed around the vaginal vault. There was a small opening for the vagina, and it was decided that no additional narrowing was necessary. One figure-of-eight suture was needed in the stump of the right cardinal ligament near the uterine stump. This made for good hemostasis.

The pelvis was then again peritonealized, utilizing 2-0 Vicryl with a locking suture in such a manner that the infundibular and round ligament stumps were placed in a retroperitoneal manner. Having closed the peritoneum, the pelvis was irrigated with saline and then attention directed to closure of the abdomen. It was noted at this point that the appendix was visible and appeared normal.

The peritoneum was closed with a running locking suture of 3-0 Vicryl. The rectus muscle approximated with a running locking suture of 2-0 Vicryl. The fascia was closed with 2 separate running locking sutures of 0 Vicryl starting laterally and tied separately in the midline. The wound was irrigated with Betadine. The subcutaneous tissue approximated was with a running locking suture of 2-0 Vicryl and the skin closed with staples.

Transverse Cesarean Section

Preoperative Diagnosis: Full-term pregnancy.

Postoperative Diagnosis: Full-term pregnancy, delivered.

Procedure Performed: Cesarean section.

Anesthesia: Spinal.

Estimated Blood Loss: 750 mL.

Indications for Procedure: The patient is a 28-year-old, gravida 3, para 2 who has had 2 previous cesarean section deliveries. She is at full term and comes now for delivery of her fetus.

Description of Procedure: All appropriate consent forms were signed, after which the patient was wheeled into the operating room. Spinal anesthesia was administered. She was placed in the supine position, and the abdomen was prepped and draped in the usual sterile manner.

After anesthetic was found to be adequate, a transverse incision was made and carried through subcutaneous tissues. Cauterization was applied to all bleeding points. Fascia of the rectus muscle was incised transversely and dissected upward and downward from the underlying abdominal muscles. After the abdominal muscles were spread apart, the peritoneum was identified and vertically incised. A bladder blade was then inserted, and the vesicouterine peritoneum was transversely incised. A bladder flap was created, and the bladder blade was reinserted. The lower uterine segment was transversely incised.

The amniotic fluid was clear. The fetus was in the cephalic presentation. The head was delivered, then the nose and mouth were suctioned and the rest of the baby girl was delivered manually. The infant was handed to the pediatrician for further care. The placenta was then delivered manually without difficulty. The uterine incision was closed in 2 layers using #1 chromic in a running locking fashion. Hemostasis was good.

The bladder flap was repaired with 2-0 Vicryl in running fashion. The uterus was returned into the peritoneal cavity and thoroughly lavaged with lactated Ringer solution to remove remaining blood clots and amniotic fluid. The peritoneum was closed with 0 PDS continuous interlocking sutures, and the skin was closed with staples.

Instrument and sponge counts were correct x2. The patient was taken to the recovery in satisfactory condition, with stable vital signs.

VAGINAL HYSTERECTOMY, ANTERIOR COLPORRHAPHY, KELLY PLICATION OF THE URETHRA, AND POSTERIOR COLPOPERINEORRHAPHY

DESCRIPTION OF PROCEDURE: With the patient under general anesthesia in the lithotomy position, she was prepped and draped in the usual manner. Bimanual examination was performed with the findings as noted above.

Labia minora were sutured to the labia majora, using silk sutures on each side. A weighted speculum was placed in the posterior wall of the vagina, and the cervix was grasped bilaterally with 2 tenacula.

An incision was made circumferentially around the cervicovaginal junction, after which the cervicovaginal mucosa was pushed upward. An Allis clamp was then placed between the uterosacral ligaments and an opening was made into the cul-de-sac and widened. Figure-of-eight sutures of 2-0 Vicryl were taken to approximate the peritoneum to the posterior vaginal mucosa. To control oozing, the middle suture was held long. The right and then the left uterosacral ligaments were doubly clamped. The left uterosacral ligament was then suture ligated with a suture also being placed in the vaginal mucosa on its respective side to form a new fornix of the vagina.

The more distal suture was placed on the uterosacral ligament distally, and this was held long. This was repeated on the right side. The right and the left uterine pedicles were then doubly clamped, cut, and suture ligated with sutures of 0 Vicryl. The weighted speculum was then placed in the cul-de-sac. A finger was inserted in front of the uterus to a level at the vesicouterine junction to ascertain this location. This area was then dissected free. Both bladder pillars were clamped, cut, and suture ligated with suture of 2-0 Vicryl. An opening was then made in the uterovesical peritoneum.

The uterus was then delivered posteriorly, after which double clamps were placed across the right medial portion of the right broad ligament, ovarian ligament, middle portion of the fallopian tube, and another clamp was placed across the lower portion of the broad ligament, including the round ligament. This too was doubly clamped, after which the right side of the uterus was freed.

Each pedicle was doubly suture ligated with sutures of 0 Vicryl. The distal suture on the region of the round ligament was held long. This was then repeated on the left side. Oozing was noted to be present, which was controlled with figure-of-eight sutures of 2-0 Vicryl until hemostasis was noted to have been obtained.

The ovaries were palpated and found to be normal. Lap, sponge, instrument, and needle count were reported to be correct.

The peritoneum was closed with a pursestring suture of 2-0 Vicryl, after the weighted speculum had been removed. Ties on the uterosacral ligaments were tied together as well as tied across the round ligaments on each side. These were then tied to each other, so that there was contralateral and ipsilateral tying. In this way, the pedicles were exteriorized and hemostasis was noted to be obtained.

Two Allis clamps were then placed at the base of the cystocele. Another Allis clamp was placed at the apex of the cystocele. The anterior vaginal mucosa was then incised at the midline to the Allis clamp at the apex of the cystocele. The vaginal mucosa was then dissected by sharp and blunt dissection from the underlying tissue. Bleeding was encountered laterally, which was controlled using figure-of-8 sutures of 2-0 Vicryl. A series of mattress sutures of 2-0 Vicryl were then taken to imbricate the cystocele. Two Kelly plication sutures of 2-0 Vicryl were then taken, and this gave good support to the urethra. A Foley catheter was then inserted into the urethra and urine was noted to be clear. The catheter was inserted easily without any evidence of obstruction.

Excess anterior vaginal mucosa was then excised, after which the anterior vagina was approximated using interrupted sutures of 2-0 Vicryl. Hemostasis was noted to have been obtained.

Attention was then turned to the posterior wall. Two Allis clamps were placed at the mucocutaneous junction in the region of the fourchette, and another clamp was placed at the apex of the rectocele. The tissue between the distal 2 clamps and the region of fourchette was excised, and carefully measured so that the introitus would be a 3-finger introitus. The posterior vaginal mucosa was then incised in the midline by sharp and blunt dissection. The posterior vaginal mucosa was then dissected to the level at the Allis clamp at the apex of the rectocele. The posterior vaginal mucosa was dissected with blunt and sharp dissection from the underlying tissue. The rectocele was then imbricated using mattress sutures of 2-0 Vicryl. Two sutures of 0 Vicryl were then taken in the levator ani musculature. The excess posterior vaginal mucosa was then excised, after which the posterior vaginal mucosa was approximated using interrupted sutures of 2-0 Vicryl. The stitches in the levator ani muscle were then tied in the midline, after which the closure of the posterior vaginal mucosa was continued using 2-0 Vicryl. The perineal muscles were then approximated in the midline in layers, using 2-0 Vicryl, after which the perineal skin was approximated using interrupted sutures of 2-0 Vicryl.

Hemostasis was noted to be present. Lap, sponge, instrument and needle count were reported to be correct. A finger was inserted into the rectum, and no stitches were present in the rectum. A 2-inch iodoform gauze was packed into the vagina. The Foley catheter was noted to be draining clear at the close of the procedure.

VIDEO-ASSISTED LAPAROSCOPIC SALPINGECTOMY, LYSIS OF ADHESIONS, AND CHROMOPERTUBATION

DESCRIPTION OF PROCEDURE: The patient was prepped and draped and placed in the lithotomy position. Examination under anesthesia revealed long, closed posterior cervix, normal-size uterus that was anteverted, a normal adnexa on the right, and a left adnexal mass about 5 cm.

Foley catheter was placed into the bladder, drained clear yellow urine, and the vaginal speculum was inserted to visualize a normal cervix, which was grasped anteriorly. A HUMI probe was put into the uterus at 7 cm.

The surgeons changed gloves and approached the abdomen. At this point, Veress needle was inserted in an infraumbilical incision and 3-1/2 liters of carbon dioxide gas created a pneumoperitoneum. At this point, a 10-mm trocar was inserted through the pneumoperitoneum, and we immediately noted that we were in an omental space. The trocar was removed, and a Versaport was put in. Under Versaport visualization, the trocar was inserted, and we noted that we were in the peritoneal cavity.

At this point, the liver was examined and found to be normal. The gallbladder was found to be normal. Attention was turned to the pelvic cavity. Immediately noted was a normal-size uterus and a very large, 5- to 6-cm ampullary tubal pregnancy.

We then placed a 5-mm and a 10-mm port in the left and right lower quadrants, through which we inserted our instruments.

The surgical assistant was able to raise the ectopic pregnancy while the surgeon, using the Davol and electrode needle, cut along the mesenteric edge. Immediately, the ectopic pregnancy started pumping furiously and immediately about 200 mL of blood were lost. We quickly placed a 12-mm trocar in and a GIA stapler in the right lower quadrant.

At this point, the GIA stapler on the right side was grasped by the assistant while the srugeon grasped the tubal pregnancy on the left side. Raising it up, the assistant was able to use the GIA stapler and clip the ectopic pregnancy. Immediately, the bleeding stopped; however, by this time we had about 500 mL of blood in the peritoneal cavity.

We then had to remove the entire tube at the ampullary end. Upon examination, however, we noted that the fimbriae of this tube were completely enmeshed into the ectopic pregnancy and there would not have been a chance to do a salpingostomy. The ectopic pregnancy was dropped into the Endosac and removed and sent to pathology.

At this point, copious irrigation was performed to remove all the clots and clearly examine the suture site of the left ectopic pregnancy.

Chromopertubation revealed that the suture line was completely clean and hemostatic. It also revealed that there was complete tubal occlusion of the right tube, showing a completely clogged fimbrial portion. The ovaries were noted to be normal, and the uterus was noted to be normal.

At this point, we completely removed all the clots and removed the instruments to remove the entire pneumoperitoneum. All the gas was removed. We placed 0 Vicryl sutures into the fascial areas of the infraumbilical and the right lower quadrant, and 4-0 undyed Vicryl closed all the skin incisions.

At this point, the HUMI and the Foley catheter were removed, and the patient was taken to the recovery room in stable condition.

VIDEO-ASSISTED LAPAROSCOPY FOR PELVIC PAIN

PREOPERATIVE DIAGNOSIS: Pelvic pain.

POSTOPERATIVE DIAGNOSES: Endometriosis. Right ovarian endometrioma. Tuboovarian adhesions, right.

PROCEDURES PERFORMED: Video-assisted laser laparoscopy, with ablation of endometriosis and right ovarian endometrioma. Lysis of right tuboovarian and ovarian adhesions.

FINDINGS AT PROCEDURE: There were multiple typical endometriosis spots identified on the anterior abdominal wall and on the broad ligaments of the cul-de-sac. The left tube and ovary had been surgically removed. The uterus was normal size, and no fibroids or adhesions were found. There was endometriosis on the right mesosalpinx, and toward the ovary the fimbriated end revealed filmy adhesions. The ovary was of normal size, shape, and consistency. It was bound to the pelvic sidewall with dense adhesions. An endometrioma 1 cm in diameter was found after lysing these adhesions. The bowel was free of adhesions. The appendix, gallbladder, and liver were anatomically correct and normal in appearance.

DESCRIPTION OF PROCEDURE: The patient was placed in the supine position and prepped and draped in the usual sterile manner. After pelvic examination, a Jarcho cannula was attached to the cervix. An infraumbilical incision was made, and a Veress needle was inserted into the peritoneal cavity. Approximately 2500 mL of carbon dioxide was insufflated. A trocar was inserted after removal of the Veress needle. Through the trocar, a 10-mm laser laparoscope was inserted. The laser laparoscope was affixed to the carbon dioxide generator. Findings were viewed on video screen.

The carbon dioxide laser was affixed to the laparoscopic operating channel, and the endometriosis on the anterior abdominal serosa, the broad ligament, and the cul-de-sac was ablated. Next, the right mesosalpinx was freed of endometriosis. The carbon dioxide laser was then used to lyse the adhesions between the ovary and tube on the right. The right ovary was mobilized by lysing the adhesions between the right ovary, the broad ligament, and the lateral pelvic sidewall. The 1-cm endometrioma was ablated.

The abdomen was copiously irrigated with lactated Ringer solution. Instruments were removed. Carbon dioxide was removed from the abdomen, and the incision was closed with 3-0 Vicryl running sutures. A sterile gauze pad was placed over the incision site. Sponge and instrument counts were correct x3.

The patient tolerated the procedure well and was taken to the recovery suite in satisfactory condition.

Appendix 6
Common Terms by Procedure

Acute Scrotal Pain Emergency Room Report
blood on urination
cremasteric reflex
hemiscrotum
marked tenderness

Adenotonsillectomy
adenoid
adenotonsillectomy
Bovie electrocautery
chronic tonsillitis
general endotracheal anesthesia
hemostasis
Mayo stand
McIvor mouth gag
mouth breather
obstructive adenoid
red rubber catheter
Rose position
shoulder roll
slotted tongue depressor
soft palate
suction cautery
superior constrictor muscle
tonsillar capsule

Bilateral Laparoscopic Tubal Ligation
adnexa
bipolar forceps
carbon dioxide
catheterized
Cefotan
cervix
cul-de-sac
3-0 Dexon suture
Foley catheter
Hegar dilator

Harris-Kronner uterine
manipulator/injector (HUMI)
HUMI cannula
laparoscope
laparoscopy
lithotomy position
multiparous
perineum
pneumoperitoneum
prepped and draped
routine fashion
Sims speculum
single-toothed tenaculum
trocar
umbilicus
urinary bladder
uterine cavity
vagina
Veress needle
vulva

Bilateral Tubal Ligation, Modified Pomeroy Method
abdominal cavity
abdominal wall
bilateral tubal ligation
day surgery recovery area
elective sterilization
hemostasis
knuckle of tube
peritoneum
0 plain tie
Pomeroy bilateral tubal ligation
prepped and draped
sharp dissection
sterile dressing
sterile manner
supine position
tubal ligation
3-0 Vicryl suture

Dilatation And Curettage

dilatation and curettage
dorsal lithotomy position
double-tooth tenaculum
irregular vaginal bleeding
products of conception
recovery area
retained products of conception
spontaneous abortion
suction curette
usual sterile fashion
vaginal bleeding
weighted speculum

Ectopic Pregnancy Discharge Summary

amenorrhea
cervical canal
cervical ectopic pregnancy
ectopic gestational sac
ectopic pregnancy
endometrial hypervascularity
evacuation
fetal demise
gestational sac
G4, P2, AB1
live gestation
methotrexate therapy
normal uterine cavity
potassium chloride
sonogram
transvaginal intracardiac instillation
uterine artery embolization
vaginal spotting

Endometrial Cancer History & Physical

adjuvant therapy
adnexal cyst
appendectomy
atypia
axillary dissection

benign proliferative polyp
bilateral salpingo-oophorectomy
endometrial adenocarcinoma
endometrial polyp
endometrial thickening
estrogen receptor
grade 3 infiltrating duct carcinoma
gravida 4, para 4
heterogeneous cyst
homogeneous cyst
hormonal receptor
hormonal treatment
infiltrating duct carcinoma
lumpectomy
lymph node positive
oncologic history
operative hysteroscopy
Pap smear
postmenopausal
progesterone receptor
radiotherapy
tamoxifen
tonsillectomy
vaginal hysterectomy
vaginal ultrasound

Genetics Consultation: Angelman Syndrome

Angelman syndrome
background slowing
choking
chromosome 15
developmental delay
distractible
drooling
electroencephalogram (EEG)
exon 9
full-term, uncomplicated pregnancy
gagging
global development milestone delay
gray matter
head circumference
hyperactive

incomplete myelination
involuntary hand movement
periventricular white matter
posterior region
postnatal onset microcephaly
putamen
rhythmic delta run
sequence analysis
speech impairment
temporal lobe
UBE3A gene
up-going toe
variant
white matter
wide-based gait

Henoch-Schönlein Consultation

colicky abdominal pain
erythematous lesion
Henoch-Schönlein purpura
joint pain
macular eruption
nonblanching
pinna
upper respiratory infection

Hypopituitarism in Infant History & Physical

anterior fontanelle
bilirubin
blood culture
blood sugar
cortisol
cry response
duskiness
gag reflex
gestational age
growth hormone
hyperbilirubinemia
hypoglycemia
hypopituitarism
jaundiced infant
magnetic resonance imaging (MRI)

molding of the head
Moro reflex
neonatal intensive care unit
oxygen supplementation
phototherapy
posterior fontanelle
septic workup
serum insulin
suck reflex
thyroid-stimulating hormone (TSH)
total testosterone
white blood count

Hysterectomy Discharge Summary

adnexal mass
bilateral salpingo-oophorectomy
bowel function
dilatation and curettage
electrocardiogram (EKG)
endometrium
exploratory laparotomy
fibromyoma
frozen section
gravida 2, para 2 female
pelvic examination
pelvic mass
postoperative course
total abdominal hysterectomy
uterine adenomyosis
uterine fibromyoma
vaginal ultrasound

Infant With Intrauterine and Neonatal Complications Discharge Summary

anti-Kell antibody
Apgar score
ascites
blueberry muffin spot
cesarean section
cord blood
cordocentesis

cytomegalovirus culture
direct Coombs test
erythroblast
erythropoietin concentration
fetal monitoring
gravida 3, para 2 woman
hematopoiesis
hemolytic disease
hepatitis B
hydrops
intrauterine transfusion
leukopenia
lues
mild respiratory distress
packed red blood cells
parvovirus
reticulocyte count
rubella
serological testing
tachypnea
thrombocytopenia
toxoplasmosis
transient oxygen
ultrasound study
umbilical cord blood

Infertility Referral Letter

appropriately timed intercourse
birth control pills
dysmenorrhea
endometriosis
fallopian tube
hysterosalpingogram
infertility
irregular menstrual cycles
menstrual irregularity
morphology
motility
Norinyl
ovulatory pattern
patency of the fallopian tubes bilaterally
semen analysis
unprotected intercourse

Laparoscopic Uterine Suspension

abdominal wall
cervix
Ethicon suture
fascial bridge
general anesthesia
grasper
incision site
infraumbilical incision
intraperitoneal position
laparoscope
laparoscopic trocar and sheath
laparoscopic uterine suspension
local anesthesia
MetraPass suture passer
plication
prepped and draped
pubic symphysis
round ligament
single-toothed tenaculum
speculum
Steri-Strips
straight catheter
subcuticular suture
suprapubic incision
suture passer
usual sterile manner
uterine cavity
uterine manipulator
uterine prolapse
vagina
4-0 Vicryl subcuticular suture

Newborn History & Physical Examination

amniotic fluid
anterior fontanelle
Apgar score
blood type O negative
blow-by oxygen
caput
chlamydia

clear amniotic fluid
costal margin
dietary counseling
Dubowitz exam
erythromycin ophthalmic ointment
fasting blood sugar
first stage of labor
gestational age
Glucola test
glucose level
gonorrhea
grasp reflex
hepatitis B vaccine
1-hour glucose
3-hour glucose
human immunodeficiency virus (HIV)
hypoglycemia
intact placenta
intrauterine pregnancy
large for gestational age
Moro reflex
normal female genitalia
Pap smear
per os
posterior fontanelle
prenatal laboratory
prenatal vitamins
rapid plasma reagin (RPR)
red reflex
RhoGAM
second stage of labor
spontaneous rupture of membranes
suck reflex
third stage of labor
urine culture
vaginal discharge
vitamin K

Pediatric Neuroblastoma Discharge Summary

bone scan
chemotherapy
computed tomography (CT)

cycle of chemotherapy
lymph node involvement
magnetic resonance imaging (MRI)
metastasis
metastatic spread
myoclonus
neural foramina
neuroblastoma
opsoclonus
pathological finding
posterior transsacral approach
presacral mass
sacral neural foramina
transrectal biopsy
upper sacral lymph node
whole-body CT scan

Pediatric Pulmonology Discharge Summary

abnormal chest x-ray
activity restriction
adenotonsillectomy
albuterol
anteroposterior (AP)
AP diameter
asymptomatic
bilateral myringotomy
bronchiolitis
bulla
complete blood count (CBC)
cesarean section
developmental delay
dietary restriction
Down syndrome
emphysema
erythrocyte sedimentation rate (ESR)
grade 1/6 to 2/6
hyperinflation
hypotonia
immunoglobulin E (IgE)
intermittent difficulty breathing
interstitial marking
laboratory value

Mycoplasma pneumoniae
myocardial infarction
neonatal period
normal to palpation
oxygen saturation
pectus deformity
polyethylene tube
respiratory problem
supplemental oxygen
systolic murmur
wheezing

Postpartum Ovarian Vein Thrombosis Discharge Summary

abdominal ultrasound
acute appendicitis
amoxicillin
exploratory laparotomy
exquisite tenderness
gentamicin
G1, P2
heparin
iliac fossa
magnetic resonance imaging (MRI)
metronidazole
normal vaginal delivery
retroperitoneal mass
right iliac fossa
right loin
warfarin
28 weeks' gestation

Primary Low-Flap Cesarean Section

abdominal cavity
Apgar score
bladder flap
cesarean section
1-0 chromic suture
0 Dexon suture
direct occiput posterior
imbricating stitch

locking fashion
low transverse incision
nasopharynx
oropharynx
parietal peritoneum
peritoneal cavity
Pfannenstiel incision
placenta
prepped and draped
rectus fascia
running layer
running suture
skin staples
spinal anesthesia
usual manner
uterus
vertex

Total Abdominal Hysterectomy with Bilateral Salpingo-Oophorectomy

angled suture
Betadine
bilaterally clamped, cut and suture ligated
cardinal ligament
cervix
clamped, cut and suture ligated
figure-of-eight suture
Foley catheter
general anesthesia
hemostatic
infundibulopelvic ligament
laparotomy pad
ligament stump
normal-looking small uterus
normal tubes and ovaries
O'Sullivan-O'Connor retractor
paracervical tissue
pelvic brim
peritoneum
Pfannenstiel incision
prepped and draped
pubic hair

A87

rectus muscle
retract the bowel
round ligament
running locking suture
satisfactory general anesthesia
sterile manner
subcutaneous tissue
uterine blood vessel
uterus, cervix, tubes and ovaries
vaginal mucosa
vaginal vault
vertical manner
0 Vicryl suture

Transverse Cesarean Section

abdominal muscle
amniotic fluid
bladder blade
bladder flap
bleeding point
blood clot
cauterization
cephalic presentation
cesarean section delivery
consent form
continuous interlocking suture
delivered manually
full-term pregnancy
gravida 3, para 2
hemostasis
incised transversely
instrument and sponge count
lactated Ringer solution
lower uterine segment
0 PDS continuous interlocking suture
peritoneal cavity
peritoneum
prepped and draped
running fashion
running locking fashion
satisfactory condition
spinal anesthesia
stable vital signs

staples
subcutaneous tissue
supine position
thoroughly lavaged
transverse incision
transversely incised
usual sterile manner
uterine incision
vesicouterine peritoneum

Vaginal Hysterectomy, Anterior Colporrhaphy, Kelly Plication of the Urethra, and Posterior Colpoperineorrhaphy

Allis clamp
apex
approximated
bimanual examination
bladder pillar
broad ligament
cervicovaginal junction
cervicovaginal mucosa
cervix
contralateral
cul-de-sac
cystocele
doubly clamped
exteriorized
fallopian tube
figure-of-eight suture
3-finger introitus
Foley catheter
fornix
fourchette
general anesthesia
hemostasis
imbricate
interrupted suture
introitus
iodoform gauze
ipsilateral
Kelly plication suture

labia majora
labia minora
lap, sponge, instrument and needle
   count
levator ani muscle
lithotomy position
mattress suture
mucocutaneous junction
ovarian ligament
perineal muscle
peritoneum
plication suture
posterior vaginal mucosa
posterior wall
prepped and draped
pursestring suture
rectocele
round ligament
sharp and blunt dissection
silk suture
suture ligated
tenaculum
urethra
usual manner
uterine pedicle
uterosacral ligament
uterovesical peritoneum
vagina
vaginal mucosa
vesicouterine junction
2-0 Vicryl suture
weighted speculum

Video-Assisted Laparoscopic Salpingectomy, Lysis of Adhesions, and Chromopertubation

adnexal mass
ampullary tubal pregnancy
carbon dioxide gas
chromopertubation
clear yellow urine
copious irrigation

ectopic pregnancy
electrode needle
Endosac
examination under anesthesia
fascial area
fimbrial portion
Foley catheter
GIA stapler
Harris-Kronner uterine
   manipulator/injector (HUMI)
hemostatic
HUMI probe
infraumbilical incision
lithotomy position
normal adnexa
normal-size uterus
omental space
peritoneal cavity
pneumoperitoneum
prepped and draped
recovery room
right lower quadrant
salpingostomy
stable condition
trocar
tubal pregnancy
4-0 undyed Vicryl suture
vaginal speculum
Versaport
0 Vicryl suture

Video-Assisted Laparoscopy for Pelvic Pain

abdominal serosa
ablated
ablation
adhesion
anterior abdominal wall
broad ligament
carbon dioxide generator
correct x3
cul-de-sac
dense adhesions

endometrioma
endometriosis spot
fibroid
filmy adhesion
fimbriated end
gauze pad
incision site
infraumbilical incision
insufflated
Jarcho cannula
lactated Ringer solution
laparoscopic operating channel
laser laparoscopy
lysis of adhesions
mesosalpinx
normal size, shape, and consistency

ovarian endometrioma
ovary
pelvic pain
pelvic sidewall
peritoneal cavity
prepped and draped
recovery suite
satisfactory condition
sponge and instrument counts
supine position
trocar
tube and ovary
tuboovarian adhesion
usual sterile manner
Veress needle
video-assisted laser laparoscopy

Appendix 7
Apgar Score

After 60 seconds	Score	0	1	2
heart rate	-----	absent	under 100	over 100
respiratory effort	------	absent	slow, irregular	good (screams)
muscle tone	------	limp	good in limbs	active movement
reaction to nasal catheter	------	none	makes grimaces	cough or sneezing
skin color	------	pale	rosy trunk, blue extremities	rosy
Score	------	(total points: 8-10 is normal)		

Developmental Milestones From Birth to 5 Years

Age (Months)	Adaptive/Fine Motor	Language	Gross Motor	Personal-Social
1	Grasp reflex (hands fisted)	Facial response to sounds	Lifts head in prone position	Stares at face
2	Follows object with eyes past midline	Coos (vowel sounds)	Lifts head in prone position to 45°	Smiles in response to others
4	Hands open; brings objects to mouth	Laughs and squeals; turns toward voice	Sits; head steady; rolls to supine	Smiles spontaneously
6	Palmar grasp of objects	Babbles (consonant sounds)	Sits independently; stands, hands held	Reaches for toys; recognizes strangers
9	Pincer grasp	Says "mama" and "dada" nonspecifically; comprehends "no"	Pulls to stand	Feeds self; waves bye-bye
12	Helps turn pages of book	2-4 words; follows command with gesture	Stands independently; walks, 1 hand held	Points to indicate wants
15	Scribbles	4-6 words; follows command with no gesture	Walks independently	Drinks from cup, imitates activities
18	Turns pages of book	10-20 words; points to 4 body parts	Walks up steps	Feeds self with spoon
24	Solves single-piece puzzles	Combines 2-3 words; uses "I" and "you"	Jumps; kicks ball	Removes coat; verbalizes wants
30	Imitates horizontal and vertical lines	Names all body parts	Rides tricycle using pedals	Pulls up pants; washes and dries hands
36	Copies circle; draws person with 3 parts	Gives full name, age, and sex; names 2 colors	Throws ball overhand; walks up stairs (alternating feet)	Toilet trained; puts on shirt, knows front from back
42	Copies cross	Understands "cold," "tired," "hungry"	Stands on 1 foot for 2-3 seconds	Engages in associative play
48	Counts 4 objects; identifies some numbers and letters	Understands prepositions (under, on, behind, in front of); asks "how" and "why"	Hops on 1 foot	Dresses with little assistance; shoes on correct feet

Age (Months)	Adaptive/Fine Motor	Language	Gross Motor	Personal-Social
54	Copies square; draws person with 6 parts	Understands opposites	Broad-jumps 24 inches	Bosses and criticizes; shows off
60	Prints first name; counts 10 objects	Asks meaning of words	Skips (alternating feet)	Ties shoes

Recommended Immunizations

Immunization	Recommended Age
Diphtheria, tetanus, pertussis (DTaP)	2 months 4 months 6 months 15 months to 18 months 4 years to 6 years
Haemophilus influenzae type b (Hib)	2 months 4 months 6 months 12 months to 15 months
Hepatitis A (Hep A)	24 months to 18 years (in selected areas)
Hepatitis B virus vaccine (Hep B)	#1: Birth to 1 month #2: 1 month to 4 months #3: 6 months to 18 months
Inactivated poliovirus (IPV)	2 months 4 months 6 months to 18 months 4 years to 6 years
Influenza	6 months, then yearly (in selected areas)
Measles, mumps, rubella (MMR)	12 months to 15 months 4 years to 6 years
Pneumococcal conjugate (PCV)	2 months 4 months 6 months 12 months to 15 months
Td	11 years to 12 years Every 10 years throughout life
Varicella (Var)	12 months to 18 months

For additional information, please visit the Centers for Disease Control and Prevention (CDC) National Immunization Program (NIP) web site at *http://www.cdc.gov/nip/*

Routine Immunization of HIV-Infected Children in the United States

Vaccine	Known Asymptomatic HIV Infection	Symptomatic HIV Infection
Diphtheria, tetanus, pertussis (DTaP) [or DTP]	Yes	Yes
Haemophilus influenzae type b (Hib)	Yes	Yes
Hepatitis B	Yes	Yes
Inactivated poliovirus (IPV)*	Yes	Yes
Influenza§	Yes	Yes
Measles, mumps, rubella (MMR)	Yes	Yes†
Pneumococcal conjugate vaccine (PCV)‡	Yes	Yes
Rotavirus	No	No
Streptococcus pneumoniae	Yes	Yes
Varicella‖	No	No

Adapted from the American Academy of Pediatrics. In Peter G, ed. *1997 Red Book: Report of the Committee on Infectious Diseases.* 24th ed. Elk Grove Village, IL: American Academy of Pediatrics, 1997.

*Only inactivated polio vaccine (IPV) should be used for HIV-infected children, HIV-exposed infants whose status is indeterminate, and household contacts of HIV-infected patients.

† Severely immunocompromised HIV-infected children should not receive MMR vaccine.

‡ Pneumococcal vaccine should be administered at 2 years of age to all HIV-infected children. Children who are older than 2 years of age should receive pneumococcal vaccine at the time of diagnosis. Revaccination after 3 to 5 years is recommended in either circumstance.

§ Influenza vaccine should be provided each fall and repeated annually for HIV-exposed infants 6 months of age and older, HIV-infected children and adolescents, and for household contacts of HIV-infected patients.

‖ Varicella vaccine is not currently indicated for HIV-exposed or HIV-infected patients, but studies are in progress to determine safety and possible indication.

Appendix 11
Oral Rehydration Fluids and Infant Formulas

Commercially Available Oral Rehydration Formulas

Lytren

Pedialyte

Rehydralyte

WHO Formula

Infant Formulas

Cow's milk-based standard formulas	Soy-based standard formulas	Preterm formulas	Special formulas #
Enfamil (Mead Johnson); with/without iron	Isomil (Ross)	Similac Special Care (Ross)	Nutramigen (Mead Johnson)
Similac (Ross); with/without iron	ProSobee (Mead Johnson)	Enfamil Premature (Mead Johnson); with/without iron	Pregestimil (Mead Johnson)
PM 60/40 (Ross)†		Similac NeoSure (Ross)‖	Portagen (Mead Johnson)
Gerber; with/without iron (Gerber)			Alimentum (Ross)‖
Good Start (Carnation)†			Lactofree (Mead Johnson) Neocate (Scientific Hospital Supplies, Inc.)

‖ Available only as ready-to-feed formula.

† Formula with a low renal solute load.

Indications for Special Formulas:

Name	Indications
Nutramigen	Cow's milk allergy, severe or multiple food allergies, severe or persistent diarrhea, galactosemia
Pregestimil	Malabsorption, intestinal resection, severe or persistent diarrhea, food allergies
Portagen	Steatorrhea secondary to cystic fibrosis, intestinal reactions, pancreatic insufficiency, biliary atresia, lymphatic anomalies, celiac disease
Alimentum	Problems with digestion or absorption, severe or prolonged diarrhea, cystic fibrosis, steatorrhea, food allergies, intestinal resection
Lactofree	Lactose intolerance without cow's milk mild protein intolerance
Neocate	Cow's milk mild allergy, soy and protein hydrolysate intolerance, multiple food protein intolerances

Appendix 12
Common Poisonings and Their Antidotes

Poison by Category	Antidote
acetaminophen	acetylcysteine (Mucomyst)
alcohols	
ethylene glycol, methanol, folinic acid	ethanol, folic acid (Folvite)
anticholinergics	
diphenhydramine, benztropine	physostigmine (Antilirium)
anticoagulants	
coumarin derivatives	vitamin K1 (AquaMEPHYTON, Mephyton)
heparin	protamine
benzodiazepines	flumazenil (Romazicon)
botulism	botulinum antitoxin
carbon monoxide	oxygen
carbon tetrachloride	acetylcysteine (Mucomyst)
cardiac medications	
beta-adrenergic blockers	glucagon
calcium channel blockers	calcium chloride
digoxin	digoxin immune fab (Digibind)
cholinergics	
organophosphates, carbamates	atropine, pralidoxime
cyanide	amyl nitrate, sodium nitrite, sodium thiosulfate, methylene blue, hydroxocobalamin
hydrofluoric acid	calcium gluconate
iron	deferoxamine mesylate (Desferal)
isoniazid	pyridoxine (Aminoxin)
lead	edetate calcium disodium (calcium disodium versenate)
opioids	naloxone (Narcan), nalmefene (Revex), naltrexone (ReVia)
organophosphates, anticholinesterases	atropine, pralidoxime (2-PAM, Protopam)
salicylates	sodium bicarbonate (Neut)
tricyclic antidepressants	sodium bicarbonate (Neut)

Appendix 13
Drugs by Indication

ABDOMINAL DISTENTION (POSTOPERATIVE)
Hormone, Posterior Pituitary
  Pitressin® [US]
  Pressyn® AR [Can]
  Pressyn® [Can]
  vasopressin

ABETALIPOPROTEINEMIA
Vitamin, Fat Soluble
  Amino-Opti-E® [US-OTC]
  Aquasol A® [US]
  Aquasol E® [US-OTC]
  E-Complex-600® [US-OTC]
  E-Vitamin® [US-OTC]
  Palmitate-A® [US-OTC]
  vitamin A
  vitamin E
  Vita-Plus® E Softgels® [US-OTC]
  Vitec® [US-OTC]
  Vite E® Creme [US-OTC]

ABORTION
Antiprogestin
  Mifeprex® [US]
  mifepristone
Electrolyte Supplement, Oral
  sodium chloride
Oxytocic Agent
  oxytocin
  Pitocin® [US/Can]
Prostaglandin
  carboprost tromethamine
  Cervidil® Vaginal Insert
    [US/Can]
  dinoprostone
  Hemabate™ [US/Can]
  Prepidil® Vaginal Gel [US/Can]
  Prostin E2® Vaginal Suppository
    [US/Can]

ACETAMINOPHEN POISONING
Mucolytic Agent
  acetylcysteine
  Acys-5® [US]
  Mucomyst® [US/Can]
  Parvolex® [Can]

ACNE
Acne Products
  Acetoxyl® [Can]
  adapalene
  Akne-Mycin® [US]
  Alti-Clindamycin [Can]
  Apo®-Clindamycin [Can]
  A/T/S® [US]
  Benoxyl® [Can]
  Benzac® AC Wash [US]
  Benzac® [US]
  Benzac® W Wash [US/Can]
  Benzagel® [US]
  Benzagel® Wash [US]
  Benzamycin® [US]
  Benzashave® [US]
  benzoyl peroxide
  benzoyl peroxide and
    hydrocortisone
  Brevoxyl® Cleansing [US]
  Brevoxyl® [US]
  Brevoxyl® Wash [US]
  Cleocin HCl® [US]
  Cleocin Pediatric® [US]
  Cleocin Phosphate® [US]
  Cleocin T® [US]
  Cleocin® [US]
  Clinac™ BPO [US]
  Clindagel™ [US]
  Clindamax [US]
  clindamycin
  Clindets® [US]

Clindoxyl® Gel [Can]
cyproterone and ethinyl estradiol
(Canada only)
Dalacin® C [Can]
Dalacin® T [Can]
Del Aqua® [US]
Desquam-E™ [US]
Desquam-X® [US/Can]
Diane®-35 [Can]
Differin® [US/Can]
Emgel® [US]
Erycette® [US]
EryDerm® [US]
Erygel® [US]
Erythra-Derm™ [US]
erythromycin and benzoyl peroxide
erythromycin (ophthalmic/topical)
Exact® Acne Medication [US-OTC]
Fostex® 10% BPO [US-OTC]
Loroxide® [US-OTC]
Neutrogena® Acne Mask [US-OTC]
Neutrogena® On The Spot® Acne
Treatment [US-OTC]
Novo-Clindamycin [Can]
Oxy 10® Balanced Medicated Face
Wash [US-OTC]
Oxyderm™ [Can]
Palmer's® Skin Success Acne
[US-OTC]
PanOxyl®-AQ [US]
PanOxyl® Bar [US-OTC]
PanOxyl® [US/Can]
ratio-Clindamycin [Can]
Romycin® [US]
Seba-Gel™ [US]
Solugel® [Can]
Staticin® [US]
Theramycin Z® [US]
Triaz® Cleanser [US]
Triaz® [US]
T-Stat® [US]
Vanoxide-HC® [US/Can]
Zapzyt® [US-OTC]

Antibiotic, Topical
Apo®-Metronidazole [Can]
Flagyl ER® [US]
Flagyl® [US/Can]
Florazole ER® [Can]
MetroCream® [US/Can]
MetroGel® Topical [US/Can]
MetroLotion® [US]
metronidazole
Nidagel™ [Can]
Noritate® [US/Can]
Novo-Nidazol [Can]
Trikacide® [Can]
Antiseborrheic Agent, Topical
AVAR™ Cleanser [US]
AVAR™ Green [US]
AVAR™ [US]
Aveeno® Cleansing Bar [US-OTC]
Clenia™ [US]
Fostex® [US-OTC]
Nocosyn™ [US]
Pernox® [US-OTC]
Plexion SCT™ [US]
Plexion™ TS [US]
Plexion® [US]
Rosanil™ [US]
Rosula® [US]
Sastid® Plain Therapeutic Shampoo
and Acne Wash [US-OTC]
Sulfacet-R® [US]
sulfur and salicylic acid
sulfur and sulfacetamide
Zetacet® [US]
Estrogen and Androgen Combination
cyproterone and ethinyl estradiol
(Canada only)
Diane®-35 [Can]
Keratolytic Agent
Avage™ [US]
Compound W® One Step Wart
Remover [US-OTC]
Compound W® [US-OTC]
DHS™ Sal [US-OTC]

A99

Dr. Scholl's® Callus Remover [US-OTC]

Dr. Scholl's® Clear Away [US-OTC]

Duoforte® 27 [Can]

Freezone® [US-OTC]

Fung-O® [US-OTC]

Gordofilm® [US-OTC]

Hydrisalic™ [US-OTC]

Ionil® Plus [US-OTC]

Ionil® [US-OTC]

Keralyt® [US-OTC]

LupiCare™ Dandruff [US-OTC]

LupiCare™ II Psoriasis [US-OTC]

LupiCare™ Psoriasis [US-OTC]

Mediplast® [US-OTC]

MG217 Sal-Acid® [US-OTC]

Mosco® Corn and Callus Remover [US-OTC]

NeoCeuticals™ Acne Spot Treatment [US-OTC]

Neutrogena® Acne Wash [US-OTC]

Neutrogena® Body Clear™ [US-OTC]

Neutrogena® Clear Pore Shine Control [US-OTC]

Neutrogena® Clear Pore [US-OTC]

Neutrogena® Healthy Scalp [US-OTC]

Neutrogena® Maximum Strength T/Sal® [US-OTC]

Neutrogena® On The Spot® Acne Patch [US-OTC]

Occlusal™ [Can]

Occlusal®-HP [US/Can]

Oxy® Balance Deep Pore [US-OTC]

Oxy Balance® [US-OTC]

Palmer's® Skin Success Acne Cleanser [US-OTC]

Pedisilk® [US-OTC]

Propa pH [US-OTC]

Sal-Acid® [US-OTC]

Salactic® [US-OTC]

SalAc® [US-OTC]

salicylic acid

Sal-Plant® [US-OTC]

Sebcur® [Can]

Soluver® [Can]

Soluver® Plus [Can]

Stri-dex® Body Focus [US-OTC]

Stri-dex® Facewipes To Go™ [US-OTC]

Stri-dex® Maximum Strength [US-OTC]

Stri-dex® [US-OTC]

tazarotene

Tazorac® [US/Can]

Tinamed® [US-OTC]

Tiseb® [US-OTC]

Trans-Ver-Sal® [US-OTC/Can]

Wart-Off® Maximum Strength [US-OTC]

Zapzyt® Acne Wash [US-OTC]

Zapzyt® Pore Treatment [US-OTC]

Retinoic Acid Derivative

Accutane® [US/Can]

Altinac™ [US]

Amnesteem™ [US]

Avita® [US]

Claravis™ [US]

isotretinoin

Isotrex® [Can]

Rejuva-A® [Can]

Renova® [US]

Retin-A® Micro [US/Can]

Retin-A® [US/Can]

Retinova® [Can]

tretinoin (topical)

Tetracycline Derivative

Alti-Minocycline [Can]

Apo®-Minocycline [Can]

Apo®-Tetra [Can]

Brodspec® [US]

Declomycin® [US/Can]

demeclocycline
Dynacin® [US]
EmTet® [US]
Gen-Minocycline [Can]
Minocin® [US/Can]
minocycline
Novo-Minocycline [Can]
Novo-Tetra [Can]
Nu-Tetra [Can]
ratio-Minocycline [Can]
Rhoxal-minocycline [Can]
Sumycin® [US]
tetracycline
Wesmycin® [US]
Topical Skin Product
azelaic acid
Azelex® [US]
BenzaClin® [US]
clindamycin and benzoyl peroxide
Duac™ [US]
Finacea™ [US]
Finevin® [US]
Topical Skin Product, Acne
BenzaClin® [US]
clindamycin and benzoyl peroxide
Duac™ [US]

ACQUIRED IMMUNODEFICIENCY SYNDROME (AIDS)
Antiretroviral Agent, Fusion Protein
    Inhibitor
enfuvirtide
Fuzeon™ [US/Can]
Antiretroviral Agent, Non-nucleoside
    Reverse Transcriptase Inhibitor
    (NNRTI)
Kaletra™ [US/Can]
lopinavir and ritonavir
Antiretroviral Agent, Nucleoside
    Reverse Transcriptase Inhibitor
    (NRTI)
abacavir, lamivudine, and zidovudine

Trizivir® [US/Can]
Antiretroviral Agent, Protease Inhibitor
atazanavir
Reyataz™ [US]
Antiretroviral Agent, Reverse
    Transcriptase Inhibitor
    (Nucleoside)
emtricitabine
Emtriva™ [US]
Antiretroviral Agent, Reverse
    Transcriptase Inhibitor
    (Nucleotide)
tenofovir
Viread™ [US]
Antiviral Agent
Apo®-Zidovudine [Can]
AZT™ [Can]
Combivir® [US/Can]
Crixivan® [US/Can]
delavirdine
didanosine
Epivir-HBV® [US]
Epivir® [US]
Fortovase® [US/Can]
Heptovir® [Can]
Hivid® [US/Can]
indinavir
Invirase® [US/Can]
lamivudine
nelfinavir
nevirapine
Norvir® SEC [Can]
Norvir® [US/Can]
Novo-AZT [Can]
Rescriptor® [US/Can]
Retrovir® [US/Can]
ritonavir
saquinavir
stavudine
3TC® [Can]
Videx® EC [US/Can]
Videx® [US/Can]
Viracept® [US/Can]

Viramune® [US/Can]
zalcitabine
Zerit® [US/Can]
zidovudine
zidovudine and lamivudine
Nonnucleoside Reverse Transcriptase
    Inhibitor (NNRTI)
efavirenz
Sustiva® [US/Can]
Nucleoside Reverse Transcriptase
    Inhibitor (NRTI)
abacavir
Ziagen® [US/Can]
Protease Inhibitor
Agenerase® [US/Can]
amprenavir

ADRENOCORTICAL FUNCTION ABNORMALITY

Adrenal Corticosteroid
    Acthar® [US]
    A-HydroCort® [US]
    A-methapred® [US]
    Apo®-Prednisone [Can]
    Aristocort® Forte Injection [US]
    Aristocort® Intralesional Injection
        [US]
    Aristocort® Tablet [US/Can]
    Aristospan® Intraarticular Injection
        [US/Can]
    Aristospan® Intralesional Injection
        [US/Can]
    Betaject™ [Can]
    betamethasone (systemic)
    Betnesol® [Can]
    Celestone® Phosphate [US]
    Celestone® Soluspan® [US/Can]
    Celestone® [US]
    Cel-U-Jec® [US]
    Cortef® Tablet [US/Can]
    corticotropin
    cortisone acetate
    Cortone® [Can]

Decadron®-LA [US]
Decadron® [US/Can]
Decaject-LA® [US]
Decaject® [US]
Deltasone® [US]
Depo-Medrol® [US/Can]
Depopred® [US]
dexamethasone (systemic)
Dexasone® L.A. [US]
Dexasone® [US/Can]
Dexone® LA [US]
Dexone® [US]
Hexadrol® [US/Can]
H.P. Acthar® Gel [US]
hydrocortisone (systemic)
Kenalog® Injection [US/Can]
Medrol® Dosepak™ [US/Can]
Medrol® Tablet [US/Can]
methylprednisolone
Orapred™ [US]
Pediapred® [US/Can]
PMS-Dexamethasone [Can]
Prednicot® [US]
prednisolone (systemic)
Prednisol® TBA [US]
prednisone
Prednisone Intensol™ [US]
Prelone® [US]
ratio-Dexamethasone [Can]
Solu-Cortef® [US/Can]
Solu-Medrol® [US/Can]
Solurex L.A.® [US]
Sterapred® DS [US]
Sterapred® [US]
Tac™-3 Injection [US]
Triam-A® Injection [US]
triamcinolone (systemic)
Triam Forte® Injection [US]
Winpred™ [Can]
Adrenal Corticosteroid
    (Mineralocorticoid)
    Florinef® Acetate [US/Can]
    fludrocortisone

ALPHA-1 ANTITRYPSIN DEFICIENCY (CONGENITAL)

Antitrypsin Deficiency Agent
    alpha-1-proteinase inhibitor
    Aralast™ [US]
    Prolastin® [US/Can]
    Zemaira™ [US]

AMEBIASIS

Amebicide
    Apo®-Metronidazole [Can]
    Diodoquin® [Can]
    Diquinol® [US]
    Flagyl ER® [US]
    Flagyl® [US/Can]
    Florazole ER® [Can]
    Humatin® [US/Can]
    iodoquinol
    MetroCream® [US/Can]
    metronidazole
    Noritate® [US/Can]
    Novo-Nidazol [Can]
    paromomycin
    Trikacide® [Can]
    Yodoxin® [US]
Aminoquinoline (Antimalarial)
    Aralen® Phosphate [US/Can]
    chloroquine phosphate

AMENORRHEA

Ergot Alkaloid and Derivative
    Apo® Bromocriptine [Can]
    bromocriptine
    Parlodel® [US/Can]
    PMS-Bromocriptine [Can]
Gonadotropin
    Factrel® [US]
    gonadorelin
    Lutrepulse™ [Can]
Progestin
    Alti-MPA [Can]
    Apo®-Medroxy [Can]
    Aygestin® [US]
    Camila™ [US]
    Crinone® [US/Can]
    Depo-Provera® [US/Can]
    Errin™ [US]
    Gen-Medroxy [Can]
    hydroxyprogesterone caproate
    Hylutin® [US]
    Jolivette™ [US]
    medroxyprogesterone acetate
    Micronor® [US/Can]
    Nora-BE™ [US]
    norethindrone
    Norlutate® [Can]
    Nor-QD® [US]
    Novo-Medrone [Can]
    Prochieve™ [US]
    Prodrox® [US]
    Progestasert® [US]
    progesterone
    Prometrium® [US/Can]
    Provera® [US/Can]
    ratio-MPA [Can]

ANAPHYLACTIC SHOCK

Adrenergic Agonist Agent
    Adrenalin® Chloride [US/Can]
    epinephrine

ANAPHYLACTIC SHOCK (PROPHYLAXIS)

Plasma Volume Expander
    dextran 1
    Promit® [US]

APNEA (NEONATAL IDIOPATHIC)

Theophylline Derivative
    aminophylline
    theophylline

APNEA OF PREMATURITY

Respiratory Stimulant
    Cafcit® [US/Can]

caffeine (citrated)
Stimulant
   Cafcit® [US/Can]
   caffeine (citrated)

ATTENTION DEFICIT/HYPERACTIVITY DISORDER (ADHD)
Amphetamine
   Adderall® [US]
   Adderall XR™ [US]
   Desoxyn® [US/Can]
   Dexedrine® Spansule® [US/Can]
   Dexedrine® Tablet [US/Can]
   dextroamphetamine
   dextroamphetamine and amphetamine
   Dextrostat® [US]
   methamphetamine
Central Nervous System Stimulant, Nonamphetamine
   Concerta® [US]
   Cylert® [US]
   dexmethylphenidate
   Focalin™ [US]
   Metadate® CD [US]
   Metadate™ ER [US]
   Methylin™ ER [US]
   Methylin™ [US]
   methylphenidate
   PemADD® CT [US]
   PemADD® [US]
   pemoline
   PMS-Methylphenidate [Can]
   ratio-Methylphenidate [Can]
   Ritalin® LA [US]
   Ritalin-SR® [US/Can]
   Ritalin® [US/Can]
Norepinephrine Reuptake Inhibitor, Selective
   atomoxetine
   Strattera™ [US]

AUTISM
Antidepressant, Selective Serotonin Reuptake Inhibitor
   Apo®-Fluoxetine [Can]
   fluoxetine
   FXT® [Can]
   Gen-Fluoxetine [Can]
   Novo-Fluoxetine [Can]
   Nu-Fluoxetine [Can]
   PMS-Fluoxetine [Can]
   Prozac® [US/Can]
   Prozac® Weekly™ [US]
   ratio-Fluoxetine [Can]
   Rhoxal-fluoxetine [Can]
   Sarafem™ [US]
Antipsychotic Agent, Butyrophenone
   Apo®-Haloperidol [Can]
   Haldol® Decanoate [US]
   Haldol® [US]
   haloperidol
   Novo-Peridol [Can]
   PMS-Haloperidol LA [Can]
   ratio-Haloperidol [Can]
   Rho®-Haloperidol Decanoate [Can]

BIRTH CONTROL
Contraceptive
   estradiol cypionate and medroxyprogesterone acetate
   ethinyl estradiol and drospirenone
   ethinyl estradiol and etonogestrel
   ethinyl estradiol and norelgestromin
   Evra® [Can]
   Lunelle™ [US]
   NuvaRing® [US]
   Ortho Evra™ [US]
   Yasmin® [US]
Contraceptive, Implant (Progestin)
   levonorgestrel
   Mirena® [US]
   Norplant® Implant [Can]
   Plan B® [US/Can]
Contraceptive, Oral

Alesse® [US/Can]
Apri® [US]
Aviane™ [US]
Brevicon® [US]
Cryselle™ [US]
Cyclessa® [US]
Demulen® 30 [Can]
Demulen® [US]
Desogen® [US]
Enpresse™ [US]
Estrostep® Fe [US]
ethinyl estradiol and desogestrel
ethinyl estradiol and ethynodiol
    diacetate
ethinyl estradiol and levonorgestrel
ethinyl estradiol and norethindrone
ethinyl estradiol and norgestimate
ethinyl estradiol and norgestrel
femhrt® [US/Can]
Kariva™ [US]
Lessina™ [US]
Levlen® [US]
Levlite™ [US]
Levora® [US]
Loestrin® Fe [US]
Loestrin® [US/Can]
Lo/Ovral® [US]
Low-Ogestrel® [US]
Marvelon® [Can]
mestranol and norethindrone
Microgestin™ Fe [US]
Minestrin™ 1/20 [Can]
Min-Ovral® [Can]
Mircette® [US]
Modicon® [US]
MonoNessa™ [US]
Necon® 0.5/35 [US]
Necon® 1/35 [US]
Necon® 1/50 [US]
Necon® 7/7/7 [US]
Necon® 10/11 [US]
Nordette® [US]
Norinyl® 1+35 [US]

Norinyl® 1+50 [US]
Nortrel™ [US]
Ogestrel®
Ortho-Cept® [US/Can]
Ortho-Cyclen® [US/Can]
Ortho-Novum® 1/50 [US/Can]
Ortho-Novum® [US]
Ortho-Tri-Cyclen® Lo [US]
Ortho Tri-Cyclen® [US/Can]
Ovcon® [US]
Ovral® [US/Can]
Portia™ [US]
PREVEN® [US]
Select™ 1/35 [Can]
Sprintec™ [US]
Synphasic® [Can]
Tri-Levlen® [US]
Tri-Norinyl® [US]
Triphasil® [US/Can]
Triquilar® [Can]
Trivora® [US]
Zovia™ [US]
Contraceptive, Progestin Only
    Alti-MPA [Can]
    Apo®-Medroxy [Can]
    Aygestin® [US]
    Camila™ [US]
    Depo-Provera® [US/Can]
    Errin™ [US]
    Gen-Medroxy [Can]
    Jolivette™ [US]
    levonorgestrel
    medroxyprogesterone acetate
    Micronor® [US/Can]
    Mirena® [US]
    Nora-BE™ [US]
    norethindrone
    norgestrel
    Norlutate® [Can]
    Norplant® Implant [Can]
    Nor-QD® [US]
    Novo-Medrone [Can]
    Ovrette® [US/Can]

Plan B® [US/Can]
Provera® [US/Can]
ratio-MPA [Can]
Estrogen and Progestin Combination
ethinyl estradiol and etonogestrel
ethinyl estradiol and norelgestromin
Evra® [Can]
NuvaRing® [US]
Ortho Evra™ [US]
Spermicide
Advantage 24™ [Can]
Advantage-S™ [US-OTC]
Aqua Lube Plus [US-OTC]
Conceptrol® [US-OTC]
Delfen® [US-OTC]
Emko® [US-OTC]
Encare® [US-OTC]
Gynol II® [US-OTC]
nonoxynol 9
Semicid® [US-OTC]
Shur-Seal® [US-OTC]
VCF™ [US-OTC]

BREAST ENGORGEMENT (POSTPARTUM)

Estrogen and Androgen Combination
Climacteron® [Can]
estradiol and testosterone
Estrogen Derivative
Alora® [US]
Cenestin™ [US/Can]
Climara® [US/Can]
Congest [Can]
Delestrogen® [US/Can]
Depo®-Estradiol [US/Can]
Esclim® [US]
Estrace® [US/Can]
Estraderm® [US/Can]
estradiol
Estring® [US/Can]
Estrogel® [Can]
estrogens (conjugated A/synthetic)
estrogens (conjugated/equine)

Femring™ [US]
Gynodiol® [US]
Oesclim® [Can]
Premarin® [US/Can]
Vagifem® [US/Can]
Vivelle-Dot® [US]
Vivelle® [US/Can]

CANDIDIASIS

Antifungal Agent
Abelcet® [US/Can]
Absorbine Jr.® Antifungal
[US-OTC]
Aftate® Antifungal [US-OTC]
Aloe Vesta® 2-n-1 Antifungal
[US-OTC]
Amphocin® [US]
Amphotec® [US/Can]
amphotericin B cholesteryl sulfate
complex
amphotericin B (conventional)
amphotericin B lipid complex
Ancobon® [US/Can]
Apo®-Fluconazole [Can]
Apo®-Ketoconazole [Can]
Baza® Antifungal [US-OTC]
Bio-Statin® [US]
Blis-To-Sol® [US-OTC]
butoconazole
Candistatin® [Can]
Canesten® Topical [Can]
Canesten® Vaginal [Can]
Carrington Antifungal [US-OTC]
ciclopirox
Clotrimaderm [Can]
clotrimazole
Cruex® [US-OTC]
1-Day™ [US-OTC]
Dermasept Antifungal [US-OTC]
Diflucan® [US/Can]
econazole
Ecostatin® [Can]
Exelderm® [US/Can]

Femizol-M™ [US-OTC]
Femstat® One [Can]
fluconazole
flucytosine
Fungi-Guard [US-OTC]
Fungizone® [US/Can]
Fungoid® Tincture [US-OTC]
Gen-Fluconazole [Can]
Gold Bond® Antifungal [US-OTC]
Gynazole-1™ [US]
Gyne-Lotrimin® 3 [US-OTC]
Gyne-Lotrimin® [US-OTC]
Gynix® [US-OTC]
itraconazole
ketoconazole
Ketoderm® [Can]
Lamisil® Cream [US]
Loprox® [US/Can]
Lotrimin® AF Athlete's Foot Cream
  [US-OTC]
Lotrimin® AF Athlete's Foot
  Solution [US-OTC]
Lotrimin® AF Jock Itch Cream
  [US-OTC]
Lotrimin® AF Powder/Spray
  [US-OTC]
Micaderm® [US-OTC]
Micatin® [US/Can]
miconazole
Micozole [Can]
Micro-Guard® [US-OTC]
Mitrazol™ [US-OTC]
Monistat® 1 Combination Pack
  [US-OTC]
Monistat® 3 [US-OTC]
Monistat® 7 [US-OTC]
Monistat® [Can]
Monistat-Derm® [US]
Mycelex®-3 [US-OTC]
Mycelex®-7 [US-OTC]
Mycelex® Twin Pack [US-OTC]
Mycostatin® [US/Can]
naftifine

Naftin® [US]
Nizoral® A-D [US-OTC]
Nizoral® [US/Can]
Novo-Fluconazole [Can]
Novo-Ketoconazole [Can]
Nyaderm [Can]
nystatin
Nystat-Rx® [US]
Nystop® [US]
oxiconazole
Oxistat® [US/Can]
Pedi-Dri® [US]
Penlac™ [US/Can]
Pitrex [CAN]
PMS-Nystatin [Can]
ratio-Nystatin [Can]
Spectazole™ [US/Can]
Sporanox® [US/Can]
sulconazole
Terazol® 3 [US/Can]
Terazol® 7 [US/Can]
terbinafine (topical)
terconazole
Tinactin® Antifungal Jock Itch
  [US-OTC]
Tinactin® Antifungal [US-OTC]
Tinaderm [US-OTC]
Ting® [US-OTC]
tioconazole
TipTapToe [US-OTC]
tolnaftate
Triple Care® Antifungal [OTC]
Trosyd™ AF [Can]
Trosyd™ J [Can]
Vagistat®-1 [US-OTC]
Zeasorb®-AF [US-OTC]
Antifungal Agent, Systemic
  AmBisome® [US/Can]
  amphotericin B liposomal
Antifungal/Corticosteroid
  Mycolog®-II [US]
  Mytrex® [US]
  nystatin and triamcinolone

CHICKENPOX
Antiviral Agent
  acyclovir
  Apo®-Acyclovir [Can]
  Gen-Acyclovir [Can]
  Nu-Acyclovir [Can]
  Zovirax® [US/Can]
Vaccine, Live Virus
  varicella virus vaccine
  Varivax® [US/Can]

CONDYLOMA ACUMINATUM
Antiviral Agent
  interferon alfa-2b and ribavirin
    combination pack
  Rebetron™ [US/Can]
Biological Response Modulator
  Alferon® N [US/Can]
  interferon alfa-2a
  interferon alfa-2b
  interferon alfa-2b and ribavirin
    combination pack
  interferon alfa-n3
  Intron® A [US/Can]
  Rebetron™ [US/Can]
  Roferon-A® [US/Can]
Immune Response Modifier
  Aldara™ [US/Can]
  imiquimod
Keratolytic Agent
  Condyline™ [Can]
  Condylox® [US]
  Podocon-25™ [US]
  Podofilm® [Can]
  podofilox
  podophyllum resin
  Wartec® [Can]

CONTRACEPTION
Contraceptive
  estradiol cypionate and
    medroxyprogesterone acetate

  ethinyl estradiol and drospirenone
  ethinyl estradiol and etonogestrel
  ethinyl estradiol and norelgestromin
  Evra® [Can]
  Lunelle™ [US]
  NuvaRing® [US]
  Ortho Evra™ [US]
  Yasmin® [US]
Contraceptive, Implant (Progestin)
  levonorgestrel
  Mirena® [US]
  Norplant® Implant [Can]
  Plan B® [US/Can]
Contraceptive, Oral
  Alesse® [US/Can]
  Apri® [US]
  Aviane™ [US]
  Brevicon® [US]
  Cryselle™ [US]
  Cyclessa® [US]
  Demulen® 30 [Can]
  Demulen® [US]
  Desogen® [US]
  Enpresse™ [US]
  Estrostep® Fe [US]
  ethinyl estradiol and desogestrel
  ethinyl estradiol and ethynodiol
    diacetate
  ethinyl estradiol and levonorgestrel
  ethinyl estradiol and norethindrone
  ethinyl estradiol and norgestimate
  ethinyl estradiol and norgestrel
  femhrt® [US/Can]
  Kariva™ [US]
  Lessina™ [US]
  Levlen® [US]
  Levlite™ [US]
  Levora® [US]
  Loestrin® Fe [US]
  Loestrin® [US/Can]
  Lo/Ovral® [US]
  Low-Ogestrel® [US]
  Marvelon® [Can]

mestranol and norethindrone
Microgestin™ Fe [US]
Minestrin™ 1/20 [Can]
Min-Ovral® [Can]
Mircette® [US]
Modicon® [US]
MonoNessa™ [US]
Necon® 0.5/35 [US]
Necon® 1/35 [US]
Necon® 1/50 [US]
Necon® 7/7/7 [US]
Necon® 10/11 [US]
Nordette® [US]
Norinyl® 1+35 [US]
Norinyl® 1+50 [US]
Nortrel™ [US]
Ogestrel®
Ortho-Cept® [US/Can]
Ortho-Cyclen® [US/Can]
Ortho-Novum® 1/50 [US/Can]
Ortho-Novum® [US]
Ortho-Tri-Cyclen® Lo [US]
Ortho Tri-Cyclen® [US/Can]
Ovcon® [US]
Ovral® [US/Can]
Portia™ [US]
PREVEN® [US]
Select™ 1/35 [Can]
Sprintec™ [US]
Synphasic® [Can]
Tri-Levlen® [US]
Tri-Norinyl® [US]
Triphasil® [US/Can]
Triquilar® [Can]
Trivora® [US]
Zovia™ [US]
Contraceptive, Progestin Only
  Alti-MPA [Can]
  Apo®-Medroxy [Can]
  Aygestin® [US]
  Camila™ [US]
  Depo-Provera® [US/Can]
  Errin™ [US]

Gen-Medroxy [Can]
Jolivette™ [US]
levonorgestrel
medroxyprogesterone acetate
Micronor® [US/Can]
Mirena® [US]
Nora-BE™ [US]
norethindrone
norgestrel
Norlutate® [Can]
Norplant® Implant [Can]
Nor-QD® [US]
Novo-Medrone [Can]
Ovrette® [US/Can]
Plan B® [US/Can]
Provera® [US/Can]
ratio-MPA [Can]
Estrogen and Progestin Combination
  ethinyl estradiol and etonogestrel
  ethinyl estradiol and norelgestromin
  Evra® [Can]
  NuvaRing® [US]
  Ortho Evra™ [US]
Spermicide
  Advantage 24™ [Can]
  Advantage-S™ [US-OTC]
  Aqua Lube Plus [US-OTC]
  Conceptrol® [US-OTC]
  Delfen® [US-OTC]
  Emko® [US-OTC]
  Encare® [US-OTC]
  Gynol II® [US-OTC]
  nonoxynol 9
  Semicid® [US-OTC]
  Shur-Seal® [US-OTC]
  VCF™ [US-OTC]

CRYPTORCHISM
Gonadotropin
  chorionic gonadotropin (human)
  Novarel™ [US]
  Pregnyl® [US/Can]

Profasi® HP [Can]
Profasi® [US]

CYSTIC FIBROSIS
Enzyme
  dornase alfa
  Pulmozyme® [US/Can]

DIAPER RASH
Dietary Supplement
  ME-500® [US]
  methionine
  Pedameth® [US]
Protectant, Topical
  A and D® Ointment [US-OTC]
  Baza® Clear [US-OTC]
  Clocream® [US-OTC]
  Desitin® [US-OTC]
  vitamin A and vitamin D
  zinc oxide, cod liver oil, and talc
Topical Skin Product
  Ammens® Medicated Deodorant
    [US-OTC]
  Balmex® [US-OTC]
  Boudreaux's® Butt Paste [US-OTC]
  Critic-Aid Skin Care® [US-OTC]
  Desitin® Creamy [US-OTC]
  Zincofax® [Can]
  zinc oxide

DUCTUS ARTERIOSUS (CLOSURE)
Nonsteroidal Antiinflammatory Drug
  (NSAID)
  Indocin® I.V. [US]
  indomethacin

DUCTUS ARTERIOSUS (TEMPORARY MAINTENANCE OF PATENCY)
Prostaglandin
  alprostadil
  Prostin VR Pediatric® [US/Can]

DWARFISM
Growth Hormone
  Genotropin Miniquick® [US]
  Genotropin® [US]
  human growth hormone
  Humatrope® [US/Can]
  Norditropin® Cartridges [US]
  Norditropin® [US/Can]
  Nutropin AQ® [US/Can]
  Nutropin Depot® [US]
  Nutropin® [US]
  Protropin® [US/Can]
  Saizen® [US/Can]
  Serostim® [US/Can]

DYSBETALIPOPROTEIN-EMIA (FAMILIAL)
Antihyperlipidemic Agent,
  Miscellaneous
  bezafibrate (Canada only)
  Bezalip® [Can]
  PMS-Bezafibrate [Can]
Vitamin, Water Soluble
  niacin
  Niacor® [US]
  Niaspan® [US/Can]
  Nicotinex [US-OTC]
  Slo-Niacin® [US-OTC]

DYSMENORRHEA
Nonsteroidal Antiinflammatory Drug
  (NSAID)
  Advil® [US/Can]
  Aleve® [US-OTC]
  Anaprox® DS [US/Can]
  Anaprox® [US/Can]
  Ansaid® Oral [US/Can]
  Apo®-Diclo [Can]
  Apo®-Diclo SR [Can]
  Apo®-Diflunisal [Can]
  Apo®-Flurbiprofen [Can]
  Apo®-Ibuprofen [Can]
  Apo®-Keto [Can]

Apo®-Keto-E [Can]
Apo®-Keto SR [Can]
Apo®-Mefenamic [Can]
Apo®-Napro-Na [Can]
Apo®-Napro-Na DS [Can]
Apo®-Naproxen [Can]
Apo®-Naproxen SR [Can]
Cataflam® [US/Can]
diclofenac
diflunisal
Dolobid® [US]
EC-Naprosyn® [US]
Feldene® [US/Can]
flurbiprofen
Froben® [Can]
Froben-SR® [Can]
Gen-Naproxen EC [Can]
Gen-Piroxicam [Can]
Genpril® [US-OTC]
Haltran® [US-OTC]
ibuprofen
Ibu-Tab® [US]
I-Prin [US-OTC]
ketoprofen
mefenamic acid
Menadol® [US-OTC]
Midol® Maximum Strength Cramp
    Formula [US-OTC]
Motrin® IB [US/Can]
Motrin® [US/Can]
Naprelan® [US]
Naprosyn® [US/Can]
naproxen
Naxen® [Can]
Novo-Difenac® [Can]
Novo-Difenac-K [Can]
Novo-Difenac® SR [Can]
Novo-Diflunisal [Can]
Novo-Flurprofen [Can]
Novo-Keto [Can]
Novo-Keto-EC [Can]
Novo-Naprox [Can]
Novo-Naprox Sodium [Can]

Novo-Naprox Sodium DS [Can]
Novo-Naprox SR [Can]
Novo-Pirocam® [Can]
Novo-Profen® [Can]
Nu-Diclo [Can]
Nu-Diclo-SR [Can]
Nu-Diflunisal [Can]
Nu-Flurprofen [Can]
Nu-Ibuprofen [Can]
Nu-Ketoprofen [Can]
Nu-Ketoprofen-E [Can]
Nu-Mefenamic [Can]
Nu-Naprox [Can]
Nu-Pirox [Can]
Orudis® KT [US-OTC]
Orudis® SR [Can]
Oruvail® [US/Can]
Pexicam® [Can]
piroxicam
PMS-Diclofenac [Can]
PMS-Diclofenac SR [Can]
PMS-Mefenamic Acid [Can]
Ponstan® [Can]
Ponstel® [US/Can]
ratio-Flurbiprofen [Can]
Rhodis™ [Can]
Rhodis-EC™ [Can]
Rhodis SR™ [Can]
Riva-Diclofenac [Can]
Riva-Diclofenac-K [Can]
Riva-Naproxen [Can]
Voltaren Rapide® [Can]
Voltaren® [US/Can]
Voltaren®-XR [US]
Voltare Ophtha® [Can]
Nonsteroidal Antiinflammatory Drug
    (NSAID), COX-2 Selective
rofecoxib
Vioxx® [US/Can]

EAR WAX
Otic Agent, Ceruminolytic
A/B® Otic [US]

Allergan® Ear Drops [US]
antipyrine and benzocaine
Auralgan® [US/Can]
Aurodex® [US]
Auroto® [US]
Bausch & Lomb Earwax Removal
[US-OTC]
Benzotic® [US]
carbamide peroxide
Cerumenex® [US/Can]
Debrox® [OTC]
Debrox® Otic [US-OTC]
Dec-Agesic® A.B. [US]
Dent's Ear Wax [US-OTC]
Dolotic® [US]
E*R*O Ear [US-OTC]
Mollifene® Ear Wax Removing
Formula [US-OTC]
Murine® Ear Drops [US-OTC]
Rx-Otic® Drops [US]
triethanolamine polypeptide oleate-
condensate

ECLAMPSIA
Barbiturate
Luminal® Sodium [US]
phenobarbital
PMS-Phenobarbital [Can]
Benzodiazepine
Apo®-Diazepam [Can]
Diastat® [US/Can]
Diazemuls® [Can]
diazepam
Diazepam Intensol® [US]
Valium® [US/Can]

ENDOMETRIOSIS
Androgen
Cyclomen® [Can]
danazol
Danocrine® [US/Can]
Contraceptive, Oral
Alesse® [US/Can]
Apri® [US]

Aviane™ [US]
Brevicon® [US]
Cryselle™ [US]
Cyclessa® [US]
Demulen® 30 [Can]
Demulen® [US]
Desogen® [US]
Enpresse™ [US]
Estrostep® Fe [US]
ethinyl estradiol and desogestrel
ethinyl estradiol and ethynodiol
diacetate
ethinyl estradiol and levonorgestrel
ethinyl estradiol and norethindrone
ethinyl estradiol and norgestimate
ethinyl estradiol and norgestrel
femhrt® [US/Can]
Kariva™ [US]
Lessina™ [US]
Levlen® [US]
Levlite™ [US]
Levora® [US]
Loestrin® Fe [US]
Loestrin® [US/Can]
Lo/Ovral® [US]
Low-Ogestrel® [US]
Marvelon® [Can]
mestranol and norethindrone
Microgestin™ Fe [US]
Minestrin™ 1/20 [Can]
Min-Ovral® [Can]
Mircette® [US]
Modicon® [US]
MonoNessa™ [US]
Necon® 0.5/35 [US]
Necon® 1/35 [US]
Necon® 1/50 [US]
Necon® 7/7/7 [US]
Necon® 10/11 [US]
Nordette® [US]
Norinyl® 1+35 [US]
Norinyl® 1+50 [US]
Nortrel™ [US]

Ogestrel®
Ortho-Cept® [US/Can]
Ortho-Cyclen® [US/Can]
Ortho-Novum® 1/50 [US/Can]
Ortho-Novum® [US]
Ortho-Tri-Cyclen® Lo [US]
Ortho Tri-Cyclen® [US/Can]
Ovcon® [US]
Ovral® [US/Can]
Portia™ [US]
PREVEN® [US]
Select™ 1/35 [Can]
Sprintec™ [US]
Synphasic® [Can]
Tri-Levlen® [US]
Tri-Norinyl® [US]
Triphasil® [US/Can]
Triquilar® [Can]
Trivora® [US]
Zovia™ [US]
Contraceptive, Progestin Only
Aygestin® [US]
Camila™ [US]
Errin™ [US]
Jolivette™ [US]
Micronor® [US/Can]
Nora-BE™ [US]
norethindrone
norgestrel
Norlutate® [Can]
Nor-QD® [US]
Ovrette® [US/Can]
Hormone, Posterior Pituitary
nafarelin
Synarel® [US/Can]
Progestin
hydroxyprogesterone caproate
Hylutin® [US]
Prodrox® [US]

FACTOR IX DEFICIENCY
Antihemophilic Agent
AlphaNine® SD [US]

Bebulin® VH [US]
factor IX complex (human)
Hemonyne® [US]
Konyne® 80 [US]
Profilnine® SD [US]
Proplex® T [US]

FACTOR VIII DEFICIENCY
Blood Product Derivative
Alphanate® [US]
antihemophilic factor (human)
Hemofil® M [US/Can]
Humate-P® [US/Can]
Koaate®-DVI [US]
Monarc® M [US]
Monoclate-P® [US]
Hemophilic Agent
antiinhibitor coagulant complex
Autoplex® T [US]
Feiba VH Immuno® [US/Can]

FAMILIAL ADENOMATOUS POLYPOSIS
Nonsteroidal Antiinflammatory Drug
(NSAID), COX-2 Selective
Celebrex® [US/Can]
celecoxib

FEVER
Antipyretic
Abenol® [Can]
Acephen® [US-OTC]
acetaminophen
Advil® Children's [US-OTC]
Advil® Infants' Concentrated Drops [US-OTC]
Advil® Junior [US-OTC]
Advil® [US/Can]
Aleve® [US-OTC]
Amigesic® [US/Can]
Anaprox® DS [US/Can]
Anaprox® [US/Can]
Apo®-Acetaminophen [Can]
Apo®-Ibuprofen [Can]

Apo®-Napro-Na [Can]
Apo®-Napro-Na DS [Can]
Apo®-Naproxen [Can]
Apo®-Naproxen SR [Can]
Argesic®-SA [US]
Asaphen [Can]
Asaphen E.C. [Can]
Ascriptin® Enteric [US-OTC]
Ascriptin® Extra Strength
  [US-OTC]
Ascriptin® [US-OTC]
Aspercin Extra [US-OTC]
Aspercin [US-OTC]
aspirin
Atasol® [Can]
Bayer® Aspirin Extra Strength [US-OTC]
Bayer® Aspirin Regimen Children's
  [US-OTC]
Bayer® Aspirin Regimen Regular
  Strength [US-OTC]
Bayer® Aspirin [US-OTC]
Bayer® Plus Extra Strength
  [US-OTC]
Bufferin® Arthritis Strength
  [US-OTC]
Bufferin® Extra Strength [US-OTC]
Bufferin® [US-OTC]
Cetafen Extra® [US-OTC]
Cetafen® [US-OTC]
Easprin® [US]
EC-Naprosyn® [US]
Ecotrin® Maximum Strength
  [US-OTC]
Ecotrin® [US-OTC]
Entrophen® [Can]
Feverall® [US-OTC]
Genapap® Children [US-OTC]
Genapap® Extra Strength [US-OTC]
Genapap® Infant [US-OTC]
Genapap® [US-OTC]
Genebs® Extra Strength [US-OTC]
Genebs® [US-OTC]

Gen-Naproxen EC [Can]
Genpril® [US-OTC]
Halfprin® [US-OTC]
Haltran® [US-OTC]
ibuprofen
Ibu-Tab® [US]
Infantaire [US-OTC]
I-Prin [US-OTC]
Liquiprin® for Children [US-OTC]
Mapap® Children's [US-OTC]
Mapap® Extra Strength [US-OTC]
Mapap® Infants [US-OTC]
Mapap® [US-OTC]
Menadol® [US-OTC]
Mono-Gesic® [US]
Motrin® Children's [US/Can]
Motrin® IB [US/Can]
Motrin® Infants' [US-OTC]
Motrin® Junior Strength
  [US-OTC]
Motrin® [US/Can]
Naprelan® [US]
Naprosyn® [US/Can]
naproxen
Naxen® [Can]
Novasen [Can]
Novo-Naprox [Can]
Novo-Naprox Sodium [Can]
Novo-Naprox Sodium DS [Can]
Novo-Naprox SR [Can]
Novo-Profen® [Can]
Nu-Ibuprofen [Can]
Nu-Naprox [Can]
Pediatrix [Can]
Redutemp® [US-OTC]
Riva-Naproxen [Can]
Salflex® [US/Can]
salsalate
Silapap® Children's [US-OTC]
Silapap® Infants [US-OTC]
sodium salicylate
St. Joseph® Pain Reliever [US-OTC]
Tempra® [Can]

Tylenol® Extra Strength [US-OTC]
Tylenol® Infants [US-OTC]
Tylenol® Junior Strength [US-OTC]
Tylenol® [US/Can]
Valorin Extra [US-OTC]
Valorin [US-OTC]
ZORprin® [US]

FIBROCYSTIC BREAST DISEASE
Androgen
Cyclomen® [Can]
danazol
Danocrine® [US/Can]

FIBROCYSTIC DISEASE
Vitamin, Fat Soluble
Aquasol E® [US-OTC]
vitamin E

FOLLICLE STIMULATION
Ovulation Stimulator
Bravelle® [US]
Fertinex® [US]
urofollitropin

GENITAL HERPES
Antiviral Agent
famciclovir
Famvir™ [US/Can]
valacyclovir
Valtrex® [US/Can]

GENITAL WART
Immune Response Modifier
Aldara™ [US/Can]
imiquimod

GIARDIASIS
Amebicide
Apo®-Metronidazole [Can]
Flagyl ER® [US]
Flagyl® [US/Can]
Florazole ER® [Can]
Humatin® [US/Can]

metronidazole
Noritate® [US/Can]
Novo-Nidazol [Can]
paromomycin
Trikacide® [Can]
Anthelmintic
albendazole
Albenza® [US]

GONOCOCCAL OPHTHALMIA NEONATORUM
Topical Skin Product
silver nitrate

GONORRHEA
Antibiotic, Macrolide
Rovamycine® [Can]
spiramycin (Canada only)
Antibiotic, Miscellaneous
spectinomycin
Trobicin® [US]
Antibiotic, Quinolone
gatifloxacin
Tequin® [US/Can]
Zymar™ [US]
Cephalosporin (Second Generation)
Apo®-Cefuroxime [Can]
cefoxitin
Ceftin® [US/Can]
cefuroxime
Mefoxin® [US/Can]
ratio-Cefuroxime [Can]
Zinacef® [US/Can]
Cephalosporin (Third Generation)
cefixime
ceftriaxone
Rocephin® [US/Can]
Suprax® [Can]
Quinolone
Apo®-Oflox [Can]
ciprofloxacin
Cipro® [US/Can]

Cipro® XR [US/Can]
Floxin® [US/Can]
ofloxacin
Tetracycline Derivative
Adoxa™ [US]
Apo®-Doxy [Can]
Apo®-Doxy Tabs [Can]
Apo®-Tetra [Can]
Brodspec® [US]
Doryx® [US]
Doxy-100® [US]
Doxycin [Can]
doxycycline
EmTet® [US]
Monodox® [US]
Novo-Doxylin [Can]
Novo-Tetra [Can]
Nu-Doxycycline [Can]
Nu-Tetra [Can]
ratio-Doxycycline [Can]
Sumycin® [US]
tetracycline
Vibramycin® [US]
Vibra-Tabs® [US/Can]
Wesmycin® [US]

GROWTH HORMONE DEFICIENCY

Diagnostic Agent
levodopa
Growth Hormone
Genotropin Miniquick® [US]
Genotropin® [US]
human growth hormone
Humatrope® [US/Can]
Norditropin® Cartridges [US]
Norditropin® [US/Can]
Nutropin AQ® [US/Can]
Nutropin Depot® [US]
Nutropin® [US]
Protropin® [US/Can]
Saizen® [US/Can]
Serostim® [US/Can]

GROWTH HORMONE (DIAGNOSTIC)

Diagnostic Agent
Geref® Diagnostic [US]
sermorelin acetate

HEMOLYTIC DISEASE OF THE NEWBORN

Immune Globulin
BayRho-D® Full-Dose [US]
BayRho-D® Mini-Dose [US]
MICRhoGAM® [US]
Rho(D) immune globulin
RhoGAM® [US]
WinRho SDF® [US]

HEMORRHAGE (POSTPARTUM)

Ergot Alkaloid and Derivative
ergonovine
Methergine® [US/Can]
methylergonovine
Oxytocic Agent
oxytocin
Pitocin® [US/Can]
Prostaglandin
carboprost tromethamine
Hemabate™ [US/Can]

HERPES SIMPLEX

Antiviral Agent
acyclovir
Apo®-Acyclovir [Can]
Cytovene® [US/Can]
famciclovir
Famvir™ [US/Can]
foscarnet
Foscavir® [US/Can]
ganciclovir
Gen-Acyclovir [Can]
Nu-Acyclovir [Can]
trifluridine
Viroptic® [US/Can]

Vitrasert® [US/Can]
Zovirax® [US/Can]
Antiviral Agent, Topical
Abreva™ [US-OTC]
docosanol

HERPES ZOSTER
Analgesic, Topical
Antiphlogistine Rub A-535 Capsaicin [Can]
ArthriCare® for Women Extra Moisturizing [US-OTC]
ArthriCare® for Women Silky Dry [US-OTC]
Capsagel® [US-OTC]
capsaicin
Capzasin-HP® [US-OTC]
TheraPatch® Warm [US-OTC]
Zostrix®-HP [US/Can]
Zostrix® [US/Can]
Antiviral Agent
acyclovir
Apo®-Acyclovir [Can]
famciclovir
Famvir™ [US/Can]
Gen-Acyclovir [Can]
Nu-Acyclovir [Can]
valacyclovir
Valtrex® [US/Can]
Zovirax® [US/Can]

HICCUPS
Phenothiazine Derivative
chlorpromazine
Largactil® [Can]
Thorazine® [US]

HAEMOPHILUS INFLUENZAE
Toxoid
diphtheria, tetanus toxoids, and acellular pertussis vaccine and *Haemophilus influenzae* type b conjugate vaccine

TriHIBit® [US]
Vaccine, Inactivated Bacteria
ActHIB® [US/Can]
diphtheria, tetanus toxoids, and acellular pertussis vaccine and *Haemophilus influenzae* type b conjugate vaccine
Haemophilus influenzae type b conjugate vaccine
HibTITER® [US]
PedvaxHIB® [US/Can]
TriHIBit® [US]
Vaccine, Inactivated Virus
Comvax® [US]
Haemophilus influenzae type b conjugate and hepatitis B vaccine

HORMONAL IMBALANCE (FEMALE)
Progestin
Alti-MPA [Can]
Apo®-Medroxy [Can]
Aygestin® [US]
Camila™ [US]
Crinone® [US/Can]
Depo-Provera® [US/Can]
Errin™ [US]
Gen-Medroxy [Can]
hydroxyprogesterone caproate
Hylutin® [US]
Jolivette™ [US]
medroxyprogesterone acetate
Micronor® [US/Can]
Nora-BE™ [US]
norethindrone
Norlutate® [Can]
Nor-QD® [US]
Novo-Medrone [Can]
Prochieve™ [US]
Prodrox® [US]
Progestasert® [US]
progesterone
Prometrium® [US/Can]

Provera® [US/Can]
ratio-MPA [Can]

HYDATIDIFORM MOLE (BENIGN)

Prostaglandin
Cervidil® Vaginal Insert [US/Can]
dinoprostone
Prepidil® Vaginal Gel [US/Can]
Prostin E2® Vaginal Suppository [US/Can]

HYPERPLASIA, VULVAR SQUAMOUS

Estrogen Derivative
Alora® [US]
Cenestin™ [US/Can]
Climara® [US/Can]
Congest [Can]
Delestrogen® [US/Can]
Depo®-Estradiol [US/Can]
Esclim® [US]
Estrace® [US/Can]
Estraderm® [US/Can]
estradiol
Estring® [US/Can]
Estrogel® [Can]
estrogens (conjugated A/synthetic)
estrogens (conjugated/equine)
estrogens (esterified)
estrone
estropipate
Femring™ [US]
Gynodiol® [US]
Kestrone® [US/Can]
Menest® [US]
Oesclim® [Can]
Oestrilin [Can]
Ogen® [US/Can]
Ortho-Est® [US]
Premarin® [US/Can]
Vagifem® [US/Can]
Vivelle-Dot® [US]
Vivelle® [US/Can]

HYPOGONADISM

Androgen
Andriol® [Can]
Androderm® [US]
AndroGel® [US/Can]
Android® [US]
Delatestryl® [US/Can]
Depo®-Testosterone [US]
Methitest® [US]
methyltestosterone
Striant™ [US]
Testim™ [US]
Testoderm® [US]
Testoderm® with Adhesive [US]
Testopel® [US]
testosterone
Testred® [US]
Virilon® [US]
Diagnostic Agent
Factrel® [US]
gonadorelin
Lutrepulse™ [Can]
Estrogen Derivative
Alora® [US]
Cenestin™ [US/Can]
Climara® [US/Can]
Congest [Can]
Delestrogen® [US/Can]
Depo®-Estradiol [US/Can]
diethylstilbestrol
Esclim® [US]
Estinyl® [US]
Estrace® [US/Can]
Estraderm® [US/Can]
estradiol
Estring® [US/Can]
Estrogel® [Can]
estrogens (conjugated A/synthetic)
estrogens (conjugated/equine)
estrogens (esterified)
estrone
estropipate
ethinyl estradiol

Femring™ [US]
Gynodiol® [US]
Honvol® [Can]
Kestrone® [US/Can]
Menest® [US]
Oesclim® [Can]
Oestrilin [Can]
Ogen® [US/Can]
Ortho-Est® [US]
Premarin® [US/Can]
Vagifem® [US/Can]
Vivelle-Dot® [US]
Vivelle® [US/Can]

IMPETIGO
Antibiotic, Topical
bacitracin, neomycin, and
polymyxin B
Bactroban® Nasal [US]
Bactroban® [US/Can]
mupirocin
Mycitracin® [US-OTC]
Neosporin® Ophthalmic Ointment
[US/Can]
Neosporin® Topical [US/Can]
Triple Antibiotic® [US]
Penicillin
Apo®-Pen VK [Can]
Nadopen-V® [Can]
Novo-Pen-VK® [Can]
Nu-Pen-VK® [Can]
penicillin G procaine
penicillin V potassium
PVF® K [Can]
Suspen® [US]
Truxcillin® [US]
Veetids® [US]
Wycillin® [US/Can]

INFERTILITY (FEMALE)
Ergot Alkaloid and Derivative
Apo® Bromocriptine [Can]
bromocriptine
Parlodel® [US/Can]

PMS-Bromocriptine [Can]
Gonadotropin
chorionic gonadotropin (human)
menotropins
Novarel™ [US]
Pergonal® [US/Can]
Pregnyl® [US/Can]
Profasi® HP [Can]
Profasi® [US]
Repronex® [US/Can]
Ovulation Stimulator
Clomid® [US/Can]
clomiphene
Serophene® [US/Can]
Progestin
Crinone® [US/Can]
Prochieve™ [US]
Progestasert® [US]
progesterone
Prometrium® [US/Can]

LABOR INDUCTION
Oxytocic Agent
oxytocin
Pitocin® [US/Can]
Prostaglandin
carboprost tromethamine
Cervidil® Vaginal Insert [US/Can]
dinoprostone
Hemabate™ [US/Can]
Prepidil® Vaginal Gel [US/Can]
Prostin E2® Vaginal Suppository
[US/Can]

LABOR (PREMATURE)
Adrenergic Agonist Agent
Brethine® [US]
Bricanyl® [Can]
terbutaline

LACTATION (SUPPRESSION)
Ergot Alkaloid and Derivative
Apo® Bromocriptine [Can]

bromocriptine
Parlodel® [US/Can]
PMS-Bromocriptine [Can]

LACTOSE INTOLERANCE

Nutritional Supplement
Dairyaid® [Can]
Lactaid® Extra Strength [US-OTC]
Lactaid® Ultra [US-OTC]
Lactaid® [US-OTC]
lactase
Lactrase® [US-OTC]

LEAD POISONING

Chelating Agent
BAL in Oil® [US]
Calcium Disodium Versenate® [US]
Chemet® [US/Can]
Cuprimine® [US/Can]
Depen® [US/Can]
dimercaprol
edetate calcium disodium
penicillamine
succimer

LICE

Scabicides/Pediculicides
A-200™ [US-OTC]
Acticin® [US]
Elimite® [US]
End Lice® [US-OTC]
Hexit™ [Can]
Kwellada-P™ [Can]
lindane
malathion
Nix® Dermal Cream [Can]
Nix® [US/Can]
Ovide™ [US]
permethrin
PMS-Lindane [Can]
Pronto® [US-OTC]
pyrethrins
Pyrinex® Pediculicide [US-OTC]
Pyrinyl Plus® [US-OTC]

Pyrinyl® [US-OTC]
R & C™ II [Can]
R & C™ Shampoo/Conditioner
  [Can]
R & C® [US-OTC]
RID® Mousse [Can]
Rid® Spray [US-OTC]
Tisit® Blue Gel [US-OTC]
Tisit® [US-OTC]

LUNG SURFACTANT

Lung Surfactant
beractant
Survanta® [US/Can]

MAPLE SYRUP URINE DISEASE

Vitamin, Water Soluble
Betaxin® [Can]
Thiamilate® [US]
thiamine

MEASLES

Vaccine, Live Virus
Attenuvax® [US]
measles, mumps, and rubella
  vaccines, combined
measles virus vaccine (live)
M-M-R® II [US/Can]
Priorix™ [Can]

MEASLES (RUBEOLA)

Immune Globulin
BayGam® [US/Can]
immune globulin (intramuscular)

MECONIUM ILEUS

Mucolytic Agent
acetylcysteine
Acys-5® [US]
Mucomyst® [US/Can]
Parvolex® [Can]

MELASMA (FACIAL)

Corticosteroid, Topical

fluocinolone, hydroquinone, and
   tretinoin
Tri-Luma™ [US]
Depigmenting Agent
fluocinolone, hydroquinone, and
   tretinoin
Tri-Luma™ [US]
Retinoic Acid Derivative
fluocinolone, hydroquinone, and
   tretinoin
Tri-Luma™ [US]

MENOPAUSE
Ergot Alkaloid and Derivative
belladonna, phenobarbital, and
   ergotamine tartrate
Bellamine S [US]
Bellergal® Spacetabs® [Can]
Bel-Phen-Ergot S® [US]
Bel-Tabs [US]
Estrogen and Androgen Combination
Climacteron® [Can]
estradiol and testosterone
Estrogen and Progestin Combination
Activella™ [US]
CombiPatch® [US]
estradiol and norethindrone
estradiol and norgestimate
estrogens and medroxyprogesterone
Ortho-Prefest® [US]
Premphase® [US/Can]
Prempro™ [US/Can]
Estrogen Derivative
Alora® [US]
Cenestin™ [US/Can]
Climara® [US/Can]
Congest [Can]
Delestrogen® [US/Can]
Depo®-Estradiol [US/Can]
diethylstilbestrol
Esclim® [US]
Estinyl® [US]
Estrace® [US/Can]

Estraderm® [US/Can]
estradiol
Estring® [US/Can]
Estrogel® [Can]
estrogens (conjugated A/synthetic)
estrogens (conjugated/equine)
estrogens (esterified)
ethinyl estradiol
Femring™ [US]
Gynodiol® [US]
Honvol® [Can]
Menest® [US]
Oesclim® [Can]
Premarin® [US/Can]
Vagifem® [US/Can]
Vivelle-Dot® [US]
Vivelle® [US/Can]

MENORRHAGIA
Androgen
Cyclomen® [Can]
danazol
Danocrine® [US/Can]

MERCURY POISONING
Chelating Agent
BAL in Oil® [US]
dimercaprol

MUMPS
Vaccine, Live Virus
measles, mumps, and rubella
   vaccines, combined
M-M-R® II [US/Can]
Mumpsvax® [US/Can]
mumps virus vaccine, live, attenuated
Priorix™ [Can]

MUMPS (DIAGNOSTIC)
Diagnostic Agent
MSTA® Mumps [US/Can]
mumps skin test antigen

NIPPLE CARE
Topical Skin Product

glycerin, lanolin, and peanut oil
Masse® Breast Cream [US-OTC]

OBSESSIVE-COMPULSIVE DISORDER (OCD)

Antidepressant, Selective Serotonin
    Reuptake Inhibitor
    Alti-Fluvoxamine [Can]
    Apo®-Fluoxetine [Can]
    Apo®-Fluvoxamine [Can]
    Apo®-Sertraline [Can]
    fluoxetine
    fluvoxamine
    FXT® [Can]
    Gen-Fluoxetine [Can]
    Luvox® [Can]
    Novo-Fluoxetine [Can]
    Novo-Fluvoxamine [Can]
    Novo-Sertraline [Can]
    Nu-Fluoxetine [Can]
    Nu-Fluvoxamine [Can]
    Nu-Sertraline [Can]
    paroxetine
    Paxil® CR™ [US/Can]
    Paxil® [US/Can]
    PMS-Fluoxetine [Can]
    PMS-Fluvoxamine [Can]
    PMS-Sertraline [Can]
    Prozac® [US/Can]
    Prozac® Weekly™ [US]
    ratio-Fluoxetine [Can]
    ratio-fluvoxamine [Can]
    ratio-Sertraline [Can]
    Rhoxal-fluoxetine [Can]
    Rhoxal-Fluvoxamine [Can]
    Rhoxal-sertraline [Can]
    Sarafem™ [US]
    sertraline
    Zoloft® [US/Can]
Antidepressant, Tricyclic (Tertiary
    Amine)
    Anafranil® [US/Can]
    Apo®-Clomipramine [Can]
    clomipramine
    CO Clomipramine [Can]
    Gen-Clomipramine [Can]
    Novo-Clopramine [Can]

OILY SKIN

Antiseborrheic Agent, Topical
    Aveeno® Cleansing Bar [US-OTC]
    Fostex® [US-OTC]
    Pernox® [US-OTC]
    Sastid® Plain Therapeutic Shampoo
      and Acne Wash [US-OTC]
    sulfur and salicylic acid

OPIATE WITHDRAWAL (NEONATAL)

Analgesic, Narcotic
    paregoric

OTITIS EXTERNA

Aminoglycoside (Antibiotic)
    AKTob® [US]
    Alcomicin® [Can]
    amikacin
    Amikin® [Can]
    Apo®-Tobramycin [Can]
    Diogent® [Can]
    Garamycin® [US/Can]
    gentamicin
    kanamycin
    Kantrex® [US/Can]
    Myciguent [US-OTC]
    Neo-Fradin™ [US]
    neomycin
    Neo-Rx [US]
    PMS-Tobramycin [Can]
    ratio-Gentamicin [Can]
    tobramycin
    Tobrex® [US/Can]
Antibacterial, Otic
    acetic acid
    VoSol® [US]
Antibiotic/Corticosteroid, Otic
    Acetasol® HC [US]

acetic acid, propylene glycol
   diacetate, and hydrocortisone
AntibiOtic® Ear [US]
ciprofloxacin and hydrocortisone
Cipro® HC Otic [US/Can]
Coly-Mycin® S Otic [US]
Cortimyxin® [Can]
Cortisporin® Otic [US/Can]
Cortisporin®-TC Otic [US]
neomycin, colistin, hydrocortisone,
   and thonzonium
neomycin, polymyxin B, and
   hydrocortisone
PediOtic® [US]
VoSol® HC [US/Can]
Antibiotic, Otic
   Apo®-Oflox [Can]
   chloramphenicol
   Chloromycetin® Parenteral [US/Can]
   Floxin® [US/Can]
   ofloxacin
   Pentamycetin® [Can]
Antifungal/Corticosteroid
   Dermazene® [US]
   iodoquinol and hydrocortisone
   Vytone® [US]
Cephalosporin (Third Generation)
   ceftazidime
   Fortaz® [US/Can]
   Tazicef® [US]
   Tazidime® [US/Can]
Corticosteroid, Topical
   Aclovate® [US]
   Acticort® [US]
   Aeroseb-HC® [US]
   alclometasone
   Alphatrex® [US]
   amcinonide
   Aquacort® [Can]
   Aristocort® A Topical [US]
   Aristocort® Topical [US]
   Betaderm® [Can]
   Betamethacot® [US]

betamethasone (topical)
Betatrex® [US]
Beta-Val® [US]
Betnovate® [Can]
CaldeCORT® [US-OTC]
Capex™ [US/Can]
Carmol-HC® [US]
Celestoderm®-EV/2 [Can]
Celestoderm®-V [Can]
Cetacort®
clobetasol
Clocort® Maximum Strength
   [US-OTC]
clocortolone
Cloderm® [US/Can]
Cordran® SP [US]
Cordran® [US/Can]
Cormax® [US]
CortaGel® [US-OTC]
Cortaid® Maximum Strength
   [US-OTC]
Cortaid® with Aloe [US-OTC]
Cort-Dome® [US]
Cortizone®-5 [US-OTC]
Cortizone®-10 [US-OTC]
Cortoderm [Can]
Cutivate™ [US]
Cyclocort® [US/Can]
Del-Beta® [US]
Delcort® [US]
Dermacort® [US]
Dermarest Dricort® [US]
Derma-Smoothe/FS® [US/Can]
Dermatop® [US/Can]
Dermolate® [US-OTC]
Dermovate® [Can]
Dermtex® HC with Aloe
   [US-OTC]
Desocort® [Can]
desonide
DesOwen® [US]
Desoxi® [Can]
desoximetasone

diflorasone
Diprolene® AF [US]
Diprolene® [US/Can]
Diprosone® [Can]
Eldecort® [US]
Elocon® [US/Can]
Embeline™ E [US]
fluocinolone
fluocinonide
Fluoderm [Can]
flurandrenolide
fluticasone (topical)
Gen-Clobetasol [Can]
Gynecort® [US-OTC]
halcinonide
halobetasol
Halog®-E [US]
Halog® [US/Can]
Hi-Cor-1.0® [US]
Hi-Cor-2.5® [US]
Hyderm [Can]
hydrocortisone (topical)
Hydrocort® [US]
Hydro-Tex® [US-OTC]
Hytone® [US]
Kenalog® Topical [US/Can]
LactiCare-HC® [US]
Lanacort® [US-OTC]
Lidemol® [Can]
Lidex-E® [US]
Lidex® [US/Can]
Locoid® [US/Can]
Luxiq™ [US]
Lyderm® [Can]
Maxiflor® [US]
Maxivate® [US]
mometasone furoate
Novo-Clobetasol [Can]
Nutracort® [US]
Olux® [US]
Orabase® HCA [US]
Oracort [Can]
Penecort® [US]

PMS-Desonide [Can]
prednicarbate
Prevex® [Can]
Prevex® HC [Can]
Psorcon™ E [US]
Psorcon™ [US/Can]
Qualisone® [US]
ratio-Clobetasol [Can]
ratio-Ectosone [Can]
ratio-Topilene® [Can]
ratio-Topisone® [Can]
Sarna® HC [Can]
Scalpicin® [US]
S-T Cort® [US]
Synacort® [US]
Synalar® [US/Can]
Taro-Desoximetasone [Can]
Taro-Sone® [Can]
Tegrin®-HC [US-OTC]
Temovate E® [US]
Temovate® [US]
Tiamol® [Can]
Ti-U-Lac® H [Can]
Topicort®-LP [US]
Topicort® [US/Can]
Topsyn® [Can]
Triacet™ Topical [US]
Triaderm [Can]
triamcinolone (topical)
Tridesilon® [US]
U-Cort™ [US]
Ultravate™ [US/Can]
urea and hydrocortisone
Uremol® HC [Can]
Westcort® [US/Can]
Otic Agent, Analgesic
A/B® Otic [US]
Allergan® Ear Drops [US]
antipyrine and benzocaine
Auralgan® [US/Can]
Aurodex® [US]
Auroto® [US]
Benzotic® [US]

Dec-Agesic® A.B. [US]
Dolotic® [US]
Rx-Otic® Drops [US]
Otic Agent, Antiinfective
Cresylate® [US]
m-cresyl acetate
Quinolone
ciprofloxacin
Cipro® [US/Can]
Cipro® XR [US/Can]
lomefloxacin
Maxaquin® [US]
nalidixic acid
NegGram® [US/Can]

OTITIS MEDIA

Antibiotic, Carbacephem
Lorabid™ [US/Can]
loracarbef
Antibiotic, Miscellaneous
Apo®-Trimethoprim [Can]
Primsol® [US]
Proloprim® [US/Can]
trimethoprim
Antibiotic, Otic
Apo®-Oflox [Can]
Floxin® [US/Can]
ofloxacin
Antibiotic, Penicillin
pivampicillin (Canada only)
Pondocillin® [Can]
Cephalosporin (First Generation)
Apo®-Cefadroxil [Can]
Apo®-Cephalex [Can]
Biocef® [US]
cefadroxil
cephalexin
Duricef® [US/Can]
Keflex® [US]
Keftab® [US/Can]
Novo-Cefadroxil [Can]
Novo-Lexin® [Can]
Nu-Cephalex® [Can]

Cephalosporin (Second Generation)
Apo®-Cefaclor [Can]
Apo®-Cefuroxime [Can]
Ceclor® CD [US]
Ceclor® [US/Can]
cefaclor
cefpodoxime
cefprozil
Ceftin® [US/Can]
cefuroxime
Cefzil® [US/Can]
Novo-Cefaclor [Can]
Nu-Cefaclor [Can]
PMS-Cefaclor [Can]
ratio-Cefuroxime [Can]
Vantin® [US/Can]
Zinacef® [US/Can]
Cephalosporin (Third Generation)
Cedax® [US]
cefdinir
cefixime
ceftibuten
Omnicef® [US/Can]
Suprax® [Can]
Macrolide (Antibiotic)
Apo®-Erythro Base [Can]
Apo®-Erythro E-C [Can]
Apo®-Erythro-ES [Can]
Apo®-Erythro-S [Can]
Diomycin® [Can]
E.E.S.® [US/Can]
Erybid™ [Can]
Eryc® [US/Can]
EryPed® [US]
Ery-Tab® [US]
Erythrocin® [US]
erythromycin and sulfisoxazole
erythromycin (systemic)
Eryzole® [US]
Nu-Erythromycin-S [Can]
PCE® [US/Can]
Pediazole® [US/Can]
PMS-Erythromycin [Can]

Otic Agent, Analgesic
  A/B® Otic [US]
  Allergan® Ear Drops [US]
  antipyrine and benzocaine
  Auralgan® [US/Can]
  Aurodex® [US]
  Auroto® [US]
  Benzotic® [US]
  Dec-Agesic® A.B. [US]
  Dolotic® [US]
  Rx-Otic® Drops [US]
Penicillin
  Alti-Amoxi-Clav® [Can]
  amoxicillin
  amoxicillin and clavulanate
    potassium
  Amoxicot® [US]
  Amoxil® [US]
  ampicillin
  Apo®-Amoxi [Can]
  Apo®-Amoxi-Clav® [Can]
  Apo®-Ampi [Can]
  Augmentin ES-600™ [US]
  Augmentin® [US/Can]
  Augmentin XR™ [US]
  Clavulin® [Can]
  Gen-Amoxicillin [Can]
  Lin-Amox [Can]
  Marcillin® [US]
  Moxilin® [US]
  Novamoxin® [Can]
  Novo-Ampicillin [Can]
  Nu-Amoxi [Can]
  Nu-Ampi [Can]
  PMS-Amoxicillin [Can]
  Principen® [US]
  ratio-AmoxiClav
  Trimox® [US]
Sulfonamide
  Apo®-Sulfatrim [Can]
  Bactrim™ DS [US]
  Bactrim™ [US]
  erythromycin and sulfisoxazole

Eryzole® [US]
Gantrisin® Pediatric Suspension
    [US]
Novo-Trimel [Can]
Novo-Trimel D.S. [Can]
Nu-Cotrimox® [Can]
Pediazole® [US/Can]
Septra® DS [US/Can]
Septra® [US/Can]
sulfamethoxazole and
    trimethoprim
Sulfatrim® DS [US]
Sulfatrim® [US]
sulfisoxazole
Sulfizole® [Can]
Truxazole® [US]
Tetracycline Derivative
  Adoxa™ [US]
  Alti-Minocycline [Can]
  Apo®-Doxy [Can]
  Apo®-Doxy Tabs [Can]
  Apo®-Minocycline [Can]
  Apo®-Tetra [Can]
  Brodspec® [US]
  Doryx® [US]
  Doxy-100® [US]
  Doxycin [Can]
  doxycycline
  Dynacin® [US]
  EmTet® [US]
  Gen-Minocycline [Can]
  Minocin® [US/Can]
  minocycline
  Monodox® [US]
  Novo-Doxylin [Can]
  Novo-Minocycline [Can]
  Novo-Tetra [Can]
  Nu-Doxycycline [Can]
  Nu-Tetra [Can]
  oxytetracycline
  Periostat® [US]
  ratio-Doxycycline [Can]
  ratio-Minocycline [Can]

Rhoxal-minocycline [Can]
Sumycin® [US]
Terramycin® I.M. [US/Can]
tetracycline
Vibramycin® [US]
Vibra-Tabs® [US/Can]
Wesmycin® [US]

OVARIAN FAILURE

Estrogen and Progestin Combination
  estrogens and medroxyprogesterone
  Premphase® [US/Can]
  Prempro™ [US/Can]
Estrogen Derivative
  Alora® [US]
  Cenestin™ [US/Can]
  Climara® [US/Can]
  Congest [Can]
  Delestrogen® [US/Can]
  Depo®-Estradiol [US/Can]
  Esclim® [US]
  Estrace® [US/Can]
  Estraderm® [US/Can]
  estradiol
  Estring® [US/Can]
  Estrogel® [Can]
  estrogens (conjugated A/synthetic)
  estrogens (conjugated/equine)
  estrogens (esterified)
  estrone
  estropipate
  Femring™ [US]
  Gynodiol® [US]
  Kestrone® [US/Can]
  Menest® [US]
  Oesclim® [Can]
  Oestrilin [Can]
  Ogen® [US/Can]
  Ortho-Est® [US]
  Premarin® [US/Can]
  Vagifem® [US/Can]
  Vivelle-Dot® [US]
  Vivelle® [US/Can]

OVULATION INDUCTION

Gonadotropin
  chorionic gonadotropin (human)
  chorionic gonadotropin
   (recombinant)
  menotropins
  Novarel™ [US]
  Ovidrel® [US]
  Pergonal® [US/Can]
  Pregnyl® [US/Can]
  Profasi® HP [Can]
  Profasi® [US]
  Repronex® [US/Can]
Ovulation Stimulator
  Bravelle® [US]
  chorionic gonadotropin
   (recombinant)
  Clomid® [US/Can]
  clomiphene
  Fertinex® [US]
  Ovidrel® [US]
  Serophene® [US/Can]
  urofollitropin

PAIN (ANOGENITAL)

Anesthetic/Corticosteroid
  Analpram-HC® [US]
  Enzone® [US]
  Epifoam® [US]
  Pramosone® [US]
  Pramox® HC [Can]
  pramoxine and hydrocortisone
  ProctoFoam®-HC [US/Can]
  Zone-A Forte® [US]
  Zone-A® [US]
Local Anesthetic
  benzocaine
  dibucaine
  dyclonine
  Fleet® Pain Relief [US-OTC]
  Foille® [US-OTC]
  Hurricaine® [US]
  Mycinettes® [US-OTC]

Nupercainal® [US-OTC]
Pontocaine® [US/Can]
pramoxine
Prax® [US-OTC]
ProctoFoam® NS [US-OTC]
tetracaine
Trocaine® [US-OTC]
Tronolane® [US-OTC]
Tronothane® [US-OTC]

PELVIC INFLAMMATORY DISEASE (PID)

Aminoglycoside (Antibiotic)
  AKTob® [US]
  Alcomicin® [Can]
  amikacin
  Amikin® [Can]
  Apo®-Tobramycin [Can]
  Diogent® [Can]
  Garamycin® [US/Can]
  gentamicin
  Nebcin® [US/Can]
  PMS-Tobramycin [Can]
  ratio-Gentamicin [Can]
  tobramycin
Cephalosporin (Second Generation)
  Cefotan® [US/Can]
  cefotetan
  cefoxitin
  Mefoxin® [US/Can]
Cephalosporin (Third Generation)
  Cefizox® [US/Can]
  cefotaxime
  ceftizoxime
  ceftriaxone
  Claforan® [US/Can]
  Rocephin® [US/Can]
Macrolide (Antibiotic)
  Apo®-Erythro Base [Can]
  Apo®-Erythro E-C [Can]
  Apo®-Erythro-ES [Can]
  Apo®-Erythro-S [Can]
  azithromycin

Diomycin® [Can]
E.E.S.® [US/Can]
Erybid™ [Can]
Eryc® [US/Can]
EryPed® [US]
Ery-Tab® [US]
Erythrocin® [US]
erythromycin (systemic)
Nu-Erythromycin-S [Can]
PCE® [US/Can]
PMS-Erythromycin [Can]
Zithromax® [US/Can]
Z-PAK® [US/Can]
Penicillin
  ampicillin and sulbactam
  piperacillin
  piperacillin and tazobactam
    sodium
  Pipracil® [Can]
  Tazocin® [Can]
  ticarcillin
  ticarcillin and clavulanate
    potassium
  Ticar® [US]
  Timentin® [US/Can]
  Unasyn® [US/Can]
  Zosyn® [US]
Quinolone
  Apo®-Oflox [Can]
  Ciloxan® [US/Can]
  ciprofloxacin
  Cipro® [US/Can]
  Cipro® XR [US/Can]
  Floxin® [US/Can]
  Ocuflox® [US/Can]
  ofloxacin
Tetracycline Derivative
  Adoxa™ [US]
  Apo®-Doxy [Can]
  Apo®-Doxy Tabs [Can]
  Apo®-Tetra [Can]
  Brodspec® [US]
  Doryx® [US]

Doxy-100® [US]
Doxycin [Can]
doxycycline
EmTet® [US]
Monodox® [US]
Novo-Doxylin [Can]
Novo-Tetra [Can]
Nu-Doxycycline [Can]
Nu-Tetra [Can]
Periostat® [US]
ratio-Doxycycline [Can]
Sumycin® [US]
tetracycline
Vibramycin® [US]
Vibra-Tabs® [US/Can]
Wesmycin® [US]

PERTUSSIS
Toxoid
Adacel® [Can]
Daptacel™ [US]
diphtheria, tetanus toxoids, and
acellular pertussis vaccine
diphtheria, tetanus toxoids, and
acellular pertussis vaccine and
Haemophilus influenzae type b
conjugate vaccine
diphtheria, tetanus toxoids, and
whole-cell pertussis vaccine
diphtheria, tetanus toxoids, whole-
cell pertussis, and *Haemophilus
influenzae* type b
conjugate vaccine
Infanrix® [US]
Pentacel™ [Can]
TriHIBit® [US]
Tripedia® [US]
Vaccine, Inactivated Bacteria
diphtheria, tetanus toxoids, and
acellular pertussis vaccine and
Haemophilus influenzae type b
conjugate vaccine
TriHIBit® [US]

PINWORMS
Anthelmintic
Combantrin™ [Can]
mebendazole
Pin-X® [US-OTC]
pyrantel pamoate
Reese's® Pinworm Medicine
[US-OTC]
Vermox® [US/Can]

PITUITARY FUNCTION TEST (GROWTH HORMONE)
Diagnostic Agent
arginine
R-Gene® [US]

PITYRIASIS (ROSEA)
Corticosteroid, Topical
Aclovate® [US]
Acticort® [US]
Aeroseb-HC® [US]
alclometasone
Alphatrex® [US]
amcinonide
Amcort® [Can]
Anusol® HC-1 [US-OTC]
Anusol® HC-2.5% [US-OTC]
Aquacort® [Can]
Aristocort® A Topical [US]
Aristocort® Topical [US]
Bactine® Hydrocortisone [US-OTC]
Betaderm® [Can]
Betamethacot® [US]
betamethasone (topical)
Betatrex® [US]
Beta-Val® [US]
Betnovate® [Can]
CaldeCORT® Anti-Itch Spray [US]
CaldeCORT® [US-OTC]
Capex™ [US/Can]
Carmol-HC® [US]
Celestoderm®-EV/2 [Can]

Celestoderm®-V [Can]
Cetacort®
clobetasol
Clocort® Maximum Strength
  [US-OTC]
clocortolone
Cloderm® [US/Can]
Cordran® SP [US]
Cordran® [US/Can]
Cormax® [US]
CortaGel® [US-OTC]
Cortaid® Maximum Strength
  [US-OTC]
Cortaid® with Aloe [US-OTC]
Cort-Dome® [US]
Cortizone®-5 [US-OTC]
Cortizone®-10 [US-OTC]
Cortoderm [Can]
Cutivate™ [US]
Cyclocort® [US/Can]
Del-Beta® [US]
Delcort® [US]
Dermacort® [US]
Dermarest Dricort® [US]
Derma-Smoothe/FS® [US/Can]
Dermatop® [US/Can]
Dermolate® [US-OTC]
Dermovate® [Can]
Dermtex® HC with Aloe [US-OTC]
Desocort® [Can]
desonide
DesOwen® [US]
Desoxi® [Can]
desoximetasone
diflorasone
Diprolene® AF [US]
Diprolene® [US/Can]
Diprosone® [Can]
Eldecort® [US]
Elocon® [US/Can]
Embeline™ E [US]
fluocinolone
fluocinonide

Fluoderm [Can]
flurandrenolide
fluticasone (topical)
Gen-Clobetasol [Can]
Gynecort® [US-OTC]
halcinonide
halobetasol
Halog®-E [US]
Halog® [US/Can]
Hi-Cor-1.0® [US]
Hi-Cor-2.5® [US]
Hyderm [Can]
hydrocortisone (topical)
Hydrocort® [US]
Hydro-Tex® [US-OTC]
Hytone® [US]
Kenalog® in Orabase® [US/Can]
Kenalog® Topical [US/Can]
LactiCare-HC® [US]
Lanacort® [US-OTC]
Lidemol® [Can]
Lidex-E® [US]
Lidex® [US/Can]
Locoid® [US/Can]
Luxiq™ [US]
Lyderm® [Can]
Maxiflor® [US]
Maxivate® [US]
mometasone furoate
Nasonex® [US/Can]
Novo-Clobetasol [Can]
Nutracort® [US]
Olux® [US]
Orabase® HCA [US]
Oracort [Can]
Penecort® [US]
PMS-Desonide [Can]
prednicarbate
Prevex® [Can]
Prevex® HC [Can]
Psorcon™ E [US]
Psorcon™ [US/Can]
Qualisone® [US]

ratio-Clobetasol [Can]
ratio-Ectosone [Can]
ratio-Topilene® [Can]
ratio-Topisone® [Can]
Sarna® HC [Can]
Scalpicin® [US]
S-T Cort® [US]
Synacort® [US]
Synalar® [US/Can]
Taro-Desoximetasone [Can]
Taro-Sone® [Can]
Tegrin®-HC [US-OTC]
Temovate E® [US]
Temovate® [US]
Tiamol® [Can]
Ti-U-Lac® H [Can]
Topicort®-LP [US]
Topicort® [US/Can]
Topsyn® [Can]
Triacet™ Topical [US]
Triaderm [Can]
triamcinolone (topical)
Tridesilon® [US]
U-Cort™ [US]
Ultravate™ [US/Can]
urea and hydrocortisone
Uremol® HC [Can]
Valisone® Scalp Lotion [Can]
Westcort® [US/Can]

PLANTAR WARTS
Keratolytic Agent
Duofilm® Solution [US]
salicylic acid and lactic acid
Topical Skin Product
silver nitrate

POISON IVY
Protectant, Topical
bentoquatam
IvyBlock® [US-OTC]

POISON OAK
Protectant, Topical
bentoquatam
IvyBlock® [US-OTC]

POISON SUMAC
Protectant, Topical
bentoquatam
IvyBlock® [US-OTC]

POLIOMYELITIS
Vaccine, Live Virus and Inactivated
Virus
IPOL™ [US/Can]
poliovirus vaccine (inactivated)

POSTPARTUM HEMORRHAGE
Uteronic Agent
carbetocin (Canada only)
Duratocin™ [Can]

PREECLAMPSIA
Electrolyte Supplement, Oral
magnesium sulfate

PREGNANCY (PROPHYLAXIS)
Contraceptive
estradiol cypionate and
medroxyprogesterone acetate
ethinyl estradiol and drospirenone
ethinyl estradiol and etonogestrel
ethinyl estradiol and norelgestromin
Evra® [Can]
Lunelle™ [US]
NuvaRing® [US]
Ortho Evra™ [US]
Yasmin® [US]
Contraceptive, Implant (Progestin)
levonorgestrel
Mirena® [US]
Norplant® Implant [Can]
Plan B® [US/Can]
Contraceptive, Oral
Alesse® [US/Can]

Apri® [US]
Aviane™ [US]
Brevicon® [US]
Cryselle™ [US]
Cyclessa® [US]
Demulen® 30 [Can]
Demulen® [US]
Desogen® [US]
Enpresse™ [US]
Estrostep® Fe [US]
ethinyl estradiol and desogestrel
ethinyl estradiol and ethynodiol
   diacetate
ethinyl estradiol and levonorgestrel
ethinyl estradiol and norethindrone
ethinyl estradiol and norgestimate
ethinyl estradiol and norgestrel
femhrt® [US/Can]
Kariva™ [US]
Lessina™ [US]
Levlen® [US]
Levlite™ [US]
Levora® [US]
Loestrin® Fe [US]
Loestrin® [US/Can]
Lo/Ovral® [US]
Low-Ogestrel® [US]
Marvelon® [Can]
mestranol and norethindrone
Microgestin™ Fe [US]
Minestrin™ 1/20 [Can]
Min-Ovral® [Can]
Mircette® [US]
Modicon® [US]
MonoNessa™ [US]
Necon® 0.5/35 [US]
Necon® 1/35 [US]
Necon® 1/50 [US]
Necon® 7/7/7 [US]
Necon® 10/11 [US]
Nordette® [US]
Norinyl® 1+35 [US]
Norinyl® 1+50 [US]

Nortrel™ [US]
Ogestrel®
Ortho-Cept® [US/Can]
Ortho-Cyclen® [US/Can]
Ortho-Novum® 1/50 [US/Can]
Ortho-Novum® [US]
Ortho-Tri-Cyclen® Lo [US]
Ortho Tri-Cyclen® [US/Can]
Ovcon® [US]
Ovral® [US/Can]
Portia™ [US]
PREVEN® [US]
Select™ 1/35 [Can]
Sprintec™ [US]
Synphasic® [Can]
Tri-Levlen® [US]
Tri-Norinyl® [US]
Triphasil® [US/Can]
Triquilar® [Can]
Trivora® [US]
Zovia™ [US]
Contraceptive, Progestin Only
   Alti-MPA [Can]
   Apo®-Medroxy [Can]
   Aygestin® [US]
   Camila™ [US]
   Depo-Provera® [US/Can]
   Errin™ [US]
   Gen-Medroxy [Can]
   Jolivette™ [US]
   levonorgestrel
   medroxyprogesterone acetate
   Micronor® [US/Can]
   Mirena® [US]
   Nora-BE™ [US]
   norethindrone
   norgestrel
   Norlutate® [Can]
   Norplant® Implant [Can]
   Nor-QD® [US]
   Novo-Medrone [Can]
   Ovrette® [US/Can]
   Plan B® [US/Can]

Provera® [US/Can]
ratio-MPA [Can]
Estrogen and Progestin Combination
ethinyl estradiol and etonogestrel
ethinyl estradiol and norelgestromin
Evra® [Can]
NuvaRing® [US]
Ortho Evra™ [US]
Spermicide
Advantage 24™ [Can]
Advantage-S™ [US-OTC]
Aqua Lube Plus [US-OTC]
Conceptrol® [US-OTC]
Delfen® [US-OTC]
Emko® [US-OTC]
Encare® [US-OTC]
Gynol II® [US-OTC]
nonoxynol 9
Semicid® [US-OTC]
Shur-Seal® [US-OTC]
VCF™ [US-OTC]

PREMATURE LUTEINIZING HORMONE (LH) SURGE

Antigonadotropic Agent
cetrorelix
Cetrotide™ [US/Can]

PREMENSTRUAL DYSPHORIC DISORDER (PMDD)

Antidepressant, Selective Serotonin
Reuptake Inhibitor
Apo®-Fluoxetine [Can]
fluoxetine
FXT® [Can]
Gen-Fluoxetine [Can]
Novo-Fluoxetine [Can]
Nu-Fluoxetine [Can]
PMS-Fluoxetine [Can]
Prozac® [US/Can]
Prozac® Weekly™ [US]
ratio-Fluoxetine [Can]

Rhoxal-fluoxetine [Can]
Sarafem™ [US]

PUBERTY (PRECOCIOUS)

Hormone, Posterior Pituitary
nafarelin
Synarel® [US/Can]
Luteinizing Hormone-Releasing
Hormone Analog
Eligard™ [US]
leuprolide acetate
Lupron Depot-Ped® [US]
Lupron Depot® [US/Can]
Lupron® [US/Can]
Viadur® [US/Can]

REYE SYNDROME

Diuretic, Osmotic
mannitol
Osmitrol® [US/Can]
Resectisol® Irrigation Solution [US]
Ophthalmic Agent, Miscellaneous
glycerin
Vitamin, Fat Soluble
AquaMEPHYTON® [US/Can]
Mephyton® [US/Can]
phytonadione

RUBELLA

Vaccine, Live Virus
measles, mumps, and rubella
vaccines, combined
Meruvax® II [US]
M-M-R® II [US/Can]
Priorix™ [Can]
rubella virus vaccine (live)

SWIMMER'S EAR

Antibiotic/Corticosteroid, Otic
AntibiOtic® Ear [US]
ciprofloxacin and hydrocortisone
Cipro® HC Otic [US/Can]
Cortimyxin® [Can]
Cortisporin® Otic [US/Can]

neomycin, polymyxin B, and
hydrocortisone
PediOtic® [US]
Otic Agent, Analgesic
A/B® Otic [US]
Allergan® Ear Drops [US]
antipyrine and benzocaine
Auralgan® [US/Can]
Aurodex® [US]
Auroto® [US]
Benzotic® [US]
Dec-Agesic® A.B. [US]
Dolotic® [US]
Rx-Otic® Drops [US]

SYPHILIS
Antibiotic, Miscellaneous
chloramphenicol
Chloromycetin® Parenteral [US/Can]
Diochloram® [Can]
Pentamycetin® [Can]
Penicillin
Bicillin® L-A [US]
penicillin G benzathine
penicillin G (parenteral/aqueous)
penicillin G procaine
Permapen® Isoject® [US]
Pfizerpen® [US/Can]
Wycillin® [US/Can]
Tetracycline Derivative
Adoxa™ [US]
Apo®-Doxy [Can]
Apo®-Doxy Tabs [Can]
Apo®-Tetra [Can]
Brodspec® [US]
Doryx® [US]
Doxy-100® [US]
Doxycin [Can]
doxycycline
EmTet® [US]
Monodox® [US]
Novo-Doxylin [Can]
Novo-Tetra [Can]

Nu-Doxycycline [Can]
Nu-Tetra [Can]
Periostat® [US]
ratio-Doxycycline [Can]
Sumycin® [US]
tetracycline
Vibramycin® [US]
Vibra-Tabs® [US/Can]
Wesmycin® [US]

TETANUS
Antibiotic, Miscellaneous
Apo®-Metronidazole [Can]
Flagyl ER® [US]
Flagyl® [US/Can]
Florazole ER® [Can]
metronidazole
Noritate® [US/Can]
Novo-Nidazol [Can]
Trikacide® [Can]
Immune Globulin
BayTet™ [US/Can]
tetanus immune globulin (human)
Toxoid
Adacel® [Can]
Daptacel™ [US]
diphtheria and tetanus toxoid
diphtheria, tetanus toxoids, and
acellular pertussis vaccine
diphtheria, tetanus toxoids, and
acellular pertussis vaccine and
Haemophilus influenzae type b
conjugate vaccine
diphtheria, tetanus toxoids, and
whole-cell pertussis vaccine
diphtheria, tetanus toxoids, whole-
cell pertussis, and *Haemophilus
influenzae* type b
conjugate vaccine
Infanrix® [US]
Pentacel™ [Can]
tetanus toxoid (adsorbed)
tetanus toxoid (fluid)

TriHIBit® [US]
Tripedia® [US]
Vaccine, Inactivated Bacteria
  diphtheria, tetanus toxoids, and
    acellular pertussis vaccine and
    Haemophilus influenzae type b
    conjugate vaccine
  TriHIBit® [US]

TETANUS (PROPHYLAXIS)
Antitoxin
  tetanus antitoxin

THROAT INFECTION
Antibacterial, Topical
  Dequadin® [Can]
  dequalinium (Canada only)
Antifungal Agent, Topical
  Dequadin® [Can]
  dequalinium (Canada only)

VAGINAL ATROPHY
Estrogen and Progestin Combination
  Activella™ [US]
  CombiPatch® [US]
  estradiol and norethindrone

VAGINITIS
Antibiotic, Vaginal
  sulfabenzamide, sulfacetamide, and
    sulfathiazole
  V.V.S.® [US]
Estrogen and Progestin Combination
  estrogens and medroxyprogesterone
  Premphase® [US/Can]
  Prempro™ [US/Can]
Estrogen Derivative
  Alora® [US]
  Cenestin™ [US/Can]

Climara® [US/Can]
Congest [Can]
Delestrogen® [US/Can]
Depo®-Estradiol [US/Can]
diethylstilbestrol
Esclim® [US]
Estinyl® [US]
Estrace® [US/Can]
Estraderm® [US/Can]
estradiol
Estring® [US/Can]
Estrogel® [Can]
estrogens (conjugated A/synthetic)
estrogens (conjugated/equine)
estrone
ethinyl estradiol
Femring™ [US]
Gynodiol® [US]
Honvol® [Can]
Kestrone® [US/Can]
Oesclim® [Can]
Oestrilin [Can]
Premarin® [US/Can]
Vagifem® [US/Can]
Vivelle-Dot® [US]
Vivelle® [US/Can]

VITILIGO
Psoralen
  methoxsalen
  8-MOP® [US/Can]
  Oxsoralen® Lotion [US/Can]
  Oxsoralen-Ultra® [US/Can]
  Ultramop™ [Can]
  Uvadex® [US/Can]
Topical Skin Product
  Benoquin® [US]
  monobenzone